KU-370-249

Gynaecology

To our wives, Mae, Winnie and Julia, for their patience, understanding and support

For Churchill Livingstone:

Publisher: Peter Richardson
Project Editor: Elif Fincanci-Smith
Production Controller: Neil Dickson
Design: Design Resources Unit
Sales Promotion Executive: Kathy Crawford

Gynaecology

Edited by

Robert W. Shaw MD MRCOG FRCS(Edin)
Professor of Obstetrics and Gynaecology
University Hospital of Wales
Cardiff
UK

W. Patrick Soutter MD MSc FRCOG
Reader in Gynaecological Oncology
Institute of Obstetrics and Gynaecology
Royal Postgraduate Medical School
Hammersmith Hospital
London
UK

Stuart L. Stanton FRCS FRCOG
Consultant Gynaecologist and Urogynaecologist
St George's Hospital
London
UK

CHURCHILL LIVINGSTONE
EDINBURGH LONDON MADRID MELBOURNE NEW YORK TOKYO 1992

CHURCHILL LIVINGSTONE
Medical Division of Longman Group UK Limited

Distributed in the United States of America by Churchill Livingstone Inc., 650 Avenue of the Americas, New York, N.Y. 10011, and by associated companies, branches and representatives throughout the world.

First published 1992
Reprinted 1993

ISBN 0-443-04139-3

British Library Cataloguing in Publication Data

A catalogue record for this book is available from the British Library.

Library of Congress Cataloging in Publication Data

Gynaecology / edited by Robert W. Shaw, W. Patrick Soutter, Stuart L. Stanton.
p. cm.
Includes index.
ISBN 0-443-04139-3
1. Gynecology. I. Shaw, Robert W. (Robert Wayne) II. Soutter, W. P. (W. Pat) III. Stanton, Stuart L.
[DNLM: 1. Genital Diseases, Female. WP 140 G9951]
RG101.G867 1992
618.1 — dc20
DNLM/DLC
for Library of Congress 92-6864
CIP

The publisher's policy is to use **paper manufactured from sustainable forests**

Printed and bound in Great Britain by
William Clowes Limited, Beccles and London

Preface

Why another gynaecological textbook? Not just the many advances in gynaecology, although that is reason enough for any new book, but a combination of the advent of subspecialization with the major changes in gynaecology which are not reflected in the current textbooks.

There has been a swing towards medical treatments using highly specific agents such as hormone analogues, anti-hormones, biosynthetic hormones and selective anti-mitotics. This has resulted in a reduction in certain types of gynaecological surgery with the utilization of a medical approach instead.

The development of better instrumentation has allowed endoscopic surgery to be applied to many situations and conditions which hitherto would have required laparotomy and major surgical procedures. This has allowed a move towards more daycare and outpatient operations.

Within the sphere of fertility treatment, the assisted reproduction techniques have now become well established and can offer hope to many otherwise childless couples provided appropriate choices are made.

The increasing prevalence and importance of topics such as HIV disease, medicolegal issues and forensic gynaecology have been thought to be important enough to justify separate sections or chapters.

The interdependence of gynaecology on other specialties such as general surgery, oncology, psychiatry and anaesthetics is reflected in the basis of many of these chapters.

All of these developments and the vast changes in practice they have produced make the publication of *Gynaecology* timely.

The editors, who are subspecialists in reproductive endocrinology, oncology and urogynaecology respectively, have chosen authors whose chapters reflect their widespread experience.

They have reviewed their topics to provide a text which reflects the higher standards of practice in our specialty in the 1990s.

The keypoints at the end of each chapter endeavour to encompass the salient points which we hope will serve as a succinct revision and thus be useful to trainees.

We hope that the division of the text into the major sections of basic anatomy, physiology and biochemistry, and the specialty interest subdivisions of reproductive endocrinology, oncology and urogynaecology will appeal to general trainees preparing for the MRCOG or equivalent as well as serving as a definitive text for specialists within gynaecology generally.

Finally, we hope this will complement the companion textbook *Obstetrics* by the late Alec Turnbull and Geoffrey Chamberlain.

London — R.W.S.
1992 — W.P.S.
S.L.S.

Contributors

M. I. M. Abuzeid MD MRCOG
Lecturer in Reproductive Medicine, Department of Obstetrics and Gynaecology, University of Bristol, Bristol, UK

Alan G. Amias FRCS FRCOG
Consultant Gynaecologist, St George's Hospital, London, UK

Nazar N. Amso MB ChB MRCOG
Clinical Research Fellow, Academic Department of Obstetrics and Gynaecology, Royal Free Hospital School of Medicine, London, UK

Malcom C. Anderson FRCOG FRCPath
Senior Lecturer in Histopathology, Queens Medical Centre, University of Nottingham, Nottingham, UK

R. Baber MRCOG FRACOG
Research Fellow in Obstetrics and Gynaecology, King's College Hospital, London, UK

Michael Baum ChM FRCS MD(h.c.)
Professor of Surgery, Institute of Cancer Research, The Royal Marsden Hospital, London, UK

Richard W. Beard MD FRCOG
Professor of Obstetrics and Gynaecology, St Mary's Hospital Medical School, London, UK

R. P. Brettle MB ChB FRCP
Consultant Physician and Part-time Senior Lecturer, City Hospital, Edinburgh, UK

Michael Brooks MRCS
Lecturer in Surgery, King's College Hospital, London, UK

William G. Brose MD
Assistant Professor of Anesthesia, Pain Management Services, Stanford University Medical Center, Stanford, California, USA

Linda Cardozo MD FRCOG
Consultant Gynaecologist, King's College Hospital, London, UK

Anne Clark
Research Registrar in Obstetrics and Gynaecology, The Royal London Hospital, London, UK

Roger V. Clements MA(Oxon) BM BCh FRCS(Ed) FRCOG
Medical Executive Director, North Middlesex Hospital NHS Trust; Honorary Lecturer in Obstetrics and Gynaecology, Royal Free Hospital Medical School; Assistant Professor UK Faculty, St George's Hospital Medical School, Grenada

Carmel A. E. Coulter FRCP FRCR
Consultant in Radiotherapy and Oncology, St Mary's and The Middlesex Hospitals, London, UK

Michael Cousins MBBS MD(Syd) FFARACS FFARCS
Head of Department of Anaesthesia and Pain Management, Royal North Shore Hospital, St Leonards; Chair of Anaesthesia, Faculty of Medicine, University of Sydney, Sydney, NSW, Australia

Sarah Creighton MB BS MRCOG
Registrar in Obstetrics and Gynaecology, King's College Hospital, London, UK

N. E. Day BA PhD
Professor of Public Health, University of Cambridge; Director, Medical Research Council, Biostatistics Unit, Cambridge, UK

N. Duignan MD MAO FRCOG
Associate Professor of Obstetrics and Gynaecology, University College Dublin; Consultant Obstetrician and Gynaecologist, Coombe Lying-in Hospital and St Vincent's Hospital, Dublin, Eire

Sheila L. B. Duncan MD FRCOG
Reader and Honorary Consultant in Obstetrics and Gynaecology, Jessop Hospital for Women, Sheffield, UK

Stephen R. Ebbs MS FRCS
Senior Registrar and Consultant Surgeon, Mayday University Hospital, Surrey, UK

D. Keith Edmonds MB ChB FRCOG FRACOG
Consultant Obstetrician and Gynaecologist, Queen Charlotte's and Chelsea Hospital, London, UK

Anthony France MA MB BChir MRCP
Consultant Physician, Immunodeficiency Unit, King's Cross Hospital, Dundee, UK

Jonathan M. Frappell FRCS FRCS(Ed) MRCOG
Consultant Obstetrician and Gynaecologist, Freedom Fields Hospital, Plymouth, UK

Simon C. A. Fraser MB ChB(Ed) FRCS(Ed) FRCS(Eng)
Research Fellow, King's College Hospital, London, UK

Anna Glasier MD MRCOG BSc
Director of Family Planning and Well Woman Services, Lothian Health Board; Consultant Gynaecologist and Part-time Senior Lecturer, University of Edinburgh, Edinburgh, UK

Lawrence Goldie MB ChB DPM MD FRCPsych Grad Memb Brit Psychol Soc
Director, British Postgraduate Medical Federation Course 'Caring for the Dying and Bereaved'; Course Director, Institute of Obstetrics and Gynaecology: Psychosexual Problems; Physician, The Lister Hospital, London, UK

James A. Gray MB ChB FRCPE
Consultant in Communicable Diseases, Regional Infectious Diseases Unit, City Hospital; Part-time Senior Lecturer in Medicine, University of Edinburgh, Edinburgh, UK

J. G. Grudzinskas BSc MB BS MD FRCOG FRACOG
Professor and Head of the Academic Unit of Obstetrics and Gynaecology, The Royal London Hospital Medical College and St Bartholomew's Hospital Medical College, London, UK

R. N. Heasley MD MRCOG
Consultant Obstetrician and Gynaecologist, Craigavon Area Hospital; *Formerly* Senior Lecturer, Department of Obstetrics and Gynaecology, Queen's University, Belfast, UK

M. M. Henry MB FRCS
Consultant Surgeon, Central Middlesex Hospital; Senior Lecturer in Surgery, St Mary's Hospital, Honorary Consultant Surgeon, St Mark's Hospital, London, UK

Paul Hilton MD BS MRCOG
Consultant Gynaecologist (sub-specialist in Urogynaecology), Newcastle Health Authority; Honorary Senior Lecturer, University of Newcastle, Newcastle-upon-Tyne, UK

David M. Holmes BSc MD MRCOG
Consultant Obstetrician and Gynaecologist, St Paul's Hospital, Cheltenham, UK

Elizabeth Houang MB ChB FRCPath
Consultant Microbiologist, Queen Charlotte's and Chelsea Hospital, London, UK

C. N. Hudson MChir, FRCS FRCOG FRACOG
Consultant Obstetrician and Gynaecologist, St Bartholomew's Hospital, London, UK

Michael Hull MD FRCOG
Professor of Reproductive Medicine and Surgery, University of Bristol Department of Obstetrics and Gynaecology, Bristol Maternity Hospital, Bristol, UK

G. R. Kinghorn MD FRCP
Clinical Director of Communicable Diseases in the Department of Genitourinary Medicine, Royal Hallamshire Hospital, Sheffield, UK

Hannah E. Lambert FRCOG FRCR
Consultant Clinical Oncologist and Honorary Senior Lecturer, Hammersmith Hospital, London, UK

Frances Lewington BSc PhD
Principal Scientific Officer, Metropolitan Police Forensic Science Laboratory, London, UK

Barry Victor Lewis MD FRCOG FRCS
Senior Consultant Gynaecologist, Watford General Hospital; Vice President, British Society of Gynaecological Endoscopy; Treasurer, European Society of Hysteroscopy, London, UK

Mary Ann Lumsden BSc MB MD FRCOG
Registrar in Obstetrics and Gynaecology, Royal Infirmary of Edinburgh, Edinburgh, UK

Sir Malcolm MacNaughton MD LLD FRCP(Glas) FRCOG FRSE
Emeritus Professor of Obstetrics and Gynaecology, University of Glasgow, Glasgow, UK

Raul A. Margara MD
Consultant and Senior Lecturer, Royal Postgraduate Medical School, Hammersmith Hospital, London, UK

W. P. Mason FRCS FRCOG
Consultant Obstetrician and Gynaecological Oncologist, The Samaritan Hospital for Women, London, UK

J. Moodley MD
Professor of Obstetrics and Gynaecology, Faculty of Medicine, University of Natal, South Africa

A. R. Mundy MS FRCS MRCP
Professor of Urology, University of London at Guy's Hospital and Institute of Urology, London, UK

John Newton MD FRCOG
Head of Department of Obstetrics and Gynaecology, Birmingham Maternity Hospital, Birmingham, UK

Shaughn O'Brien MB BCh MD FRCOG
Professor and Head of Department of Obstetrics and Gynaecology, Keele University; Consultant Obstetrician and Gynaecologist, North Staffordshire Hospital Centre, Stoke-on-Trent, Staffordshire, UK

Anthony D. Parsons MB BS MA FRCOG
Senior Lecturer of Obstetrics and Gynaecology, University of Warwick; Consultant Obstetrician and Gynaecologist, Rugby NHS Trust, Rugby, UK

R. John Parsons BScTech, PhD, FIPSM
Director, Humberside Medical Physics Service, The Princess Royal Hospital, Hull, UK

Alison C. Peattie MB ChB MRCOG
Honorary Consultant and Senior Lecturer in Obstetrics and Gynaecology, St George's Hospital and Medical School, London UK

Alan C. Perkins BSc MSc PhD FIPSM
Consultant Medical Physicist, Department of Medical Physics, University Hospital, Queens Medical Centre, Nottingham, UK

Martin Charles Powell MD FRCS MRCOG
Senior Registrar in Obstetrics and Gynaecology, City Hospital, Nottingham, UK

Margaret Puxon, QC MRCS LRCP MB ChB(Hons) MD(Obst) FRCOG
Member of Her Majesty's Counsel of the Inner Temple, London, UK

Michael A. Quinn MB ChB MGO(Melb) MRCP(UK) MRCOG FRACOG CGO
Associate Professor of Obstetrics and Gynaecology, University of Melbourne; Director of Oncology, Royal Women's Hospital; Consultant Gynaecologist, Peter MacCallum Cancer Institute, Melbourne, Australia

P. W. Reginald MD MRCOG
Consultant Obstetrician and Gynaecologist, Wexham Park and Windsor Hospitals, Slough; Honorary Senior Lecturer, St Mary's Hospital, London, UK

Raine E. I. Roberts MB ChB DCH DMJ(Clin) FRCGP
Clinical Director of the Sexual Assault Referral Centre, St Mary's Hospital, Manchester, UK

P. Robson MB BS BA(Hons)Psychol MRCOG
Senior Registrar in Obstetrics and Gynaecology, Hammersmith Hospital, London, UK

Gordon J. S. Rustin MD MSc MRCP
Senior Lecturer in Medical Oncology and Honorary Consultant, Charing Cross Hospital, London; Consultant, Mount Vernon Hospital, Middlesex, UK

J. M. Sackier MD FRCS
Associate Clinical Professor of Surgery, UCLA School of Medicine, Cedars–Sinai Medical Center, Los Angeles, California, USA

Robert W. Shaw MD MRCOG FRCS(Edin)
Professor of Obstetrics and Gynaecology, University Hospital of Wales, Cardiff, UK

Stephen K. Smith MD MRCOG
Professor of Obstetrics and Gynaecology, University of Cambridge, Rosie Maternity Hospital, Cambridge, UK

W. Patrick Soutter MD MSc FRCOG
Reader in Gynaecological Oncology, Institute of Obstetrics and Gynaecology, Royal Postgraduate Medical School, Hammersmith Hospital, London, UK

Stuart L. Stanton FRCS FRCOG
Consultant Gynaecologist and Urogynaecologist, St George's Hospital, London, UK

John W. W. Studd MD FRCOG
Consultant Gynaecologist, King's College Hospital; Director, Fertility and Endocrinology Centre, Lister Hospital, London, UK

Malcolm Symonds MD FRCOG
Foundation Professor of Obstetrics and Gynaecology, University of Nottingham, Nottingham, UK

William Thompson BSc MD FRCOG
Professor of Obstetrics and Gynaecology, Queen's University, Belfast, UK

John Tidy MRCOG BSc MD
Registrar in Obstetrics and Gynaecology, The Samaritan Hospital for Women, London, UK

Jean-Pierre Van Besouw BSc(Hons) MB BS FCAnaes
Consultant Anaesthetist, St George's Hospital, London, UK

Ian Vellacott MRCOG
Consultant Obstetrician and Gynaecologist, The Counts Hospital, Lincoln, UK

C. P. West MBChB MRCOG DCH
Consultant Obstetrician and Gynaecologist, Simpson Memorial Maternity Pavilion, Edinburgh, UK

C. B. Wood MD FRCS
Senior Lecturer in Surgery, Royal Postgraduate Medical School, Hammersmith Hospital, London, UK

F. C. W. Wu BSc MD FRCP(Edin)
Clinical Consultant, MRC Reproductive Biology Unit; Honorary Senior Lecturer in Medicine, Western General Hospital, Edinburgh, UK

Contents

* The drug terodiline mentioned in these chapters has now been withdrawn.

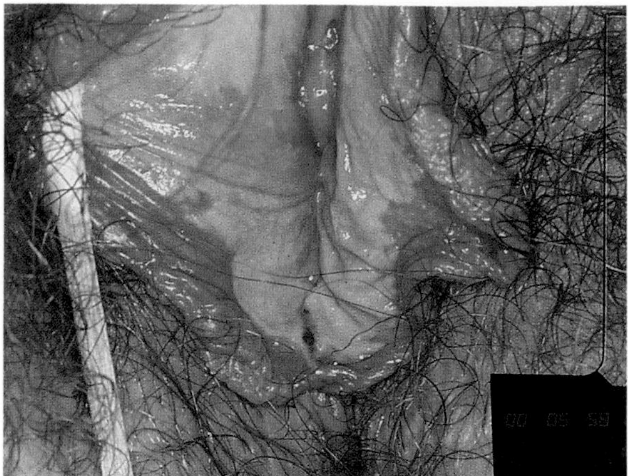
Extensive area of acetowhite change.

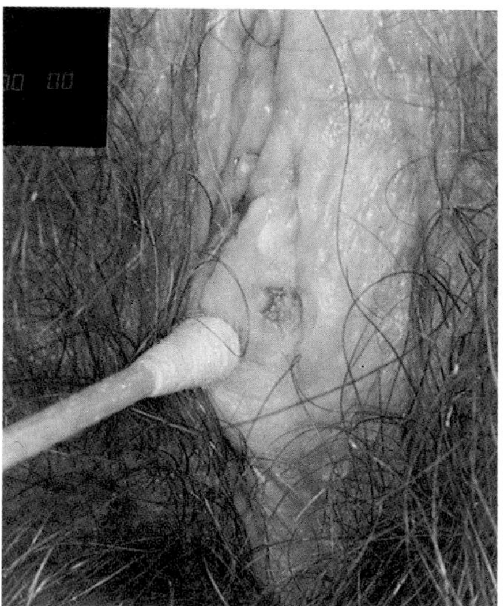
Squamous hyperplasia with a small ulcer caused by scratching.

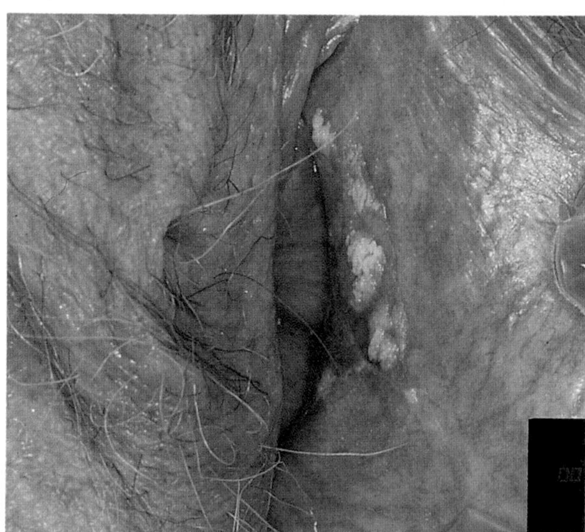
VIN III appearing as leukoplakia.

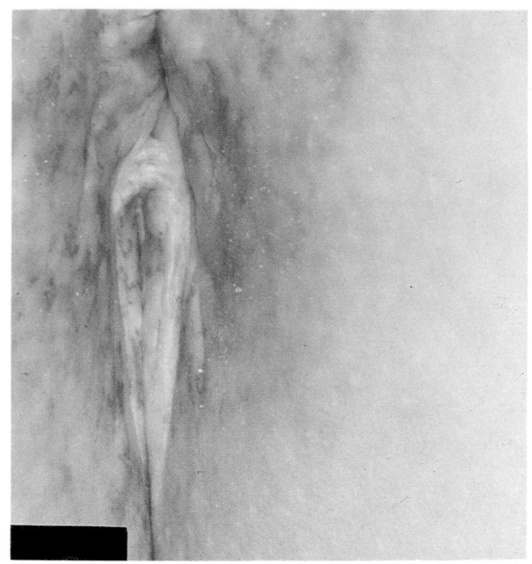
Lichen sclerosus.

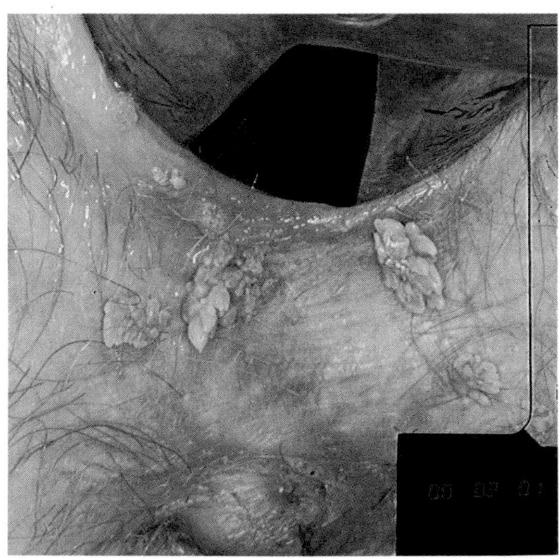
Small genital warts at the fourchette.

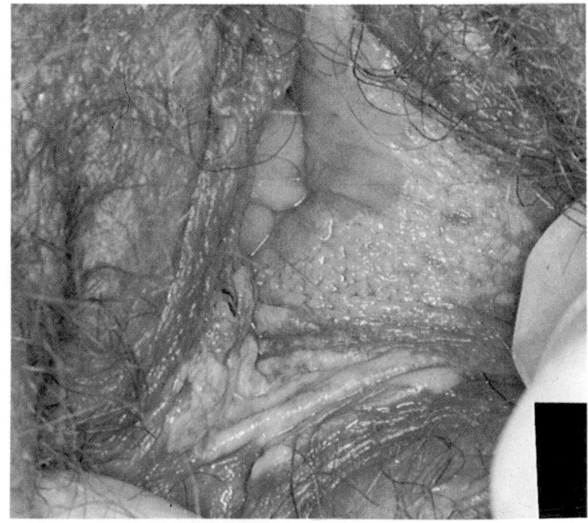
VIN III on labium minorum.

Uterus bicornis bicollis with double vagina (A. Auderbert).

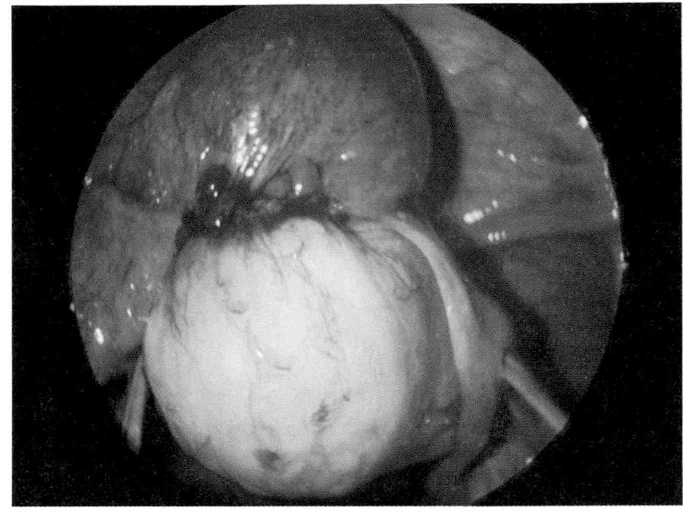

Large right endometriotic cyst adherent to the uterus (H. Frangenheim).

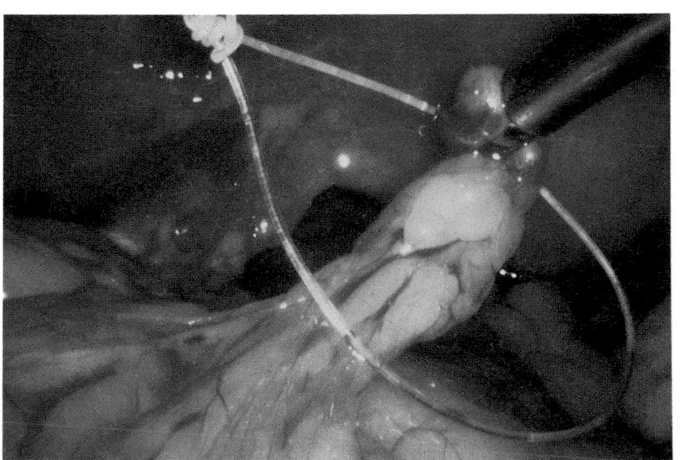

Ligation of vascular omentum with roeder loop (Ethicon) (K. Semm).

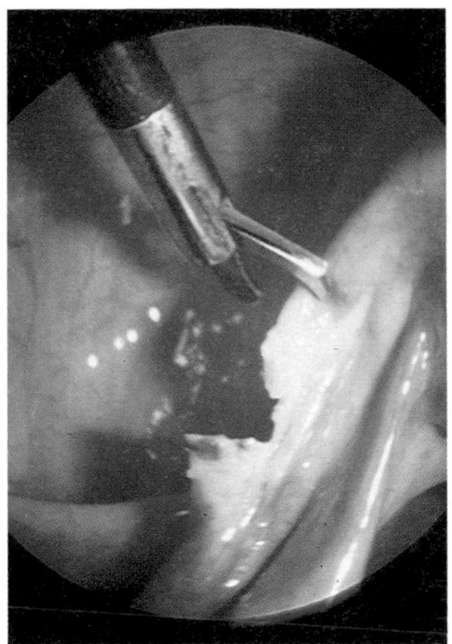

Hook scissors cutting fallopian tube following bipolar diathermy (H. Frangenheim).

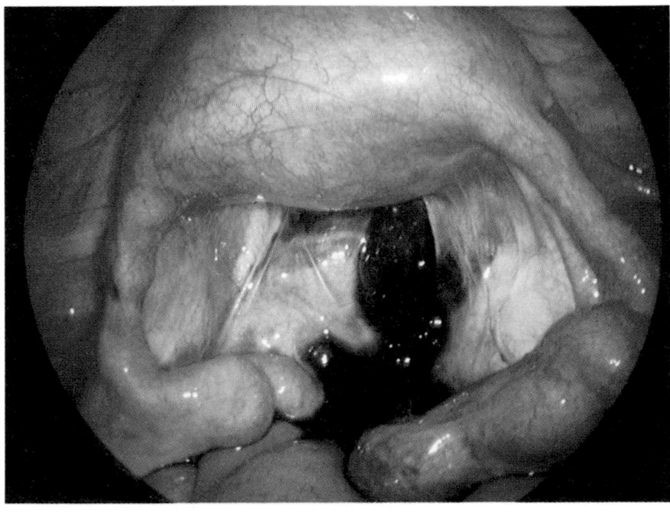

Extensive peritubal and periovarian adhesions. Spill and loculation of methylene blue dye (H. Frangenheim).

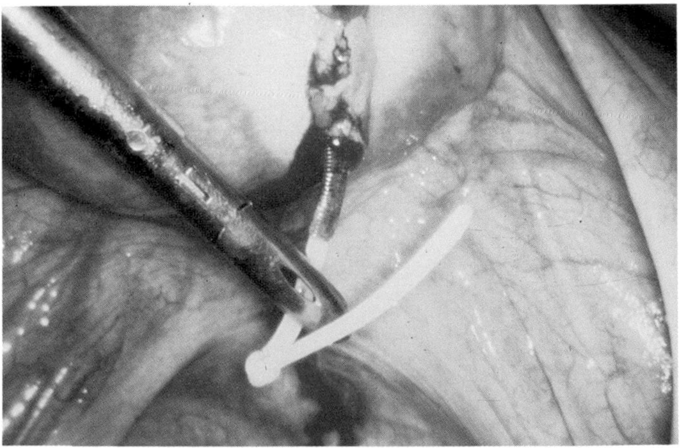

Perforation of fundus of the uterus by a Copper-7 contraceptive device. Laparoscopic recovery (K. Semm).

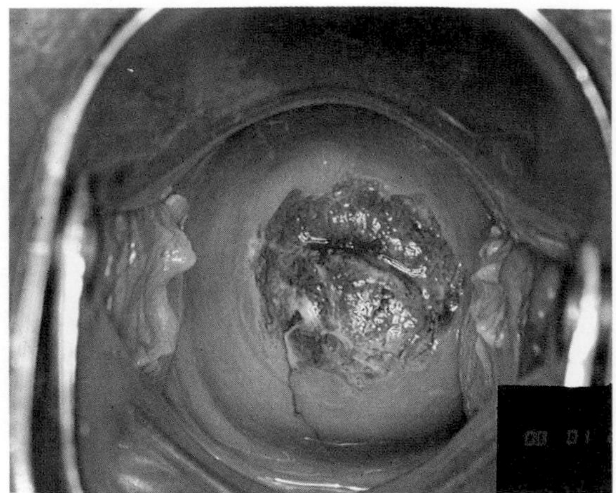

Normal cervix with ectropion.

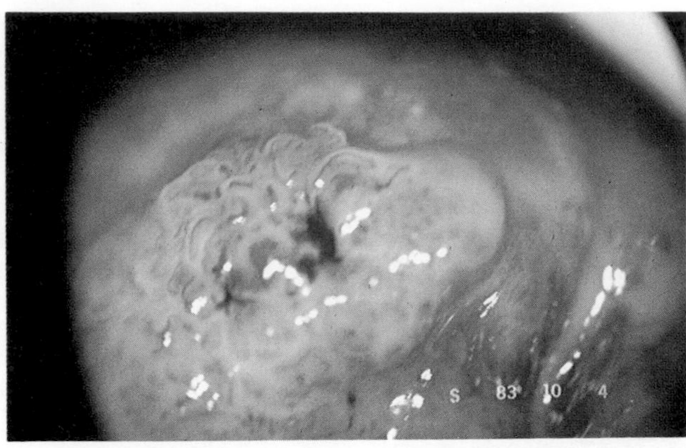

Large cervical condyloma showing microvilli and looped capillaries.

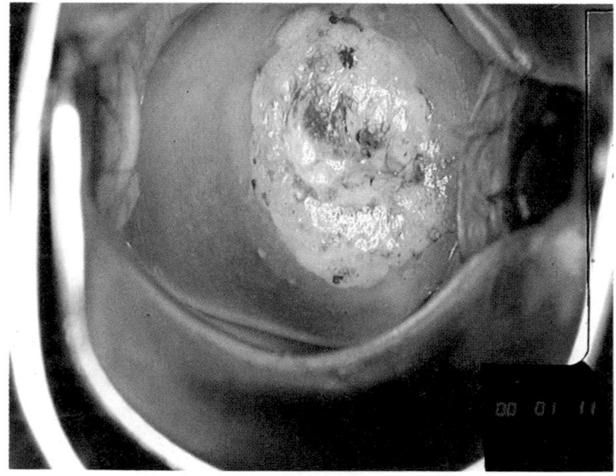

CIN III showing strong acetowhite with clear, regular edges.

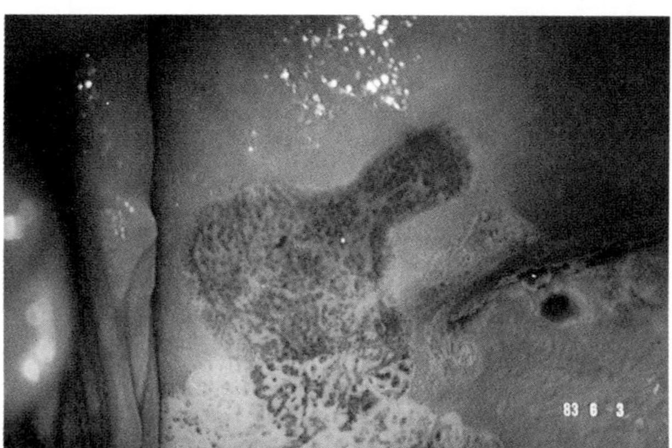

Microinvasion with coarse punctation.

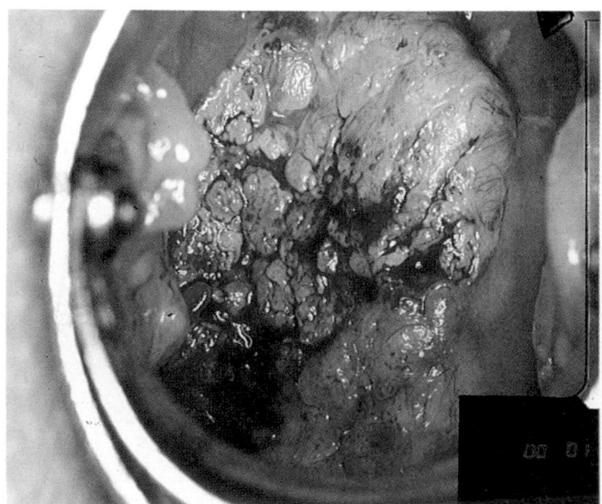

Stage Ib cervical cancer—irregular surface.

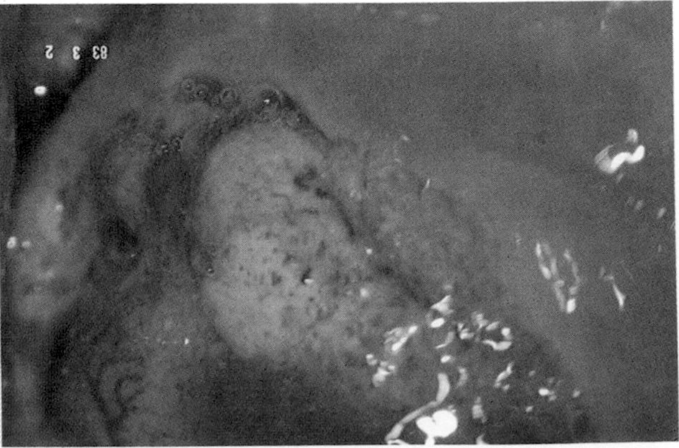

Atypical vessels and irregular surface of invasion.

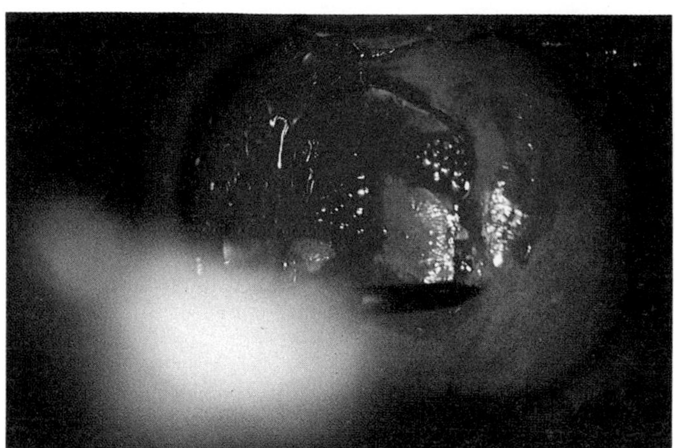
Cone biopsy being performed with LLETZ.

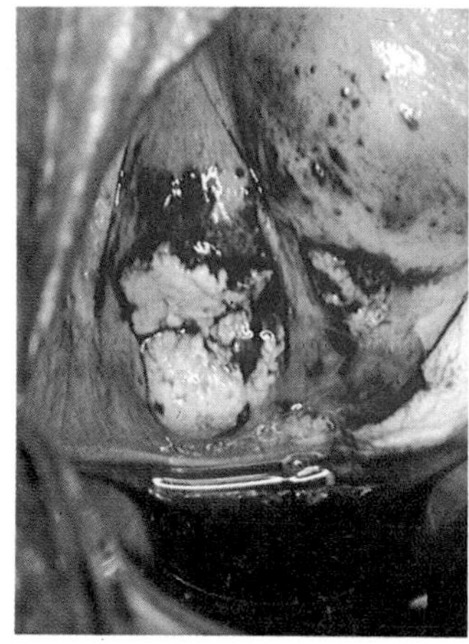
VAIN III after hysterectomy.

SEXUALLY TRANSMITTED DISEASES

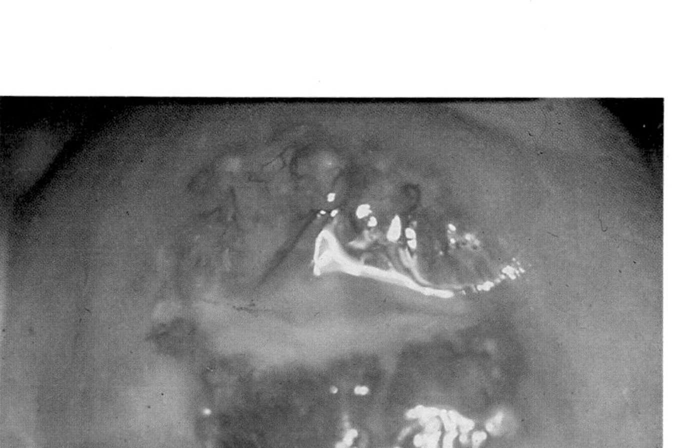
Chlamydial cervicitis.

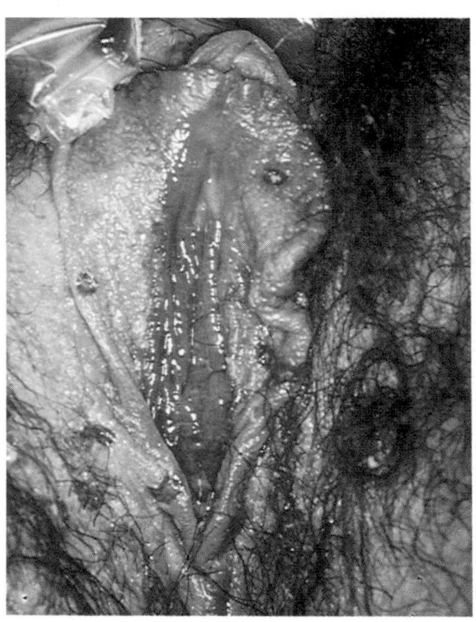
Primary genital herpes—multiple ulcers on labia minora.

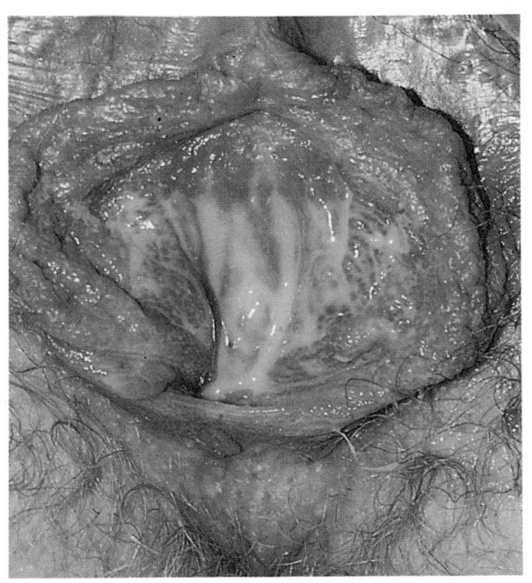
Bacterial vaginosis.

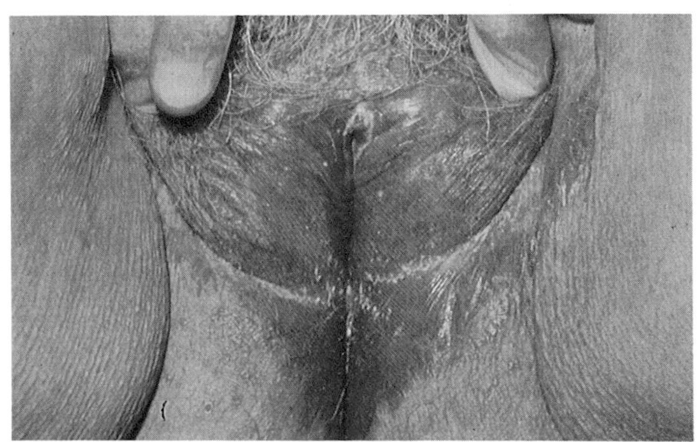
Candida vulvitis.

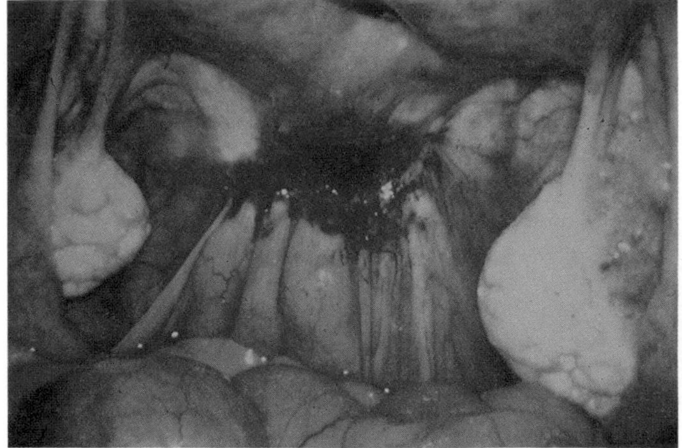

Haemorrhagic endometriosis in pouch of Douglas involving serosal surface of rectum.

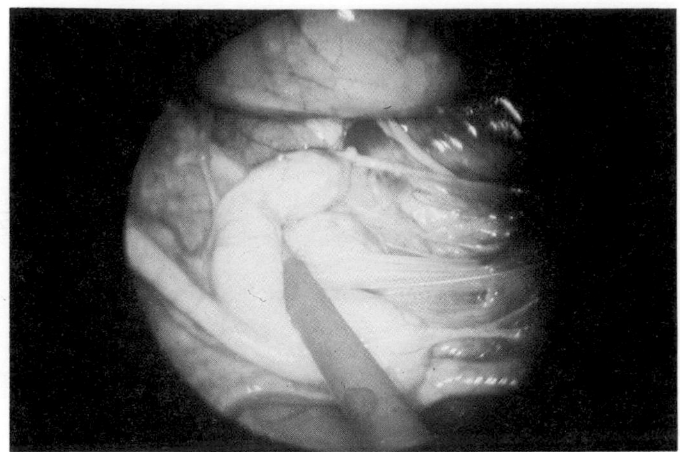

Peritubal and pelvic adhesions — endpoint in long-standing endometriosis producing infertility.

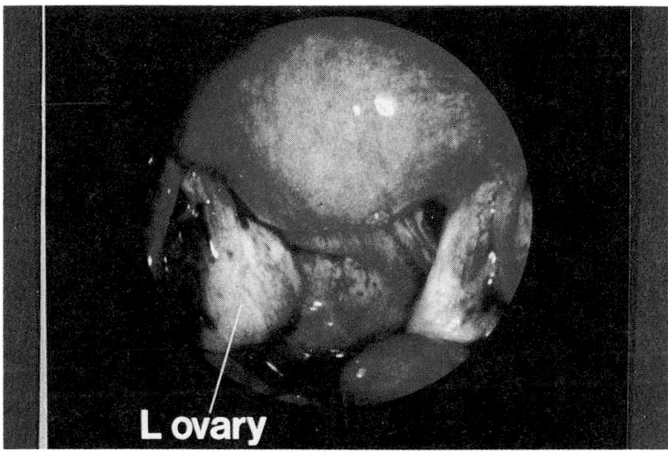

Endometrioma in left ovary, superficial deposits on both ovaries and on uterosacral ligaments.

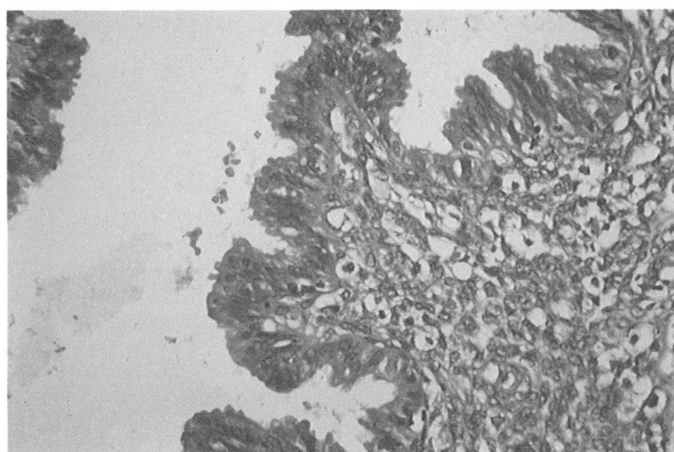

Histopathological confirmation of endometriosis in lesions excised from umbilicus.

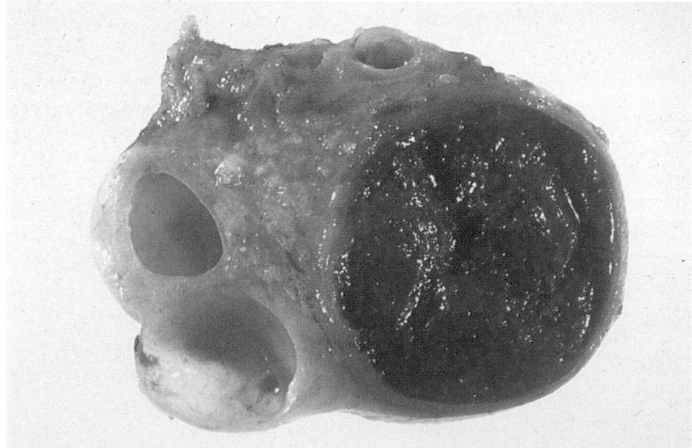

Chocolate cyst in ovary removed at radical surgery for recurrent endometriosis.

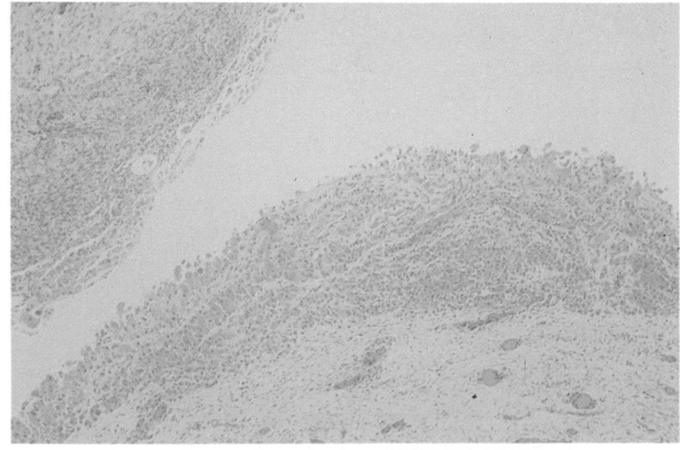

Histology of endometriotic cyst wall — evidence of fibrosis, haemorrhage, macrophages, etc. but no definable glandular elements — often the finding with long-standing endometriosis.

SECTION 1

Basic Principles and Investigations

1. Embryology of the female genital tract: its genetic defects and congenital anomalies

S. L. B. Duncan

An understanding of the development of the female genital tract is important in the practice of gynaecology. The mechanisms by which sexual differentiation is established long before birth are complex and remarkable. They are also easily perturbed. Advances in genetics and in our understanding of steroidogenesis together with painstaking experimental work on mammalian embryos have combined to improve our understanding of some of the derangements of the female genital tract seen in clinical practice. Errors of development which result in intersex states, though rare, are distressing but careful study of sporadic cases has provided knowledge out of proportion to their frequency.

In this chapter are discussed some of the key events in the development of the female genital tract especially where these relate to clinical abnormalities. Genetic conditions and congenital abnormalities of the genital tract affecting gynaecological practice are outlined. A basic understanding of the development of the gut and urogenital system is assumed as is an understanding of the formation of gametes, cell division and of female and male chromosome complements. This chapter does not include discussion of disorders where development is so disorganized that it is incompatible with life, nor does it deal with conditions diagnosed in infancy and primarily dealt with by the paediatric surgeon. Reference is made to male development only in so far as it is of relevance in understanding congenital anomalies in the female or where the phenotype is female. Thus, disorders of virilization or of spermatogenesis in phenotypic males are not discussed.

EMBRYOLOGY

Development of the mesonephros and kidneys

Both the urinary and genital systems develop from a common mesodermal ridge running along the posterior abdominal wall. Although the systems are less intimately connected in the female compared with the male, the external openings eventually reach the same urogenital sinus.

During the fifth week of embryonic life (i.e. from fertilization) the nephrogenic cord develops from the mesoderm and forms the urogenital ridge and mesonephric duct (later to form the wolffian duct). The mesonephros consists of a comparatively large ovoid organ on each side of the midline with the developing gonad on the medial side of its lower portion. The paramesonephric duct, later to form the müllerian system, develops as an ingrowth of coelomic epithelium anterolateral to the mesonephric duct. The primordial germ cells migrate from the yolk sac along the dorsal mesentery of the hindgut and reach the primitive gonad by the end of the sixth week (42 days; Fig. 1.1). The fate of the mesonephric and paramesonephric ducts is critically dependent on gonadal secretion (see Section 2). Assuming female development, the two paramesonephric ducts extend caudally to project into the posterior wall of the urogenital sinus as the müllerian tubercle. There is degeneration of the wolffian system. The lower ends of the müllerian system fuse, later to form the uterus, cervix and upper vagina while the cephalic ends remain separate, forming the fallopian tubes (Fig. 1.2).

The ureter develops as an outgrowth of the mesonephric

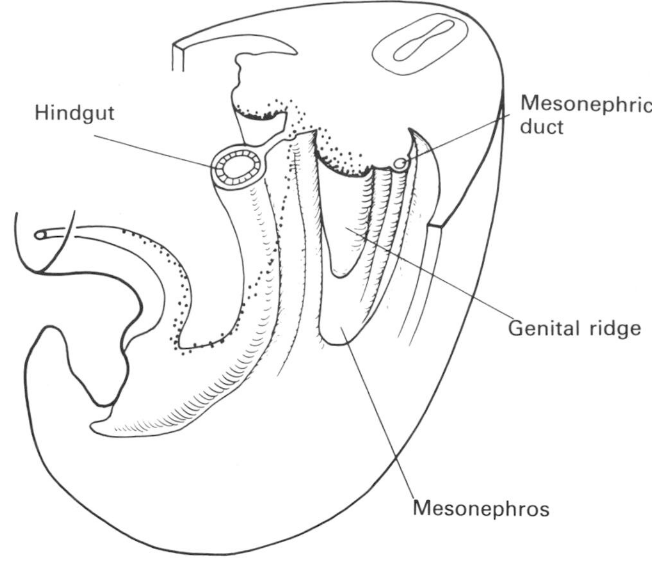

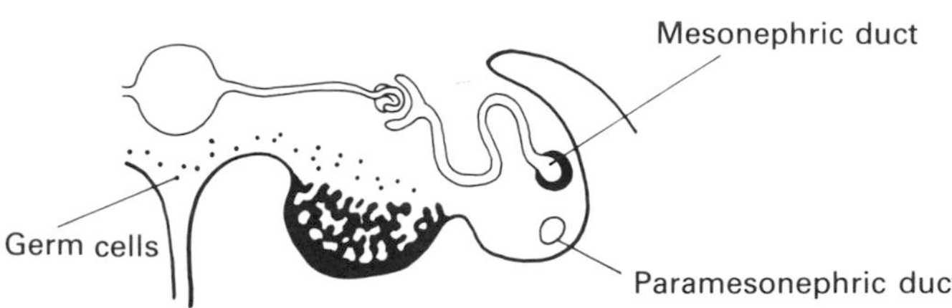

Fig. 1.1 Cross-sectional diagram of posterior abdominal wall in embryo.
Top: migration of germ cells into genital ridge, overlying the mesonephros, with mesonephric duct on lateral aspect;
bottom: paramesonephric (müllerian) duct lying anterolaterally to the mesonephric duct.

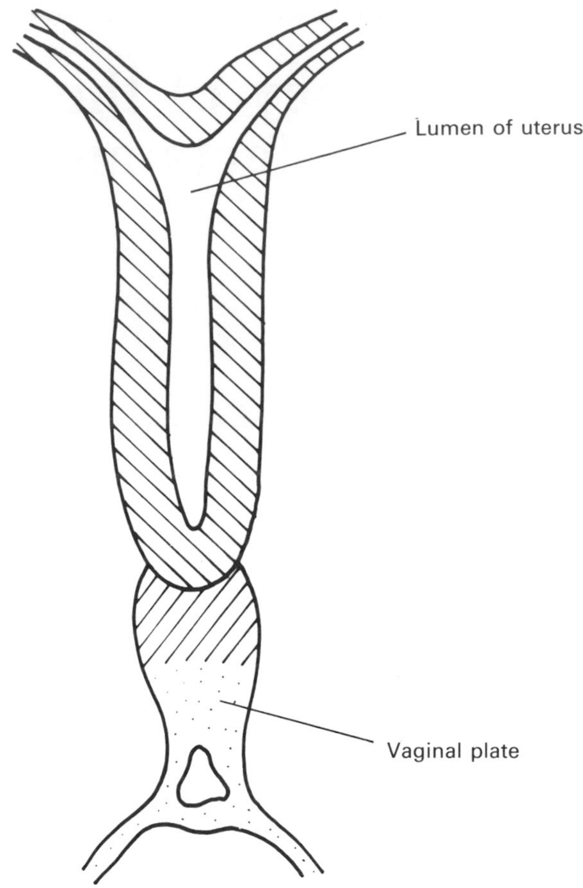

Fig. 1.2 The fused lower paramesonephric ducts later form the uterus, cervix and upper vagina. The müllerian tubercle has invaginated but not opened into the urogenital sinus.

duct close to its lower end and grows outward and upward to penetrate the metanephric mesoderm which ultimately forms the definitive kidney. Unilateral renal aplasia is usually due to degeneration of the ureteric bud and this failure is frequently associated with failure of müllerian development on the same side since both are dependent on adequate development of the mesonephric system. Splitting of the ureteric bud results in partial or complete duplication of the ureter. If a developing ureter fails to connect with the bladder it may retain its connection with the wolffian duct and thus open into the vagina or vestibule. This is more likely to occur if there has been splitting of the bud and abnormal ureteric development. The kidney starts off much more caudally than the gonads and failure to ascend accounts for its occasional pelvic location and for supernumerary renal vessels which result from the persistence of embryonic vessels.

The cloaca

Meanwhile, and usually before the seventh week, the urorectal septum divides the cloaca into the urogenital sinus and the anorectal canal. When the urogenital septum reaches the cloacal membrane, the perineum is formed (Figs 1.3 and 1.4). An ectodermal anal pit forms to meet the anorectal canal and an opening forms here during the ninth embryonic week. Thus, the lower third of the anal canal forms from ectoderm and consists of stratified squamous epithelium and is supplied by the internal pudendal artery. Where the anal pit fails to form or there is atresia of the lower end of the rectum, the thickness of the intervening layer is very variable. Sometimes the rectal opening is in the perineum or even in the vagina (Fig. 1.5).

The urogenital sinus may be divided into:

1. An upper part which forms the urinary bladder. The early connection superiorly with the allantois obliterates and forms the urachus which connects the apex of the bladder to the umbilicus. If mesoderm fails to invade the cloacal membrane anteriorly, extrophy of the bladder results.
2. A pelvic part which forms the urethra and lower vagina. This is intimately connected with the development of the lower part of the müllerian system.

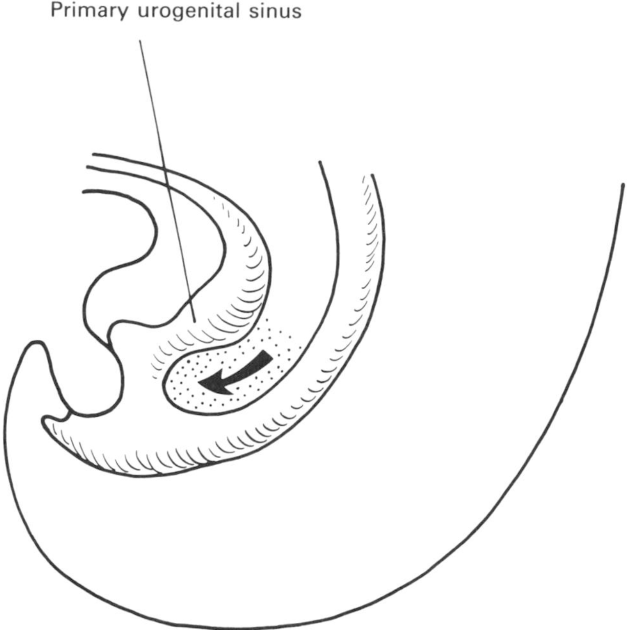

Fig. 1.3 Development of the urorectal septum (arrowed), eventually separating the bladder and vagina from the rectum.

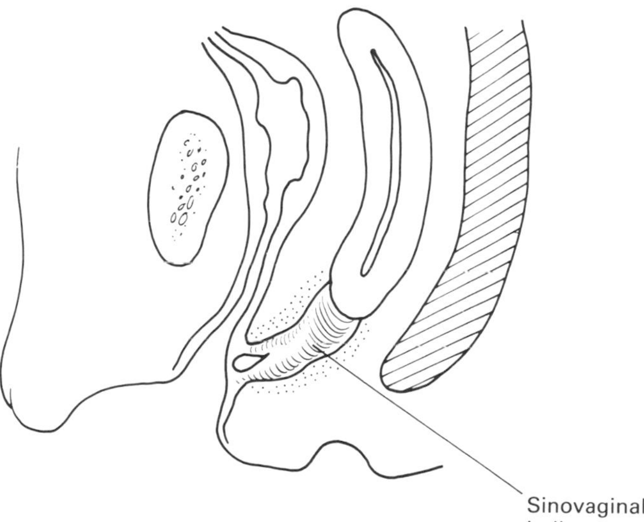

Fig. 1.4 A later stage in development where the müllerian tubercle and the sinovaginal bulbs (not yet canalized) are elongating and lying within the urorectal septum. In this diagram the anorectal canal has failed to connect with the anal pit; this would later present as an imperforate anus.

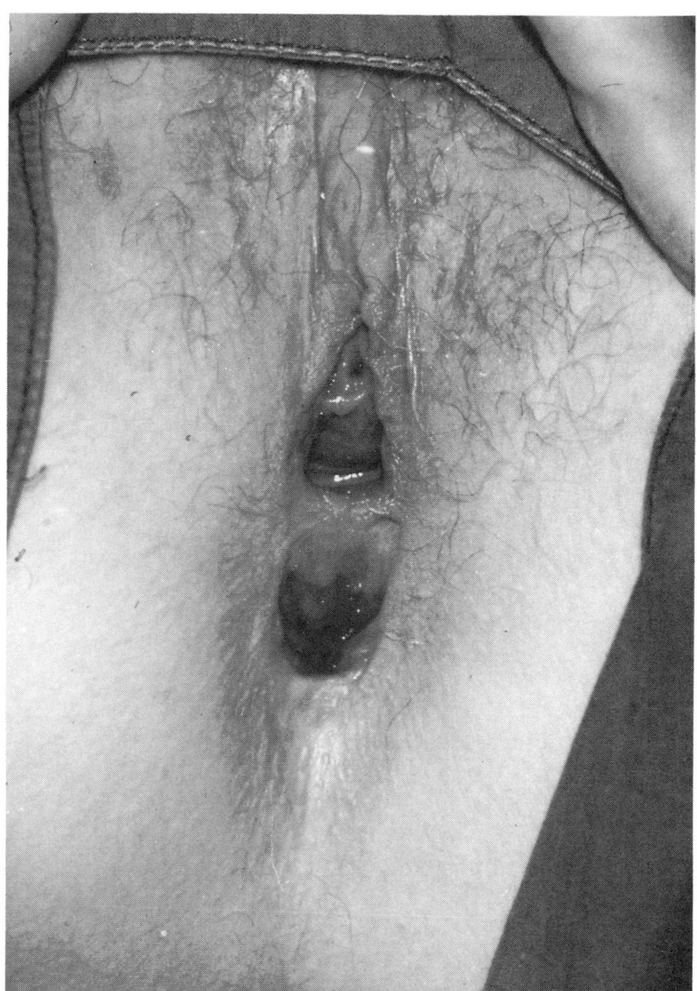

Fig. 1.5 Incomplete development of urorectal septum resulting in perineal anus with deficient perineum.

Development of the müllerian system

The müllerian ducts, which have fused in their lower part, reach and invaginate the urogenital sinus in the ninth week (30 mm stage). The end is solid and single and forms the müllerian tubercle which does not open into the sinus but makes contact with sinovaginal bulbs which are solid outgrowths from the sinus. As the hind part of the fetus unfolds and the pelvic region elongates, the sinus and the müllerian tubercle become increasingly distanced from the tubular portion of the ducts and a solid epithelial cord forms which provides length for the future vagina (Fig. 1.4). Thereafter lacunae appear which eventually join up to canalize the future vagina. How much of the original solid plate and epithelium of the vagina comes from the original urogenital sinus has long been a matter of dispute among embryologists. The current view is that most of the upper vagina is of müllerian origin and that there is metaplasia of müllerian epithelium to form its stratified squamous epithelium (Gray & Skandalakis 1972). The solid sinovaginal bulbs also have to canalize to form the lower vagina and this occurs above the level of the eventual hymen so that the epithelia of both surfaces of the hymen are of urogenital sinus origin.

Complete canalization of the vagina is a comparatively late event (occurring in the sixth and seventh month) and failure may occur at a variety of levels and for variable

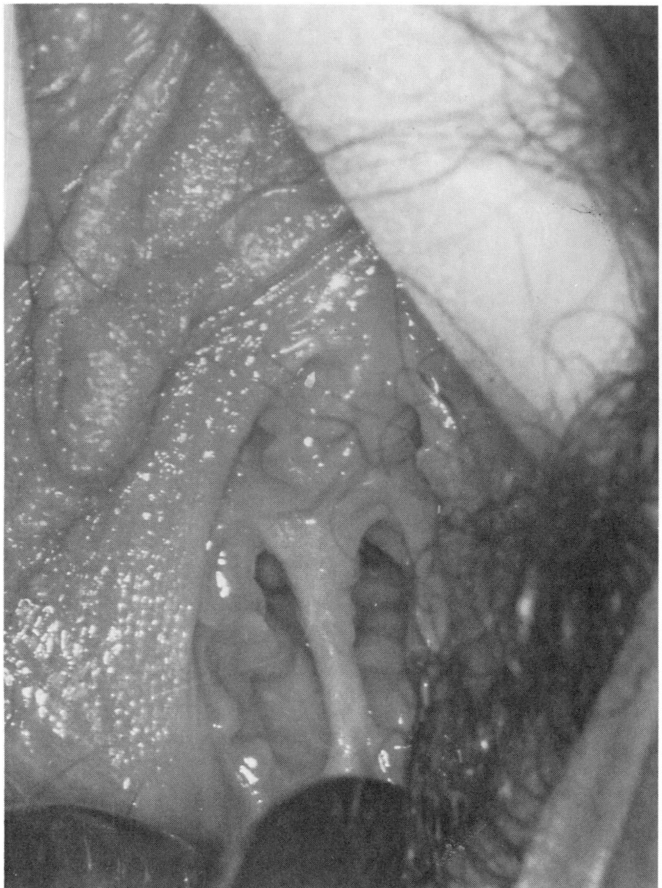

Fig. 1.6 Anteroposterior septum at introitus.

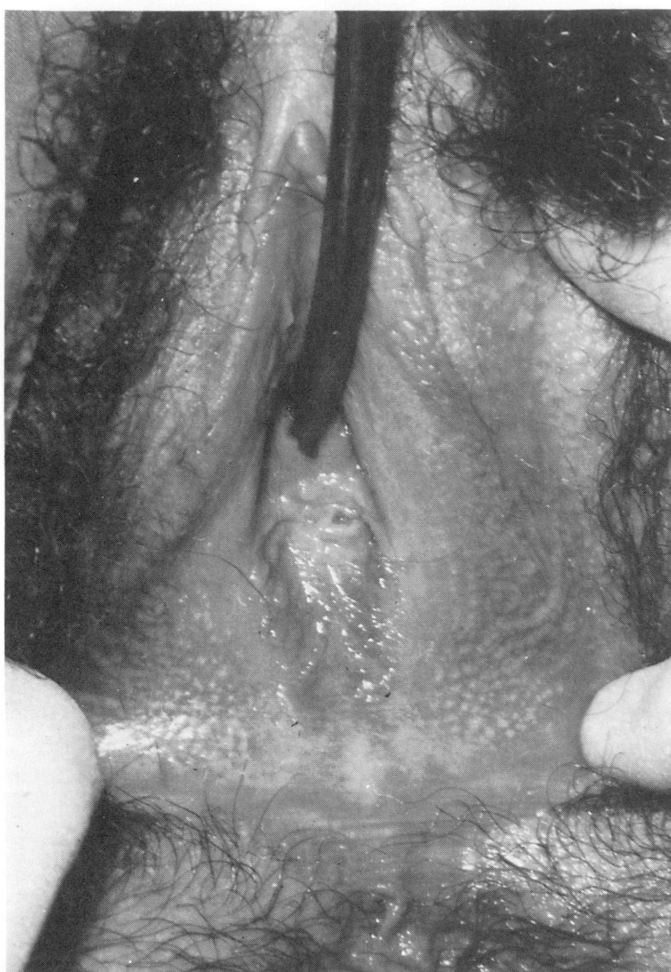

Fig. 1.7 Almost complete occlusion of introitus with small opening about 2 cm posterior to the urethra and slightly to the left. There had been no obstruction to menstrual flow but there was apareunia and inability to insert a tampon.

depth. If the tubular portions of the müllerian ducts develop to form a uterus and cervix, there is usually a patent upper vagina. If there is no development of the urogenital sinus, the subsequent vaginal atresia involves most of the vagina. Where there is müllerian agenesis, the urogenital sinus still forms but does not lengthen as much as normally and the vagina is short though of variable length. Correct early formation with failure of complete canalization (essentially failure of the lacunae to join up fully) can leave a variety of septae: transverse, sagittal, coronal or oblique of varying thicknesses (Fig. 1.6). The mildest abnormality of this sort to cause complete obstruction is a lower vaginal transverse membrane (imperforate hymen) which is generally just above the anatomical hymen. Partial obstruction may result in apareunia or inability to insert a tampon but no obstruction to menstrual flow (Fig. 1.7).

Duplication or failure of fusion at uterine level

Fusion of the ducts occurs at an early stage of müllerian development before organ differentiation into cervix or uterine body. Thus, there is no point at which a formed uterus and cervix fuse. A true duplication of the uterus, cervix and tubes can occur but this involves splitting of the müllerian duct at an early stage. This can occur on one or both sides but is rare. More common is incomplete development of the fused ducts indicating their bilateral origin, i.e. incomplete fusion of two halves. These variations form a series of well recognized uterine anomalies of varying clinical significance (see below; Gray & Skandalakis 1972).

Remnants of the mesonephric duct

The distal portion of the regressing wolffian duct may leave remnants in the mesovarium (epoopheron) or in the cervical or vaginal walls (Gartner's duct). These may form cysts. The incidence of some remnant is estimated to be about 20% but they are less often of clinical significance.

Mechanism and timescale of gonadal development

To understand the development of the external genitalia and some of the derangements of internal structures, it is necessary to consider some of the factors which control gonadal development. This complex area has been much clarified by the studies of many workers in the last decades, notably Jost & Wachtel (Wilson et al 1981a). This aspect is more fully dealt with in Chapter 12 but some reference to this area is necessary to understand the importance of timing in deviations of embryological development. The basic sequence is chromosomal sex, gonadal differentiation and phenotype. Essentially, whatever chromosome complement is present, it is the endocrine effects of the gonads which determine phenotype.

The germ cells arise outside the gonad and if they do not arrive at the genital ridge during the sixth week of embryonic development, the gonad only forms a fibrous streak. By this stage the gonad is bipotential and consists essentially of primordial germ cells, connective tissue of the genital ridge and covering epithelium. It is a structure with cortical and medullary potential.

What happens then depends on whether there is sufficient testicular component to induce somatic cells to form all or part of a male system. Normally this occurs when there is a Y chromosome and the relevant genes are carried in the pericentric region of the short arm. Exceptions to this situation are recognized, e.g. 46 XX males where there is no recognizable Y chromosome.

The precise connection between the Y chromosome and the somatic cells is not clear. It is certain that formation of the testis precedes any other sexual development. Some years ago a serologically determined male antigen, found on the plasma membrane of the cells of the male embryo, was recognized as a Y-induced histocompatibility antigen (H–Y; Wachtel 1983). This substance is essential for the organization of seminiferous tubules and subsequent male development. Without it, no male gonadal development proceeds. Recent monoclonal antibody techniques have shown that this Y-inducer substance is not necessarily contained in the Y chromosome, as it is present in XX males, but the concept of its presence to induce male development is still valid. Interchange of material and copy of the testis-determining gene on an X chromosome are being studied by DNA techniques (Ferguson-Smith 1988). The subsequent testicular development is one of cortical regression and medullary growth leading to the development of spermatic cords, seminiferous tubules and Leydig cells. Human chorionic gonadotrophin stimulates the Leydig cells and testosterone synthesis is well under way by 9 weeks from fertilization.

The differentiation of the gonad determines the hormonal environment and in turn the differentiation of the internal duct system, the external genitalia and perhaps the embryonic brain. (Wilson et al 1981b). The timing of these steps is shown in Figure 1.8.

Mechanism and timescale of ovarian development

Morphological development of the ovary starts about

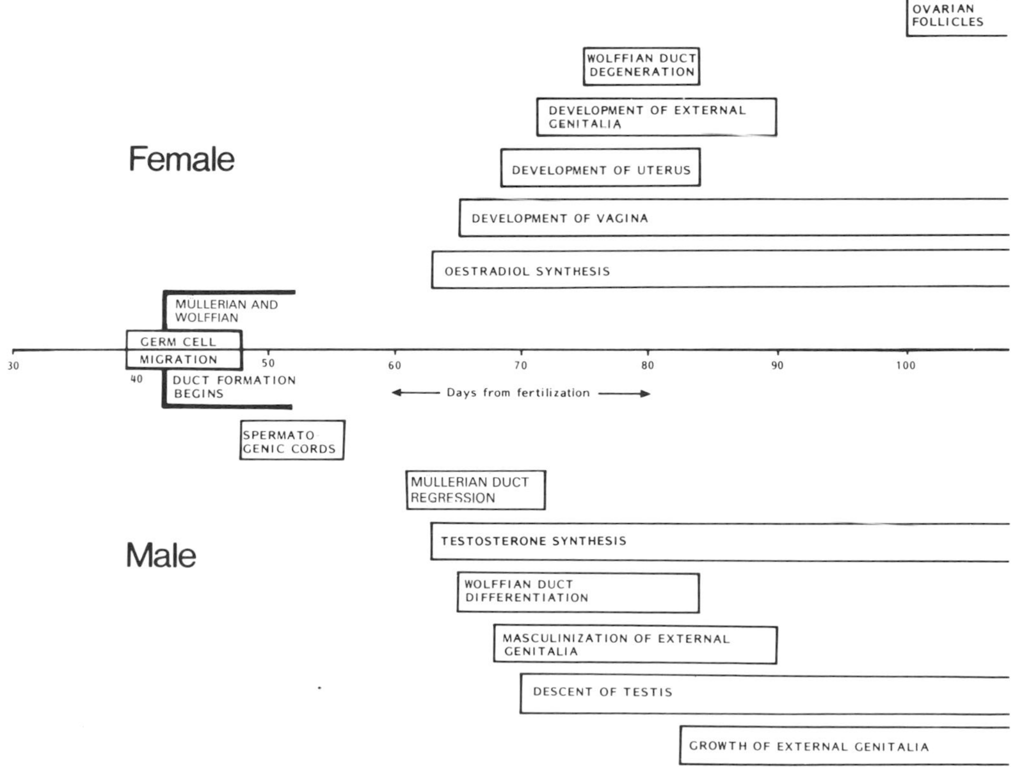

Fig. 1.8 Timing of anatomical, gonadal and endocrine events. Data from Coulam (1979) and Wilson et al (1981b).

2 weeks later than the testis and proceeds more slowly. Development of the female internal duct system is not dependent on ovarian formation and proceeds ahead of development of the germ cells. Nevertheless, oestrogen is produced from the ovary prior to germ cell growth and it is presumed that the primitive Leydig cells produce oestrogen by conversion from testosterone — a process that has been shown to occur before differentiation.

If no H–Y antigen is formed, the cortical zone of the gonad develops and contains the germ cells, whereas the medullary zone regresses to form a compressed aggregation of tubules and Leydig cells in the hilus of the ovary. The germ cells divide and by 20 weeks of gestation there are primordial follicles with oocytes. The peak formation of primordial follicles is about this time and is about 5–7 million by 20 weeks. Atresia starts about then and by birth there are about 1–2 million germ cells surrounded by a layer of follicular cells. The germ cells enter the first meiotic division and are arrested in prophase.

Development of the duct systems

Provided that the genital ridge develops, all embryos have wolffian and müllerian systems. Normally one system develops and the other regresses. Whatever the chromosomal sex, it is the production of androgen that controls development of the wolffian system.

This process is accomplished by the production of müllerian inhibiting factor which is the initial product of the testis and the first interactive event between the gonad and the duct system. MIF is a glycoprotein of about 70 000 molecular weight and it appears to be formed by the spermatogenic tubules very early in their development. The process of inhibition of the müllerian ducts is an active one and if this early function of the testis fails, then a female genital tract will develop. The production of MIF is quite separate from that of androgen production. It acts locally and deficiency can be unilateral. A hereditary disorder of persistent müllerian duct syndrome exists where a fallopian tube and hemiuterus may occur on one or both sides and coexist with normal wolffian development in otherwise normal genetic and phenotypic males. It is not clear whether this results from failure to produce MIF or from tissue unresponsiveness. Suboptimal testicular function is probable since there is often failure of testicular descent.

Another feature indicative of the independence of these processes is that there is usually regression of the müllerian ducts even when defective testosterone synthesis results in an under-masculinized male. If there is no functional testis, no MIF is produced, the müllerian system develops and there is no stimulation of the wolffian system. This is the normal event in the female but proceeds whether there is a normal ovary or not. The two genital duct systems and the urinary tract have a common opening between the genital folds. Their fate depends on the formation of the external genitalia.

Development of the external genitalia

There is overlap in timing of the formation of the external genitalia and the internal duct system (Fig. 1.9). There is a common indifferent stage, consisting of two genital folds, two genital swellings and a midline, anterior genital tubercle. The female development is a simple progression from these structures.

Genital tubercle → clitoris
Genital folds → labia minora
Genital swellings → labia majora

In the male, the genital folds elongate and fuse to form:

Genital tubercle → glans
Genital folds → penis and urethra
Genital swelling → scrotum

This process is normally dependent on fetal testosterone production. Agents or inborn errors that prevent the synthesis or action of androgens inhibit formation of the external genitalia.

By the end of the first trimester of pregnancy, fusion of

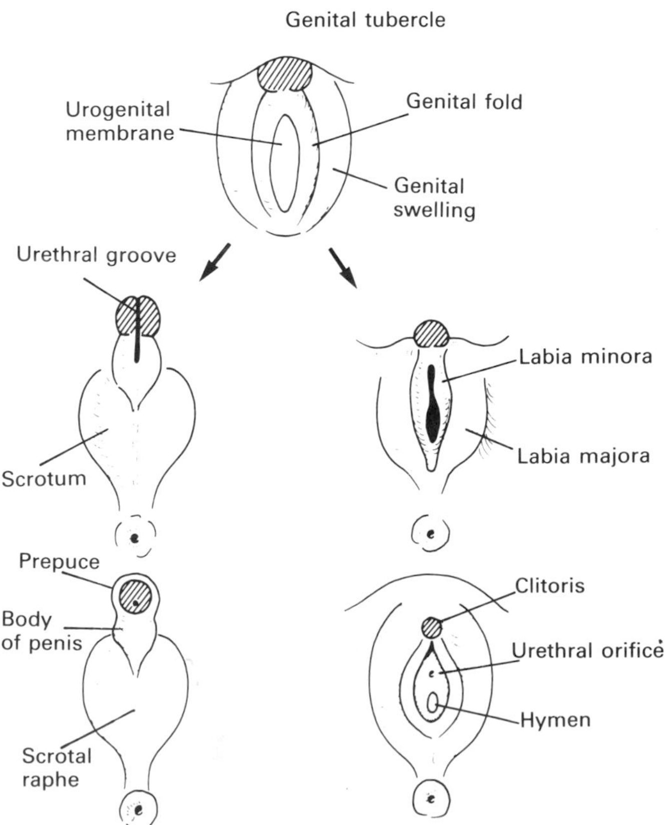

Fig. 1.9 Development of female and male external genitalia from the different stages.

the genital folds has occurred in the male but with little differential growth. Hence at this stage of gestation inspection of the genitalia may be misleading. It is during the second trimester that most of the differential male growth occurs.

The external genitalia are very sensitive to androgen effects during development, the end-result depending on both androgen availability and local tissue sensitivity. This can account for a variable degree of ambiguity of the basic female phenotype. If sufficient local androgen activity is not achieved by the 10th week from fertilization, incompletely masculinized genitalia will result in the male. Equally, exposure to sufficient androgens can result in a very similar appearance in the female. In congenital adrenal hyperplasia in the female, the degree of masculinization is variable (Fig. 1.10) but full scrotal and penile development may take place. However, the timing of adrenal development means that the androgenic stimulus arrives too late to affect the internal duct system. Once the external genitalia are fully developed, future androgen stimulus in the female will cause clitoral hypertrophy but not fusion of the labia.

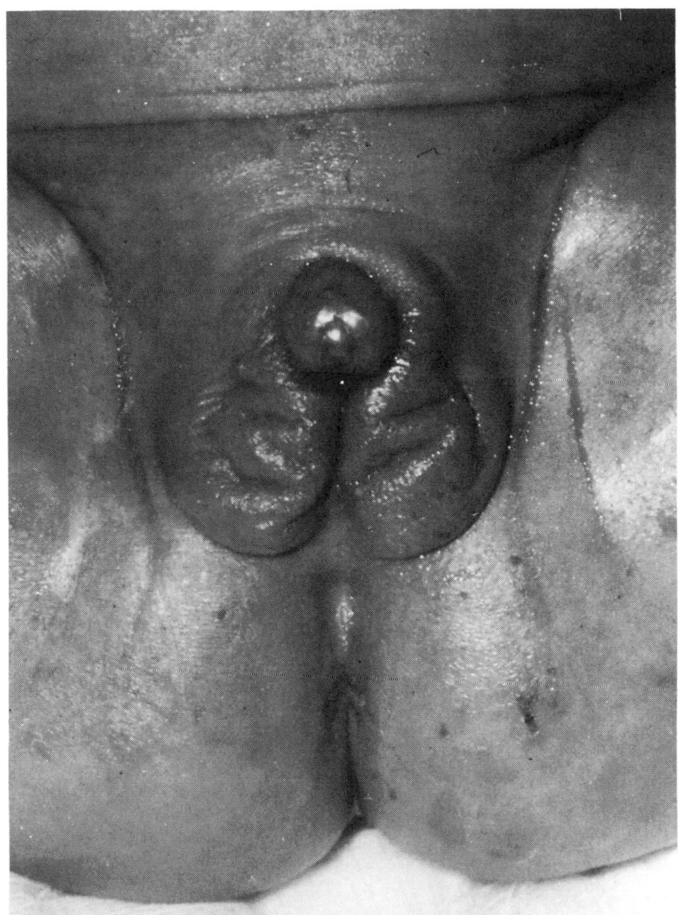

Fig. 1.10 Masculinized female genitalia in congenital adrenal hyperplasia.

Defective virilization resulting in female phenotype

There are several mechanisms by which defective virilization in a genetic male may occur. Although this range of conditions is quite uncommon, their existence has helped elucidation of the mechanism of differentiation. They are of importance to the gynaecologist where the end-result is one of female or ambiguous external genitalia. Because awareness of these conditions arose by sporadic reports in different countries, an assortment of terminology developed including XY gonadal dysgenesis, agonadism, vanishing testes, anatomical testicular failure, male pseudohermaphrodism, and testicular feminization. There are several subgroups:

1. Chromosomal anomaly, e.g. some cases of 45 X/46 XY.
2. Gonadal failure: testicular regression due to, for example, viral infection or vascular accident.
3. Defect of testosterone biosynthesis: enzyme defects.
4. End-organ resistance: complete androgen insensitivity; incomplete androgen insensitivity; 5_{α}-reductase deficiency; androgen receptor failure.

Better sense can be made of the component of gonadal failure in this spectrum of conditions, by recognition of critical stages in testicular development with the final effect depending on the embryonic stage at the time of testicular failure (Coulam 1979). It is important to distinguish testicular failure from androgen insensitivity (see Ch. 12) and this section refers only to individuals who are agonadal by the time of birth.

The spectrum of clinical effect depends on whether the fetal testis produced enough MIF to suppress the müllerian system, and whether there was enough androgen production to develop both the wolffian system and male external genitalia. There are seven different clinical entities (Table 1.1). In this group of conditions, to have a female phenotype there has to be failure of testicular development before androgen is secreted, but not necessarily before MIF is produced. Therefore such a girl would not be expected to have wolffian duct development. Whether or not there is a female genital tract depends on whether there was MIF (or enough MIF) before gonadal failure occurred. To have ambiguous or male genitalia, there must have been some secretion of androgen before gonadal failure occurred. The amount and duration of androgen production determines the anatomical result. Müllerian and wolffian ducts can coexist if gonadal failure occurred before müllerian regression was complete yet after androgen secretion had started. The clinical effects can be seen as a consequence of loss of testicular function at different stages of intrauterine development. The possible range extends from complete failure of development of the genital ridge (and therefore no internal duct system of either kind) to a male phenotype with anorchia.

Table 1.1 Classification of XY agonadal individuals

	Embryonic testicular regression		Fetal testicular regression				
Timing	Early	Late	Early			Mid	Late
Days from fertilization		43	60	69	75	84	120
Embryological consequence of testicular failure	No genital ridge development	Müllerian regression not yet started; no testosterone production	Müllerian regression not complete; testosterone synthesis *just* started	Müllerian regression still not complete; testosterone enough for duct development	Müllerian regression complete; testosterone production too little to develop duct system but some for external genitalia	Müllerian regression complete; wolffian development complete; incomplete external genitalia; rudimentary testes	Complete wolffian duct system; complete external genitalia; no testes or epididymis
Müllerian system	–	+	+	+	–	–	–
Wolffian system	–	–	–	+	–	+	+
External genitalia	Female	Female	Ambiguous	Ambiguous	Ambiguous	Ambiguous Male	Male

Adapted from Coulam (1979).

The cause of these testicular insults is not usually known. They can be experimentally induced by drugs such as cyproterone acetate. In the human situation some may be viral or a consequence of torsion or vascular occlusion. This group of conditions is best called the testicular regression syndrome, classified further according to the timing of the failure in development (Table 1.1).

Testosterone failure

The group of individuals with a Y chromosome, gonadal formation but some abnormality of testosterone production or effect are not discussed further here. Some however, result in an entirely female phenotype (e.g. androgen insensitivity syndrome) and are relevant to disorders of puberty (see Ch. 13).

GENETICS — SEX CHROMOSOME ANOMALIES

Although sexual development is essentially gonadal, this is influenced by the sex chromosome complement. There are many derangements of the X and Y chromosomes and some of these have important anatomical and functional effects. The problem may reside in the number or in the structure of the chromosomes and variations may occur in mosaic or non-mosaic form. The main non-mosaic forms are summarized in Table 1.2 in order of the number of X chromosomes and of extra Y chromosomes.

Aneuploidy

Aneuploidy may result from non-disjunction of either meiotic division in either parent or in an early cleavage of the zygote. Some are more common in older women (e.g. 47 XXX and 47 XXY) and the non-disjunction is presumed to arise mainly in maternal meiosis. The occurrence of 45 X does not seem to be related to maternal age (Therman 1986).

Although there is a wide range of clinical effects, some generalizations can be made:

1. If there is a Y chromosome, the phenotype is usually male.
2. If the number of sex chromosomes increases beyond three (i.e. more than one extra) there is a strong tendency to some degree of mental retardation.
3. Additional Y chromosome material tends to increase height.

Table 1.2 Identified non-mosaic patterns of sex chromosomes. Normal male and female karyotypes highlighted.

Female phenotype	Male phenotype	Barr bodies
45 X	**46 XY** 47 XYY 48 XYYY	0
46 XX	46 XX 47 XXY 48 XXYY 49 XXYYY	1
47 XXX	48 XXXY 49 XXXYY	2
48 XXXX	49 XXXXY	3
49 XXXXX		4

4. Provided there is at least one Y chromosome, one or more extra chromosomes result in hypogonadism.
5. In each somatic cell, all but one X chromosomes are inactivated (lyonized).

Both Kleinefelter's syndrome (XXY) and XYY occur in about 1 in 700 newborn males. The clinical features are well recognized but are outside the scope of this chapter. The higher-order anomalies with a male phenotype are very rare.

X chromosome aneuploidy with a female phenotype

Many of the abnormal X chromosomal complements are associated with gonadal dysgenesis and abnormalities of stature.

One X less

The 45 X chromosome constitution accounts for more than half of the number of girls with Turner's syndrome. The overall incidence of this condition is about 1 in 2500 live female births but nearly half have a mosaic pattern or some other X chromosome aberration (de la Chapelle 1983). Short stature is invariable in 45 X; sexual infantilism is usual, and other somatic features such as webbed neck, low hairline, cubitus valgus, pigmented naevi and cardiovascular anomalies are variably expressed but useful diagnostically. There is no systematic impairment of IQ, at least by verbal testing, but scoring on spatial ability tends to be lower. Classically, by the time of birth (or puberty) the gonads are non-functioning streaks but ovarian function has been described in about 3% and even fertility (especially in those with mosaicism or structural anomalies of a second X). Pregnancy loss and karyotype anomalies of the fetus are common when pregnancy does occur.

One extra X

Triple X arises in about 1 in 1200 live female births and often passes unnoticed. There is no consistent clinical syndrome, thus accounting for the lack of ascertainment, but an increased incidence of psychosis has been noted. Phenotype, puberty and fertility are normal though there is a higher incidence of secondary amenorrhoea and early menopause. There is a tendency to increased height. Conception may result in XXX or XXY (or mosaic) progeny, but this occurs much less often than the predicted 50% and it is clear that in the meiotic division of the oocyte, the extra X chromosome ends up in the polar body more often than would be predicted by chance.

More than one extra X

This is rare. Dysmorphism and mental retardation are usual but psychosis and aggression are not features. There may be some resemblance to Down's syndrome (Grouchy & Turleau 1984). Phenotype, external genitalia and puberty are usually normal. Menstrual disorders are common. Fertility is possible and the incidence of chromosomal abnormalities in the progeny, though not well assessed, is likely to be high.

Mosaicism

This is more common for sex chromosomes than for autosomes. Two cell lines can arise from a single zygote due to non-disjunction in an early mitosis. The commonest are 46 XX or 46 XY accompanied by a 45 X cell line but an enormous variety is possible and there can be more than two cell lines. The mechanisms which control their origin are extremely complicated and not well understood (Simpson et al 1982).

The clinical effects are wide-ranging and especially complex when there is both an XX and an XY cell line. The relative proportion of the different cell lines tends to determine the phenotype but this can vary in different organs and some result in hermaphrodite or intersex states.

Structural abnormalities of X chromosomes

Apart from the number of X chromosomes and mosaic cell lines, there are many possible variations in the X chromosome pattern in the female. Developments in banding techniques and in other methods of studying DNA sequences have enabled the locations on the X chromosome of genes determining gonadal and somatic features to be identified (Fig. 1.11). Development in techniques has necessitated frequent revision of concepts of karyotype/phenotype correlation and this process is still continuing. Undetected mosaicism is always a possibility and any generalizations are subject to early revision. The basic conventions of banding and nomenclature of chromosomes with

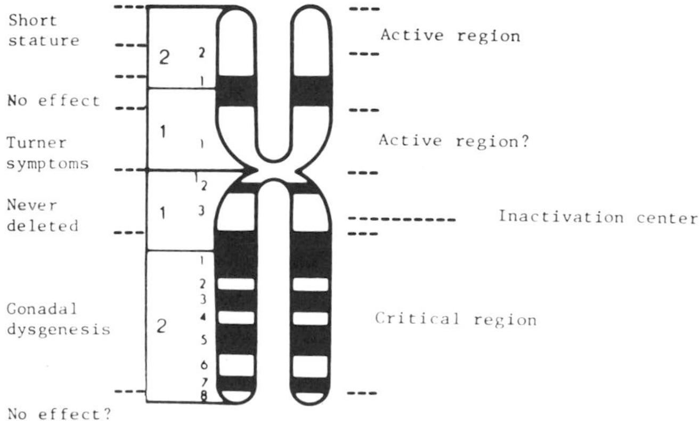

Fig. 1.11 Diagram of X chromosome showing the main active regions. On the left, the main phenotypic effects of various deletions are shown (from Therman 1986 with permission).

respect to deletion and isochromy should be understood (Fig. 1.12).

The generalizations given in Table 1.3 are relevant to an understanding of the clinical effects.

Table 1.3 General effects of structural abnormalities of X chromosomes

	Aspects of phenotype affected	Effect of loss of material	Effect of extra material
Short arm	Ovarian function	Gonadal dysgenesis	
	Somatic features of Turner's	Turner's phenotype	
	Growth	Short stature	
Long arm	Ovarian function	Gonadal dysgenesis	
	Growth	Reduced growth	Increased growth

If there is one normal X and the other is abnormal, inactivation of the abnormal one occurs in the somatic cells and this tends to diminish the effect of the abnormality.

Gonadal function, stature and the stigmata of Turner's syndrome depend on the nature of the second X chromosome and this clinical effect is further varied by the existence of a mosaic cell line (usually 45 X). Despite the fact that the second X is usually inactivated, both X chromosomes are required for female fertility. Whether deletion of portions of either arm of one X chromosome results in gonadal dysgenesis depends critically on exactly what genetic material is missing. Deletion of all or part of the short or long arm can occur. If most or all of the short arm is deleted, then short stature and Turner's features are usual. Deletion of most or all of the long arm is nearly always associated with gonadal dysgenesis.

A ring chromosome can form if part of both ends are missing. The clinical effect will depend on the amount of genetic material lost but the effect tends to be less than if a whole arm is absent. Isochromy, due to misdivision at the centromere, can result in two long arms i(Xq) instead of a short (p) and a long (q) arm. In effect this results in three long arms and one short one and the effect on gonadal function and stature is the same as 45 X.

Gonadal determinants appear to be located on both arms but it is not a question of total amount, since duplication of one fails to compensate for loss of the other and each arm must carry different functions. There appear to be components determining stature on both arms but loss of short arm material seems to result more consistently in short stature.

Although this area remains complex and only partially understood, a reasonable prediction of stature and potential for gonadal function can be made from consideration of the karyotype (Table 1.4).

XX gonadal dysgenesis

There need not be a demonstrable abnormality of sex chromosome pattern for gonadal dysgenesis to occur. The

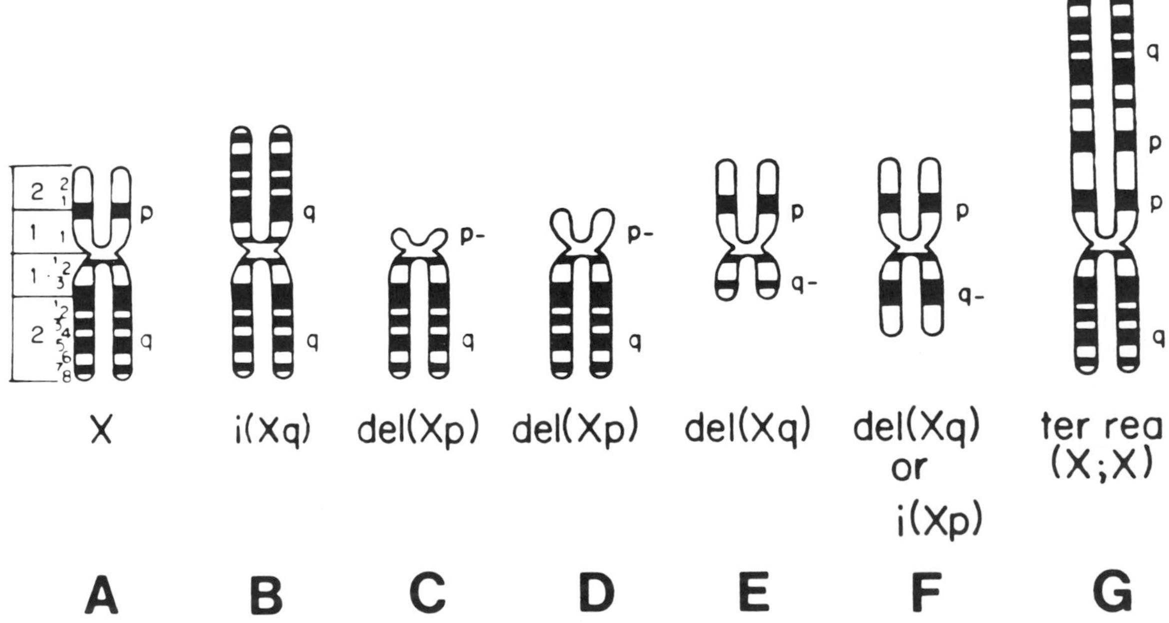

Fig. 1.12 Schematic diagram of some structural abnormalities of the X chromosome. **A** normal; **B** isochrome for long arm; **C** deletion of most of the short arm; **D** probable interstitial deletion of the middle portion of the short arm; **E** interstitial deletion of the long arm; **F** deletion of a portion of the long arm; G short arm end-to-end terminal rearrangement (from de la Chapelle 1983 with permission).

Table 1.4 Correlation of X karyotype, phenotype and gonadal development

Sex chromosomes				
Problem	Example of karyotype	Stature	Primary amenorrhoea	Breast development
Monosomy for X	45 X	Short	Almost certain	Absent or minimal
Short arm material missing				
Isochromy of long arm	46 X, i(Xq) or 45 X/46 X, I(Xq)	Short	Almost certain	Absent or minimal
Most of short arm	46 X, del(X)(p11)	Short	Variable	May be some
Terminal part of short arm	46 X, del(X)(P22)	Short	Not likely	Usually some
Long arm material missing				
Isochromy of short arm (rare or doubtful mosaic)	46 X, i(Xp)	Reduced	Certain	None
Most of long arm	46 X, del(X)(q13)	Reduced	Likely	Mininal
Terminal part of long arm	46 X, del(X)(q22)	Reduced	Likely	Minimal
Mosaic	45 X/46 XX	Variable	Variable	Variable*
	46 XX/range of deletions/isochromy	Variable	Variable	Variable*

* The effect of these depends very much on the proportion and distribution of the normal cell line.

Compiled from data in Simpson et al (1982).

gonads and genitalia look exactly the same in this condition as in 45 X though most such girls are of normal stature without Turner features. This condition is usually autosomal recessive and developments in genetics may clarify the mechanism in the future.

Translocations

Translocation can occur between an X chromosome and an autosome. The effect on ovarian function and phenotype varies (position effect). The normal X is inactivated and the parts of the other X attached to the autosomal segments remain active (Zakharov & Baranovskaya 1983). If the translocation is unbalanced there is mental retardation and ovarian failure. If balanced, mental retardation is still likely.

X–X translocations

One X chromosome may be replaced by a very long X consisting of two X chromosomes attached by either their long or short arms. This results in a variable amount of X genetic material being deleted or being present in a double dose. Where long arm material is lost there is usually gonadal dysgenesis, despite the extra X material. The translocation X is late replicating and it is the structurally normal X which is genetically active (Fig. 1.13; Dewald & Spurbeck 1983).

True hermaphrodites

This condition is characterized by the demonstration of both ovarian and testicular tissue. From the genetic point of view it is heterogeneous. The commonest single chromosome pattern is 46 XX but there is often more than one cell line and this may be due to chimerism (two cell lines at fertilization) or mitotic non-disjunction. Recognized cell lines include 46 XX/46 XY and 46 XX/47 XXY. Essentially, the more testicular tissue there is, the more likely is gonadal descent. Usually there is at least a hemiuterus and if ovarian tissue is present it is more likely to be on the left side.

The management depends on the phenotype (see Ch. 12). Ovulation and, where the anatomy is appropriate, conception and delivery can occur.

CONGENITAL ABNORMALITIES OF FEMALE DEVELOPMENT

Anomalies of female development may present to the gynaecologist in many ways and at different stages of life. The preceding sections have aimed to set out a basis for understanding variations in terms of chromosomal sex, gonadal development (including inappropriate hormone production), sex duct development and external genitalia. Some of the resulting conditions are mainly the concern of the paediatric surgeon, e.g. cloacal anomalies; the urologist, e.g. bladder extrophy, abnormal ureters; the paediatrician, e.g. disorders of growth. There is necessarily overlap in the specialties in conditions such as ambiguous genitalia (see Ch. 12) and disorders of puberty (see Ch. 13).

This section deals with anatomical disorders of the genital tract in the phenotypic female. Fetal diagnosis, although possible for some conditions, is not considered further here. Conditions with a genetic but no anatomical genital abnormality, e.g. 45 X, and other conditions pre-

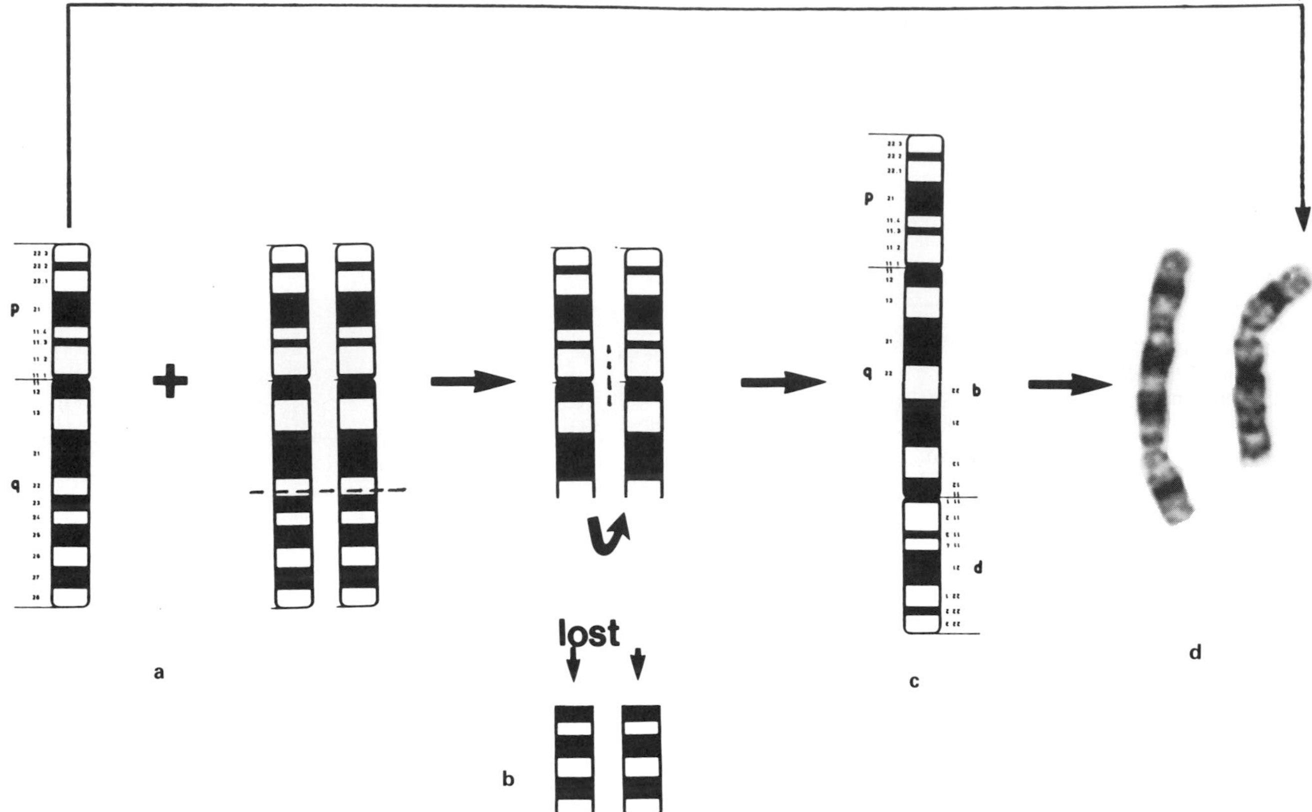

Fig. 1.13 Formation of an isodicentric X chromosome idic(X) (q22). (**a**) chromatid breakage at band q22; (**b**) reunion of sister chromatids with loss of acentric segment; (**c**) division of centromere to form end-to-end fusion chromosome. One centromere becomes inactive. (**d**) chromosomes from a 46 X idic(X)(q22) cell.

senting with primary amenorrhoea, e.g. complete androgen insensitivity, are discussed later (see Ch. 13).

Some of the anatomical abnormalities seen are an arrest of a stage of normal development, e.g. vaginal atresia, while others, e.g. bladder extrophy, do not represent a stage which the normal fetus ever passes through.

The most common times of presentation of abnormalities of the genital tract are:

1. *Newborn* — if there are external abnormalities or obstruction of bladder or bowel;
2. *Childhood* — if there is no external abnormality but there is disturbance of function;
3. *Puberty* — particularly if menstrual function is affected;
4. *Coitarche* — relative obstruction during intercourse;
5. *Adult* — infertility or during pregnancy or parturition.

It is not possible to estimate the incidence of genital tract anomalies accurately since the age of ascertainment, the thoroughness of surveillance and the inclusion of minor anomalies will influence this. In pregnancy, an incidence of müllerian anomalies of 1 in 600 women has been estimated but this excludes the very important groups who cannot conceive. Perhaps a reasonable estimate would be some abnormality of the genital tract in 1% of phenotypic females.

The neonate or child

Neonates and children with congenital abnormalities of female development may present in one of several ways:

1. Ambiguous genitalia.
2. Imperforate vagina, with a large abdominal mass due to mucocolpos.
3. Duplication of the vulva.
4. Cloaca (often involving spinal defects).
5. Ectopia vesicae.
6. Imperforate anus.
7. Disorders of renal system affecting micturition or drainage.

Need for gynaecological assessment

Although recognition, diagnosis and management are the province of the paediatrician and paediatric surgeon there are several reasons why a gynaecologist should be involved:

1. Study of the original anatomy aids comprehension of the problem.
2. Familiarity with the surgery on the infant helps with reconstructive surgery at puberty or later.
3. Where there are anomalies of the urinary or bowel systems, liaison improves the investigation of the anatomy of the genital tract.
4. Diagnosis of the abnormal vulva is not easy and improves with practice.

Where there are abnormalities of the urinary or bowel systems in the female, concomitant anomalies of the genital tract are quite common. However, the need to consider the function of the genital tract is less pressing and its investigation in these conditions presenting early in life is often incomplete (Fleming et al 1986).

Multiple abnormalities

These include persistent cloaca (Fig. 1.14), bladder extrophy and ectopic ureter. The anatomy of the genital tract can be clarified in the course of investigation using endoscopy, ultrasound, contrast vaginogram (or sinogram) and, where necessary, laparotomy. The primary concern is function of the bladder and bowel but free drainage of the genital tract is also important as obstruction is often a feature. Careful recording of the genital anatomy is valuable for prognosis and later reference (Ducan 1989).

Imperforate vagina

Mucocolpos due to an imperforate vagina may cause a large abdominal mass in the newborn. It is not clear why this occurs only occasionally when there is obstruction or whether a minor degree occurs in all girls with an imperforate vagina but passes unnoticed. Although the clinical problem is rare in the newborn, nevertheless it is important in the differential diagnosis of an abdominal mass in a newborn girl.

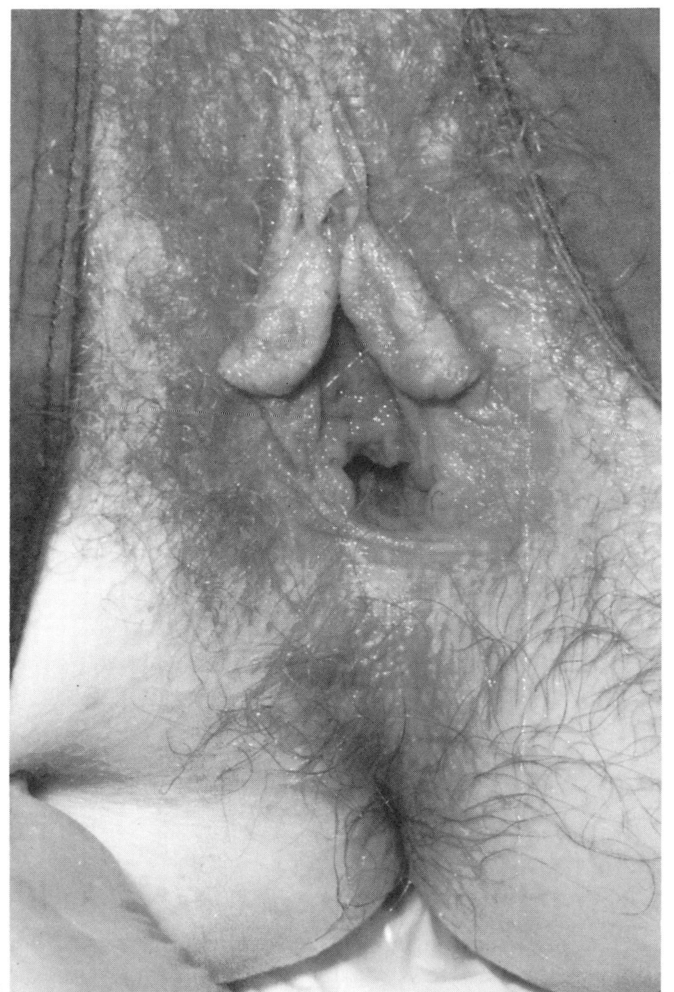
a

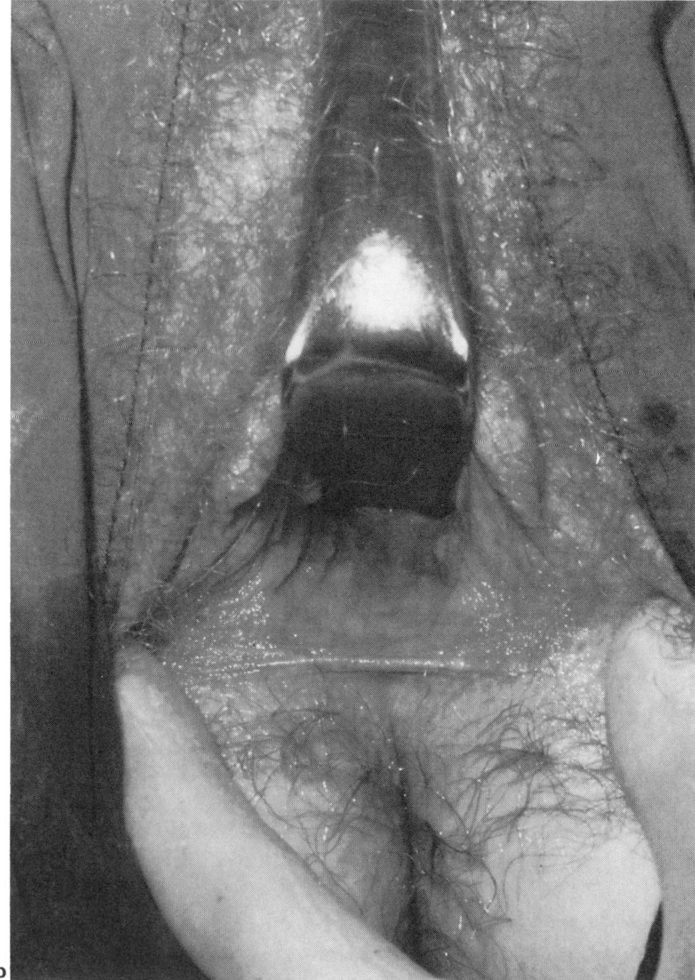
b

Fig. 1.14 Cloaca. (**a**) Single opening with absence of anus; (**b**) rectal columns posteriorly in cloaca.

Duplication of vulva

This is rare and full paediatric surgical investigation is required to establish other abnormalities and effective drainage. A didelphic uterus is likely. If there is no functional problem then an acceptable cosmetic effect would be the aim.

Ambiguous genitalia

This conditions arises in:

1. Virilized females, e.g. congenital adrenal hyperplasia; high maternal androgen levels; maternal drug ingestion.
2. Undermasculinized male;
3. True hermaphrodite.

The diagnosis and management are essentially paediatric and clinical aspects of abnormal sexual development are discussed in Chapter 12. At birth, ambiguity is a management problem requiring high priority. The best available advice should be obtained.

Puberty or later

Of the conditions with gynaecological relevance considered here some result from embryological failure, some are a consequence of mutant genes and in others a genetic factor is suspected but not certain. Reporting of these conditions has not been systematic and has been more likely where there have been family aggregates. The close relation between urinary tract and genital anomalies should be remembered.

In müllerian agenesis, there is no corpus or cervix and no upper vagina (Fig. 1.15). There may or may not be fallopian tubes representing the upper separate ends of the müllerian duct system. The condition has been reported in siblings but not with enough consistency to suggest that it is due to single gene defect. Müllerian agenesis accounts for over 80% of girls with no vagina.

Vaginal atresia with development of the müllerian system is a distinct condition with no reporting of family aggregates except where the atresia is part of multiple anomalies (Simpson et al 1982). The failure of the urogenital sinus to form the lower vagina may be complete or there may be a lower vagina with an obstruction of variable thickness in the mid-portion. True duplication due to splitting of the müllerian duct or even of the genital ridge early in embryogenesis does not have any family aggregates whereas incomplete fusion may be one component of a congenitally determined malformation. Even if it occurs as the only abnormality, incomplete fusion seems to have a polygenic or multifactorial basis resulting in some family aggregation.

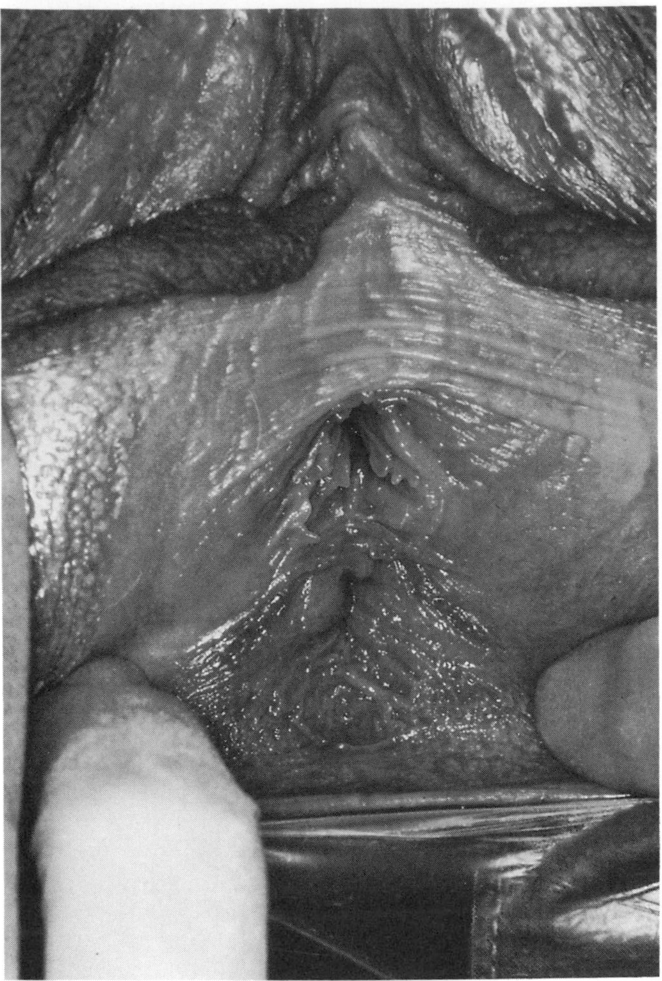

Fig. 1.15 Vulva (labia widely retracted) of a girl with müllerian agenesis. The urethra is abnormally patulous and there is very little formation of the urogenital sinus portion of the vagina.

Presentation

Abnormalities not diagnosed in infancy may become of clinical relevance around the time of puberty or later and are more likely to affect the vagina or upper genital tract. Vulvar abnormalities, however, may become evident because of hormonal stimulation. Failure of puberty development is discussed in Chapter 13. Where there is primary amenorrhoea with secondary sexual development, absence of the uterus or obstruction to menstrual flow should be considered. Other presenting complaints include apareunia or inability to insert a tampon.

Vaginal atresia or obstruction

Where this condition has not been diagnosed in infancy, failure to menstruate is the likeliest presenting symptom. The crucial clinical question is whether or not there is haematocolpos. Higher levels of obstruction, at the cervix

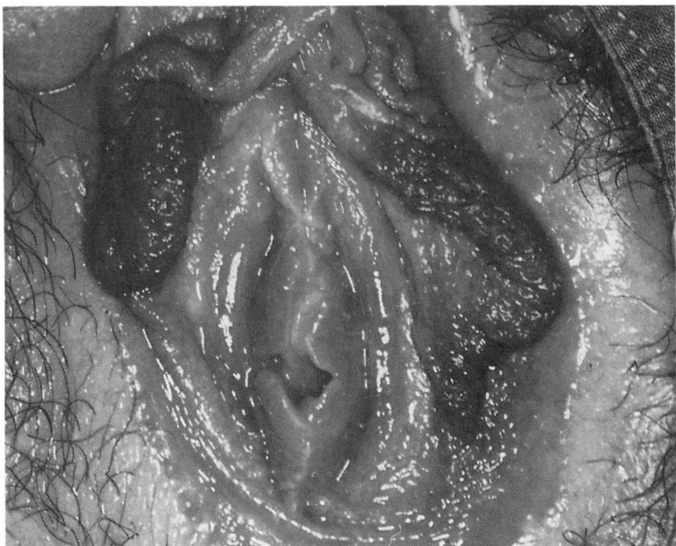

Fig. 1.16 Normal-looking vulva of a girl with vaginal atresia and haematocolpos and haematometra. There was a short lower vagina.

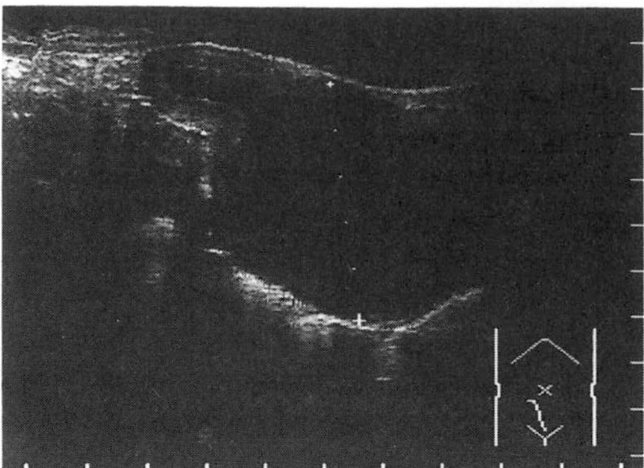

Fig. 1.17 Ultrasound scan of the same girl showing distended upper vagina and distended uterus.

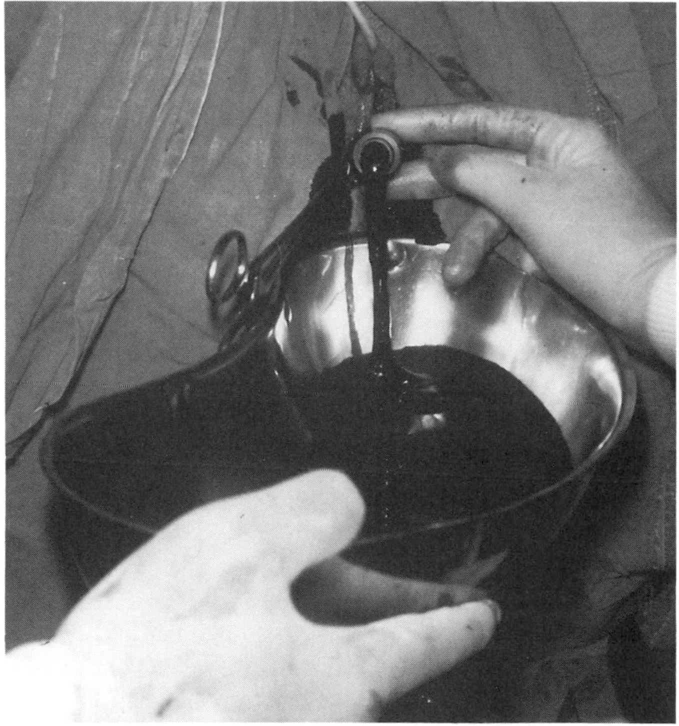

Fig. 1.18 Drainage of haematocolpos required dissection and insertion of a trocar.

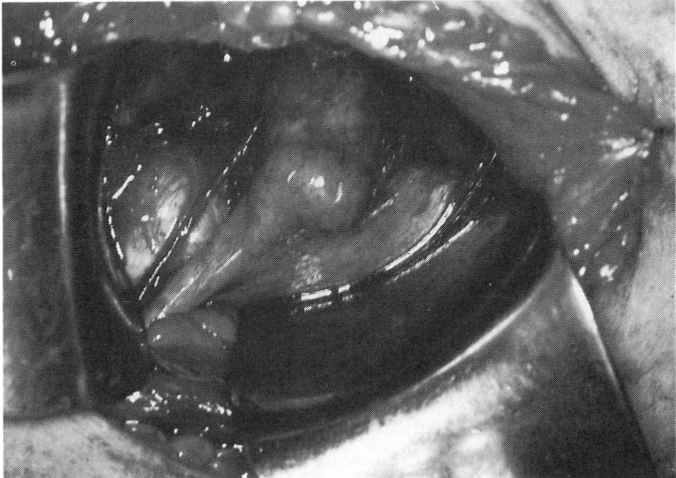

Fig. 1.19 Associated haematosalpinx.

or upper vagina, will tend to cause symptoms sooner and also cause more serious backflow and endometriosis. Any recurrent abdominal pain (not necessarily regular or monthly) in pubertal girl with some secondary sexual development should be investigated sooner rather than later. Ultrasound of the pelvis and kidneys is very useful. Inspection of the introitus, although important, may be misleading where there is a high obstruction (Fig. 1.16–1.19).

Where the obstruction is low and thin, usually just above the hymen, a simple cruciate incision to allow free drainage of retained menses is all that is required initially. After two or three further periods, by which time the anatomy will probably be restored to normal, laparoscopy is indicated to diagnose and treat any endometriosis. The anatomy of the renal tract should be established.

Where there is vaginal atresia, management can be difficult. If it is not possible to reach the upper vagina from the perineum, an abdominoperineal approach may be required. Achieving drainage is not usually difficult and should be effected from the vagina if possible. The difficulty is to maintain subsequent patency. Much patience and ingenuity may be required. Continuous oestrogen-progestogen treatment may provide a respite (Duncan 1989).

Atresia of the cervix

This condition is due to failure of development of the cervical portion of the fused müllerian ducts. It is rare and serious. The uterus may be normal or didelphic. If initial attempts to create a cervical opening are not effective it may be better to resort to hysterectomy before serious intraperitoneal infection occurs since the resulting tubo-ovarian masses and peritonitis may become life-threatening (Geary & Weed 1973). Unless this condition is diagnosed and treated very early, the tubes are unlikely to function. Indeed, access to the uterus and ovaries may be quite impossible after episodes of peritonitis. In one of my own cases with large, bilateral hydrosalpinges after years of conservative efforts, removal of the diseased tubes because of severe peritonitis led to quiescence with continuing ovarian and uterine function and at least a prospect of in vitro or donor egg fertility.

Vaginal agenesis

Where vaginal agenesis is part of müllerian duct failure the clinical picture is different. The introitus may look normal or there may be hypoplasia of the entire urogenital component. Usually there is a short (1–2 cm) vagina. The incidence is about 1 in 10 000 female births. Ureterorenal anomalies occur in about 50%. A rudimentary uterus is quite common but it may be just a thin band of tissue on one or both sides and is not canalized. The appearances on ultrasound have sometimes been deceptive but with better resolution a false impression of canalization is less likely. However, it should be noted that ultrasound of the uterus is more difficult where there is no vagina.

The presentation is generally with amenorrhoea and well developed secondary sex characteristics. Care is required if the girl is seen soon after the time of expected menarche to establish for certain whether or not there is a functioning uterus. If not, the question of a neovagina is best deferred until there is an interest in sexual activity. A range of techniques are available (Lesavony 1985; Edmonds 1988) but the extent to which a small vagina can be enlarged by non-surgical means should not be underestimated where motivation is high.

Where there is a short blind vagina and müllerian agenesis, androgen insensitivity must be included in the differential diagnosis. Small breasts and poorly developed axillary and pubic hair are important accompanying features. There may be a family history. Virilization at puberty is a feature of partial androgen insensitivity. Chromosome analysis is helpful in these circumstances and should be done when there is müllerian agenesis without well developed secondary sexual characteristics.

Persistent urogenital sinus

A common genitourinary channel is the normal arrangement in a male infant and occurs to some degree during development in all female infants. Failure of development and caudal movement of the lower vagina results in a higher common channel than usual. The confluence of the vagina and urethra may be at a very variable level. The condition is present in most girls with infantile congenital adrenal hyperplasia; all individuals with an intersex condition brought up as girls, and spontaneous incomplete development (see Ch. 13).

The presentation depends on whether there is, or has been, masculinization (which is not necessarily a feature) and on prior surgery, possibly in infancy. The typical feature is a small, single opening with no visible separate urethra and fusion of the labia majora. A minor degree of the condition may interfere with coitus or use of tampons. In a severe degree, surgery is necessary to enable coitus.

Virilization occurring at puberty

There are a number of causes:

1. An intersex problem rectified in infancy but leaving a slightly enlarged clitoris. This tends to enlarge at

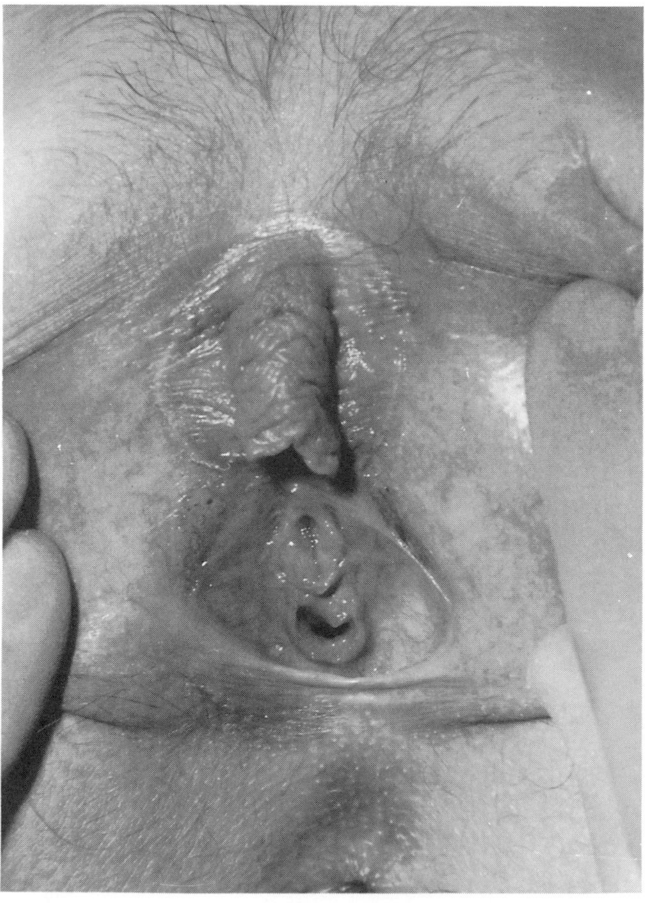

Fig. 1.20 Hypertrophy of clitoris occurring at puberty due to oestrogen administration in an otherwise phenotypic female (XY). There had been minimal hypertrophy in infancy associated with intersex (mainly scrotal development with testes) and the gonads had been removed in the neonatal period. Note that the androgenic stimulus in utero had not been sufficient to fuse the genital folds.

puberty during spontaneous or replacement hormone stimulation — even just oestrogens (Fig. 1.20).
2. Incomplete androgen insensitivity. There may have been only slight clitoral enlargement which responds further to the greater androgen boost at puberty.
3. 5_{α}-reductase deficiency — this is always relative and again the puberty levels of testosterone cause growth.
4. Gonadoblastoma in a dysgenetic gonad.

The hormonal, gonadal and anatomical status must be completely evaluated. Inappropriate androgen secretion must be removed, except in some cases of 5_{α}-reductase deficiency where reinforcement of the male gender has been successful. If clitoral hypertrophy remains a problem — and it will not tend to regress much if oestrogen replacement is effected — some form of clitoral reduction should be offered (Duncan 1989).

Uterine anomalies

Absence of the uterus is an important cause of primary amenorrhoea and is discussed more fully in Chapter 13. Since it is essentially due to failure of development of the lower part of the paramesonephric (müllerian) ducts, the cervix and upper vagina are also absent. There may be a vestigial uterus and cervix without canalization and without function.

True duplication of the müllerian ducts with doubling of reproductive structures on one or both sides is rare.

Fusion anomalies are more common and result in a variety of well recognized uterine shapes (Fig. 1.21). Where there is atresia of one of the paramesonephric ducts there is a unicornuate uterus with a single tube. The kidney on the side of the defective duct is often absent. If the unilateral atresia is partial, the rudimentary part may be an appendage to the well developed side and, if it fails to communicate, the rudimentary horn causes complications. Where there is a didelphic uterus, the uterine cavities are completely separate (Fig. 1.22) but the two cervices are often united externally. The vagina may or may not be septate. In this condition, asymmetry of the vagina may result in complete closure of only one-half with subsequent cryptomenorrhoea and haematometra but with apparently normal menstrual function (Figs 1.23–1.25). Curiously, when this condition occurs, the occluded side is nearly always on the right. There is ipsilateral absence of the kidney (Rock & Jones 1980). Failure of complete müllerian duct fusion and failure to form a ureter are both a consequence of a defective mesonephric duct.

Provided there is no obstruction to menstrual flow, these uterine anomalies present few problems in the absence of pregnancy. An increased incidence of miscarriage, poor fetal growth, malpresentation and placental adherence is recognized. The incidence of abnormalities and the complication rate are ill defined since ascertainment is higher where there are complications and operative delivery. Pregnancy may occur in a non-communicating rudimentary horn by transperitoneal sperm passage and can result in a difficult diagnostic and management problem.

For many of the anatomical congenital anomalies, the

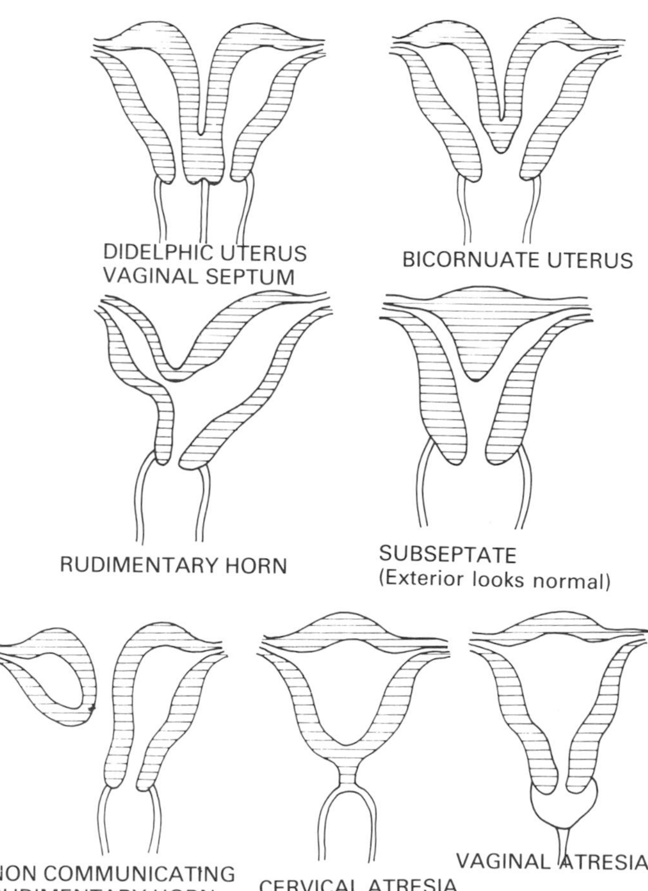

Fig. 1.21 Varieties of uterine anomaly.

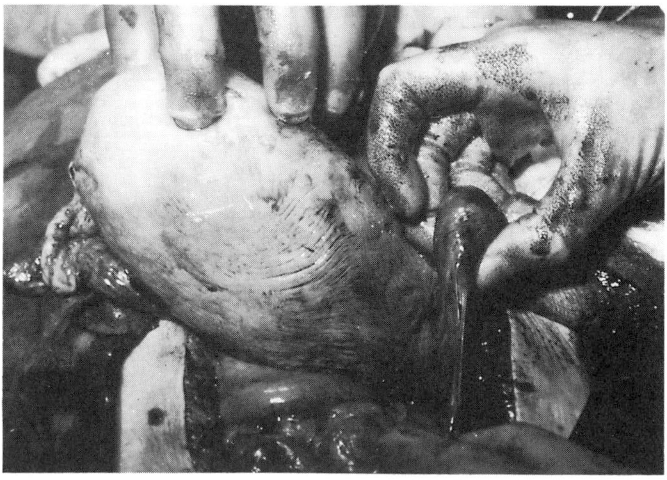

Fig. 1.22 Didelphic uterus at the time of caesarean section. The non-pregnant right uterus is attached externally at the cervix.

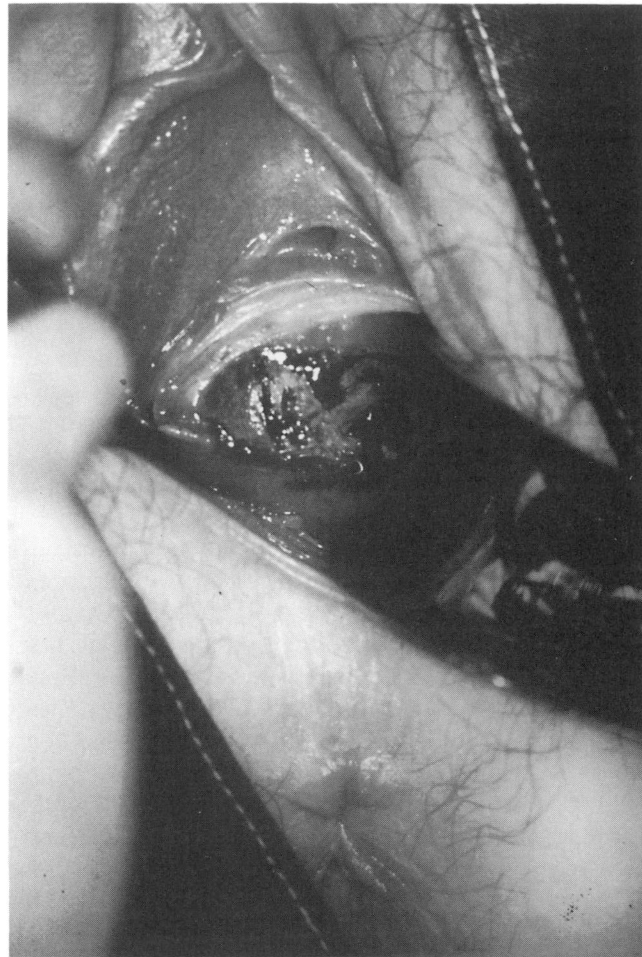

Fig. 1.23 Partially exposed haematocolpos of right hemivagina. The speculum is in the normal left hemivagina.

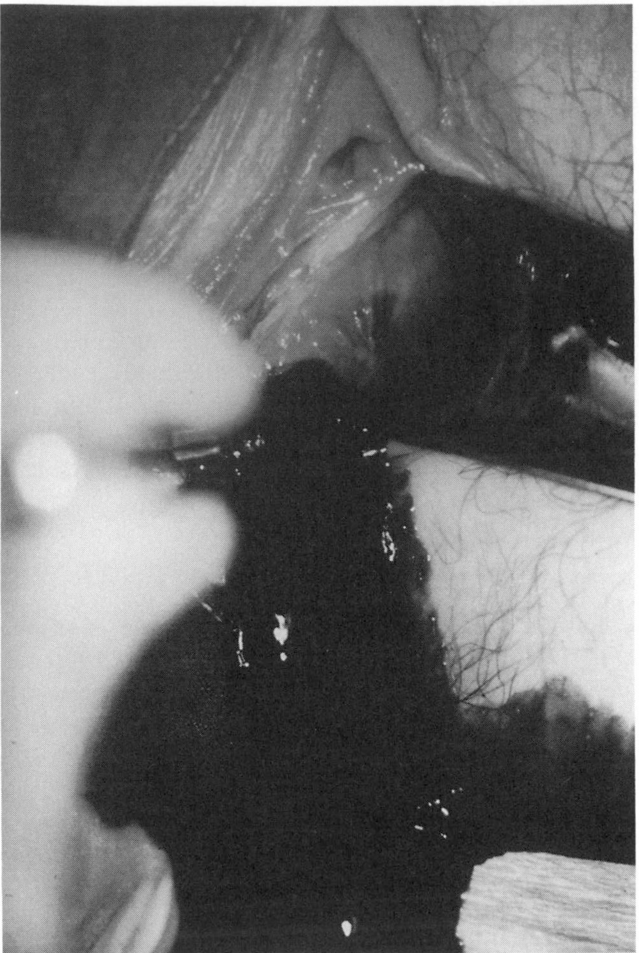

Fig. 1.24 Incision and drainage.

event which caused developmental failure is not clear even if the stage of arrest can be recognized. Much has been discovered about the controlling mechanisms in recent decades and further elucidation is likely.

KEY POINTS

1. The nephrogenic cord develops from the mesoderm and forms the urogenital ridge and mesonephric duct (later to form the wolffian duct).
2. The paramesonephric duct, later to form the müllerian system, develops as an ingrowth of coelomic epithelium anterolateral to the mesonephric duct.
3. In the normal female, the wolffian system degenerates and the lower ends of the müllerian system fuse to form the uterus, cervix and upper vagina while the cephalic ends remain separate, forming the fallopian tubes.
4. Unilateral renal aplasia is frequently associated with failure of müllerian development on the same side since both are dependent on adequate development of the mesonephric system.
5. If the tubular portions of the müllerian ducts develop to form a uterus and cervix, there is usually a patent upper vagina.
6. If there is no development of the urogenital sinus, the subsequent vaginal atresia involves most of the vagina.
7. Where there is müllerian agenesis, the urogenital sinus still forms but does not lengthen as much as normally and the vagina is short though of variable length.
8. Chromosomal sex determines the development of the gonad and this, in turn, ordains the sexual phenotype.
9. The wolffian system is dependent upon androgens for its development.
10. The müllerian system will develop in the absence of a glycoprotein secreted by the fetal testis called müllerian inhibiting factor (MIF) and does not require a normal ovary.

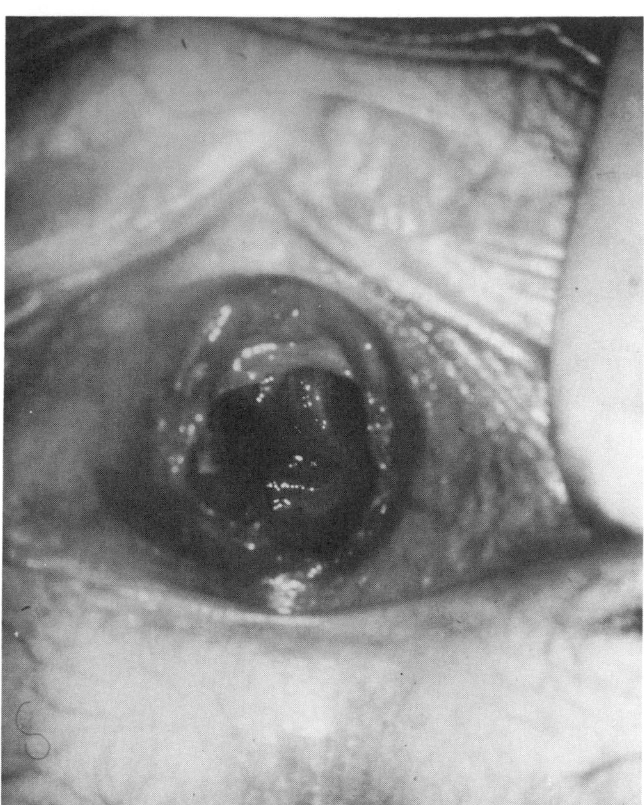

Fig. 1.25 Septum in the same girl after drainage.

11. The development of external genitalia depends upon both the presence of androgens and local tissue sensitivity to androgens.
12. If a Y chromosome is present, the phenotype is usually male.
13. Although the second X chromosome is usually inactivated, both X chromosomes are required for fertility.
14. Gonadal dysgenesis can occur in an XX individual.
15. The primary concern in the management of abnormalities recognized in childhood is function of the bladder and bowel but free drainage of the genital tract is also important as obstruction is often a feature and permanent damage may result if this is not corrected before puberty.
16. Müllerian agenesis is the commonest cause for an absent vagina in girls.
17. Any recurrent abdominal pain in a pubertal girl with some secondary sexual development should be investigated sooner rather than later with a view to excluding haematocolpos. Ultrasound of the pelvis and kidneys is very useful.
18. If correction of cervical atresia is unsuccessful, hysterectomy should be employed to avoid the potentially lethal peritonitis that may result.

REFERENCES

Coulam C B 1979 Testicular regression syndrome. Obstetrics and Gynecology 53: 44–49

de la Chapelle A 1983 Sex chromosome anomalies. In: Emery A E H, Rimoin D L (eds) Principles and practice of medical genetics. Churchill Livingstone, Edinburgh, p 197

Dewald G W, Spurbeck J L 1983 Sex chromosome anomalies associated with premature gonadal failure. Seminars in Reproductive Endocrinology 1: 79–90

Duncan S L B 1989 Gynaecological aspects of congenital anomalies. In: Stanton S (ed) Clinical gynaecological urology. Churchill Livingstone, London

Edmonds D K 1988 Congenital malformations of the vagina and their management. Seminars in Reproductive Endocrinology 6: 91–98

Ferguson-Smith M 1988 Genes on the X and Y chromosomes controlling sex. British Medical Journal 297: 635–636

Fleming S E, Hall R, Gysler M, McLorie G A 1986 Imperforate anus in females. Frequency of genital tract involvement. Incidence of associated anomalies and functional outcome. Journal of Paediatric Surgery 21: 146–150

Geary W L, Weed J C 1973 Congenital atresia of the uterine cervix. Obstetrics and Gynecology 42: 213–217

Gray S W, Skandalakis J E 1972 The female reproductive tract. In: Embryology for surgeons. W B Saunders, Philadelphia, pp 633–664

Grouchy J, Turleau C 1984 Sex chromosomes. In: Clinical atlas of human chromosomes, 2nd edn. John Wiley, New York, pp 375–409

Lesavony M A 1985 Vaginal reconstruction. Urological Clinics of North America 12: 369–379

Rock J A, Jones H W 1980 The double uterus associated with an obstructed hemivagina and ipsilateral renal agenesis. American Journal of Obstetrics and Gynecology 138: 339–342

Simpson J L, Golbus M S, Martin A, Sarto G E 1982 Disorders of sex chromosomes and sexual differentiation. In: Genetics in obstetrics and gynecology, Grune & Stratton, New York

Therman E 1986 Numerical sex chromosome abnormalities. In: Human chromosomes; structure, behavior, effects, 2nd edn. Springer-Verlag, New York, pp 176–181

Wachtel S S 1983 H–Y antigen and the biology of sex determination. Grune & Stratton, New York

Wilson J D, Griffin J E, George F W, Leshin M 1981a The role of gonadal steroids in sexual differentiation. Recent Progress in Hormone Research 37: 1–39

Wilson J D, George F W, Griffin J E 1981b The hormonal control of sexual development. Science 211: 1278–1284

Zakharov A F, Baranovskaya 1983 X–X chromosome translocations and their karyotype–phenotype correlations. In: Sandbert A A (ed) Cytogenetics of the mammalian X chromosome part B. Alan R Liss, New York

FURTHER READING

Gray S W, Skandalakis J E 1972 Embryology for surgeons — the embryological basis for the treatment of congenital defects. W B Saunders, Philadelphia

Sadler T W 1985 Langman's medical embryology, 5th edn. Williams & Wilkins, Baltimore

Westenfelder M, Whitaker R H 1981 Malformations of the external genitalia. Monographs in paediatrics 12. Karger, Basel

2. Pelvic anatomy

I. Vellacott

THE OVARY

The size and appearance of the ovaries depends on both age and the stage of the menstrual cycle. In the young adult, they are almond-shaped, solid and grayish-pink in colour; 3 cm long, 1.5 cm wide and about 1 cm thick. The long axis is normally vertical before childbirth; after this there is a wide range of variation, presumably due to considerable displacement in the first pregnancy.

The ovary is the only intra-abdominal structure not to be covered by peritoneum. Each ovary is attached to the cornu of the uterus by the ovarian ligament, and at the hilum to the broad ligament by the mesovarium, which contains its supply of vessels and nerves. Laterally, each is attached to the suspensory ligament of the ovary with folds of peritoneum which become continuous with that over the psoas major.

Structure (Fig. 2.1)

The ovary has a central vascular medulla consisting of loose connective tissue containing many elastin fibres and non-striated muscle cells, and an outer thicker cortex, denser than the medulla and consisting of networks of reticular fibres and fusiform cells, although there is no clear-cut demarcation between the two. The surface of the ovary is covered by a single layer of cuboidal cells, the germinal epithelium. Beneath this is an ill defined layer of condensed connective tissue, the tunica albuginea, which increases in density with age. At birth, numerous primordial follicles are found, mostly in the cortex but some in the medulla. With puberty, some form each month into graafian follicles which at later stages of their development

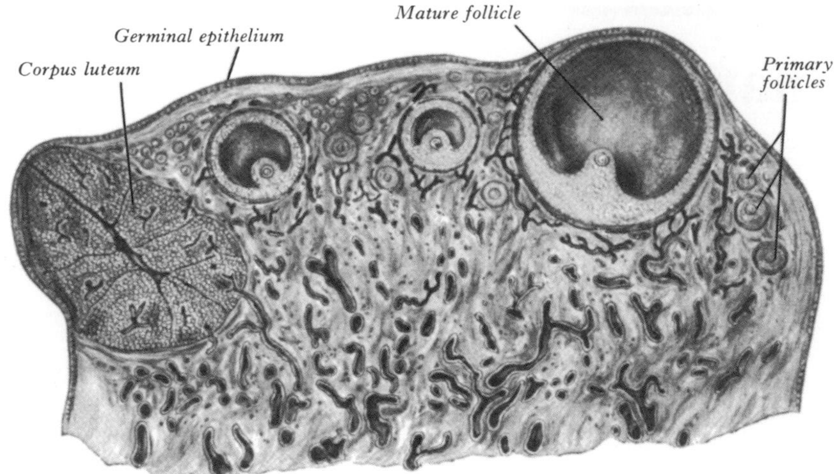

Fig. 2.1 Semi-diagrammatic section of an ovary.

form corpora lutea and ultimately atretic follicles, the corpora albicantes.

Relations

Anteriorly lie the fallopian tubes, the superior portion of bladder and uterovesical pouch; posteriorly is the pouch of Douglas. The broad ligament and its content are related inferiorly whilst superior to the ovaries are bowel and omentum. The lateral surface of the ovary is in contact with the parietal peritoneum and the pelvic side walls.

Vestigal structures

The vestigal remains of the mesonephric duct and tubules are always present in young children, but are variable structures in adults. The epoophoron, a series of parallel blind tubules, lies in that part of the broad ligament between the mesovarium and the fallopian tube, the mesosalpinx. The tubules run to the rudimentary duct of the epoophoron, which runs parallel to the lateral fallopian tube. Situated in the broad ligament, between the epoophoron and the uterus, are occasionally seen a few rudimentary tubules, the paroophoron.

In a few individuals, the caudal part of the mesonephric duct is well developed, running alongside the uterus to the internal os. This is the duct of Gartner.

Age-changes

During early fetal life, the ovaries are situated in the lumbar region near the kidneys. They gradually descend into

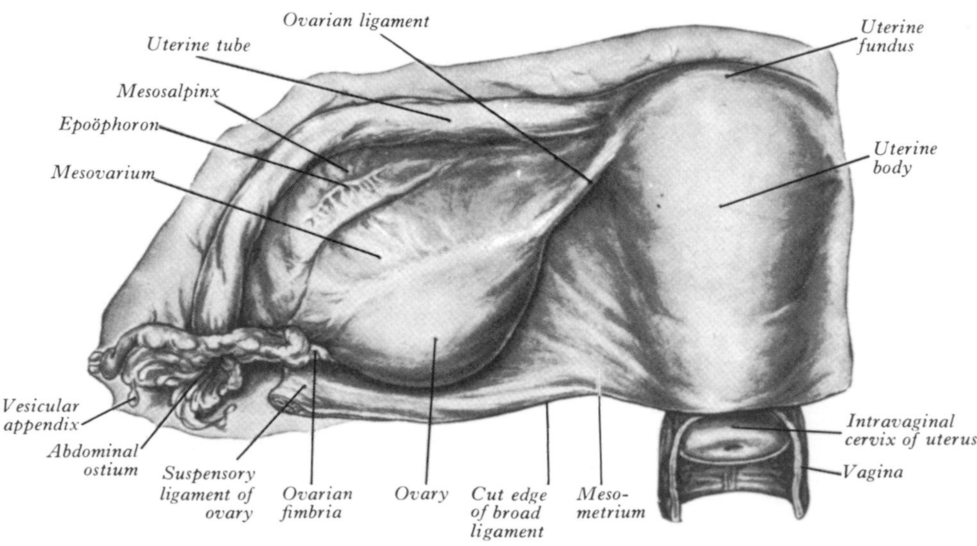

Fig. 2.2 Posterosuperior aspect of the uterus and the left broad ligament. The 'ligament' has been spread out and the ovary is displaced downwards.

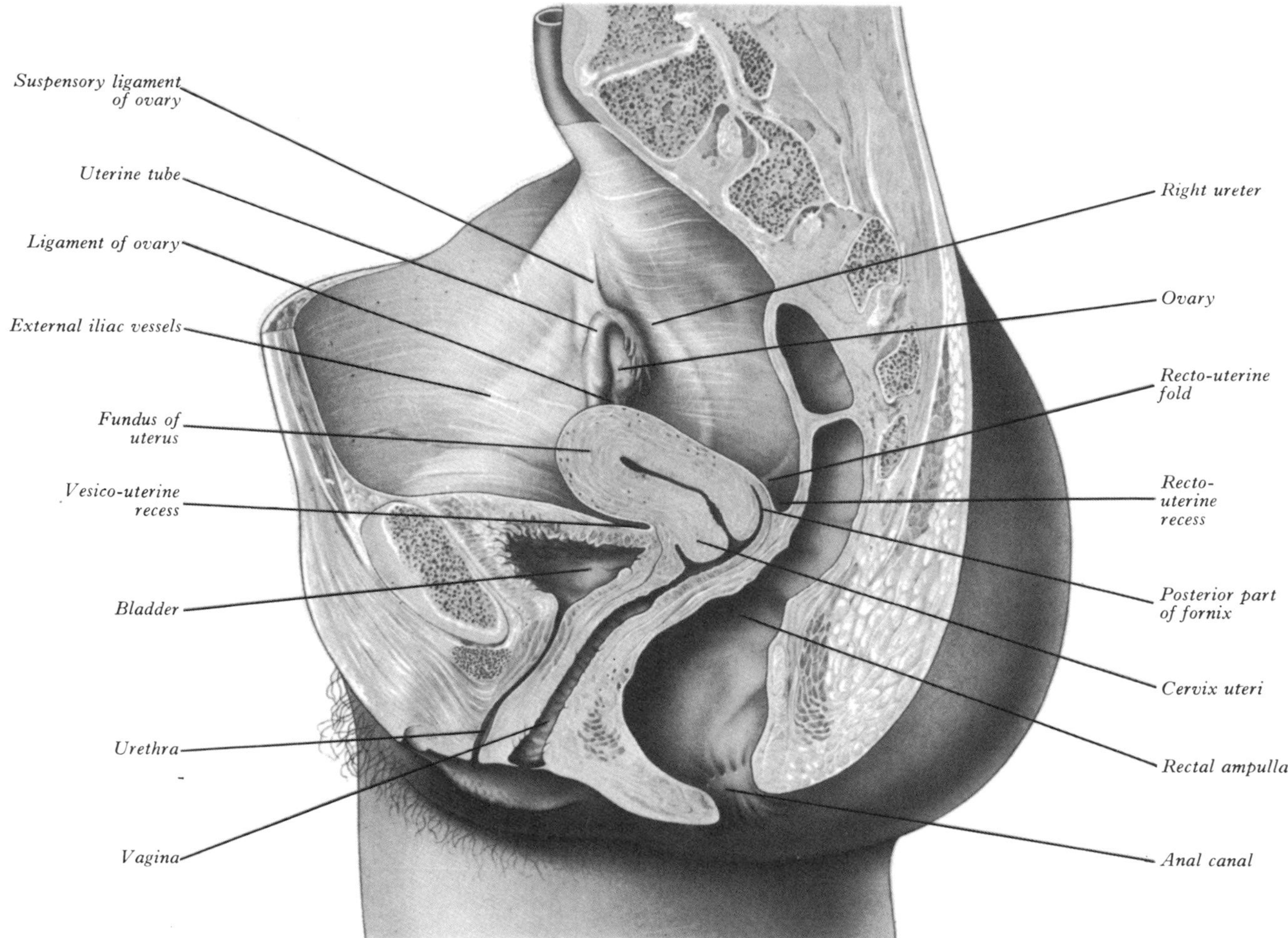

Fig. 2.3 Median sagittal section through a human female pelvis. The peritoneum is shown in blue.

the lesser pelvis and during childhood they are small and situated near the pelvic brim. They are packed with primordial follicles. The ovary grows in size until puberty by an increase in the stroma. Ova are first shed around the time of onset of menstruation and ovulation is usually established within a couple of years.

After the menopause, the ovary atrophies and assumes a smaller shrivelled appearance. The fully involuted ovary of old age contains practically no germinal elements.

THE FALLOPIAN TUBE

The uterine or fallopian tubes are two oviducts originating at the cornu of the uterus which travel a rather tortuous course along the upper margins of the broad ligament. They are around 10 cm in length and end in the peritoneal cavity close to the ovary. This abdominal opening is situated at the end of a trumpet-shaped lateral portion of tube, the infundibulum. This opening is fringed by a number of petal-like processes, the fimbriae, one of which closely embraces the tubal end of the ovary, the ovarian fimbria. This fimbriated end has an important role in fertility.

Medial to the infundibulum is the ampulla which is thin-walled and tortuous and comprises at least half the length of the tube. The medial third of the tube, the isthmus, is relatively straight. The tube has narrowed at this point, from around 3 mm at the abdominal opening to 1–2 mm. The final centimetre is within the uterine wall, the interstitial portion.

Structure (Fig. 2.2)

The tubes are typical of many hollow viscera in that they contain three layers. The outer serosal layer consists of peritoneum and underlying areolar tissue. This covers the whole tube apart from the fimbriae at one end, and the interstitial portion at the other. The middle muscular layer consists of outer longitudinal fibres and inner circular ones. This is fairly thick at the isthmus and thins at the ampulla.

The mucous membrane is thrown into a series of plicae or folds, especially at the infundibular end. It is lined with columnar epithelium, much of which contains cilia, which, together with the peristaltic action of the tube, help in sperm and ovum transport. Secretory cells are also present as well as a third group of intercalary cells of uncertain function.

Relations

These are similar to those of the ovary (see above). Medially, the fallopian tube, after arching over the ovary, curves around its tubal extremity and passes down its free border.

THE UTERUS

The uterus is shaped like an inverted pear tapering inferiorly to the cervix and, in the non-pregnant state, is situated entirely within the lesser pelvis. It is hollow and has thick muscular walls. Its maximal external dimensions are about 9 cm long, 6 cm wide and 4 cm thick. The upper expanded part of the uterus is termed the body or corpus. The area of insertion of each fallopian tube is termed the cornu and that part of the body above the cornu, the fundus. The uterus tapers to a small central constricted area, the isthmus, and below this is the cervix, which projects obliquely into the vagina and can be divided into vaginal and supravaginal portions (Fig. 2.3)

The cavity of the uterus has the shape of an inverted triangle when sectioned coronally; the fallopian tubes open at the upper lateral angles. The lumen is apposed anteroposteriorly. The constriction at the isthmus where the corpus joins the cervix is the anatomical internal os. Seen microscopically, where the mucous membrane of the isthmus becomes that of the cervix is the histological internal os.

Structure (Fig 2.4)

The uterus consists of three layers — the outer serous layer (peritoneum); the middle muscular layer (myometrium) and the inner mucous layer (endometrium).

The peritoneum covers the body of the uterus and posteriorly, the supravaginal portion of cervix. This serous coat is intimately attached to a subserous fibrous layer, except laterally where it spreads out to form the leaves of the broad ligament.

The muscular myometrium forms the main bulk of the uterus and comprises interlacing smooth muscle fibres intermingling with areolar tissue, blood vessels, nerves and lymphatics. Externally these are mostly longitudinal but the larger intermediate layer has interlacing longitudinal, oblique and transverse fibres. Internally, they are mainly longitudinal and circular.

The inner endometrial layer is not sharply separated from the myometrium: the tubular glands dip into the innermost muscle fibres. This is covered by a single layer of columnar epithelium. Ciliated prior to puberty, this columnar epithelium is mostly lost due to the effects of pregnancy and menstruation. The endometrium undergoes cyclical histological changes during menstruation and varies in thickness between 1 and 5 mm.

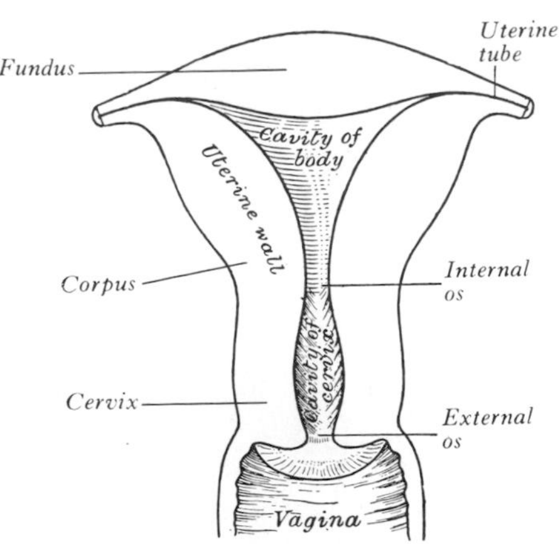

Fig. 2.4 Sectional diagram showing the interior divisions of the uterus and its continuity with the vagina.

The cervix

The cervix is cylindrical in shape, narrower than the body of the uterus and around 2.5 cm in length. It can be divided into the upper, supravaginal and lower vaginal portions. Due to anteflexion or retroflexion, the long axis of the cervix is rarely the same as the long axis of the body. Anterior and lateral to the supravaginal portion is cellular connective tissue, the parametrium. The posterior aspect is covered by peritoneum of the pouch of Douglas. The ureter runs about 1 cm laterally to the supravaginal cervix. The vaginal portion projects into the vagina to form the fornices.

The upper part of the cervix mostly consists of involuntary muscle, whereas the lower part is mainly fibrous connective tissue.

The mucous membrane of the endocervix has anterior and posterior columns from which folds radiate out, the arbor vitae. It has numerous deep glandular follicles which secrete a clear alkaline mucus, the main component of physiological vaginal discharge. The epithelium of the endocervix is cylindrical and also ciliated in its upper two-thirds, and changes to stratified squamous epithelium around the region of the external os. This change may be abrupt or there may be a transitional zone up to 1 cm in width.

Position

The longitudinal axis of the uterus is approximately at right-angles to the vagina and normally tilts forwards: this is termed anteversion. The uterus is usually also flexed forwards on itself at the isthmus — anteflexion. In around 20% of women, this tilt is not forwards but backward — retroversion and retroflexion, respectively. In most cases, this does not have a pathological significance and the uterus is mobile.

Relations

Anteriorly, the uterus is related to the bladder, and is separated from it by the uterovesical pouch of peritoneum. Posteriorly is the pouch of Douglas plus coils of small intestine, pelvic colon and upper rectum. Laterally, the relations are the broad ligaments and that contained within it. Of special importance are the uterine artery and also the ureter, running close to the supravaginal cervix.

Age-changes

The disappearance of maternal oestrogenic stimulation after birth causes the uterus to decrease in length by around one-third and in weight by about one-half. The cervix is then around twice the length of the body. At puberty, however, the corpus grows much faster and the size ratio reverses; the body becomes twice the length of the cervix. After the menopause, the uterus undergoes atrophy, the mucosa becomes very thin, the glands almost disappear and the walls become relatively less muscular. These changes affect the cervix more than the corpus so that the cervical lips disappear and the external os becomes more or less flush with the vault.

THE VAGINA

The vagina is a fibromuscular tube which extends posterosuperiorly from the vestibule to the uterine cervix. It is longer in its posterior wall (around 9 cm) than anteriorly (around 7.5 cm). The vaginal walls are normally in contact except superiorly, at the vault, where they are separated by the cervix. The vault of the vagina is divided into four fornices — posterior, anterior and two lateral. These increase in depth posteriorly. The mid-vagina is a transverse slit, and the lower portion has an H-shape in transverse section.

Structure

The mucous membrane of the vagina is firmly attached to the underlying muscle and consists of stratified squamous epithelium. There are no glands present and the vagina is lubricated by mucus secretion from the cervix. The epithelium is thick and rich in glycogen, which increases in the postovulatory phase of the cycle. Doderlein's bacillus is a normal commensal of the vagina, breaking down the glycogen to form lactic acid and producing a pH of around 4.5. This pH has a protective role for the vagina in decreasing the incidence of pyogenic infection.

The muscle layers consist of an outer longitudinal and inner circular layer, but these are not distinctly separarate and are mostly spirally arranged and interspersed with elastic fibres.

The hymen

The hymen is a thin fold of mucous membrane across the entrance to the vagina. It has no known function. There are usually one or more openings in it to allow menses to escape. If these are not present a haematocolpos will form with the commencement of menstruation. The hymen is usually, but not always, torn with first intercourse but can also be torn digitally or with tampons. It is certainly destroyed in childbirth and only small tags remain — carunculae myrtiformes.

Relations

The upper posterior vaginal wall forms the anterior peritoneal reflection of the pouch of Douglas. The middle third is separated from the rectum by pelvic fascia and the lower third abuts the perineal body.

Anteriorly, the upper vagina is in direct contact with the base of the bladder whilst the urethra runs down the lower half in the midline to open into the vestibule; its muscles fuse with the anterior vaginal wall.

Laterally, at the fornices, the vagina is related to the attachment of the cardinal ligaments. Below this are levator ani muscles and the ischiorectal fossa. Near the vaginal orifice, the lateral relations include the vestibular bulb, bulbospongiosus muscles and Bartholin's gland.

Age-changes

Immediately after birth, the vagina is under the influence of maternal oestrogen so the epithelium is well developed. Acidity is similar to that of an adult and Doderlein's bacilli are present. After a couple of weeks, the effects of maternal oestrogen disappear, the pH rises to 7 and the epithelium atrophies.

At puberty, the reverse occurs. The pH becomes acid again, the epithelium undergoes oestrogenization and the numbers of Doderlein's bacilli markedly increase. The vagina undergoes stretching during coitus, and especially childbirth, and the rugae tend to disappear.

At the menopause, the vagina tends to shrink and the epithelium atrophies.

THE VULVA

The female external genitalia, commonly referred to as the vulva, include the mons pubis, the labia majora and mi-

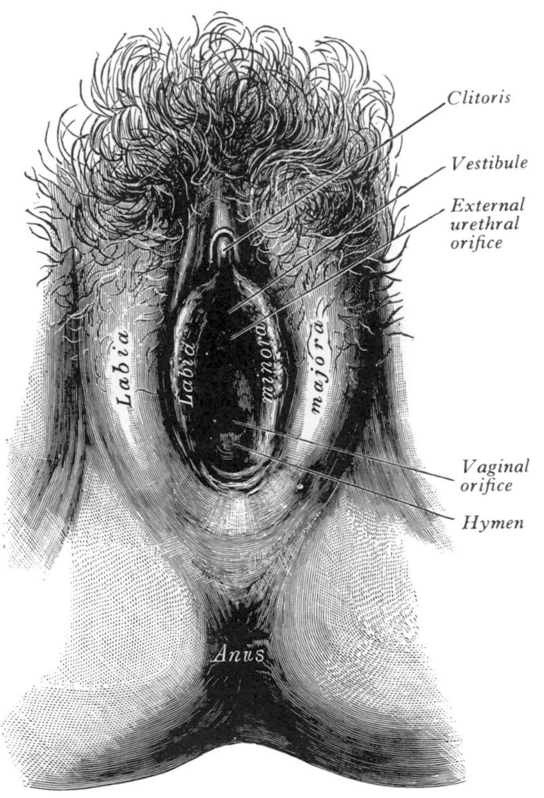

Fig. 2.5 Female external genitalia, with the labia majora et minora separated.

nora, the vestibule, the clitoris, and the greater vestibular glands (Fig. 2.5).

Labia majora

The labia majora are two prominent folds of skin with underlying adipose tissue bounding either side of the vaginal opening. They contain numerous sweat and sebaceous glands and correspond to the scrotum of the male. Anteriorly, they fuse together over the symphysis pubis to form a deposition of fat known as the mons pubis. Posteriorly, they merge with the perineum. From puberty onwards, the lateral aspects of the labia majora and the mons pubis are covered with coarse hair. The inner aspects are smooth but have numerous sebaceous follicles.

Labia minora

The labia minora are two small vascular folds of skin, containing sebaceous glands but devoid of adipose tissue, which lie within the labia majors. Anteriorly they divide into two to form the prepuce and frenulum of the clitoris. Posteriorly they fuse to form a fold of skin called the fourchette. They are not well developed before puberty and atrophy after the menopause. Their vascularity allows them to become turgid during sexual excitement.

Clitoris

This is a small erectile structure, about 2.5 cm long, homologous with the penis but not containing the urethra. The body of the clitoris contains two crura, the corpora cavernosa, which are attached to the inferior border of the pubic rami. The clitoris is covered by ischiocavernosus muscle, whilst bulbospongiosus muscle inserts into its root. The clitoris has a highly developed cutaneous nerve supply and is the most sensitive organ during sexual arousal.

Vestibule (Fig 2.6)

The vestibule is the cleft between the labia minora. Into it open the vagina, urethra, the paraurethral (Skene's) ducts and the ducts of the greater vestibular (Bartholin's) glands. The vestibular bulbs are two masses of erectile tissue on either side of the vaginal opening and contain a rich plexus of veins within bulbospongiosus muscle. Bartholin's glands, each about the size of a small pea, lie at the base of each bulb and open via a 2 cm duct into the vestibule between the hymen and the labia minora. These are mucus-secreting, producing copious amounts during intercourse to act as a lubricant. They are compressed by contraction of bulbospongiosus muscle.

Perineal body

This is a fibromuscular mass occupying the area between the vagina and the anal canal. It supports the lower part of the vagina and is of variable length. It is frequently torn during childbirth.

Age-changes

In infancy, the vulva is devoid of hair and there is considerable adipose tissue in the labia majora and mons pubis which is lost during childhood but reappears during puberty, at which time hair grows. The vaginal opening tends to widen and sometimes shorten after childbirth. After the menopause, the skin atrophies and becomes thinner and drier. The labia minora shrink, subcutaneous fat is lost and the vaginal orifice becomes smaller.

THE URETER

The ureters are a pair of muscular tubes which convey urine to the bladder by peristaltic action. They are between 25 and 30 cm in length, about half abdominally and half within the pelvis. Each has a diameter of around 3 mm but there are slight constrictions as they cross both the brim of the lesser pelvis and when they enter the bladder.

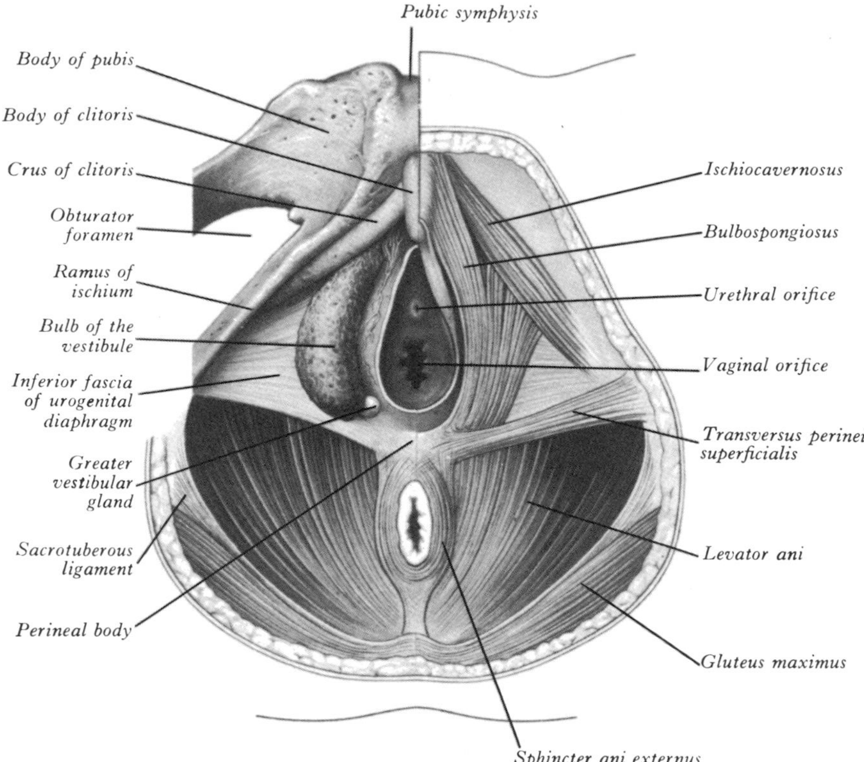

Fig. 2.6 Dissection of the female perineum to show the bulb of the vestibule and greater vestibular gland on the right; on the left side of the body the muscles superficial to these structures have been left in situ.

Structure

The ureter has three layers. The outer fibrous coat merges inferiorly with the bladder wall. The middle muscular one has outer circular and inner longitudinal non-striated fibres plus a further outer longitudinal layer along the lower third of the ureter. The inner mucous coat is lined with transitional epithelium and is continuous with the mucous membrane of the bladder below.

Relations and course

Throughout its abdominal course, the ureter travels retroperitoneally along the anteromedial aspect of psoas major and is crossed by the ovarian vessels. The right ureter passes down just laterally to the inferior vena cava and must be carefully retracted away if dissection of the nodes of the inferior vena cava is necessary.

The ureter enters the pelvis anterior to the sacroiliac joints and crosses the bifurcation of the common iliac artery. It then passes along the posterolateral aspect of the pelvis, running in front of and below the internal iliac artery and its anterior division, medial to the obturator vessels and nerves.

On reaching the true pelvis, the ureter turns forwards and medially, passing lateral to the uterosacral ligaments. It then travels through the base of the broad ligament and, lateral to the cervix, is crossed superiorly from the lateral to the medial side by the uterine artery. It continues, running about 1.5 cm lateral to the cervix, anterolateral to the upper part of the vagina and, passing slightly medially, enters the bladder at the trigone.

Surgical injury

The ureter can be damaged during gynaecological surgery at a number of points in its course. It can be injured near the pelvic brim where it is adjacent to the ovarian vessels or lower, near the cervix, where it crosses the uterine vessels. The dangers are greater when the pelvis is distorted by fibroids or ovarian cysts or the ureter's course is displaced by a broad ligament cyst. Damage can occur through the ureter being cut, crushed, or ligated and occasionally it may be devitalized by extensive dissection, especially at Wertheim's hysterectomy. Occasionally, it is injured by high sutures near the cervix in a pelvic floor repair.

THE BLADDER

The bladder is a muscular reservoir capable of altering its size and shape depending on the amount of fluid within it. It is a retroperitoneal viscus and lies behind the symphysis pubis. When empty it is the shape of a tetrahedron, with a triangular base or fundus, and a superior and two inferolateral surfaces. The two inferolateral surfaces meet to form the rounded border which joins the superior surface at the apex. The base and the inferolateral surface meet at the urethral orifice to form the bladder neck. As the bladder fills, it expands upwards and outwards and becomes more rounded. Normal bladder capacity is between 300 and 600 ml but it can, in cases of urinary retention, contain several litres and extend as far as the umbilicus.

Vesical interior

The mucous membrane of the bladder is only loosely attached to the underlying muscular coat, so that it becomes irregularly folded when the bladder is empty. A triangular area, the trigone, is immediately above and behind the urethral openings; the posterolateral angles are formed by the ureteric orifices. The mucous membrane here is redder in colour, smooth and attached firmly to the underlying muscle. The superior boundary is slightly curved — the interureteric ridge.

The ureteric orifices are slit-like and about 2.5 cm apart in the contracted bladder. They enter the bladder at an oblique angle which helps to prevent reflux of urine during filling.

Structure (Fig. 2.7)

The wall of the bladder is in three layers. The outer serous coat, the peritoneal covering, is only present over the fundus. The muscular layer, the detrusor muscle, consists of three layers of non-striated muscle, inner and outer longitudinal layers and a middle circular layer.

The mucous membrane is entirely covered by transitional epithelium which is responsive to ovarian hormonal stimulation. There are no true glands in this layer.

Relations

Superiorly, the bladder is covered by peritoneum. This extends forwards on to the anterior abdominal wall and sideways on to the pelvic side walls where there is a peritoneal depression, the paravesical fossa. As the bladder fills the peritoneum is displaced upwards anteriorly, so that suprapubic catheterization of the full bladder can take place without the peritoneal cavity being entered. Anteriorly, below the peritoneal reflection is the loose cellular tissue of the cave of Retzius.

Posteriorly the base of the bladder is separated from the upper vagina by pubocervical fascia. Above this is the supravaginal portion of cervix. The peritoneal reflection is at the isthmus of the uterus to form a slight recess, the uterovesical pouch, which often contains coils of intestine.

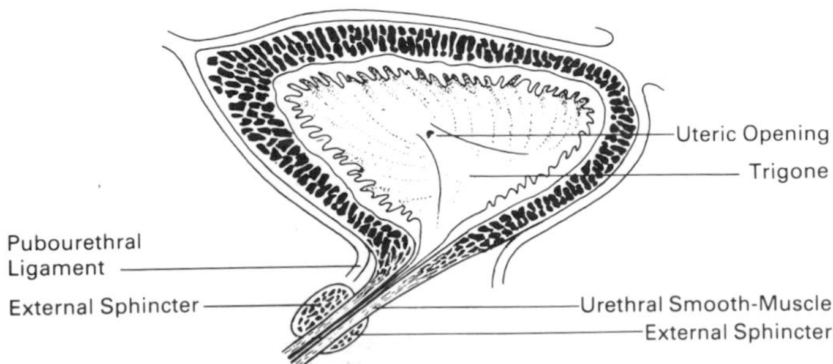

Fig. 2.7 Except where it is fixed at its based, the bladder is a highly distensible structure, and urinary continence probably depends upon the physical relations of the fixed/mobile junction.

Surgical injury

The bladder may occasionally be opened during abdominal hysterectomy. The trigone, being in close relation with the upper vagina and anterior fornix, is fortunately rarely damaged and perforation is usually 3–4 cm above it and can be easily repaired without damage to the ureter. If the injury is not noted, however, a vesicovaginal fistula may result. Damage may also occur during anterior colporrhaphy or vaginal hysterectomy, especially if a previous repair has been performed.

THE URETHRA

The urethra begins at the internal meatus of the bladder and runs anteroinferiorly behind the symphysis pubis, immediately related to the anterior vaginal wall. It is around 4 cm long and about 6 mm in diameter. It crosses the perineal membrane and ends at the external urethral orifice in the vestibule, about 2.5 cm behind the clitoris. Skene's tubules, draining the paraurethral glands, open into the lower urethra. These glands are homologous to the male prostate.

There are no true anatomical sphincters to the urethra. The decussation of vesical muscle fibres at the urethrovesical junction acts as a form of internal sphincter and continence is normally maintained at this level. Urethral resistance is mostly due to the tone and elasticity of the involuntary muscles of the urethral wall, and this keeps it closed except during micturition. About 1 cm from its lower end, before it crosses the perineal membrane, the urethra is encircled by voluntary muscle fibres, arising from the inferior pubic ramus, to form the so-called external sphincter. This sphincter allows the voluntary arrest of urine flow.

Structure

The urethra has mucous and muscular coats. Near the bladder the mucous membrane is lined by transitional epithelium which gradually converts into non-keratinizing stratified squamous epithelium as it approaches the external urethral meatus. The muscular layer, consisting of inner longitudinal and outer circular fibres, is continuous with those of the bladder.

Relations

Anteriorly, the urethra is separated from the symphysis pubis by loose cellular tissue. Posteriorly is the anterior vaginal wall plus Skene's tubules. Laterally is the urogenital diaphragm, bulbospongiosus muscle and the vestibular bulb.

THE SIGMOID COLON

The pelvic or sigmoid colon is continuous with the descending colon and commences at the brim of the pelvis. It forms a loop around 40 cm in length and lies in the lesser pelvis behind the broad ligament. It is entirely covered by peritoneum, which forms a mesentery, the sigmoid mesocolon, which diminishes in length at either end and is largest at mid-segment. The lower end of the colon is continuous with the rectum at the level of the third sacral vertebra.

Structure

The mucous membrane of the colon is thrown into irregular folds and is covered by non-ciliated columnar epithelium. Separated from this layer by areolar tissue is the muscle layer. This is arranged as an inner circular layer and outer longitudinal layer which has three narrow bands, the taeniae coli. These bands are shorter than the general surface of the colon and therefore give it its typical sacculated appearance. The serous coat has attached a series of small pieces of fat, the appendices epiploicae.

Relations

The position and shape of the pelvic colon vary considerably and hence so do its relations. Inferiorly it rests on the uterus and bladder. Above and on the right are the coils of ileum; below and on the left is the rectum. Posterior relations also include the ureter, the internal iliac vessels, piriformis muscle and the sacral plexus, all on the left side. Lateral relations include the ovary, external iliac vessels and the obturator nerve.

THE RECTUM

The rectum, which begins at the level of the third sacral vertebra, moulds to the concavity of the sacrum and coccyx: its anteroposterior curve forms the sacral flexure of the rectum. It is around 12 cm in length. The lower end dilates to form the ampulla which bulges into the posterior vaginal wall and then continues as the anal canal. When distended, the rectum has three lateral curves, the upper and lower are usually convex to the right and the middle convex to the left. Peritoneum covers the front and sides of the upper third of rectum, and the front of the middle third. The lower third is devoid of peritoneum.

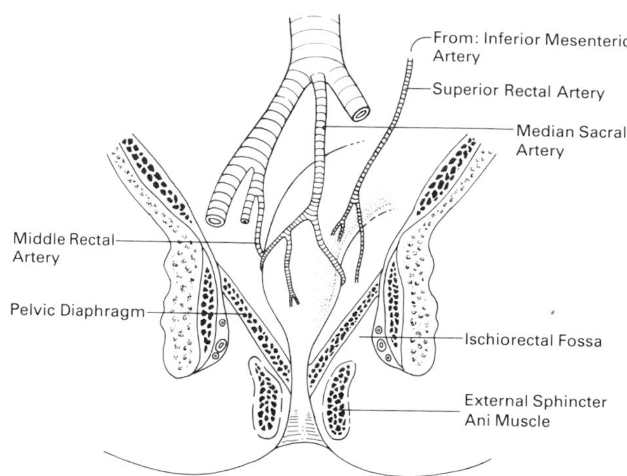

Fig. 2.8 The rectum has a rich anastomotic blood supply, from the median sacral, the internal iliac and the inferior mesenteric arteries and this arrangement is reflected in its venous drainage.

Structure (Fig. 2.8)

Unlike the sigmoid colon, there are no sacculations, appendices epiploicae or mesentery. The taeniae coli blend about 5 cm above the junction of the rectum and colon and form two bands, anterior and posterior, which descend the rectal wall. When the rectum is empty the mucous membrane is thrown into longitudinal folds which disappear with distension. Permanent horizontal folds are also present and are more pronounced during distension. The lining is of mucus-secreting columnar epithelium.

Anal canal

The anal canal is around 3 cm long and passes downwards and backwards from the rectum. It is slit-like when empty but distends greatly during defecation. This is aided by the presence of fat laterally in the ischiorectal fossa. Anteriorly the anal canal is related to the perineal body and lower vagina; posteriorly to the anococcygeal body.

For most of its length it is surrounded by sphincteric muscles which are involved in the control of defecation. The action of the levator ani muscles which surround it are also important in the control mechanism. The internal sphincter is involuntary and is a thickening of the circular muscle of the gut wall enclosing the anal canal just above the anorectal junction. The external sphincter is voluntary and composed of three layers of striated muscle.

Relations

The relations of the rectum are particularly important because they can be felt on digital examination. Posteriorly are related the lower three sacral vertebrae, the coccyx, median sacral and superior rectal vessels. Posterolateral relations are piriformis, coccygeus and levator ani muscles, plus third, fourth and fifth sacral and coccygeal nerves. Below and lateral to the levator ani muscle is the ischiorectal fossa.

Anteriorly, above the peritoneal reflection lie the uterus and adnexa, upper vagina and pouch of Douglas with its contents. Below the reflection it is related to the lower vagina.

PELVIC MUSCULOFASCIAL SUPPORT

Pelvic peritoneum

Posteriorly, the peritoneum is reflected from the rectum on to the posterior wall of the vagina, at which point it is in close contact with the outside world, a fact that can be used both diagnostically and therapeutically. It then passes upwards over the cervix and uterus to form the rectouterine pouch, the pouch of Douglas.

The peritoneum then passes over the fundus of the uterus and down its anterior wall to reach the junction of the body and cervix, where it reflects over the anterior wall of the bladder, forming a shallow recess, the uterovesical pouch. The peritoneum in front of the bladder is loosely applied to the anterior abdominal wall so that it strips away as the bladder fills. Suprapubic catheterization of the distended bladder can therefore be performed without entering the peritoneal cavity.

On either side of the uterus a double fold of peritoneum passes to the lateral pelvic side walls, the broad ligament. These two layers, anteroinferior and posterosuperior, enclose loose connective tissue, the parametrium. At the upper border, between the two layers, is the fallopian tube. The mesentery between the broad ligament and the fallopian tube is the mesosalpinx, and to the ovary, the mesovarium. Beyond the fallopian tube, the upper edge of the broad ligament as it passes to the pelvic side wall forms the infundibulopelvic ligament, or suspensory ligament of ovary, and contains the ovarian blood vessels and nerves. Between the fallopian tube and the ovary, the mesosalpinx contains the vestigial epoophoron and paroophoron. After crossing the ureter, the uterine vessels pass between the layers of the broad ligament at its inferior border. They then ascend the ligament medially and anastomose with the ovarian vessels.

Pelvic ligaments

The round ligaments, a mixture of smooth muscle and fibrous tissue, are two narrow flat bands which arise from the lateral angles of the uterus and then pass laterally, deep to the anterior layer of the broad ligament, towards the lateral pelvic side wall. They then turn forwards towards the deep inguinal ring, crossing medial to the vesical vessels, obturator vessels and nerve, obliterated umbilical artery and the external iliac vessels. They finally pass through the inguinal canal to end in the subcutaneous tissue of the labia majora. Together with the uterosacral ligaments, the round ligaments help to keep the uterus in a position of anteversion and anteflexion.

The ovarian ligaments, which are fibromuscular cords of similar structure to the round ligament, lie within the broad ligament and each runs from the cornu of the uterus to the medial border of the ovary. The round and ovarian ligaments together form the homologue of the gubernaculum testis of the male.

In addition, there are also condensations of pelvic fascia on the upper surface of the levator ani muscles, the so-called 'fascial ligaments', comprised of elastic tissue and smooth muscle. They are attached to the uterus at the level of the supravaginal cervix and, being extensive and strong, have an important supporting role. The transverse cervical or cardinal ligaments pass laterally to the pelvic side walls, and their posterior reflection continues around the lateral margins of the rectum as the uterosacral ligaments. They insert into the periostium of the fourth sacral vertebra. These ligaments provide the major support to the uterus above the pelvic diaphragm, helping to prevent uterine descent. The uterosacrals also help to pull the supravaginal cervix backwards in the pelvis, to assist in anteflexion. Anteriorly, the pubocervical fascia is more of a fascial plane than a distinct ligament. It extends beneath the base of the bladder, passing around the urethra and inserting into the body of the pubis. It supports the bladder base and the anterior vaginal wall.

Pelvic musculature (Figs 2.9, 2.10)

The levator ani and coccygeus muscles on either side, together with their fascial coverings, form the pelvic diaphragm which separates the structures in the pelvis from the perineum and ischiorectal fossa. This diaphragm together with all the tissue between the pelvic cavity and the perineum make up the pelvic floor. In lower mammals, the diaphragm represents the abductor and flexor muscles of the tail; in humans, who have an erect attitude, these muscles help provide support to the pelvic viscera.

Levator ani muscle is a wide, thin curved sheet of muscle which arises anteriorly from the pelvic surface of the body of the pubic bone, the ischial spine and the tendinous arch of the obturator fascia between the two. The muscle fibres converge across the midline. Levator ani can be divided into three parts: *puborectalis*, which is most medial, encircling the rectum and vagina and acting as support and additional sphincter for both; *pubococcygeus*, the

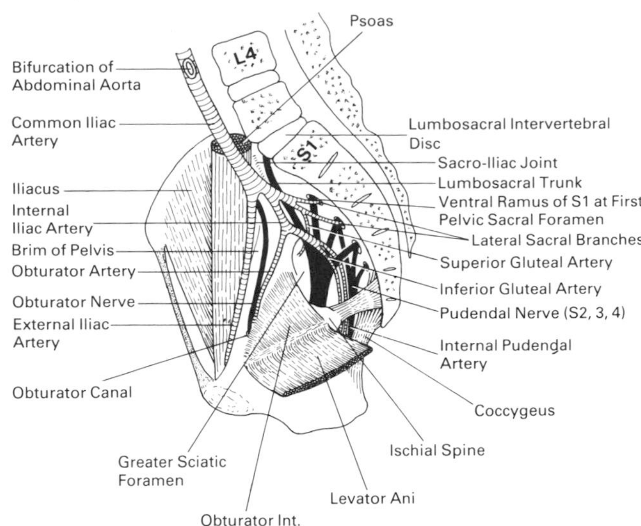

Fig. 2.9 Pelvic musculature. Muscles leave the pelvis either above the superior ramus of the pubis or through the greater or lesser sciatic foramina. Nerves and vessels also leave via the obturator foramen.

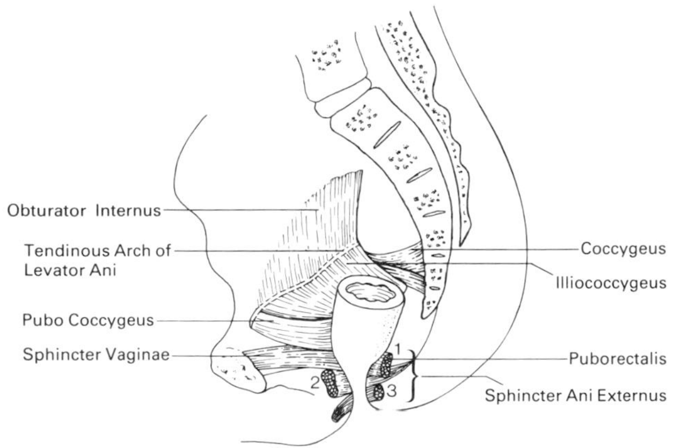

Fig. 2.10 Muscles of the pelvic floor. The slings of muscle that surround and separate the major body effluents have an important role as sphincters.

strongest part of the muscular component, which is slung from the pubis to the coccyx; and *iliococcygeus*, the most posterior, also attached to the coccyx.

The posterior part of the pelvic floor is made up of coccygeus muscle, a thin flat triangular muscle, lying on the same plane as the iliococcygeal portion of levator ani. It arises from the ischial spine and inserts into lower sacrum and upper coccyx. Like levator ani, it acts by supporting the pelvic viscera.

Most of the side wall of the lesser pelvis is covered by the fan-shaped obturator internus muscle which is attached to the obturator membrane and the neighbouring bone. The fibres run backwards and turn laterally at a right angle to emerge through the lesser sciatic foramen. The side wall is covered medially by obturator fascia (Fig. 2.11).

The ischiorectal fossa, the wedge-shaped space lateral to

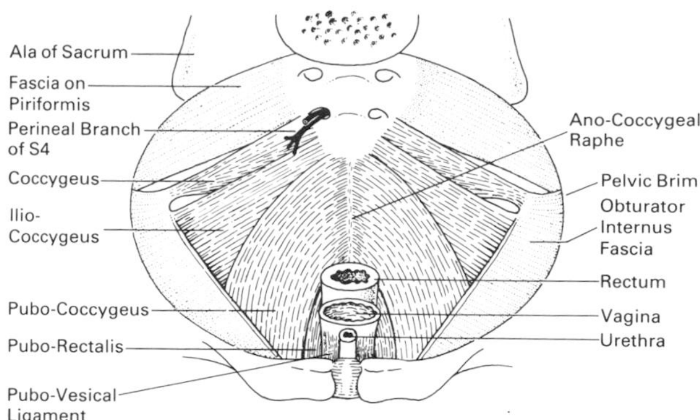

Fig. 2.11 The urogenital diaphragm. The floor of the pelvis slopes steeply forwards and plays an important role in continence and childbirth.

the anus, is bounded laterally by obturator internus and superomedially by the external surface of levator ani. The base is the perineal skin. The fossa extends forwards, almost to the pubis and backwards almost to the sacrum, where it is widest and deepest. The posterior boundary is made up by sacrotuberous ligament and gluteus maximus muscle, and the anterior boundary by the upper surface of the deep fascia of the sphincter urethrae muscle. It crosses the midline in front of the anal canal.

The musculature of the urogenital region can be divided into two groups, the superficial and deep muscles. Superficially, there are three: *bulbospongiosus*, the sphincter vaginae, which surrounds the vaginal orifice, posteriorly being continuous with the perineal body and anteriorly attaching to the corpora cavernosa of the clitoris; *ischiocavernosus*, covering the unattached surface of the crus of the clitoris; and *superficial transverse perineal* muscle. More deeply are the deep transverse perineal muscle, starting from the inner surface of the ischial ramus and passing to the perineal body, and sphincter urethrae, surrounding the membranous urethra. These layers, and their fascial component, constitute the urogenital diaphragm.

The perineal body or central perineal tendon is a fibromuscular mass lying between the anal canal and the vagina. Superficially it contains insertions of transverse perineal muscles and fibres of the external anal sphincter, and on a deeper plane levator ani muscle. It supports the lower part of vagina, and is frequently torn during childbirth.

BLOOD SUPPLY TO THE PELVIS

Abdominal aorta

The abdominal portion of the aorta commences as it passes between the crura of the diaphragm at the level of the body of the 12th thoracic vertebra. It runs downwards to the left of the midline along the front of the vertebral column and bifurcates at the level of the body of the fourth lumbar vertebra to form the right and left common iliac arteries.

The inferior vena cava runs immediately on its right. In the lower part of its course, ovarian and inferior mesenteric branches arise from the front of the aorta, and median sacral and lumbar branches arise from the back.

Ovarian artery

The ovarian arteries are long slender vessels which arise from the anterolateral aspect of the aorta just below the origin of the renal arteries. The right artery crosses the anterior surface of the vena cava, the lower part of abdominal ureter and then, lateral to the ureter, enters the pelvis via the infundibulopelvic ligament. The left artery crosses the ureter almost immediately after its origin and then travels lateral to it, crossing the bifurcation of the common iliac artery at the pelvic brim to enter the infundibulopelvic ligament. Both arteries then divide to send branches to the ovaries through the mesovarium. Small branches pass to the ureter and fallopian tube and one branch passes to the cornu of the uterus where it freely anastomoses with branches of the uterine artery to produce a continuous arterial arch (Fig. 2.12).

The ovarian and uterine trunks drain into a pampiniform plexus of veins in the broad ligament near the mesovarium, which can occasionally become varicose. The right ovarian vein drains into the inferior vena cava, the left usually into the left renal vein.

Inferior mesenteric artery

The inferior mesenteric artery arises 3–4 cm above the bifurcation of the aorta. It descends at first in front of the aorta, then to the left of it, to cross the left common iliac artery medial to the left ureter and continue in the mesentery of the sigmoid colon into the lesser pelvis. During its course, it gives off a left colic branch which supplies the left half of the transverse colon and descending colon and a sigmoid branch supplying the sigmoid colon. In the lesser pelvis, it continues as the superior rectal artery, supplying upper rectum and anastomosing with the middle and inferior rectal branches. The inferior mesenteric artery can occasionally be traumatized during para-aortic lymph node dissection and will bleed freely. Transection however is not of serious consequence to the blood supply to the lower bowel due to considerable anastomotic connections.

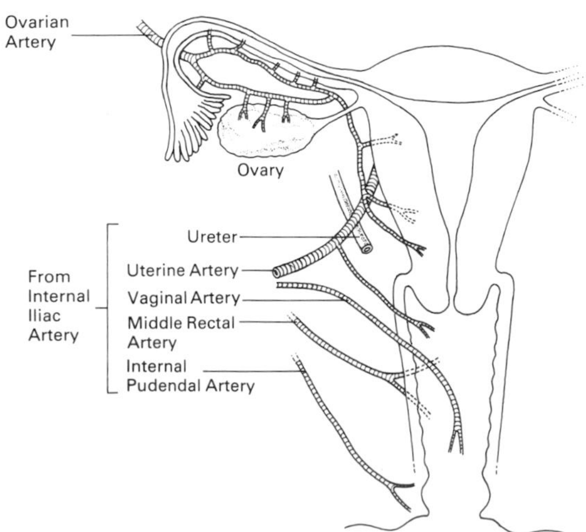

Fig. 2.12 Blood supply of the genitalia. The uterus has an anastomotic supply from both the ovarian and uterine arteries, both vessels running in the broad ligament.

Common iliac artery

After the aortic bifurcation, the two common iliac arteries run a distance of 4–5 cm before again bifurcating to form internal and external iliac branches on either side. The left artery runs partly lateral and partly in front of the corresponding iliac vein. On the right side, the slightly longer artery runs in front of the lowermost portion of inferior vena cava and the terminations of the two common iliac veins, and then lateral to the left common iliac vein. The bifurcation of the common iliac artery is in front of the sacroiliac joint. The ureter lies in front of the bifurcation at this point.

External iliac artery and its branches

These are larger than the internal iliac vessels and run obliquely and laterally down the medial border of psoas major. At a point midway between the anterior superior iliac spine and the symphysis pubis it enters the thigh behind the inguinal ligament and becomes the femoral artery. At this point it is lateral to the femoral vein but medial to the nerve. The ovarian vessels cross in front of the artery just below the bifurcation, as does the round ligament. The external iliac vein is partly behind the upper part of the artery, but medial in its lower part.

The external iliac artery gives off two main branches. The inferior epigastric artery ascends obliquely along the medial margin of the deep inguinal ring, pierces transversalis fascia and runs up between rectus abdominis muscle and its posterior sheath, supplying the muscle and sending branches to the skin. It anastomoses with the superior epigastric artery above the level of the umbilicus. The deep circumflex artery runs posteroinferior to the inguinal ligament to the anterior superior iliac spine and then pierces transversus abdominis muscle to supply that muscle and internal oblique.

Once the external iliac artery has pierced the thigh and become the femoral artery it almost immediately gives off an external pudendal branch which supplies much of the skin of the vulva, anastomosing with the labial branches of the internal pudendal artery.

Internal iliac artery and its branches

The internal iliac arteries are both 4 cm long and descend to the upper margin of the greater sciatic foramen where they divide into anterior and posterior divisions (Fig. 2.13). In the fetus they are twice as large as the external iliac vessels and ascend the anterior wall to the umbilicus to form the umbilical artery. After birth, with the cessation of the placental circulation, only the pelvic portion remains patent; the remainder becomes a fibrous cord, the lateral umbilical ligament. The ureter runs anteriorly down the artery and the internal iliac vein runs behind.

The posterior division has three branches which mainly supply the musculature of the buttocks. The iliolumbar artery ascends deep to psoas muscle and divides to supply iliacus and quadratus lumborum. The lateral sacral arteries descend in front of the sacral rami and supply the structures of the sacral canal. The superior gluteal artery is the direct continuation and leaves the lesser pelvis through the greater sciatic foramen to supply much of the gluteal musculature.

The anterior division has seven main branches. The superior vesical artery runs anteroinferiorly between the side of the bladder and the pelvic side wall to supply the upper part of the bladder. The obturator artery passes to the obturator canal and thence to the adductor compartment of the thigh. Inside the pelvis it sends off iliac, vesical and pubic branches (Table 2.1).

The vaginal artery corresponds to the inferior vesical artery of the male. It descends inwards, low in the broad ligament to supply the upper vagina, base of the bladder and adjacent rectum. It anastomoses with branches of the uterine artery to form two median longitudinal vessels, the azygos arteries of the vagina, one descending in front and the other behind.

The uterine artery passes along the root of the broad ligament and about 2 cm from the cervix crosses above and in front of the ureter. It then runs tortuously along the lateral margin of the uterus between the layers of the broad ligament. It supplies the cervix and body of the uterus, part of the bladder, and one branch anastomoses with the vaginal artery to produce the azygos arteries. It ends by anastomosing with the ovarian artery. The branches of the uterine artery pass circumferentially around the myometrium, giving off coiled radial branches which end as basal arteries supplying the endometrium.

The middle rectal artery is a small branch passing medially to the rectum to vascularize the muscular tissue of the lower rectum and anastomose with the superior and inferior rectal arteries.

The internal pudendal artery, the smaller of the two terminal trunks of the internal iliac artery, descends anterior to piriformis and, piercing the pelvic fascia, leaves the pelvis through the inferior part of the greater sciatic foramen, crosses the gluteal aspect of the ischial spine and enters the perineum through the lesser sciatic foramen (Fig. 2.14). It then traverses the pudendal canal, with the pudendal nerve, about 4 cm above the ischial tuberosity. It then proceeds forwards above the inferior fascia of the urogenital diaphragm and divides into a number of branches. The inferior rectal branch supplies skin and musculature of the anus and anastomoses with the superior and middle rectal arteries: the perineal artery supplies much of the perineum, and small branches supply the labia, vestibular bulbs and

Table 2.1 Arterial supply of the pelvic organs

Organ	Artery	Origin
Ovary	Ovarian Uterine	Aorta Internal iliac
Fallopian tube	Ovarian Uterine	Aorta Internal iliac
Uterus	Uterine Ovarian	Internal iliac Aorta
Vagina	Vaginal Uterine Internal pudendal Middle rectal	Internal iliac Internal iliac Internal iliac Internal iliac
Vulva	Internal pudendal External pudendal	Internal iliac Femoral
Ureter	Renal Ovarian Uterine Superior vesical Inferior vesical	Aorta Aorta Internal iliac Internal iliac Internal iliac
Bladder	Superior vesical Inferior vesical	Internal iliac Internal iliac
Urethra	Inferior vesical Internal pudendal	Internal iliac Internal iliac
Sigmoid colon	Left colic	Inferior mesenteric
Rectum	Superior rectal Middle rectal Inferior rectal	Inferior mesenteric Internal iliac Internal pudendal (internal iliac)

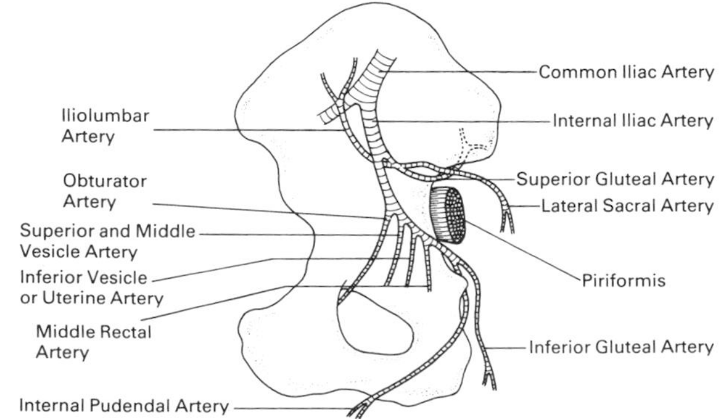

Fig. 2.13 The blood supply to the pelvic viscera is derived in the main from the internal iliac artery.

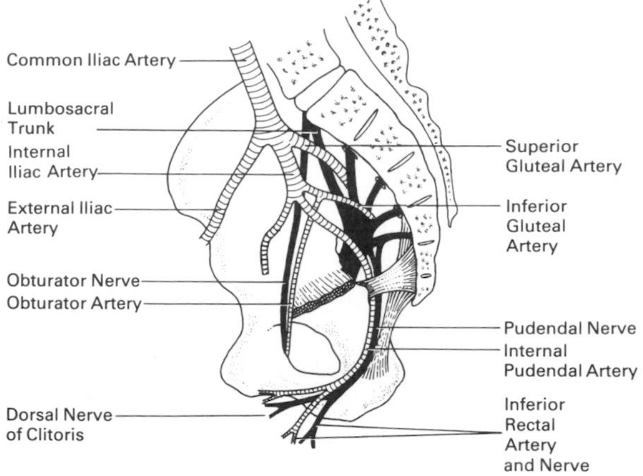

Fig. 2.14 Pelvic nerves and blood supply of the pudenda. The major nerve is the pudendal, but it is supplemented by the posterior cutaneous nerve of the thigh and the ilioinguinal and genitofemoral nerves.

vagina. The artery terminates as the dorsal artery of the clitoris.

The inferior gluteal artery, the larger terminal trunk, descends behind the internal pudendal artery, traverses the lower part of the greater sciatic foramen and with the superior gluteal artery supplies much of the buttock and back of the thigh.

NERVE SUPPLY TO THE PELVIS

Autonomic nerves (see Fig. 2.14)

The internal pelvic organs are supplied by both the sympathetic and the parasympathetic autonomic nervous system, and this is their sole innervation. As they descend into the pelvis, branches from the lower part of the lumbar sympathetic trunk join the aortic plexus of sympathetic

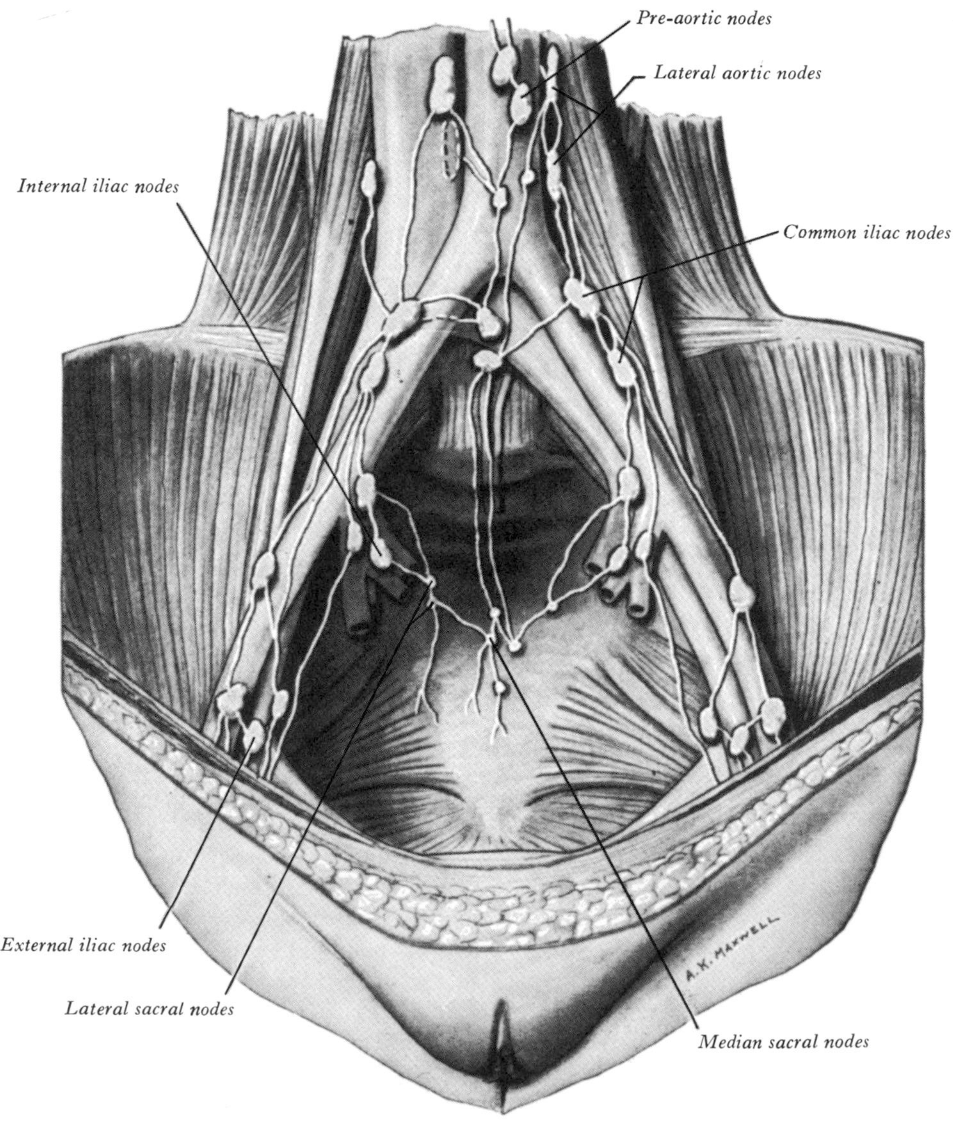

Fig. 2.15 The lymph vessels and nodes of the pelvis.

nerves and ganglia as it continues downwards over the bifurcation of the aorta to form the superior hypogastric plexus. This then divides to form the right and left inferior hypogastric or pelvic plexuses, which lie lateral to the rectum and further subdivide into two — anterior innervating the base of the bladder and urethra and posterior innervating the uterus, cervix, vagina, sigmoid colon and rectum.

The parasympathetic nerves enter the pelvis through the second, third and fourth sacral nerves. The preganglionic fibres are distributed through the pelvic plexus and the parasympathetic ganglia are situated close to, or in the walls of, the viscera concerned. With the exception of the ovaries and fallopian tube which are supplied directly by nerves from the preaortic plexus travelling along the ovarian vessels, all internal pelvic organs are supplied via the pelvic plexuses.

Somatic nerves

The lumbar plexus is formed by the anterior primary rami of the first three lumbar nerves, part of the fourth and a contribution from the 12th thoracic (subcostal) nerve. It lies on the surface of psoas major and gives off a number of major branches.

The iliohypogastric and ilioinguinal nerves both arise from the first lumbar nerve. The former gives branches to the buttock, while the latter supplies the skin of the mons pubis and surrounding vulva. The genitofemoral nerve arises from the first and second lumbar nerves, its femoral branch supplying the upper thigh, whilst its genital branch supplies the skin of the labium majus. The lateral femoral cutaneous nerve arises from the second and third lumbar nerves and also supplies the thigh.

The femoral nerve is the largest branch, coming from second, third and fourth lumbar nerves. It descends in the groove between psoas and iliacus muscles and enters the thigh deep to the inguinal ligament, lateral to the femoral sheath, to supply the flexors of the hip, the extensors of the knee and numerous cutaneous branches including the saphenous nerve. The obturator nerve also comes from the second, third and fourth lumbar nerves and passes downwards medial to psoas into the pelvis, to supply the adductor muscles of the hip.

The lumbosacral trunk comes from the fourth and fifth lumbar nerves and passes medial to psoas into the pelvis to join the anterior primary rami of the first three sacral nerves to form the sacral plexus in front of piriformis muscle. From this plexus, a number of branches emerge. The most important of these are the sciatic nerve — a large nerve formed from the fourth and fifth lumbar and the first, second and third sacral nerves — which leaves the pelvis through the lower part of the greater sciatic foramen to supply the muscles of the back of the thigh and the lower limb, and the pudendal nerve, which forms from the second, third and fourth sacral nerves.

The pudendal nerve leaves the pelvis between piriformis and coccygeus muscles and curls around the ischial spine to re-enter the pelvis through the lesser sciatic foramen, where medial to the internal pudendal artery, it lies in the pudendal canal on the lateral wall of the ischiorectal fossa. The point where the nerve circles the ischial spine is the region in which a pudendal block of local anaesthetic is injected.

The pudendal nerve gives a number of terminal branches. The inferior rectal nerve gives motor and sensory fibres to the external anal sphincter, anal canal and skin around the anus. The perineal nerve passes forwards below the internal pudendal artery to give labial branches, supplying the skin of the labia majora, the deep perineal nerve supplying the perineal muscles and the bulb of the vestibule. The dorsal vein of the clitoris passes through the pudendal canal, giving a branch to the crus and piercing the perineal membrane 1–2 cm from the symphysis pubis. It supplies the clitoris and surrounding skin.

LYMPHATIC DRAINAGE TO THE PELVIS

In the pelvis, as elsewhere in the body, the lymph nodes

Table 2.2 Lymphatic drainage of the pelvic

Organ	Lymph nodes
Ovary	Lateral aortic nodes
Fallopian tube	Lateral aortic nodes Superficial inguinal nodes External and internal iliac nodes
Corpus uteri	External and internal iliac nodes Superficial inguinal nodes Lateral aortic nodes
Cervix	External and internal iliac nodes Obturator node Sacral nodes
Upper vagina	External and internal iliac nodes Obturator node Sacral nodes
Lower vagina	Superficial inguinal nodes
Vulva	Superficial inguinal nodes Internal iliac nodes (deep tissues)
Ureter	Lateral aortic nodes Internal iliac nodes
Bladder	External and internal iliac nodes
Urethra	Internal iliac nodes
Sigmoid colon	Preaortic nodes
Upper rectum	Preaortic nodes
Lower rectum and canal	Internal iliac nodes
Anal orifice	Superficial inguinal nodes

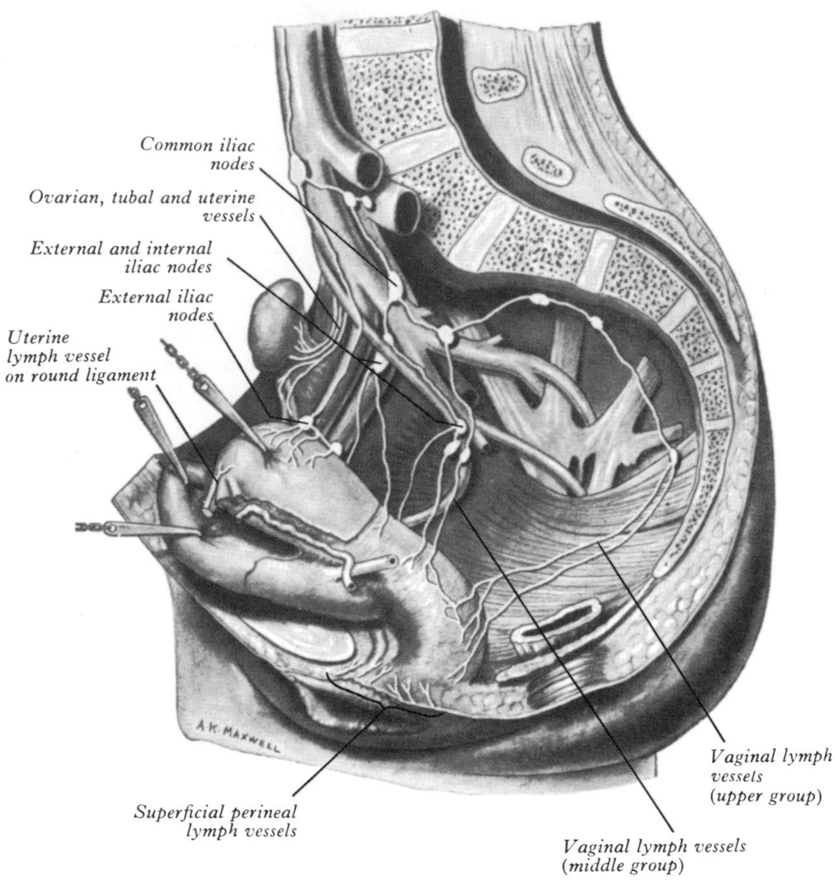

Fig. 2.16 The lymphatic drainage of the female reproductive organs (semi-diagrammatic, after Cunéo & Marcille).

are arranged along the blood vessels. The lateral aortic lymph nodes lie on either side of the aorta; their efferents form a lumbar trunk on either side which terminates at the cisterna chyli. Those structures which receive their blood supply directly from branches of the aorta, i.e. ovary, fallopian tube, upper ureter and, in view of arterial anastomoses, uterine fundus, drain directly into the lateral aortic group of nodes.

The lymph drainage of most other structures within the pelvis is via more outlying groups of lymph nodes associated with the iliac vessels. The common iliac lymph nodes are grouped around the common iliac artery and usually arranged in medial, lateral and intermediate chains. They receive efferents from the external and internal iliac nodes and send efferents to the lateral aortics (Fig. 2.15). The external iliac nodes lie on the external iliac vessels and are in three groups, lateral, medial and anterior. They collect from the cervix, upper vagina, bladder, deeper lower abdominal wall and from the inguinal lymph nodes. Inferior epigastric and circumflex iliac nodes are associated with these vessels and can be considered to be outlying members of the external iliac group (Table 2.2)

The internal iliac nodes, which surround the internal iliac artery, receive afferents from all the pelvic viscera, deeper perineum and muscles of the thigh and buttock. The obturator lymph node, sometimes present in the obturator canal, and the sacral lymph nodes on the median and lateral sacral vessels can be considered to be outlying members of this group (Fig. 2.16).

The upper group of superficial inguinal lymph nodes forms a chain immediately below the inguinal ligament. The lateral members receive afferents from the gluteal region and ajoining lower anterior abdominal wall. The medial members drain the vulva and perineum, lower vagina, lower anal canal, ajoining anterior abdominal wall and also from the uterus owing to lymph vessels that accompany the round ligament to the anterior abdominal wall. The lymphatics on either side of the vulva communicate freely, emphasizing the importance of removing the whole vulva in cases of malignant disease. The superficial lymph nodes send their efferents to the external iliac lymph nodes, passing around the femoral vessels or traversing the femoral canal.

The deep inguinal (femoral) lymph nodes, varying from one to three, are on the medial side of the femoral vein. They receive efferents from the deep femoral vessels, some from the superficial inguinal nodes; one, the node of Cloquet, is thought to drain the clitoris. Efferents from the deep nodes pass through the femoral canal to the external iliac group.

KEY POINTS

1. The course of pelvic migration of the ovaries is important to understand their site in mal descent.
2. The mucous membrane of the endocervix has anterior and posterior columns from which folds radiate out, the arbor vitae.
3. The ureter runs close (1.5 cm) lateral to the cervix, anterior lateral to the upper part of the vagina.
4. At the pelvic brim the ureter passes anteriorly to the sacro-iliac joints and crosses the bifurcation of the common iliac artery. Here it is at risk of injury during oophorectomy.
5. The size and ratio of the cervix to uterus change with age and parity.
6. Doderlein's bacillus is important in maintaining the acid pH in the vagina and thus preventing vaginal infections.
7. There are no true anatomical sphincters to the urethra.
8. The round and ovarian ligaments together form the homologue of the gubernaculum testis in the male.
9. The ovarian arteries arise from the aorta; whilst the right ovarian vein drains into the vena cava the left ovarian vein usually drains into the left renal vein.
10. The pudendal nerve leaves the pelvis between the piriformis and coccygens muscles, curls around the ischial spine and re-enters the pelvis via the lesser sciatic foramen lying medial to the internal pudendal artery in the lateral wall of the ischiorectal fossa.

ACKNOWLEDGEMENTS

Figures 2.1–2.6, 2.15 and 2.16 are reproduced from *Gray's Anatomy*, 37th edn (eds: Williams P L et al 1989), and Figures 2.7–2.14 are reproduced from *Obstetrics* (eds: Turnbull A, Chamberlain G 1989), with permission of the authors and the publishers, Churchill Livingstone, Edinburgh.

3. Endoscopy

B. V. Lewis

The gynaecological surgeon should be skilful in using not only the laparoscope but also the hysteroscope, the cystoscope, the proctoscope and the sigmoidoscope (Table 3.1). These instruments will sometimes be needed in the evaluation of malignant disease. Most gynaecologists limit the use of the laparoscope to the investigation of pelvic pain, infertility and sterilization. However laparoscopic surgery now routinely includes adhesiolysis, destruction of endometriosis with heat or laser, and conservative surgery for tubal pregnancy. Laparoscopic surgery is also used for ovarian cystectomy and the removal of small subperitoneal fibroids, but these operations require special skill and training.

Table 3.1 Gynaecological endoscopy

Procedure	Investigation
Laparoscopy	Diagnostic Operative Oocyte collection — gamete intrafallopian transfer and in vitro fertilization
Hysteroscopy	Diagnostic Operative
Tuboscopy	
Cystoscopy	Evaluation of malignant disease and fistulae Haematuria, urgency, incontinence and detrusor instability
Sigmoidoscopy and proctoscopy	Rectal bleeding Faecal incontinence Radiation proctitis

The new operation of tuboscopy allows study of the physiology and anatomy of the tubal epithelium and permits more accurate selection of patients for in vitro fertilization rather than tubal surgery.

Diagnostic hysteroscopy is being complemented by intrauterine surgery such as myomectomy, polypectomy, detection and removal of lost intrauterine devices and the division of synechiae. Hysteroscopic treatment of menorrhagia by laser ablation or loop resection of the endometrium is becoming available in specialized centres and it is hoped that simple hysteroscopic sterilization will become more effective. Thus endoscopy requires a considerable and growing proportion of surgical time (Gordon & Lewis 1988).

LAPAROSCOPY

In the last 20 years laparoscopy has become the pre-eminent method of gynaecological diagnosis and today at least 20% of gynaecological operations are laparoscopies. The major technological advances which have contributed to this dramatic rise in number are a high-power light source, a fibreoptic or fluid cable for light transmission, and the Hopkins rod lens system of telescopes which provide a bright, clear undistorted image and a wide angle of view.

Instruments

Rigid telescopes are manufactured in several diameters but a 10 mm telescope is probably the most common with a choice of 30, 45, or 0° angle of view. For photography, 11 mm telescopes should be used; smaller 5 mm telescopes are available but offer few advantages, except in children. The pneumoperitoneum is established using a 7 cm or

12 cm long Verres needle. The shorter Verres needles are safer but 12 cm needles are necessary in fat patients. A pyramidal trocar is easy to insert but there is a risk of puncturing an abdominal wall vessel; a conical trocar is safer but needs a stronger thrust.

Diagnostic laparoscopy should always be performed using a second puncture so that a Verres needle or a probe can manipulate the bowel and elevate the ovaries. The uterus must be manipulated into anteversion with a single tooth tenaculum applied to the anterior lip of the cervix and an intrauterine cannula which has a channel for hydropertubation.

Carbon dioxide should be insufflated into the peritoneum from a specially designed machine which gives a continuous gas flow varying between 1 and 3 l/min. The intra-abdominal pressure is automatically regulated and loss of carbon dioxide by leakage is automatically compensated. The surgeon can see the pressure and gas flow rates at all times during the operation. Not more than 3 litres of gas is needed for diagnostic laparoscopy and often the volume required is less, but during operative laparoscopy more gas may be needed. It is helpful to have facilities for teaching students and recording the findings. A beam splitter fixed to the ocular part of the telescope allows an assistant to observe the anatomy using a rigid or flexible teaching aid. Photographs can be taken with a 35 mm camera body fitted to the telescope with flash supplied from an endocomputer which gives the correct exposure and reduces blurring of the photograph due to movement of the camera. Closed circuit television should be available in every operating theatre. This system is essential when operative laparoscopy is being performed so that the nurses and assistants can help the surgeon by manipulating the ancillary instruments. A television system consists of a light-weight chip camera, a large monitor, a colour control unit and a high-quality video recorder. The surgeon can either use a beam splitter so that he or she can see directly through the telescope or alternatively can operate while viewing the television monitor.

Laparoscopic instruments are shown in Figures 3.1–3.4.

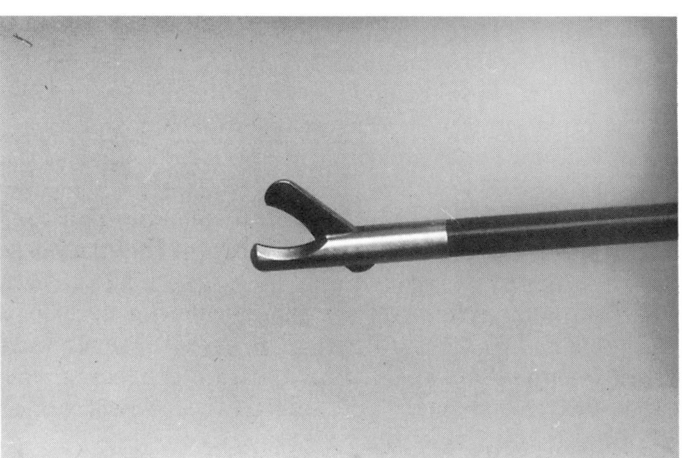

Fig. 3.1 Laparoscopic scissors.

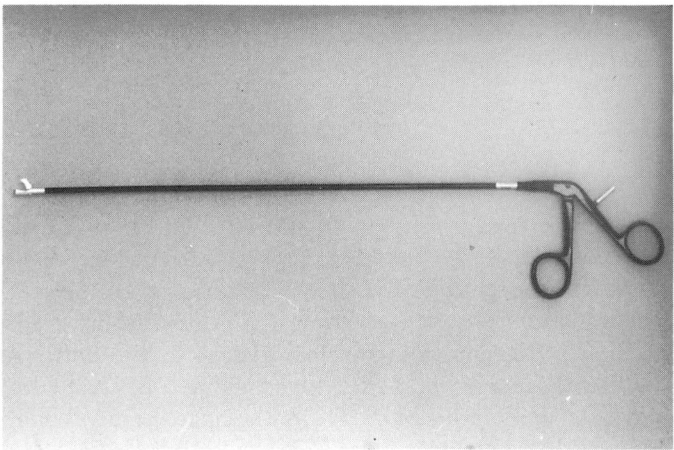

Fig. 3.2 Laparoscopic biopsy forceps (from Gordon & Lewis 1988).

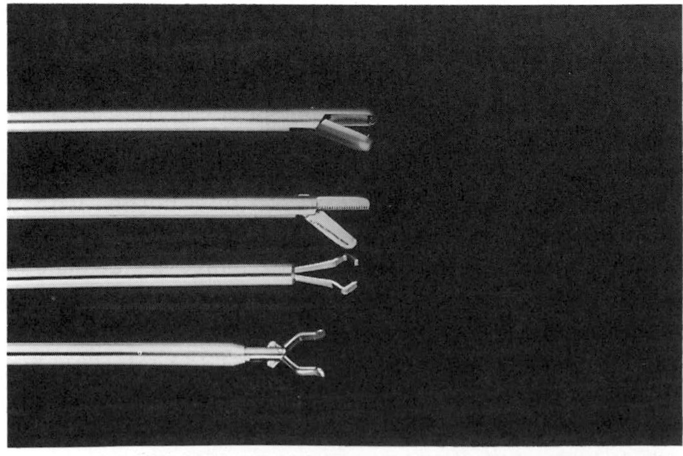

Fig. 3.3 Laparoscopic biopsy and holding forceps.

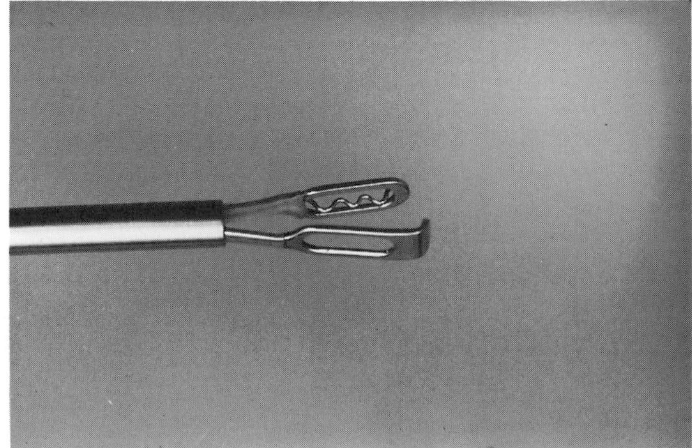

Fig. 3.4 Laparoscopic unipolar diathermy forceps (from Gordon & Lewis 1988).

Surgical technique

Laparoscopy usually requires 1 night in hospital but can be performed as a day-case. The patient should void prior to surgery or the bladder is emptied by catheterization. General anaesthesia is induced with a short-acting intravenous barbiturate and ventilation is maintained through an endotracheal or laryngeal tube, after intravenous muscle relaxants have been administered. Suxamethonium often causes muscle pains for 48 hours but atracurium or vecuronium do not. Anaesthesia is maintained with halothane or nitrous oxide. Sometimes local anaesthetic can be used for diagnostic laparoscopy or sterilization but the patients must be co-operative and are usually given premedication and 1 mg of intravenous fentanyl prior to the subumbilical infiltration of 20 ml 0.5% lignocaine.

As the surgeon becomes more experienced, the operation can be performed quickly using a smaller pneumoperitoneum, with the result that more laparoscopies can be carried out with patients breathing spontaneously through a mask but always with strict monitoring of the pulse and blood pressure. The patient is placed in a modified lithotomy position with her legs flexed to 45° and a Trendelenburg tilt of 15°. The Verres needle is inserted through a subumbilical incision with the abdominal wall manually elevated to prevent damage to the bowel or the retroperitoneal vessels. If there has been previous surgery or if intraperitoneal adhesions are expected, the position of the needle within the peritoneum is checked by the aspiration test. The trocar and cannula are then inserted into the abdomen with the point of the cannula directed into the pelvis. When the warmed telescope is in position the abdominal wall is transilluminated prior to the second puncture to avoid damaging the inferior epigastric artery. The Verres needle may be difficult to insert in an obese woman and in such patients it is helpful to introduce the needle just above the pubic symphysis where the fascial layers of the abdominal wall are adherent and the fat is less. Alternatively the Verres needle can be inserted through the pouch of Douglas. When the operation is complete, as much carbon dioxide as possible is released from the abdomen to reduce distension and diaphragmatic irritation.

Diagnostic laparoscopy (Table 3.2)

Infertility is probably the most frequent indication for laparoscopy in order to assess tubal patency, exclude other pelvic pathology and for oocyte collection and gamete intrafallopian transfer (Table 3.3). A probe through a secondary incision is essential to lift and elevate each tube and ovary so that the fimbria can be seen free from bowel, and so that the medial surface of each ovary can be examined for endometriosis and periovarian adhesions. Dilute methylene blue (10 or 20 ml) is then injected through the cervix, and should leak into the peritoneal cavity without resistance. Laparoscopy in the postmenstrual phase avoids the risk of disturbing an early pregnancy, but mid-cycle laparoscopy allows a developing follicle or ovulation stigma to be seen. Premenstrual laparoscopy should be avoided because the oedematous secretory endometrium can occlude the cornual orifice, suggesting tubal blockage.

Table 3.2 Diagnostic laparoscopy

Indications
Infertility
Endometriosis
Acute pelvic inflammatory disease
Ectopic pregnancy
Unexplained pelvic pain
Ovarian cysts and fibroids
Location of lost intrauterine devices
Prior to in vitro fertilization or reversal of sterilization
Primary amenorrhoea and congenital abnormalities
Polycystic ovarian disease
Possible indications
Malignant disease — response to therapy
Subacute appendicitis
Pelvic varicocele
Hirsutism

Table 3.3 Laparoscopy in infertility

Hydropertubation to assess tubal patency
Diagnosis of endometriosis before and after treatment
Recognition of peritubal or periovarian adhesions
Recognition of a developing follicle or corpus luteum
Follicle puncture and oocyte collection
Gamete intrafallopian transfer
Tuboscopy or salpingoscopy for studying tubal mucosa

Endometriosis is common. In this disease laparoscopy may be usefully performed in the premenstrual phase because a small endometrioma deep in the pelvis may be inconspicuous immediately after menstruation. Conversely a large endometriotic cyst may fill the pelvis and be adherent to the uterus or bowel. A tense cyst will often rupture with manipulation and the released blood will stimulate more adhesions.

Sometimes pelvic inflammatory disease cannot be distinguished clinically from a leaking tubal abortion without laparoscopy. Acute gonococcal salpingitis produces distended oedematous tubes with a haemorrhagic exudate on their surface and, often, pus leaking into the pelvis. A sample of pus should be aspirated and cultured. Chlamydial salpingitis does not produce pus but there may be adhesions in the upper abdomen between the liver and the diaphragm. This is the Fitz–Hugh–Curtis syndrome (Fig. 3.5).

If inadequately treated, acute salpingitis leads to ad-

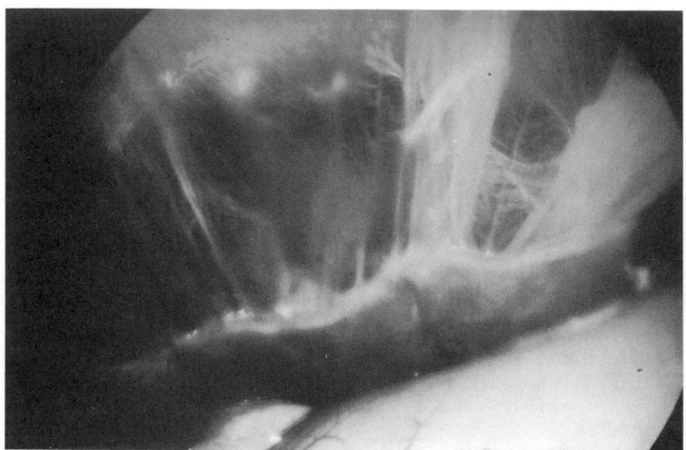

Fig. 3.5 Fitz–Hugh–Curtis Syndrome seen on laparoscopy (photo courtesy of A Auderbert).

hesions, hydrosalpinx, infertility and chronic pelvic pain; therefore high-dose broad-spectrum antibiotics plus metronidazole are essential. Pelvic tuberculosis is now rare in Europe but should be suspected in emigrants from developing countries. Caseous nodules produce a typical appearance in an advanced case, but the nodules should not be biopsied because of the risk of intraperitoneal spread. An unruptured tubal pregnancy may be suspected clinically but can only be diagnosed with certainty by laparoscopy, where the finding of blood in the pouch of Douglas with a distended fallopian tube is typical. Tubal pregnancy with bleeding must be distinguished from intraperitoneal haemorrhage due to a ruptured follicular or luteal cyst.

Uncomplicated ovarian cysts, functional cysts, endometriotic cysts, polycystic ovarian syndrome, fimbrial cysts and subperitoneal fibroids can only be distinguished from each other with certainty by direct endoscopic visualization, while complications such as haemorrhage, rupture or torsion causing acute abdominal pain can always be diagnosed and often treated using the laparoscope and ancillary instruments.

One of the most common indications for laparoscopy is unexplained or atypical pelvic pain and often a negative finding helps with the management of difficult clinical problems. Sometimes wholly unexpected findings may be found, such as acute or chronic retrocaecal or pelvic appendicitis, sigmoid tumours or an inflammatory bowel mass. Preliminary laparoscopy is essential prior to reversal of sterilization in order to determine the length of viable tube, the appearance of the fimbria, and the site of obstruction. Laparoscopy is often the only way of recognizing ovarian and müllerian tissue in amenorrhoea due to chromosomal abnormalities. In hirsutism the gonad can be biopsied.

The value of laparoscopy in assessing malignant disease is limited to stage 1A and 1B ovarian cancer, but is perhaps of some value in estimating the response to cisplatin or carboplatin chemotherapy in more advanced tumours. However there is a risk of perforation of a viscus after primary treatment for ovarian cancer and adhesions often limit the view of metastatic deposits which may be more accurately assessed by computerized tomography or magnetic resonance imaging.

Operative laparoscopy (Table 3.4)

In the past decade major advances have been made in operative laparoscopy using conventional surgical techniques pioneered by Semm in Kiel, West Germany (Semm & Mettler 1980; Semm 1983), or laser surgery with a carbon dioxide or a neodymium YAG laser modified for use via the laparoscope. Semm calls this new surgical operation 'pelviscopy' to distinguish it from conventional laparoscopy while Nezhat has coined the term 'videolaseroscopy' to describe the technique of laser surgery while viewing the intra-abdominal manipulations on a television screen (Nezaat 1986).

Pelviscopy or surgical laparoscopy is not necessarily quicker, but results at least as good as conventional laparotomy are claimed and in the case of ectopic pregnancy superior results have been reported. The main advantage is short hospitalization with major savings in cost. These advanced surgical techniques require special training and a surgeon familiar with diagnostic laparoscopy should not commence pelviscopy without attending training courses or assisting an expert surgeon. Pelviscopy should never be

Table 3.4 Operative laparoscopy

Sterilization
Mechanical block
Fallope rings
Hulka clips
Filshie clips
Heat
Unipolar diathermy
Bipolar diathermy
Endocoagulation
Adhesiolysis
Scissors
Carbon dioxide or neodymium YAG laser
Videolaseroscopy
Salpingolysis and salpingostomy
Recovery of lost contraceptive devices
Conservative treatment of tubal pregnancy
Destruction of endometriosis
Ovariectomy and ovarian cystectomy
Ovarian biopsy
Salpingoscopy or tuboscopy
Gamete intrafallopian transfer and in vitro fertilization
Ventrosuspension
Division of the uterosacral ligaments

performed without adequate instruments specially developed for this specific purpose. These include rigid scissors with straight or concave blades, non-crushing grasping forceps, palpation probes with centimetre markings, dissecting forceps and insulated bipolar diathermy forceps (Figs 3.1–3.4). Many variations of these instruments are manufactured. In addition there are biopsy forceps, needles for puncturing and draining cysts, hollow manipulating probes which hold the tube in place by suction and specially designed applicators for loop and clip sterilization.

Semm (1988) has designed instruments for tying knots around vascular pedicles using special Ethibinder ligatures or endoligatures but these are used by a minority of surgeons. The technique of tying knots can be practised on a model pelvic trainer, which consists of a rectangular plastic box with portals of entry for instruments on the surface and a model of the pelvic viscera enclosed within.

No pelviscopic surgery should be commenced without two additional pieces of equipment. These are an Acupurator to wash the pelvis free of blood and debris by infusing saline or Ringer's solution under pressure and then aspirating until the pelvis is clean, and an instrument to stop bleeding. An endocoagulator applies heat (100–120°) to the jaws of a crocodile forceps which grasps a vessel, or to a point coagulator to stop bleeding from small arteries (Fig. 3.6). The machine is controlled by the surgeon who uses a foot pedal to start the current flowing. Surgical diathermy can also be used and although unipolar electrocoagulation is still practised, bipolar diathermy is safer because the current passes between the jaws of the forceps rather than through the patient with the risk of burning bowel. When diathermy is being used all the trocars must be insulated to prevent skin burns.

The carbon dioxide laser cuts tissue very well but gives poor haemostasis, whereas the light from the neodymium YAG laser is absorbed by blood and therefore seals vessels as it cuts.

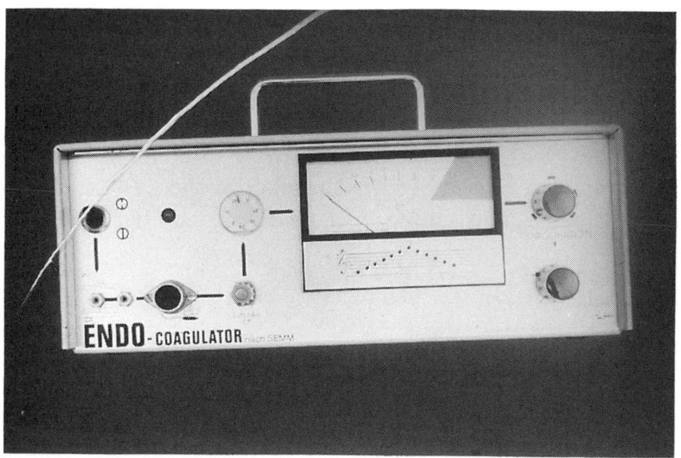

Fig. 3.6 Endocoagulator (from Gordon & Lewis 1988).

Indications for laparoscopic surgery

Sterilization

The commonest laparoscopic operation is female sterilization. A more detailed discussion of sterilization is considered in Chapter 21.

In the original method of unipolar electrocoagulation, the tube was grasped by a Palmer biopsy forceps through a second incision and an electric current applied until the tube turned white. The avascular area was then cut with hook scissors. In this technique it is vital to identify the fimbria before electrocoagulation to ensure the tube is correctly identified. Unfortunately the electric current spreads outside the immediate operation site and therefore causes extensive destruction of the tube, which makes surgical reversal of sterilization impossible. Therefore unipolar diathermy should be abandoned.

Bipolar electrocoagulation or endocoagulation using a low-voltage current carries less risk of damaging bowel and causes only local destruction where the forceps hold the tube. The coagulated area should still be cut but reversal of sterilization remains technically possible.

Mechanical blockage of the tube using special applicating forceps is now widely practised. The three most common devices used for sterilization are the Fallope or Lay Loop (a 1 mm silastic ring applied over a loop of tube), the Hulka clip made of plastic with a gold-plated steel spring, and the Filshie clip which has an outer frame of titanium and a silastic lining which crushes the tubes when the clip is closed. No method of laparoscope sterilization is totally free from risk of failure and subsequent intrauterine or ectopic pregnancy. Failure can occur because of recanalization or fistula formation, and is more likely within 3 months of confinement or when performed immediately after termination of pregnancy. Provided the patient has been counselled before surgery, claims for subsequent failure can be defended in law if the original operation was correctly performed and documented.

Adhesiolysis

In infertility there are often extensive adhesions between the tubes and ovaries and the pelvic side wall resulting from old pelvic inflammatory disease. Perifimbial, peritubal or periovarian adhesions are usually thin and avascular so that adhesiolysis is easy with the hook scissors. Thicker adhesions should be coagulated with the insulated bipolar forceps before cutting with scissors. An alternative method is to use the carbon dioxide laser with a backstop to prevent scatter of laser light and a smoke extractor to permit clear vision. Adhesions behind the ovary which are difficult to see can be safely divided by directing the laser beam on to the adhesion with a mirror.

More advanced endoscopic surgery can be used for

salpingolysis and salpingostomy. In the Semm technique three or four portals of entry are needed for ancillary instruments. The laparoscope is inserted in the usual way via a subumbilical incision and the hydrosalpinx is held by atraumatic grasping forceps. Methylene blue is first injected through the cervix to distend the tube, and the terminal obstruction is then opened with straight scissors so that the dye leaks into the abdomen. The opening can then be widened by inserting closed scissors into the tube, opening the blades, and then withdrawing the instrument. The cut edges are usually left open, but Semm describes a method of suturing the fimbria to the peritoneal surface of the tube as in conventional surgery, but only a minority of surgeons consider this necessary. Alternatively the hydrosalpinx can be opened by a carbon dioxide or neodymium YAG laser which also stops bleeding from small vessels. At the completion of these laparoscopic operations the pelvis must be washed clean by repeated irrigation with normal saline or Hartmann's solution.

Laparoscopic salpingostomy gives results comparable to laparotomy and microsurgery because the bowel is not handled and ileus does not occur, so further adhesion formation is less common (Semm 1988).

Salpingoscopy or tuboscopy

Terminal salpingostomy often fails because high pressure in the distended hydrosalpinx destroys the fimbria and the ciliated mucosa of the tube. In salpingoscopy a fine telescope is inserted through the terminal ostium so that the tubal mucosa can be examined when the lumen is distended by a saline infusion. Mucosal lesions such as flattening or adhesions of the epithelial folds, the presence of polyps and loss of cilia have all been observed. When major epithelial folds in the ampulla of the tube are flattened and the tube itself is thin-walled and atrophic, the prognosis for successful reconstructive surgery is poor and the patient should be referred for in vitro fertilization. However, if the major and the minor folds are preserved, simple salpingostomy may be followed by an intrauterine pregnancy. Salpingoscopy was originally carried out with the abdomen open but is now performed through a separate incision during laparoscopy. The tuboscope may be rigid or flexible, which helps in manipulating the tip through the tubal ostium (Figs 3.7 and 3.8).

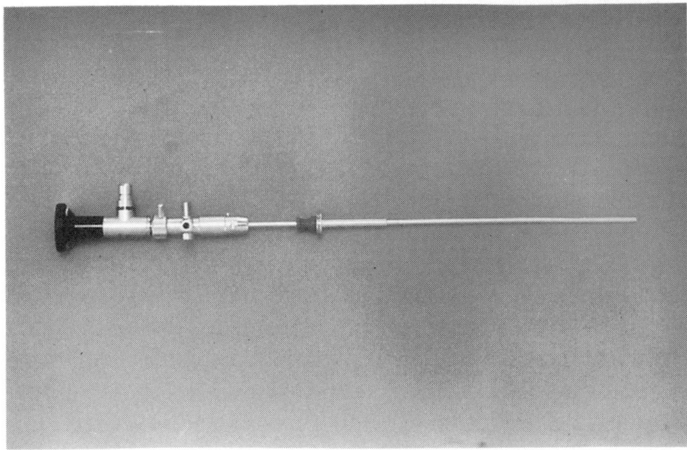

Fig. 3.7 Rigid tuboscope.

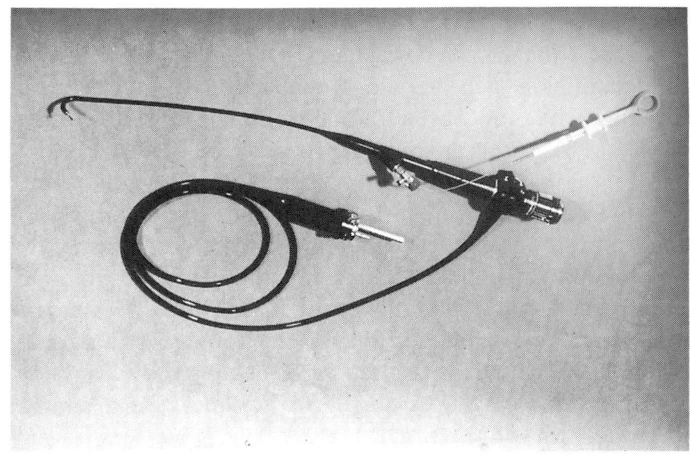

Fig. 3.8 Flexible tuboscope.

Recovery of lost intrauterine devices and laparoscopic ovarian surgery

A lost intrauterine device located in the abdomen by ultrasound can be recovered at laparoscopy using a Palmer grasping forceps. The coil may be embedded in the myometrium or may lie free in the pouch of Douglas or paracolic gutter. Occasionally it may be adherent to or entangled in omentum and in this case laparotomy is safer.

Minor operations on the ovary include ovarian biopsy in women with hirsutism, the polycystic ovarian syndrome, or in women with amenorrhoea and a streak gonad. The Palmer forceps has a screw to withdraw the biopsy into the sheath. Alternatively a punch forceps can be used to obtain an adequate biopsy. Bleeding is stopped with diathermy.

Simple fimbrial or functional cysts can be aspirated with a needle, and a simple benign cystadenoma or endometrioma can be removed by incision of the cyst, traction on its capsule, and cautery or laser to provide haemostasis.

Endometriosis

An increasing number of patients with endometriosis are being treated laparoscopically as surgical techniques improve. Conventional laparoscopy allows destruction of endometriotic deposits in the pouch of Douglas, uterosacral ligaments and ovaries using grasping forceps, bipolar diathermy or endocoagulation.

Light from a carbon dioxide laser was originally directed down the operating sheath of the laparoscope, but it proved difficult to align the telescope with the aiming beam so a second puncture is now advised. The laser beam can be either focused or defocused. The focused beam incises tissue like a knife and is ideal for cutting adhesions, whereas the defocused beam vaporizes endometriotic spots. Variable power densities are necessary for large and small deposits of endometriosis and the intraperitoneal smoke plume produced by the laser must be evacuated by suction. The extent of vaporization is easy to control and may be limited to a depth of 1 mm, which enables endometriosis to be destroyed even on the surface of the bladder, free from the risk of damaging the mucosa. Small ovarian endometriomas are first incised with the laser and the contents aspirated before the interior of the cyst is vaporized. Bruhat and his colleagues in Clermont-Ferrand, France have considerable experience in this technique and describe high pregnancy rates following carbon dioxide vaporization (Pouly et al 1986).

Nezhat (1989) has described the technique of videolaseroscopy which allows the surgeon to operate with a carbon dioxide laser in a more upright position; the operation is done while watching the video monitor, and therefore surgical fatigue is reduced. Because the carbon dioxide laser beam is absorbed by water there is rapid dispersion of heat and a low risk of thermal damage to surrounding organs so that surgery is safe, even in the vicinity of the ureter and bowel. Even extensive endometriotic deposits can be operated on with this method and although the operating time may be prolonged — up to 2 hours in some patients — most of the operations can be performed on a day-case basis. Nezhat reported on 156 patients with mild to extensive endometriosis treated by videolaseroscopy: 102 (65%) became pregnant within 18 months (Table 3.5).

Second-generation lasers such as the neodymium YAG, argon or KTP are now used with increasing frequency. The neodymium YAG is especially useful — although more expensive — as there is a significant reduction in the amount of smoke and as the flexible probe with a sapphire tip is in contact with the endometrioma and is easier to manipulate. Because the power density is high at the tip of the probe and then rapidly decreases, there is little danger of deep penetration and damage to normal tissue (Lomano 1987).

Table 3.5 Pregnancy rate in 24 months in 156 patients with endometriosis and infertility after 18-month follow-up

Stage (AFS)	No. of patients	No. of pregnancies	%
I	31	24	77
II	63	39	62
III	41	25	61
IV	21	14	66
Total	156	102	65

From Nezhat 1989.

Conservative surgery for tubal pregnancy

One of the major advances in laparoscopy has been conservative surgery for ectopic pregnancy, pioneered especially by the Groupe de Recherche pour l'Avancement de la Laparoscopie in France (Bruhat et al 1980; Pouly et al 1986). Pouly et al (1986) report 400 ectopic pregnancies in 367 patients between 1974 and 1986, of which 95% were treated through the laparoscope. Similar results have been reported in the USA and West Germany. Lubke (1988) in Berlin reported 290 patients treated by laparoscopy out of a total of 399 ectopic pregnancies (72.7%; Table 3.6). In this series 52% of ectopic pregnancies were in the ampulla of the tube, 30.8% had had a previous ectopic and the mean operation time was 58 minutes in 195 cases.

Table 3.6 Conservative treatment of ectopic pregnancy

Author	No. of patients	No. of ectopic pregnancies	Laparoscopic treatments
Pouly et al 1986	367	400	95%
Lubke 1988	290	399	72.7%

While endoscopic surgery is technically possible in most patients, there are contraindications to conservative treatment which must be followed for safe surgery. These include shock, major bleeding into the peritoneum, cornual or interstitial pregnancy, adhesions, obesity and a large haematosalpinx. It is also wise to use laparotomy if the human chorionic gonadotrophin levels are very high.

The operation commences by suction lavage until the pelvis is free from blood and a clear view of the tube is obtained. A solution of adrenaline 1:100 000 or Pitressin is next injected into the antimesenteric border of the tube which is then incised with a carbon dioxide laser or hook scissors. The tube then contracts and the pregnancy sac is

Table 3.7 Contraindications to conservative laparoscopic surgery for ectopic pregnancy

Absolute
Shock
Haemoperitoneum > 2000 ml
Interstitial pregnancy
Encysted haematocele
Haematosalpinx > 6 cm

Relative
Haemoperitoneum > 500 ml
Haematosalpinx > 4 cm
Obesity
Adhesions
Total human chorionic gonadotrophin > 20 000 iu/l

extruded, removed by suction, or teased out with grasping forceps. The edges of the tube may be left open. The results compare favourably with laparotomy and intrauterine pregnancy rates of 65% have been reported.

Gamete intrafallopian transfer and in vitro fertilization

Laparoscopic oocyte recovery is now less frequently performed than ultrasound-directed oocyte recovery but is still essential for intrafallopian gamete or zygote replacement. During oocyte collection each follicle should first be punctured from the lateral side and then alternately aspirated and washed with buffered heparinized culture medium until the oocyte is identified. An automatic suction machine helps. Gamete intrafallopian transfer is performed with a 60 mm catheter with a mobile stop at its tip to prevent deep penetration of the fimbria. The fallopian tubes must be steadied with an atraumatic grasping forceps prior to insertion of the gametes and mobilized into the axis of the catheter for ease of insertion.

Ventrosuspension and division of the uterosacral ligaments

These procedures are not commonly performed but a mobile retroversion can easily be brought into anteversion at laparoscopy. A 2 cm incision is made in each iliac fossa down to the level of the external oblique aponeurosis. A Palmer forceps is inserted; the round ligament is grasped and drawn into the incision and is then stitched and sutured to the fascia with absorbable sutures.

Division of the uterosacral ligament can be carried out for severe secondary dysmenorrhoea usually at the same time as the treatment of endometriosis. The ligaments are divided close to the uterus using a carbon dioxide or neodymium YAG laser. The operation is quickly performed and has some success in relieving pain.

Complications of laparoscopy

Most of the major complications of laparoscopy can be avoided by good technique (Table 3.8). It is especially important to exercise care while inserting the Verres needle and for transillumination of the abdominal wall prior to the second incision to protect the inferior epigastric artery. Puncture of a small vessel can be controlled by diathermy, sutures or heat, but serious haemorrhage requires immediate laparotomy.

Table 3.8 Complications of laparoscopy

Trauma
Bowel
Retroperitoneal vessels
Bladder
Omental vessels
Salpingitis
Abdominal wall
Bleeding from inferior epigastric artery
Umbilical infection and haematoma formation
Paraumbilical hernia
Surgical emphysema
Gas embolus
Anaesthetic

The major anaesthetic complications are entirely avoidable. A small volume of carbon dioxide gas should be insufflated into the abdomen; steep Trendelenburg tilt should be avoided to prevent respiratory embarrassment. It is essential that the anaesthetist monitors the pulse and blood pressure so that major respiratory or cardiovascular problems can be recognized at a stage when they are completely reversible.

Advances in surgical techniques will ensure that the number of laparoscopies continues to increase, maintaining the pre-eminent position this operation now occupies in gynaecological surgery.

HYSTEROSCOPY

Hysteroscopy is the examination of the uterine cavity using a narrow rigid telescope inserted through the cervix. However, the widespread clinical use of hysteroscopy only became practical with the development of high-powered light sources together with a method of distension to separate the walls of the uterine cavity (Lewis 1988).

Instruments

Diagnostic hysteroscopy is performed with a 4 mm telescope contained in a sheath which has a channel for gas or fluid distension. The Hopkins rod lens system allows a clear undistorted image. Most telescopes for hysteroscopy have a 25° or 30° lens.

A simple telescope is used for diagnosis only (Fig. 3.9). More complex instruments include the Hamou colpo-

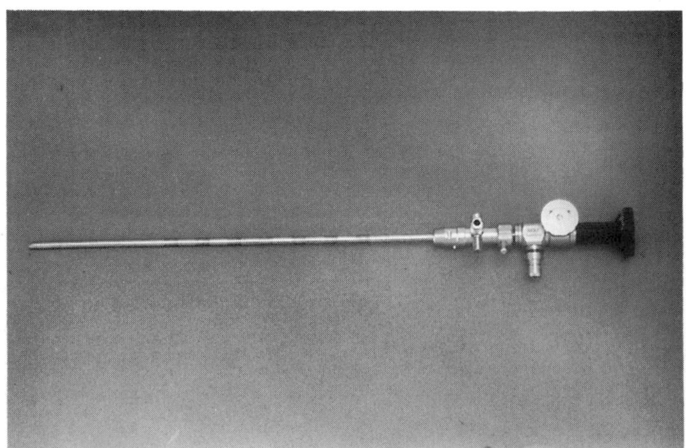

Fig. 3.9 Simple hysteroscope with a focusing wheel (from Gordon & Lewis 1988).

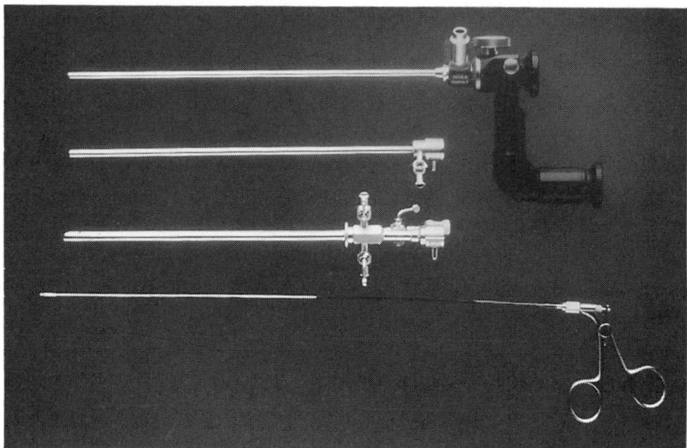

Fig. 3.10 Hamou hysteroscope and operating sheath with biopsy forceps.

microhysteroscope which has a direct ocular piece with two magnifications and an offset ocular piece with a further two magnifications (Taylor & Hamou 1983; Fig. 3.10). Alternatively a microview telescope has a proximal wheel for adjusting the focus and magnification. For intrauterine surgery a wider outer sheath of 7 mm diameter is required; this has a separate channel for the introduction of instruments, including scissors, suction tubes, biopsy forceps, laser fibres and catheters. The sheath normally blocks the cervix and prevents the escape of gas or fluid but if leaks do occur, a special portio adaptor can be placed over the cervix and held by suction.

The fluid used to distend the cavity is Hyskon, a viscous solution of 30% dextran which has good optical properties and is non-miscible with blood. Hyskon is sticky when dry and can block the taps unless the telescope is thoroughly washed. Dextrose (5%) is cheaper but less effective unless there is active bleeding. In laser surgery or endometrial resection either saline or glycine is irrigated under pressure to maintain a clear view. Carbon dioxide hysteroscopy is the choice for diagnostic examinations and minor surgery. The gas is insufflated from a specially designed Hysteroflator or Metromat machine which electronically monitors the pressure and limits the gas flow to a maximum of 100 ml/min.

A low flow of gas reduces the danger of gas embolus or cardiac arrhythmia. Insufflating machines for laparoscopy are dangerous and must never be used.

Technique

Office hysteroscopy is usually performed without dilation or local anaesthetic but operative hysteroscopy requires a paracervical block anaesthetic, and laser surgery or endometrial ablation should be performed under general anaesthesia. In postmenopausal women or in nulliparae, gentle dilation of the cervix may be needed but to avoid bleeding the dilators should not be inserted deeply. Hysteroscopy should be performed in the postmenstrual phase of the cycle because a clear view is usually obtained with no bleeding and no risk of pregnancy.

A single toothed vulselleum forceps is first attached to the cervix and the telescope is then inserted without pressure and under direct vision until it passes through the smooth endocervix and enters the uterine cavity. The telescope is advanced towards the fundus and then rotated to bring the cornual orifices into view. Magnification from × 20 to × 150 is possible; this allows the glandular and cellular structures of the endocervix and endometrium to be examined when the lens is in contact with the endometrium.

Diagnostic hysteroscopy

Panoramic hysteroscopy is especially useful in diagnosing submucous fibroids or mucous polyps causing dysmenorrhoea or menorrhagia (Table 3.9). Congenital uterine abnormalities causing recurrent abortions can easily be seen and adhesions causing Asherman's syndrome and secondary amenorrhoea can be diagnosed. Hysteroscopy is also useful when a contraceptive coil is lost or broken and helps to confirm the diagnosis of dysfunctional bleeding. The operation may be helpful in diagnosing retained products of conception, and in adenocarcinoma it can exclude involvement of the endocervix. Concern about the intraperitoneal spread of malignant cells has not been confirmed because malignant cells have not been recovered from the peritoneum in women undergoing hysterectomy immediately after hysteroscopy (Parent et al 1985).

Table 3.9 Diagnostic hysteroscopy

Panoramic hysteroscopy
(unit magnification)
Submucous fibroids
Submucous polyps
Congenital septa
Intrauterine adhesions
Lost intrauterine devices
Carcinoma
Retained products of conception
Microhysteroscopy
(magnification ×20–150)
Transformation zone

The colpomicrohysteroscope allows examination of the transformation zone when it lies inside the endocervical canal. This area can be examined at × 20 magnification with the squamous epithelium stained with Lugol's iodine and the columnar epithelium stained with Waterman's Blue (Hamou & Taylor 1982).

Operative hysteroscopy (Table 3.10)

Dividing adhesions in Asherman's syndrome is usually easy with scissors or by pressure from the bevelled end of the telescope. Major degrees of congenital abnormality of the uterus cannot be repaired through the hysteroscope but fusion defects such as septa are best treated by cutting the septum with strong scissors or with the laser (Perino et al 1987). Simple directed endometrial biopsy and recovery of lost pieces of a broken intrauterine device can be performed with grasping forceps.

Table 3.10 The role of operative hysteroscopy

Division of synechiae
Division of septa
Recovery of intrauterine devices
Laser photocoagulation of endometrium
Loop electroresection of endometrium
Roller ball electrocoagulation of endometrium
Radiofrequency induced thermal endometrial ablation
Sterilization

Several mechanical devices have been designed to sterilize women by occluding the cornual end of the tubes. These include the P Block, a hydrogelic intratubal device, or a nylon *dispositif* held in place with a hook and inserted into the cornua using the operating sheath of the hysteroscope (Fig. 3.11). These devices do not give complete security because they may become dislodged. The most promising method of hysteroscopic sterilization is the ovabloc system where liquid silicone is injected into the fallopian tube and then solidifies as a formed-in-place plug. Loffer (1984) reports successful sterilization in 80% of women at the first attempt. Patients can be treated on an outpatient basis with local anaesthesia; however, sterilization is not secure until an X-ray 3 months later confirms that the silicone plugs are in place.

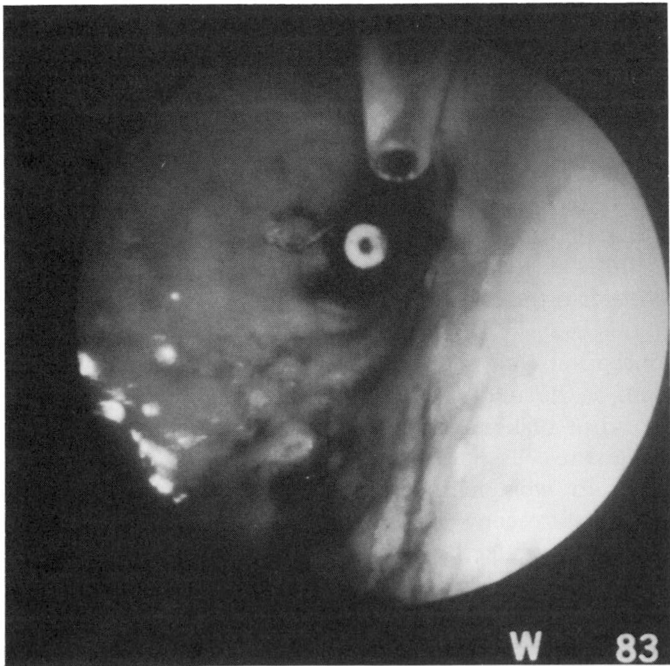

Fig. 3.11 Hysteroscopy; silastic plug in the cornua of the tube with loop for removal (photo courtesy of Joris De Mayer).

There is considerable interest in the technique of laser photovaporization of the endometrium for the treatment of menorrhagia using neodymium YAG and a disposable fibre to direct the light down the operating channel of the hysteroscope (Goldrath et al 1981; Cornier 1986). The sapphire tip of the fibre can be either in contact with the endometrium or very close to its surface. The operation is performed on women with severe functional menorrhagia and, if successful, results in absent or light periods. This selective destruction of the endometrium is performed under direct vision with the object of inducing intrauterine adhesions. Not all women will have amenorrhoea after this procedure; only about 50% have permanent amenorrhoea but a significant minority develop a normal period which is acceptable in women with severe menorrhagia. The failure rate is about 10%.

The operation should be limited to women with a normal sized uterus and should be preceded by a diagnostic hysteroscopy to exclude intrauterine pathology such as submucous fibroids or endometrial hyperplasia. Pretreatment with Danazol for 4–6 weeks prior to ablation causes the endometrium to atrophy and improves vision during surgery.

The operating hysteroscope has a sheath with two channels — one for the fibre carrying the laser beam and the second for infusion of fluid, which distends the cavity and washes out blood and debris. A solution of glycine is usually used but this can be absorbed into the circulation with a risk of cerebral or pulmonary oedema. Ringer lactate solution is safer but a strict record of fluid infused and fluid collected must be kept so that a deficit can be recognized (Loffer 1987).

The infusion fluid should be under positive pressure from a pump or a plastic bag compressed with a tourniquet. Positive pressure reduces bleeding from the endometrium by compressing the veins. Endometrial fragments, bubbles or debris are washed out by opening the outflow channel in the operative sheath of the hysteroscope (Loffer 1988) (Table 3.11).

Because laser energy is limited to the superficial layers of the endometrium, deep penetration into the myometrium is unlikely so the risk of damage to the abdominal contents is small. However, the telescope itself may perforate the uterus unless it is inserted gently and under direct vision. Another major risk that has been identified is gas

Table 3.11 Results of Nd: YAG laser hysteroscopic endometrial ablation

	No. of patients (%)		
	Goldrath et al 1981	Loffer 1988	Multicentre
Total number	260	60	45
Amenorrhoea	103 (48)	11 (20)	1 (4)
Hypomenorrhoea	103 (48)	27 (49)	17 (74)
Normal flow	4 (2)	6 (11)	2 (9)
Not known (<2 months follow up)	44	5	22

From Loffer 1988

embolus when a coaxial quartz fibre is used as opposed to a bare fibre. With a coaxial fibre, gas rather than fluid can be used to cool the sapphire tip of the fibre, and gas under pressure can enter the circulation causing a fatal embolus.

The laser machines are expensive and therefore an alternative simpler method of endometrial resection has been developed using a resectoscope as used in transurethral prostatectomy (DeCherney et al 1987, Hallez et al 1987).

Endometrial resection is performed under general anaesthesia but can be carried out under paracervical block. Although it is usually performed on women with a normal uterus with functional menorrhagia, submucous fibroids can also be satisfactorily resected, but careful patient selection is essential and large fibroids or intramural fibroids, should not be treated because of the danger of uterine perforation and damage to bowel.

High frequency diathermy is used with a mixture of cutting and coagulating current and strips of endometrium are resected down to the level of the myometrium. The anterior wall of the uterus is more difficult to resect than the posterior wall and the endocervical canal should usually be spared because of the risk of haemorrhage from branches of the uterine artery. Unlike the bladder, the uterine cavity is small and therefore manipulation of the resectoscope is more difficult. There is considerable danger of perforation unless a clear view is constantly maintained with a continuous flow irrigation system using glycine or Ringer/lactate infused into the uterus under pressure from a pump. A high intrauterine pressure reduces bleeding and a continuous flow washes out chips of endometrium and debris.

Large volumes of fluid may be used (up to several litres) and very strict input/output charts must be maintained because of the risk of intravascular absorption and pulmonary or cerebral oedema. This risk is 1 or 2%. If excessive fluid is retained, the operation should be abandoned and a diuretic given.

There are few published results of endometrial resection because the technique is new and follow-up is incomplete. Preliminary results suggest they are comparable to laser photovaporization with about 50% amenorrhoea, a significant proportion of oligomenorrhoea or normal menses and 10–15% failures due to technical difficulty or adenomyosis (Magos 1989). The publication of long-term results in larger series is awaited with interest.

Because of the potential danger and technical difficulty of the technique, there is a long learning curve for the surgeon. With experience, operating time can be reduced to about 20 minutes with a rapid improvement in results. Training is essential and all surgeons should first be experienced hysteroscopists.

Alternative methods of endometrial destruction with heat are being explored.

Electro-coagulation of the endometrium with the ball end resectoscope offers a simple alternative in women with functional menorrhagia (Vancaillie 1989). The aim of the procedure is to inflict thermal damage to the basal layer of the endometrium and therefore patients are pretreated with Danazol or Provera, to cause endometrial atrophy. The electrode consists of two insulated arms along the optic of the operating hysteroscope connected at the apex by a metal bar holding a 2 mm metal ball which can roll freely. A unipolar coagulating current of 40–70 W is applied and the roller ball moved at a speed of about 10 mm/s over the endometrium. Only a small volume of distension medium (maximum 30 ml Dextran or dextrose) is needed.

A novel method of endometrial destruction using microwave energy to heat the endometrium has recently been described (Phipps et al 1990, 1991). The cervix is dilated and then a specially designed probe is inserted into the uterine cavity. Microwave energy at a power of 400 W is applied which raises the temperature at the probe surface to about 55°C (Menostat, Rocket of London). Electromagnetic radiation relies on the interaction between the endometrium and an electric field generated around the treatment applicator and is thus not direct heating.

Preliminary results suggest that the incidence of amenorrhoea and oligomenorrhoea compare favourably with laser ablation or electroresection. Although simple to use and easy to learn, the technique is still undergoing clinical trials and long-term results are not available. The method is only suitable for women with functional bleeding and a normal uterus. A large endometrial cavity is less easy to treat so preoperative assessment by hysteroscopy, curettage and possibly ultrasound scans to measure the width between the cornua is essential.

Complications

Hysteroscopy is a safe procedure with minimal risks. Gas embolism is a rare complication which can almost completely be avoided if the correct insufflation apparatus is used with a maximum flow rate of 100 ml carbon dioxide per minute. A small quantity of carbon dioxide in the peritoneum is rapidly absorbed. During operative hysteroscopy under anaesthesia, the anaesthetist should listen to the heart sounds with a stethoscope. Even a small quantity of carbon dioxide in the heart can be detected by a grinding noise which ceases when the carbon dioxide inflow is switched off (Brundin, personal communication). Very rarely dextran causes anaphylaxis.

Perforation of the uterus with a rigid telescope should be eliminated if minimal force is used during insertion and especially if the telescope is inserted under direct vision. Laser ablation or loop resection carries a risk of perforation if the resection is deep and the operation should not continue when the circular muscle fibres are exposed.

Acute pelvic sepsis is a contraindication for hysteroscopy, but postoperative infection is possible, especially if the original indication for the operation is removal of products of conception or a retained contraceptive device.

Pregnancy is also a contraindication for hysteroscopy, except in the rare instances of removal of a lost intrauterine device or for chorion villus biopsy.

Finally, there is a small but significant risk of pulmonary or cerebral oedema during operative hysteroscopy when glycine or saline is used to distend and flush the uterine cavity because of fluid intravasation. Therefore, the volume of fluid infused should be measured and compared to the volume collected and any major discrepancy should be carefully noted. Immediate treatment with diuretics, oxygen and steroids should be started.

CYSTOSCOPY, PROCTOSCOPY AND SIGMOIDOSCOPY

The main use of the cystoscope in gynaecology is to evaluate cervical cancer and to investigate urinary symptoms including haematuria and incontinence or fistulae. All patients with invasive cervical cancer should undergo cystoscopy prior to therapy as part of clinical staging.

The earliest indication of bladder involvement by tumour is bullous oedema but if present it does not indicate Stage II disease. Ridges and furrows into the bladder wall should be interpreted as signs of submucous involvement of the bladder, especially if the bladder is fixed to the growth. A finding of malignant cells in cytological washings from the urinary bladder requires further examination and biopsy (International Federation of Gynaecology and Obstetrics 1988).

Patients with urge incontinence or detrus or instability should be cystoscoped before commencing medical treatment to exclude bladder calculi, polyps, tumours, diverticulae, basal trigonitis or atrophic changes which could respond to oestrogen therapy. It is important to culture the urine and to observe the bladder capacity which may be increased due to muscle atony or markedly reduced due to spasm.

Post radiation cystitis is a delayed complication of pelvic irradiation for cancer and in this case bladder capacity can be very small because of radiation fibrosis.

Obstetric urinary fistulae are still common in developing countries but most fistulae seen in industrialized countries are due to surgical trauma or cancer. All bladder fistulae should be assessed by cystoscopy with particular attention to the size of the fistula and its proximity to the ureteric orifices.

Ureteric fistula should always be investigated by cystoscopy and retrograde catheterization prior to planned reconstructive surgery.

The proctoscope and sigmoidoscope are less frequently used by the gynaecological surgeon. Women presenting with rectal bleeding, tenesmus or blood-stained mucous must have their lower bowel examined to exclude cancer of the rectum. A digital examination or proctoscopy is usually adequate to examine the rectum. Sigmoidoscopy up to 25 cm should only be performed after a bowel washout otherwise the view will be obscured by faeces. Common bowel diseases which may first present to the gynaecologist include haemorrhoids, fissure-in-ano, diverticulitis, ulcerative colitis, radiation proctitis and occasionally Crohn's disease.

KEY POINTS

1. Diagnostic laparoscopy is used for unexplained pelvic pain and to detect endometriosis, acute pelvic inflammatory disease, ectopic pregnancy, to investigate infertility, and prior to in vitro fertilization.
2. Therapeutic laparoscopy is used for salpingolysis, salpingostomy, adhesiolysis, conservative surgery for tubal pregnancy, ovarian cystectomy, recovery of lost intrauterine contraceptive devices, GIFT, IVF and ventro suspension. Laser laparoscopy is used for destruction of endometriomas, and removal of subperintoneal fibroids.
3. Tuboscopy is used to study physiology and anatomy of the tube and for selection of patients for IVF.
4. Hysteroscopy is used to diagnose submucous fibroids, polyps, congenital septa, and endometrial carcinoma, for transcervical endometrial resection, myomectomy and polypectomy, and for laser coagulation of the endometrium.
5. Endometrial destruction is indicated in menorrhagia with a normal sized uterus. The techniques used include laser, photocoagulation, loop electroresection, roller ball electro-coagulation, and radiofrequency induced thermal endometrial ablation.
6. Main uses of cystoscopy are to stage cervical cancer, evaluate fistulae and urinary symptoms including haematuria, incontinence, urgency and frequency.
7. Proctoscopy and sigmoidoscopy are used to evaluate patients with bleeding, tenesmus, and painful anal and rectal lesions.

REFERENCES

International Federation of Gynaecology and Obstetrics 1988 Radiumhemmet, Stockholm Annual Report on the results of treatment of gynaecological cancer, vol 20.

Bruhat M A, Manhes H, Mage G, Pouly J L 1980 Treatment of ectopic pregnancy by means of laparoscopy. Fertility and Sterility 33: 411–414

Cornier E 1986 Traitement hystérofibroscopique ambulatoire des métrorragies rebelles par laser Nd:YAG. Journal de Gynaecologie, Obstétrique et Biologie de la Réproduction 15: 661–664

DeCherney A, Diamond M P, Lary G, Polani M L 1987 Endometrial ablation for intractable uterine bleeding: hysteroscopic resection. Obstetrics and Gynecology 70: 664–670

Goldrath M H, Fuller T A, Segal S 1981 Laser photovaporization of endometrium for the treatment of menorrhagia. American Journal of Obstetrics and Gynecology 140: 14–19

Gordon A G, Lewis B V 1988 Gynaecological endoscopy. Chapman & Hall, London

Hallez J P, Netter A, Cartier R 1987 Methodical intrauterine resection. American Journal of Obstetrics and Gynecology 156: 1080–1084

Hamou J, Taylor P J 1982 Panoramic, contact and microcolpohysteroscopy in gynecologic practice. Current Problems in Obstetrics and Gynecology 6

Lewis B V 1988 Hysteroscopy in clinical practice. Journal of Obstetrics and Gynaecology 9: 47–55

Loffer F D 1987 Hysteroscopic sterilisation with the use of formed in-place silicone plugs. American Journal of Obstetrics and Gynecology 149: 261–270

Loffer F D 1987 Hysteroscopic endometrial ablation with the Nd:YAG laser using a non-touch technique. Obstetrics and Gynecology 69: 679–682

Loffer F D 1988 Obstetrics and Gynecology Clinics of North America 15: 77–89

Lomano J M 1987 Nd:YAG laser ablation of early pelvic endometriosis. Lasers in Surgery and Medicine 7: 56–60

Lubke T 1988 Proceedings of IIIrd European Congress on Hysteroscopy and Endoscopic Surgery. Amsterdam

Magos A L, Bauman R, Turnbull A C 1989 Transcervical resection of endometrium in women with menorrhagia. British Medical Journal 1: 1209–1212

Nezhat C 1986 Videolaseroscopy. Colposcopy and Gynecologic Laser Surgery 2: 221–224

Nezhat C 1989 In: Studd J (ed) Progress in obstetrics and gynaecology, vol 7. Churchill Livingstone, Edinburgh, pp 293–303

Parent B, Guedj H, Barbot J, Nodarian P 1985 Hysteroscopie panoramique. Maloine, Paris

Perino A, Mencaglia L, Hamou J, Cittadini E 1987 Hysteroscopy for metroplasty of uterine septa. Fertility and Sterility 48: 321–323

Phipps J, Lewis B V, Roberts T et al 1990 Treatment of functional menorrhagia by radiofrequency induced thermal endometrial ablation. Lancet i: 374–376

Phipps J, Lewis B V, Prior M V, Roberts T 1991 Clinical and experimental studies with radiofrequency induced thermal endometrial ablation. Obstetrics and Gynecology (in press)

Pouly J L, Manhes H, Mage G, Canis M, Bruhat M A 1986 Le traitement conservateur coelioscopique de la grossesse extra-uterine. Contraception, Fertilité, Sexualité 14: 543–551

Pouly J L, Fournier L, Manhes H, Mage G, Bruhat M 1988 Groupe de recherche pour l'avancement de la laparoscopie. Clermont-Ferrand, France

Semm K 1983 Endoskopische intra abdominal Chirurgie in der Gynäkalogie. Wiener Klinische Wochenschrift 95: 353–367

Semm K 1988 Pelviscopic surgery in gynaecological endoscopy. In: Gordon A G, Lewis B V Gynaecological endoscopy. Chapman & Hall, London

Semm K, Mettler 1980 Technical progress in pelvic surgery via operative laparoscopy. American Journal of Obstetrics and Gynecology 138: 121–127

Taylor P J, Hamou J E 1983 Hysteroscopy. Journal of Reproductive Medicine 28: 359–389

Vancaillie T G 1989 Electrocoagulation of the endometrium with the ball end resectoscope. Obstetrics and Gynecology 74: 425–427

4. Laser theory, practice and safety

R. J. Parsons

INTRODUCTION

A laser is a device capable of producing near-parallel beams of monochromatic light, both visible and invisible, at controlled intensities. This light can be focused, thus concentrating its energy, so that it can then be utilized to treat various conditions. The term 'laser' is an acronym for *l*ight *a*mplification by the *s*timulated *e*mission of *r*adiation. The process of stimulated emission was foreshadowed by Einstein at the turn of the century but it was not until 1960 that the first optical device was constructed (Maiman 1960). Since that time many lasers have been made but comparatively few have found their way into gynaecological practice. The aim of this chapter is to explain briefly the operation of a laser, the effects of laser energy on tissue, the common laser types, the practical clinical use of such lasers in gynaecology and laser safety.

BASIC LASER PHYSICS

At the molecular and atomic level, particles can only possess discrete amounts of energy — there is no continuum. Transition between these energy states is achieved by the absorption of a quantum of energy (a photon) necessary to raise the particle to a higher energy level (Fig. 4.1a) or by

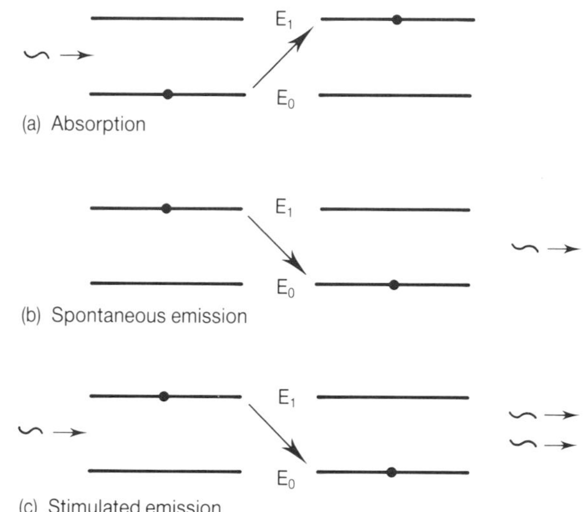

Fig. 4.1 Basic atomic processes. (**a**) Absorption of a photon of energy; (**b**) spontaneous emission of a photon; (**c**) stimulated emission of an additional photon of energy.
~ = Photon; E_0 = lower energy state; E_1 = higher energy state; • = particle.

emitting a photon and falling back to the lower energy state (Fig. 4.1b). In a normal substance these two processes are in balance and the number of particles in each energy state remains constant and less than the number in any state below (Fig. 4.2a). The process of stimulated emission is when the arrival of a photon causes the energy state to decay, rather than rise to a higher state, with the consequent emission of a second photon, in phase and at the same frequency, as the stimulating photon (Fig. 4.1c). For this process to occur the normal relationship between the numbers of particles at various energy states must be reversed — the number of particles at one energy state must be greater than those at the energy state below. This is called population inversion (Fig. 4.2b).

In order for this process of stimulated emission to become self-sustaining as in a laser, most of the emitted photons must be kept within the system and allowed to go on stimulating further emissions. Only a small percentage

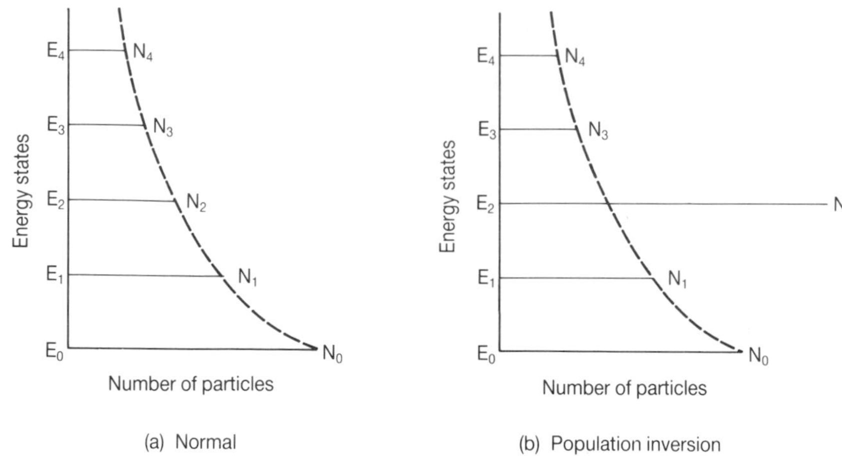

Fig. 4.2 Relationship between energy states and populations. (**a**) Normal population distribution; (**b**) population inversion.

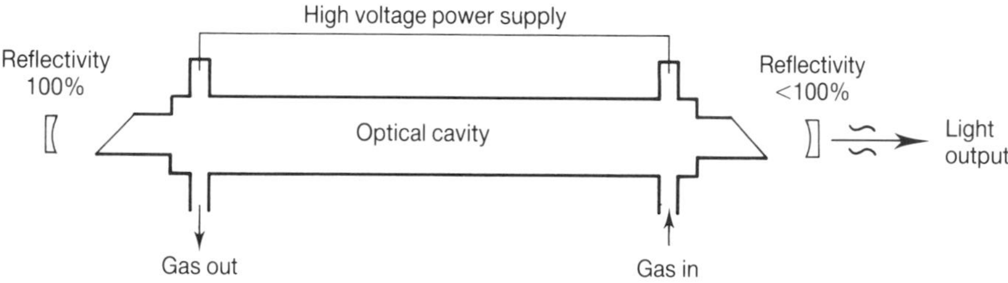

Fig. 4.3 Block diagram of a typical flowing gas laser system.

of photons should be allowed to escape to become the laser output.

A typical flowing gas laser system is shown in Figure 4.3. The gas mixture within which the population inversion will take place flows through an electrical discharge tube which is fed by a high-voltage potential. This excites the particles above the inversion level required and normal decay to this lower state takes place (state N_2, Fig. 4.2b). Provided that the rate of decay to a lower state is less than the rate of arrival at the upper state, a population inversion will be created and stimulated emission becomes possible. Photons are retained within the system by mirrors outside the discharge tube but a small percentage is allowed to escape through one of the mirrors.

There are many variations on this theme, ranging from solid-state lasers to liquid dye lasers, but the basic principles remain the same. There is a pumping mechanism to create the population inversion, an optical mechanism to retain photons and a means of allowing some of the radiation to escape from the system. A more detailed explanation of laser physics is provided elsewhere (Carruth & McKenzie 1986).

The radiation emitted is monochromatic (if only one decay path is involved), coherent and collimated. Collimation, or the near-parallel nature of laser light, can be exploited in many ways and it is the main feature which makes such devices useful in the medical world. A single convex lens placed in the beam will bring it to a focus, the size of which is dependent upon the width of the collimated beam. The use of different lenses or varying the lens-to-tissue distance alters the diameter of the beam at the point of contact with the tissue (Fig. 4.4). This is referred to as

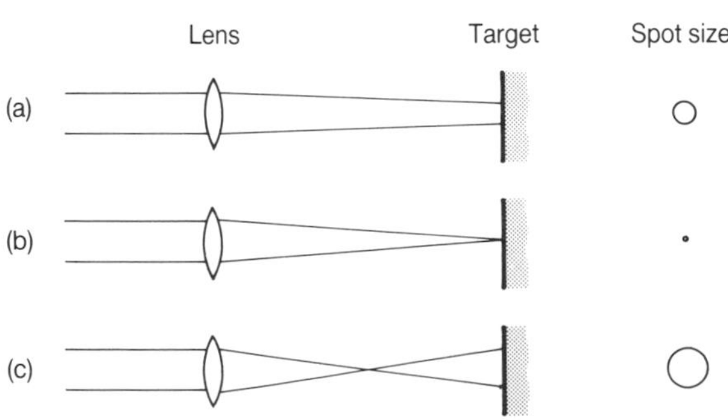

Fig. 4.4 Changing the focal length of the focusing lens while keeping the lens-to-tissue distance constant alters the spot size — the diameter of the beam at the point of contact with the tissue.
(**a**) The focal length of the lens is greater than the lens-to-tissue distance; (**b**) the focal length of the lens is the same as the lens-to-tissue distance — the laser is focused on the tissue; (**c**) the focal length of the lens is less than the lens-to-tissue distance.

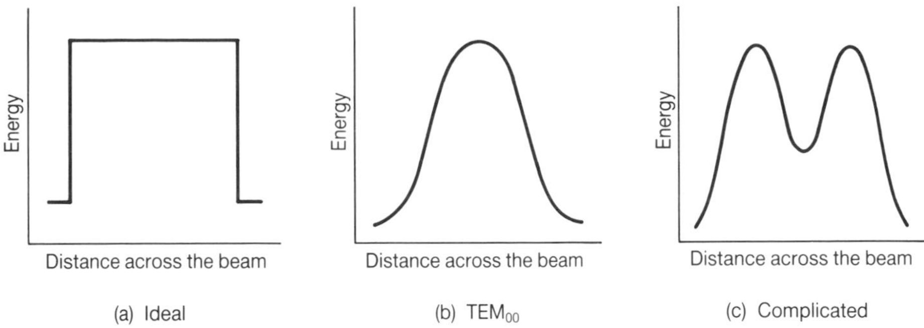

Fig. 4.5 Laser beam profiles. (**a**) Ideal; (**b**) TEM_{00}; (**c**) complicated.

changing the spot size. In carbon dioxide (CO_2) lasers the size of the visible helium–neon spot will not always be the same as the CO_2 spot because the lens will not focus in the same way as these beams of different wavelengths.

The most important determinant of the effects of a laser upon tissue is the power density (PD). This can be calculated roughly as:

$$PD = 100 \times W/D^2 \text{ watts/cm}^2$$

where PD is power density, W is power output in watts and D is the effective diameter of the spot in millimetres. D can be measured by firing a short low-power pulse at a wooden tongue depressor. The power density can be altered by changing either the power or the spot size but the latter has the greater effect.

A further property of the light output which is often quoted is that of transverse excitational mode (TEM). This can be described as the energy profile of the beam across its width. The ideal mode is one of a step change in power (Fig. 4.5a) but the nearest practical profile is that resembling a gaussian distribution or TEM_{00} as shown in Figure 4.5b. However, many lasers have a more complicated profile, an example of which is shown in Figure 4.5c. Modern lasers are much more stable than previously but if the surgeon requires quantitative light–tissue interaction (Sharp et al 1981) then mode stability becomes very important.

LIGHT–TISSUE INTERACTION

Light impinging on tissue is subject to the normal laws of physics. Some of the light is reflected and some is transmitted through the air–tissue barrier and passes into the tissue where it is scattered or absorbed. Obviously the extent to which each process dominates is dependent upon the physical properties of the light and the tissue. The theory of light–tissue interaction is not as well developed as that of ionizing radiation (Wall et al 1988) but enough is known to explain the macroeffects upon which most laser treatments depend.

At very low energy density levels (power density × time), say below 4 J/cm², a stimulating effect on cells has been observed but above this level the effect is reversed and suppression occurs (Mester et al 1968). As the energy density rises to 40 J/cm², indirect cell damage can take place if any sensitizing agents present become activated (e.g. haematoporphorin derivative). Direct tissue damage does not take place until about 400 J/cm² when the first thermal effects appear and photocoagulation occurs. Another 10-fold increase in energy density results in complete tissue destruction as it is sufficient to raise the cell temperature rapidly to 100°C causing total cell destruction and tissue vaporization. Obviously these are general observations and other properties of the incident beam will have an influence but the general 10-fold relationship alluded to above holds even though other parameters may be varied. Amongst the most important of these are the wavelength and the pulsatile nature of the radiation involved.

The wavelength absorption characteristics of various body tissues are reasonably well understood, qualitatively if not quantitatively. Figure 4.6 shows the absorption curves for water, melanin and haemoglobin which, to a large extent, will determine the curves for tissue as a

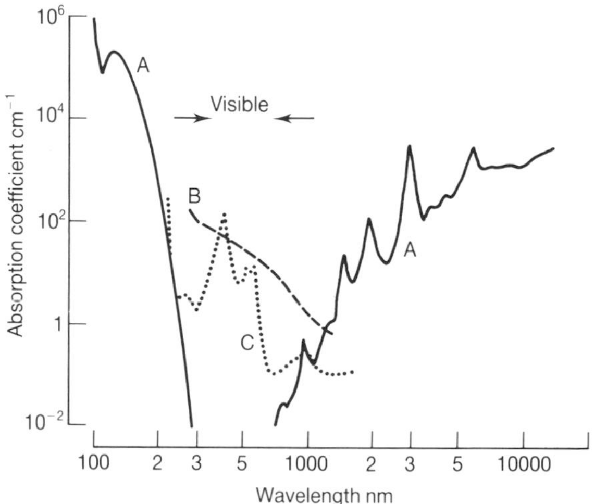

Fig. 4.6 Absorption characteristics of (**A**) water; (**B**) melanin; (**C**) haemoglobin at different wavelengths. After Boulnosis (1986).

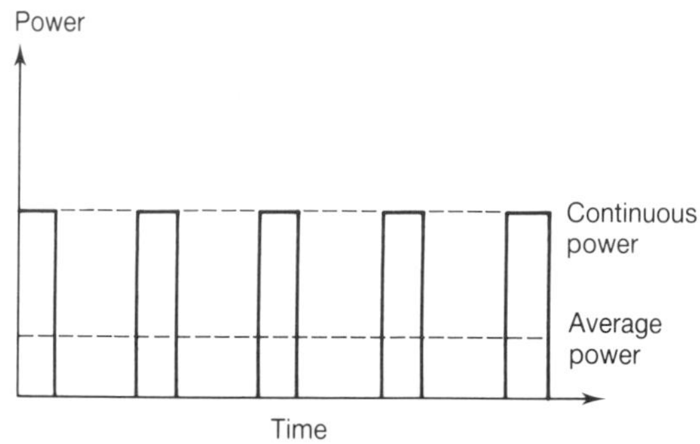

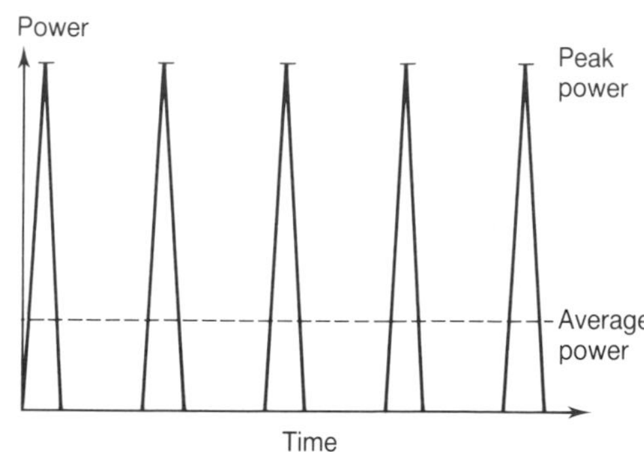

Fig. 4.7 The effects of pulse irradiation.

whole. In the ultraviolet and the middle-to-far infrared spectrum, absorption by water predominates whereas melanin and haemoglobin effects take over in the visible range. From this graph it is easy to see that a particular laser, operating at a fixed wavelength, will be preferentially absorbed by one tissue constituent and its effects will be different to another laser with a different wavelength.

So far it is implied that the laser is operated continuously for long enough for thermal effects to appear (continuous wave or CW mode). However, it is relatively simple, by means of a shutter or a controllable power supply, to switch the energy on and off rapidly — the pulse mode. In general the medical definition of a pulse is a burst of energy lasting 0.25 s or less. This does not correspond to the physics definition of a pulse and care must be taken to avoid confusion. Methods of generating these pulses differ between lasers and the tissue effects can also vary. The reason for this phenomenon is shown in Figure 4.7.

Figure 4.7a shows the output from a CW laser which is modulated by a perfect shutter. The average power delivered to the tissue can be calculated from a knowledge of the CW power, the pulse repetition rate and width. In the case of an electronically controlled high-pulse power system where the time–power curve is not so closely defined (Fig. 4.7b), it is much more difficult to determine the average power delivered. It is necessary to measure the energy of the pulse and the pulse repetition rate. The peak power, although impressive, is almost irrelevant.

The effects on tissue of this pulsatile radiation are to reduce the pure thermal effects (lower average power input) whilst maintaining and sometimes enhancing the vaporization potential. Provided the pulse repetition rate is sufficiently low to allow heat conduction to take place between pulses, the tissue temperature will stabilize at a lower value.

Very short pulses, such as those produced by Q-switched lasers, can cause electromechanical breakdown in tissues because of the extremely high energy densities obtainable. In the early days these lasers were tested in gynaecology but untoward side-effects were noted (Minton et al 1965).

COMMON LASER SYSTEMS

Three main lasers have found a place in gynaecological practice:

1. The CO_2 laser.
2. The neodymium: yttrium aluminium garnet (Nd:YAG) laser.
3. The argon ion (Ar^+) laser.

These will be described in detail with a further section devoted to other types which have been used in research and could possibly enter general usage in a short time depending on their availability, price, reliability and clinical results.

The CO_2 laser

This system is the one which has been most used in gynaecology since its introduction in the early 1970s. This has been because of its clinical suitability, ease of use, reliability and easy serviceability. Although a major drawback is that it cannot be transmitted by fibres, it has so far not been displaced by other lasers.

As the name implies, the active lasing medium is CO_2 dioxide gas. Efficiencies of 15% energy conversion to light output have been achieved. In fact, an analyser has used this ability for detecting CO_2 in the breath! The first generation of CO_2 lasers used a flowing gas system such as that shown in Figure 4.3, with high voltage direct-current excitation. A gas mixture of CO_2, nitrogen and helium was used to help achieve and maintain the population inversion. Sealed tube lasers are now available with radiofrequency low-voltage discharges being used for excitation. This has made the machines smaller and removed the need for gas bottles.

The output radiation of 10.6 μm wavelength is well into

the infrared region of the spectrum. From the earlier discussion, it would be expected that this radiation would be absorbed rapidly by tissue water and should therefore cut and vaporize more easily than coagulate. This is indeed the case as 90% of the incident radiation is absorbed within about 0.03 mm of the surface and intense heating occurs. Coagulation will only take place in small blood vessels less than 0.5 mm in diameter, but haemostasis can be facilitated by reducing the power density so that the zone of thermal damage around the central crater is wider.

As yet there is no commercially available fibre which can transmit 10.6 μm light efficiently so all commercial systems use some form of articulated arm. At each joint there is a mirror which is adjusted so that the beam stays central despite movement between the two adjacent limbs of the arm. The choice of the mirror material is limited because of the need to reflect two beams of widely differing wavelengths. Because 10.6 μm is invisible, an aiming beam must be used so that the operator can see where the therapeutic beam is going to have its effect. A helium–neon (HeNe) laser emitting at 628 nm (red) is incorporated into the system and optically aligned so that it coincides with the therapeutic beam. (*Note*: this alignment can degenerate and should be checked regularly.) The mirrors must therefore be chosen to reflect both the infrared CO_2 beam and the red HeNe aiming beam.

The final delivery to the operation site can be carried out in two ways, both incorporating a focusing lens. For hand-held surgery the lens at the end of a straight delivery tube focuses the beam on the operative field about 1 cm from the end of the tube. The lens-to-tissue distance can thus be varied at will so that the spot size will be changed within a narrow range (Fig. 4.8a). Colposcopic delivery involves a mirror after the focusing lens which brings the beam into line with the viewing axis of the colposcope. This mirror is at the end of a joystick so that the beam may be moved around within the viewed area (Fig 48.b). Originally the spot size was changed by altering the power of this lens and so was limited to three or four predetermined sizes. Now the use of zoom optics allows infinite adjustment over a limited range (0.5–4 mm).

Power outputs of these lasers can be from a few watts up to 100 W. Most commercial systems in gynaecology produce up to 25–35 W as this, coupled with a variable spot size, provides power densities of up to 6000 W/cm^2, sufficient for tissue-cutting and vaporization at a controllable rate. The extra power provided by instruments producing 40–60 W is useful for dealing with patients who bleed during the procedure.

The Neodymium:YAG laser

This device is a solid-state laser with the active neodymium ions being incorporated in an artificial crystal of YAG. Pumping is achieved by energy input from a parallel gas discharge lamp, usually a water-cooled krypton tube, with the output radiation being refocused into the laser crystal. Output power levels up to 100 W continuous can be achieved but with a conversion efficiency of 1% or so, nearly 10 kW of input power is needed.

The CW energy produced is at a wavelength of 1.06 μm and is thus in the near infrared. As such, it can be trans-

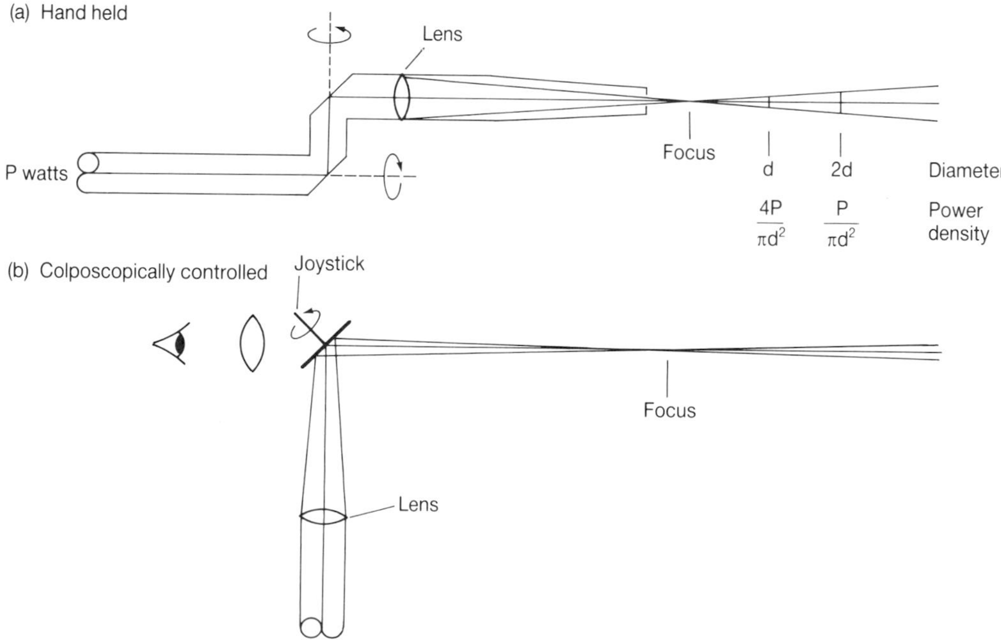

Fig. 4.8 Laser delivery systems. (**a**) Hand-held; (**b**) colposcopically controlled.

mitted easily down a flexible fibreoptic delivery system and delivered to many more anatomical sites than the CO_2 laser. The emergent radiation has lost its collimation and will diverge quite rapidly. However, sapphire tips can be added to the fibres, thus controlling the emerging beam to a certain extent and adding another dimension to laser surgery. Most fibres also have a coaxial flow of gas, usually CO_2, to keep debris away from the end of the fibre. This is particularly necessary where contamination with blood or blood products may make continuous operation difficult.

As with the CO_2 laser, 1.6 μm Nd:YAG radiation is invisible. A HeNe laser (or other light source) needs to be incorporated into the device to show where the treatment site will be. This is also a very useful safety feature as near infrared radiation can be focused on the retina and cause irreparable damage. The Nd:YAG laser is easy to operate as a Q-switched laser. An optoelectronic switch is incorporated inside the laser cavity and the lasing action prevented for a large percentage of the time. The population inversion therefore builds up to an even higher level than normal and when the switch is eventually opened a massive pulse of energy is delivered. The switch can then be closed and the process repeated. This type of action has found a use in ophthalmology where, by focusing the pulse to a very small spot, electromechanical breakdown of tissue can be induced with minimal surrounding damage.

The argon laser

This laser system employs argon as the active gas which has to become ionized before a population inversion will occur. Even then lasing is still difficult as the ions must be excited to still higher levels before a usable inversion results. This means that the overall efficiency of the system is low — less than 0.1% — with a 5 W output of light being typical. Two transitions occur simultaneously at 488 nm (blue) and 514.5 nm (blue-green), thus giving the operator a choice of wavelengths, although there is very little difference in their therapeutic effects. The output beam can be delivered by fibreoptics and can act as its own aiming beam after suitable attenuation. In fact it is better for the tube to operate continuously and rely upon mechanical shutters to control the output.

The major use for this laser has been in ophthalmology where it has reigned supreme since the early 1970s because of its ability to penetrate and be focused on most parts of the eye. The argon can be replaced by other noble gases, such as krypton, and commercial dual tube systems are available. Krypton produces two beams in the visible at 568 nm (yellow) and 647 nm (red) and therefore has somewhat different penetration characteristics to its more popular brother.

Other laser systems

There are many other laser systems now being used in medicine and the time period from research to common usage seems to be getting shorter. It is neither possible nor desirable to give a complete list but the following few examples may soon find an accepted place in gynaecological surgery.

Metal vapour lasers, as their name implies, consist of a container filled with a heated and vaporized metal in an inert gas atmosphere at low pressure. The electrical discharge used must be pulsed because the population inversion cannot be sustained long enough for true CW operation to take place. Two types of metal vapour laser have found a use in medicine — copper and gold. The copper vapour laser produces two beams at 510 and 578 nm at up to 25 W power output. These by themselves are not particularly useful, although the green can be used as a substitute for the argon laser in dermatology. The output is ideally suited to act as an optical pumping source for a dye laser, which can be tuned to provide radiation for photodynamic therapy.

Photodynamic therapy is a rapidly evolving treatment for certain tumours (Spikes & Jori 1987). It relies upon selective retention in tumour tissues of a drug, such as haematoporphyrin derivative, which only becomes active on exposure to light of a particular wavelength. This can vary from drug to drug and the most suitable drug–wavelength combination is still being sought. The dye laser offers help to this research effort because the wavelength of its beam can be altered. Various dyes can be excited to form a population inversion between groups of energy states — not individual states as in a true laser — but which allow a laser output to be generated. As there are many decay pathways available the output is multiwavelength but with suitable optical devices a narrow wavelength range can be selected. The copper vapour and dye laser combination can produce over 5 W of red light at 630 nm which is an absorption peak of haematoporphyrin derivative.

The other metal vapour device being investigated is the gold laser. The output of this is at 627.8 nm, a close match to the dye laser, without the added complication of two devices in series.

So far only visible and infrared lasers have been considered but research into ultraviolet lasers has produced systems which seem to rely on non-thermal mechanisms for tissue destruction. These are the excimer lasers, a term derived from excited dimer, where the active medium is made from a combination of two substances which do not normally combine, such as a rare gas and a halide. These lasers have found a place in ophthalmology and their potential for precise tissue removal could offer the microsurgeon a very powerful tool.

PRACTICAL LASER TECHNIQUES

The early use of lasers in gynaecology was in the treatment of cervical intraepithelial neoplasia but has subsequently spread to most other areas of the lower reproductive tract. The use of the laser in treatment of intraepithelial neoplasia of the genital tract is described in Chapter 34.

The uterus

The uterus presents two main problems for the CO_2 laser: firstly, its relative inaccessibility and secondly, the treatments to be considered are mainly coagulative rather then destructive. The instrument of choice is therefore the Nd:YAG or the Ar^+ laser. The former has been utilized successfully for the hysteroscopic ablation of the endometrium for the treatment of menorrhagia.

The cervix is dilated sufficiently to allow the introduction of a hysteroscope and a coaxial outflow of sufficient distending fluid to keep the operating field visible. A 5% dextrose solution in saline is employed rather than the thicker 50% solution ideal for hysteroscopy as this tends to caramelize when exposed to Nd:YAG radiation and visibility is soon lost. Hysteroscopes with a separate aspiration channel make over-dilatation unnecessary.

The pioneers of the technique employed tubal ligation to prevent subsequent pregnancy but they have now abandoned this procedure (Goldrath 1985). However, Davis (1987) still recommends its use to stop fluid flow into the abdominal cavity during treatment.

The laser delivery fibre is introduced down the hysteroscope and brought into view. Two alternative delivery techniques have been developed with similar results (Lomano 1988). Contact surgery was the obvious way to start, the end of the fibre being kept in close contact with the endometrium as it was moved backwards and forwards over the whole surface of the uterus. A power delivery of some 50–60 W continuous (giving a PD in the order of 2000 W/cm^2 at the fibre tip) is necessary to achieve adequate ablation. A second technique has evolved where the fibre is kept at a distance from the endometrium and the end result is judged by the appearance of endometrial blanching. Slightly higher powers must be used as the beam diverges on leaving the fibre. In both cases destruction must be stopped at the endocervical canal and it is preferable to mark this margin at the beginning of the procedure.

Great care must be taken to avoid fluid overload as inevitably some is absorbed through the ablated surface of the uterus. The blanching technique has been found to result in lower absorption rates (Lomano 1988). No problems have been found with temperature in the uterus or adjacent organs and postoperative complications are low. Careful evaluation of results is still required as the number of reported cases is low but growing rapidly.

Laparoscopic and other abdominal techniques

The CO_2 and Nd:YAG and argon lasers have been used laparoscopically for some time (Tadir & Ovadia 1986). Recently other solid-state lasers such as the potassium-titanyl-phosphate laser emitting at 532 nm (KTP 532) have been tried (Daniell et al 1986). The CO_2 laser can pass only through a rigid laparoscope and then may have to be reflected on to target structures. The other systems use flexible fibres for delivery.

All tissue destruction techniques lead to smoke production and efficient evacuation must be employed. This should be connected to the insufflation apparatus as, if the rate of evacuation is too high, deflation of the abdominal cavity will result. Adequate beam stops must be employed as it is very easy to damage adjacent organs, some of which are out of view to the operator. The less penetrating CO_2 has the edge in this respect as thermal damage is immediately obvious.

Endometriosis has been the main target for laser laparoscopy treatment because of its multi-focal nature and the varying types of structures affected. A choice must be made between the fine control possible with a CO_2 laser and the other devices which coagulate before finally ablating if the PD is high enough. Large endometriomas need to be enucleated with extensive manipulation which will suggest the use of the CO_2 laser. Using a CO_2 laser for the laparoscopic excision of benign ovarian cysts in young women has some advantages over scissors and diathermy. Laparoscopic adhesiolysis has been carried out with the CO_2 laser. The problems with back-stops and orientation of CO_2 devices have he contributed to trials of the argon and KTP 532 lasers for this purpose. However, the CO_2 laser causes less thermal damage and is preferable when removing adhesions from the ovary or tubes.

Open tubal surgery, salpingostomy and the treatment of uterine anomalies have all been undertaken by the laser specialist (Bellina 1986) but this use is still confined to a small group and should be viewed with some caution by those entering the field.

LASER SAFETY

All laser systems currently in use have no way of distinguishing between patient and operator. The desired effect on a patient can be a serious accident to the surgeon. The subject of the safe construction and operation of lasers in medicine and surgery is thus very important and must be understood by all involved. This section is biased in favour of UK regulations but the situation is similar in most European countries and the USA although, of course, regulatory bodies and documents will have different guises.

As from January 1989 all lasers sold in the UK must conform to two basic standards. Electrical safety requirements are detailed in BS 5724 (British Standards Institution 1979) and non-ionizing radiation hazards are covered by IEC 825 (International Electrotechnical Commission 1984). A further publication by the Department of Health and Social Security (1984) outlines good laser practice together with some additional equipment safety features. All of these publications should be considered by a laser protection adviser (a health authority appointee) who will assist each user in specifying and installing lasers in clinical surroundings. Although the requirements will vary from laser to laser and from site to site, the following sections outline the major considerations involved.

Nature of the hazard

The body is divided into two regions for hazard analysis: the eye and skin. In the visible region, which extends into the near infrared, the eye is the organ most at risk. Outside this range the eye is no different to skin except that corneal damage can lead to visual loss although the retina itself may be undamaged.

Radiation entering the eye is focused on to the retina and the PD can increase by up to 5×10^5 times so that a 50 W/m^2 corneal incident beam can become 25 MW/m^2 on the retina, with disastrous and irreparable results. Maximum permitted exposure (MPE) levels are laid down by the regulations and are set well below known damage thresholds. Manufacturing and administrative controls are written to prevent operators, assistants and patients from accidentally receiving radiation in excess of these limits. There are separate values for the skin and eye, with the latter being the more stringent.

Control of hazards

Lasers are currently classified into four groups from class 1 to 4, with class 1 being the least and class 4 the most hazardous. Class 3 is also subdivided into two classes, 3A and 3B. It is the manufacturers' responsibility to classify a laser but once this is done, it will rarely be changed. Stringent safety precautions must be introduced when class 3 and 4 lasers are in use. Most medical lasers are class 3B or 4 and so need such safeguards. Aiming beams are usually class 1 or 2 and present a minimal hazard.

In addition to classifying the laser, manufacturers must ensure that the equipment complies with the specification for its particular class. Generally all systems will have a key control and some way of monitoring the power being delivered to the patient. It should also indicate either visually or audibly when the laser shutter is opened and levels in excess of the MPE are being emitted.

Administrative controls are framed to ensure that the equipment is then used safely. A set of local rules must be drawn up which specify who is allowed to use a laser and where it can be used. A laser controlled area (LCA) must be defined and the activities within that area controlled. There must be no possibility of radiation in excess of the MPE passing out of the area, even if this means blocking windows and doors. Warning signs must be exhibited at the entrance to the LCA and door interlocks can be used but are not obligatory for CO_2 lasers. Examples of such local rules can be found in other texts (Stamp 1983; Department of Health and Social Security 1984).

All personnel within the LCA *must* either be protected from the radiation by the inherent optical properties of operating equipment or must wear appropriate spectacles. For example, any common translucent glass is impervious to CO_2 laser radiation. Precautions for the Nd:YAG laser must be more complicated and special eyewear for observers and filters to protect the operator from back-reflection through a delivery system are required. Obviously such devices cannot be used when the aiming beam is derived from the therapeutic beam. In this case an additional safety shutter is required to protect the surgeon during treatment. Precautions against eye damage must be rigorously implemented for all present, including the patient.

Fire is an ever-present hazard with the use of class 4 lasers and simple precautions must be observed. Aqueous instead of spirit-based solutions should be used and paper drapes should be avoided. CO_2 radiation is readily absorbed by water and by keeping swabs soaked in water or saline, tissues adjacent to the operation site can be protected. A suitable fire extinguisher should always be available. Great care must be exercised in the presence of inflammable anaesthetic gases. Endotracheal tubes have been ignited by a laser, with serious results (Bandle & Holyoak 1987). While this situation is not likely to be encountered in gynaecology, inflammable gases may be passed rectally by the patient during laser treatment of the lower genital tract, posing a theoretical risk of explosion.

A by-product of laser treatment is a plume of smoke and debris, with a characteristic odour. This must be evacuated and collected from as near as possible to the impact zone for two important reasons. Firstly, the emission of smoke is likely to obscure the operating site. This is particularly true in cervical or vaginal surgery. Secondly, doubts have been raised over the viability of particles contained within the plume (Garden et al 1988). Although the evidence is not overwhelming, it is essential that the smoke should be adequately extracted and filtered.

Unintentional reflections of the laser beam striking an instrument can be dangerous. Although it is very unlikely that radiation reflected in this way will be sufficiently focused to cause damage it is sensible to ensure that the instruments are not highly polished and scatter any incident radiation. It should not be assumed that the reflecting qualities of a surface are the same at visible and far infrared wavelengths, so care should be exercised in the choice of specula and other operating instruments.

CONCLUSIONS

The use of lasers in gynaecology has come a long way since their introduction in the 1970s. Many different types have been used but the CO_2 laser is the most common. This is because of its ability to cut and vaporize tissue at a controllable rate, with minimum adjacent thermal damage. However, as newer devices are made available they will open up many new fields of treatment based on as yet unknown light–tissue interactions, possibly with concomitant drugs.

KEY POINTS

1. Lasers produce nearly parallel beams of monochromatic light.
2. The beam can be focused by a lens to alter the diameter of the beam at the point of contact with the tissue (the spot size).
3. The power density (PD) is the most important determinant of the effects of the laser upon tissue.
4. The greater the power density the less the thermal effect and the less the haemostatic property of the beam.
5. The beam of a CO_2 or a Nd:YAG laser is invisible so a guiding HeNe laser is required.
6. The eye must be protected from accidental exposure to laser energy. This is especially important with Nd:YAG endoscopic systems.

REFERENCES

Bandle A M Holyoak B 1987 Laser incidents. In: Moseley H, Haywood J K (eds) Medical laser safety. Institute of Physical Sciences in Medicine, London, pp 47–57

Bellina J H 1986 Tubal surgery. In: Sharp F, Jordan J A (eds) Gynaecological laser surgery. Perinatology Press, Ithaca, pp 217–236

Boulnois J 1986 Photophysical processes in recent medical laser developments: a review. Lasers in Medical Science 1: 47–66

British Standards Institution 1979 Medical electrical equipment part 1: specification for general safety requirements. BS 5724. British Standards Institution, London

Carruth J A S, McKenzie A L 1986 Medical lasers, science and clinical practice. Adam Hilger, Bristol

Daniell J F, Miller W, Tosh R 1986 Initial evaluation of the use of the potassium-titanyl-phosphate (KTP 532) laser in gynecologic laparoscopy. Fertility and Sterility 46: 373–377

Davis J 1987 The principles and use of the neodynium-YAG laser in gynaecological surgery. Clinical Obstetrics and Gynaecology 1: 331–352

Department of Health and Social Security 1984 Guidance on the safe use of lasers in medical practice. HMSO, London

Garden J M, O'Banion M K, Shelnitz L S et al 1988 Papillomavirus in the vapour of carbon dioxide laser treated verrucae. Journal of the American Medical Association 259: 1199–1202

Goldrath M H 1985 Hysteroscopic laser ablation of the endometrium. In: Baggish M S (ed) Basic and advanced laser surgery in gynecology. Appleton-Century-Crofts, Norwalk, Connecticut

International Electrotechnical Commission 1984 Radiation safety of laser products, equipment classification, requirements and user's guide. IEC standard 825. International Electrotechnical Commission, Geneva

Lomano J M 1988 Dragging technique versus blanching technique for endometrial ablation with the Nd:YAG laser in the treatment of chronic menorrhagia. American Journal of Obstetrics and Gynecology 159: 152–155

Maiman T H 1960 Stimulated optical radiation in the ruby. Nature 187: 493–494

Mester E, Ludany G, Vajda J et al 1968 Uber die Wirkung von Laser-Strahlen auf die Bakteriemphagozytose der Leukozyten. Acta Biologica et Medica Germanica 21: 317–321

Minton J P, Carlton D M, Dearman J R et al 1965 An evaluation of the physical response of malignant tumour implants to pulsed laser radiation. Surgery, Gynecology and Obstetrics 121: 538–544

Sharp F, Maclean A B, Moir I A R et al 1981 Quantitated laser tissue destruction and the development of a technique for treating cervical intraepithelial neoplasia. In: Bellina J H (ed) Gynecologic laser surgery. Plenum, New York, pp 231–244

Spikes J D, Jori G 1987 Photodynamic therapy of tumours and other diseases using porphyrins. Lasers in Medical Science 2: 3–15

Stamp J M 1983 An introduction to medical lasers. Clinical Physics and Physiological Measurement 4: 267–290

Tadir Y, Ovadia J 1986 Laser endoscopy in gynaecology. In: Sharp F, Jordan J A (eds) Gynaecological laser surgery. Perinatology Press, Ithaca, pp 241–249

Wall B F, Harrison R M, Spiers F N 1988 Patient dosimetry techniques in diagnostic radiology. Institute of Physical Sciences in Medicine, York

5. Imaging techniques in gynaecology

M. C. Powell   A. Perkins

INTRODUCTION

The discipline of radiology exists today because of the discovery of bands of radiation mainly in the electromagnetic spectrum which can penetrate human tissue and thus can be exploited for imaging. X-rays and gamma photons are at one end of this spectrum and radio waves at the other. The majority of imaging work within a radiology department involves the use of X-rays. Magnetic resonance imaging (MRI) employs high-strength magnetic fields and radiofrequency radiation, representing almost certainly the final such window in the electromagnetic spectrum. Ultrasound is a mechanical vibration used to produce images from echoes returned from within the body (Table 5.1).

X-ray computerized tomography (CT) made a considerable impact on the world of medicine in the 1970s and acted as an impetus for the development of other techniques such as MRI. CT demonstrated the potential value of high-resolution tomographic sections through the body hitherto not available with other X-ray techniques but the impact of MRI may exceed that of ultrasound in the 1960s. MRI is similar to CT in providing a cross-sectional display of body anatomy with excellent resolution of soft tissue detail. The images are essentially a map of the distribution density of hydrogen nuclei (protons) and parameters reflecting their motion in cellular water and lipids. The total avoidance of ionizing radiation, its lack of known hazard and the penetration of bone and air with little attenuation make it a particularly attractive non-invasive imaging technique. It will be without doubt the imaging technique of

Table 5.1 Diagnostic imaging systems

Modality	Source	Imaging basis	Viewing system
X-ray	X-ray tube	Photoelectric effect	X-ray film, screen, TV system
X-ray CT	X-ray tube	Photoelectric and Compton effect	Computer TV system
Scintigraphy	Radionuclide	Photoelectric and Compton effect	Gamma camera, computer
Ultrasound	Transducer	Reflection of sound	Oscilloscope, scan converter, TV system
Doppler ultrasound	Transducer	Frequency shift	Frequency spectrum analyser
MRI	Magnetic moments of protons ^{1}H, ^{31}P	Radiofrequency excitation of nuclear paramagnetism	Computer display of intensity distribution

CT = computerized tomography; MRI = magnetic resonance imaging.

the 1990s and has already radically altered the radiological approach to the central nervous system. Its role in gynaecology has still to be evaluated.

Radionuclide imaging of gynaecological tumours with radiolabelled monoclonal antibodies is also a recent imaging innovation. Originally a research tool, it has potential as an imaging method and may eventually be used for drug-targeting.

ULTRASOUND

The introduction of ultrasound imaging by Donald in the 1950s is considered by many to be a major milestone in the development of our specialty. The production of real-time ultrasound scanners has reduced the cost of the equipment which has also become lighter, smaller and easier to use. The addition of pulsed Doppler ultrasound has also made possible the measurement of fetal and uteroplacental blood flow, thereby producing physiological information from what was previously an anatomical imaging technique. With better signal-processing techniques, image resolution has been further improved. Ultrasound has now become an integral diagnostic technique in both obstetrics and gynaecology. Although the indications for ultrasound in obstetrics have become clear-cut, there remains controversy about its role in gynaecology.

Ultrasound examination is dependent on both the technical expertise of the ultrasonographer and an understanding of the history and clinical findings of the patient being assessed. Bone and gas interfere with the transmission of ultrasound and in abdominal ultrasound a full bladder is required for pelvic examinations. However, errors may arise if the bladder is overdistended displacing a mass out of the pelvis into the lower or mid-abdomen. Highly echogenic masses such as dermoids may be obscured by loops of bowel containing gas.

The introduction of the vaginal ultrasound probe has overcome some of these problems, as it avoids the need for a full bladder. Obesity is not a restricting factor and the deeper parts of the pelvis may be visualized easily. This new technique is well accepted by patients (Timor-Tritsch et al 1988). The drawbacks consist mainly of an initial lack of observer familiarity with the anatomy as seen in the transvaginal coronal and sagittal planes and a scan depth of view limited to 20–70 mm. Hence, an abdominal approach may be required for ovaries high in the pelvis. The large-calibre probe employed in vaginal ultrasound may prove difficult for some postmenopausal women and those patients in whom extensive surgery or radiotherapy to the pelvis has led to some vaginal stenosis. However, transabdominal ultrasound is also limited in such patients due to poor bladder filling. The transrectal approach is superior in patients with suspected recurrent pelvic cancer.

Ultrasound, although flexible and inexpensive, is limited by poor tissue differentiation characteristics and relies mainly on the identification of structural changes. The use of texture analysis for determining tissue signatures has proved to be more difficult than was initially envisaged.

Methodology

Ultrasound may be defined as a mechanical vibration above the audible range, this generally being of the order of 20 000 Hz (1 Hz = 1 cycle/s). The range of ultrasonic frequencies used in medicine is generally between 1 and 10 MHz. In ultrasonic imaging, the source of the ultrasound is a transducer which is designed to produce a narrow focused beam of ultrasound. A transducer is any device which converts one form of energy into another and in ultrasound equipment this is usually a crystal of an artificially produced piezoelectric material, commonly lead zirconate titanate (PZT). An oscillator circuit in the ultrasound scanner produces a series of electrical pulses which are applied to the crystal causing it to resonate at its fundamental frequency. For the majority of the scanning time the transducer is listening for the returned echoes which are reflected back from structures within the patient. In real-time scanners the piezoelectric crystal is mounted either as a linear or curvilinear array of 60–200, elements or as a mechanically oscillating transducer which produces a series of rapidly changing image frames. In general, 15–30 frames per second are required to produce a flicker-free image. The image is generally presented in the form of a grey scale display varying between black and white with dynamic range of the order of 30–40 dB.

During scanning, the probe is placed on the skin and a layer of jelly is used as an acoustic couplant facilitating the transmission of the sound from the transducer to the patient. The physical dimensions of the crystal dictate the frequency of the ultrasound: the thinner the crystal, the higher the frequency of the ultrasound beam.

The choice of frequency for a particular investigation is usually a compromise between the image resolution and the depth of penetration required. The higher the frequency, the better the resolution but the greater the attenuation of the beam within the tissues. Hence, for abdominal scanning, frequencies of between 2.5 and 3.5 MHz are commonly employed. Probes are now available for intracavity (endoprobes) and intraoperative use. The main advantages with these systems is that organs of interest are closer to the transducer, thus allowing higher frequencies (6–8 MHz) to be employed.

Diagnosis of ectopic pregnancy

Traditionally, ultrasound has been used to exclude an ectopic pregnancy by demonstrating an intrauterine pregnancy. Its secondary role comprises the detection of an adnexal mass and free fluid in the pelvis, and the measurement of endometrial thickness. By a combination of these features the negative predictive value of an ultrasound examination may be 96%. This figured is improved further with the addition of the measurement of β-human chorionic gonadotrophin (>25 iu/l). Significant problems arise in distinguishing an ectopic pregnancy without a pseudogestational sac from an early normal or failed intrauterine pregnancy where no gestational sac can be seen. The positive diagnosis of ectopic pregnancy requires the demonstration of an extrauterine fetal heart. With abdominal ultrasound this is detected in less than 5% of patients but in 23% with a vaginal probe. In one study, the overall sensitivity of diagnosing an ectopic pregnancy by the transvaginal approach was 100% with a specificity of 98.2% (Timor-Tritsch et al 1989).

Investigation of female infertility

A major advance is the assessment and monitoring of ovulation. Using transabdominal scanning, ovarian follicles can be visualized from a diameter of 3–5 mm. They appear as echo-free structures amidst the more echogenic ovarian tissue (Fig. 5.1). The rate of growth of follicular size is linear and the mean diameter prior to ovulation is 20.2 mm (range 18–24 mm; Bryce et al 1982). Structures within the follicle such as the cumulus oophorous can also be visualized. Following ovulation, internal echoes appear. Free fluid may also be observed in the pouch of Douglas.

Ultrasound can only provide presumptive evidence of ovulation. Definitive evidence requires the occurrence of pregnancy or the collection of secondary oocytes from the female genital tract. The features associated with follicular failure include the appearance of internal echoes before the follicle reaches 18 mm or continuous enlargement to 30–40 mm.

Ultrasound can be employed to time more accurately artificial insemination. Correct timing of a postcoital test can help differentiate between inadequate sperm penetration and poor mucus production in the presence of a mature follicles. Ultrasound scanning is also employed to monitor patients on clomiphene citrate therapy and a good correlation is reported between follicular diameters and plasma oestradiol concentrations. The hyperstimulation syndrome is uncommon if gonadotrophin therapy is monitored by ultrasound in conjunction with the measurement of plasma oestradiol levels. The success of in vitro fertilization (IVF) has been due .in part to the correct timing of ovulation and subsequent oocyte recovery which ultrasound can provide.

Transvaginal sonography has largely replaced the transabdominal approach in infertility practice. Follicular aspiration is possible with a needle guide attachment to the vaginal probe, as is fine-needle aspiration of fluid in the pouch of Douglas. A more precise measurement of follicular size is possible and the corpus luteum is easily recognized. In the mid luteal phase it appears as an oblong structure of 30–35 mm in length and 20–25 mm wide. A wide variety of sonographic appearances are described (Timor-Tritsch et al 1988). In addition, endometrial thickness can be more clearly evaluated. Endometrial reflectivity patterns have been proposed as another variable for the assessment of ovulation (Randall et al 1989). The waveforms of blood flow in vessels supplying the ovaries of women undergoing IVF have been studied using transvaginal pulsed Doppler ultrasound (Barber et al 1988). Blood flow patterns so observed may help in the prediction of implantation failure. The corpus luteum is easily recognized (Fig. 5.2).

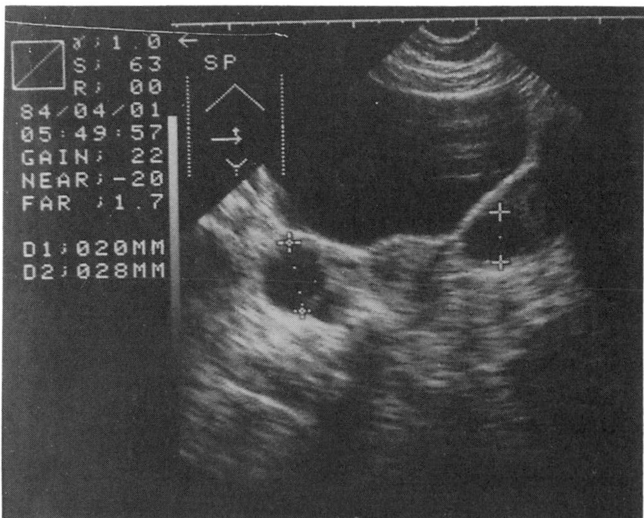

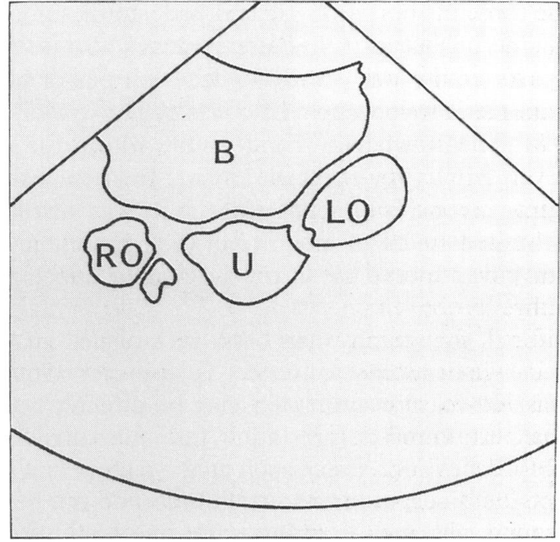

Fig. 5.1 Transabdominal ultrasound demonstrating ovarian follicles. B = Bladder; U = uterus; LO = left ovary; RO = right ovary.

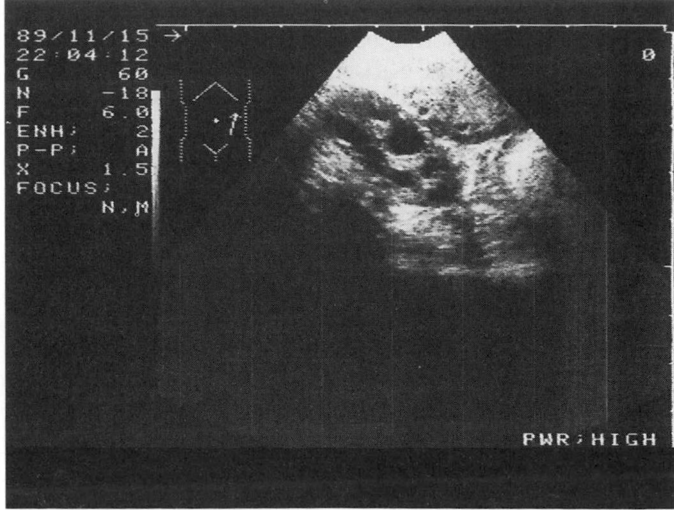

Fig. 5.2 Transvaginal ultrasound of ovarian follicles.

Endometrial and cervical cancer

There are few reports in the literature describing the use of ultrasound in the assessment of these tumours. One suggested that up to one-third of patients with endometrial cancer will appear sonographically normal (Requard et al 1981). The demonstration of fluid in the pouch of Douglas in postmenopausal women has been reported as having a high correlation with the presence of endometrial malignancy (Breckenridge et al 1982). However, ultrasound is unable to differentiate malignant from benign causes of uterine enlargement.

In patients already proven to have an endometrial cancer, it may be possible to assess the depth of myometrial invasion with high-resolution probes. In a study involving 20 cases, 70% of the ultrasound estimations of invasion depth were within 10% of the actual pathological measurement (Fleischer et al 1987). Errors of estimation occurred when the tumour was exophytic and had significant extension into the uterine cavity. False positives also occurred if the uterine cavity was overdistended with pus or blood. A subendometrial hypoechoic halo was demonstrated comparable to the low-intensity band visible within the myometrium on MRI (Powell et al 1986a). In those patients with deeply invasive tumours this layer was disrupted. Ultrasound assessment of integrity of the hypoechoic layer can be improved by the use of transvaginal or transluminal sonography.

Transrectal sonography has been investigated in cases where recurrent endometrial cancer is suspected (Squillaci et al 1988). Physical examination may be difficult because of postsurgical fibrosis. Infiltration into the surrounding connective tissues and organs such as the rectum and bladder can be identified and transrectal ultrasound can be used to guide transvaginal or transperitoneal fine-needle biopsy.

Transabdominal ultrasound is of little value in the assessment of patients with cervical cancer. Poor image quality and a difficulty in interpretation appear to be the major problems. However transrectal ultrasound can produce clear views of the parametrial tissues and is useful in assessing parametrial spread. In a reported series of 180 patients, a good correlation was found between the ultrasound and surgical findings, but significant problems arose in distinguishing between inflammatory or fibrotic change and tumour invasion (Yuhara et al 1987).

Benign and malignant ovarian disease

One of the commonest reason for requesting pelvic ultrasound is in the investigation of a patient with a suspected pelvic mass. Ultrasound provides information leading to a correct diagnosis in 56% of cases, contributory data in 23%, and non-specific information in 14%. Errors occur in 6%. The incidence of the different ultrasound characteristics of benign and malignant tumours was described by Meire at al (1978). They concluded that benign lesions are unilocular or multilocular with thin septae and no nodules, whereas malignant lesions are often multilocular with thin septae and nodules, or multilocular with thick septae with or without nodules. However benign teratomas may possess very echogenic foci, and totally echogenic lesions are less likely to be malignant than mixed echogenic lesions. In postmenopausal women, lesions less than 5 cm in diameter which are anechoic are unlikely to be malignant. However, in lesions greater than 5 cm in diameter there were three malignancies in a group of 30 anechoic lesions (Andolf & Jorgenson 1989). Campbell et al (1989) were unable to identify any morphological characteristics to differentiate reliably between ovarian tumour-like conditions, benign ovarian tumours and early malignant tumours.

Ultrasound has been proposed as a possible early screening method for ovarian cancer (Campbell et al 1982). Out of 5479 women screened, in a recent study (Campbell et al 1989), 5 women with primary stage I cancer were diagnosed and 4 with metastatic disease to the ovary. Overall the rate of false positives was 2.3%, and the likelihood of a positive scan being a primary ovarian cancer was 1 in 67. Bourne et al (1989) have proposed that the false positive rate may be reduced by the use of transvaginal colour flow imaging.

In the assessment of advanced or recurrent disease, ascites is reliably detected by ultrasound but even large masses in the peritoneal cavity escape detection. Liver and right hemi-diaphragmatic metastases are more often identified correctly.

RADIONUCLIDE IMAGING

With the development of high-resolution anatomical imaging devices such as ultrasound, CT and MRI, nuclear medicine imaging has progressively changed to provide physiological rather than anatomical detail. Modern gamma cameras are capable of accurately imaging the distribution of administered radiopharmaceuticals and the use of tomographic systems for single photon emission tomography (SPECT) has improved the display of internal processes. The use of radionuclide imaging techniques is not restricted to oncology, although this area of investigation is especially promising. Bone imaging remains the most widely performed investigation in the USA and Europe, mainly because the physiological process involved in changing bone development may be seen at an earlier stage than any anatomical change on radiographs. More recently, radiolabelled monoclonal antibodies have been employed in the localization of gynaecological cancers (radioimmunoscintigraphy) and in their treatment (radioimmunotherapy).

The purity and specificity of monoclonal antibodies give them the potential to play an important role in tumour detection and possibly in the targeting of anti-tumour agents. Tumour localization by a radiolabelled monoclonal antibody was first described in the UK in 1982 in patients with colorectal cancer. This murine monoclonal antibody (791T/36) has subsequently been shown to localize in gynaecological cancers (Powell et al 1987a). Other monoclonal antibodies produced against cell surface antigens also undergoing evaluation for imaging purposes include CA 125, placental alkaline phosphatase (PLAP) and human milk fat globule (HMFG) antigen. Different malignancies may express the same antigens, which may also be found in normal epithelial tissues, as is the case with HMFG. A monoclonal antibody OVLT3 is claimed to be specific for ovarian cancer.

Methodology

The antibodies or antibody fragments are radiolabelled with a gamma-emitting radionuclide such as Tc^{99m}, I^{131}, I^{123} or In^{111}. A subcutaneous test dose is no longer given because of the immune response it may generate in the patient. If I^{131} or I^{123} is employed, oral potassium iodide is given to block thyroid uptake of free radioactive iodide. In addition, blood pool subtraction techniques are required for I^{131} studies to simulate the non-tumour distribution of

a

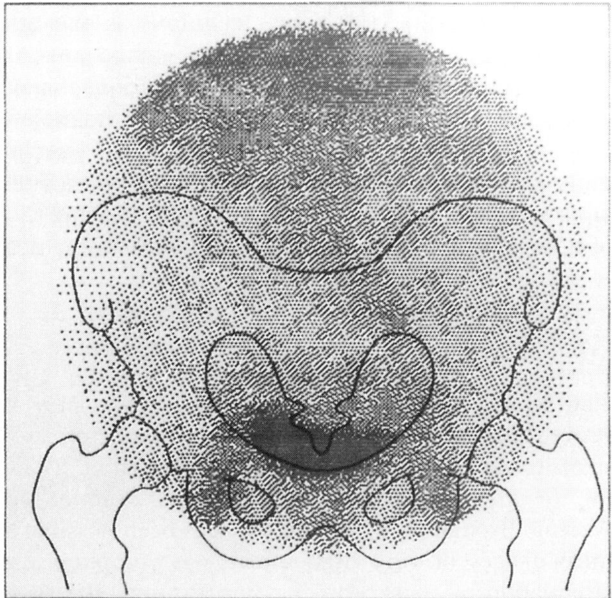

b

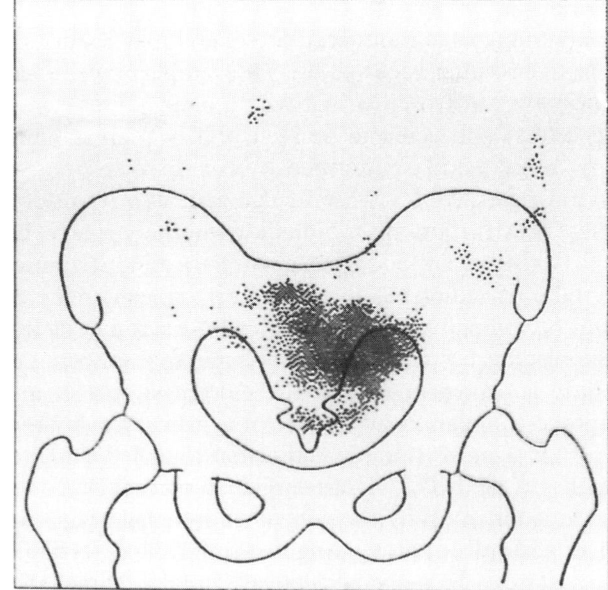

c

Fig. 5.3 Radionuclide scan: recurrent ovarian cancer — anterior views of the pelvis with 80 MBq I^{131} 791T/36. (**a**) The image before (**b**) subtraction of the Tc^{99m}-labelled blood pool image; (**c**) after subtraction with an area of increased antibody uptake on the patient's left.

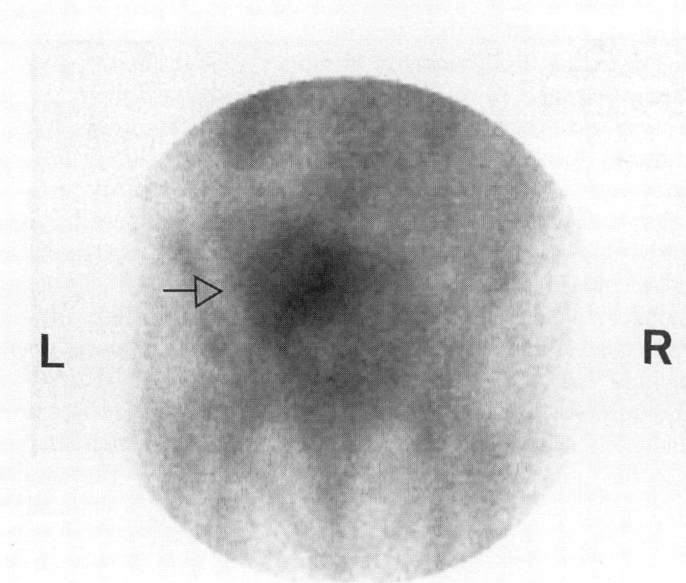

Fig. 5.4 Radionuclide scan: primary ovarian carcinoma. Anterior view of the pelvis: 80 MBq In^{111} OC–125.

labelled antibody. This is not necessary for I^{123}- or In^{111}-labelled preparations.

Following infusion of the antibody a gamma camera provides serial images of the distribution and uptake of the radiolabelled antibody between 18 and 72 h after the antibody has been administered. In^{111} is ideally suited for tomographic studies using images produced by a gamma camera mounted on a gantry which rotates through 360°. The images are reconstructed by computer in the same manner as X-ray CT. In^{111} tomography localizes the antibody uptake site more accurately, and may reduce the false positive results. Figure 5.3 is an example of an I^{131}-labelled antibody study of a patient with a palpable mass in the left iliac fossa suspected to be recurrent ovarian tumour. This was subsequently confirmed by laparoscopy.

False positive I^{131} imaging can arise as a result of incomplete subtraction of radioiodide in the urinary bladder. In^{111}-labelled antibody has a different biodistribution with uptake of radiolabel into the liver, spleen, bone marrow and occasionally the adrenal glands. Excretion of In^{111} into the bladder has not been a problem. An example of an In^{111} study is shown in Figure 5.4. A central area of increased uptake is apparent at the site of a primary ovarian cancer. In^{111} is a more suitable radiolabel than I^{131} and, together with I^{123} and Tc^{99m}, has largely replaced I^{131}. However, In^{111} is taken up by the reticuloendothelial system into the liver and spleen, preventing its use for the detection of liver metastases. Non-specific bowel uptake sometimes seen with In^{111} may account for some false positive results.

Ovarian carcinoma

In spite of a sensitivity of 87% and a specificity of 75% in ovarian cancer (Powell et al 1987a), the clinical value of this technique in primary disease is limited because the resolution is insufficient to show the involvement of surrounding organs. Radionuclide imaging may be more applicable to situations where recurrent cancer is clinically suspected as laparoscopic assessment is often inaccurate and second-look laparotomy carries a morbidity with no definite benefit to patient survival. Repeated injection of imaging doses of antibody may stimulate the development of anti-mouse antibodies. This may severely limit the use of immunoscintigraphy for repeat diagnostic imaging.

Radioimmunotherapy

Monoclonal antibodies have also been proposed for use in the targeting of cytotoxic agents or therapeutic doses of radioisotopes. This would increase the concentration at the tumour site and reduce normal tissue toxicity. Intraperitoneal injections of In^{111} and I^{131}-labelled antibodies have been used (Perkins et al 1989). 791T/36 antibody conjugates with conventional cytotoxic agents such as methotrexate, Adriamycin and with ricin A chain immunotoxin have been constructed and have been shown to be effective against human tumour xenografts in immunodeprived mice. The specificity and sensitivity of the antibody 791T/36 in gynaecological cancers is appropriate for the therapeutic application of such drug conjugates.

X-RAY TECHNIQUES AND CT

Standard radiographs are obtained by placing the patient between an X-ray source and photographic film. The images produced are essentially shadow graphs of the attenuation of X-ray photons by the patient. As a result, the structures of interest are very often obscured by the shadows cast by other overlying structures. A basic limitation of the standard X-ray technique is the effect of scattered X-ray photons adding to the image noise and degrading the quality of the final image. Various manoeuvres have been adopted to reduce this effect, for example scatter grids. The linear tomograph obtained by the synchronous movement of the X-ray tube and the film causes a blurring of the overlying and underlying structures leaving the plane of interest in focus. This procedure increases the detection of lesions such as chest metastases.

Methodology

The sensitivity of conventional radiography may be improved by using a sensitive radiation detector such as a scintillation crystal and a photomultiplier tube. By measuring the attenuation of a finely collimated beam of radiation passing through multiple angles it has been possible to produce images of very high quality. A computer uses the attenuation of each beam passing through the patient to calculate the attenuation coefficient for each area of tissue in the cross-section of interest. The final images are reconstructed using a filtered back-projection technique and then displayed in a grey scale as a series of attenuation units (with values between +500 and −500) in a matrix of 512 × 512 or 1024 × 1024 elements. Unlike MRI, the reconstruction of data is limited to the transaxial or transverse planes. This technique of imaging revolutionized modern medicine in the 1970s but the value of CT in gynaecology is less clear.

Cervical carcinoma

An intravenous urogram is a mandatory part of the FIGO staging of cervical carcinoma. The incidence of abnormalities in stage I is reported to be 2.1%; in stage II is 5.1%; in stage III is 26.8% and stage IV is 48.9% (Griffin et al 1976). The abnormalities recorded are unilateral or bilateral, partial or complete ureteric obstruction, with or without displacement, and distortion of the bladder outline. The presence of a hydronephrosis or non-functioning kidney due to stenosis from tumour invasion of the ureter puts the patient into stage III even if according to the other findings the case should be allotted to an earlier stage.

A chest X-ray is a routine pretreatment investigation but the yield of lung metastases at first presentation is likely to be no more than 2%. Barium enema abnormalities are rare in cervical cancer and proctoscopy is also positive if an abnormality is observed on the enema.

The role of lymphangiography in the staging of cervical cancer is controversial with up to 71% false positives and 16% false negatives. Percutaneous fine-needle aspiration nodal biopsy may improve the results that can be obtained with pelvic lymphangiography. CT has proved to be a reliable method for staging and following lymph node disease in patients with lymphoma but the major drawback for epithelial tumours is that the nodes require to be enlarged to be detected. Thus metastases less than 2 cm will not be identified.

Since the introduction of CT in the early 1970s, several authors have recommended its routine use in patients with cervical cancer (Fig. 5.5). While some say that infiltration of the parametrium may be easily recognizable, it is difficult to differentiate fibrosis after treatment from tumour recurrence. Both the normal cervix and cervical carcinoma have similar attenuation values with CT, so the primary tumour can only be recognized if it sufficiently alters the contour or size of the normal cervix. False positive CT diagnoses are often due to misinterpreting normal inflammatory parametrial soft tissue strands as tumour invasion or mistaking enlarged lymph nodes due to inflammation as neoplastic. It would seem that CT is not indicated as a routine staging procedure in patients with cervical cancer, but may be the examination of choice in the patient with suspected recurrent disease.

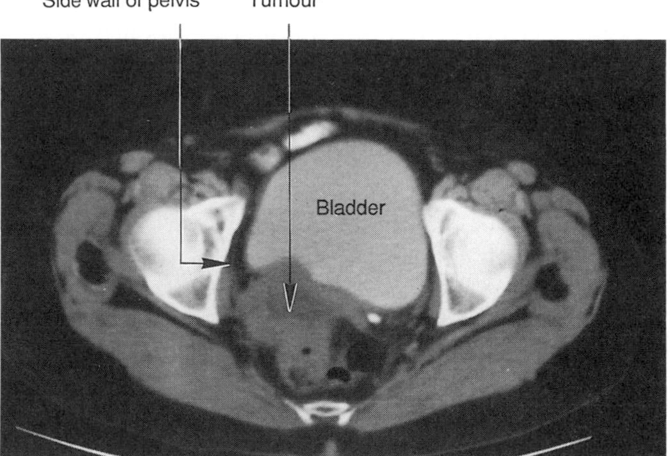

Fig. 5.5 CT scan of a stage IIIb cervical carcinoma.

Uterine carcinoma

Current radiological techniques for the assessment of patients with endometrial cancer are of limited value and are employed to assist in staging of the tumour and rarely contribute to its detection. The yield of tumour-related abnormalities that can be detected by an intravenous urogram, chest X-ray, and skeletal X-rays is low. The use of lymphangiography has the same limitations as in cervical cancer.

CT depicts an endometrial cancer as a hypodense lesion in the uterine parenchyma or as a fluid-filled uterus due to tumour obstruction of the endocervical canal or vagina. These findings however are non-specific and are easily confused with leiomyomata, intrauterine fluid collections and extension of a cervical carcinoma into the uterine body. In addition, the central lucency occurs in normal postmenopausal women. Balfe et al (1986) concluded that CT was of limited value in stage I–II disease, where clinical examination was slightly better, but was superior to clinical staging in detecting metastatic carcinoma to omentum, lymph nodes, and recurrent disease.

Ovarian carcinoma

A plain abdominal X-ray of the pelvis and abdomen may demonstrate a soft tissue mass, with or without calcification. A large benign cyst will lead to lateral displacement of small bowel loops. Calcification may occur in 12% of cystadenocarcinomas. It is said to be less dense than common calcification and due to its microscopic nature may appear as little more than a hazy shadow.

Intravenous urography is primarily indicated to ascertain the course and number of ureters prior to laparotomy. Ureteric obstruction is said to occur in 58–69% of women with ovarian carcinoma and in 32–58% with benign ovarian masses (Long & Montgomery 1950). In most instances the changes are minor. Barium studies may be indicated where there is a suspicion of a primary colonic tumour, or to exclude bowel involvement.

Lymph node metastases are thought to occur early in the course of the disease. Little importance has been attached to this as the treatment plan is generally determined by the extent of local and peritoneal spread. However lymphangiography has been employed in an attempt to stage the disease more accurately. The importance of lymphatic spread in ovarian cancer has undergone a recent reappraisal and imaging methods to assess lymphatic spread may become more important.

CT is now employed more frequently but has not been shown to influence the overall management of the patient with ovarian cancer. CT cannot differentiate benign disease from stage I cancer nor malignancy from adhesions. In addition, small peritoneal deposits are commonly missed if less than 2 cm in diameter. However CT is able to reveal intrahepatic metastases and lymphatic involvement by tumour which may not be apparent at a staging laparotomy. In most centres there would appear to be at most a limited utility for preoperative CT staging of epithelial ovarian cancer. An exception to this is the evaluation of dysgerminoma with its predilection for lymphatic spread. CT scans of the mediastinum and upper abdomen are recommended in all patients with ovarian dysgerminomas.

MAGNETIC RESONANCE IMAGING (MRI)

MRI depends upon the magnetic properties of certain nuclei which, when placed within a magnetic field and stimulated by radio waves of a specific frequency, will absorb and then re-emit some of this energy as a radio signal. This is the phenomenon of nuclear magnetic resonance (NMR) which was first described by Felix Bloch and Edward Purcell in 1946. NMR as a basis for an imaging technique was proposed some 30 years later by Lauterbur.

Methodology

Most of the images published to date have been based on the hydrogen nucleus or proton which is favourable from the NMR standpoint because it gives a relatively high signal due to its abundance in biological tissues. Other potential NMR isotopes include ^{13}C, ^{23}Na, ^{19}F and ^{31}P. ^{19}F is the only one of these with an NMR signal comparable to hydrogen but it is found in significant amounts only in teeth.

Nuclei possessing magnetic properties have an odd number of protons or neutrons. These charged particles are spinning and therefore can be considered to behave as tiny bar magnets. If placed within a magnetic field, a majority of protons will line up in the direction of the magnetic field. In addition their axes are both tilted and caused to rotate like small gyroscopes. The frequency of this so-called precessional movement is directly proportional to the strength of the applied field and is called the Larmor frequency.

If a pulse of radio waves is then imposed on the protons a strong interaction or resonance will occur when the frequency coincides with the precessional frequency of the protons. The energy absorbed by the protons is then re-emitted as a tiny nuclear signal that can be detected in a receiver coil situated around the sample. The initial size of this signal is proportional to the proton density of the sample. It will then decay in an exponential fashion as the disturbed protons relax back to their original position. The so-called T1 relaxation time is described as the time taken for the protons to return to their positions prior to stimulation by the radio waves. The T2 relaxation time is that taken for the precessing nuclei to get out of step with one another. Different sequences of radio waves have been devised so that the resulting nuclear signal is weighted to different degrees by the proton density and the T1 and T2 relaxation times. The nuclear signal is also influenced by the bulk flow of protons and MRI therefore offers the potential to gain useful insights into blood flow by a non-invasive technique.

Display of soft tissue detail is very important and with MRI the contrast between different tissues can be manipulated by altering the pattern of radio waves applied. This is done by changing the time constants associated with the different sequences of radio waves: inversion time (TI); echo time (TE); or repetition time (TR). A further advantage of MRI is the ability to obtain additional perspectives

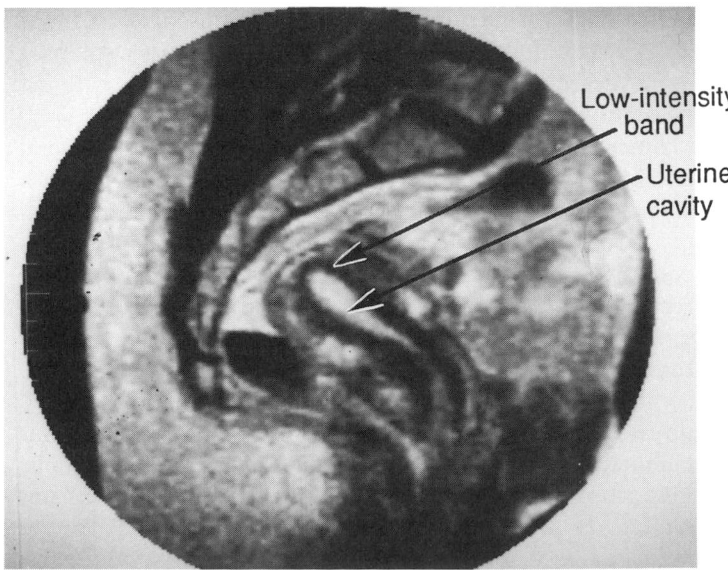

Fig. 5.6 MRI scan: sagittal view, T2 weighted. Normal retroverted uterus.

such as sagittal or coronal views without moving the patient.

The female pelvis is suitable for MRI examination because of the minimal effect of respiratory motion on the pelvic organs. Examination of the liver and upper abdomen is not possible unless fast imaging or respiratory gating is available. As the data to produce a series of images are accumulated over upwards of 20 min, patients are required to remain still during a pulse sequence. If multiple sequences are employed, the total imaging time may exceed 60 min. More elderly patients may be unable to tolerate this, particularly as they are positioned completely inside the bore of the scanner. However, recently introduced pulse sequences and improved computer software have greatly reduced the times required for a scan to take place.

Normal uterus

The uterus is easy to differentiate from the surrounding pelvic organs particularly in the sagittal plane. Even myometrium and endometrium may be distinguishable. The myometrium has a distinctive appearance with longer T2 weighted sequences, which is quite unique to this imaging method. There is within the inner aspect of the myometrium a band of low signal intensity adjacent to the endometrium, running around the uterine cavity and into the cervix as far as the external os (Fig. 5.6). The true

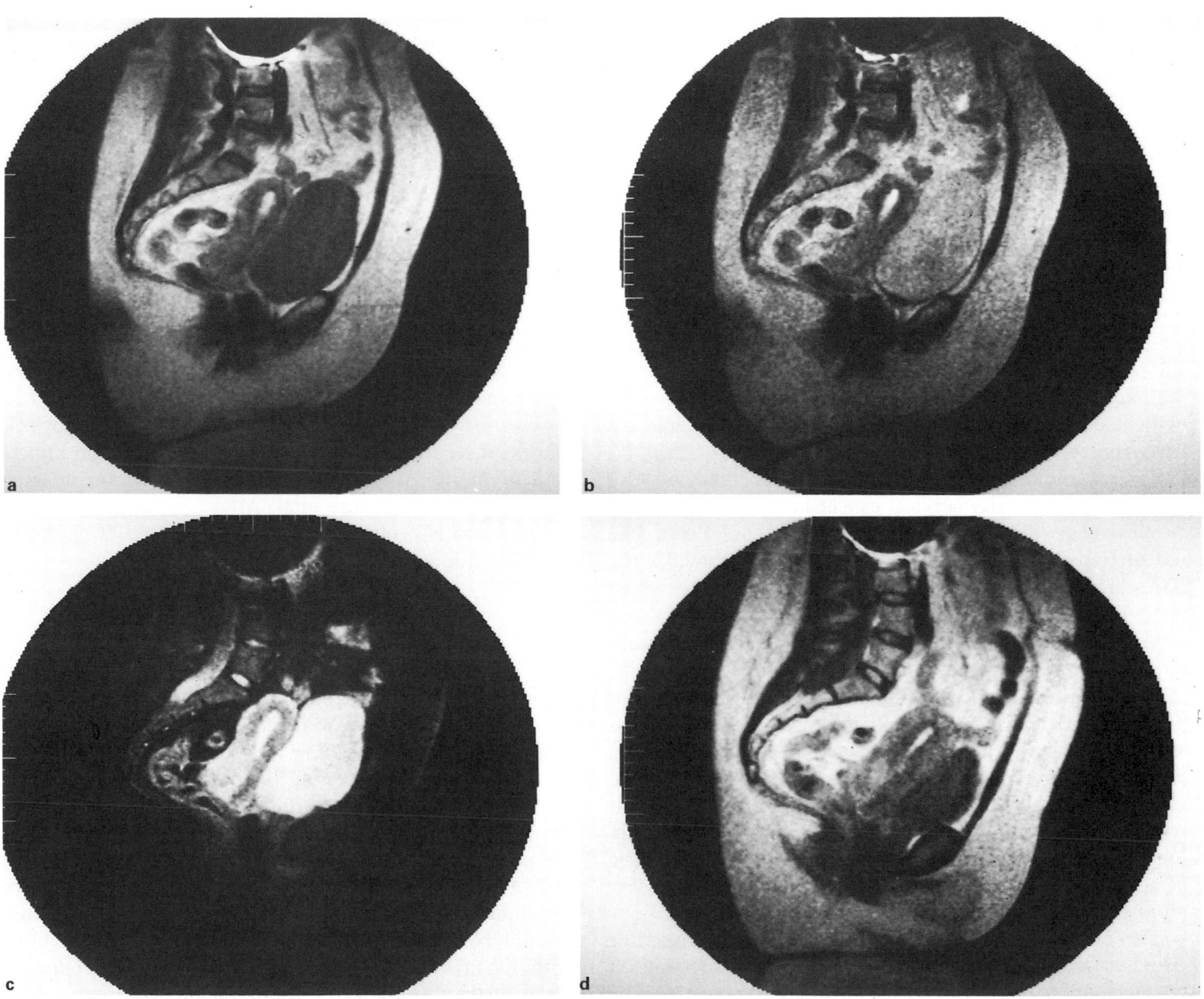

Fig. 5.7 MRI scan, sagittal view. (**a**) TI/T2; (**b**) T2; (**c**) STIR; (**d**) T2. Cervical cancer involving posterior lip of the cervix, invading the myometrium.

nature of the low-intensity band remains uncertain but its appearance in the neoplastic uterus can be helpful in determining the extent of tumour spread. The outer zone of the myometrium has an intermediate signal intensity, the two layers being quite distinct. The endometrium has a high signal intensity with T2 weighted sequences. MRI can demonstrate effectively the physiological changes which the uterus undergoes during the menstrual cycle in relationship to age and parity.

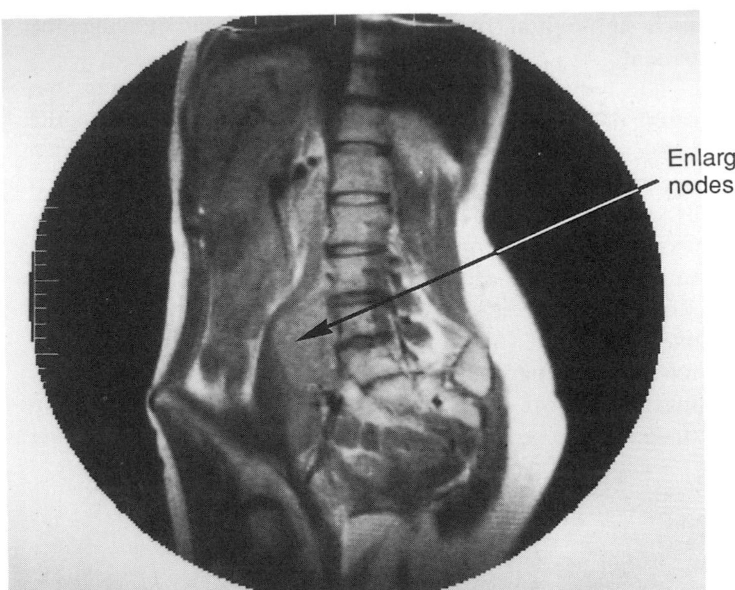

Fig. 5.8 MRI scan, oblique coronal view (Tl/T2), showing a large collection of para-aortic nodes (arrowed) resulting from an advanced cervical carcinoma.

Cervical carcinoma

The clinical assessment of cervical cancer is notoriously poor. As the size of the tumour determines the therapy, accurate staging is of paramount importance. Precise staging of primary disease provides a prognosis, allows the institution of correct treatment, and permits comparison of different treatment protocols. Both CT and ultrasound have shortcomings and are not regularly employed to stage the primary disease.

The normal cervix has a characteristic appearance with MRI. The low-intensity band on the inner aspect of the myometrium continues into the cervix. Although less marked due to the relatively lower signal from the cervix, disruption of the band indicates early invasion. Both coronal and transverse axial views show clearly the parametrial anatomy, whereas the sagittal planes demonstrate invasion into the myometrium, rectum and bladder. Figure 5.7 is an example of a squamous cell tumour on the posterior lip of the cervix which has invaded the myometrium. Although initially unclear on a Tl/T2 scan, the tumour is evident on T2 weighted scan and on the STIR (short tau inversion recovery) sequence.

Several studies have now confirmed the accuracy of MRI in the staging of early cervical cancer in comparison to the surgical stage (Powell et al 1986b; Togashi et al 1987). The use of transverse, coronal and sagittal planes provides the necessary information to calculate tumour volumes, which is of prognostic significance.

MRI is no better than CT in detecting metastatic disease to the lymph nodes as it relies on changes in the size of the lymph nodes in a similar way to CT (Fig. 5.8). The tumour deposits are not highlighted in T2 weighted sequences, as is the case with endometrial cancer, so alterations in lymph node architecture are needed to reveal metastases. Although an in vitro study has shown that lymph nodes containing metastases have a significantly longer T2 than do normal or hyperplastic nodes (Weiner et al 1986), in vivo tissue characterization based on relaxation times or signal intensities is not yet possible.

The only hope for improving the dismal prognosis for patients with recurrent cervical cancer is to detect the recurrence at an early stage when cytotoxic therapy may be of value. Clinical or radiological examination of the pelvis following radical surgery or radiotherapy can be difficult to evaluate if a recurrence is suspected. CT and ultrasound have known limitations which essentially relate to their inability to differentiate between fibrosis and tumour. In a recent report MRI effectively distinguished post-treatment fibrosis and recurrent pelvic neoplasm by measuring signal intensities from the different tissues on T2 weighted pulse sequences (Ebner et al 1988).

With the increased use of new cytotoxic regimes for primary and recurrent tumour and a move away from radical surgery to rely more on radiotherapy, accurate imaging techniques become more vital. MRI has fulfilled its early promise and is probably the imaging method of choice in patients with cervical carcinoma.

Uterine carcinoma

There have been few published studies with regard to the application of MRI to the staging of endometrial cancer. The Nottingham group were the first to highlight the potential of MRI for assessing the depth of invasion of the tumour into the myometrium (Powell et al 1986a). A series of MRI scans of patients with endometrial cancer is demonstrated in Figure 5.9. On a T2 weighted pulse sequence, endometrial cancer has a high signal intensity, similar to that of normal endometrium, but showing some degree of variability. This depends on whether the tumour is diffuse or polypoid and if the uterine cavity is distended with blood or pus. The high signal makes the tumour quite distinct from the surrounding myometrium which possesses an intermediate signal intensity.

The sagittal plane is the most appropriate for examina-

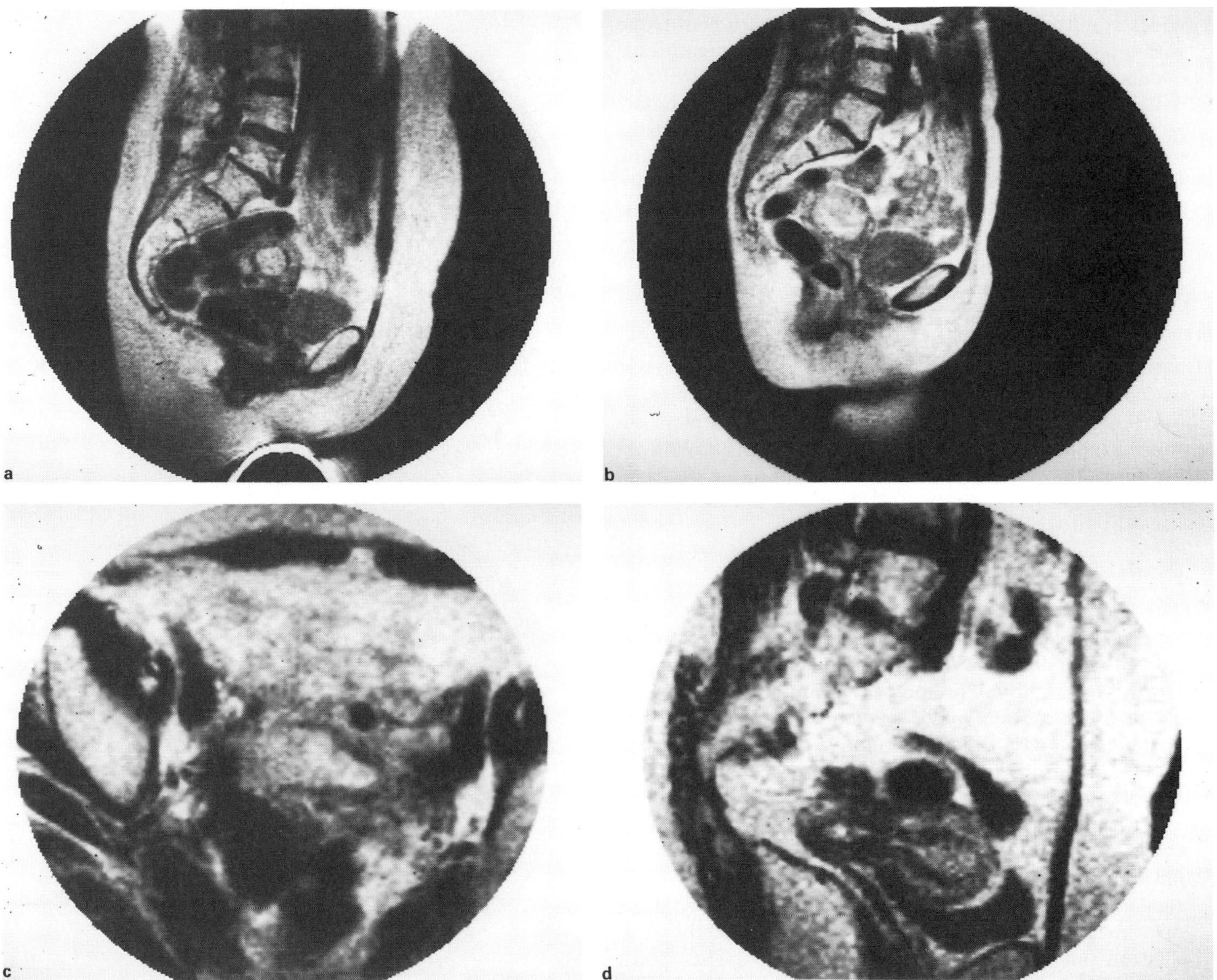

Fig. 5.9 MRI scans (T2) of 4 patients with endometrial cancer. (**a, b**) These sagittal views show the low-intensity band intact. (**c**) Transverse view: the low-intensity band is breached laterally on the figure. (**d**) Sagittal view of an acutely anteverted uterus. The low-intensity band is breached at the uterine fundus.

tion of a patient with primary endometrial cancer as this provides a longitudinal view of the uterus which will include both corpus and cervix. The sagittal plane of view also provides the opportunity to assess anterior invasion of the tumour into the bladder and posteriorly to the rectum. In patients with a small postmenopausal uterus, if image slices are taken at 10 mm intervals, small lesions may be overlooked if they lie between adjacent slices. This risk is reduced by taking images at 5 mm gaps.

In a premenopausal uterus it may be impossible to differentiate tumour from adenomatous hyperplasia or indeed normal endometrium. The low-intensity band may still be evident in the postmenopausal woman and is important in the MRI assessment of tumour invasion. Powell et al (1986a) found the band to be thinned or absent in those patients with deeply invasive tumours (Fig. 5.9c, d). MRI was also found in this study to have a good correlation with the pathological measurement of myometrial invasion. MRI can therefore provide information with regard to this important prognostic sign before surgery takes place.

More advanced tumours are also well visualized with MRI. The metastatic lesions maintain the high signal characteristic of the primary growth. This is particularly the case with metastases to the lymphatics where lymph nodes of normal architecture are replaced by tumour tissue with a high signal. A similar pattern of signal intensities is obtained from recurrent endometrial cancer.

Leiomyosarcomata are relatively uncommon and only recurrent lesions have so far been reported. The signal pattern is more intermediate on a T2 weighted pulse sequence, and not dissimilar to that from a benign leiomyoma or normal myometrium. Therefore the detection of early malignant change in a leiomyoma does not seem feasible at present. In those patients presenting with more advanced disease, alterations in the uterine configuration could well suggest malignant change.

MRI appears to represent a unique method of assessing a patient with an endometrial cancer, possessing advantages over other radiological techniques in stage I and II disease, but probably equal to CT in the patient with a more advanced tumour. MRI is superior to CT in the assessment of lymphatic metastases and the recognition of recurrent disease.

Ovarian carcinoma

The first reported use of MRI in the evaluation of primary ovarian cancer came from Nottingham (Johnson et al 1984). This study consisted of 12 patients and was performed on a clinical prototype system, using the steady state free precession pulse sequence. The authors concluded that MRI scanning had unique tissue-differentiating capabilities which may be of benefit in the staging of this gynaecological cancer.

A further study from the same centre was the first to evaluate MRI in both primary and recurrent ovarian cancer on a commercial imaging system (Powell et al 1987b). A total of 49 patients were examined with a clinical suspicion of primary ovarian cancer, of which MRI correctly identified 38 out of 39 as having a malignancy. The clinical diagnosis was correct in only 78.7% (Fig. 5.10). In this study it was impossible to distinguish between the different epithelial cancers; however, large bowel cancers had a different pattern of signal intensities as well as structural differences. Large bowel metastases on the ovary were indistinguishable from primary ovarian cancer. MRI identified ascites and capsular invasion in all cases. Peritoneal metastases less than 1 cm in diameter were commonly overlooked. Extension of the tumour on to the large bowel and bladder was also not well demonstrated.

MRI is probably comparable to both CT and ultrasound in its usefulness in the staging of ovarian cancer. None to date have been shown to be sufficiently accurate to replace surgical laparotomy. The appearances of recurrent ovarian cancer were comparable to those seen with the primary disease although the cystic elements were less prevalent. MRI was compared to laparoscopy in the detection of recurrent disease. MRI was superior to laparoscopy and detected lesions clinically impalpable but also invisible to the laparoscope because of adhesions in the pelvis. An example of such a case is shown in Figure 5.11. A mass is apparent over the presacral region, which could not be palpated or seen with the laparoscope. The nature of this lesion was confirmed by a subsequent laparotomy. A sensitivity and specificity of 96 and 100% respectively was recorded for MRI in the detection of recurrent tumour compared to 100 and 81% for laparoscopy. MRI correctly identified recurrent tumour but often missed peritoneal metastases.

The multiplanar imaging facility and tissue differentiation capacity offered by MRI make it ideal for monitoring chemotherapy and for early detection of recurrent disease.

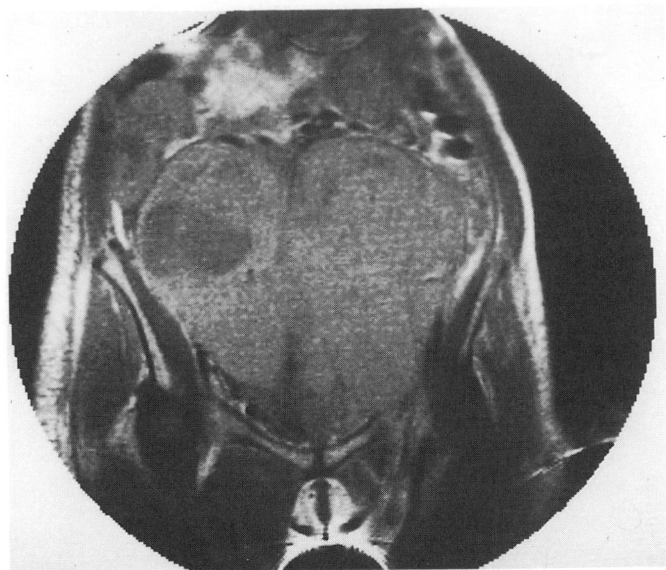

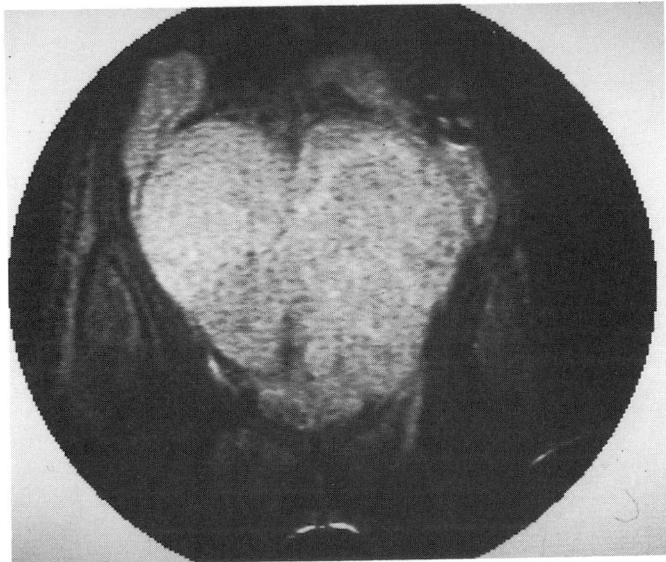

Fig. 5.10 MRI scan, coronal view. Primary ovarian cancer with a predominantly solid element. An area of necrosis is visible. (**a**) T1/T2; (**b**) STIR.

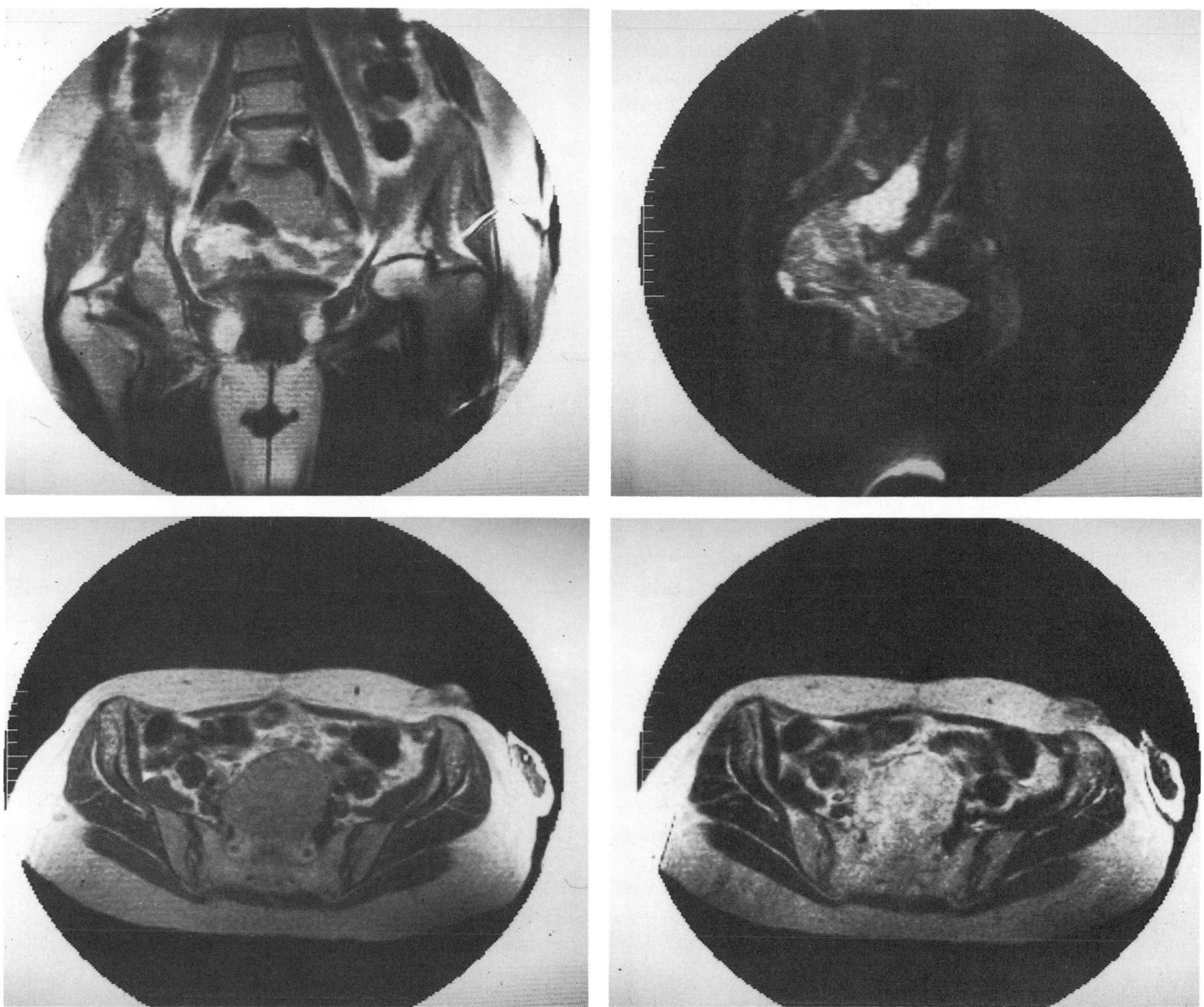

Fig. 5.11 MRI scans recurrent ovarian cancer. A presacral recurrence is shown (**a**) in coronal view (T1/T2) and (**b**) in sagittal view (STIR). Six months after second-look surgery, the tumour has recurred at the same site as shown in these transverse views; (**c**) T1/T2 and (**d**) T2.

HAZARDS ASSOCIATED WITH IMAGING INVESTIGATIONS

Although the majority of imaging procedures described are largely non-invasive, in some cases (eg. X-ray and radionuclide imaging) the procedure involves exposing the patient to ionizing radiation. This is one of the reasons why techniques such as ultrasound and MRI have received so much attention in obstetrics and gynaecology. Nevertheless, ultrasound necessitates irradiation of the patient with sound waves (mechanical vibrations) and MRI involves the application of strong and rapidly changing magnetic fields combined with radio waves. Research has shown that no real harm results from the clinical use of ultrasound or MRI investigations but each modality has an associated risk which must be appreciated. In the case of ultrasound and MRI the main biological effect is of the conversion of the interrogating source of energy (sound, magnetic flux, radio waves) into heat. The American Institute for Ultrasound in Medicine has issued the following guideline: 'In the low megahertz frequency range there have been no demonstrated significant biological effects of ultrasound in mammalian tissues exposed *in vivo* to intensities below 100 mW/cm^2.'

As early as 1896 reports were made of the visual sensation of light flashes induced by exposure to changing magnetic fields. However the main hazards associated with rapidly changing magnetic fields are those of electroconvulsion and atrial fibrillation, hence caution should be exercised with epileptic patients and those who have recently suffered from myocardial infarction. Guidelines for the use of MRI are laid down by the National British Radiological Protection Board (1984).

Before deciding to carry out any imaging investigation a clinical decision has to be made whether the benefits accrued from the results of the investigation outweigh any possible risk to the patient from the procedure to be undertaken.

CONCLUSIONS

Advances in medical imaging are occurring at such a rapid rate that our whole attitude to disease processes may alter. This is in the main due to development of sophisticated imaging techniques, computer software and display systems. Ultrasound, due to its greater flexibility and relative low cost, will retain an integral diagnostic role in gynaecology with vaginal sonography a routine adjunct to a bimanual pelvic examination. MRI is perhaps the perfect technique and may eventually replace X-rays. MRI will lead to an increase in the detection, staging and assessment of a range of disease processes including cancer. The technology needed to overcome the major disadvantages of long scanning times and relative inflexibility due to size is well advanced. Magnetic resonance spectroscopy remains largely unexplored in gynaecology, but is an exciting prospect for the future. There must be an appreciation of the high cost of these new technologies and the need for careful evaluation of their diagnostic return. At the present time there have been few trials evaluating complementary imaging techniques and these should be carried out prior to a widespread introduction of newer imaging methods.

KEY POINTS

1. Ultrasound examination is dependent on both the technical expertise of the ultrasonographer and an understanding of the history and clinical findings of the patient being assessed.
2. Vaginal ultrasound has a high sensitivity and specificity in the diagnosis of ectopic pregnancy.
3. Hyperstimulation syndrome is uncommon if gonadotrophin therapy is monitored by ultrasound and plasma oestradiol levels.
4. Vaginal ultrasound plays an important role in timing of ovulation and oocyte recovery.
5. Transrectal ultrasound is of value in identifying parametrial spread of cervical cancer.
6. Real-time ultrasound cannot reliably distinguish between benign and malignant ovarian disease.
7. Ultrasound screening for ovarian cancer remains experimental.
8. Radionuclide imaging may have some value in detecting recurrent or residual ovarian cancer.
9. A chest X-ray and intravenous urogram are essential investigations for women with cervical cancer but seldom show abnormalities in women with endometrial cancer.
10. Lymphangiography lacks precision in the identification of nodal metastases.
11. CT scanning may have a role in recurrent cervical cancer but is of limited value in other gynaecological tumours.
12. MRI accurately shows parametrial invasion of cervical cancer but does not identify lymph node metastases reliably.
13. MRI allows the depth of myometrial penetration of endometrial cancer to be measured preoperatively.

REFERENCES

Andolf E, Jorgensen C 1989 Cystic lesions in elderly women, diagnosed by ultrasound. British Journal of Obstetrics and Gynaecology 96: 1076–1079.

Balfe D M, Heiken J P, McClennan B L 1986 Oncologic imaging of carcinoma of the cervix, ovary and endometrium. In: Bragg D G, Rubin P, Youker J E (eds) Oncologic imaging. Pergamon Press, Oxford, pp 439–477

Barber R J, McSweeney M B, Gill R W et al 1988 Transvaginal pulsed doppler ultrasound assessment of blood flow to the corpus luteum in IVF patients following embryo transfer. British Journal of Obstetrics and Gynaecology 95: 1226–1230

Bourne T, Campbell S, Steer C, Whitehead M I, Collins W P 1989 Transvaginal colour flow imaging: a possible new screening technique for ovarian cancer. British Medical Journal 299: 1367–1370

Breckenridge J, Kurtz A, Ritchie W 1982 Postmenopausal uterine fluid collection: indicator of carcinoma. American Journal of Radiology 156: 725-730

Bryce R L, Shuter B, Sinosich M J 1982 The value of ultrasound, gonadotrophin and oestradiol measurements for precise ovulation prediction. Fertility and Sterility 37: 42–45

Campbell S, Goessens L, Goswamy R, Whitehead M 1982 Real-time ultrasonography for determination of ovarian morphology and volume. A possible early screening test for ovarian cancer? Lancet i: 425–426

Campbell S, Bhan V, Royston P, Whitehead M I, Collins W P 1989 Transabdominal ultrasound screening for early ovarian cancer. British Medical Journal 299: 1363–1366

Ebner F, Kressel H Y, Mintz M C et al 1988 Tumour recurrence versus fibrosis in the female pelvis: differentiation with MR imaging at 1.5T. Radiology 166: 333–340

Fleisher A C, Dudley S B, Entman S S, Baxter J W, Kalemeris G E, Everette J A 1987 Myometrial invasion by endometrial carcinoma: sonographic assessment. Radiology 162: 307–310

Griffin J W, Parker R G, Taylor W J 1976 An evaluation of procedures used in staging carcinoma of the cervix. American Journal of Radiology 127: 825–827

Johnson I R, Symonds E M, Kean D M, Worthington B S 1984 Imaging of ovarian tumours by nuclear magnetic resonance. British Journal of Obstetrics and Gynaecology 91: 260–264

Long J P, Montgomery J B 1950 The incidence of ureteral obstruction in benign and malignant gynaecologic lesions American Journal of Obstetrics and Gynecology 59: 552–562

Meire H B, Farrant P, Guha T 1978 Distinction of benign from malignant ovarian cysts by ultrasound. British Journal of Obstetrics and Gynaecology 85: 893–899

National British Radiological Protection Board 1984 Revised guidelines on acceptable limits of exposure during nuclear magnetic clinical imaging. British Journal of Radiology 56: 974–977

Perkins A C, Pimm M V, Gie C, Marksman R A, Symonds E M, Baldwin R W 1989 Intraperitoneal I^{131} and In^{111} 791T/36 monoclonal antibody in recurrent ovarian cancer: imaging and biodistribution. Nuclear Medicine Communications 10: 577–584

Powell M C, Womack C, Buckley J H, Worthington B S, Symonds E M 1986a Pre-operative magnetic resonance imaging of stage I endometrial adenocarcinoma. British Journal of Obstetrics and Gynaecology 93: 353–360

Powell M C, Buckley J H, Wastie M, Worthington B S, Sokal M, Symonds E M 1986b The application of magnetic resonance imaging to cervical carcinoma. British Journal of Obstetrics and Gynaecology 93: 1276–1285

Powell M C, Perkins A C, Pimm M V et al 1987a Diagnostic imaging of gynaecological tumours using the monoclonal antibody 791T/36. American Journal of Obstetrics and Gynecology 157: 28–34

Powell M C, Worthington B S, Symonds E M 1987b The application of MRI to ovarian cancer. In: Sharp F, Soutter W P (eds) Ovarian cancer — the way ahead. Chameleon Press, London, pp 141–158

Randall J M, Fisk N M, McTavish A 1989 Transvaginal ultrasonic assessment of endometrial growth in spontaneous and hyperstimulated menstrual cycles. British Journal of Obstetrics and Gynaecology 96: 954–959

Requard C, Wicks J, Mettler F 1981 Ultrasonography in the staging of endometrial adenocarcinoma. Radiology 140: 781–785

Squillaci E, Salzani M C, Grandireth M L et al 1988 Recurrence of ovarian and uterine neoplasms: diagnosis with transrectal US. Radiology 169: 355–358

Timor-Tritsch I E, Bar-Yam Y, Elgali S, Rotlem S 1988 The technique of transvaginal sonography with the use of a 65MHz probe. American Journal of Obstetrics and Gynecology 158: 1019–1024

Timor-Tritsch I E, Peisner D B, Lesser K B, Slanik T A 1989 The use of transvaginal ultrasonography in the diagnosis of ectopic pregnancy. American Journal of Obstetrics and Gynecology 161: 157-161

Togashi K, Nishimura K, Itoh K 1987 Uterine cervical cancer: assessment with high filed MR imaging. Radiology 160: 431–435

Weiner J L, Chako A C, Merten C W, Gross S, Coffey E L, Stein H L 1986 Breast and axillary tissue MR imaging correlation of signal intensities and relaxation times with pathologic findings. Radiology 160: 229–305

Yuhara A, Akamatsu N, Sekiba K 1987 Use of transrectal radial scan ultrasonography in evaluating the extent of uterine cervical cancer. Journal of Clinical Ultrasound 15: 507–517

6. Hormones: their action and measurement in gynaecological practice

A. Clark J. G. Grudzinskas

Hormones are one of the important means by which cells communicate with each other. They ensure that the body's physiological systems are co-ordinated appropriately. Impaired communication leads to abnormal function. Classically, hormones are secreted by a gland and transported through the circulation to a distant site of action. However, as cellular communication also occurs at a local level, it is evident that several factors can combine to modulate and co-ordinate function. The types of communication to be considered are endocrine, paracrine and autocrine.

1. *Endocrine*: Intergland or structure communication involves secretion from a gland into the circulatory system (blood or lymph) of a regulatory substance that has a specific effect on another gland or structure, e.g. pituitary secretion of follicle-stimulating hormone (FSH) stimulating ovarian activity (Fig. 6.1).
2. *Paracrine*: Intercellular communication involves the local diffusion of regulating substances from a cell to contiguous cells, e.g. insulin-like growth factor (IGF-1) secretion by granulosa cells in the ovary (Fig. 6.1).
3. *Autocrine*: Intracellular communication involves the production of regulating substances by a single cell which binds to receptors on or within the same cell, e.g. oestradiol, modulating granulosa cell action (Fig. 6.1).

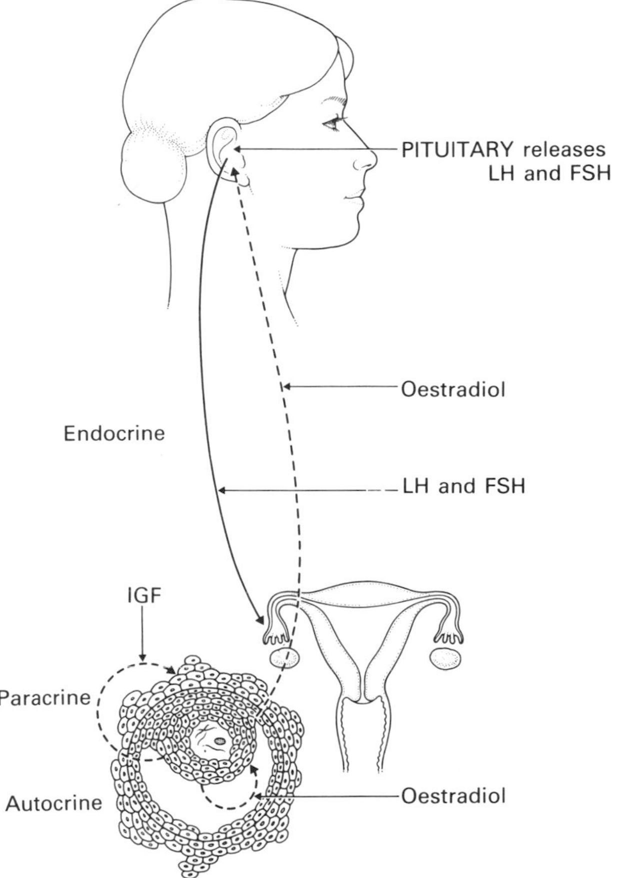

Fig. 6.1 Examples of endocrine, paracrine and autocrine hormonal communication. LH = luteinizing hormone; FSH = follicle-stimulating hormone; IGF-1 = insulin-like growth factor.

Hormones comprise two chemical groups — steroid hormones and trophic hormones. Steroid hormones include oestrogens, progestogens and androgens. Trophic hormones include the releasing hormones originating in the hypothalamus, and a variety of hormones released by the pituitary gland and trophoblast. The composition of these substances is summarized here:

Steroids

Steroids are a group of lipids composed of four linked carbon rings (hydrogenated cyclopentophenanthrene ring system). Steroid hormones, which are derived from cholesterol, can be classified according to the number of carbon atoms they possess: C-21 (progestogens, cortisol, aldosterone), C-19 (androgens) and C-18 (oestrogens).

Peptides

Peptides are compounds which yield two or more amino acids on hydrolysis. Linked together they form polypeptide hormones, e.g. gonadotrophin-releasing hormone (GnRH).

Glycoproteins

Glycoproteins consist of a protein (combination of amino acids in peptide linkages) to which carbohydrate groups (CHO-) are bound, e.g. luteinizing hormone (LH).

Hormones often circulate in extremely low concentrations and, in order to respond in a specific manner, target cells require specific receptors which recognize and bind the hormone and thereby alter cell function. Hormones act at the cellular level in two ways. Steroid hormones enter the cell and mediate action via receptors within the nucleus (King 1988). By contrast trophic hormones bind to receptors on the cell membrane which then activate 'second messenger' systems within the cell (Segaloff & Ascoli 1988). It is the affinity, specificity and concentration of receptors for a particular hormone which allow a small amount of hormone to produce a biological response.

MECHANISM OF ACTION OF STEROID HORMONES

The specificity of the tissue reaction to steroid hormones is due to the presence of specific intracellular receptor proteins for each hormone. The mechanism, illustrated in Figure 6.2, is common to the five main classes of steroid hormone: oestrogens, progestogens, androgens, glucocorticoids and mineralocorticoids (Speroff et al 1989).

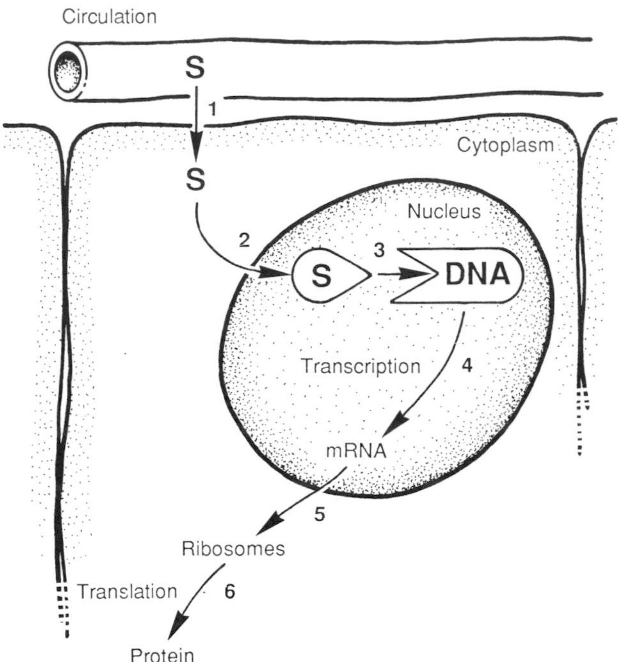

Fig. 6.2 Mechanism of action of steroid hormones. See text for details.

Stage 1: Transfer across the cell membrane

Circulating free (unbound) hormone is able to diffuse across cell membranes. However, most steroid hormone is bound with low affinity to albumin, or with high affinity to a specific binding globulin: sex hormone-binding globulin (SHBG) or cortisol-binding globulin (CBG). The concentration of free (unbound) hormone in the blood stream seems to be an important determinant of the rate of diffusion but there may be specific membrane-bound receptors which transport hormone into the cell.

Stages 2 and 3: Transfer into the nucleus and binding to receptor protein

Once in the cell, the hormone dissociates from the binding globulin and is transported across the nuclear membrane. The hormone binds with the receptor causing a conformational change that allows the receptor to bind directly with DNA (activation).

Stages 4 and 5: Synthesis of messenger RNA (mRNA)

Once bound to the nuclear receptor, the hormone-receptor complex then moves down the DNA molecule, binding with a specific gene. The mechanism by which hormone-receptor binding activates a gene is poorly understood but leads to a modification of mRNA synthesis (transcription). The RNA is synthesized and then transported to the ribosome.

Stage 6: Protein synthesis

Transfer of mRNA to the cytoplasmic ribosome results in the synthesis of protein (translation). The proteins produced, e.g. enzymes, have specific intracellular effects, the endpoint of the hormone action. For example, high midcycle levels of oestradiol from the ovary lead to the increase in LH synthesis and secretion by the anterior pituitary that results in ovulation (Yen & Lein 1976).

Regulation of steroid hormone action

Regulation of hormone action is required to enhance or reduce target tissue response and is used in clinical therapy. There are six major components:

1. Availability of hormone to cell.
2. Hormone specificity of receptor.
3. Availability of receptor.
4. Binding of hormone-receptor complex.
5. Protein synthesis.
6. Agonism/antagonism.

Availability of hormone to cell

Even if a cell has multiple receptors it will not be active in the absence of its specific hormone. For example, uterine epithelial cells have receptors for oestrogen, androgen, glucocorticoid and progestogen but because progesterone is not produced in the first half of the menstrual cycle, there is no progestational response (Robertson 1982). In addition, a hormone can be present in the blood stream but unavailable to the target cell. A hormone circulating in the blood stream, not attached to a binding protein, readily enters cells by diffusion. However, most of a circulating hormone is bound to protein carriers, such as SHBG, and therefore unavailable (King 1988). Consequently, alterations in the amount of circulating binding globulins can modulate the biological activities of their respective hormones. For example, about 80% of circulating testosterone is bound to SHBG, approximately 19% is loosely bound to albumin, and about 1% is unbound. Androgenicity is mainly dependent upon the unbound fraction and partly upon the fraction associated with albumin (Siiteri 1986). SHBG production in the liver is decreased by androgens, hence the binding capacity in men is lower than in normal women. In a hirsute woman, the SHBG level is depressed by the excess androgen, and the percentage of free and therefore active testosterone is elevated (Rosenfeld 1971).

Hormone specificity of receptor

This is the most important factor which determine specificity of action and occurs at two levels (King 1988). Presence or absence of a given receptor determines whether a cell will respond to a given class of steroids whilst hormone specificity controls which particular compound is active. For example, the oestrogen receptor which has the greatest specificity binds oestradiol 10 times more efficiently than oestrone and about 1000 times more than the androgen, testosterone; progesterone and cortisol are not recognized at all (Garcia & Rochefort 1977). This recognition specificity is a reflection of the different affinities the receptor has for the different hormone structures (Fig. 6.3). In biological terms, this means that oestradiol is more active than oestrone whilst testosterone can have oestrogenic effects but only at pharmacological concentrations (Fig. 6.4).

Androgen, glucocorticoid, progestogen and mineralocorticoid receptors are less precise in their binding require-

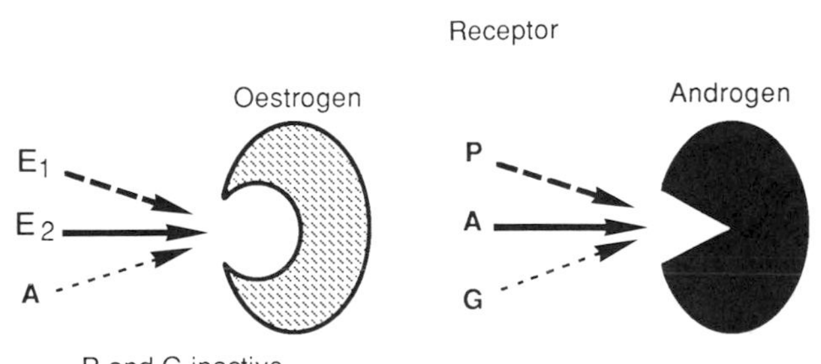

Fig. 6.3 Specificity determined by structural specificity of receptor. Oestradiol receptor has a higher affinity for oestradiol (E_2) than oestrone (E_1); androgens (A) such as testosterone have very low affinity whilst progestogens (P) and glucocorticoids (G) are inactive. Androgen receptor has less precise specificity, recognizing both P and G, albeit with less affinity than androgens.

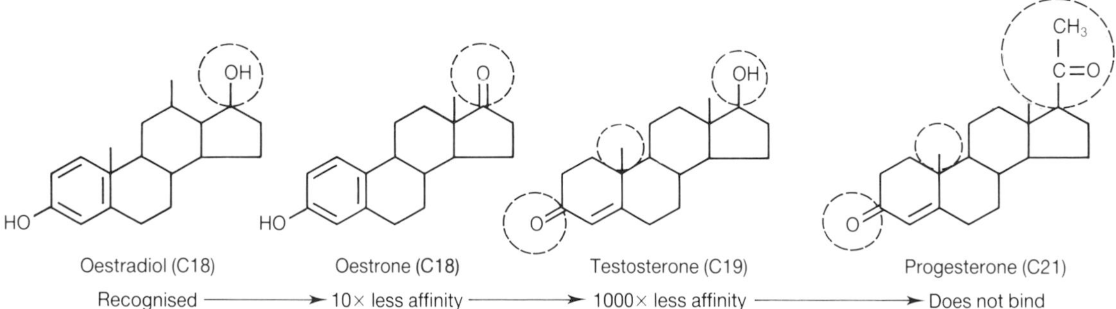

Fig. 6.4 Oestrogen receptor recognition is influenced by the differing side chains of hormones, e.g. oestrogens, testosterone and progesterone.

ments than the oestrogen receptor (Raynaud et al 1981). For example, many progestogens, especially the synthetic ones, bind to both progestogen and androgen receptors when present in pharmacological concentrations. This dual specificity is reflected in the biological activities of the compounds. For example, the practice of giving synthetic progestogens to pregnant women to prevent miscarriage resulted in some of their offspring having clinical features associated with androgen exposure (Aarskog 1979). The androgenic side-effects of the synthetic progestogens used in the oral contraceptive pill are another example.

Availability of receptor

A hormone can modify its own and/or another steroid hormone's activity by regulating the concentration of receptors in a cell. This has the biological effect of increasing tissue response to the hormone if the receptor number is increased, and vice versa if the receptor number is decreased. Oestrogen, for example, increases target tissue responsiveness to itself by increasing the concentration of FSH receptors in granulosa cells (Hillier et al 1981). This process is important in the selection and maintenance of the dominant ovarian follicle in the menstrual cycle. In order to respond to the ovulatory surge and become a 'successful' corpus luteum, the granulosa cells must acquire LH receptors. FSH induces LH receptor development on the granulosa cells of large antral follicles with oestrogen acting as chief co-ordinator (Erikson 1986).

Progesterone, on the other hand, limits the tissue response to oestrogen by reducing over time the concentration of oestrogen receptors (Tseng & Gurpide 1975), hence its use in the prevention of endometrial hyperplasia.

Binding of hormone-receptor complex

Biological activity is maintained only while the nuclear site is occupied with the hormone-receptor complex (Scholl & Lippman 1984; King 1988). The dissociation rate of the hormone and its receptor is therefore an important component of the biological response. Only low circulating levels of oestrogen are necessary for biological activity because of the long half-life of the oestrogen hormone-receptor complex (Sutherland et al 1988). As a consequence of a lower affinity for the oestrogen receptor, the less potent oestrogens (oestrone, oestriol) also have higher rates of dissociation from the receptor and therefore the oestrogen-receptor complex occupies the nucleus for a short period of time (Katzenellenbogen 1984). The higher rate of dissociation with a weak oestrogen can be compensated for by continuous application to allow prolonged nuclear-binding activity. Cortisol and progesterone circulate in higher concentrations because their receptor complexes have short half-lives in the nucleus. This regulatory mechanism is used clinically in the induction of ovulation with clomiphene citrate (Adashi 1986). The structural similarity between clomiphene citrate and oestrogen is sufficient to achieve uptake and binding of clomiphene citrate by oestrogen receptors. It has a very weak oestrogenic effect but occupies the nuclear receptor for long periods of time — weeks rather than hours (Mickkelson et al 1986).

Protein synthesis

The limited ability of receptors for progestogens, glucocorticoids and mineralocorticoids to discriminate between these hormones reduces their biological specificity. However, this effect could be counteracted if a gene's response to a hormone could be determined by specificity requirements in the DNA. Multiple regulatory units are present in the DNA proximal to the site when RNA transcription is initiated and interactions between these units and hormone-receptor complexes occur (Yamamoto 1985). It is generally agreed that these interactions are involved in the regulation of protein synthesis by steroids.

Agonism/antagonism

When a compound binds to a receptor, it can act as an agonist or antagonist. An agonist is a substance that has affinity for cell receptors of a naturally occurring substance and stimulates the same type of physiological activity. An antagonist tends to nullify the action of another substance, binding to its receptor without eliciting a biological response. In the case of the steroid hormones these activities do not necessarily require the compound to have the four-ring steroid structure. For example, diethylstilboestrol is a non-steroidal oestrogen agonist, while tamoxifen is a non-steroidal oestrogen antagonist (Fig. 6.5). Cyproterone acetate and RU486 (Mifepristone; Roussel) are the steroidal antagonists of testosterone and progesterone, respectively (Fig. 6.6). In these cases the conversion of agonists to antagonists is achieved by the addition of side chains. Each of these compounds blocks hormone action at the receptor level. Some clinical uses of steroid antagonists are listed in Table 6.1.

There are problems, however, in the clinical application of antagonists, related to the regulatory mechanisms described above. Firstly, because of the relative lack of receptor specificity, an antagonist for one class of hormone can have antagonistic effects on another class of hormone (Wakeling 1988). For example, the progesterone antagonist RU486 has affinity for the glucocorticoid receptor as well as the progesterone receptor and therefore is a potent anti-glucocorticoid. Secondly, hormones have central and peripheral actions, mediated by specific receptors. Therefore an antagonist may have adverse effects apart from the intended use. Cyproterone acetate, for example, an androgen antagonist, illustrates this diversity. It has effects

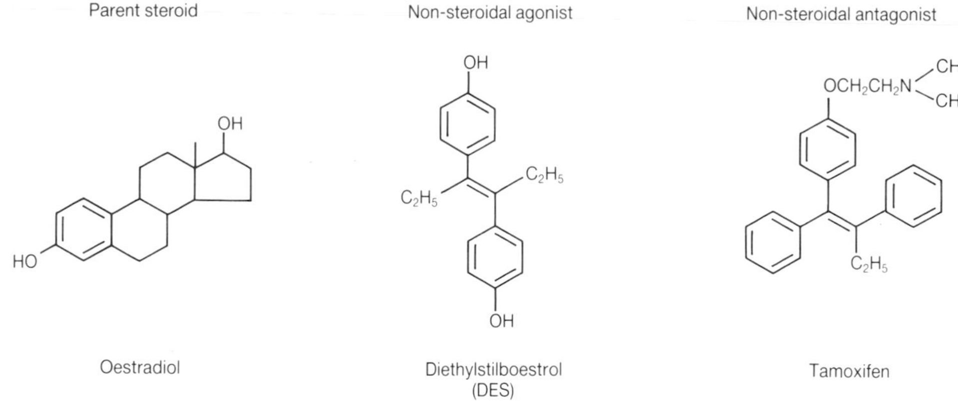

Fig. 6.5 Oestradiol with examples of a non-steroidal agonist (diethylstilboestrol) and antagonist (tamoxifen).

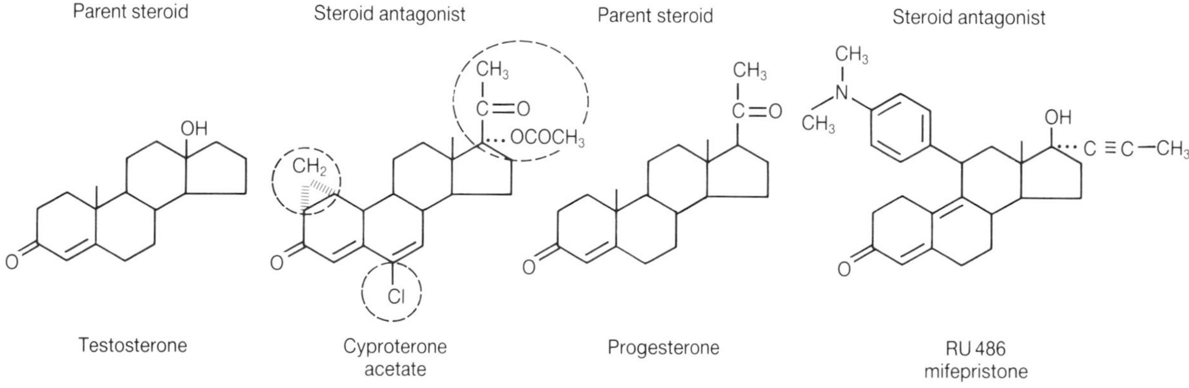

Fig. 6.6 Steroids with examples of steroid antagonists (e.g. cyproterone acetate; Mifepristone).

as diverse as suppression of libido and regression of the prostate gland. In addition cyproterone acetate may act as agonist for other chemically related hormones. It acts as a potent progestogen having agonist effects on the progesterone receptor. Hence it is used as a contraceptive agent in combination with ethinyl oestradiol.

Table 6.1 Clinical uses of steroid hormone antagonists

Drug	Clinical use
Antiprogestogens	Contraception Termination of pregnancy
Antiandrogens	Acne Benign prostatic hypertrophy Hirsutism Prostate cancer
Antioestrogens	Breast cancer Benign breast disease Endometriosis Uterine disease
Antiglucocorticoids	Adrenocortical carcinoma Cushing's syndrome
Antimineralocorticoids	Essential hypertension Oedema/ascites

MECHANISM OF ACTION OF TROPHIC HORMONES

As trophic hormones cannot enter the cell, they stimulate physiological events by uniting with a receptor on the surface of the cell and activating a sequence of communications using a second messenger system within the cell. The most widely studied and best understood of these systems is adenylate cyclase/cyclic adenosine monophosphate (cAMP); (Fig. 6.7; Rodbell 1980).

Stage 1: Binding to the cell membrane

The hormone, sometimes called the 'first messenger', binds to a receptor on the cell surface.

Stage 2: Activation of adenyl cyclase in the cell membrane

Binding of the hormone to the receptor activates the enzyme, adenylate cyclase, within the membrane wall which catalyses the conversion of adenosine 5′-triphosphate (ATP) within the cell to cyclic AMP, the second messenger. Some hormones, such as GnRH, use other second messengers, such as calcium.

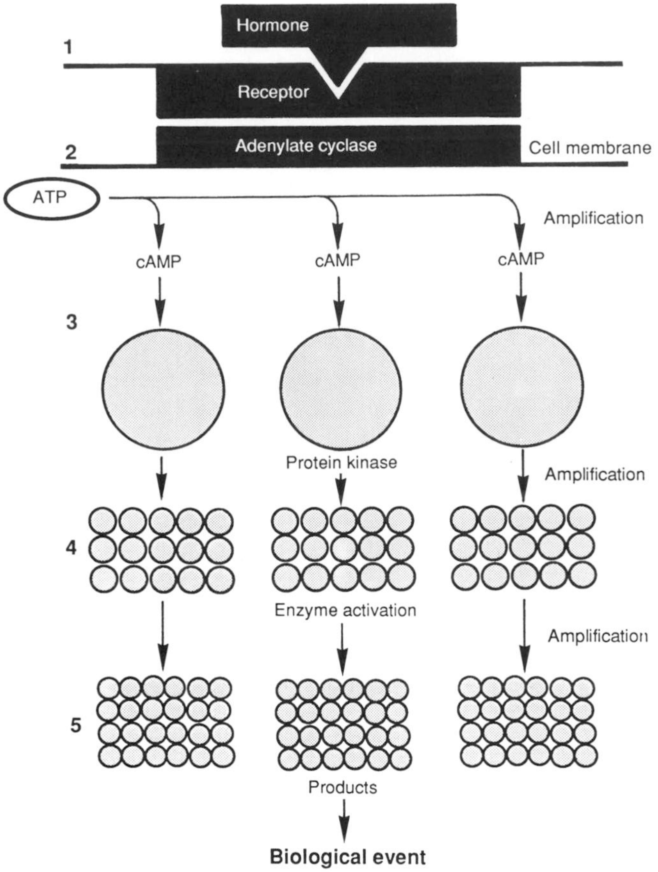

Fig. 6.7 Mechanism of action of trophic hormones. ATP = adenosine triphosphate; cAMP = cyclic adenosine monophosphate. See text for details.

Stage 3: Activation of protein kinase

The cAMP is bound to a cytoplasmic receptor protein which activates a protein kinase.

Stages 4 and 5: Activation of enzymes

The protein kinase causes phosphorylation and thereby activation of specific enzymes. These enzymes catalyse specific intracellular processes which give rise to the observed physiological effect of the hormone. The cAMP system provides a method for amplification of the hormonal signal in the circulation. Each cyclase molecule produces a lot of cAMP; the protein kinases activate a large number of molecules which in turn lead to the production of an even greater number of cellular products.

Regulation of trophic hormone action

Regulation of hormone action is required for enhancing or reducing target tissue response and is used in clinical therapy. There are five major components:

1. Availability of the hormone to the cell.
2. Hormone specificity of the receptor.
3. Availability of the receptor (up- and down-regulation).
4. Regulation of second messengers.
5. Agonism/antagonism.

Availability of hormone to cell

An effect can only occur if a cell carries a receptor for that hormone and the hormone is available to the cell receptor.

Hormone specificity of receptor

The specificity of a hormone's action and/or intensity of stimulation are dependent upon the configuration of the cell membrane receptor (Hwang & Menon 1984). It can be altered by changes in the structure or concentration of the receptor in the cell membrane. Similarly, changes in the molecular structure of a trophic hormone can interfere with cellular binding and therefore physiological action. Hormones that are structurally similar may have some overlap in biological activity. For example, the similarity in structure between growth hormone and prolactin means that growth hormone has a lactogenic action whilst prolactin has some growth-promoting activity and stimulates somatomedin production (Speroff et al 1989).

The glycoprotein hormones [LH, FSH, thyroid-stimulating hormone (TSH) and human chorionic gonadotrophin (hCG)] share an identical alpha-chain and require another portion, the beta-chain, to confer the specificity inherent in the relationship between hormones and their receptors. The beta subunits differ in both amino acid and carbohydrate content and the chemical composition may be altered under certain conditions, thereby affecting the affinity of the hormone and its receptor.

Availability of the receptor (up- and down-regulation)

The cell's mechanism for sensing the low concentrations of circulating trophic hormone is to have an extremely large number of receptors but to require only a very small percentage (as little as 1%) to be occupied by the hormone for its action to be evident (Sairam & Bhargavi 1985). Positive and negative modulation of receptor numbers by hormones is known as up- and down-regulation. The mechanism of up-regulation is unclear, but prolactin and GnRH, for example, can increase the concentration of their own receptors in the cell membrane (Katt et al 1985).

In down-regulation, an excess concentration of a trophic hormone such as LH or GnRH results in a loss of receptors on the cell membrane and therefore a decrease in biological response. This process occurs by internalization of the receptors, and is the main biological mechanism by which the activity of polypeptide hormones is limited (Segaloff & Ascoli 1988). Thus the formation of the hormone-receptor complex on the cell surface initiates the cellular response,

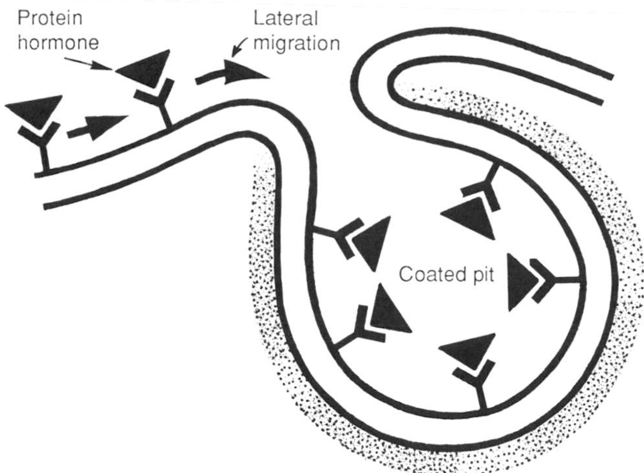

Fig. 6.8 Structure of a coated pit illustrating lateral migration.

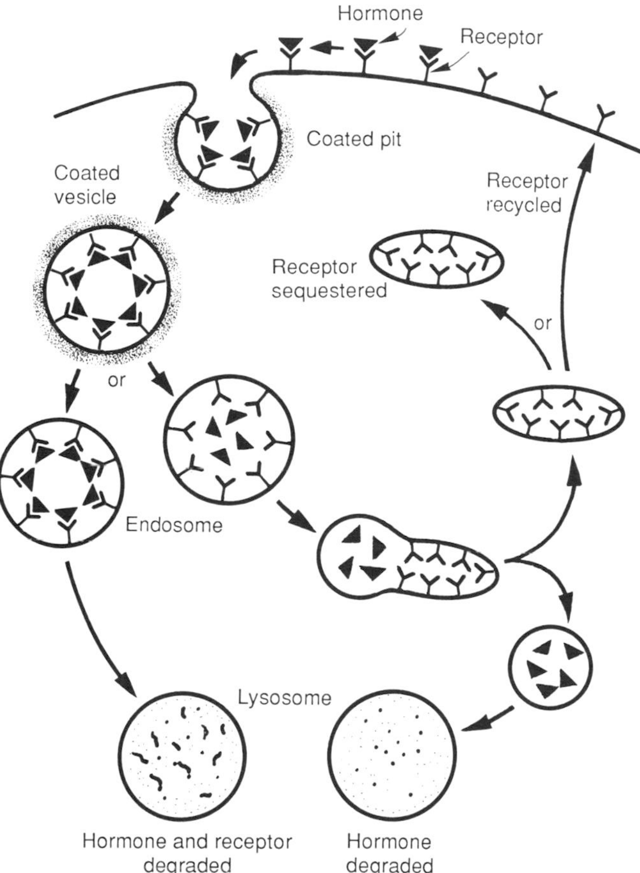

Fig. 6.9 Possible routes of receptor and hormone during receptor-mediated endocytosis.

and the internalization of the complex (with eventual degradation of the hormone) terminates the response. It therefore appears that the principal reason for the pulsatile secretion of trophic hormones is to avoid down-regulation and to maintain adequate receptor numbers. The pulse frequency, therefore, is a key factor in regulating receptor number.

It is believed that receptors are randomly inserted into the cell membrane after intracellular synthesis. They have two important sites — an external binding site which is specific for a polypeptide hormone, and an internal site which plays a role in the process of internalization (Kaplan 1981; Segaloff & Ascoli 1988). When a hormone binds to the receptor and high concentrations of the hormone are present in the circulation, the hormone-receptor complex moves laterally in the cell membrane in a process called lateral migration to a specialized area, the coated pit, the internal margin of which has a brush border (Goldstein et al 1979). Lateral migration, which takes minutes rather than seconds, thus concentrates hormone-receptor complexes in the coated pit, a process referred to as 'clustering' (Fig. 6.8). When fully occupied, the coated pit invaginates, pinches off, and enters the cell as a vesicle. The coated vesicle is delivered to the lysosomes where it undergoes degradation, releasing the hormones and receptors. The receptor may be recycled to the cell membranes and used again or the receptor and hormone may be metabolized, thus decreasing the hormone's biological activity. This process is called receptor-mediated endocytosis (Goldstein et al 1979; Fig. 6.9).

Besides down-regulation of polypeptide hormone-receptors, the process of internalization can be utilized for other cellular metabolic events, including the transfer into the cell of vital substances such as iron and vitamins. Hence, cell membrane receptors can be separated into two classes. The class I receptors are distributed in the cell membrane and transmit information to modify cell behaviour for these receptors. Internalization is a method for down-regulation and recycling is not usually a feature. Hormones which utilize this category of receptor include FSH, LH, hCG, GnRH, TSH and insulin (Kaplan 1981). The class II receptors are located in the coated pits. Binding leads to internalization which provides the cell with required facts or removes noxious agents from the biological fluid bathing the cell. These receptors are spared from degradation and can be recycled. Examples of this category include low-density lipoproteins which supply cholesterol to steroid-producing cells (Parinaud et al 1987) and transfer of immunoglobulins across the placenta to provide fetal immunity.

Regulation of second messengers

The second messenger system provides amplification of a small hormone signal in the blood stream and only a small percentage of the cell membrane receptors need to be occupied in order to generate a response. The regulation of adenylate cyclase and cyclic AMP production is important in regulating intracellular metabolic activity (Gilman 1984). Prostaglandins, guanine nucleotides, calmodulin and calcium all appear to participate in controlling the second messenger cascade (Segaloff & Ascoli 1988). The ability of the hormone-receptor complex to work through a common messenger (cAMP) and produce contrasting actions (stimulation and inhibition) is thought to be due to the presence of both stimulatory and inhibitory regulatory units (Rodbell 1980; Gilman 1984). For example, LH stimulates steroidogenesis in the corpus luteum through the coupling of stimulatory regulatory units to adenylate cyclase, stimulating the production of cAMP. Prostaglandin $F_{2\alpha}$ is directly luteolytic, inhibiting luteal steroidogenesis, and this action may be exerted via inhibitory units that block the production of cAMP (Rojas & Asch 1985).

Increasing concentrations of trophic hormones, such as gonadotrophins, are directly associated with desensitization of adenylate cyclase. There are some exceptions, namely the trophic hormones which do not utilize the adenylate cyclase mechanism (oxytocin, insulin, growth hormone, prolactin and human placental lactogen). The message of these hormones is passed directly to nuclear and cytoplasmic metabolic sites (Rasmussen 1986; Speroff et al 1989). GnRH is calcium-dependent in its mechanism of action (Jennes & Conn 1988).

Agonism/antagonism

In common with the steroid hormones, compounds can have agonist or antagonist effects. So far, only synthetic peptide agonists have come into clinical usage, analogues to GnRH being those most commonly known. The potency of the analogues is up to 200 times greater than GnRH, due to an increased affinity for pituitary GnRH receptors and a prolonged association with the receptor compared to GnRH. Though the analogues act as agonists, chronic administration stops the normal pulsatile pattern of GnRH, leading to a loss of pituitary LHRH receptors and, therefore, down-regulation. This has profound effects on the pituitary, leading to a fall in serum LH and FSH and consequently gonadal steroid secretion.

The mode of action of GnRH antagonists at the GnRH receptor is quite different from that of the agonists. Although the antagonists bind to the receptor, the down-regulation characteristic of agonist action does not occur (Clayton 1984). Rather, there is continuous occupancy of a large proportion of the receptors. Clinical application of antagonists has been delayed by the occurrence of significant toxicity.

CLINICAL ASSAYS

This section considers assay methodology for the endocrinological investigations commonly used in gynaecological practice. An understanding of basic methodology permits the clinician to have confidence in the selection of specific laboratory tests, and leads to a greater understanding of the assay for better interpretation of results (Chard 1987).

An assay determines the amount of a particular constituent of a mixture. The three types of analytical procedure commonly available in clinical practice are physicochemical assays, bioassays and binding assays.

Physicochemical assays

Some aspect of the physicochemical properties of a compound is utilized for its quantification. These are the assays used to measure electrolytes.

Bioassays

Detection or quantification is dependent on the biological actions of the compound. This was the original method of hormone assay. For example, human pregnancy could be diagnosed by the injection of maternal urine into the Black African Toad. If a high concentration of hCG was present in the urine, the toad would lay eggs.

Very recently, bioassays have stimulated interest with the development of very sensitive systems. For example, in the bioassay of prolactin, when neural tumour cells grown in culture are exposed to prolactin they replicate.

Binding assays

These assays involve the combination of the compound, for example, an antigen, with a binding substance, for example, an antibody, which is added in a fixed amount to the solution. The distribution of the antigen between the bound and free phases is directly related to the total amount of antigen present and provides a means for quantifying the latter (Fig. 6.10). Binding assays can be further subdivided into three groups: receptor assays, competitive protein-binding assays and immunoassays.

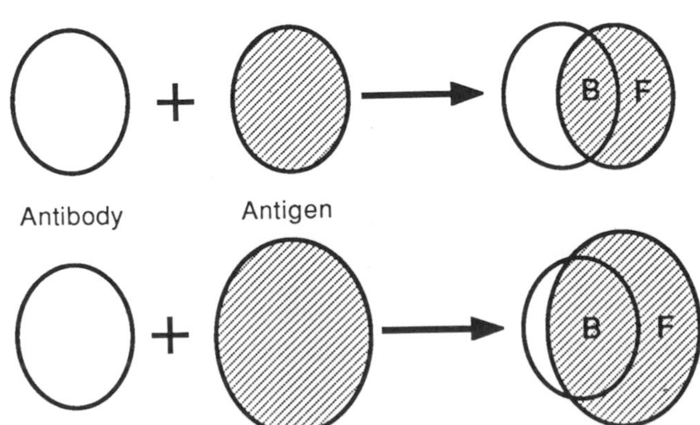

Fig. 6.10 Distribution of free (F) and bound (B) antigen in the presence of a fixed amount of antibody.

Receptor assays

A specific site on the surface of a tissue acts as the binding agent for a particular hormone, for example oestrogen receptors in breast tissue.

Competitive protein-binding assays

A naturally occurring binding protein, for example, SHBG, is used as the binder to quantify the amount of hormone present.

Immunoassays

A reaction which reaches equilibrium occurs between the hormone to be measured (antigen) and an antibody to monitor the reaction. A 'tracer' is attached to either the antigen or antibody. This tracer can be isotopic (radioactive), e.g. ^{125}I, or non-isotopic, e.g. based on fluorescence, or enzymatic action.

The basic principle of an immunoassay and how a result is obtained is described below:

1. A tracer such as a radioactive-labelled antigen (★Ag) is added to a fixed but *limited* quantity of antibody (Ab);

   Ab + ★Ag

   When the reaction commences the two reagents react quickly to form a complex. The reverse action is slow. This is the basis of a radioimmunoassay.

   Ab + ★Ag ⇌ Ab★Ag

   If the amount of antibody (Ab) is kept constant and a known amount of tracer (e.g. ★Ag 10 000 u) is added, by leaving the reaction long enough to reach equilibrium 100% binding is reached.

   Ab + ★AG ⇌ Ab★Ag
   10 000 u ⇌ 10 000 u

2. If a small quantity of the antigen (#Ag) we wish to measure is added to the same quantity of antibody (Ab) and tracer (★Ag) then labelled antigen (★Ag) and unlabelled antigen (Ag) will compete for the same limited number of binding sites offered by the antibody (Ab). Consequently, at equilibrium not all the labelled antigen (★Ag) will be bound by the antibody (Ab). Some will be displaced by the antigen (Ag) to be measured.

   Ab + Ag / ★Ag (10 000 u) ⇌ [Ab < Ag / ★Ag] (8000 u) + ★Ag (2000 u)

   Now only 80% of the ★Ag is antibody-bound, while 20% is 'free' and can be separated from the bound antibody by quantification.

3. If we now introduce more unlabelled antigen (Ag) to the reaction:

   Ab + AgAg / ★AgAb (10 000 u) ⇌ [Ab < Ag / ★Ag] (5000 u) + ★Ag (5000 u)

   there is even greater competition for the limited number of binding sites, so now only 50% of the added tracer is antibody-bound. This can be repeated for differing amounts of unlabelled antigen. The percentage of bound labelled antigen (★Ag) is progressively reduced with increasing concentrations of added unlabelled antigen (Ag).

   If it is known how much unlabelled antigen is added each time to the fixed quantities of antibody (Ab) and labelled antigen (★Ag) then a standard curve can be derived (Fig. 6.11).

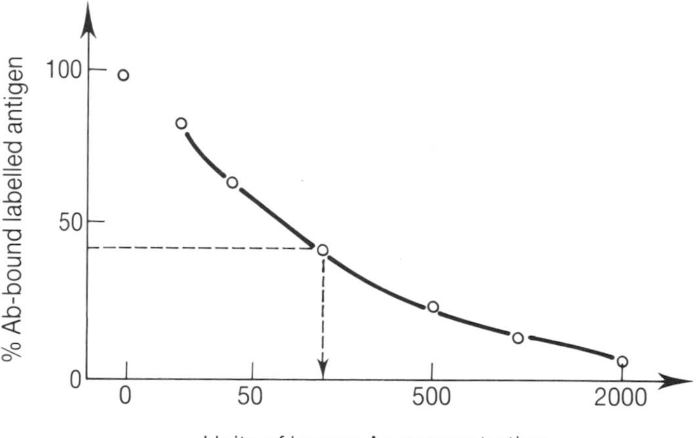

Fig. 6.11 Relationship between bound radiolabelled antigen and concentration of antigen in a dose–response curve.

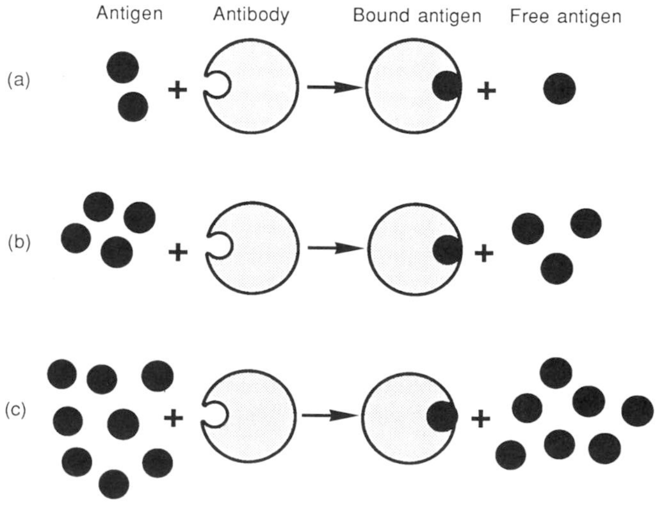

Fig. 6.12 Immunoassay: with a 'limited' concentration of antibody, varying concentrations of antigen give rise to increasing proportions of antigen in the free fraction.

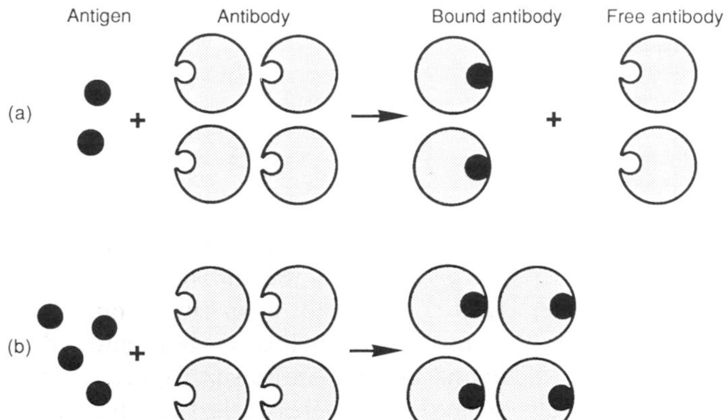

Fig. 6.13 Immunometric assay: with an 'excess' of antibody, increasing concentrations of antigen give rise to a corresponding increase in bound antibody.

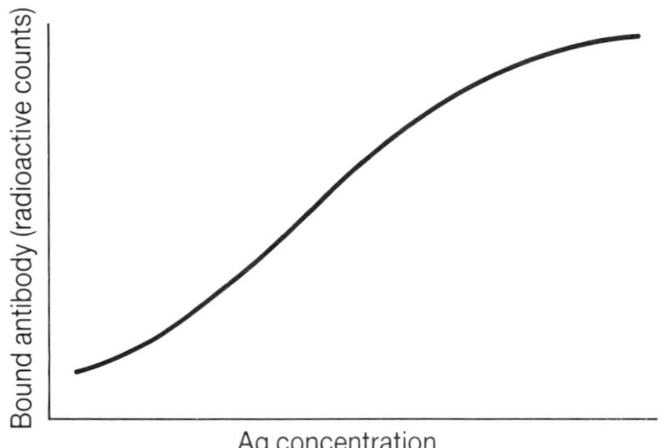

Fig. 6.14 Relationship between bound radiolabelled antibody and concentration of antigen in the immunoradiometric assay.

Hence, when a patient specimen containing an unknown amount of antigen is to be measured, the percentage of bound labelled antigen (shown by the dashed line in Fig. 6.11) left after equilibrium with the sample will then relate to the unknown amount of antigen in the sample.

This basic binding reaction can be subdivided into two categories, based on whether the antibody is present in a limited concentration or whether it is present in excess. When labelled antigen acts as the tracer, as in radioimmunoassay, the amount of antibody is constant but limited (Fig. 6.12).

If varying concentrations of the labelled antigen are to react with a constant but excess amount of antibody (Fig. 6.13) it can be termed an 'immunometric assay'. This is the type of assay used when labelled antibody, rather than antigen, acts as the tracer. In this case, the standard curve slopes in the reverse direction (Fig. 6.14) to that above because the amount of antigen is measured by the binding of the labelled antibody. As the concentration of antigen increases, so does the amount of

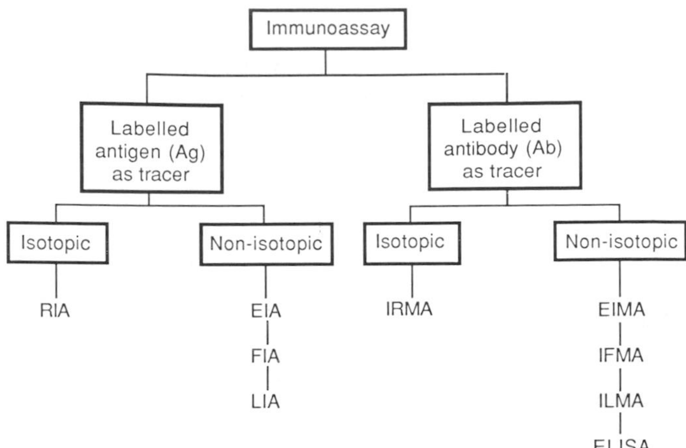

Fig. 6.15 Types of immunoassay used in clinical practice. RIA = radioimmunoassay; EIA = enzymoimmunoassay; FIA = fluoroimmunoassay; LIA = luminoimmunoassay; IRMA = immunometric assay; EIMA = enzymoimmunometric assay; IFMA, ILMA = immunofluorometric assay; ELISA = enzyme-labelled immunosorbent assay.

complexed labelled antibody. Many factors can influence the construction of the standard curve, hence every time a sample analysis is performed, a standard curve is also constructed. The acceptance of the results on the patient sample is dictated by quality control specimens containing known amounts of the antigen to be measured.

TYPES OF IMMUNOASSAY

Immunoassays are divided into two basic groups — those that use a radioactive label (isotopic assays) and those that use a non-radioactive label (non-isotopic assays). They can also be divided on the basis of whether the tracer or label is on the antigen or the antibody, as indicated in Figure 6.15.

Isotopic assays

Isotopic tracers can be divided into two types: those with an internal label and those with an external label. With an internal label, an existing atom in the molecule is replaced by a radioactive isotope of that atom (e.g. ^{3}H for ^{1}H — called a tritiated sample) and the tracer should be identical with that of the unlabelled molecule. With an external label, an atom or atoms of a radioactive isotope (e.g. ^{125}I) is covalently linked to an existing atom on the molecule. A tracer with an external label, by definition, is not identical to the unlabelled ligand though in practice its behaviour may not be distinguishable from the latter. Tracers with an internal label are commonly used in the case of small molecules such as steroid hormones and drugs. Tracers with an external label are commonly used in the case of larger peptide and protein hormones.

Radioimmunoassay (RIA)

This was the earliest form of immunoassay developed and is still the major immunoassay procedure. The tracer is a radioactive antigen, originally ^3H but superseded by ^{125}I. The antibody used in the reaction tube is polyclonal (derived from different cells) and is present in a restricted amount.

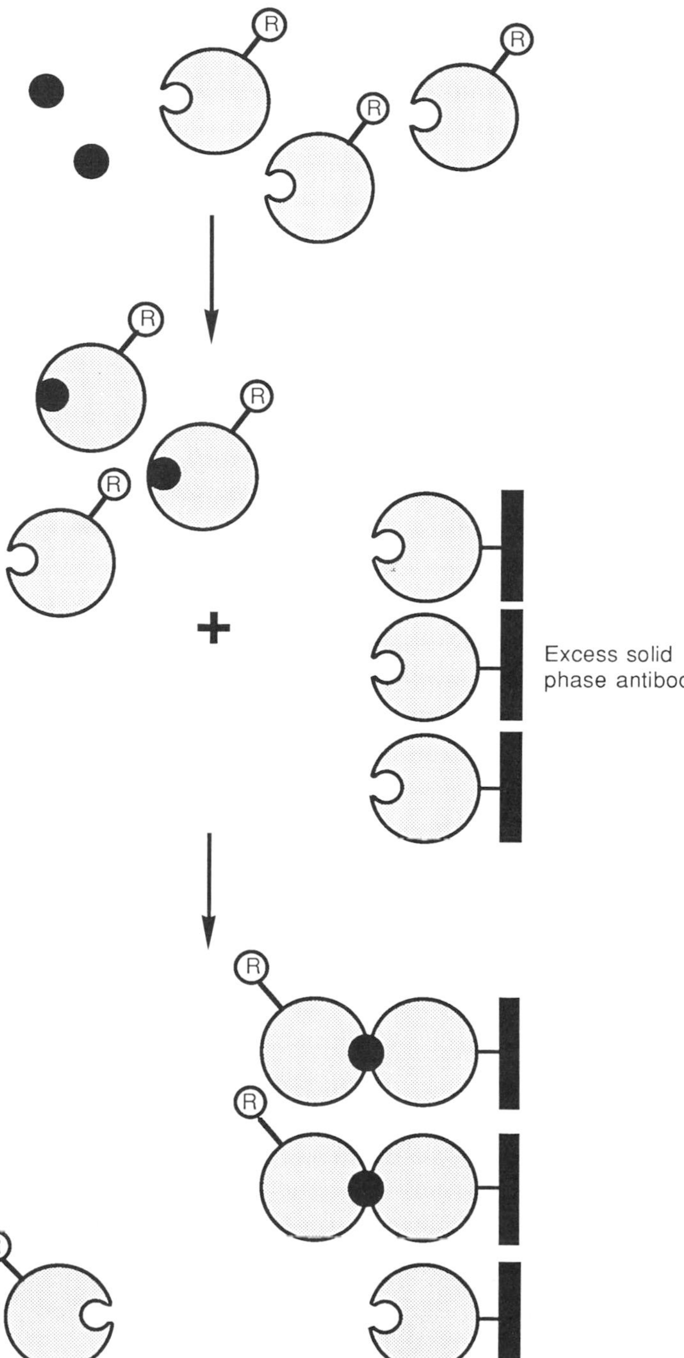

Fig. 6.16 'Two-site' immunoradiometric assay technique: the antigen is bound by two antibodies, therefore two binding sites on the antigen are involved. This technique is also referred to as a 'sandwich' assay.

Immunometric assay (IRMA)

This is a new breed of immunoassay with distinct advantages over RIA. The major application of IRMA has been in the quantification of proteins and peptides. The radioactive label is attached to the antibody, which is present in excess, and is a highly specific monoclonal antibody. The production technique of these antibodies results in a virtually limitless uniform supply of the reagent. One advantage of an IRMA is that the excess amount of radioactive antibody enables a wider range of antigen concentrations to be measured. Another advantage is that it may be performed by the 'two-site' immunometric method. This procedure is illustrated in Figure 6.16. It is also referred to as the 'sandwich' assay. The complex of the radiolabelled antibody and antigen is precipitated from the reaction mixture by the addition of another antibody directed against a second antigenic site on the antigen. This sandwich technique increases the accuracy of the assay compared to RIA.

Non-isotopic assays

In this group, the second marker antibody has an enzymatic, fluorescent or chemiluminescent tag. Assay systems that require separation of bound and free phases after incubation are referred to as heterogeneous and are more sensitive than those that do not require separation (homogeneous).

Enzyme

Enzymoimmunoassay (EIA), enzymoimmunometric assay (EIMA), enzyme-labelled immunosorbent assay (ELISA). These are currently the most widely used non-isotopic labels. Small quantities of antigen can be quantified by studying enzymatic substrate conversion that leads to a colour change. The colour formation can be a simple yes/no answer (Fig. 6.17) as in a rapid pregnancy test, or the intensity of colour can be used to quantify the

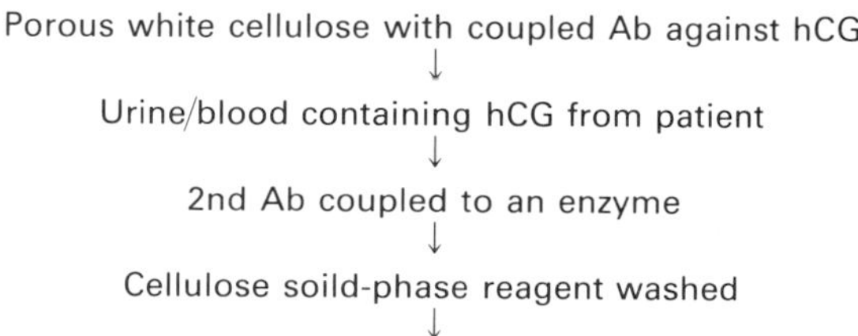

Fig. 6.17 Principle of rapid pregnancy test (tube test) using non-isotopic reagents. hCG = Human chorionic gonadotrophin.

patient sample. The second marker antibody will not be bound, so following the wash-step will not be present to react with its substrate.

Fluorescence

Fluoroimmunoassay (FIA), immunofluorometric assay (IFMA). Fluorescence is the property of certain molecules to absorb light at one wavelength and emit light at a longer wavelength. The incident light excites the molecule to a higher level of vibrational energy: as the molecule returns to the ground state it emits a photon which is the fluorescence emission. The potential sensitivity of fluorescence determination is very high but in practice is often limited by background noise. As with EIA, FIA can be divided according to whether a separation step is required into heterogeneous and homogeneous assays.

Chemiluminescence

Luminoimmunoassay (LIA), immunofluorometric assay (ILMA). Luminescence is a very similar phenomenon to fluorescence. Whereas the exciting energy in fluorescence is in the form of light, in luminescence it is provided by a chemical reaction. Chemiluminescent reactions produce light from simple chemical reactions, involving the action of oxygen or a peroxide on certain oxidation organic substances. Because there is high sensitivity inherent in the techniques, and the instrumentation is potentially simple, the application of luminescent labels in immunoassays should increase dramatically.

Agglutination assays

Agglutination assays are another type of immunoassay, using the principle that if the antigen–antibody reaction is coupled with visible compounds, such as red blood cells (haemagglutination) or latex particles (latex particle immunoassay) the presence or absence of a specific antigen or antibody can be detected in a patient sample by the presence or absence of agglutination of the cells or particles. These assays lack the sensitivity of the assays described above but can be used without any sophisticated instrumentation. The results are evaluated by eye, although the endpoint is subjective.

Haemagglutination immunoassays

Red blood cells can be used to determine the presence of specific antibodies, for example, the detection of rubella antibodies. They can also be used in the detection of antigens, for example, hepatitis B, and in blood group analysis (Fig. 6.18).

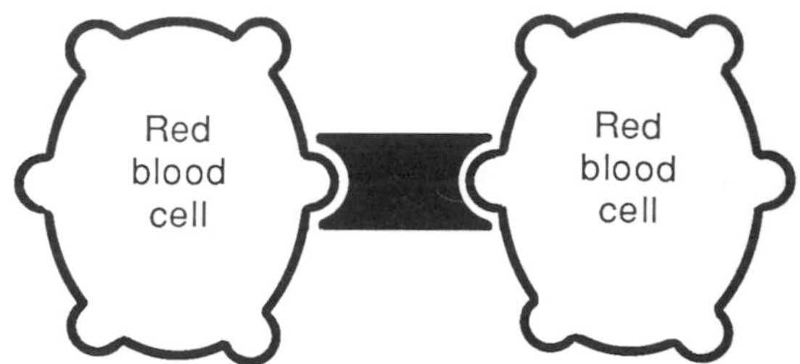

Fig. 6.18 Haemagglutination: specific antibodies to endogenous antigenic sites on red blood cells cause the cells to agglutinate. The degree of agglutination is a measure of the specific antibodies.

Latex agglutination immunoassays

This is the method utilized in slide pregnancy tests. In an analogous way to the use of cells, latex particles can be used as labels for antibodies or antigens. The advantages of latex particles over the use of red blood cells for agglutination are the stability of the reagents and a reduction in non-specific reactions.

Agglutination of the particles can mean a positive or negative result. If the particles are pretreated with hCG, agglutination on addition of the antibody solution indicates a negative result, i.e. no hCG was present in the woman's urine. If the particles had been coated with antibody and the urine containing no hCG had been added, then no agglutination would occur and lack of agglutination would be the negative result. These tests are now superseded by the tube tests using solid-phase reagents and monoclonal antibodies.

The future

Since the advent of RIA, immunoassays have played a major role in the quantification of many compounds and enabled the development of endocrinology as a medical science. As the number and variety of applications increase, the goal of assay technology remains the development of assays that give a high degree of sensitivity and specificity with ease, speed, and without the hazards of radioactivity. The new breed of non-isotopic assays, which utilize enzymes, fluorescence and chemiluminescence, are fulfilling these hopes. As budgeting continues to be a problem for all institutions, cost, which is related to personnel, reagents and equipment required for an assay, will also play a part in determining the assay of choice in the future.

Table 6.2 illustrates some of the advantages and disadvantages of the types of assay currently available, including the type of equipment and time required to obtain a result.

ACTION AND MEASUREMENT OF INDIVIDUAL HORMONES

In any assay, the precision and accuracy of the results

Table 6.2 Advantages and disadvantages of assays

Type of immunoassay	Degree of instrumentation	Time needed to do assay	Uses radiolabel
Latex agglutination	None necessary	2–30 min	No
ELISA (semi-quantitative)	None necessary	10 min–4 h	No
Enzyme-labelled assay	Colorimeter ± centrifuge*	6–12 h	No
Radiolabelled assay	Counter and centrifuge*	6–48 h	Yes
Fluoroimmunoassay	Fluorimeter ± centrifuge*	4–12 h	No
Chemiluminescent assay	Luminometer and centrifuge*	4–12 h	No

* Alternatively, other method of separation, e.g. magnets or filtration. ELISA = enzyme-labelled immunosorbent assay.

Table 6.3 Chemical composition and assay methods of hormones

Site	Hormone	Steroid	Peptide	Assay
Hypothalamus	GnRH		Decapeptide	RIA
	TRH		Tripeptide	RIA
Anterior pituitary	FSH		Glycoprotein	RIA, IRMA
	LH		Glycoprotein	RIA, IRMA, IFMA
	ACTH		Polypeptide	RIA, IRMA
	TSH		Glycoprotein	RIA, IRMA, LIA
	Growth hormone		Protein	IFMA, RIA, IRMA
	Prolactin		Protein	RIA, IRMA, bioassay
Posterior pituitary	Oxytocin		Nonapeptide	RIA
	Vasopressin (ADH)		Nonapeptide	RIA
Thyroid	T_3		Iodinated amino acid (tyrosine)	RIA, IRMA, bioassay
	T_4		Iodinated amino acid (tyrosine)	RIA, IRMA
Pancreas	Glucagon		Polypeptide	RIA
	Insulin		Polypeptide	RIA
Adrenal	Cortisol	Steroid		RIA, FIA
	Aldosterone	Steroid		RIA
	Androgens	Steroid		RIA
Ovary/testis	Oestradiol	Steroid		RIA, LIA (plasma)
	Oestrone	Steroid		LIA (urine)
	Progesterone	Steroid		RIA, LIA, FIA
	Testosterone	Steroid		RIA, LIA
	Inhibin		Peptide	RIA, bioassay
Endometrium	IGF-1, PP12		Glycoprotein	RIA,
	PEP, PP14		Glycoprotein	RIA
Trophoblast	hCG		Glycoprotein	RIA, IRMA, ELISA, latex agglutination, FIA, IFMA
	PAPP-A		Glycoprotein	RIA
	Oestriol	Steroid		RIA
	hPL		Glycoprotein	RIA, FIA
	SP1		Protein	RIA, EIA
Fetus	AFP		Glycoprotein	RIA, EIA, IFMA

GnRH = gonadotrophin-releasing hormone; TRH = thyrotrophin-releasing hormone; FSH = follicle-stimulating hormone; LH = luteinizing hormone; ACTH = adrenocorticotrophic hormone; TSH = thyroid-stimulating hormone; ADH = antidiuretic hormone; T_3 = triiodothyronine; T_4 = tetraiodothyronine; IGF-1 = insulin-like growth factor 1; PP12 = placental protein 12; PEP = progesterone-dependent endometrial protein; PP14 = placental protein 14; hCG = human chorionic gonadotrophin; PAPP-A = pregnancy-associated plasma protein A; hPL = human placental lactogen; SP1 = schwangerschafts protein 1; AFP = alpha-fetoprotein. RIA = radioimmunoassay; IRMA = immunometric assay; IFMA = immunofluorometric hormone; LIA = luminoimmunoassay; FIA = fluoroimmunoassay. ELISA = enzyme-linked immunosorbent assay; EIA = enzymoimmunoassay.

depend upon the antibody and reference standard for the antigen used, so the results on the same sample can vary from laboratory to laboratory depending upon the reagent used. When interpreting results on a patient sample, the normal ranges for the laboratory must be consulted. The chemical composition and assay methods of the hormone measured in endocrinological practice are summarized in Table 6.3. Only those hormones most relevant to gynaecological practice are considered in detail below.

Anterior pituitary hormones

Normal levels of FSH are shown in Table 6.4.

Because of the marked fluctuations in levels in a normal ovulatory cycle, timing of the blood sample in relation to ovulation is required to interpret results. The level can be as low as 0.5 iu/l at the luteal phase nadir and as high as 20 iu/l at the mid-cycle peak. However, values below 1 iu/l are associated with hypothalamic pituitary failure and values of 20 iu/l or above indicate ovarian failure, as in the menopause. In addition, FSH values within the wide range of normal can be associated with absent ovarian function if the production is below the threshold of follicular development for that patient, i.e. a normal result does not guarantee a normal endocrinological pattern in an individual patient. Fluctuating FSH levels mean the investigation might need to be repeated, in particular in a perimenopausal patient.

Luteinizing hormone

As for FSH, timing the sample in relation to the phase of the ovulatory cycle is vital. For example, the ovulatory surge is taken as above 20 iu/l. However, in polycystic ovarian disease, a raised LH (13–25 iu/l) with normal FSH values is characteristic. Therefore, a raised LH in the early to midfollicular phase is of more significance than a mid-cycle raised LH. The LH level is within the normal range in a significant number of women with polycystic ovarian disease and the diagnosis requires the use of other tests.

The prospective timing of ovulation using the LH peak presents the difficulty that the peak cannot be identified until the next value significantly lower than the peak is observed. Thus, although rapid assays for LH are now available, it is still necessary to plan the action to be taken on the basis of the first definite rise in LH values rather than on the peak, which usually occurs a day later.

As discussed earlier, unless the assay uses an antibody that is specific for the beta subunit of LH, cross-reaction can occur in the assay with the other glycoproteins of the anterior pituitary (FSH, TSH) and hCG.

Prolactin

Prolactin levels are influenced by the time of day when blood is collected and are increased by stress (including venepuncture). Transient rises can occur at ovulation. Therefore a small elevation above the normal range can occur in normal women. Such a rise should be judged in the clinical setting. If a woman has a normal menstrual cycle, the result is unlikely to be significant. However, if she is amenorrhoeic she should be investigated further.

Growth hormone

Growth hormone is secreted in short bursts, most of which occur in the first part of the night. These bursts are more frequent in children, so the results vary depending upon timing and age. Secretion is also stimulated by stress and hypoglycaemia and is inhibited by glucose and corticosteroids.

Thyrotrophin-stimulating hormone

Normal levels of TSH range from 0.4 to 5 mmol/l. The measurement of tetraiodothyronine (T_4) and TSH provides the most accurate assessment of thyroid function. When using thyroid hormone replacement therapy, both TSH and T_4 should be measured because TSH alone cannot detect overdosage.

Thyroid gland hormone

Deficiency of thyroid hormones triiodothyronine (T_3) and T_4 leads to anovulation associated with increased gonadotrophin levels. Therefore, it is important to assess

Table 6.4 Normal levels for follicle-stimulating hormone (FSH) and luteinizing hormone (LH)

Clinical state	Serum FSH	Serum LH
Normal adult female	5–20 u/l with the ovulatory mid-cycle peak about twice the base level	5–20 u/l with the ovulatory mid-cycle peak about three times the base level
Hypogonadotrophic state: Prepubertal, hypothalamic and pituitary dysfunction	<5 u/l	<5 u/l
Hypergonadotrophic state: Postmenopausal, castrate and ovarian failure	>40 u/l	>40 u/l

thyroid function prior to diagnosing premature ovarian failure.

Normal levels are as follows:

Free T_4: 10–25 pmol/l; T_3: 1.1–2.3 nmol/l (non-pregnant, no OCP); 1.4–4.3 nmol/l (pregnant/OCP).

Circulating thyroid hormone is tightly bound to a group of proteins, chiefly thyroxine-binding globulin. Oestrogen produces a rise in thyroxine-binding capacity and, therefore, thyroid function tests are affected by pregnancy and oestrogen-containing medications such as the contraceptive pill. Consequently, a raised thyroxine level does not mean that the free thyroxine concentration (the unbound and metabolically active hormone) is above the normal range.

Because of the peripheral source of T_3, its levels are not a direct reflection of thyroid secretion. In addition T_3 levels may be normal despite the presence of a goitre with elevated TSH and depressed T_4 concentrations, as T_4 plays the instrumental role in TSH regulation. Therefore, measurement of free T_4 and TSH provides the most accurate assessment of thyroid function. RIA of T_3 is important for the occasional case of hyperthyroidism due to excessive production of T_3 with normal T_4 levels (T_3 toxicosis). Drugs taken orally for cholecystograms inhibit the peripheral conversion of T_4 to T_3, and can disrupt normal thyroid levels (giving elevated T_4) for up to 30 days after administration.

Adrenal cortex

The adrenal cortex comprises three morphologically and functionally distinct regions. The outmost region (zona glomerulosa) secretes aldosterone. The zona fasciculata is the intermediate region and produces cortisol, which will be dealt with here. The zona reticularis encircles the medulla and synthesizes oestrogens and androgens.

Cortisol

Normal levels of cortisol in adults at 09.00 hours range from 300 to 700 nmol/l.

If a 24-h urine collection is used, it is necessary to ensure that a complete collection has been obtained. The measurement of creatinine excretion will identify whether a collection is incomplete. As blood levels of cortisol vary greatly throughout a 24-h period, sample timing is important. Blood levels are highest in the morning and lowest in the evening. Most laboratories' normal values are based on 09.00 hours sampling.

Ovarian hormones

Oestradiol

Normal levels of oestradiol are shown in Table 6.5.

There is a variation in oestradiol levels throughout the menstrual cycle. Results, therefore, need to be interpreted in relation to the timing of the sample in the cycle.

Progesterone

Levels in the mother during pregnancy increase in parallel with the growth of the placenta (Table 6.5). Maternal progesterone levels are related to the weight of the fetus and placenta at term.

Variations throughout the menstrual cycle can lead to difficulties in interpretation if the result is taken at an unidentified time in the cycle, particularly if a single progesterone level is taken as a marker of ovulation. Normally results taken 5–8 days prior to the next menstruation are suitable for the detection of ovulation, so the patient should be asked to keep a record of the timing of the blood sample and her next last menstrual period. A result >30 nmol/l indicates ovulation, even if timing is not known.

Testosterone

Normal levels (Table 6.5).

Testosterone:	female 0.5–3.0 nmol/l
	male 9–35 nmol/l
Androstenedione:	female/male 3–8 nmol/l
SHBG:	female 38–103 nmol/l
	male 17–50 nmol/l

Testosterone arises from a variety of sources in the female. Approximately 50% is derived from peripheral conversion of androstenedione (secreted by the adrenal cortex), while

Table 6.5 Normal ranges for oestradiol, progesterone and testosterone

	Oestradiol	Progesterone (nmol/l)	Testosterone (nmol/l)
Follicular phase	200–400 pmol/l	<4	0.5–3.0
Mid-cycle peak	400–1200 pmol/l	4–10	0.5–3.0
Luteal phase	2–10 nmol/l	30–45	0.5–3.0
Pregnancy			
First trimester	2–10 nmol/l	30–45	
Second trimester	10–30 nmol/l	70–150	
Third trimester	20–80 nmol/l	150–600	
Postmenopause	<100 pmol/l	<4	0.5–1.5

the adrenal gland and ovary contribute approximately equal amounts (25%) to the circulating levels of testosterone, except at mid-cycle when the ovarian contribution increases by 10–15%. About 80% of circulating testosterone is bound to SHBG.

hCG is secreted by the blastocyst and appears in maternal blood shortly after implantation and then rises rapidly until 8 weeks' gestation. Levels show little change at 8–12 weeks, then decline to 18 weeks and remain fairly constant until term. There is some short-term variation in blood hCG levels but no circadian rhythm. At term, the levels in the female fetus are substantially higher than those in the male (Obiekwe & Chard 1983). The mechanisms which determine the levels of hCG in maternal blood are unknown.

hCG is similar to LH in structure and thus antibodies to one cross-react with the other unless an assay for the beta subunit of hCG is used. The sensitivity of most commercial assays in the past had to be limited in order to avoid false-positive tests due to LH cross-reaction. Peak levels of hCG (approximately 100 000 iu/l) occur at 10 weeks' gestation. A patient can continue to have a positive pregnancy test for at least a week after a spontaneous or therapeutic abortion due to the prolonged half-life of hCG; hCG may be detected up to 20 weeks later if sensitive assays are used.

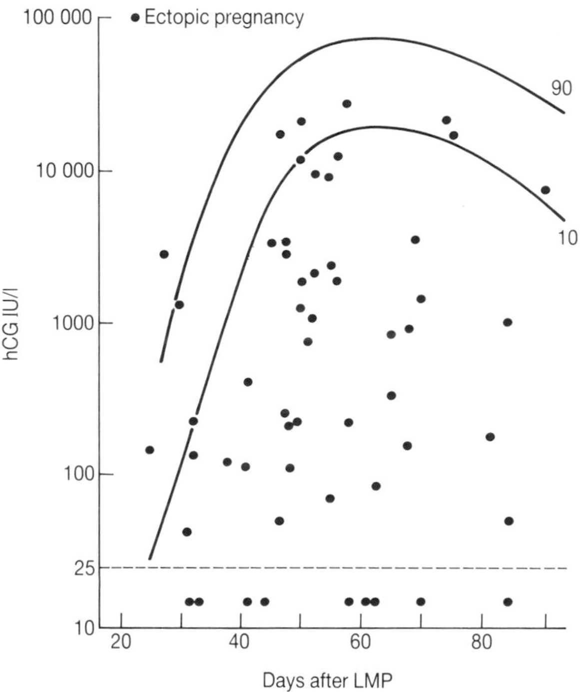

Fig. 6.19 Serum human chorionic gonadotrophin (hCG) levels in women with an ectopic pregnancy in relation to the range in normal intrauterine pregnancy. LMP = last menstrual period.

The range of serum hCG levels in ectopic pregnancy is very wide (Stabile et al 1989) so that a negative result does not rule out an ectopic nor does a result in the normal range guarantee an intrauterine pregnancy (Fig. 6.19). Quantification of hCG is usually only of value when monitoring postoperative progress in trophoblastic disease.

Fetus

Alphafetoprotein (AFP)

AFP is synthesized by yolk sac, fetal liver and gastrointestinal tract. Its function is unknown. It is used as a marker in clinical practice for the identification of congenital abnormalities.

Neural tube defects are associated with raised mid-trimester levels of AFP while Down's syndrome is associated with reduced mid-trimester AFP levels.

Normal levels. The value of AFP varies with gestation and number of fetuses present. The concentration of AFP in fetal serum rises rapidly to reach a peak at 12–14 weeks' gestation, at which time the levels are 2–3 g/l. Thereafter it falls until term with a sharp drop at 32–34 weeks. In the mother circulating AFP levels rise progressively to reach a peak at 32 weeks, then decrease towards term. Check with the local laboratory as levels also vary from one type of assay to another.

The interpretation of normality of levels depends upon gestation. Therefore incorrect assessment of gestation could lead to an erroneous conclusion on the normality of the fetus. Levels are also raised in obstetric problems (threatened miscarriage, intrauterine growth retardation, perinatal death and antepartum haemorrhage) and some congenital abnormalities (exomphalos, nephrosis, Turner's syndrome, trisomy 13).

KEY POINTS

1. Steroids exert their action through intracellular receptors whereas trophic hormones act through receptors located on the cell membrane, then through a second messenger system within the cell.
2. Androgen, progesterone and glucocorticoid receptors are less precise than oestrogen receptors in their binding affinity.
3. Synthetic progestogens can bind to both androgen and progesterone receptors reflecting the dual biological activities of progestogens.
4. Hormone potency is directly related to the duration the hormone–receptor complex occupies the nucleus.
5. Due to structural similarity with oestrogen, clomiphene citrate binds to oestrogen receptors and occupies the nucleus for long periods.
6. Agonists are substances that occupy cell receptors and stimulate natural physiological activities.

7. Antagonists are substances that can occupy receptors without being internalised, hence blocking the cell function.
8. An antagonist may block different classes of hormones due to the lack of receptor specificity.
9. Due to amplification of hormone signals by the second messenger system, only 1% of the cell receptors need to be occupied by the hormone for its action to be evident.
10. Down regulation by internalization of hormone receptors is a unique mechanism for limiting polypeptide hormone activity.
11. Depending upon the reagent used, hormone analysis results vary from one laboratory to another.
12. Endocrine investigations should be timed early in the follicular phase and repeated testing may be necessary to guard against false results.
13. The use of TSH estimation only cannot detect over-dosage and T_4 should be measured as well in women receiving thyroxine replacement therapy.
14. T_3 measurement is necessary only in patients suspected to be thyrotoxic yet with normal T_4 values.
15. Due to its long half-life, hCG can be detected in blood or urine for a few weeks after a miscarriage using a sensitive assay method.
16. Oestrogen increases target tissue responsiveness to itself by increasing FSH receptors in granulosa cells whereas progesterone limits the tissue response to oestrogen by reducing the concentrations of oestrogen receptors.

REFERENCES

Aarskog D 1979 Maternal progestins as a possible cause of hypospadias. New England Journal of Medicine 300: 75

Adashi E Y 1986 Clomiphene citrate-initiated ovulation: a clinical update. Seminars in Reproductive Endocrinology 4: 255

Chard T 1987 An introduction to radioimmunoassay and related techniques. Elsevier, Amsterdam

Clayton R N 1984 LH-RH and its analogs. In: Vickery B H, Nestor J J, Hafez E S E (eds) MTP Press, Lancaster, p 35

Erikson G F 1986 An analysis of follicle development and ovum maturation. Seminars in Reproductive Endocrinology 4: 233

Garcia M, Rochefort H 1977 Androgens on the oestrogen receptor. II. Correlation between nuclear translocation and uterine protein sysnthesis. Steroids 29: 11

Gilman A G 1984 Guanine nucleotide-binding regulatory proteins and dual control of adenylate cyclase. Journal of Clinical Investigation 73: 1

Goldstein J L, Anderson R G W, Brown M S 1979 Coated pits, coated vesicles, and receptor-mediated endocytosis. Nature 279: 679

Hillier S G, Reichert L E, Van Hall E V 1981 Control of preovulatory follicular estrogen biosynthesis in the human ovary. Journal of Clinical Endocrinology and Metabolism 52: 847

Hwang J, Menon K M J 1984 Spatial relationships of the human chorionic gonadotropin (hCG) subunits in the assembly of the hCG-receptor complex in the luteinized ovary. Proceedings of the National Academy of Science 81: 4667

Jennes L, Conn P M (1988) Mechanism of gonadotropin releasing hormone action. In: Cooke B A, King R J B, van der Molen H J (eds) Hormones and their action part II. Elsevier Science, Amsterdam, p 135

Kaplan J 1981 Polypeptide-binding membrane receptors: analysis and classification. Science 212: 14

Katt J A, Duncan J A, Herbon L et al 1985 The frequency of gonadotrophin-releasing hormone stimulation determines the number of pituitary gonadotropin-releasing hormone receptors. Endocrinology 116: 2113

Katzenellenbogen G S 1984 Biology and receptor interactions of estriol and estriol derivatives in vitro and in vivo. Journal of Steroid Biochemistry 20: 1033

King R J B 1988 An overview of molecular aspects of steroid hormone action. In: Cooke B A, King R J B, van der Molen J G J (eds) Hormones and their actions. Elsevier Science, Amsterdam, p 29

Mickkelson T J, Kroboth P D, Cameron W J et al 1986 Single-dose pharmacokinetics of clomiphene citrate in normal volunteers. Fertility and Sterility 46: 392

Obiekwe B C, Chard T 1983 Placental proteins in late pregnancy: relation to fetal sex. Journal of Obstetrics and Gynaecology 3: 163

Parinaud J, Perret B, Ribbes H et al 1987 High density lipoprotein and low density lipoprotein utilization by human granulosa cells for progesterone synthesis in serum-free culture: respective contributions of free and esterified cholesterol. Journal of Clinical Endocrinology and Metabolism 64: 409

Rasmussen H 1986 The calcium messenger system. New England Journal of Medicine 314: 1094

Raynaud J P, Ojasso T, Labrie F 1981 Steroid receptors. In: Lewis G P, Ginsburg M (eds) Mechanisms of steroid action. Macmillan, London, p 145

Robertson W B 1982 The endometrium. Butterworths, London

Rodbell M 1980 The role of hormone receptors and GTP-regulatory protiens in membrane transduction. Nature 284: 17

Rojas R J, Asch R H 1985 Effects of luteinizing hormone-releasing hormone agonist and calcium upon adenyl cyclase activity of human corpus luteum membranes. Life Sciences 36: 841

Rosenfeld R L 1971 Plasma testosterone binding globulin and indexes of the concentration of unbound plasma androgens in normal and hirsute subjects. Journal of Clinical Endocrinology and Metabolism 32: 717

Sairam M R, Bhargavi G N 1985 A role for glycosylation of the alpha subunit in transduction of biological signal in glycoprotein hormones. Science 229: 65

Scholl S, Lippman M E 1984 The estrogen receptor in MCF-7 cells: evidence from dense amino acid labelling for rapid turnover and a dimeric model of activated nucleic receptor. Endocrinology 115: 1295

Segaloff D L, Ascoli M 1988 Internalization of peptide hormones and hormone receptors. In: Cooke B A, King R J B, van der Molen J G J (eds) Hormones and their actions. Elsevier Science, Amsterdam, p 133

Siiteri P K 1986 Androgen binding proteins. In: Foret M G, Pugeat M (eds) Binding proteins of steroid hormones. John Libbey, London, p 593

Speroff L, Glass R H, Kase N G (eds) 1989 Clinical gynecologic endocrinology and fertility. Williams & Wilkins, Baltimore

Stabile I, Campbell S, Grudzinskas J G 1989 Ultrasound and circulating placental protein measurements in complications of early pregnancy. British Journal of Obstetrics and Gynaecology 96: 1182–1191

Sutherland R L, Watts C K W, Clarke C L 1988 Oestrogen actions. In: Cooke B A, King R J B, van der Molen H J (eds) Hormones and their actions. Elsevier Science, Amsterdam, p 193

Tseng L, Gurpide E 1975 Effects of progestins on estradiol receptor levels in human endometrium. Journal of Clinical Ednocrinology and Metabolism 41: 402

Wakeling A E 1988 Physiological aspects of luteinizing hormone releasing factor and sex steroid actions: the interrelationship of agonist and antagonist activities. In; Cooke B A, King R J B, van der Molen H J (eds) Hormones and their actions. Elsevier Science, Amsterdam, p 151

Yamamoto K R 1985 Steroid receptor regulated transcription of specific genes and gene networks. Annual Review of Genetics 19: 209

Yen S C, Lein A 1976 The apparent paradox of the negative and positive feedback control system on gonadotrophin secretion. American journal of Obstetrics and Gynecology 126: 942

FURTHER READING

Chard T 1987 An introduction to radioimmunoassay and related techniques. Elsevier/North Holland Biomedical Press, Amsterdam

Edwards R 1985 Immunoassay: an introduction. Heinemann Medical Books, London

Lagone J J, Van Vunakis H (eds) 1982 Methods in Enzymology, vol 84: Immunochemical techniques. Academic Press, London

Voller A, Bartlett A, Bidwell D (eds) 1981 Immunoassays for the 80s. MTP Press, Lancaster

7. Symptoms and signs in gynaecology

A. G. Amias

APPROACH TO THE GYNAECOLOGICAL PATIENT

There are a number of different circumstances in which a woman may find herself consulting a doctor for gynaecological purposes and undergoing a clinical examination. Most commonly the first encounter is with the general practitioner either at a surgery or health centre but occasionally in the patient's home if acute symptoms have developed. Attendance at hospital for a specialist opinion usually follows a general practitioner referral though sometimes this may be requested by consultants from other disciplines within the hospital or elsewhere. Increasingly nowadays a woman may prefer to discuss gynaecological matters at a family planning or well woman clinic or when attending a Department of Genitourinary Medicine. Patients with acute symptoms may present themselves or be referred to an Accident and Emergency Department where a pelvic examination may be necessary and gynaecological problems either of an acute or semi-urgent nature may require the attention of a wide variety of non-specialists either in primary health care or in the hospital service.

General practitioner

A woman with a gynaecological problem should be encouraged to seek the advice of her general practitioner in the first instance as the doctor will in most cases have some background knowledge of the woman and her family relationships, which are almost invariably relevant to the elucidation of gynaecological disorders or concerns.

Furthermore, a woman is less likely to feel shy or embarrassed with her family doctor than when confronting total strangers with what may be a very personal problem. Sometimes however the reverse may apply, especially if the general practitioner is a family friend of many years' standing.

Nevertheless, in most circumstances the general practitioner is in the best position to elucidate symptoms, to advise the patient and if a referral to a gynaecologist is thought to be indicated, to provide the specialist with relevant details and an informed view of the patient's condition.

Family planning/well woman clinics

In times past it was relatively rare for a young woman to seek gynaecological advice other than in connection with pregnancy. In all probability the first time she would have undergone a pelvic examination would have been in early pregnancy and the examination would have been carried out either by the general practitioner or at an antenatal clinic. For the vast majority of healthy women, the postnatal examination would therefore have been the first occasion when the condition of the pelvic organs had been assessed in their non-pregnant state, albeit within a short time after confinement. These circumstances may explain certain traditional misapprehensions about the effect of pregnancy on pelvic anatomy.

It was the changing social climate, the wishes and justifiable demands of women themselves and the development of a comprehensive free family planning and screening service which led young women to seek advice and reassurance about their gynaecological health at the beginning of their reproductive career and at regular intervals thereafter. As a result many young women have their first experience of gynaecological consultation and examination not under the stress of worrying symptoms and fear of disease but in the calmer context of seeking contraceptive advice, cervical and breast screening or, perhaps, prepregnancy counselling. Apart from the advantages to the woman of an early familiarity with what is involved in a gynaecological consultation and examination, the information gained from the counselling and examination of populations of basically normal young women has proved invaluable in a number of different areas. Knowledge of the background pattern of cervical cytology early in a woman's sexual career is an obvious example as is the discovery of symptomless congenital anomalies of the genital tract and variations in normal anatomy. But the principal value of a network of family planning and well woman clinics is clearly the service that they render to the individual woman; population studies and epidemiological information are a vital but secondary byproduct.

HOSPITAL CONSULTATIONS

Gynaecological outpatient clinics

In 'ideal' circumstances women referred to a gynaecological outpatient clinic will be those with a specific gynaecological problem for which a general practitioner is seeking specialist advice. In such cases the patient will already have had an opportunity to explain her symptoms in the more informal atmosphere of her doctor's surgery and in many cases, though not invariably, will also have undergone a pelvic examination. According to circumstances a doctor might find it preferable to avoid a gynaecological examination in the surgery due perhaps to the difficulty of providing a chaperone or because the patient feels shy or embarrassed. Such a problem is also likely to arise if a male doctor visits a patient at home even though early examination of a patient with acute symptoms could be highly informative.

A visit to a gynaecological outpatient clinic is a daunting experience for any woman of whatever age and by whichever means she has been advised to see a gynaecologist. Depending on the reasons for the referral she is already likely, before coming to the hospital, to be anxious about her symptoms and their significance. This can be said to be true of any patient sent to see a specialist but there are particular fears surrounding a gynaecological referral which must be appreciated by all the staff involved including receptionists, nurses, laboratory and X-ray staff as well as the clinicians themselves. A woman with gynaecological symptoms which are often of an intimate nature may have deep inner worries about their effects upon her sexuality, marital relationship and fertility. Older women in particular will be fearful of the possibility of cancer which, in the gynaecological field, carries frightening overtones of loss of womanhood due to the disease itself and also its treatment. Similar considerations apply to patients referred with possible malignant disease of the breast, and workers in that field need also to be aware of the woman's anxiety, as well as other doctors, including gynaecologists, who may see the patient first.

A patient referred to a hospital gynaecologist for the first time will also be uneasy about the prospect of discussing details of her personal history with a total stranger — probably male — in unfamiliar surroundings and possibly in the presence of medical students. Much of this anticipatory apprehension can be dispelled by providing the patient with adequate information well in advance of the outpatient appointment. A clear explanation by the general practitioner of the reason for the hospital referral, together with a 'thumbnail sketch' of the consultant concerned will help to allay anxiety. In addition most hospitals now supply an information leaflet when sending details of the appointment. Such a leaflet can be attractively produced, conveying in clear welcoming terms the flavour of the hospital, the layout of the outpatient clinic and precise details of when and where the patient is to attend.

Many institutions in addition to designated teaching hospitals are involved in the training of undergraduate and postgraduate students and this should be specifically mentioned in the information leaflet so that the patient can be prepared in advance and is aware that she can be seen without students if she so desires. This point should also be raised by the general practitioner, but if the need for the training of students is put across in a positive and constructive way most patients, even those attending gynaecological clinics, are willing to take part. In the same way that decisions over management are increasingly being seen as a partnership between patient and doctor, this sharing of roles can be extended into the parallel process of medical education where the patient can be seen to play as vital a part as the medical teacher in helping to produce the next generation of doctors and specialists.

For many women the thought of being examined gynaecologically by a male doctor is another burden to bear when attending a hospital clinic for the first time. For a few the prospect is unacceptable for religious or cultural reasons or on the grounds of women's rights. In the former category are women, usually of the Muslim faith, for whom personal modesty is intrinsically bound up with their religious upbringing and in such cases every effort should be made to provide the services of a female doctor who has the requisite specialist experience. It is preferable for these matters to be discussed with the general practitioner before an appointment is made in case special arrangements are required or even for referral to another clinic or hospital.

The consultation

The special circumstances of a gynaecological consultation compared with other hospital attendances demand extra care on the part of all concerned with the running of the clinic.

A gynaecological patient, already perhaps consumed with fear and worry, will agonize still more if she has to wait an inordinate length of time before seeing a doctor. Sometimes delays are inevitable but a simple and reassuring explanation to waiting patients can do much to alleviate stress.

The history

The taking of a gynaecological history is an exercise requiring tact, experience and skill in equal measure. It is estimated that in over 70% of cases careful evaluation of symptoms alone will enable a confident gynaecological diagnosis to be made before any physical examination is carried out. History-taking therefore is all-important and should be conducted in a calm and unhurried manner so as to put a nervous and anxious patient at her ease. Disorders of the female genital tract give rise to a relatively small range of gynaecological symptoms, e.g. menstrual disorders, pain and discharge, but their effects upon the patient's general physical and emotional health may be profound and also quite different from one patient to another, even though superficially the gynaecological complaint is identical. The similarity in the brief details given in referral letters for a symptom such as menorrhagia may conceal a wide variety of clinical states and the way in which a patient describes her symptoms, her appearance and manner whilst so doing and her rapport with her questioner will enhance the value of the information obtained, which must be to the patient's ultimate benefit.

As in other branches of medicine gynaecological history-taking can be easy or difficult. At the one extreme are patients with relatively clear-cut symptoms such as the finding of a lump in the abdomen, 'something coming down' in the vagina or the sudden onset of postmenopausal bleeding. Such events are relatively easy for the patient to describe and for the doctor (or student) to set down. At the other end of the scale is the woman with a complex menstrual problem perhaps stretching back over months or even years and involving variations in cycle length and patterns of bleeding already subjected to a number of different treatments. Such a complicated history may be as taxing for a patient to put across as it is for the doctor to record in a reasonably concise form, especially as in cases which go back over a period of time the patient may understandably have difficulty in recalling the sequence of events with any accuracy. Some women, perhaps prompted by their general practitioners, will have made some written notes or marked their diaries, which can be very helpful at least for the immediate past, though even the most practised history-taker's heart will sink at the sight of a patient grasping a sheaf of closely written stationery chronicling her history in exhaustive detail. Although such documents are intended by the patient to be factually helpful to herself and the gynaecologist they are more revealing as an indication of her attitude to and preoccupation with her disorder and its effects upon her life. This may be relevant in choosing between alternative forms of treatment.

To assist in unravelling a complicated gynaecological history, it is tempting to resort to the use of an itemized history sheet so that all aspects can be covered in the form of a checklist. Such a system, though well intentioned, is not advisable as it encourages history-taking by rote, appears to give equal weight to all items and therefore results in a two-dimensional picture of the patient's condition. If on the other hand the gynaecologist (and the student in training) learns to face a gynaecological patient with an open mind and a blank sheet of paper, a more useful account of her condition is likely to emerge in which the patient's principal complaints and concerns are highlighted and other aspects of her history are given the perspective and validity that they warrant. In this regard a doctor's letter, as mentioned above, may give little indication of the strength of a patient's complaint if several factors, e.g. bleeding, pain, discharge etc. are set down with no indication of their relative significance.

A further issue peculiar to gynaecological patients is that women may seek a consultant referral in the hope of obtaining help for deep-seated emotional, sexual and marital problems even if they have no overt physical disorder. For various reasons such patients may feel that a specialist can help them more easily than a general practitioner either because the latter is too familiar a figure or because a hospital clinician is seen to have more easy access to counselling services, psychiatrists etc. Such a situation will soon be revealed to an experienced gynaecologist who will discover that the patient has obtained a referral from her general practitioner on the spurious grounds of, say, a minor menstrual disturbance as a 'cry for help'.

Two recent examples in the author's experience relating to events long past illustrate this use of a gynaecological referral by the patient to obtain access to a therapeutic environment. The first is a patient aged 48 with eight living children and a history of three or four first-trimester miscarriages. In addition, between the sixth and seventh successful pregnancies there was an intrauterine death of the fetus at 24 weeks. The doctor's letter mentioned that the patient was worried about an increase in the length of her cycle from 28 to 40 days and also occasional hot flushes. After being seen, examined and reassured the woman, who had not attended the hospital since the birth of her eighth child 13 years earlier, revealed the genuine reason for her visit which was to ask for a further explanation for the fetal death at 24 weeks. Despite the subsequent births of her seventh and eighth children and the lapse of almost 20 years this woman had been unable to resolve the loss of her baby and was at last seeking to do so.

The second example of a contrived referral is a patient

aged 23 referred with a complaint of a non-offensive, non-irritant white vaginal discharge. The initial history taken by a medical student noted a termination of pregnancy at the age of 18, a spontaneous first-trimester abortion at the age of 20 and an attack of presumed pelvic inflammation at the age of 22. During the consultation the patient was asked whether she had made a rapid recovery from the termination of pregnancy and in replying she made the almost casual observation that she knew she was 'damned forever' for what she had done. This vehement and startling phrase uncovered the real as opposed to the spurious reason for the hospital attendance, and after being interviewed at length by the departmental nurse counsellor the patient was referred for psychiatric and psychotherapeutic help.

Such cases, in which a relatively trivial complaint is used as a lever towards a specialist consultation, have to be distinguished from the many patients with gynaecological symptoms which are known to be stress-related or to have an emotional basis in some cases. These include disorders of menstruation, abdominal and pelvic pain, non-infective vaginal discharge, dyspareunia and certain urinary symptoms.

A sensitive and experienced clinician will be aware of all these factors which could have a profound influence on the pattern of this first encounter with an anxious patient. Setting aside for the moment the information available from other sources, including any notes that the patient may have previously made, the doctor should encourage her to describe her symptoms or problems in the order of their importance or significance to her.

The order in which a patient chooses to 'state her business' is not necessarily the most convenient for the doctor to set down. Scientific training encourages a logical and sequential approach to a problem but the form in which the patient gives her history may be as significant as its content and this should be reflected in the doctor's written notes. A truthful summary of what the patient actually said is more likely to emerge from open note-taking than from the use of printed forms which, though superficially convenient, are limiting and restrictive.

The symptoms

The diagnostic significance of individual gynaecological symptoms is discussed in appropriate detail in the relevant sections of this work. As part of this survey of clinical method in gynaecology some general comments are offered as an aid to the clinical approach to the patient at her first visit rather than during the later processes of investigation and management.

Certain symptoms and complaints are seen by the general public and doctors alike as being unquestionably the province of the gynaecologist. These include disorders of menstruation; complications of pregnancy and childbirth; questions relating to contraception and abortion; fertility problems; symptoms and signs originating in the pelvis and lower genital tract; menopausal symptoms, and certain sexual problems if thought to be of a physical rather than a psychological nature, such as coital pain and difficulty, and possibly loss of libido. The latter symptoms, which merge with the allied fields of psychiatry and psychosexual medicine, are an appropriate bridge into complaints which may be more or less relevant to other specialties. Abdominal pain for example is an extremely common reason for a gynaecological referral either before or after the patient has been seen by a general surgeon or physician or other specialist. This also applies to the finding of a lump in the abdomen either by the patient herself or by a doctor examining her for another purpose. A patient may sometimes reach the gynaecologist with symptoms apparently due to disorders of gastric or intestinal function, including heartburn and alterations in bowel habit, in which pain is not a prominent symptom but which might nevertheless be related to or caused by gynaecological disease. A notorious example is the commonplace symptom of dyspepsia which may be the first presentation of ovarian cancer.

Disorders of urinary function in women are increasingly associated both in the public and professional mind with diseases or displacements of the female genital tract as evidenced by the development of urological gynaecology as a gynaecological subspecialty. Consequently there is common ground between urologists and gynaecologists in evaluating the significance of urinary symptoms in women, who may present themselves or be referred initially to either specialty for investigation.

In certain countries of the world, notably North America and Europe, management of disease of the breast is seen as a part of routine gynaecological practice. Fortunately this is not so in the UK where such an important field of practice is seen to merit the undivided attention of specialist surgeons. Nevertheless a woman who has found a lump in her breast is sometimes seen first by a gynaecologist who would be wise to refer the patient onwards with all speed if any pathology is suspected. Apart from the presentation of a patient complaining of a lump, a gynaecological examination should always include examination of the breasts even in the absence of any relevant symptoms (see below). Patients with mastalgia and mastitis are 'shared' more commonly between breast surgeons and gynaecologists who can learn from each other's experience in the management of these difficult clinical problems (see Chapters 26 and 35).

These observations on the inter-relationship between gynaecology and allied specialties serve to illustrate that far from practising in a restricted field, the gynaecologist requires a wide understanding of the ways in which disorders of other systems may present with symptoms suggesting a gynaecological origin, for example, endocrine disease, certain psychiatric disorders and chronic infections presenting as primary disorders of menstrual function. Furthermore the genital tract may become involved in disease processes originating elsewhere, such as direct spread of infection or cancer from other intra-abdominal structures, or by secondary tumours. Conversely, the experienced gynaecologist is aware that disorders of the female genital tract including cancer may first present with symptoms and signs referable to other body systems (e.g. skin, hair, digestive and urinary tracts). This awareness must be shared with general practitioner and other specialist colleagues to avoid undue delay in the diagnosis and treatment of conditions such as functioning ovarian tumours and cancer of the ovary, endometrium and cervix.

To complete this discussion of gynaecological history-taking the commonly encountered group of symptoms loosely covered by the term 'disorders of menstrual function' can be used to illustrate some of the problems and pitfalls in unravelling and interpreting gynaecological symptoms. A complaint of heavy periods is the commonest abnormality of menstrual bleeding for which a woman seeks medical advice. Menorrhagia may take the form of heavier than usual loss without an alteration in the length of her period, the usual daily flow continuing for longer or a combination of the two. Although heavy flooding with the passage of clots is the more dramatic event a woman may be more inconvenienced by a prolongation of her period from say 5 to 10 days, even if the daily loss is no greater than before, because of the disturbance to her daily life and interference with sexual activity. It is important to establish whether the menstrual cycle has remained regular despite the increased bleeding in view of the more serious pathological significance of irregular loss. An accurate description of the last 6 months of her cycles or a menstrual chart or diary kept for this period of time is very helpful. Accompanying symptoms suggestive of anaemia should be sought but if none are present and the woman is found to have a normal haemoglobin concentration it does not mean that her story should be doubted or disbelieved.

The amount and type of sanitary protection required during a given period is an indication of blood loss but is largely dependent upon a woman's fastidiousness and personal hygiene and therefore of limited objective value. In a classic menorrhagia due say to uterine fibroids the monthly loss is usually similar from period to period though there is likely to be a worsening over time. In such cases it is relatively easy for a woman to be certain that the cycle remains regular which she will sometimes judge not by the date of commencement of each period but by the number of 'clear' days in between. The difficulty arises when the amount and duration of bleeding varies from month to month so the patient may find it impossible to be sure of the overall cycle length. In these circumstances it is wiser to assume an irregular bleeding pattern and to investigate the case accordingly.

The gynaecologist should remember that the majority of women will tend to regard any form of vaginal bleeding, however bizarre, in menstrual terms. 'My periods are more frequent', 'I am getting two periods every month', 'My periods are all over the place', 'I don't know where I am with my periods' are commonly heard phrases used by women in describing irregular bleeding for which the explanation may range from the trivial to the deadly. Rather than trying to disentangle the cases of irregular but 'normal' menstruation from the rest it is far wiser to assume that any patient with irregular bleeding requires further investigation, including in most cases curettage. This need not include a brief irregularity in young women and girls or cases where the cycle has slightly shortened resulting in minor inconvenience only.

A similar approach should be used for women with perimenopausal and postmenopausal bleeding for whom further investigation including diagnostic curettage is obligatory. It is pointless to intellectualize as to whether a given episode of bleeding within a few weeks or months of what was thought to be the last period is or is not a return to menstruation. Even if the description is suggestive of a period the endometrium must be explored without delay. When bleeding has occurred many months or years after the menopause no doubts about the need for curettage are entertained even if there are obvious signs of atrophic vaginitis. It is incidentally sometimes the case that a woman will ignore persistent postmenopausal bleeding, assuming that her recent smear test has excluded uterine as well as cervical cancer—a salutary failure of health education.

'Dysfunctional' menstrual abnormalities tend to be variable, intermittent and often self-limiting. Many general practitioners are aware of this and will have assessed, observed and treated women with these conditions. In other circumstances a woman may be referred for a gynaecological opinion as soon as she goes to see her doctor either because the doctor prefers to avoid examining and treating women with gynaecological complaints for reasons already discussed or because the patient is similarly unwilling to be treated at the surgery. Sometimes the patient's symptoms have resolved by the time of consultation and although it is regrettable that delays occur, there is no doubt that the passage of time can resolve many minor disorders of menstruation as well as other symptoms including abdominal and pelvic pain and vaginal discharge. What is perhaps surprising is that a woman who is no longer complaining usually still prefers to keep the appointment in order to be seen, examined and reassured by a specialist.

The cycle length and any irregularity or intermenstrual bleeding together with dysmenorrhoea should be enquired about. Any oral contraception, hormones or other drugs should be recorded. Pathological features of vaginal discharge, such as colour, odour or pruritus should be noted. The presence of superficial or deep dyspareunia and symptoms related to prolapse should also be recorded.

Often, acute or chronic abdominal pain is a presenting symptom. The length of history, duration of pain, frequency, character, localization, aggravation or improvement by bowel action, micturition or menstruation and interference with work and analgesia which relieves it should all be noted.

Prolapse, in addition to producing backache and a feeling of something coming down, may produce bladder symptoms of stress incontinence and recurrent urinary tract infection (if incomplete emptying occurs) and occasionally frequency and urgency, and bowel symptoms with incomplete bowel emptying.

Finally the past history should include all pregnancies and major abdominal and pelvic surgery. With bowel or urinary symptoms, a history of spinal injury or surgery is important.

It is a popular myth that women who are menstruating should not attend the gynaecological clinic but should defer the appointment to a more appropriate time in the month. In most circumstances this is a reasonable decision as a woman who is having her period will naturally prefer not to undergo a pelvic examination at a time when she will be particularly sensitive and embarrassed.

She will also assume that it is distasteful for a doctor to have to carry out an examination when she is menstruating. A cervical smear and colposcopy have to be postponed. But this 'menstrual taboo' carries great potential danger of delayed diagnosis where there is abnormal vaginal bleeding. All gynaecologists can quote examples of the consequences of postponing consultations on these grounds, such as the author's recollection of a woman aged 51 who had been bleeding from a carcinoma of the cervix for 5 months before coming to hospital and a younger woman who, on being eventually seen in the gynaecological clinic, was found to have intermittent claudication due to profound anaemia (haemoglobin 5 g/dl) from prolonged bleeding, albeit of benign aetiology.

Gynaecological examination

Care should be taken to reduce embarrassment by conducting the examination in a quiet and thoughtful manner, in the presence only of a nurse chaperone and, with the patient's consent, one other person receiving instructions, usually the student who has taken the history. It should not be necessary to stress the need for the examination to be conducted in privacy in a single clinic room set aside for the purpose.

For a satisfactory gynaecological examination sufficient clothing should be loosened or removed to enable the supraclavicular region, the breasts and axillae, the abdomen and the pelvis to be inspected and examined fully. In many cases an entirely satisfactory examination can take place without the need for the patient to remove much of her own clothing other than her underwear. Elementary sensitivity on the part of the doctor and nurse would also ensure that the patient is not needlessly exposed during the course of the examination. It is unnecessary for example for the breasts to remain uncovered whilst the abdomen is being examined; similarly the simple gesture of keeping the patient's legs covered whilst she is lying on the couch will be much appreciated.

Before beginning the examination the doctor must explain to the patient exactly what is to be done, also asking permission for the student or other trainee to be present and, if appropriate, to take part in the examination. During the examination of the upper part of the body the patient should be sitting or semi-recumbent with the upper end of the couch elevated.

A great deal can be learned by preliminary observation of the patient with regard to her general appearance, build and nutritional state and also her mood, degree of anxiety and attitude to her gynaecological complaint. Much of the latter will have been gathered during the taking of her history but if this was carried out by another person the doctor should spend a few moments going over the main points with the patient, not necessarily to obtain further information but principally to enter into a dialogue and to gauge her feelings. Observation is also very important for patients with subacute and acute gynaecological symptom with respect to the degree of pain, additional factors such as shortness of breath and also the emotional state.

For patients referred with acute problems to the Accident and Emergency Department or admitted at once to the gynaecological ward the examination will necessarily focus on the area concerned, usually the abdomen, for such conditions as acute pelvic infection, ruptured ectopic pregnancy, torsion etc.

Examination of the breasts

This is an essential part of any gynaecological examination and should only be omitted if they have recently been examined either at a well woman or family planning clinic or if the patient is under regular surveillance at a breast clinic. It is also unnecessary to increase the embarrassment of a young girl by exposing the breasts for examination unless she has relevant symptoms. Palpation of the axillae is an integral part of breast examination but it takes very little extra effort also to palpate the supraclavicular regions: an obligatory step for any patient known or suspected to have malignant disease, especially of the ovary.

Abdominal examination

Systematic abdominal examination should be carried out with the patient lying almost flat; the head end of the couch remains slightly raised or higher if the patient is elderly or has a cardiac or respiratory problem. A good deal can be learned from abdominal inspection alone. If pain is a symptom the patient is asked to indicate its approximate site even if she is currently painfree. It is also helpful to know at the outset of areas of probable tenderness. Before palpation the examiner should spend a few moments observing the abdomen to note its shape and size, the degree of distension, the presence and condition of operation scars and also the movement of the abdomen with respiration. The latter is particularly relevant in acute abdominal conditions which often cause restriction of abdominal movement due to pain but may also serve as a pointer to the presence of ascites or tumours affecting the normal excursion of the diaphragm and abdominal wall with respiration. Typically, space-occupying lesions arising in the pelvis will produce lower abdominal distension either from the presence of the tumour itself or as a result of upward displacement of bladder or bowel. Such distension is commonly uniform (symmetrical) even with lesions arising unilaterally as adnexal masses tend to grow towards the midline as they increase in size. In the case of large tumours abdominal distension will be immediately obvious, the entire abdomen being occupied with what at first sight would pass for a full-term pregnancy.

In times past, before abdominal surgery was commonplace, the term ovarian cachexia was used to describe the appearance of a woman with all the hallmarks of advanced malnutrition—namely hollow, sunken features and spindly arms and legs with gross abdominal distension—due to a vast but, typically, benign ovarian cyst seriously interfering with all bodily activity including respiration and digestion. Such sights are rare in the developed world; but all too common is the woman with advanced ovarian carcinoma whose appearance resembles the ovarian cachexia of old but with the addition of a tense, shiny abdominal wall with its tracery of dilated vessels, and not infrequently a visible mass in the (left) supraclavicular fossa.

Whether or not such dramatic signs are present, the gynaecologist now proceeds to a systematic palpation of the abdomen, bearing in mind the patient's complaint and sites of pain or likely tenderness. Areas of tenderness or swelling which are likely to be due to lesions originating in the pelvis are delineated. Gynaecologists should have an easy familiarity with palpation of the liver edge and the area of the kidneys, both of which are highly relevant in the diagnosis and follow-up of gynaecological cancer, but upper abdominal palpation is also important as an omental mass may be the most prominent sign of ovarian malignancy. Palpation of the spleen is not part of a routine gynaecological examination but may be relevant with certain tropical diseases and haematological disorders.

It is usual to palpate the abdomen with the flat of the hand, lightly at first, proceeding from above downwards, leaving areas of pain or suspected tenderness to the last. In many cases light palpation will be sufficient to outline significant abdominal masses and the presence of ascites, the latter reinforced by the classic signs of eversion of the umbilicus, shifting dullness and a fluid 'thrill'. Deeper palpation, which should be performed slowly and deliberately rather than with a disconcerting jabbing movement, is then used to detect less obvious swellings at or just above the pubic symphysis, to explore the iliac fossae and the para-aortic regions. Abdominal examination is not complete without palpation of the inguinofemoral regions and the hernial orifices.

Characteristically an abdominal mass originating in the pelvis is usually lower abdominal, mainly midline, with a margin definable laterally and above but not below, and which does not move on respiration. Apart from the last, these findings can vary from case to case. Very large masses will, of course, reach above the umbilicus and the largest tumours, which tend to be ovarian rather than uterine, may fill the abdomen so completely that it is not possible to define the borders accurately or to decide whether the origin is pelvic, upper abdominal or retroperitoneal. In these cases the absence of movement on respiration is especially useful to distinguish a mass arising from below rather than above.

Most pelvic swellings adopt a midline position as they rise into the abdomen even if their origin is adnexal. This applies particularly to benign, mobile ovarian cysts which tend to float medially on their pedicles as they enlarge upwards. Unilateral swellings are characteristic of certain subserous fibroids, malignant lesions which have become fixed to surrounding structures and also, notably, broad ligament cysts which can rarely be distinguished from ovarian lesions before surgery apart from this one characteristic feature. The inability to 'get below' a pelvic tumour on abdominal palpation is a reasonably constant finding but it may not apply in the case of an ovarian mass of moderate size which may be sufficiently mobile on its pedicle to float upwards out of the pelvis leaving a well defined lower border which can be easily outlined. This mobility is most striking under general anaesthesia when the relaxation of the abdominal wall increases the prominence of such tumours which on palpation can be 'chased' around the abdominal cavity as if free from any internal attachments. A classic example of this is the dysgerminoma, a solid germ cell tumour occurring predominantly in young girls and which may be associated with immature sexual development. Palpation of this lesion under anaesthesia gives the odd impression of chasing a children's ball around the abdominal cavity.

Percussion of the abdomen is often neglected. Apart from the detection of ascites by the sign of shifting dullness or mapping out the liver margin there is a reluctance to use percussion as a natural extension of palpation in outlining any abdominal swelling, whether due to a pregnancy or otherwise. In early pregnancy, the soft border of a uterus which has just begun to rise up into the abdomen may be difficult to feel but easily defined by percussion; in late pregnancy when the uterus, at first sight, appears to occupy the whole abdomen, percussion may be more helpful than palpation in identifying the upper edge of the uterus as it merges with the resonant bowel above. The gynaecologist should percuss the abdomen as a matter of course and as an automatic adjunct to palpation and should pass on the easily acquired skill to students and trainees. Differential diagnosis, though a serious matter, can occasionally provide an opportunity for lighthearted rivalry between clinicians and the demonstration that an 'ovarian cyst' is, in reality, a volvulus of the bowel can provide the occasional small but resonant triumph over a general surgical colleague.

Pelvic examination

Clinical examination of the pelvis is of central significance in gynaecological practice. For the doctor it is the key to gynaecological diagnosis; for the patient it symbolizes her vulnerability as a woman placing herself, quite literally, in medical hands.

Historically, illustrations of the methods of vaginal examination whether for obstetric or gynaecological purposes invariably depicted the patient fully clothed, often with voluminous skirts, beneath which the respectful doctor, ceremoniously posed, proceeded with the examination without laying eyes on the genitalia: the woman meanwhile, often richly dressed and wearing a bonnet, would be looking away with an air of supreme indifference (Figs 7.1 and 7.2). Whether these charming and more than faintly comical illustrations truly reflect gynaecological practice of a bygone era is a matter of conjecture.

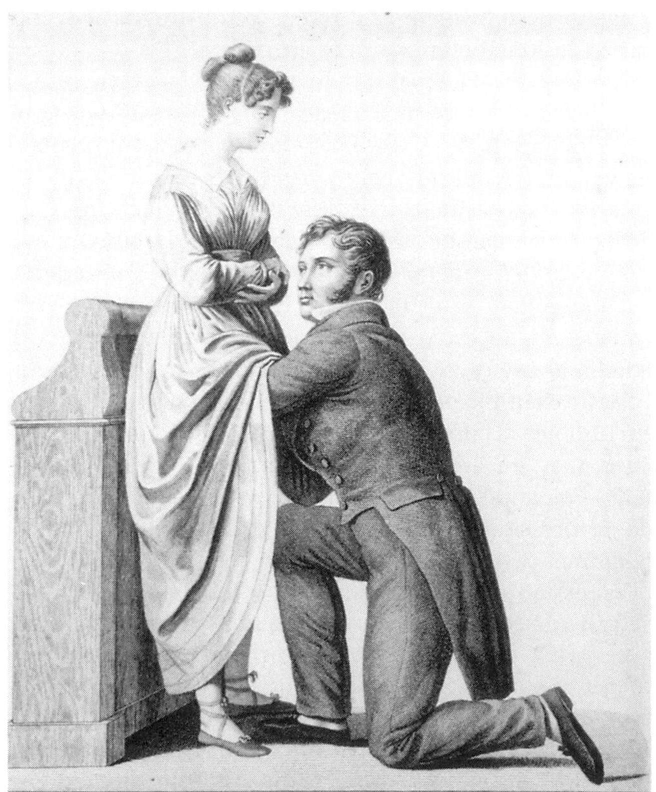

Fig. 7.1 *Toucher la femme debout*: examination of the woman standing up. From Maygrier (1822) with permission.

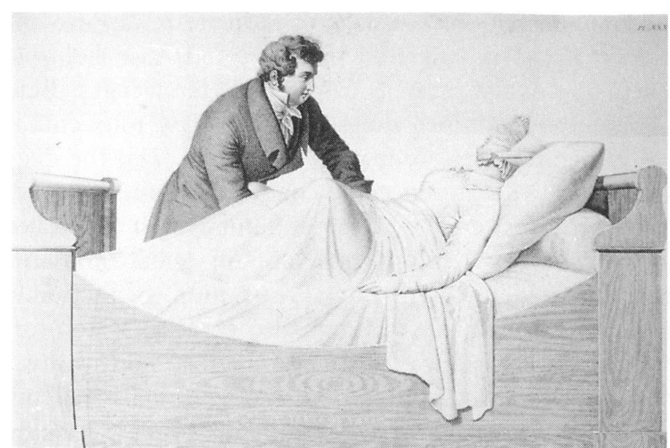

Fig. 7.2 *Toucher en position horizontale*: examination in the horizontal position. From Maygrier (1822) with permission.

Although current attitudes have displaced Victorian prudery, exposure of the vulva will remain an acutely uncomfortable experience for most women and should therefore be minimized yet sufficient to allow an adequate visual inspection of the pubic, vulval and perineal areas. In the author's view, this can best be achieved with the patient lying on her left side with the right hip and knee flexed to 90° and the left hip and knee flexed a few degrees only. When the patient is lying in this way in what is sometimes described as the modified Sims' position it is possible to carry out a full inspection of the vulva and perineum during which the patient can lie in relative comfort with her hips and thighs covered and without needing to 'open her legs' as would be the case if she were lying on her back. The latter position, which is preferred by three-quarters of the gynaecologists in the UK (Amias 1987), gives the fullest exposure of the vulva, as well as allowing access for a bimanual examination.

Speculum examination

The ability to use a vaginal speculum with skill and gentleness is a fundamental requirement for any doctor undertaking clinical gynaecology. For many women the speculum represents the most distasteful aspect of pelvic examination which can be minimized by prior explanation and a confident but gentle technique. Whilst inspecting the vulva and adjacent structures for abnormalities of the labia, perineum and introitus a judgement is made of the size of speculum required based on the appearance of the introitus and also taking into account the patient's age and parity. Sometimes it is helpful to insert a finger a short distance

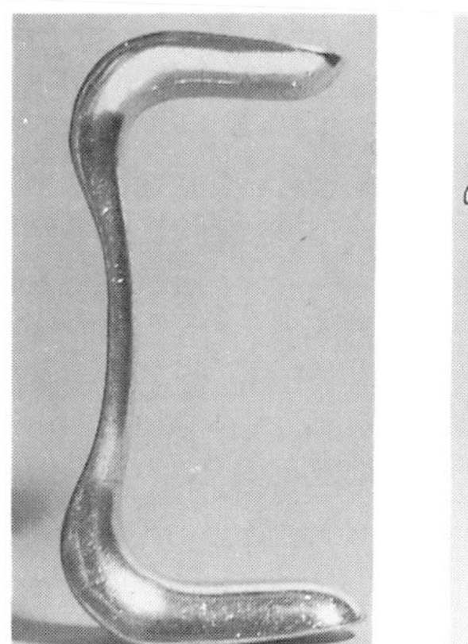

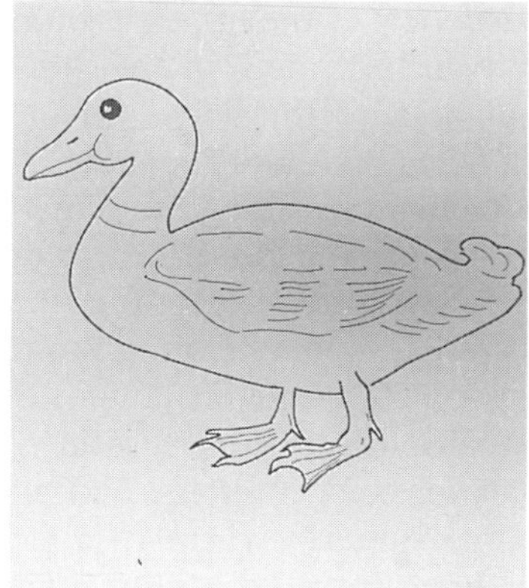

Fig. 7.3 Sims' (duck-billed) speculum.

into the vagina to make sure that the choice of instrument is appropriate.

Choice of speculum is a question of type of instrument as well as size. From a survey of British gynaecological practice, the author estimates that about 85% of consultants regularly use some form of bivalve (Cusco-type) speculum with only a small minority preferring the duck-billed (Sims'-type) as their instrument of first choice (Fig. 7.3). Both of these instruments are found in all gynaecological clinics, variously modified from the traditional pattern. In the British survey six varieties of bivalve speculum in current use were described, three of which are shown in Figure 7.4, the others being relatively minor modifications of those illustrated. The common feature of all these instruments, whether the traditional Cusco's, the plastic disposable type or the Brewer or Semm illuminated speculum, is that the handle and opening mechanism are designed to be held against the perineum rather than the pubis. The instruments are constructed so that the intended posterior blade rotates, swivels or slides

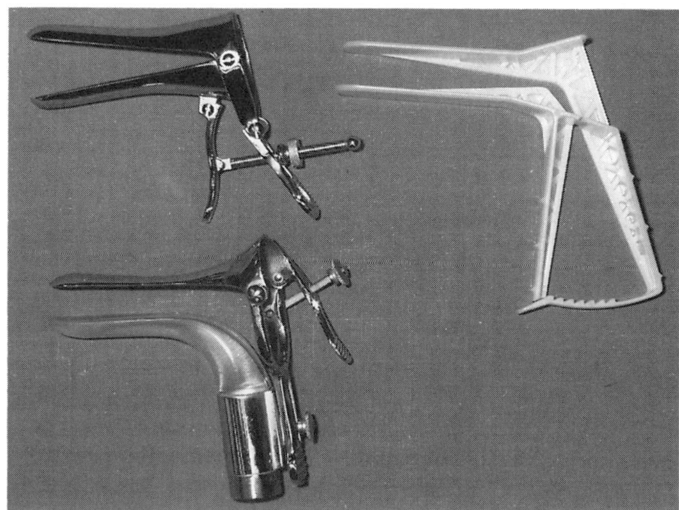

Fig. 7.4 Three varieties of bivalve speculum.

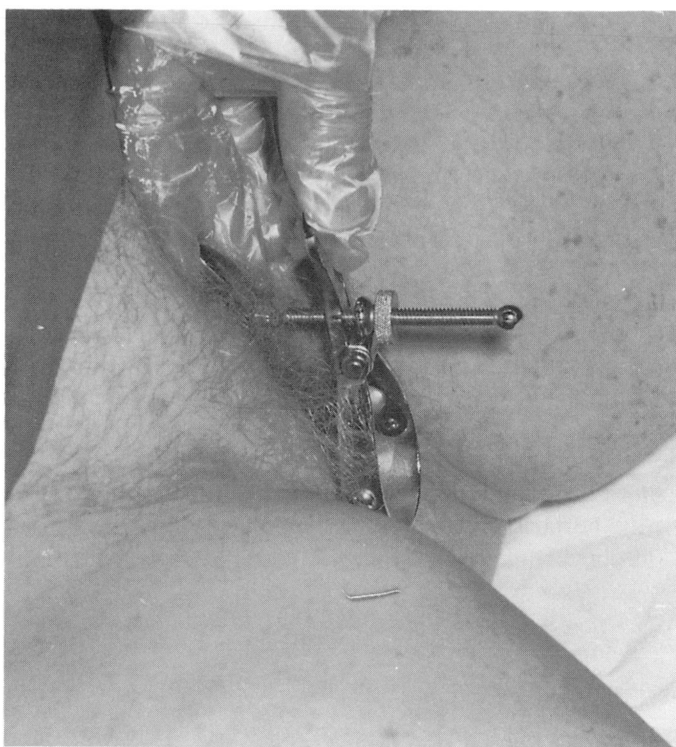

Fig. 7.5 Bivalve speculum inserted with the patient in the dorsal position.

on the relatively fixed anterior blade which is in one piece with the viewing aperture. Thus, when the instrument is correctly placed with the handle rearwards the pressure of the widening blades is exerted not forwards against the highly sensitive urethra, clitoris and mons pubis but against the less sensitive posterior vaginal wall and perineum (Amias 1984, 1987). This is most naturally achieved with the patient lying on her left side but is the practice adopted by only one-quarter of British gynaecologists.

Most commonly the bivalve speculum is inserted with the patient lying in the dorsal (supine position) with the handles 'back to front' held against part of the vulva and pubis (Fig. 7.5). Unless great care is taken this can be extremely uncomfortable for the patient, especially when the blades are widened and the opening mechanism is pressed against the clitoris and pubic hair.

The bivalve speculum suitably warmed and of appropriate size is the most generally used instrument for naked-eye inspection of the vagina and cervix and also for certain minor procedures including colposcopy, cryocautery or 'cold' coagulation of the cervix and the insertion of intrauterine contraceptive devices. A convenient method of warming speculums is to use a small waterbath of the type used to heat a baby's feeding bottle.

Before passing the speculum, the examiner should take care to part the labia with the left hand so that the warmed and lubricated instrument can be inserted through the introitus without catching or pulling in any skin edges in the process. This technique avoids the unpleasant practice of placing the blades along the line of the labia and then twisting the instrument 90° into position.

For the purposes of inspection of the vagina and cervix and the taking of cervical smears the speculum does not need to be locked in an open position and there is more to be gained by varying the pressure on the handles to bring into view all parts of the vagina as the instrument is slowly withdrawn. Used in this way the bivalve speculum is an all-purpose single-handed instrument, unlike the Sims' speculum which requires both hands or the assistance of another person.

In 1845 James Marion Sims (1813–1883) suspecting a major pelvic injury in a woman thrown from her horse hurriedly purchased a pewter spoon from the local general store, bent it to a right angle and used it to obtain an unimpeded view of the upper vagina and cervix. This event was the twin birth both of the Sims' speculum and Sims' position because the horsewoman lay semi-prone where she had fallen and the ballooning of the vagina due to negative abdominal pressure gave to this inspired American country practitioner the key at last to operative access for the cure of vesicovaginal fistula (Fig. 7.6).

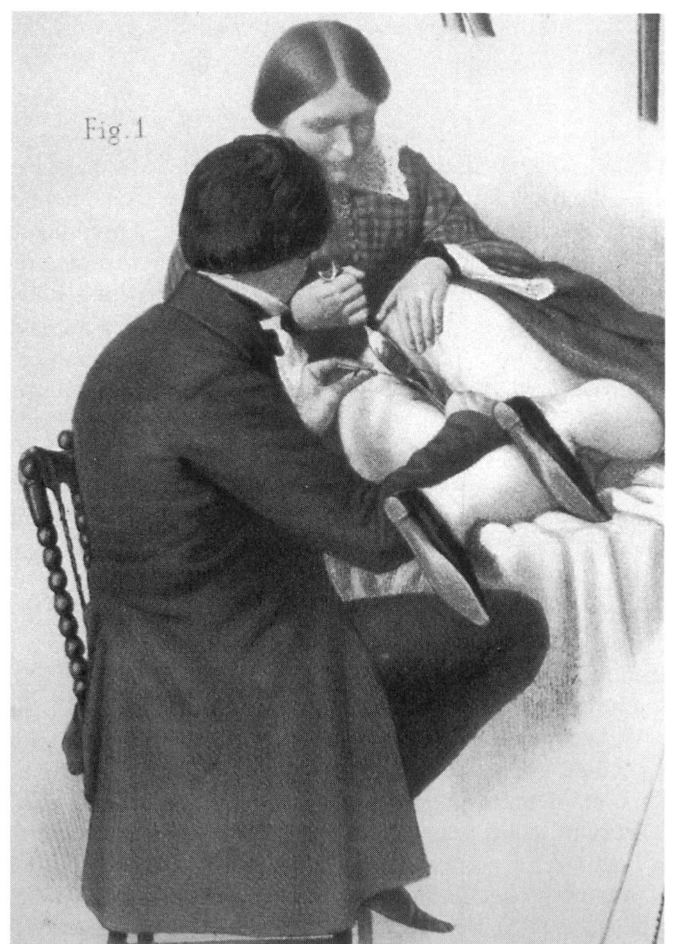

Fig. 7.6 Sims' position for repair of vesicovaginal fistula, using a Sims' speculum. From Savage (1876) with permission.

Nowadays, in operating rooms throughout the world the duck-billed speculum (Fig. 7.3), double- or single-ended and variously modified, is in constant daily use for every dilatation and curettage and all forms of major or minor vaginal surgery, where it is vastly to be preferred to the weighted Auvard speculum, surely now obsolete. Although similarly available in all outpatient clinics, Sims' speculum is rarely the instrument of first choice for clinical examination, being less adaptable than the bivalve speculum, especially for viewing the cervix, because of the need to retract the anterior vaginal wall separately with sponge-holding forceps. For prolapse however Sims' speculum has advantage over Cusco's and even amongst the 'dorsalist majority' of British gynaecologists about one-third will choose the left lateral position to examine a patient with a complaint of prolapse and will change to a Sims' speculum for the purpose.

Fergusson's speculum (Fig. 7.7), now rarely used, was at one time part of the trio of instruments available in most outpatient clinics. Basically a simple metal tube, flanged at the viewing end and cut at an angle at the other, Fergusson's speculum was used to view the cervix rather than the vaginal walls but is now superseded by the other types. It had its heyday in times past when it was the custom to cauterize cervical erosions at the slightest provocation, usually in the postnatal clinic; the speculum afforded much-needed protection of the vaginal walls as the junior doctor moved from couch to couch with the white-hot electrocautery.

Bimanual examination

The final stage of gynaecological examination is bimanual palpation of the pelvis. As for speculum examination, this can be carried out with the patient either in the dorsal or left lateral position according to preference. Flimsy

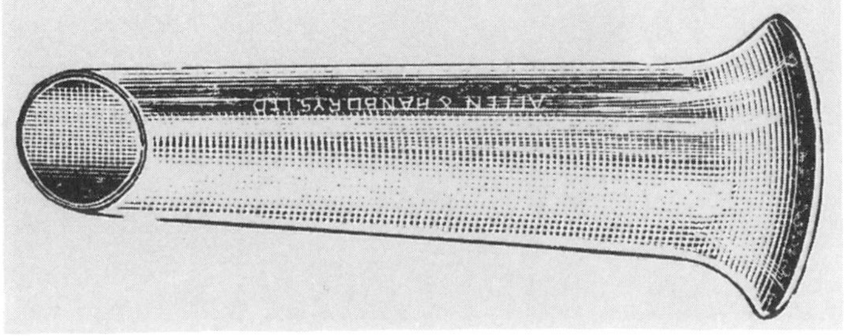

Fig. 7.7 Fergusson's speculum.

transparent plastic gloves have been used for gynaecological examination but in view of the risk of human immunodeficiency virus infection it is now strongly recommended that rubber gloves of operating room quality are used instead.

A well conducted bimanual examination will identify and localize areas of tenderness within the pelvis and lower genital tract, will demonstrate the size, shape, position and mobility of the uterus and cervix and will determine the size and nature of ovarian and other adnexal swellings as well as masses which may be palpable in the pouch of Douglas. In some cases, notably in the diagnosis, assessment and follow-up of pelvic cancer, rectal examination should also be performed. In the case of cervical carcinoma for example it is easier to assess the degree of parametrial involvement by rectal rather than vaginal examination as the examining finger in the rectum has a greater excursion from side to side behind rather than below the cervix, so that each uterosacral ligament can be palpated for its full extent from cervix to lateral pelvic wall.

The relative merits of the dorsal and left lateral positions for gynaecological pelvic examinations have been debated by the author and others (Amias 1984, 1987; Drife 1988). In the British survey conducted by the author, 74% of consultants preferred the supine position for both bimanual and speculum examination, though within this large majority nearly 40% did use the lateral position in special circumstances, notably prolapse.

Within the 26% of consultants favouring the lateral position for speculum examination half of these also conducted bimanual examination with their patients in the same position. The arguments for speculum examination in the left lateral position have been outlined above, particularly in relation to the construction of the instrument and its handling. In addition, the view obtained of the upper vagina due to the slight ballooning effect is especially useful for examination of the vault of the vagina, in assessing prolapse, in planning the route for hysterectomy and in seeking causes for urinary incontinence, including fistulae. Clinicians in the survey also found that the lateral position was helpful in the postoperative review of gynaecological procedures, in recurrent prolapse and, most importantly, for cancer follow-up when a rectal examination is also necessary. The left lateral position is much appreciated by women with limited hip abduction due to arthritis or injury, those with cardiac or respiratory disease or the very elderly who may become very uncomfortable if required to lie on their backs even for a relatively short period of time. Although palpation of the pelvic structures with the patient lying on the left side is more difficult at first, it is a skill worth acquiring as part of the training of all gynaecologists. Even though women have come to expect that they will be examined in the dorsal position when attending a gynaecologist or family planning clinic, clinicians who have been 'brought up' to use this position should be prepared and able to adapt their skills to use the lateral position if circumstances dictate. This will particularly apply in the case of shy or nervous women, including young girls, older nulliparae and members of certain ethnic minorities.

In the final analysis clinical method is an amalgam of upbringing, acquired skills, fashion and habit. In the field of gynaecological examination the method adopted is less important than the manner in which it is performed. If the patient is aware that her doctor is sensitive and understanding she is less likely to find this most intimate of all clinical examinations the unwelcome ordeal that she had anticipated.

KEY POINTS

1. Early screening rather than when the disease is fully developed is important.
2. Pre-consultation information is helpful to allay fears.
3. Minor symptoms may disguise deeper underlying reasons for gynaecological consultation.
4. Inter-relationship with other disciplines is important in the recognition of presentation of other diseases by gynaecological symptoms and conversely, presentation of gynaecological disease by non-gynaecological symptoms.

REFERENCES

Amias A G 1984 Left lateral, please. Lancet ii: 220

Amias A G 1987 Pelvic examination: a survey of British practice. British Journal of Obstetrics and Gynaecology 94: 975–978

Drife J O 1988 Lateral thinking in gynaecology. British Medical Journal 296: 807–808

8. Preoperative care and assessment

J. P. Van Besouw

'Inside every adult is a child afraid of the dark.'
Anonymous

OBJECTIVES

Preoperative preparation for surgery should begin once the surgeon has placed the patient's name on the waiting list. In an ideal world this would involve close co-operation between surgeon and anaesthetist with patient assessment, relevant investigations and the modification of treatment regimens appropriate to the course of surgery and anaesthesia carried out prior to admission; potentially difficult problems should be assessed in an anaesthetic or surgical outpatient clinic (Burn 1976).

Unfortunately the more common practice in the UK is for patients to be admitted the day before surgery, subjected to blanket and often inappropriate investigations with insufficient time to act on results or to change therapies where necessary prior to surgery. It is therefore of paramount importance that the gynaecologist is aware of the precepts of preoperative assessment and the relevant course of action to take in order to improve the efficiency and safety of the system. Preoperative preparation revolves around the following objectives:

1. The evaluation of physical status.
2. Investigations relevant to the course of surgery and anaesthesia.
3. The evaluation of current medication and the modification of therapy where indicated.
4. Consent and counselling prior to surgery.

EVALUATION OF PHYSICAL STATUS

The assignment of a physical status category to patients based upon history and examination can act as a useful language when conferring information to the anaesthetists on their preoperative visit. The most widely used system at present is that recommended by the American Society of Anaesthesiologists (ASA; Table 8.1). In this system patients are placed into one of five categories. Although this is a good indicator of the physical status of the patient prior to surgery, because the nature of the intended surgery is not taken into consideration it is not a good prognosticator of postoperative morbidity and has been criticized (Keats 1978).

Table 8.1 Classification of physical status

Status	Definition
ASA 1	Normal healthy patient — no known organic, biochemical or psychiatric disease
ASA 2	Patient with mild to moderate systemic disease
ASA 3	Patient with severe systemic disease that limits normal activity
ASA 4	Patient with severe systemic disease that is a consistent threat to life
ASA 5	Patient who is moribund and unlikely to survive 24 h

The addition of the letter E, e.g. 2(E), indicates those patients in whom emergency surgery is undertaken.
After American Society of Anaesthesiologists (ASA) 1963.

History

It is important in the preoperative preparation to take a detailed history with particular emphasis on those points relevant to the course of surgery and anaesthesia. This should include details of the presenting complaint, current medication, past medical history etc. The anaesthetist will be interested in any cardiorespiratory problems as well as any adverse reactions to anaesthesia that the patient may have suffered during previous surgery. Some of the more important questions are outlined in Table 8.2 and their relevance to the course of surgery and anaesthesia is detailed in subsequent sections.

Table 8.2 Important questions in an anaesthetic preoperative assessment

System or organ	Condition
Cardiovascular	Angina pectoris Myocardial infarction Rheumatic fever Systemic vascular disease
Respiratory	Acute coryza Exercise tolerance Dyspnoea and orthopnoea Asthma and allergic lung diseases Bronchitis; cough and sputum production Pulmonary infection Pulmonary surgery Smoking
Nervous system	Epilepsy Neuromuscular disease Neuropathy Psychiatric disease including treatment
Liver	Alcohol consumption Hepatitis
Endocrine	Diabetes mellitus Thyroid disease Adrenal disease
Genitourinary	Renal disease Sexually transmitted diseases Menstrual history
Previous anaesthesia	Nausea and vomiting Adverse reactions Postspinal headache Familial problems with anaesthesia

Examination

The importance of a full examination documented in the notes by the house surgeon cannot be overemphasized. The anaesthetist will be interested in signs of respiratory disease including the nature and pattern of respiration, the presence of abnormal breath sounds plus additional signs of respiratory incapacity, e.g. tracheal deviation, cyanosis etc. Simple bedside tests of respiratory function, such as peak expiratory flow measurements, may be useful indicators of respiratory reserve. Cardiovascular examination should include assessment of heart rate and rhythm, auscultation for cardiac murmurs with particular emphasis on diastolic murmurs or the presence of a third or fourth heart sound. The measurement of arterial blood pressure is essential and should be repeated at least twice at intervals if it is found to be elevated. The gynaecologist will obviously be interested in examination pertinent to the presenting complaint. More detailed examination of other systems is dictated by the presence of intercurrent disease. For example, neurological assessment of the patient with multiple sclerosis or assessment of joint mobility in the patient with rheumatoid arthritis is of particular importance if leg stirrups are to be employed.

Intercurrent medical disease

It is not possible or intended to give a comprehensive account of the effects of medical conditions on the course of surgery and anaesthesia but rather to give an overview of problems which are commonly found in patients presenting for surgery and the measures which can be taken in order to ensure that perioperative morbidity is kept to a minimum.

Cardiovascular disease (Foex 1981)

The presence of cardiovascular disease is associated with increased morbidity and mortality following anaesthesia. Evaluation of the severity of the condition and instigation of measures to reduce the incidence of complications is therefore an essential part of preoperative assessment. A number of attempts have been made to identify perioperative risk factors in order to try and improve perioperative morbidity. The most widely known is the cardiac risk index score (Goldman et al 1977; Table 8.3). Patients with a score greater than 13 should receive further medical treatment prior to surgery. The value of this system has however been questioned (Jeffery et al 1983; Pace 1984).

Coronary artery disease. The incidence of coronary

Table 8.3 Preoperative factors relating to the development of postoperative cardiac complications

Factors	Points
Gallop rhythm or elevated jugular venous pressure	11
Myocardial infarction in preceding 6 months	10
Rhythm other than sinus or premature atrial contractions on preoperative electrocardiogram	7
> 5 premature ventricular contractions per minute	7
Age > 70 years	5
Emergency surgery	4
Intraperitoneal, intrathoracic or aortic operation	3
Poor general physical status	3
Significant aortic stenosis	3

After Goldman et al 1977.

artery disease in this country is high and patients may present with a spectrum of conditions from angina pectoris to myocardial infarction. The presence of coronary artery disease is associated with a significant increase in perioperative morbidity and mortality, including an increased incident risk of postoperative reinfarction in individuals presenting for surgery within 3 months of myocardial infarction (Rao et al 1983). The development of angina is indicative of an imbalance between the oxygen demands of the myocardium and the oxygen supply — although not necessarily the severity of coronary arteriosclerosis (Patterson 1985) — and is aggravated by perioperative hypertension or hypotension and tachycardia. Hypertension and tachycardia increase heart work whilst hypotension and tachycardia reduce myocardial perfusion. In the preoperative assessment of these patients it is therefore essential to assess the nature, frequency and duration of the anginal attacks, the efficacy of current medication and where control of symptoms is inadequate a cardiological opinion should be sought. Where possible, elective surgery is best postponed for at least 3 months in individuals who have suffered recent myocardial infarction.

Hypertension. Hypertension has been defined by the World Health Organization as a persistently elevated systolic pressure >160 mmHg and/or a diastolic pressure >95 mmHg. Severe hypertension is present when blood pressure exceeds 180/100 mmHg and is found in 11% of patients presenting for surgery (Foex 1982). Anaesthesia in the presence of uncontrolled hypertension has a significant morbidity and mortality (Goldman & Caldera 1979). Therefore preoperative assessment should determine the adequacy of blood pressure control, the nature of current therapy and assessment of any major organ dysfunction associated with sustained hypertensive disease, notably coronary artery disease, renal disease and cerebrovascular disease. Where hypertension is present then instigation of appropriate treatment is indicated. Where patients have diastolic blood pressure in excess of 120 mmHg, surgery should be postponed as, untreated, they have been shown to exhibit extreme lability of pressure perioperatively (Prys-Roberts 1984).

Valvular heart disease. Valvular heart disease may be congenital or acquired and more commonly affects the left side of the heart, resulting in haemodynamic disturbances in left ventricular function and producing pressure-related disorders secondary to stenotic lesions of the aortic or mitral valves, or volume-related disorders secondary to regurgitant lesions of the same valves. In the preoperative assessment the degree of cardiac reserve must be ascertained by evaluation of patient exercise tolerance and the role of compensatory mechanisms, e.g. increased sympathetic activity and myocardial hypertrophy, in the maintenance of normal cardiac output should be noted. All patients should have prophylactic antibiotics before surgery in order to prevent the development of bacterial endocarditis. The current recommendations for gynaecological surgery are gentamicin 1.5 mg/kg intravenously and ampicillin 1 g intravenously 30 minutes prior to surgery (or on induction of anaesthesia) followed by two further doses at 8 and 16 hours postoperatively. In those individuals who are penicillin-sensitive, erythromycin 500 mg intravenously is given by infusion over 30 minutes before the induction of anaesthesia.

Dysrhythmias. The presence of dysrhythmias may be associated with cardiovascular, renal, pulmonary or metabolic disease or may occur secondary to drug therapy, e.g. digoxin, and may if untreated result in marked haemodynamic disturbance. The frequency of dysrhythmia is increased by perioperative events, such as hypoxia, hypercarbia, alterations in acid–base status or potassium homeostasis. Preoperative assessment should focus on the nature and frequency — whether supraventricular or ventricular — of the dysrhythmia, the correction of any exacerbating conditions and the initiation of appropriate therapy. Heart block of any kind is always due to organic damage to the conducting system and if third-degree or second-degree Mobitz type 2 should be treated with transvenous pacing prior to surgery.

Respiratory disease

The primary function of the lungs is to provide an interface for the exchange of oxygen and carbon dioxide between blood and the atmosphere, a necessary part of the metabolic process. Pulmonary disease has the effect of decreasing the efficiency of this exchange which, in combination with the respiratory depressant effects of anaesthesia and surgery on pulmonary function, results in an increase in postoperative morbidity and mortality (Fowkes et al 1982). Preoperative pulmonary evaluation is mandatory for all patients scheduled for surgery. Preoperative tests of respiratory reserve are dictated by the severity of the presenting symptoms.

Upper respiratory tract infections. It is seldom necessary for patients with upper respiratory tract infections to undergo elective surgery. The infection, combined with the immunosuppressive effects of anaesthesia, the postoperative inhibition of coughing and the sedative effects of narcotic agents used to relieve postoperative pain, increases the risk of developing postoperative viral pneumonia. It is therefore advisable to withhold surgery for at least 2 weeks until recovery is complete.

Obstructive lung disease. This is a heterogeneous group of conditions ranging from bronchitis to asthma which may be chronic or acute, reversible or irreversible and which together constitute the largest single group of respiratory diseases. Preoperative preparation should aim to assess the severity of the condition using a combination of clinical judgement, simple spirometry such as the measurement of vital capacity, forced expiratory volume in one second

(FEV_1) and blood gas analysis where indicated (Rigg & Jones 1978). From the results of those tests appropriate therapy may be instigated. This should include advice on stopping smoking, preoperative physiotherapy, and breathing exercises, the use of bronchodilators in those cases where reversibility is demonstrated and antibiotics for the treatment of any acute exacerbations of chronic bronchitis. It is advisable to repeat these tests following treatment and if necessary to delay surgery until the patient is in an optimum condition. In those patients with severe pulmonary disease where the FEV_1 is $<25\%$ of that predicted, and arterial oxygen tensions are <7.3 kPa in air, the possibility of surgery under regional or local anaesthesia should be entertained.

Restrictive lung disease. This group of pulmonary diseases includes fibrosing alveolitis, sarcoidosis, asbestosis and the pulmonary manifestations of systemic disease, e.g. rheumatoid arthritis and systemic lupus erythematosus and is characterized by a decreased transfer capacity with a restrictive lung volume. The clinical features are of dyspnoea and hypoxia on mild exertion with a normal sensitivity to carbon dioxide; patients are frequently on steroid therapy. Most cases will not be a problem to the anaesthetist; however, any chest infection should be treated before surgery and postoperative oxygen therapy may be necessary.

Diseases of the nervous system

Although there are a large number of neurological diseases, few are of consequence to the course of surgery and anaesthesia; however, problems may be encountered with the following.

Epilepsy. Epilepsy is an expression of a disorder of neuronal function resulting from the excessive synchronous discharge from a focal area of neuronal hyperexcitability. This may present as an expression of a local event, e.g. temporal lobe epilepsy, or spread to the entire cerebral cortex resulting in a generalized seizure. It is advisable for patients to continue with anticonvulsant therapy in the perioperative period and for the anaesthetist to be informed of the epilepsy, as a number of anaesthetic agents predispose to seizure activity.

Multiple sclerosis. This is a progressive disease of young adults (15–40 years) characterized by random multiple sites of demyelination of neurones within the brain and spinal cord. It is manifest by visual disturbance, cerebellar problems with resulting disturbances of gait and spinal cord demyelination with limb paraesthesiae and urinary incontinence for which the patient may be referred to the gynaecologist. It is important to document the degree of neurological impairment before surgery and to explain to the patient that the stress associated with surgery has been shown to exacerbate the condition in the postoperative period.

Renal disease

The most important feature in the preoperative preparation of patients with renal disease is the assessment of the biochemical abnormality relative to the therapeutic manoeuvres taken to correct it. Patients on dialysis with established renal failure presenting for elective surgery should be dialysed 12–24 hours prior to surgery to correct any hyperkalaemia or acid–base abnormality. In patients with chronic anaemia, correction by preoperative transfusion is generally unnecessary; however, the detection of postoperative cyanosis is impaired by low haemoglobin levels. Non-renally excreted drugs should be used where possible. Infusions of morphine should be used cautiously as its active metabolite, morphine-6-glucuronamide, is renally excreted and may accumulate in sufficient concentrations to produce respiratory depression (Osbourne et al 1986).

Hepatic disease

Patients with moderate to severe hepatic disease are at considerable risk of developing perioperative problems following surgery and anaesthesia (Aranha et al 1982, Garrison et al 1984). Hepatic failure is associated with alterations of renal, pulmonary and cardiovascular physiology, impaired metabolic and haematological homeostasis and altered pharmacokinetics. Preoperative assessment is aimed at identifying the severity of the hepatic disease both clinically and biochemically. In the preoperative preparation it is necessary to give prophylactic antibiotics, vitamin K and possibly diuretics for ascites. Clotting abnormalities should be corrected with the appropriate blood products. The tendency to develop renal failure postoperatively is high and it is frequently fatal.

Endocrine disease and obesity

Patients presenting for surgery may exhibit a number of endocrine abnormalities. Perioperative problems tend to arise as a result of mismanagement of hormone replacement therapy and as such are dealt with in the section on the influence of pre-existing medication. One important condition to consider however is the effect of obesity on the course of surgery and anaesthesia.

Obesity can be defined as body fat content in excess of 30% in the female or where the ratio of weight (in kg) over height (m^2) is greater than 30. Patients in this category present with considerable risk in surgery, associated with abnormalities of respiratory and cardiovascular physiology. There are also technical problems with access for surgery and problems with postoperative mobilization. Appropriate dietary advice in the outpatient clinic with regular follow-up by a dietician prior to surgery is advocated in order to reduce some of these problems.

Haematological disorders

Anaemia. Anaemia is an acute or chronic reduction in the number of circulating erythrocytes manifest by a decrease in the concentration of haemoglobin and a concomitant reduction in the oxygen-carrying capacity of the blood. In most cases the cause may be known, e.g. menorrhagia. However where this is unclear, relevant investigations to elucidate the cause before surgery are essential. In patients with chronic anaemia (for example, chronic renal failure) compensatory changes include a shift to the right of the oxyhaemoglobin dissociation curve (thus increasing oxygen release at a tissue level) and an increase in cardiac output to maintain oxygen availability. The necessity for a minimum preoperative haemoglobin of 10 g/dl is based on a physiological necessity for a minimum oxygen availability of 250 ml of oxygen per minute. Oxygen availability is the product of the cardiac output, the haemoglobin concentration, the haemoglobin saturation and ability to carry oxygen. Therefore in patients with a normal cardiac output and a normal haemoglobin, the oxygen availability is in the region of 1000 ml of oxygen per minute. A reduction of the haemoglobin to 10 g/dl decreases this to around 650 ml of oxygen per minute. If during the course of surgery any of the other variables such as cardiac output secondary to hypovolaemia or the myocardial depressant effects of the anaesthetics are taken into account, this will further reduce and approach a level where tissue oxygen availability will be impaired. Therefore in individuals whose haemoglobin level is less than 10 g/dl — for which the cause has been identified — preoperative transfusion 48 hours prior to surgery may be indicated.

Defective haemoglobin synthesis.

Sickle cell haemoglobin (Anonymous 1989). Described by Herrick in 1910, sickle cell disease is an inherited group of disorders ranging from benign sickle cell trait to a severe form of sickle cell anaemia characterized by the substitution of normal haemoglobin A by abnormal haemoglobin S. The symptoms of the disease are related to the inability of the haemoglobin S to withstand hypoxia which results in the reduced haemoglobin forming tactoids which cause disruption and eventual rupture of the red cell. This leads to microvascular occlusion with infarction and organ damage.

Sickle cell trait, the heterozygous form of the condition, generally presents few problems as far as surgery and anaesthesia are concerned. Conversely, sickle cell anaemia presents a grave threat to the patient in the perioperative period and preoperative exchange transfusion is indicated in those individuals with a haemoglobin of <8 g/dl, preferably with freshly donated blood. It is desirable to achieve a figure of $>70\%$ normal red cells in a peripheral blood film. The preoperative administration of alkaline to increase blood pH to prevent sickling is not indicated as it promotes a left shift of the oxyhaemoglobin dissociation curve, thereby decreasing the availability of oxygen to the tissues.

Thalassaemia. This is a collective term for a group of inherited disorders associated with a reduction or lack of production of the structurally normal components of the haemoglobin molecule, i.e. beta thalassaemia, a diminution of beta globulin production, or alpha thalassaemia, a reduction of alpha globulin synthesis. Patients should be treated in a similar way to those who have sickle cell disease.

RELEVANT INVESTIGATIONS PRIOR TO SURGERY

All patients scheduled for major surgery should have basic haematological and biochemical screening beforehand. In ASA grade 1 patients without evidence of intercurrent disease undergoing minor surgery the value of such tests is more contentious.

Haematology

A full blood count is considered to be a minimum preoperative requirement prior to surgery, supplemented in patients of negroid or Mediterranean extraction by sickle cell test and if necessary haemoglobin electrophoresis. Where perioperative transfusion is envisaged, blood should be sent for grouping, including Rhesus group and cross-match, preferably 24 hours before surgery. In those patients with abnormalities of clotting, e.g. on anticoagulant therapy or with liver disease, full clotting profiles should be sent and appropriate corrective therapy instituted prior to surgery.

Biochemistry

Biochemical analysis of a patient's urine is generally performed by the nursing staff on admission or in the outpatient clinic using one of the many multitest dipstick kits. These can detect glycosuria, proteinuria etc. and if results are abnormal, further investigation is warranted. Serum multiple analysis for abnormalities of urea, electrolytes and liver function are indicated in the following circumstances.

1. If renal function may be impaired by virtue of the primary gynaecological pathology, such as late-stage carcinoma of the cervix, or secondary to systemic disease.
2. If current medication includes drugs likely to affect serum electrolytes, e.g. diuretic therapy or corticosteroids.
3. If hepatic or bony secondaries are suspected.

4. If postoperative nephrotoxic cytotoxic therapy is contemplated.
5. If postoperative enteral or parenteral nutrition is envisaged.

Microbiology

A midstream urine specimen should be sent for microscopic examination and culture to exclude urinary tract infection before any gynaecological procedure is carried out. In those patients in whom pelvic inflammatory disease is suspected or where tubal surgery is to be undertaken with a known previous history of pelvic inflammatory disease, swabs from the vagina, cervix and urethra should be sent for microscopic culture and sensitivity studies.

Virology

In those individuals where hepatitis B virus infection is suspected e.g. drug abusers or those with a previous history of hepatitis, testing for hepatitis surface antigen is necessary.

Human immunodeficiency virus (HIV) is a lente virus and the aetiologic agent responsible for causing the acquired immune deficiency syndrome. The screening of at-risk individuals for HIV antibodies, e.g. prostitutes, intravenous drug abusers and partners of bisexual males, can only be undertaken with a patient's permission and following counselling. At-risk individuals should be managed according to local hospital policy following the Department of Health guidelines (DHSS 1985, 1986, HMSO Circular 1990).

Imaging and electrocardiogram

Many of these procedures are indicated by the nature of the presenting complaint and the anticipated surgery, e.g. lymphangiography and pelvic carcinoma, ultrasound of the liver where hepatic secondaries are suspected. Preoperative chest X-ray is only necessary in those patients where underlying pulmonary or cardiac disease is present or in those individuals such as immigrants where exposure to chest diseases such as tuberculosis is suspected. Routine electrocardiographic examination is only necessary in the elderly or if cardiovascular disease is present. An abnormal electrocardiogram is associated with an increased perioperative risk.

INFLUENCES OF PRE-EXISTING MEDICATION

Corticosteroids

Patients treated with systemic corticosteroids develop suppression of the hypothalamic pituitary adrenal axis. High circulating levels of corticosteroids suppress hypothalamic production of corticotrophin-releasing factor and result in depression of anterior pituitary release of adrenocorticotrophic hormone. The degree of suppression is dependent on the dosage and duration of treatment but some adrenal suppression can occur within 1 week of starting corticosteroids. Following the cessation of corticosteroid therapy it may be some months before complete recovery in the hypothalamic pituitary axis occurs.

A surgical operation promotes a stress response in an individual leading to an increased output of corticosteroids. It has been estimated that a major surgical operation results in an increase of around 200–400 mg cortisol. Therefore in patients undergoing surgery with a potentially suppressed hypothalamic pituitary axis, it is essential that additional corticosteroids be given in order to avoid the risk of adrenal cortical insufficiency. Patients undergoing minor surgery can be managed by a small increase in the daily dose of corticosteroids or by monitoring vital signs and treating with incremental hydrocortisone if features suggestive of adrenal cortical insufficiency arise. For major surgery it is usual to give increased cover in the form of hydrocortisone 100–200 mg intramuscularly with the premedication, and then 50–100 mg four times daily reducing to a daily maintenance dose after several days. However it has been questioned whether such additional steroids are always necessary (Lloyd 1981). Patients treated with topical steroids (e.g. to the skin or rectum) occasionally absorb sufficient quantities to cause adrenal suppression and those patients who use high-dose beclomethasone inhalers to treat their asthma have also been reported to have a degree of adrenocortical insufficiency.

Oral contraceptives

Women taking the combined oral contraceptive pill have a higher incidence of deep venous thrombosis when compared with non-pill users. This risk is increased by anaesthesia and surgery with its accompanying immobilization. It has been estimated that among pill takers undergoing major surgery, the relative risk of deep vein thrombosis was twice that of non-users (Stadel 1981). However the reduction in the dosage of the oestrogen component of the preparation since this work suggests that the real risk may now be less. Oestrogens have been shown to increase the plasma concentration of several clotting factors as well as decreasing antifibrinolytic activity and the level of antithrombin 3, factors which all increase the tendency to deep vein thrombosis. Six weeks after discontinuation of the oestrogen pill these changes in the coagulation and fibrinolytic systems have reverted entirely (Von Kallua et al 1971) but epidemiological evidence suggests that the excess risk of deep vein thrombosis reverts to normal in less than a month (Vessey 1970). Current opinion therefore is that the combined oral contraceptive pill should be discontinued 1 month before major surgery and restarted at the first menses at least 2 weeks postoperatively (Guillebaud 1985). It is important that the patient is counselled in alternative contraceptive measures or unwanted pregnancy may result (Carter & Pryce 1985).

The risk of deep vein thrombosis following minor surgery, including laparoscopy, is however extremely small and any risk from the oral contraceptive pill is more than outweighed by the risk of pregnancy. It is therefore recommended that the pill should be continued in these circumstances. Where patients continue to take the pill up until the time of surgery (particularly emergency surgery) prophylactic low-dose heparin should be considered, particularly if there are other risk factors such as obesity and smoking. Those oestrogens given for hormone replacement therapy in postmenopausal patients should similarly be discontinued. Progestogens however do not cause the changes which favour venous thrombosis and therefore the constraints of the combined pill do not apply to those individuals taking the progestogen-only pill.

Insulin and oral hypoglycaemic agents

As previously stated the effects of anaesthesia and surgery result in a stress reaction resulting in an outpouring of catabolic hormones such as catecholamines, corticosteroids, glucagon and thyroxin. One of the metabolic effects of these is to stimulate glycogenolysis and gluconeogenesis, resulting in increased glucose liberation. These hormones also promote an increase in lipolysis which under normal circumstances is offset by the antilipolytic effect of the increased secretion of insulin which occurs as a result of the hypoglycaemia. The resultant effect is a depletion of liver glycogen and protein catabolism. In patients with untreated type 1 insulin-dependent diabetes, such a stress response results in hyperglycaemia and ketoacidosis. In the type 2 diabetic where some residual insulin secretion is retained, these effects may be less profound and the tendency to ketoacidosis is less marked. The perioperative management of the diabetic patient aims to avoid these problems by exogenous control of glucose homeostasis.

Type 1 diabetics. For all surgery involving general anaesthesia the patients should be admitted several days prior to operation and stabilized on short-acting insulins. Numerous different regimens for perioperative management have been advocated; however, the simplest consists of omission of the insulin dose on the day of operation; instead, an infusion of 10% glucose with potassium and soluble insulin is established. Alternatively an infusion of glucose and potassium may be supplemented by soluble insulin administered separately intravenously by a pump or by regular small subcutaneous injections. These are continued until the patient is into the perioperative period and re-established on her normal insulin regimen. All such regimens require regular and careful monitoring of glucose and potassium. Suitable regimens are suggested by Alberti & Hockaday (1983).

Type 2 diabetes. For minor surgery it is often sufficient to omit the oral hypoglycaemic agent on the morning of the operation with perioperative measurement of the blood sugar using dextrosticks. The hyperglycaemic effect of the operation is usually counteracted by the residual effect of the previous day's dose of hypoglycaemic agents. If there are problems or the operation becomes prolonged the patient is managed as for type 1 diabetes. For major surgery patients should be treated as for type 1 diabetes with conversion from oral hypoglycaemic control to short-acting insulin therapy.

Drugs acting on the cardiovascular system

Patients whose cardiovascular disease is controlled with drugs should in general continue on their medication in the perioperative period. The abrupt withdrawal of clonidine, used in the treatment of hypertension, can cause profound rebound sympathetic overactivity with anxiety, sweating, tremor and severe hypertension. This can occur even after the omission of a single dose. It is therefore essential that clonidine is continued over the perioperative period, parenterally if necessary.

Many patients with cardiovascular disease will be on beta-adrenergic blocking drugs and/or calcium channel blocking agents. In general these should be continued through the perioperative period as their abrupt withdrawal may be associated with the precipitation of myocardial infarction. The myocardial depressant nature of these agents however is of importance to the anaesthetist as some volatile anaesthetic agents may be synergistic with these drugs, with a resultant adverse effect on cardiovascular haemodynamics.

Patients on potassium-losing diuretics, whether or not being given potassium supplements, should have their plasma potassium estimated and hypokalaemia corrected preoperatively, particularly in the presence of concurrent digoxin therapy. Patients on short-term anticoagulation treatment, e.g. for deep vein thrombosis, should have their surgery postponed until full anticoagulation is stopped. When the patient need for coagulation however is long term, for example those with prosthetic heart valves, it is important to liaise with the physician supervising such treatment. In general the patient should be admitted several days before surgery to allow adjustment to the degree of anticoagulation. A British corrected ratio in a range of 2 to 3 is considered suitable for surgery. Postoperatively, anticoagulation should be maintained with intravenous heparin until the patient is once again able to take the oral agent. Where an anticoagulated patient requires emergency surgery the British corrected ratio is adjusted to the suitable range by the administration of fresh frozen plasma or a small amount of vitamin K (1 mg).

Drugs acting on the nervous system

Monoamine oxidase inhibitors

Drugs of this group are used in the treatment of depression which is resistant to other agents and their therapeutic effects are believed to result from the inhibition of the central nervous system monoamine oxidase, leading to an increase in the central nervous system catecholamine and 5-hydroxytriptamine concentrations. Their peripheral effects however include monoamine oxidase inhibition, inhibition of hepatic drug oxygenation and a variable degree of sympathetic blockade. Sympathomimetic agents may promote a hypertensive crisis, opiates (in particular pethidine) may cause profound hypotension, and barbiturates are metabolized at a variable and unpredictable rate. Although these problems can be overcome by withdrawing the drug at least 2 weeks before surgery, this can only be done in liaison with the prescribing psychiatrist.

Tricyclic, quadricyclic antidepressants and major tranquillizers

It is generally safe for patients to continue on these drugs provided that the anaesthetist is made aware that they are being given so that the anaesthetic may be varied appropriately. The sudden cessation of administration of these agents may result in an acute exacerbation of the psychiatric illness. In the case of patients suffering from a psychotic illness stabilized on an oral major tranquillizer, it may be worth considering giving it parenterally over the operative period.

Lithium

It is the usual practice to withdraw lithium 1 week before major surgery because of the risk of toxicity should there be an electrolyte imbalance or a deterioration in renal function. This risk however must be balanced against the possible relapse of the affective disorder for which the drug is being prescribed and again liaison with the psychiatrist is important.

Anticonvulsants

As mentioned previously, it is vital that patients continue to receive anticonvulsant medication over the operative period. It is usual to give the dose orally on the day of surgery and then parenterally until such time as the patient is able once again to take oral tablets. Sodium valproate deserves particular mention because in addition to its anticonvulsant properties it interferes with haemostasis. This drug causes depression of platelet count including frank thrombocytopenia in a dose-related fashion and it has been reported on occasions to cause impairment of platelet aggregation and minor defects of coagulation, including hypofibrinogenaemia. It is therefore recommended that patients taking this agent who require surgery should have a platelet and coagulation screen beforehand.

SMOKING (Jones 1985)

Although not strictly medication, the effects of smoking on perioperative events and the necessity to encourage patients to stop smoking before surgery is important in the preoperative preparation of the patient. Cigarettes have a number of deleterious effects, including:

1. Cardiovascular system: reduction in oxygen availability secondary to carbon monoxide binding to haemoglobin.
2. Respiratory system: the impairment of mucociliary clearance and hyper-reactivity of small airways increase the predisposition to postoperative chest infections.
3. Immune system: a reduction in neutrophil chemotaxis and immunoglobin concentration.
4. An increase in platelet aggregatibility.

Patients should be encouraged to stop smoking at least 6 weeks before surgery in order to improve pulmonary function. If this is not possible then they should be definitely encouraged to stop for at least 48 hours prior to surgery in order to eliminate carbon monoxide and thereby improve oxygen availability.

ALCOHOL (Edwards 1985)

It is important to appreciate the effects of alcohol on surgical morbidity and to ascertain any alcohol-related problems in the preoperative preparation of the patient. Surgery is associated with an increased risk to the heavy drinker due to diminution of the stress response, an impaired immunity, abnormalities of electrolyte control etc. The development of the alcohol withdrawal syndrome can occur within 8 hours of abstention and treatment with infusions of alcohol is sometimes necessary. In the alcoholic with systemic manifestations of the condition secondary to severe hepatic disease (e.g. bleeding diathesis), pretreatment with parenteral vitamins and the correction of clotting abnormalities are essential. The preoperative administration of steroids in alcoholics with severe impairment of the stress response may also be necessary.

COUNSELLING AND CONSENT

The objective of preoperative counselling is to present the patient with sufficient information to enable her to make a reasoned choice regarding her treatment. It is necessary for the doctor to inform the patient of the nature of her medical condition, the available treatment regimens, including the necessity for surgery, and the success or prognosis associated with these options. In doing so the nature and extent of potential complications must be outlined and any patient anxiety or apprehension should be discussed and, where appropriate, allayed. Armed with this information the patient will then be in a position to give her expressed rather than implied consent.

Counselling is very much a multistage procedure, allowing constant reinforcement and giving the patient ample opportunity to voice any concern. It begins the moment the patient is told that treatment is necessary and is continued in the preoperative period: both medical and nursing staff have important roles to play. The value of counselling in allaying preoperative anxiety is well known (Wilson-Barnett 1984). It is constantly being reviewed as new techniques emerge to cope with the influences of personality variability on behavioural responses in the postoperative period (Mathews & Ridgeway 1981). The value of such techniques (for example, cognitive coping) which encourage patients to focus on positive aspects of their treatment is well recognized (Ridgeway & Mathews 1982).

The role of the patient is also important. Factors such as her physical and mental state, intellectual capacity, prior knowledge and expectations of the treatment will dictate the extent and the nature of the counselling process. The extent to which treatment procedures, complications and side-effects are explained is also influenced by the society in which she lives. In the highly litigious-conscious American society, counselling may be protracted and patient anxiety increased by the discussion of every conceivable complication. Coupled with this there may be a very defensive medical practice associated with inappropriate investigations and monitoring, with their inherent risks. Within the UK there is an increasing level of compensation for medical negligence; however there is as yet no statutory medical requirement for doctors to discuss every potential complication or side-effect associated with a procedure. The legal precedent (Sidaway 1985) regarding the degree of disclosure of risk allows for doctors to make an assessment of the information they should disclose to the patient and limit it to that amount which will allow the patient to make a rational choice about treatment. The level of information should not deter the patient from undergoing treatment to the ultimate detriment of her health.

It may be pertinent to involve the patient's relatives in counselling — provided she consents — particularly where the elderly or mentally ill are concerned or where malignancy is present and where special provisions need to be made for terminal care. In addition to the patient–doctor relationship, information can also be imparted by the use of local or nationally produced information pamphlets and videos from hospitals, Royal Colleges, public institutions, charitable and patient organizations. The information should be presented in a lucid fashion, in clear language and should not be patronizing. It is advisable to include a disclaimer such as the one used by the American College of Obstetricians and Gynecologists: 'the information in this pamphlet does not indicate an exclusive course of treatment or procedure to be followed and should not be considered as excluding other acceptable methods of practice'. The Royal College of Obstetricians and Gynaecologists' study group on litigation in obstetrics and gynaecology (1985) made the following recommendations:

1. Communication between doctors and patients must be adequate.
2. Preoperative discussion with the patient should be full and noted in the hospital records.
3. The patient should be informed of likely operative complications. Not every conceivable complication should be discussed but the patient's questions should be answered truthfully.
4. A postoperative appointment should be offered to discuss any problems which may have arisen.
5. The opinions of senior staff and operative notes including details of any complications must be fully documented.

Informed consent

Failure to obtain consent may result in a doctor facing a criminal prosecution for assault or a civil claim for damages. The nature in which consent is obtained is also of importance: failure to give the patient sufficient information regarding the possible complications of a given procedure leaves the doctor open to a potential claim for damages for negligence. UK law allows the doctor to set that level of information although it must be one which is acceptable to the majority of practitioners within the field. However the ultimate decision as to whether or not the patient was sufficiently well informed lies within the courts. In England anyone of sound mind and over 16 years of age can give legally valid consent for surgical or medical treatment, provided that at the time it was obtained the patient was not under the influence of alcohol or drugs, including premedication. Under the age of 16 years, a parent, guardian or local authority (for children in care) or High Court (for children who are wards of court) can give consent provided the necessary explanations have been given.

Consent in relation to a child only allows for diagnostic or therapeutic procedures which will benefit the child. Therefore consent to non-therapeutic sterilization or experimentation without benefit is unlawful. In the case of contraception and termination of pregnancy, the General Medical Council advise that parental consent should be obtained. However patient confidentiality must be respected and the doctor should use his or her judgement prior to agreeing to contraception or termination in a minor, if necessary following discussion with a colleague. Where a doctor feels it necessary to obtain parental consent against a patient's expressed wish, he or she should inform the patient accordingly.

Consent from mentally handicapped people is more complex and is governed by the provisions of the Mental Health Act 1983. However, this Act only provides statutory powers covering formal consent for treatment in respect of mental illness and does not allow the undertaking of elective surgery for any other condition unless it is a threat to the patient's life. Therefore the consent of a mentally handicapped person should be sought as for a normal individual. The validity of the consent will however be determined by the underlying degree of mental handicap and should involve a full discussion with all the interested parties. In those who are severely handicapped a guardianship order should be obtained, although a guardian may not give consent to medical treatment without the patient's permission. It is therefore wise to seek legal advice in situations involving mentally handicapped patients where informed consent is unobtainable.

A ruling by the Court of Appeal in 1989 has clarified some of the points regarding sterilization in mentally handicapped women. In an extreme emergency where the patient's condition renders it impossible to obtain consent, then a doctor may proceed to carry out treatment in order to protect the patient's life without her prior consent. It is advisable to discuss the situation with the next of kin; however they have no legal right to consent or to withhold consent for treatment for the patient. Consent may be implicit by a patient's conduct or may be given expressly in conversation. Ideally however it should be in writing in order that it can be maintained as primary evidence. Consent forms should be simple, stating the nature of the procedure intended including the consent for further or alternative procedures as deemed necessary at the time of operation; that the procedure has been fully explained and (where applicable) no specific individual will perform the surgery or anaesthesia. The form is then signed by the patient and the doctor who explained the procedure and placed in the patient's notes. Forms for sterilization procedures should carry a disclaimer stating that there is a possibility of failure.

DAY-CASE SURGERY

When considering patients for day-case surgery there are two aspects to consider. Firstly, is the procedure suitable? Ideally it should be of short duration (less than 1 hour), and associated with a low incidence of perioperative and postoperative complications, in particular a low incidence of postoperative pain and nausea. Suitable gynaecological procedures include dilatation and curettage, suction termination of pregnancy, and diagnostic laparoscopy (Thurlow 1983). The second thing to consider is patient suitability. In most cases it is limited to those within ASA category 1 and 2; however special consideration can be given to patients of ASA class 3 where the patient is well known to both surgeon and anaesthetist, e.g. check cystoscopy in the elderly.

Skilled surgery and anaesthesia are essential and these cases should not be delegated to the inexperienced house surgeon or anaesthetist. The preoperative assessment is generally undertaken in the gynaecological clinic and a knowledge of the constraints of day-case surgery is therefore essential in order to prevent unwarranted cancellation secondary to patient unsuitability. Where the surgeon is unclear whether a patient is suitable or not then prior consultation with an anaesthetic colleague is advised. The principles of preoperative assessment however are the same as those outlined for inpatients above. Adequate information about preparation for anaesthesia in surgery, including the withholding of food and drink for at least 6 hours prior to admission, and detailed instructions about discharge from hospital should be given, including the necessity to have an escort to accompany the patient home and look after her for 24 hours after surgery and anaesthesia. Day-case patients should also be told not to drive vehicles, operate machinery or take unprescribed drugs or alcohol within that period of time.

JEHOVAH'S WITNESSES

The Jehovah's Witnesses are a fundamentalist sect formed in the USA in the 1870s. In recent years their numbers have increased substantially and it is now estimated that there are in excess of 80 000 in the UK (Clarke 1982). Their beliefs are based upon their own unique interpretation of the Bible and contradict those of the major churches. A minor part of their doctrine is taken to imply that blood transfusion should be forbidden as violating God's Law. Jehovah's Witnesses accept medical treatment in all other respects and make no attempt to argue against the medical indications for blood transfusion. They are willing to take responsibility for their lives and accept that the constraints they place on their medical attendants may lead to their death. To this end, health authorities with the help and guidance of the medical defence societies have produced forms consenting to treatment but stating that blood transfusion is unacceptable and the doctor will be absolved of any consequence of its omission. The legal value of these documents has however been questioned (Casale 1979; Palmer 1980). Each individual doctor must decide if he or she is willing to treat such a patient given the constraints placed on management. Techniques of haemodilution and autotransfusion are acceptable to some Jehovah's Witnesses and have been developed to facilitate surgery. It must be remembered that to administer blood against the wishes of the patient constitutes assault.

The situation with regard to children is different by virtue of the Children and Young Persons Act 1933.

The Medical Defence Union and the Medical Protection Society stress that they are always happy to offer advice in such circumstances and that whatever decision is taken, they will give full support to the individual doctor if that decision is subsequently challenged.

KEY POINTS

1. Assignment of physical status category to patient is based on history and examination but should take account of intended surgery as well.
2. Cooperation between surgeon and anaesthetist for preoperative patient assessment is of value.
3. Preoperative stabilization for diabetic patients is important.
4. Prompt and adequate communication is vital in preventing litigation.
5. Day-case surgery requires skilled anaesthesia as well as skilled surgery.
6. Elective surgery should be delayed where a cardiac infarct has occurred within 3 months, in the presence of an upper respiratory tract infection, uncontrolled hypertension, untreated cardiac dysrhythmia, taking the oral contraceptive pill (unless the surgery is minor or intermediate) and hypokalaemia.

REFERENCES

Alberti K G M M, Hockaday T D R 1983 Diabetes mellitus. In: Weatherall D J, Ledingham J G, Warrell D A (eds) Oxford textbook of medicine, vol 1. Oxford University Press, Oxford, pp 5–48

American Society of Anaesthesiologists 1963 New classification of physical status. Anaesthesiology 24: 111

Anonymous 1989 Sickle cell disease and non specialists. Drugs and Therapeutics Bulletin 27: 3

Aranha G Y, Sontag S J, Greenlee H B 1982 Cholecystectomy in cirrhotic patients, a formidable operation. American Journal of Surgery 143: 55–60

Burn J M B 1976 Preoperative assessment clinics. Proceedings of the Royal Society of Medicine 69: 734–736

Carter R J, Pryce J 1985 Risk of pregnancy while waiting for an operation. British Medical Journal 291: 516

Casale F 1979 Blood transfusion and Jehovah's Witnesses. British Medical Journal 1: 1796

Clarke J M F 1982 Surgery in Jehovah's Witnesses. British Journal of Hospital Medicine 27: 497–500

DHSS 1985, 1986 Acquired immune deficiency syndrome

Booklet 1: AIDS General information for doctors; CMO(85)7.

Booklet 2: Information for doctors concerning the introduction of HTLV III antibody tests; CMO(85)12.

Booklet 3: Guidance for surgeons, anaesthetists, dentists and their teams in dealing with patients infected with HTLV III; CMO(86)7. Department of Health and Social Security, London

Edwards R 1985 Anaesthesia and alcohol. British Medical Journal 291: 423–424

Foex P 1981 Preoperative assessment of the patient with cardiovascular disease. British Journal of Anaesthesia 53: 731–744

Foex P 1982 Anaesthesia and cardiovascular disease. The importance of preoperative assessment. In: Atkinson R, Langton-Hewer C (eds) Recent advances in anaesthesia, vol 14. Churchill Livingstone, Edinburgh, p 7–29

Fowkes J R, Lunn J, Farrow S C 1982 Epidemiology in anaesthesia: mortality risk in patients with coexisting physical disease. British Journal of Anaesthesia 54: 819–825

Garrison R N, Cryer H M, Howard D A, Polk H C 1984 Clarification of risk factors for abdominal operations in patients with hepatic cirrhosis. Annals of Surgery 199: 648–655

Goldman L, Caldera D 1979 Risks of general anaesthesia and elective operations in the hypertensive patient. Anaesthesiology 50: 285–292

Goldman L, Caldera D, Nussbaum S R et al 1977 Multifactorial index of cardiac risk in non cardiac surgical procedures. New England Journal of Medicine 297: 845–850

Guillebaud J 1985 Surgery and the pill. British Medical Journal 291: 498–499

HMSO Circular 1990 Guidance for clinical health care workers: protection against infection with HIV and hepatitis viruses. HMSO, London

Jeffery C C, Kinsman J, Cullen D J, Brewster D C 1983 A prospective evaluation of cardiac risk index. Anaesthesiology 58: 462–464

Jones R M 1985 Smoking before surgery: the case for stopping. British Medical Journal 290: 1763–1764

Keats A S 1978 The ASA classification of physical status: a recapitulation. Anaesthesiology 49: 223–236

Lloyd E L 1981 A rational regimen for perioperative steroid supplements and a clinical assessment of the requirements. Annals of the Royal College of Surgeons of England 63: 54–57

Mathews A, Ridgeway V 1981 Personality and surgical recovery. British Journal of Clinical Psychology 20: 243–260

Osbourne R J, Joel S P, Slevin M L 1986 Morphine intoxication in renal failure. The role of morphine-6-glucuronamide. British Medical Journal 292: 1548–1549

Pace M L 1984 A reconsideration of the merits of the cardiac risk index. Anesthesiology 60: 607–608

Palmer R M 1980 Consent and confidentiality, disclosure of medical records. Medical Protection Society, London

Patterson D 1985 Angina. British Journal of Hospital Medicine 33: 8–16

Prys-Roberts C 1984 Anaesthesia and hypertension. British Journal of Anaesthesia 56: 711–724

Rao T L K, Jacob J H, El Ehs A A 1983 Reinfarction following anaesthesia in patients with myocardial infarction. Anaesthesiology 59: 499–508

Ridgeway V, Mathews A 1982 Psychological preparation for surgery: a comparison of methods. British Journal of Clinical Psychology 21: 271–280

Rigg J R, Jones N L 1978 Clinical assessment of respiratory function. British Journal of Anaesthesia 50: 3–13

Royal College of Obstetricians and Gynaecologists 14th Study Group 1985 Litigation and obstetrics and gynaecology. Chamberlain G, Orr C, Sharp F (eds) Royal College of Obstetricians and Gynaecologists, London, p 311

Sidaway 1985 Sidaway *v* Board of Governors of Bethlem Royal and Maudsley Hospital. Weekly Law Rep 2: 480

Stadel B V 1981 Oral contraceptives and cardiovascular disease. New England Journal of Medicine 305: 672–677

Thurlow A 1983 Outpatient anaesthesia: current concepts. In: Mazze

R I (ed) Clinics in Anaesthesiology, vol 1. W B Saunders, Philadelphia, pp 397–413
Vessey M P, Doll R, Fairburn A S, Globar G 1970 Post operative thromboembolism and the use of oral contraceptives. British Medical Journal iii: 123–126
Von Kaulla E, Droegmueller W, Aoki N, Von Kaulla K M 1971 Antithrombin III depression and thrombin generation acceleration in women taking oral contraceptives. American Journal of Obstetrics and Gynecology 109: 868–873
Wilson-Barnett J 1984 Intervention to alleviate patients' stress: a review. Journal of Psychosomatic Research 28: 63–72

FURTHER READING

Stevens J (ed) 1986 Preparation for anaesthesia. Clinics in Anaesthesiology 4: 3
Stoelting R K, Dierdorf F F, McCammon R C (eds) 1988 Anaesthesia and co-existing disease, 2nd edn. Churchill Livingstone, Edinburgh

SECTION 2

Reproductive Endocrinology

9. Control of hypothalamic–pituitary function

R. W. Shaw

INTRODUCTION

Over the last 30 years it has become increasingly apparent that a major component of endocrine regulation is a function of the brain and the hypothalamus in particular.

The hypothalamus lies at the base of the brain between the anterior margin of the optic chiasma anteriorly and the posterior margin of the mammillary bodies posteriorly. Precise boundaries are difficult to define but it extends from the hypothalamic sulcus above to the tuber cinereum below which itself connects the hypothalamus with the pituitary gland via its extension distally into the pituitary stalk.

ANATOMY OF THE HYPOTHALAMIC–PITUITARY AXIS

The portion of the hypothalamus of special interest in the control of reproductive function is the neurophypophysis, which can be divided into three regions:

1. the infundibulum, which constitutes the floor of the third ventricle (often termed the median eminence) and parts of the walls of the third ventricle, which is continuous with
2. the infundibular stem, or pituitary stalk, which is continuous distally with
3. the infundibular process or posterior pituitary gland (Fig. 9.1).

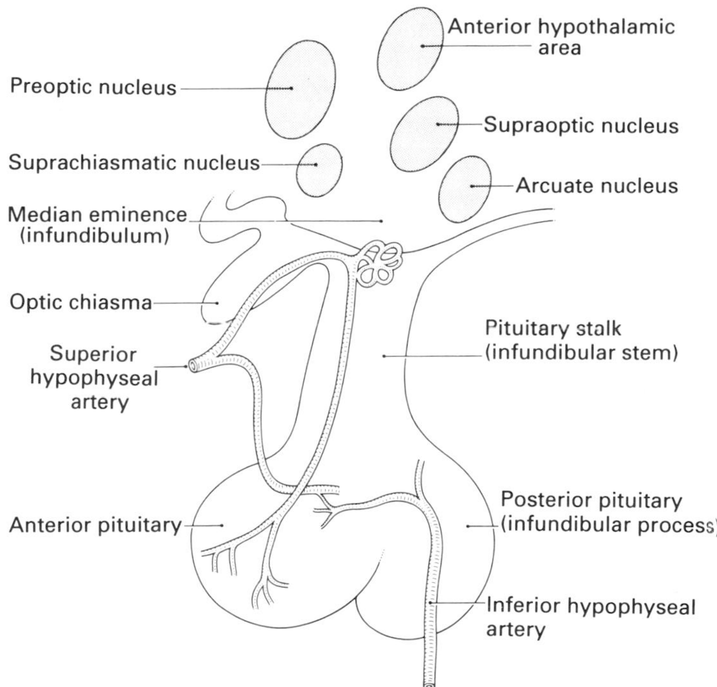

Fig. 9.1 Anatomy of the hypothalamus and pituitary.

The adenohypophysis consists of:

1. The pars distalis or anterior lobe of the pituitary;
2. The pars intermedia — intermediate lobe;
3. The pars tuberalis, which is a thin layer of adenohypophyseal cells lying on the surface of the infundibular stem and infundibulum.

The anterior pituitary does not normally receive an arterial vasculature but it receives blood through portal vessels. The arteries supplying the median eminence and infundibular stalk empty into a dense network of capillaries which are heavily innervated and drain into the portal venous plexus. In the human these are present on all sides of the infundibular stalk, particularly posteriorly. These lead to the anterior pituitary formed by vessels from the median eminence and upper stalk joined ventrally by the short portal vessels arising in the lower infundibular stalk. Some 80–90% of the blood supply to the anterior pituitary is provided by the long portal vessels; the remainder comes from the short portal veins. The sinusoids of the adenohypophysis thus receive blood that has first traversed capillaries residing in the neurohypophyseal complex and this unique relationship provides the basis for the view that the hypothalamus regulates the secretion of adenohypophyseal hormones through neurohormonal mechanisms involving hypothalamic releasing and inhibiting factors.

Neural connections

There are numerous and extensive neural pathways connecting the hypothalamus with the rest of the brain. The majority of afferent hypothalamic nerve fibres run in the lateral hypothalamic areas whilst efferent pathways are more medially placed. One important efferent connection is the supraopticohypophyseal nerve tract carrying fibres from the supraoptic and paraventricular nuclei to the infundibular process of the pituitary, whilst other fibres carry hypothalamic releasing or inhibiting factors from the medial and basal parts of the hypothalamus to the anterior pituitary (Fig. 9.2).

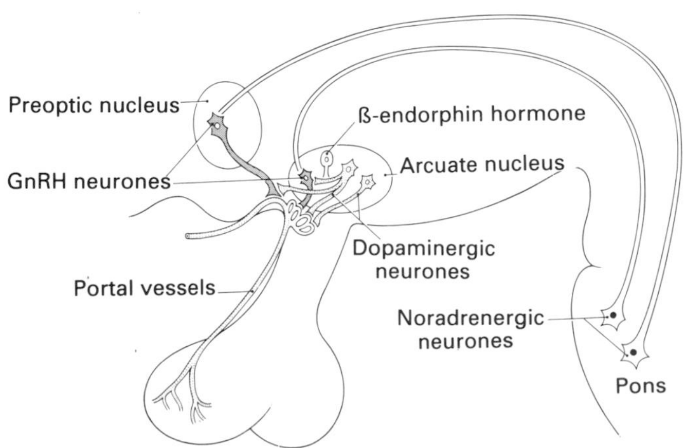

Fig. 9.2 Representation of neurochemical interactions which are important in the control of gonadotrophin-releasing hormone (GnRH) secretion.

HYPOTHALAMIC REGULATION OF PITUITARY SECRETION

Considerable effort has been made in the past two decades to identify, characterize and synthesize the substances thought to be produced in the neural elements in the infundibulum. Several substances which can either stimulate or suppress the rate of release of one or more hormones from the pituitary gland have been found in the infundibular complex. These include oxytocin, vasopressin, dopamine, adrenaline, noradrenaline, gonadotrophin-releasing hormone (GnRH, or its synonym, luteinizing hormone-releasing hormone (LHRH)), thyrotrophin-releasing hormone (TRH), somatostatin, vasoactive intestinal peptide (VIP), and neurophysins (Table 9.1). Other substances are likely to be added to this list in the future. Further discussion in this chapter will be restricted to the roles played by LHRH, and dopamine and other neurotransmitters controlling their rates of release and synthesis.

Table 9.1 Hypothalamic releasing and inhibiting factors

Hypothalamic-releasing hormone
Gonadotrophin-releasing hormone (GnRH; LHRH)
Thyrotrophin-releasing hormone (TRH)
Growth hormone-releasing hormone (GHRH)
Corticotrophin-releasing hormone (CRH)
Hypothalamic-inhibiting factors
Somatostatin
Prolactin-inhibiting factor (PIF)

LHRH

In 1971 Schally and co-workers isolated pure preparations of porcine LHRH from hypothalamic extracts and subsequently its structure was discovered and synthesis was achieved (Matsuo et al 1971a, b). The finding of follicle-stimulating hormone (FSH)-releasing activity of this

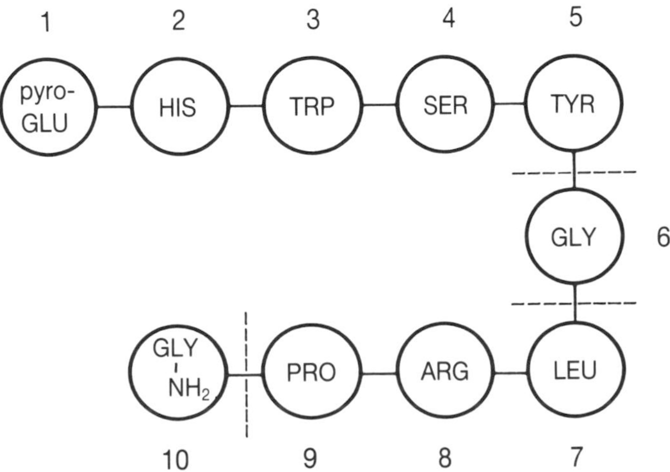

Fig. 9.3 Amino acid sequency of GnRH (mol wt 1181), synonymous with LHRH. Dashed line represents sites of enzymatic cleavage.

LHRH led to the formulation of the hypothesis for a single hypothalamic-releasing hormone controlling secretion of both luteinizing hormone (LH) and FSH from the pituitary gland, with the suggestion that sex steroids might play a role in modulating the proportions of LH and FSH released. The amino acid sequence of LHRH is shown in Figure 9.3.

LHRH neuron system

LHRH neuronal cell bodies are found principally in two areas — the preoptic anterior hypothalamic area and the tuberal hypothalamus, principally the arcuate nucleus and periventricular nucleus. Both groups of neurons project to the median eminence where the bulk of LHRH-containing terminals are found in brain tissue in close proximity to the portal capillary plexus (Fig. 9.2).

Regulation of gonadotrophin secretion by LHRH

LHRH has been demonstrated in the hypophyseal portal blood from a number of animal species using radioimmunoassays. Electrical stimulation of the preoptic area of the brain in female rats on the day of pro-oestrus increases LHRH concentration in portal blood and the stimulus induces a marked release of LH from the anterior pituitary. In contrast administration of antibodies against LHRH prevents this electrically stimulated LH release. These data provide evidence favouring a cause-and-effect relationship between LHRH release by the hypothalamus and LH release by the anterior pituitary.

It is now firmly established that LHRH can stimulate the secretion of both LH and FSH in animals and humans. Following intravenous administration of synthetic LHRH a significant rise in serum LH will be seen within 5 min, and sometimes of FSH, reaching a peak within about 30 min, but FSH peaks are often delayed further. LH release has a linear log–dose relationship up to doses of 250 μg but no such relationship can be found for FSH.

In the female the magnitude of gonadotrophin release, particularly LH, in individuals varies with the stage of the menstrual cycle, being greatest in the preovulatory phase, less marked in the luteal phase and least in the follicular phase of any individual cycle (Yen et al 1972; Shaw et al 1974; Fig. 9.4).

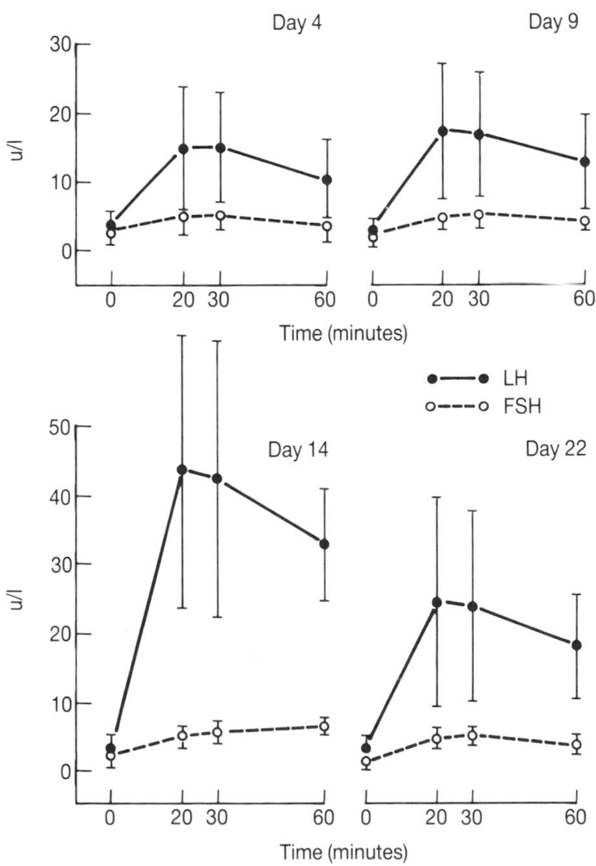

Fig. 9.4 LH and FSH release following 100 μg GnRH at different phases of the same menstrual cycle in 6 normal women (mean ± s.d.). From Shaw et al (1974).

Mechanism of action of LHRH on pituitary cells

A summary of data concerning the cellular events involved in the mechanism of action of LHRH is depicted in Figure 9.5. Within seconds of LHRH binding to and activating LHRH receptors on the pituitary gonadotrophs, intracellular free Ca^{2+} concentrations increase. This Ca^{2+} is

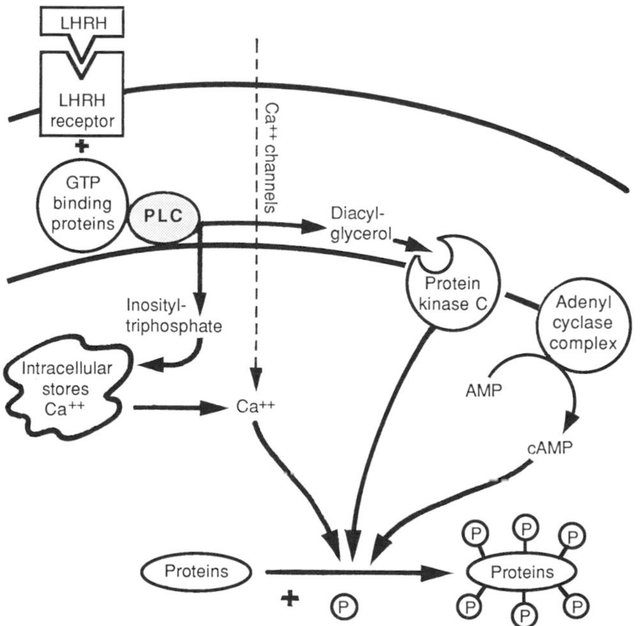

Fig. 9.5 Schematic representation of hormone LHRH-receptor signal activation. GTP = guanosine triphosphate; PLC = phospholipase-C enzyme; AMP = adenosine monophosphate; cAMP = cyclic AMP; P = phosphate group.

initially mobilized from intracellular stores (e.g. endoplasmic reticulum) but also, to maintain sustained LH release, extracellular Ca^{2+} enters the gonadotroph through receptor-regulated voltage-dependent Ca^{2+} channels.

The initial mobilization of intracellular Ca^{2+} is induced by inositol triphosphate released as a consequence of receptor activation of membrane bound phospholipase-C enzyme. Diacylglycerol is also released by the action of phospholipase-C and in turn activates the phosphorylating enzyme protein kinase C. The adenyl cyclase complex is also stimulated and cyclic adenosine monophosphate (cAMP) is generated. Ca^{2+}, protein kinase C and cAMP all then interact to stimulate release of stored LH and FSH and subsequent biosynthesis (for review see Clayton 1989).

MODULATORY ROLE OF MONOAMINES, OTHER NEUROTRANSMITTERS AND SECOND MESSENGERS ON LHRH SECRETION

Past studies have indicated that LH release and ovulation were dependent upon drug-affected neural stimuli of both cholinergic and adrenergic origins. The infundibulum contains large stores of noradrenaline, a lesser quantity of dopamine and a small amount of adrenaline (Fig. 9.6).

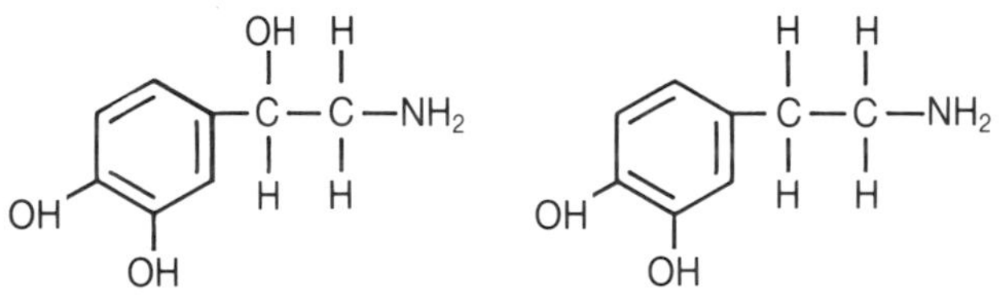

Fig. 9.6 Chemical structure of biogenic amines.

Dopamine

The hypothalamic tuberoinfundibular dopaminergic pathway is formed by neurons with cell bodies located in the arcuate nucleus and axons which project to the external layer of the median eminence in close juxtaposition to portal vessels. The coexistence of dopamine and LHRH-containing axons in the same region of the median eminence suggests the possibility of dopaminergic involvement in the control of gonadotrophin secretion.

The addition of dopamine to pituitaries coincubated with hypothalamic fragments increase the release of LH, whilst the addition of phentolamine, an alpha-receptor blocker, prevents dopamine-induced LH release. These early in vivo experiments suggested that the hormonal background was capable of modifying the response to dopamine since it seemed ineffective in ovariectomized animals or during oestrus or dioestrus day 1 of the oestrous cycle. Dopamine was more effective at pro-oestrus or in oestrogen- and progesterone-primed rats.

In humans the inhibitory role of dopamine and its agonists on LH as well as prolactin release has been demonstrated (Le Blanc et al 1976; Lachelin et al 1977). Elevated levels of prolactin can also stimulate dopamine turnover in the hypothalamus and it is postulated that the stimulated dopamine secretion in turn alters LHRH secretion and hence reduces FSH and LH release. Hence dopamine in the human may principally have an inhibitory effect on LHRH secretion.

The contradictory roles played by dopamine in LHRH release are in all likelihood the consequence of more than one action of dopamine on the LHRH-secreting neuron. The steroid environment appears to modify the components involved in the dopaminergic control of LHRH secretion with oestrogen appearing to affect the population of excitatory or inhibitory dopamine receptors and suggestive of the fact that the feedback control of LHRH output by oestrogen is partly exerted at a hypothalamic level by reducing dopamine neuronal activity.

Noradrenaline

Most experimental evidence supports a stimulatory role for noradrenaline in the control of gonadotrophin release. Turnover of hypothalamic noradrenaline is increased during the preovulatory surge of gonadotrophins at pro-oestrus, and noradrenaline synthesis in the anterior hypothalamus is enhanced in ovariectomized rats. These effects on LHRH secretion appear to be mediated by alpha -receptors since phenoxybenzamine, an alpha-blocker, suppresses the postcastration rise in gonadotrophins in male rats and phentolamine blocks the pulsatile release of LH in ovariectomized monkeys (for review see McCann & Ojeda 1976).

Selective blockade of noradrenaline synthesis prevents the preovulatory LH surge and that induced by gonadal steroids; the above data are suggestive that noradrenergic terminals in the preoptic or anterior hypothalamic area synapse with LHRH neurons involved in the control of the preovulatory surge of gonadotrophins.

Serotonin

High concentrations of serotonin are found in the median eminence with most of the serotonin-containing neurons originating from the raphe nucleus in the mid-brain–pons area. Present evidence shows that serotonin plays a predominantly inhibitory role in gonadotrophin release (see McCann & Ojeda 1976).

OTHER NEUROTRANSMITTERS AND SECOND MESSENGERS

Other neurotransmitters may play a less important role in the regulation of LHRH neurons. Acetylcholine and gamma-aminobutyric acid stimulate LH release. Both these agents are far commoner as neurotransmitting agents than dopamine or noradrenaline in central nervous system nerve terminals in general but their importance in LHRH neuronal activity seems less than that of dopamine and noradrenaline.

Prostaglandins

The role of prostaglandins in brain function is not clear, but the brain can synthesize and release prostaglandins and they do modify the adenyl cyclase–AMP system in central and peripheral neurons. Prostaglandins, particularly those of the E series, can induce gonadotrophin release in several species and prostaglandin synthetase inhibitors, e.g. indomethacin, block steroid-induced LH release (Ojeda & McCann 1978). Prostaglandin E is found in the median eminence in greater quantity than the rest of the medial basal hypothalamus; this distribution is consistent with the concept of its physiological role in the neural control of pituitary function.

The role played by prostaglandin E in LHRH release from hypothalamic secretory neurons appears to be an intracellular one. Activation of noradrenaline release from nerve terminals synapsing with LHRH neurones stimulates postsynaptic production of prostaglandin E which in turn enhances the release of LHRH. The prostaglandin E effect may either be a direct one or mediated by a cyclic nucleotide.

The control of LHRH secretion is thus highly complex and dependent upon a number of inhibitory and excitatory pathways involving various neurotransmitters. The control mechanisms are further complicated by the role of ovarian steroids in altering LHRH release and in modifying pituitary responsiveness to LHRH.

MODULATORY EFFECT OF OVARIAN STEROIDS

Negative feedback

Negative feedback control or inhibition of pituitary LH and FSH release has been postulated since 1932 when Moore & Price considered that the ovary and adenohypophysis were linked in a rigid system of hormonal interactions. The quantitative relationship between ovarian steroids and gonadotrophin release can be demonstrated by disturbing the negative feedback loop by oophorectomy which produces over a period of days an increase in circulating LH and FSH; this reaches a plateau at about 3 weeks with levels which are some 10 times preoperative

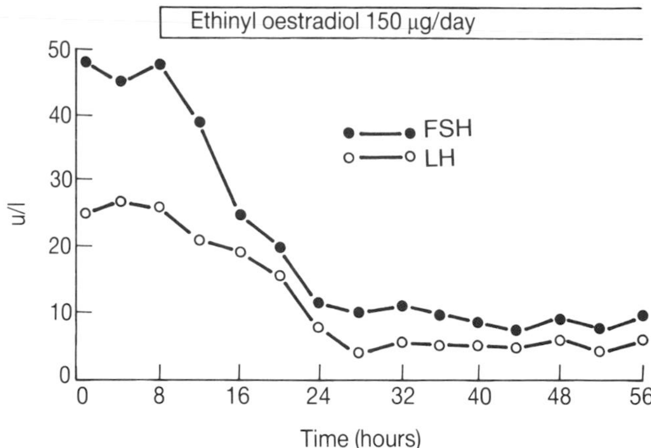

Fig. 9.7 The negative feedback effect of oestrogen on serum LH and FSH in a postmenopausal woman (unpublished data, Shaw 1975).

values. Alternatively the administration of exogenous oestrogens to oophorectomized or postmenopausal women will result in rapid suppression of circulating gonadotrophin levels (Fig. 9.7).

The negative feedback changes result from both a direct pituitary site of action of oestradiol with a decrease in sensitivity of the gonadotroph to LHRH (McCann et al 1974) and an action within the hypothalamus with a decrease in LHRH secretion, possibly via increased inhibitory dopaminergic activity.

The threshold for the negative feedback action of oestrogen is set to bring about suppression of gonadotrophin release with relatively small increases in oestradiol-17β in the normal female. This negative feedback loop is the main factor which maintains the relatively low basal concentrations of plasma LH and FSH in the normal female — circulating levels of oestradiol-17β within the range 100–200 pmol/l will suppress the early follicular phase gonadotrophin rise which initiates follicular development.

A negative feedback effect of progesterone on gonadotrophin secretion is now well established. Whilst progesterone has little effect on baseline LH release, even in large doses, it can suppress the ovulatory surge of LH as demonstrated in human females administered with synthetic progestagens (Larsson-Cohn et al 1972) and oestrogen-induced positive feedback surges cannot be produced during the luteal phase in women (Shaw 1975). The principal negative feedback action of progesterone is thus upon the mid-cycle gonadotrophin surge and it may be responsible for its short 24-h duration. It also seems likely that progesterone is an important factor in the reduced frequency of gonadotrophin pulses observed during the luteal phase of the cycle when compared to their frequency in the follicular phase (see below).

Positive feedback

The fact that under certain circumstances oestrogen may stimulate (positive feedback) rather than inhibit gonadotrophin release was first proposed by Hohlweg & Junkmann (1932). Their proposal has since been substantiated by numerous experimental reports in animals and humans. Under physiological conditions the positive feedback operates only in females; it is brought about by oestrogen and appears to be an essential component in producing the mid-cycle ovulatory surge of gonadotrophins. Administration of oestradiol-17β to females during the early or mid follicular phase of the cycle will induce a surge of gonadotrophins (Yen et al 1974; Shaw 1975; (Fig. 9.8) but treatment with the same doses of oestrogen during the mid follicular phase induces a far greater release of LH than during the early follicular phase (Yen et al 1974; (Fig. 9.8). Studies on the dynamics of this positive feedback response to oestrogen, observed in greatest detail in the rhesus monkey, demonstrate an activation delay of some 32–48 h from the commencement of oestrogen administration until the onset of the positive feedback-induced gonadotrophin surge; a minimum threshold level to be exceeded, and a strength–duration aspect of the stimulus (Karsch et al 1973).

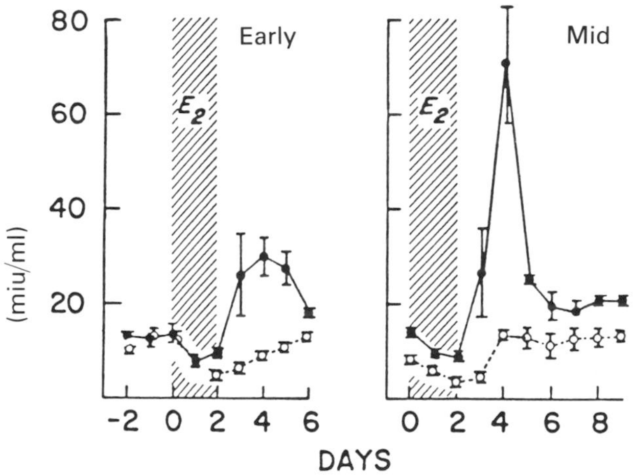

Fig. 9.8 The positive feedback effect of exogenous oestrogen (E_2 = 200 μg ethinyl oestradiol/day) on gonadotrophin release; qualitative differences in the early and mid follicular phase of the cycle. ● = LH; ○ = FSH. From Yen et al (1974) with permission.

Oestrogen elicits gonadotrophin release by increasing pituitary responsiveness to LHRH and possibly by stimulating increased LHRH secretion by the hypothalamus. In the normally menstruating female, oestrogen pretreatment produces an initial suppressive action on pituitary responsiveness to LHRH (Shaw et al 1975a) followed by a later augmenting action which is both concentration- and duration-dependent (Shaw et al 1975a; Young & Jaffe 1976). The augmenting effect of oestrogen

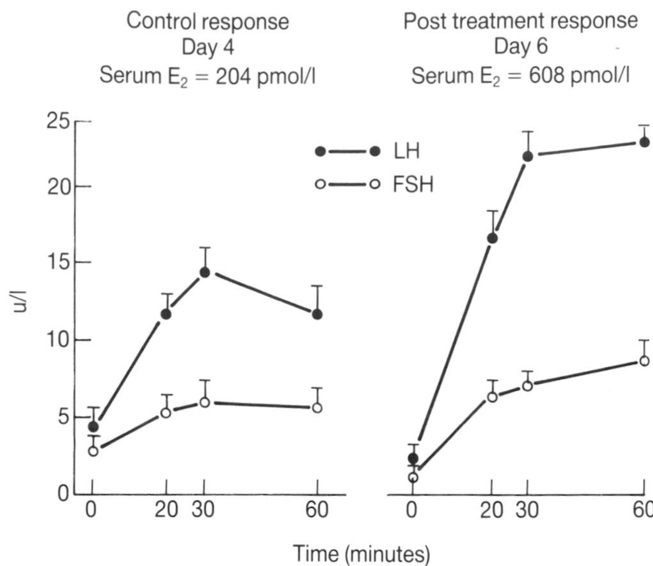

Fig. 9.9 Oestrogen augmentation of pituitary response to 100 μg LHRH bolus in 4 women receiving 2.5 mg oestradiol benzoate i.m., 2 h after initial control response on day 4 of cycle and retested 48 h later on day 6 of cycle. From Shaw (1975).

on LHRH pituitary responsiveness is demonstrated in Figure 9.9.

These data and others suggest that the mid-cycle oestrogen-induced surge of gonadotrophins may occur without any increased output of hypothalamic LHRH being necessary and indeed this occurs in patients with endogenous LHRH deficiency receiving pulsatile LHRH treatment at a constant rate.

Progesterone by itself does not appear to exert a positive feedback effect. However, when administered to females in whom the pituitary has undergone either endogenously induced or exogenously administered oestrogen priming, progesterone can induce the increased pituitary responsiveness to LHRH. (Shaw et al 1975b; Fig. 9.10). Since circulating progesterone levels are increasing significantly during the periovulatory period this action may be of importance in determining the magnitude and duration of the mid-cycle gonadotrophin surge.

SELF-PRIMING OF THE PITUITARY GONADOTROPH BY LHRH

Results from in vitro experiments with pituitary cells in culture indicate that LHRH is involved not only in release of stored LH and FSH, but is of importance in maintaining synthesis of gonadotrophins within the gonadotroph. Hence repeated exposure of the gonadotrophin-producing cells to LHRH seems essential for the maintenance of adequate pituitary stores.

Rommler & Hammerstein (1974) first demonstrated that the response to a second injection of LHRH was greater

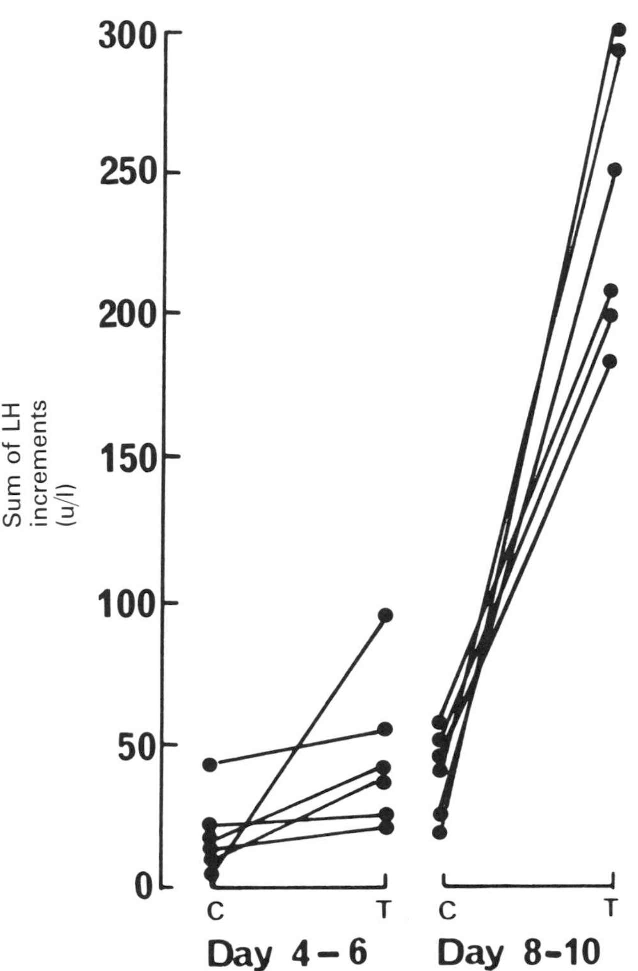

Fig. 9.10 Effect of progesterone pretreatment (12.5 mg i.m.) on LH response to 100 μg GnRH i.v. during the early and mid follicular phases of the cycle, showing the increased priming effect of oestrogen. C = control; T = after progesterone. Modified from Shaw et al (1975b).

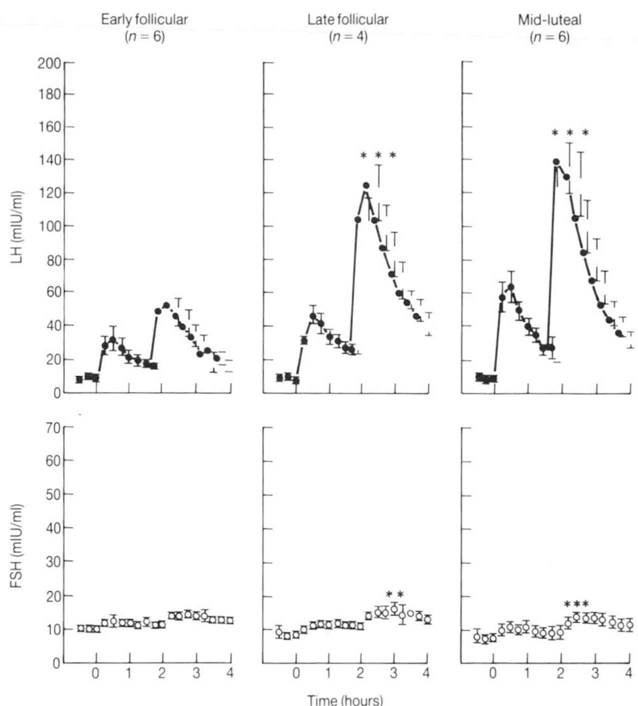

Fig. 9.11 Self-priming effect of bolus injection of GnrH: differing responses at different phases of the menstrual cycle. From Wang et al (1976) with permission.

than the initial response in females when they were retested 1–4 h following the first exposure. This response has been termed 'self-priming'.

Wang and co-workers (1976) published more intensive studies throughout the menstrual cycle and were able to demonstrate that self-priming had a definite cycle relationship which was greatest in the late follicular phase and around mid-cycle — at times of increased circulating oestrogen levels — and oestrogen preferentially induces LH rather than FSH release (Fig. 9.11).

This self-priming effect of LHRH is of importance in understanding the physiological control mechanisms of gonadotrophin release. It suggests that there are two pools of gonadotrophins, one readily releasable by initial exposure to LHRH and a second reserve pool. The exposure of this larger reserve pool to LHRH allows it to be more readily released by a subsequent exposure to LHRH and is suggestive of a transfer of gonadotrophins from one pool to the other. The stage of the cycle, i.e. the endogenous sex steroid environment prevailing — the modulators — and the degree of LHRH stimulation — the prime controller — together influence these transfer capabilities and sensitivity of the pituitary in its response to LHRH.

PULSATILE NATURE OF GONADOTROPHIN RELEASE

The manner of gonadotrophin release is of a pulsatile pattern and it has been demonstrated that there is a pulsatile pattern of LHRH concentration in the pituitary stalk effluent of the rhesus monkey (Carmel et al 1976). This suggests that the pulsatile pattern of gonadotrophin release from the anterior pituitary is probably casually related to the periodic increase in the hypothalamic LHRH system.

Further support of this hypothesis is obtained from the fact that antisera to LHRH abolish the pulsatile release of gonadotrophins and that pulsatile LH release can only be reinstated by pulsed delivery of LHRH and not by constant infusion.

Comparison of the pulsatile pattern of gonadotrophin release at different phases of the menstrual cycle demonstrates profound modulation by ovarian steroids (Fig. 9.12).

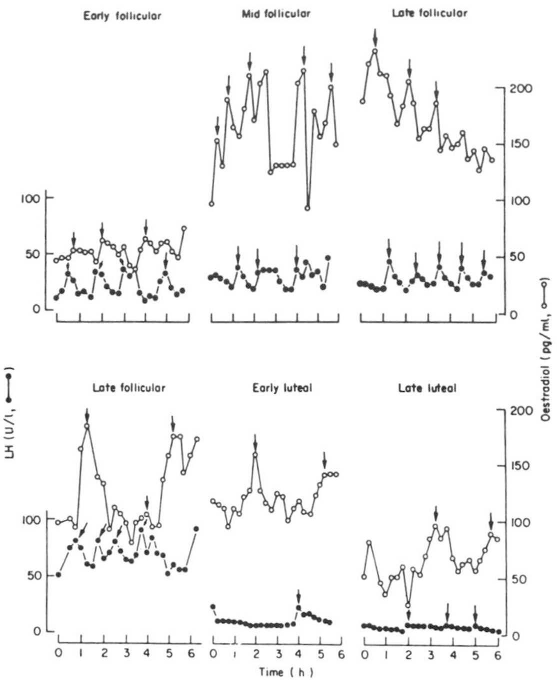

Fig. 9.12 Concentrations of LH and oestradiol at different phases of the menstrual cycle demonstrating different pulse frequency and amplitude. From Backstrom et al (1982) with permission.

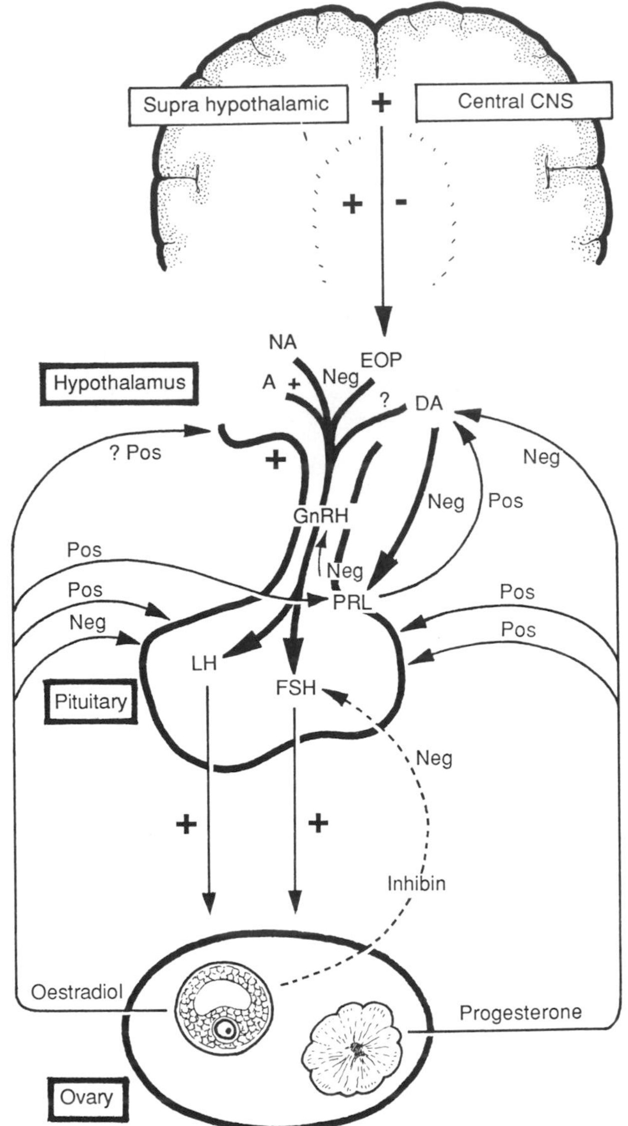

Fig. 9.13 Feedback control mechanisms in the hypothalamic–pituitary–ovarian axis. CNS = Central nervous system; NA = noradrenaline; A = adrenaline; EOP = endogenous opioids; PRL = prolactin; DA = dopamine; GnRH = gonadotrophin-releasing hormone; LH = luteinizing hormone; FSH = follicle-stimulating hormone.

In hypogonadal subjects pulses exhibit high amplitude and high frequency with reversal of the LH:FSH ratio. However, the higher circulating level of FSH is probably not due to a higher FSH secretory rate, but rather its accumulation related to its slower clearance rate (longer half-life).

In normal cycling females during the follicular phase a characteristic low-amplitude, high-frequency pulse pattern is observed. This suggests that oestrogen appears to be most effective in reducing the amplitude of gonadotrophin pulses, more markedly FSH than LH. In contrast the pulse pattern during the luteal phase is one of high amplitude and low frequency — probably modified by progesterone effect on the catecholaminergic and LHRH neuron systems (Fig. 9.12).

INTEGRATIVE CONTROL OF THE HYPOTHALAMIC–PITUITARY UNIT DURING THE MENSTRUAL CYCLE

How can the complex inter-related changes in ovarian steroids and pituitary gonadotrophins that occur within each menstrual cycle be explained on the basis of our present understanding of the control of the hypothalamic pituitary unit (Fig. 9.13).

LH and FSH are released from the anterior pituitary in an episodic, pulsatile manner and the available evidence supports a hypothalamic mechanism for this pulsatile release. Both oestradiol-17β and progesterone can induce a positive feedback release of gonadotrophins, in many respects comparable to that seen at mid-cycle, but progesterone can only induce its effect on a previously oestrogen-primed pituitary gland. There is presumptive evidence that these positive feedback stimuli involve both a direct pituitary action with alteration in synthesis of gonadotrophins and sensitivity to LHRH preceding an induced increase in hypothalamic release of LHRH.

The pattern of gonadotrophin release from the pituitary in response to repeated pulses of submaximal dose of

LHRH or constant low-dose infusion over several hours suggests the presence of two functionally related pools of gonadotrophins. The first primary pool is immediately releasable whilst the secondary pool requires a continued stimulus input and represents the effect of LHRH on synthesis and storage of gonadotrophins within the pituitary cell. The size or activity of these two pools represents pituitary sensitivity and reserve respectively which varies throughout the cycle and is regulated by the feedback action of ovarian steroids and by the self-priming action of LHRH itself. Oestradiol preferentially induces the augmentation of reserve and impedes sensitivity to LHRH with a differential effect apparent for LH release. This oestradiol effect is both dose- and time-related.

Follicular phase

In the early follicular phase both the immediately releasable and the reserve pool of gonadotrophins are at a minimum. The increased FSH release, responsible for initiating follicle development, must indicate an increased output of LHRH with the lowering of negative feedback action in the presence of low levels of oestrogen and progestrogen. As follicles develop oestrogen levels rise, and negative feedback action of oestrogen on LHRH increases suppressing FSH levels. With these progressive increases in oestradiol throughout the mid follicular phase, the quantitative estimates of the primary, immediately releasable, pool of gonadotrophins increase slightly, whilst the reserve pool increases greatly, thus demonstrating the augmentation action of oestradiol primarily upon the reserve pool. Since there is no marked increase in circulating gonadotrophin levels during this phase, secretion of LHRH must be minimal or else there is evidence of impedance of LHRH sensitivity by oestrogen.

Mechanism for preovulatory gonadotrophin surge

During the late follicular phase there is an increase in the amount of oestradiol secreted by the ovary. Under this influence the sensitivity of the gonadotroph to LHRH eventually reaches a phase when LHRH can exert its full self-priming action. The consequence is the transference of gonadotrophins from the secondary reserve pool to the releasable pool. The increased pituitary responsiveness to LHRH may be further enhanced by the slight progesterone rise which can affect its action on a fully oestrogen-primed anterior pituitary. These changes culminate in the production of the ovulatory gonadotrophin surge. It is possible that these events could occur even if the gonadotrophs were exposed to a constant level of LHRH. However, an increased secretion of LHRH, as reported in rhesus monkeys and rats (Sarker et al 1976), at mid-cycle which would act synergistically with the changes in pituitary sensitivity seems likely also in the human.

Luteal phase

The significantly lower basal gonadotrophin secretion in the face of high pituitary capacity during the mid luteal phase suggests that endogenous LHRH should be very low.

A progressive decrease in sensitivity and reserve characterizes pituitary function during the late luteal phase and into the early follicular phase of the next cycle. This is probably due to a progressive decline in oestrogen and progesterone on which sensitivity and reserve are dependent. The role played by the proposed ovarian inhibin on preferentially controlling FSH secretion has still to be determined.

It is therefore apparent that the functional state of the pituitary gonadotroph as a target cell is ultimately determined by the modulating effect of ovarian steroid hormones via their influence on the gonadotroph's sensitivity and reserves and upon the hypophysiotrophic effect of LHRH itself.

With such a complex inter-related control mechanism, it is perhaps not surprising that many drugs which affect neurotransmitters, ill health and associated endocrine disorders can disrupt normal hypothalamic–pituitary–ovarian function, resulting in disordered follicular growth and suppression of ovulation (see Ch. 18).

KEY POINTS

1. The unique portal blood supply to the pituitary gland provides the basis of hypothalamic regulation of the pituitary secretion. It also explains the vulnerability of the gland to hypotension.
2. LHRH controls the secretion of both FSH and LH with ovarian sex steroids playing the role in modulating the proportions of each hormone secreted.
3. The final step in the release of stored LH and FSH, and subsequent induction of further biosynthesis of both hormones following LHRH stimulation involves Ca^{2+}, protein Kinase C and cAMP.
4. The control of LHRH secretion is highly complex and depends upon a number of inhibitory (dopamine) and excitatory (noradrenaline, prostaglandins) neurotransmitters modulated by ovarian steroids.
5. The response of the pituitary gland to exogenous LHRH depends upon the ovarian sex steroid environment prevailing and the degree of LHRH stimulation.
6. Ovarian steroids modulate the pattern of gonadotrophin pulse secretion. Oestrogens are more effective in reducing the pulse amplitude (more so of FSH than LH) whereas progesterone reduces the

pulse frequency of LH as shown during the luteal phase.

7. The positive feedback of oestradiol and progesterone on gonadotrophin secretion may involve a direct pituitary action with alteration in sensitivity to LHRH preceding an induced increase in hypothalamic release of LHRH.
8. LHRH is not only necessary for the release of gonadotrophins (primary pool) but repeated exposure of the pituitary gland to LHRH is essential for adequate synthesis and storing of these hormones (secondary pool).
9. The size or activity of these primary and secondary pools and accordingly the pituitary response to infused LHRH varies throughout the menstrual cycle. It is regulated by the feedback of ovarian steroids and the level of LHRH itself. Oestrogen preferentially augments the secondary while it impedes the primary pool especially of LH release.
10. The final modulation of pituitary sensitivity as a target organ to LHRH is ultimately determined by the effect of ovarian steroids.
11. Progesterone can induce an LH surge by increasing the gonadotrophe's responsiveness to LHRH only in women previously primed by endogenous or exogenous oestrogen.
12. The role of prostaglandin E in LHRH release may be an intracellular one. Activation of noradrenaline release from nerve terminals stimulates post-synaptic production of prostaglandin E which enhances LHRH release.

REFERENCES

Backstrom C T, McNeilly A S, Leask R M, Baird D T 1982 Pulsatile secretion of LH, FSH, prolactin, oestradiol and progesterone during the human menstrual cycle. Clinical Endocrinology 17: 29–42

Carmel P D, Araki S, Ferin M 1976 Prolonged stalk portal blood collection in rhesus monkeys. Pulsatile release of gonadotrophin-releasing hormone (GnRH). Endocrinology 99: 243–248

Clayton R N 1989 Cellular actions of gonadotrophin-releasing hormone: the receptor and beyond. In: Shaw R W, Marshall J C (eds) LHRH and its analogues — their use in gynaecological practice. Wright, London, pp 19–34

Hohlweg W, Junkmann K 1932 Die hormonal-nervose Regulierung der Funktion des Hypophysenvorderlappens. Klinische Wochenschrift II: 321–323

Karsch F J, Weick R F, Butler W R et al 1973 Induced LH surges in the rhesus monkey: strength–duration characteristics of the estrogen stimulus. Endocrinology 92: 1740–1747

Lachelin G C L, LeBlanc H, Yen S S C 1977 The inhibitory effect of dopamine agonists on LH release in women. Journal of Clinical Endocrinology and Metabolism 44: 728–732

Larsson-Cohn V, Johansson E D B, Wide L, Gemzell C 1972 Effects of continuous daily administration of 0.1 mg of norethindrone on the plasma levels of progesterone and on the urinary excretion of luteinizing hormone and total oestrogens. Acta Endocrinologica (Copenhagen) 71: 551–556

LeBlanc H, Lachelin G C L, Abu-Fadil S, Yen S S C 1976 Effects of dopamine infusion on pituitary hormone secretion in humans. Journal of Clinical Endocrinology and Metabolism 43: 668–674

Matsuo H, Arimura A, Nair R M G, Schally A V 1971a Synthesis of the porcine LH- and FSH-releasing hormone by the solid phase method. Biochemical and Biophysical Research Communications 45: 822–827

Matsuo H, Baba Y, Nair R M G, Arimura A, Schally A V 1971b Structure of porcine LH- and FSH-releasing hormone. I The proposed amino acid sequence. Biochemical and Biophysical Research Communications 43: 1334–1339

McCann S M, Ojeda S R 1976 Synaptic transmitters involved in the release of hypothalamic releasing and inhibiting hormones. In: Ehrenpreis S, Kopin I J (eds) Reviews of Neuroscience, vol 2. Raven Press, New York, pp 91–110

McCann S M, Ojeda S R, Fawcett C P, Krulich L 1974 Catecholaminergic control of gonadotrophin and prolactin secretion with particular reference to the possible participation of dopamine. Advances in Neurology 5: 435

Moore C R, Price D 1932 Gonad hormone function and the reciprocal influence between gonads and hypophysis. American Journal of Anatomy 50: 13–72

Ojeda S R, McCann S M 1978 Control of LH and FSH release by LHRH: influence of putative neurotransmitters. Clinics in Obstetrics and Gynaecology 5: 283–303

Rommler A, Hammerstein J 1974 Time-dependent alterations in pituitary responsiveness caused by LH-RH stimulations in man. Acta Endocrinologica (Copenhagen) (suppl) 21: 184

Sarker D K, Chiappa S A, Fink G 1976 Gonadotrophin releasing hormone surge in proestrus rats. Nature 264: 461–463

Schally A V, Arimura A, Kastin A 1971 Gonadotrophin releasing hormone — one polypeptide regulates secretion of LH and FSH. Science 173: 1036–1038

Shaw R W 1975 A study of hypothalamic–pituitary–gonadal relationships in the female. MD Thesis, Birmingham University

Shaw R W, Butt W R, London D R, Marshall J C 1974 Variation in response to synthetic luteinizing hormone-releasing hormone (LH-RH) at different phases of the same menstrual cycle in normal women. Journal of Obstetrics and Gynaecology of the British Commonwealth 81: 632–639

Shaw R W, Butt W R, London D R 1975a Effect of oestrogen pretreatment on subsequent response to luteinizing hormone-releasing hormone (LH-RH) in normal women. Clinical Endocrinology 4: 297–304

Shaw R W, Butt W R, London D R 1975b The effect of progesterone on FSH and LH response to LH-RH in normal women. Clinical Endocrinology 4: 543–550

Wang C F, Lasley B L, Lein A, Yen S S C 1976 The functional changes of the pituitary gonadotrophs during the menstrual cycle. Journal of Clinical Endocrinology and Metabolism 42: 718–724

Yen S S C, VandenBerg G, Rebar R, Ehara Y 1972 Variations of pituitary responsiveness to synthetic LRF during different phases of the menstrual cycle. Journal of Clinical Endocrinology and Metabolism 35: 931–934

Yen S S C, VandenBerg G, Tsai C C, Siler T 1974 Causal relationship between the hormonal variables in the menstrual cycle. In: Ferin M et al (eds) Biorhythms and human reproduction. John Wiley, New York, pp 219–238

Young J R, Jaffe R B 1976 Strength duration characteristics of estrogen effects on gonadotropin response to gonadotropin-releasing hormone in women. II Effects of varying concentrations of estradiol. Journal of Clinical Endocrinology and Metabolism 42: 432–442

10. Ovarian function and ovulation induction

A. Glasier

INTRODUCTION

Ovarian function

The functioning of the ovary ensures regular folliculogenesis and ovulation during the reproductive years. It is totally dependent on the secretion of gonadotrophins from the anterior pituitary.

In the normal human female the number of oocytes is greatest at around 20 weeks of intrauterine life when almost 7 000 000 germ cells can be found within the ovaries. A total of 99% of oocytes formed in fetal life undergo atresia or degeneration. By puberty around 400 000 germ cells are present and in each subsequent normal ovarian cycle one single preovulatory follicle develops to the point of ovulation.

Follicles at all stages of development can be found distributed throughout the stroma of both ovaries at all times until the menopause. Derived from coelomic mesenchyme, the stroma is not an inert support matrix. Growing follicles induce changes in surrounding cells which differentiate into granulosa and thecal cells, and when a follicle becomes atretic many of the cells dedifferentiate to form stromal cells. Folliculogenesis can be conveniently described in different stages.

Recruitment

The ovarian follicle destined to ovulate is drawn from a pool of non-growing primordial follicles, each consisting of an oocyte, a basement membrane and a single layer of surrounding granulosa cells. Within the ovary at any one time most follicles are primordial and only a few are recruited into the growing pool. The cohort of growing follicles undergoes a process of development and differentiation which takes about 85 days and spans three ovarian cycles. It is not clear how follicles are recruited into the growing pool but the process is probably independent of pituitary control and may depend on paracrine factors. The number of follicles recruited into the growing pool is probably a function of the size of the total pool available and decreases with advancing age.

Intermediate follicular development

Once recruited, follicles undergo development and differentiation. The number of granulosa cells increases, the oocyte enlarges, a zona pellucida develops and theca cells align outside the follicle, investing it with an independent blood supply. Only a fraction of the total number of follicles that started the growth sequence reach the stage of becoming potential ovulatory follicles capable of undergoing maturation to the point of ovulation. At the start of the menstrual cycle about 20 antral follicles 2–4 mm in diameter are capable of further development depending on the appropriate gonadotrophin stimulation. The remainder of the cohort — the majority — become atretic. As the previous corpus luteum regresses there is an intercycle rise of follicle-stimulating hormone (FSH), thought to propel suitably responsive follicles into the final stages of the growth cycle.

During the early stages of follicle development granulosa cells acquire FSH receptors and thecal cells acquire luteinizing hormone (LH) receptors. Binding of the LH to receptors on the thecal cells stimulates the production of androgens; FSH binding to the granulosa cells activates the aromatase enzyme system, enabling the conversion of androgens to oestrogens, thus keeping the intrafollicular environment highly oestrogenic. The follicle which most rapidly acquires aromatase activity and LH receptors probably becomes the dominant follicle. As the dominant follicle begins to grow, oestrogen concentrations rise and through negative feedback inhibit pituitary FSH secretion. FSH concentration falls below the threshold required for follicle growth to continue, thus less mature follicles with fewer FSH receptors become atretic. The dominant follicle continues to grow in the presense of subthreshold levels of FSH. The effects of gonadotrophins on follicular development are shown in Figure 10.1.

When the dominant follicle has reached maturity the secretion of oestrogen is sufficient to induce positive feedback and a massive discharge of pituitary LH occurs. The LH surge, acting through prostaglandins, induces changes in the structure and biochemistry of the follicle resulting in rupture and extrusion of the oocyte surrounded by the cumulus mass. LH binds to granulosa cell receptors to stimulate progesterone secretion and initiates a series of morphological and functional changes known as luteinization. The main secretory product of the corpus luteum is progesterone. In the normal ovarian cycle the lifespan of the corpus luteum is 12–14 days. The mechanism of luteolysis is poorly understood in the primate, although in many other species luteal regression is induced by uterine prostaglandins. In a fertile cycle human chorionic gonadotropin (hCG) produced by the conceptus prolongs the lifespan of the corpus luteum which continues to secrete progesterone until the placenta takes over.

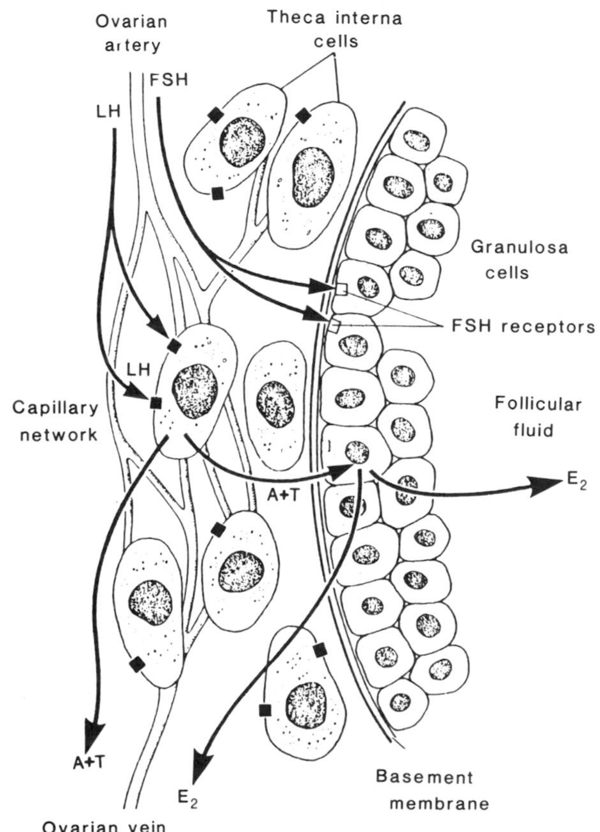

Fig. 10.1 Action of gonadotrophins on the follicle and the synthesis of oestrogens. Luteinizing hormone (LH) interacts with receptors on the theca cells (■) to stimulate production of androgens. Follicle-stimulating hormone (FSH) activates the aromatase system in the granulosa cells by interacting with receptors (□). A = androstenedione; T = testosterone; E_2 = oestradiol. From Baird (1984).

FAILURE OF OVULATION

In developed countries roughly one-third of patients presenting with infertility are suffering from some form of ovulatory dysfunction. A defect in the hypothalamus, pituitary or ovary itself will lead to a disturbance of ovarian function and ovulation accompanied by a variety of menstrual disorders including primary and secondary amenorrhoea and oligomenorrhoea. Successful treatment relies on identifying the underlying abnormality and instituting the appropriate therapy. A classification of anovulatory disorders was endorsed by the World Health Organization in 1976 (Lunenfeld & Insler 1978).

Ovarian activity is totally dependent on gonadotrophin secretion. Normal secretion of gonadotrophins depends on the pulsatile release of gonadotrophin-releasing hormone (GnRH) by the hypothalamus, as described in Chapter 9. Failure or disturbance of the pulsatile secretion of GnRH or of the secretion of LH or FSH will result in disturbances of ovulation. Women with anovulation due to these abnormalities fall into one of seven groups.

Group 1

Failure of gonadotrophin secretion results in low concentrations of serum gonadotrophins with a reduction in both the amplitude and frequency of LH pulses. This results in very low levels of oestrogen production: women present with amenorrhoea and often complain of symptoms related to oestrogen lack such as vaginal dryness. Since there is no oestrogenic stimulation of endometrial growth the administration of exogenous progestagens will not stimulate a withdrawal bleed. Serum prolactin concentrations in these women are often low as a result of oestrogen lack.

Group 2

Women in this group are characterized by normal levels of FSH with normal or elevated levels of LH but with disturbances in the pulsatile pattern of LH secretion. Prolactin concentration is normal and there is some endogenous oestrogen secretion. Patients present with a variety of menstrual disturbances including amenorrhoea, oligomenorrhoea and luteal phase insufficiency. Because there is oestrogenic stimulation of the endometrium the administration and subsequent withdrawal of progestagens will stimulate bleeding. Women with polycystic ovarian syndrome are included in this group.

Group 3

This group includes two conditions in which the ovary itself fails. All the oocytes present within the ovaries develop during intrauterine life, as discussed earlier. An ovary devoid of germ cells cannot function as an endocrine gland and ovulation will not occur. The ovary may fail to develop normally in utero and will be present in adult life as a streak of tissue with no oocytes (such as in Turner's syndrome). Acquired premature ovarian failure can occur in association with ovarian antibodies, as a result of cytotoxic drugs or radiotherapy or in association with minor autosomal abnormalities in women with an otherwise normal chromosome complement. More commonly no identifying cause can be found and ovarian failure probably results from a reduced population of germ cells developing during intrauterine life. In these women the serum oestradiol levels are low, LH levels are elevated and FSH levels are grossly elevated. In all these cases ovarian failure is irreversible; no treatment will induce the development of absent follicles.

Resistant ovary-syndrome. Women with failure of ovulation due to resistant ovary syndrome will present in a similar manner with low levels of oestrogen and elevated levels of gonadotrophins. In this condition however the ovaries do contain primordial follicles but these are apparently resistant to gonadotrophin stimulation despite apparantly normal hypothalamopituitary function. Intermittent episodes of follicular development with a lowering of serum gonadotrophins, vaginal bleeding and, very occasionally, spontaneous pregnancy may occur. Suppression of elevated gonadotrophins for some months with exogenous oestrogens may restore spontaneous ovarian cycles for a short time.

Group 4

This group comprises women with congenital or acquired genital tract disorders presenting with amenorrhoea and with no withdrawal bleeding in response to repeated courses of oestrogen administration.

Group 5

Group 5 includes women with hyperprolactinaemia. Hyperprolactinaemia will result in amenorrhoea, oligomenorrhoea, luteal phase insufficiencies or in apparantly normal ovulation. If a space-occupying lesion cannot be identified in the hypothalamus or pituitary gland women are classed in this group.

Group 6

Women with hyperprolactinaemia in whom a space-occupying lesion can be identified are classified in this group.

Group 7

The final group includes women with a space-occupying lesion but without an elevated serum prolactin.

INVESTIGATION

History

Certain aspects of the history may help to determine the underlying cause of the anovulation. In addition to a routine gynaecological history, care should be taken to ask specifically about weight loss; vegetarianism; galactorrohoea; hirsutism and acne, and excessive exercising. A family history of endocrinopathy may be of significance. The breasts and thyroid gland should be examined carefully and general physical examination should include a Ferriman Galway score for hirsutism.

Laboratory and diagnostic assessment

Laboratory tests should include the measurement of serum oestradiol, gonadotrophins, prolactin, thyroid-stimulating hormone and testosterone. Further estimations of dehydroepiandrosterone sulphate and sex hormone-binding globulin may be indicated if results suggest polycystic ovarian syndrome (see Chapter 22). A pelvic ultrasound scan may help in the diagnosis of congenital abnormalities and of polycystic ovarian syndrome when the presence of enlarged ovaries with multiple small follicles in thickened stroma may be identified.

If ovarian failure is diagnosed it is worth measuring ovarian antibodies. Diagnostic laparoscopy and ovarian biopsy will be necessary to distinguish between premature ovarian failure and resistant ovary syndrome. An X-ray of the pituitary fossa should be carried out in all women presenting with amenorrhoea or with hyperprolactinaemia. If skull X-ray is suggestive of a space-occupying lesion, computerized tomography scan of the pituitary and hypothalamus is indicated.

Dynamic test procedures

Various dynamic tests of endocrine function are available, although the value of some of them is questionable. The administration of exogenous GnRH to test the capacity of the pituitary to produce LH and FSH is commonly performed using a pharmacological amount of GnRH (usually 100 μg) and the results have little or no bearing on subsequent patient management. The administration of thyrotrophin-releasing hormone to normal women results in a significant increase in serum prolactin. A blunted response to thyrotrophin-releasing hormone stimulation has been proposed as a means of distinguishing between hyperprolactinaemia due to a pituitary tumour and idiopathic hyperprolactinaemia, but individual variation in the response makes results difficult to interpret.

The administration of an exogenous progestogen and subsequent withdrawal will serve to distinguish women with very low levels of oestrogen who fail to bleed, and may be helpful in determining whether an individual woman is likely to respond to ovulation induction with anti-oestrogens. Women who fail to bleed following a combination of oestrogen and a progestogen have an anatomical abnormality such as uterine agenesis, until proved otherwise. Other dynamic tests of endocrine function are indicated if thyroid or adrenal dysfunction is suspected.

MONITORING OF OVULATION INDUCTION

Whatever technique is used to induce ovulation, the procedure is time-consuming and often very expensive. In addition women being treated must have a high level of commitment and be prepared to comply with the need for regular monitoring. With some therapies it is enough merely to confirm that ovulation has taken place. Basal body temperature charts, mid luteal phase serum progesterone concentration and serial estimations of the urinary metabolite of progesterone — pregnanediol — are all commonly used to confirm ovulation. If there is a substantial risk of multiple pregnancy; if treatment is being administered via an indwelling intravenous cannula, or if timing for the administration of hCG or for sexual intercourse are involved, monitoring must include serial assessment of follicular growth and maturity and follicle number. Frequent if not daily estimations of oestrogen concentrations in blood or urine should be made and interpreted hand in hand with assessment of follicle growth by pelvic ultrasound scan. In our lab serum oestradiol concentrations reach a mean of around 1000 pmol/l in a spontaneous cycle in the presence of a single preovulatory follicle 20 mm in diameter. Three follicles of around 10 mm in diameter together will secrete equivalent amounts of oestrogen, which can be confusing without information from ultrasound scanning and may lead to misinterpretation. Daily measurement of LH concentrations will allow the detection of a spontaneous surge or premature luteinization.

TREATMENT

GnRH

Following the isolation and characterization of GnRH by Schally and coworkers in 1971 GnRH became available for clinical studies. Initial attempts to induce ovulation with GnRH used high doses administered infrequently and results were inconsistent. Leyendecker et al in 1980 were the first to demonstrate the effectiveness of administering GnRH in a more physiological manner with high-frequency pulsatile treatment. Since that time pulsatile GnRH has become an established technique for the induction of ovulation in certain anovulatory states. Since GnRH is a peptide it has to be administered parenterally and a pulsatile pattern is achieved by using a miniature infusion pump, of which there are a number of models available.

GnRH can be given subcutaneously or intravenously. Absorption is sometimes impaired from subcutaneous sites, resulting in a suboptimal response, perhaps because the pituitary is not receiving a pulsatile message. Results are more consistent with intravenous administration but there is a theoretical risk of infection and thromboembolism. It is logical to try the subcutaneous route in the first instance (using the upper arm rather than the anterior abdominal wall) and to switch to an intravenous route if the response is poor.

Infusion continues from the start of treatment until ovulation is confirmed. In patients with an intact pituitary an endogenous surge of LH usually occurs spontaneously when oestrogen concentrations reach the threshold to induce positive feedback. Alternatively a bolus dose of hCG may be given once a preovulatory follicle is identified by ultrasound scan. In our experience hCG administered too soon will result either in anovulation or in a short luteal phase. Giving hCG rather than waiting for a spontaneous LH surge does allow exact timing of intercourse and may be helpful if patients live too far away to enable daily monitoring.

In women with hypogonadotrophic hypogonadism, and low levels of endogenous LH, pusatile GnRH should be continued after ovulation to provide support for the corpus luteum. Premature cessation of GnRH may result in failure of the corpus luteum with a short luteal phase and menstruation.

If GnRH is being administered intravenously it may be wiser to stop the infusion with its attendant risks once ovulation has been confirmed and to support the corpus luteum with hCG. In women with normal or elevated endogenous LH concentrations, support of the corpus luteum is probably not necessary.

The dose of GnRH and the chosen pulse frequency varies between centres. A fairly standard regime is 5 μg intravenously or 10 μg subcutaneously given with one pulse every 90 minutes in a bolus of between 40 and 80 μl. It may be necessary to titrate the dose according to the patient's weight and response but rarely should it be necessary to give a dose of more than 20 μg per pulse. Since endogenous feedback mechanisms operate in most patients, inducing a spontaneous LH surge, hyperstimulation is rare but multiple pregnancies have been reported.

Ovulation induction with GnRH is most successful in women with hypogonadotrophic hypogonadism; however, in patients with organic pituitary disease treated surgically or with radiotherapy results are often poor. Patients with normogonadotrophic amenorrhoea and with polycystic ovarian syndrome — particularly those with a body mass index greater than 25 — are more resistant to treatment, perhaps because their endogenous LH secretion interferes with the pulsatile pattern achieved by the pump. Women with hyperprolactinaemia will ovulate in response to pulsatile GnRH but bromocriptine is the drug of choice and is much more practical to administer. There is however a place for its use in women who cannot tolerate or who are only partially responsive to bromocriptine and who prefer to avoid surgery.

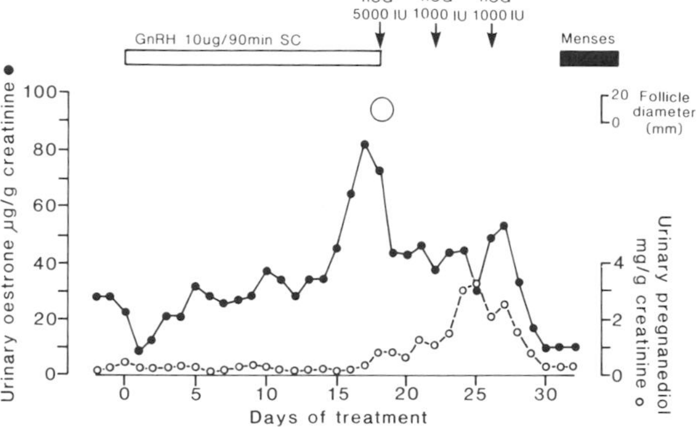

Fig. 10.2 Induction of ovulation in a woman with hypogonadotrophic hypogonadism using pulsatile GnRH. Administration of 10 μg GnRH every 90 minutes subcutaneously resulted in development of a preovulatory follicle which ovulated in response to hCG. Ovarian activity was monitored by measuring urinary oestrone (●) and pregnanediol (○) excretion daily.

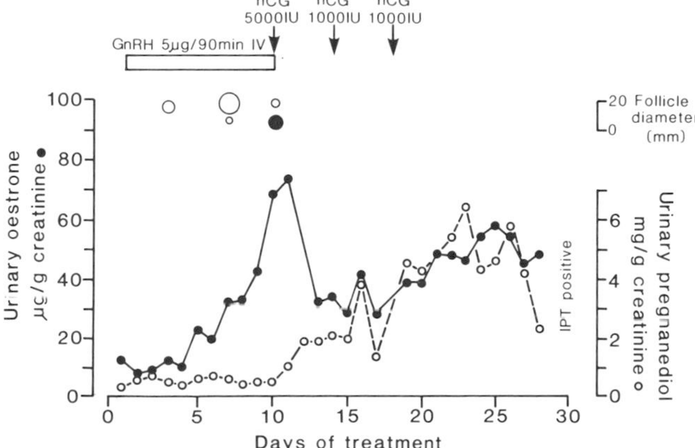

Fig. 10.3 Induction of ovulation in a hyperprolactinaemic woman using pulsatile GnRH. Administration of 5 μg GnRH every 90 minutes intravenously resulted in development of a preovulatory follicle which ovulated in response to hCG. Ovarian activity was monitored by measuring urinary oestrone (●) and pregnanediol (○) excretion. Pregnancy test was positive 29 days after starting treatment.

Two examples of successful ovulation induction using pulsatile GnRH are shown here. In Figure 10.2 GnRH was administered subcutaneously at a dose of 10 μg every 90 minutes to a 27-year-old woman with weight-related secondary amenorrhoea. Before starting treatment she had been found to have a basal LH concentration of 1.1 u/l. After 19 days of subcutaneous GnRH a preovulatory-sized follicle of 16 mm diameter was identified by pelvic ultrasound scan and 5000 iu hCG was administered intramuscularly. Two further injections of hCG (1000 iu) were given 4 and 8 days later to support the corpus luteum. Ovarian activity was monitored by the measurement of oestrone and pregnanediol excretion in urine samples collected daily. Oestrone concentrations rose rapidly from the 14th day of treatment, indicating rapid follicle growth, and urinary pregnanediol concentrations rose following the ovulating dose of hCG and remained elevated until menses 13 days later. In this cycle the patient did not conceive.

Figure 10.3 illustrates the case of a 22-year-old woman with hyperprolactinaemic amenorrhoea. Despite treatment with 17.5 mg bromocriptine daily, the patient remained amenorrhoeic with a serum prolactin concentration of 1660 mu/l — over four times the upper limit of normal. She was anxious to avoid surgery but wanted to start a family and ovulation induction was attempted using pulsatile GnRH. An initial cycle of treatment with subcutaneous GnRH resulted in an anovulatory cycle. Figure 10.3 shows the patient's second treatment cycle with 5 μg GnRH administered every 90 minutes intravenously. A sharp rise in urinary oestrone excretion indicates follicular development and 5000 iu hCG was given on day 10 in the presence of a follicle 16 mm in diameter. Urinary pregnanediol concentration rose indicating ovulation and by day 30 after the start of treatment a pregnancy test was positive.

GnRH analogues

The very short half-life of GnRH limits its use clinically and from shortly after its characterization, attempts were made to synthesize superactive and long-acting analogues which would be easier to administer and more effective. Primarily developed to stimulate pituitary gonadotrophin secretion, the long-acting analogues, after an initial brief stimulation, paradoxically resulted in the suppression of pituitary and therefore of ovarian activity. Binding to pituitary GnRH receptors the analogue prevents regeneration of new receptors in the gonadotrophe membrane and the long half-life of the analogue keeps the pituitary under constant exposure to the drug as if during a continuous GnRH infusion. The compound can be administered by subcutaneous injection or by nasal spray but in these forms has to be given daily. Recently biodegradable implants which last for over a month have been developed. The initial stimulatory effect results in increased secretion of LH and FSH and consequently of oestrogen, resulting in irregular vaginal bleeding which can be overcome if administration begins in the mid luteal phase of the cycle. Since GnRH analogues result in a so-called 'medical hypophsyectomy' they are useful in every condition negatively influenced by oestrogens. These applications will be discussed in detail in later chapters but the GnRH analogues are becoming used increasingly in two areas of ovulation induction.

GnRH analogues and in vitro fertilization

Since the first successful in vitro fertilization pregnancy over 10 years ago, it has become quite clear that higher pregnancy rates can be expected with increasing numbers of pre-embryos transferred. Thus superovulation strategies (strategies expressly designed to achieve multiple follicular development) aim to produce enough oocytes to provide three or four pre-embryos which are suitable for transfer. In women with intact pituitaries, superovulation not uncommonly provokes unpredictable responses, including cyst formation, premature luteinization, early (unexpected) ovulation and asynchrony of follicular growth. This results in the cancellation of cycles or in poor results at oocyte recovery. Suppression of endogenous pituitary gonadotrophin secretion allows good-quality stimulation with significantly higher numbers of oocytes being retrieved and significant improvements in pregnancy rates being claimed as a result of 'higher-quality' embryos being produced.

GnRH analogues with high baseline LH

Women with high endogenous levels of LH are well recognized as being more refractory to ovulation induction techniques, particularly to exogenous gonadotrophin administration. GnRH analogues can be used in a similar manner to suppress high LH levels and spontaneous LH surges, which often occur prematurely as a result of the development of many immature follicles producing oestrogen in amounts sufficient to induce positive feedback in the absence of a mature preovulatory follicle. The technique has also been employed to treat women with apparently unexplained infertility who on closer scrutiny are found to have poor luteal phase progesterone values.

For the purposes of superovulation or ovulation induction GnRH analogues are usually started in the luteal phase of the preceding cycle at a dose of between 600 and 900 μg. Given intranasally or by subcutaneous injection, the analogue is administered daily for a minimum of 14 days in order to achieve ovarian suppression. Thereafter human menopausal gonadotrophin is administered daily at high doses (3 or 4 ampoules/day) in addition to the analogue until one or more preovulatory follicle is identified. hCG is given to induce ovulation and the analogue is stopped. Either a high dose of hCG (10 000 iu) or repeated booster injections during the luteal phase must be given to overcome the persisting suppression of endogenous LH secretion.

Gonadotrophins

With the discovery that follicular development is dependent on gonadotrophin secretion, attempts started in the 1950s to induce ovulation with exogenous LH and FSH. The first pregnancy was reported in 1960 by Gemzell et al using gonadotrophins derived from human pituitaries. Shortly after, gonadotrophins derived from urine obtained from postmenopausal women became available for clinical use and this remains the source of gonadotrophins widely in use today. The most commonly used commercial preparation is Pergonal (Serono). It is marketed in ampoules containing lactose (10 mg) and hMG as a sterile freeze-dried powder with LH activity of 75 iu and FSH activity of 75 iu in each ampoule.

The roles of LH and FSH in the development of the follicle and in normal ovulation have been discussed earlier in this chapter. Many different treatment regimes have been employed for gonadotrophin therapy. These have been fairly extensively reviewed by Brown (1986) and include fixed-dose schedules with and without oestrogen monitoring, and individually tailored dosage regimes. Since it is widely recognized that individual responses to exogenous gonadotrophins vary significantly and that the risk of hyperstimulation and multiple pregnancy is high, the individually tailored dose schedule represents the optimal regime and will be described here in principle.

hMG

hMG is given by daily injection. In women with oligomenorrhoea or who are gestagen withdrawal-positive, treatment should be started within a few days of a menstrual bleed. In women with amenorrhoea treatment can be started at any time provided pregnancy has been excluded. Follicular development is monitored by the measurement of daily serum oestradiol or urinary oestrogen. The starting dose of hMG and the size of the increments vary according to the individual clinician. Because of the risk of hyperstimulation it is best to start at a low dose with small increments. In Edinburgh we start by administering only 1 ampoule (75 iu) each day for 5 days. If there is no rise in oestrogen concentrations above the baseline the dose is increased by 30% and held at that level for a further 5 days, and so on until a response is achieved. Once oestrogen levels rise above the threshold level the dose is kept constant and daily injections are continued until one or more follicles of preovulatory size (20 mm diameter) is identified at ultrasound scan and oestrogen levels are compatible with the presence of a mature follicle (>1000 pmol/l in our lab). At this stage an injection of hCG is administered and the patient advised to have sexual intercourse on a number of occasions over the next 36–72 hours. Oestrogen values at which hCG is administered will vary depending on assay methods used and on individual preferences, as will the dose of hCG administered and the time interval between the last dose of hMG before hCG is given.

There is also no universal agreement as to whether and how hCG should be given in the luteal phase. Generally speaking women with low endogenous levels of LH secretion should receive booster doses of hCG, say 1000 iu, 4 and 8 days after the ovulating dose. Women with normal or elevated levels of LH theoretically do not require luteal phase support.

If the first cycle of treatment is unsuccessful in inducing ovulation the regime can be modified. If follicular development is satisfactory but the cycle is anovulatory or the luteal phase short, the dose of hCG may be increased or boosters administered respectively. In subsequent treatment cycles the starting dose of hMG can be chosen according to the dose required to induce follicular development in the first cycle, thus shortening the treatment period for each patient.

It is widely agreed that patients with low serum gonadotrophin and oestrogen concentrations respond best to gonadotrophin therapy and that women with normal or elevated endogenous LH are more difficult to treat; hence the increasing use of GnRH analogues in combination with gonadotrophins.

Complications and side-effects

Despite years of experience with gonadotrophin administration for the induction of ovulation there is still no foolproof way to avoid hyperstimulation and multiple pregnancy. Even with the most meticulous monitoring, starting at low doses with conservative increments and adhering to strict criteria for witholding hCG, clinicians and patients still get caught out. The most critical requirement for gonadotrophin therapy is achieving the correct dose of FSH and maintaining it within precise limits, which are different for every woman. Most recent series of results report multiple pregnancy rates between 20 and 30%, the majority being twins. In addition the abortion and stillbirth rates following therapy are between 10 and 28% — figures which are inflated partly by the incidence of multiple pregnancy. There appears to be no increase in the incidence of congenital abnormalities in pregnancies induced with gonadotrophins. A case of multiple pregnancy resulting from ovulation induction with gonadotrophins is illustrated here. A 33-year-old woman with primary amenorrhoea due to hypogonadotrophic hypogonadism was treated initially with pulsatile GnRH. Despite the successful induction of ovulation the patient was unable to cope with wearing an infusion pump and — although fully aware of the risks of multiple pregnancy — opted for gonadotrophin therapy.

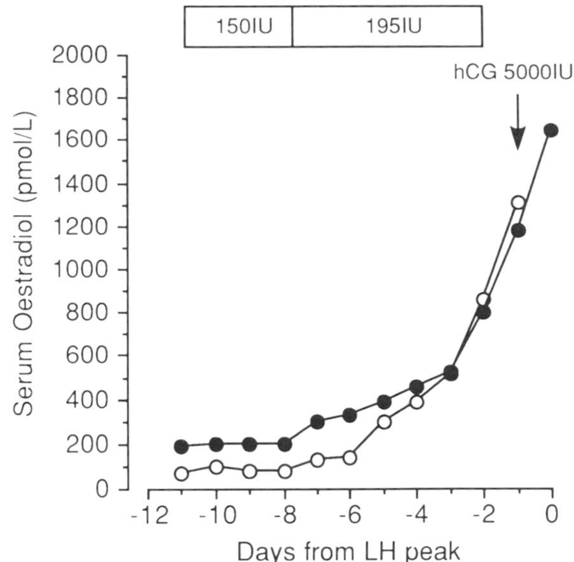

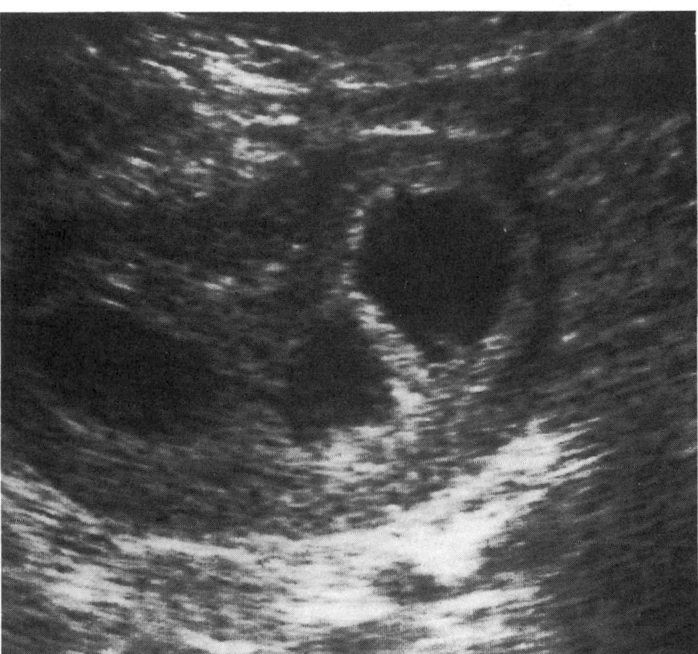

Fig. 10.4a Daily serum oestradiol concentrations (pmol/l) in a woman (○) treated with hMG 150 iu for 5 days and 195 iu for 6 days compared with mean daily concentrations from 12 women ovulating spontaneously (●). hCG was administered to the patient in the presence of two preovulatory follicles and she conceived. (**b**) Pelvic ultrasound scan at 8 weeks' gestation showed three fetal sacs.

Ovulation was successfully induced with hMG in 6 cycles. Ovarian activity was monitored with daily estimations of serum oestradiol and frequent ultrasound scans to determine the follicle number were carried out. The threshold dose of hMG, i.e. that which resulted in the growth of follicles beyond 10 mm and rise in serum oestradiol concentration above 300 pmol/l was consistently 150 iu hMG. Following a short interval without treatment hMG was recommended.

The eighth cycle of treatment is illustrated in Figure 10.4. hMG was started at the threshold dose and increased after 5 days to 195 iu/l, as there was no evidence of follicle growth. After a total of 11 days of hMG and in the presence of two follicles of 24 mm diameter and three follicles of less than 10 mm, 5000 iu hCG was given to induce ovulation and the patient was instructed to have intercourse. Two booster doses of hCG were given in the luteal phase and on this occasion the patient conceived.

Daily serum oestradiol concentrations are plotted in Figure 10.4 and compared with the mean daily concentrations obtained from 12 women who were ovulating spontaneously and undergoing donor insemination (for clarity the error bars have been excluded). Oestradiol concentrations during the treatment cycle do not differ significantly from spontaneous cycles in which single ovulation is the norm, although hCG was given in the presence of two preovulatory follicles.

An ultrasound scan performed 56 days after the start of treatment showed the presence of three gestational sacs and a later scan confirmed a triplet pregnancy. This case demonstrates that despite careful monitoring of the fertile partner it is still easy to be caught out.

Hyperstimulation syndrome

Hyperstimulation has been reported as occurring in between 1 and 20% of patients treated with gonadotrophins and is a result of multiple follicular development and ovarian enlargement. Signs and symptoms appear 3–6 days after the ovulating dose of hCG is administered. If no pregnancy intervenes ovarian enlargement decreases slowly until menses but if conception occurs the ovaries often enlarge yet more as a result of hCG production from the trophoblast and may last throughout the first trimester. Mild hyperstimulation is accompanied by bilateral ovarian enlargement causing abdominal heaviness, swelling, tension and pain. In moderate hyperstimulation the ovaries may enlarge to 12 cm in diameter. Swelling and discomfort are more pronounced and may be accompanied by nausea and vomiting and occasionally diarrhoea. Both forms settle with time and with bedrest and symptomatic treatment. If hyperstimulation is severe, massive enlargement of the ovaries is accompanied by different degrees of acute shifts in body fluids with ascites formation, hydrothorax, hypovolaemia, and shock.

The fluid shifts seem to be the result of an increase in capillary permeability and can be prevented by the prostaglandin synthetase inhibitor indomethacin. Since the derangement involves the shift of fluid from the intravascular compartment into the pleural and peritoneal cavities, management of severe hyperstimulation is aimed at treating shifts in body fluids and correcting electrolyte imbalance.

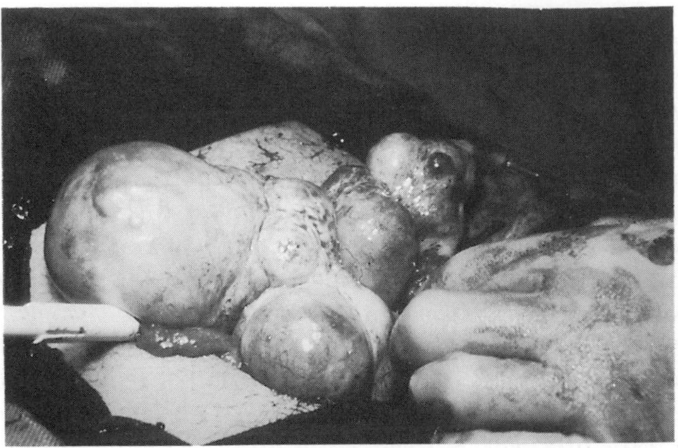

Fig. 10.5 Grossly hyperstimulated ovary in a woman treated with superovulation for in vitro fertilization. Laparotomy was performed for a ruptured ectopic pregnancy.

Severe hyperstimulation is rare but when the full-blown syndrome occurs it can be very alarming and even fatalities have been reported.

When a patient is admitted with severe hyperstimulation haemoglobin, full blood count, haematocrit and urea and electrolytes should be checked daily. A chest X-ray should be performed to exclude or monitor pleural effusion and a clotting screen should be carried out — these investigations should be repeated as indicated, particularly if the patient's condition deteriorates. If the patient is shocked a central venous pressure line may be necessary. Hypovolaemia may be corrected by administering plasma or a plasma expander such as dextran with appropriate electrolyte solutions. In extreme cases disseminated intravascular coagulation may intervene and anticoagulant therapy may be required. While pleural effusions may be safely drained many clinicians prefer to avoid abdominal paracentesis for draining ascites as puncture or rupture of an ovarian cyst may cause severe haemorrhage.

While hyperstimulation syndrome is rare following gonadotrophin therapy for the induction of ovulation, multiple follicular development is the aim of superovulation for assisted conception techniques and hyperstimulation is not an uncommon sequela of in vitro fertilization. Figure 10.5 shows a hyperstimulated ovary. The patient presented as an emergency some 2 weeks after an embryo transfer following in vitro fertilization. She was shocked and had a distended and acutely tender abdomen. Ultrasound scan showed the presence of grossly enlarged multicystic ovaries and an empty uterus. An initial diagnosis of hyperstimulation syndrome was made but serum beta human chorionic gonadotrophin measured over 1000 iu and a ruptured ectopic pregnancy was found at laparotomy.

Purified FSH preparations

Recently a highly purified preparation of human FSH has

been developed by Serono, extracted from hMG using anti-hCG antibodies to cause adsorption of LH on to gel columns. Highly purified FSH (Metrodin) was initially marketed as a more logical (and physiological) therapy for ovulation induction in women with polycystic ovarian syndrome. As well as endogenous LH levels being increased it has been suggested that there is a specific lack of adequate FSH stimulation in this group of patients. Thus treatment with FSH alone may be expected to provide the specific hormone required and to decrease the incidence of hyperstimulation which presents a particular problem in this group. A number of studies of the use of pure FSH have been carried out. Low doses (40–225 iu/day) have proven to be safe and effective but the duration of treatment is prolonged and generally results do not differ significantly from hMG.

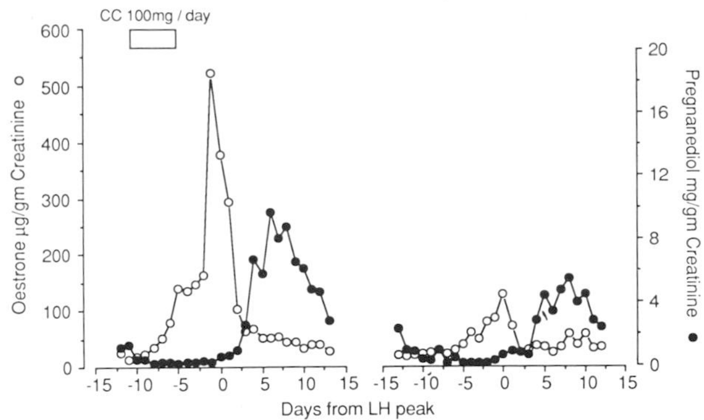

Fig. 10.6 Daily urinary oestrone (○) and pregnanediol (●) excretion in a woman treated with 100 mg/day clomiphene citrate (CC) for 5 days compared with daily measurements made in her spontaneous cycle.

Clomiphene citrate

Clomiphene citrate is a non-steroidal triphenylethylene compound with a structure similar to that of stilboestrol. First synthesized in 1956, it has been widely used for the induction of ovulation for the last 20 years. Its pharmacology and mode of action are still incompletely understood and the literature is often confusing. The commercially available form is a mixture of two isomers, enclomiphene which is a potent antioestrogen and zuclomiphene which has weak oestrogenic properties.

The main site of action of clomiphene citrate is the hypothalamus. Acting in its capacity as an anti-oestrogen it displaces endogenous oestrogen from hypothalamic receptor sites, thus removing negative feedback. The frequency of pulsatile GnRH secretion is increased, resulting in a rise in the pulse frequency of both LH and FSH release. The evidence for a direct effect of clomiphene citrate on the pituitary comes entirely from animal models in which a stimulatory effect on gonadotrophin release from the pituitary may be achieved by sensitizing the gonadotrophe to GnRH. A direct effect on the ovary has also been hypothesized but the evidence for this is unclear. Increased secretion of endogenous gonadotrophins in response to clomiphene citrate results commonly in multiple follicular development. Figure 10.6 illustrates the daily oestrone and pregnanediol excretion (timed in relation to the day of the LH peak) in a woman who ovulates spontaneously. In the spontaneous cycle only one preovulatory follicle could be identified by pelvic ultrasound on the day of the LH peak. When 100 mg clomiphene citrate was administered daily from the second day of the cycle for 5 days, three follicles of greater than 18 mm in diameter were present and mid-cycle oestrone and luteal phase pregnanediol concentrations in urine were accordingly substantially elevated.

Clomiphene is administered orally for 5 days in the follicular phase of the cycle. The actual timing of administration varies between centres, with start days varying between day 2 and day 5 of the cycle. Most centres use an initial dose of 50 mg, increasing in 50 mg steps to 150 or 200 mg if ovulation is not induced by the lower dose.

In some women follicular development occurs in response to clomiphene but failure of positive feedback results in anovulation as an LH surge is not generated. In these cases hCG can be given in combination with clomiphene: 5000 iu hCG is administered when the presence of a preovulatory sized follicle, with appropriate oestrogen levels, is confirmed.

Failure to respond to clomiphene citrate with follicular development is not uncommon, particularly in women with polycystic ovarian syndrome. Before switching to an alternative therapy it may be worth treating for a longer period of time, say 8 days of clomiphene at a reduced dose. In women with increased endogenous testosterone concentrations, supplementing with dexamethasone (0.5 mg/day) may result in an improved response. It may be that increased levels of circulating androgens inhibit aromatase activity and folliculogenesis. Dexamethasone should be stopped once ovulation has been confirmed because of the theoretical harmful effects on the fetus.

The primary indication for clomiphene citrate is in women with normogonadotrophic normoprolactinaemic disorders of ovulation (group 2). Treatment is generally unsuccessful in women who are hypo-oestrogenic.

Side-effects of clomiphene citrate include visual disturbances, hot flushes, breast tenderness, abdominal discomfort and rashes. Hyperstimulation does occur but not with such frequency nor with such alarmingly high numbers of follicles or fetuses as with gonadotrophins. As such, intensive monitoring is not usually undertaken; the confirmation that ovulation has occurred is sufficient. A multiple pregnancy rate of between 6 and 12% has been reported. In a review of 2369 pregnancies carried out by Merrell (1972), 7.9% were multiple, with 6.9% being twins and 0.5% triplets.

While most studies report successful ovulation induction in up to 70% of women, pregnancy rates are commonly less than 50%. Luteal phase inadequacies, cervical mucus hostility, and an increase in the abortion rate have long been cited as possible explanations for this discrepancy. More recently with increasing information on gamete biology becoming available from research associated with in vitro fertilization programmes, concern has been expressed over a possible detrimental effect of clomiphene on the endometrium and on oocytes and embryos.

Tamoxifen

Other anti-oestrogenic preparations are available and act in a similar manner to clomiphene. Tamoxifen is widely used for the treatment of benign breast disease but does not have a product licence for use in the induction of ovulation. Nevertheless, given for 5 days in the same way as clomiphene, 20 mg/day tamoxifen will induce ovulation in those same groups of women and may be useful in some women who are unable to tolerate clomiphene.

Cyclofenil

Cyclofenil (Rehibin) is a compound structurally similar to diethylstilboestrol. Unlike clomiphene citrate, cyclofenil has no anti-oestrogenic properties and little is known about its mechanism of action in the human. It has been reported to increase FSH levels in the rat. It is claimed that cyclofenil enhances the production of thin copious elastic mucus, favouring sperm transport and overcoming one of the well recognized drawbacks of clomiphene citrate. Multiple follicular development is not a feature of this compound. Women who are suitable for therapy with clomiphene citrate should respond to cyclofenil and there are reports of superior results in terms of pregnancy rates. The literature on cyclofenil is sparse.

Bromocriptine

Bromocriptine is a dopamine agonist widely used in the UK and Europe for the treatment of hyperprolactinaemia. Unlike the other pituitary hormones prolactin secretion is under negative control with prolactin inhibitory factor inhibiting production by the lactotrophes. Prolactin inhibitory factor is thought to be dopamine, therefore a dopamine agonist might be expected to inhibit prolactin secretion.

Given orally on a daily basis the starting dose is 2.5 mg and may be increased to doses of up to 17.5 mg. Patients often complain initially of nausea and it may be necessary to start with half a tablet taken with food at bedtime in order to get patient compliance. Once normoprolactinaemia has been achieved and regular menstruation established the pregnancy rate is of the order of 80% or more. The drug should be stopped once pregnancy has been confirmed, although from a number of studies of large populations of women conceiving on bromocriptine, the incidence of congenital malformation is no higher than that of spontaneous pregnancies. Since bromocriptine does not increase the ovulation rate there is no risk of multiple pregnancy and monitoring is only required to determine that ovulation is occurring.

Women who are unable to tolerate bromocriptine or who remain hyperprolactinaemic may be treated with other dopamine agonists such as lisuride, pergolide or metergoline but at present these are only available on a named-patient basis. If a pituitary tumour is present this may be removed surgically or treated with radiotherapy and in those women without a tumour, GnRH or hMG may be used to induce ovulation with some success.

KEY POINTS

1. The functioning of the ovary ensures regular folliculogenesis and ovulation during the reproductive years.
2. The cohort of growing follicles undergo a process of development and differentiation which takes about 85 days and spans three ovarian cycles.
3. In developed countries roughly one third of patients presenting with infertility are suffering from some form of ovulatory dysfunction.
4. Various dynamic tests of endocrine functions are available, although the value of some of them is questionable.
5. With some therapies it is enough merely to confirm that ovualation has taken place.
6. In women with hypogonadotrophic hypogonadism, and low levels of endogenous LH, pulsatile GnRH should be continued after ovulation to provide support for the corpus luteum.
7. Despite years of experience with gonadotrophin administration for the induction of ovulation there is not a foolproof way to avoid hyperstimulation and multiple pregnancy, but careful ultrasound and endocrine monitoring are mandatory.
8. Clomiphene citrate has been widely used for induction of ovulation for the last 20 years and is usually the first line of treatment in subjects who are normoprolactinaemic.
9. Careful evaluation of patients with hyperprolactinaemia to exclude a pituitary tumour is essential before prescribing bromocriptine.

REFERENCES

Baird D T 1984 The ovary. In: Austin C R, Short R V (eds) Reproduction in mammals, Vol 3. Cambridge University Press, Cambridge, pp 91–114

Brown J B 1986 Gonadotropins. In: Insler V, Lunenfeld B (eds) Infertility: male and female. Churchill Livingstone, Edinburgh, pp 359–396

Gemzell C A, Diczfalusy E, Tillinger K-G 1960 Human pituitary follicle-stimulating hormone. I. Clinical effect of a partially purified preparation. Ciba Foundation Colloquia on Endocrinology 13: 191–195

Leyendecker G, Wildt L, Hansmann M 1980 Pregnancies following chronic intermittent (pulsatile) administration of GnRH by means of a portable pump (Zyklomat): a new approach to the treatment of infertility in hypothalamic amenorrhoea. Journal of Clinical Endocrinology and Metabolism 51: 1214–1216

Lunenfeld B, Insler V 1978 Diagnosis and treatment of functional infertility. Grosse Verlag, Berlin, pp 12–13

Merrel 1972 Merrel National Laboratories product information bulletin

Schally A V, Kastin A J, Arimura A 1972 The hypothalamus and reproduction. American Journal of Obstetrics and Gynecology 114: 423–442

11. Fertilization and implantation

R. W. Shaw

INTRODUCTION

The process of fertilization and implantation is highly complex. It involves a final maturation of the gametes, transport of the gametes in the female genital tract, the establishment of the diploid number of chromosomes at fertilization, transport of the fertilized ovum (zygote) from the fallopian tube to the uterine cavity, attachment of the pre-embryo to the endometrium, and finally implantation. The process involves a number of pituitary hormones, various steroids and locally secreted hormones. The developing pre-embryo from an early stage also secretes substances which are vital for its own survival and to enable it to endure the process of successful implantation.

THE SPERMATOZOON

The testis performs two major functions: the first is the synthesis of androgens in the Leydig cells which lie between the seminiferous tubules, and the second is to produce spermatozoa which are developed within the tubules where they come in contact with the Sertoli cells. Although the process of steroid production and spermatogenesis take place in these discrete compartments, their production is an inter-related function since adequate sperm production is only possible when androgen synthesis occurs. This ensures that the mature spermatozoa are delivered into an extragonadal environment which has been suitably prepared for efficient transfer to the female genital tract. (For further details, see Ch. 25.)

Differentiation of spermatozoa

A mature spermatozoon is an elaborate and highly special-

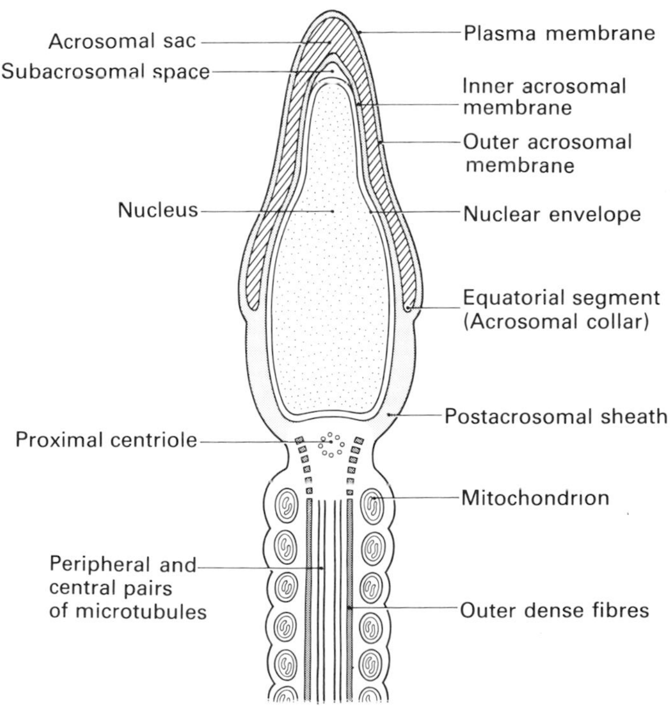

Fig. 11.1 Diagram of a human speramatozoon showing principal structures.

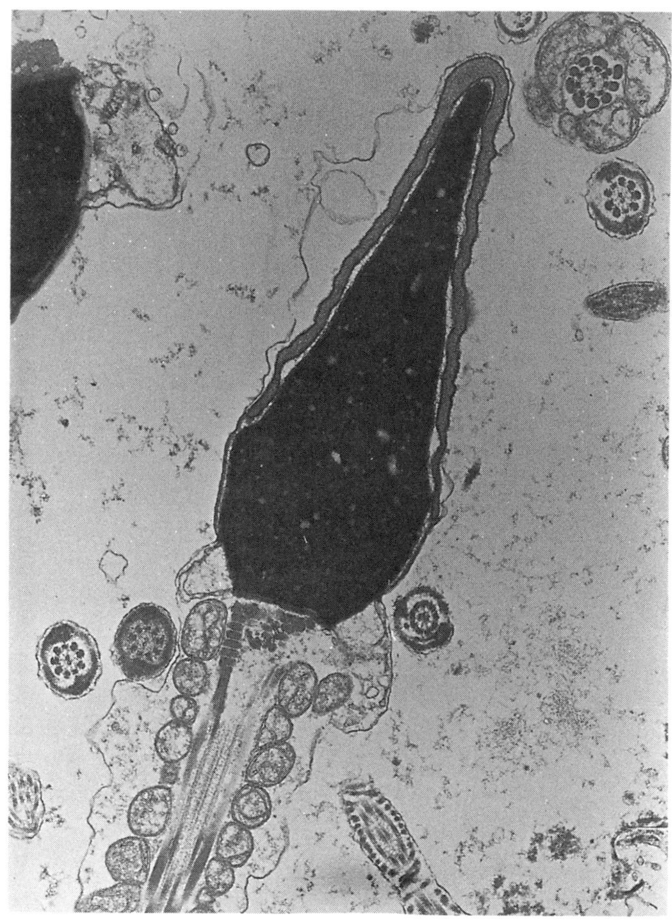

Fig. 11.2 High-power electron microscopy picture of human spermatozoon, complementing the features shown in Figure 11.1.

ized cell. It contains the basic elements common to all cells but their organization has been highly specialized. A mature spermatozoon contains the haploid number of chromosomes (22 + 1).

The major changes which occur during spermiogenesis include generation of the tail for provision of motility and forward propulsion; the mid-piece which contains the mitochondria or energy generators for the cell; the acrosome, necessary for penetration of the oocyte, and the residual body which contains other tail elements of the residue of superfluous cytoplasm. This is the final differentiation into the mature spermatozoon, whose complex structure is seen in Figures 11.1 and 11.2. These are highly complex structural changes and it is not surprising therefore that many cells commencing on this process of differentiation do not complete it successfully. It is not uncommon to find abnormally developed spermatozoa comprising 25–40% of the total contained in an ejaculate in normal fertile males.

Maturation of the spermatozoa

The spermatozoon is a few microns in length. To reach the female gamete in the tube, it must travel a distance of some 30–40 cm through the reproductive tract. It must overcome a number of obstacles in its journey; it has been estimated that less than 1 in a million spermatozoa ever complete the journey. In addition, the spermatozoa must successfully undergo a series of changes in both the male and female genital tracts before they gain full capacity to fertilize an oocyte.

Following their release from association with the Sertoli's cells, spermatozoa enter a specific fluid within seminiferous tubules which washes the spermatozoa towards the rete testis and then into the vasa efferentia and the epididymis. In the epididymis the composition and volume of the fluid undergoes major changes; the concentration of the spermatozoa increases by fluid absorption. In addition, specific secretory products from the epididymis, including various glycoproteins and carotene and glyceryl phosphoryl choline, are added. This passage through the vasa efferentia and epididymis takes some 12 days. During this process the spermatozoa gain the capability of movement as well as the potential to fertilize an oocyte. Other subtle structural changes also occur during this time. It is uncertain whether the biochemical morphological changes are critical for the functional maturity of the spermatozoa. Adequate stimulation by androgens of the epididymis is essential for this process of maturation.

The final passage of the spermatozoa from the tail of the epididymis to the vas deferens is no longer as a result of fluid movement, but due to muscular activity of the epididymis and vas.

The fluid which carries the spermatozoa into the female tract is largely derived from the major accessory sex glands, but its presence is not essential for sperm function. This is apparent from the evidence that spermatozoa taken directly from the vas deferens can fertilize oocytes.

At coitus, sperm are introduced into the female genital tract by ejaculation which expels the semen from the posterior urethra. This is achieved by contractions of the smooth muscles from the urethra and striated muscles of the bulbocavernosus and ischiocavernosus.

Transport of spermatozoa in the female tract

Following ejaculation into the vagina, the semen coagulates rapidly. The coagulating enzymes derive from the prostate acting on a fibrinogen-like substrate derived from the seminal vesicle. In normal circumstances, the coagulum is dissolved within 20–60 min by progressive activation of a proenzyme derived from the prostatic secretion component in the ejaculate. However within a minute or so of ejaculation some spermatozoa can be detected in the cervix. How the spermatozoa enter the cervix is still not clearly understood — whether by action of ciliated cells of the cervical os, or actions unknown. However, perhaps over 99% of spermatozoa from a positive ejaculation do not enter the cervix and are lost by leakage from the vagina. If they do enter the cervix successfully, they survive for many hours deep in the cervical crypts of the mucous membrane, and are nourished by cervical mucus secretions. Further progress to the uterus then depends on the consistency of the mucus. Only in the absence of progesterone domination does the mucus permit sperm penetration.

There are little data about how spermatozoa traverse the uterus to the fallopian tube. There is good evidence that major activity of the musculature of the uterus is not an important component nor prostaglandin-induced contractions. Movement through the uterus is likely to be by the spermatozoa's own motility pattern, producing their own propulsive activity and from currents of fluid set up by the action of the uterine cilia. There is evidence that the uterotubal junction may regulate entry into the oviduct via its activities as an intermittent sphincter, such that only small numbers of spermatozoa enter the fallopian tube at any one time.

Capacitation and activation

Immediately following ejaculation the spermatozoa are unable to achieve fertilization. This has been noted in studies with in-vitro fertilization. They only gain this capacity after a delay of several hours. This process of capacitation — attainment of fertilizing capacity — takes place during the journey through the female genital tract. It appears to involve the stripping from the spermatozoon of the surface coat of glycoprotein molecules which had been absorbed in the epididymis and seminal plasma. The loss of this protein coat is a result of the effects of the proteolytic enzymes and the high ionic concentration found in the secretions of an oestrogen-dominated uterus (Fig. 11.3).

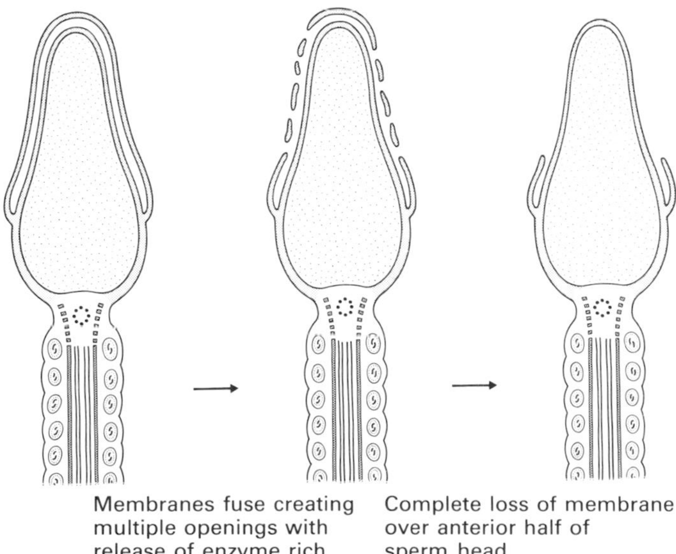

Fig. 11.3 Acrosome reactions.

Despite completing this process of capacitation, the sperms are still not fully ready to fertilize oocytes until the final process of activation has occurred. This process is calcium-dependent and involves changes throughout the spermatozoon. The first process is called 'acrosome reaction', in which the acrosome swells and its membrane fuses at a number of points, with the overlying plasma membrane taking a vesiculated appearance. A result of this process is to expose the contents of the acrosomal vesicle and the inner acrosomal membrane to the exterior. At the same time there is a change in the movement pattern of the spermatazoon. The tail movements of the spermatozoa, which previously demonstrated regular wave-like flagella beats, now become replaced by more episodic wide-amplitude whiplash movements which carry it forward.

The other apparent change occurs in the surface membrane overlying the middle and posterior half of the spermatozoon head. This membrane, previously incapable of fusion, now becomes capable of fusing with the surface membrane of the oocyte.

The exact processes involved in this process of activation are not fully determined. However, activated spermatozoa tend only to be found in close association with the oocyte and cumulus mass. This suggests that a constituent of follicular fluid, a secretion from the cumulus mass or a product in the zona pellucida itself may be responsible for this activation which facilitates the binding of the spermatozoa to the oocyte membrane.

THE OOCYTE

Structure of the ovary

The ovary consists of stromal tissue which contains the primordial follicles, and glandular tissue consisting of interstitial cells. It is the primordial follicle, consisting of the primordial germ cell surrounded by a layer of flattened mesenchymal cells, which is the fundamental functional unit within the ovary. The process of gamete production in the female consists of the processes of cell proliferation by mitosis, the process of genetic reshuffling and reduction — meiosis — and finally the reduction to the haploid number of chromosomes during oocyte maturation. One major difference between the female and the male is the vast difference between the need for proliferation by mitosis, essential in the male to maintain a massive sperm output from the testes, but less essential in the female since only one or at most a few eggs are released during each menstrual cycle.

The primordial germ cells which enter the gonad continue mitotic proliferation well after ovarian morphology is established in utero. However, unlike the situation in the male, the mitotic phase of the primordial germ cells, or oogonia, terminates finally before birth when all oogonia enter into their first meiotic division and hence become the primary oocytes. One major consequence of this early meiosis is that by the time of birth the woman has within her ovary all the oocytes that she will ever have. In the progress through the first meiotic phase, oocytes become surrounded by ovarian mesenchymal cells to form the primordial follicles. These follicles form the oocytes which become arrested in the diplotene stage of their first meiotic phase. The chromosomes remain enclosed by a nuclear membrane in the nucleus, known as the germinal vesicle. The primordial follicle remains in this arrested state within the ovary until it receives the appropriate signals to resume development.

Recruitment of follicle

The regular recruitment of primordial follicles to a pool of subsequently growing and developing follicles occurs first at puberty. Thereafter follicles recommence growth daily so that there is a continual supply of developing follicles being formed. It is on this cohort that the increased gonadotrophin secretion seen in the first few days of the menstrual cycle in the early follicular phase has its action of recruitment. If there is no appropriate gonadotrophin signal then that cohort of follicles does not develop and they undergo atresia.

Follicular development

Following puberty the integrated secretions from the hypothalamic–pituitary axis result in cyclical function in the ovary and the theca and granulosa of the ovary begin to produce oestrogens, progesterone and androgens. At each menstrual cycle several follicles are recruited and develop further as they take on the capacity to respond to gonadotrophins (see Ch. 10). As the granulosa cells multiply, fluid accumulates within the follicles converting the primordial follicles into early antral follicles. By about days 5–7 in each cycle one follicle assumes dominance and proceeds to further growth and maturation (Fig. 11.4). As follicular fluid accumulates further, the multiplying follicular cells are pushed toward the margin, the oocyte becomes surrounded by fluid and some granulosa cells and suspended in the periphery of the follicle by a small neck of granulosa cells. Thus the follicle develops into the mature graafian follicle. As this follicle further increases in size, it protrudes beyond the surface of the ovary, creating a visible projection.

Morphological changes

Once the primordial follicle is recruited to begin maturational changes, the granulosa cells surrounding the oocytes start to change from squamous to cuboidal in appearance. An increase in follicular diameter occurs in the major part of growth, resulting from an increase in diameter in the primordial oocyte from 20 μ to between 60 and 100 μ. During this critical growth phase a massive synthetic activity is occurring, particularly with the synthesis of large amounts of RNA; this activity loads the oocytes' cytoplasm with essential materials for the later stages of egg maturation. During this oocyte increase in size an acellular glycoprotein matrix termed the zona pellucida is secreted by the granulosa cells and forms an envelope surrounding the oocyte. Contact with the oocyte and the granulosa cells is maintained by cytoplasmic processes which penetrate the zona and form gap junctions at the oocyte surface. Gap junctions are also formed be-

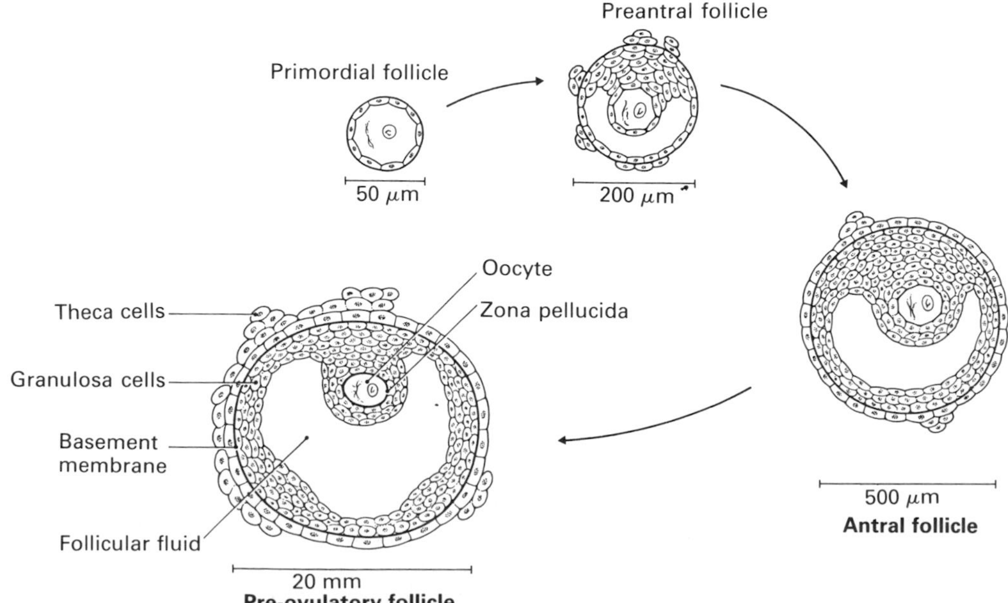

Fig. 11.4 Follicular development from primordial follicle to preovulatory stage.

tween adjacent granulosa cells, thus providing a basis for intracellular communication. Through this network, low molecular weight substrates, some amino acids and nucleotides can be passed to the growing oocyte. Meantime spindle-like stromal cells come into close proximity with the basal lamina of the granulosa cells. These theca cells and cells most proximal to the basal membrane are termed theca interna cells.

Towards the end of this critical growth and reorganization phase of the follicle, cells of the granulosa layer develop receptors for oestrogen and follicle-stimulating hormone (FSH) and the theca cells develop luteinizing hormone (LH) receptors. These are essential to gain entry into the next phase of follicular development, which becomes greatly dependent upon gonadotrophin stimulation patterns.

This gonadotrophin stimulation converts preantral follicles to antral follicles, and encourages further proliferation of granulosa and theca cells. However, there is little addition or increase in size of the oocyte itself: its chromosomes remain in the dictyate stage while RNA synthesis and protein production continue.

Steroid hormone production — two-cell theory

During this second phase of growth follicles show a steady increase in the synthesis of androgens and oestrogens. Production of these steroids is under the control of gonadotrophins; these gonadotrophins appear to facilitate effects at different locations within the follicle. Only the granulosa cells bind FSH and the theca cells bind LH. LH primarily stimulates the cells of the theca interna to synthesize androgens from acetate and cholesterol. Oestrogen synthesis by these cells, is possible to only a limited degree, particularly in the early stages of growth. In contrast, the granulosa cells are unable to form androgens. However androgen supplied to the granulosa cells from the theca cells is readily aromatized to oestrogen (Fig. 11.5). Thus androgens are produced by developing follicles from the theca cells whilst oestrogens arise via two routes — primarily thecal androgens aromatized by granulosa cells, and to a lesser degree by de novo synthesis from acetate in thecal cells.

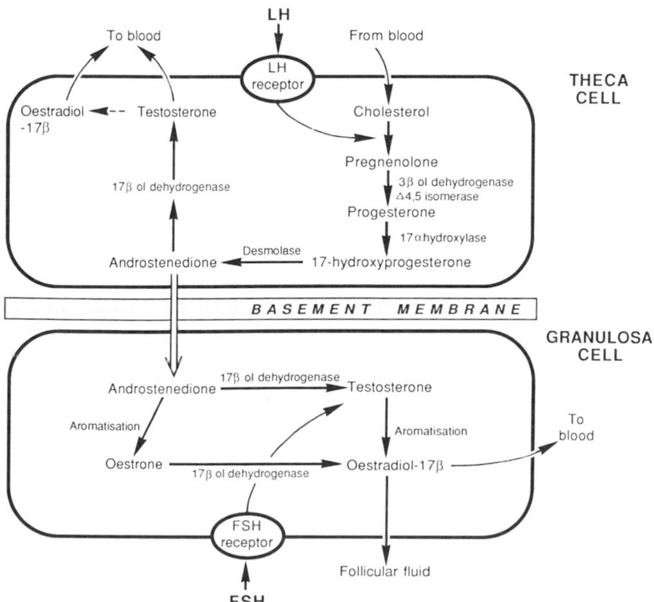

Fig. 11.5 Two-cell theory of follicular oestrogen production. LH = Luteinizing hormone; FSH = follicle-stimulating hormone.

Both the production of steroids and the increase in follicular size are interlinked. Oestrogen in conjunction with FSH plays a crucial role within the follicle towards the end of the second phase of growth. Oestrogen and FSH together stimulate the appearance of LH-binding sites in the outer layers of the granulosa cells. These LH binding sites are crucial for the antral follicle to enter the final phase of development, at least the conversion to the preovulatory follicle.

Cervical mucus

Only in the absence of a progesterone domination does the mucus permit sperm penetration. There are little data on how spermatozoa traverse the uterus to the fallopian tube, although there is good evidence that major activity of the musculature of the uterus is not an important component and passage through the uterus is likely to be achieved by the sperms' own motility pattern.

The spermatozoa then enter the ampulla of the fallopian tube by their own propulsive activity and in currents of fluid set up by the action of the uterine cilia.

Structure of the fallopian tube

After its release from the ovary, the ovum is taken up by the fallopian tube which serves a number of essential functions in the reproductive process. Firstly it is responsible for transferring the ovum into its lumen when discharged from the rupturing follicle. Secondly, it provides an environment for the ovum and spermatozoon in which fertilization can occur, and finally for transferring the fertilized cleaving embryo into the uterus after a timed interval of 3–4 days. At the distal end of the tube are the delicate finger-like projections, or fimbrie. These are lined with cilia which beat in the direction of the tubal lumen. The fimbrial cilia are capable of cyclic regeneration which occurs under the influence of oestrogen. The entire length of the fallopian tube contains cilia; ciliary beat creates a current within the tubal lumen to transport the oocyte from the peritoneal cavity into the uterus (Fig. 11.6).

It is probable that the musculature surrounding the fallopian tube also plays a role in the transport of the oocyte along its course. An increase in tubal contractility is ob-

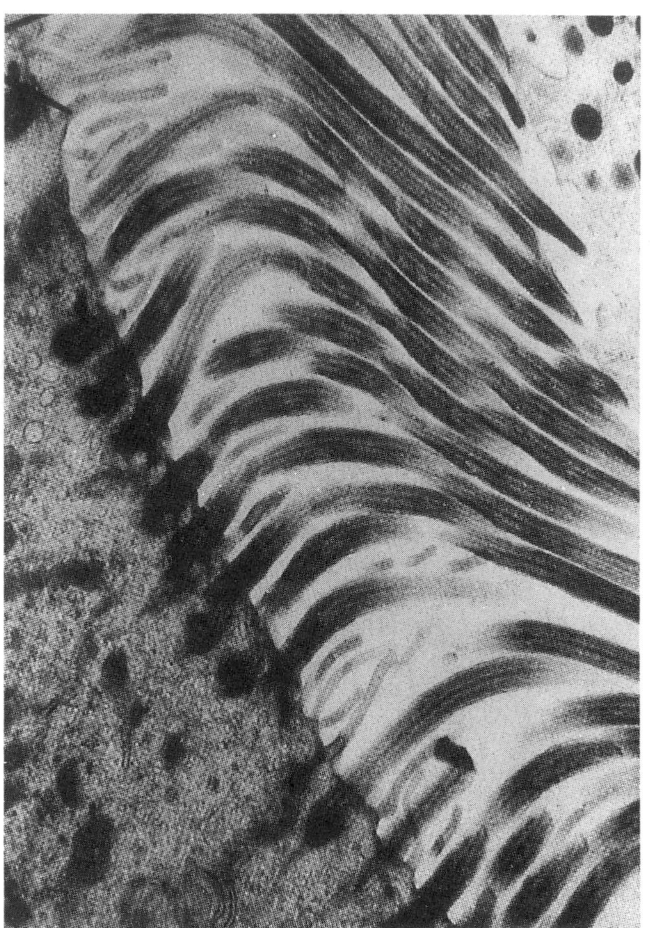

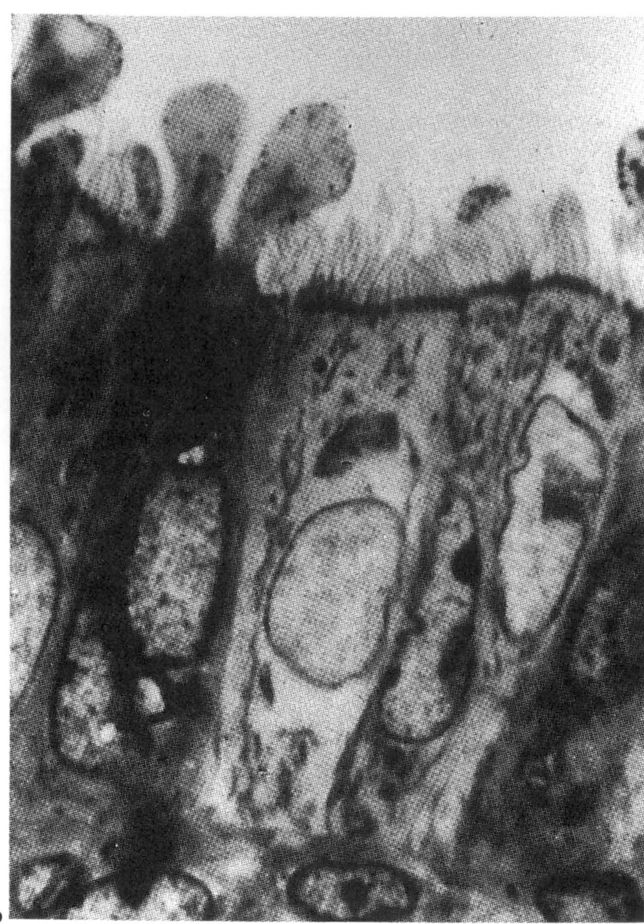

Fig. 11.6 Electron microscopy pictures of (**a**) fimbrial cilia and (**b**) the postovulatory tubal mucosa demonstrating secretory and ciliated cells. From Mastroianni & Coutifaris (1989) with permission.

served during the periovulatory phase corresponding to a fall in oestrogen secretion. Prostaglandin levels in circulation at this time have also been indicated in this tubal contractility, with prostaglandin $F_{2\alpha}$ increasing contractility.

The oocyte is retained at or near the junction between the tubal ampulla and isthmus, then delivered into the uterine cavity approximately 3–4 days after ovulation. At this time of transfer into the uterus, the embryo has developed to a morula.

Tubal secretions

Another important function of the fallopian tube is to provide a suitable environment for the spermatozoa, oocyte and the fertilization process. The secretory elements of the tubal mucosa are modified during a normal menstrual cycle. As ovulation approaches under the influence of oestrogen, the secretory cells become tall and columnar and project beyond the cilial cells, discharging secretions into the tubal lumen. The production of fluid in the fallopian tube is greatest immediately before ovulation but there are little data on the constituents of human tubal fluid or their relevance in the fertilization process.

FERTILIZATION

Fertilization is not a single event but a continuum. The fertilization process begins when the capacitated sper-

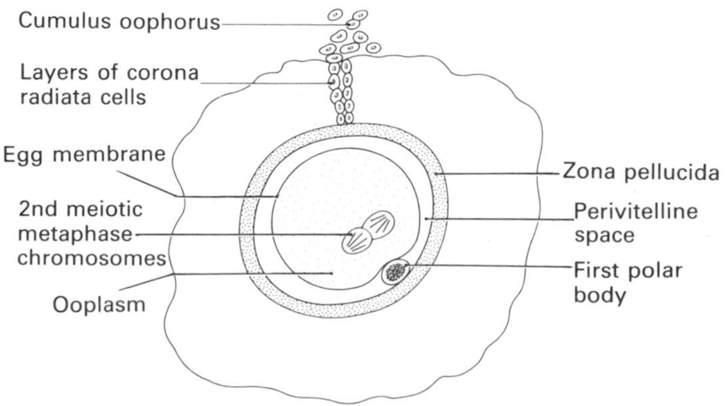

Fig. 11.7 Schematic representation of freshly ovulated oocyte.

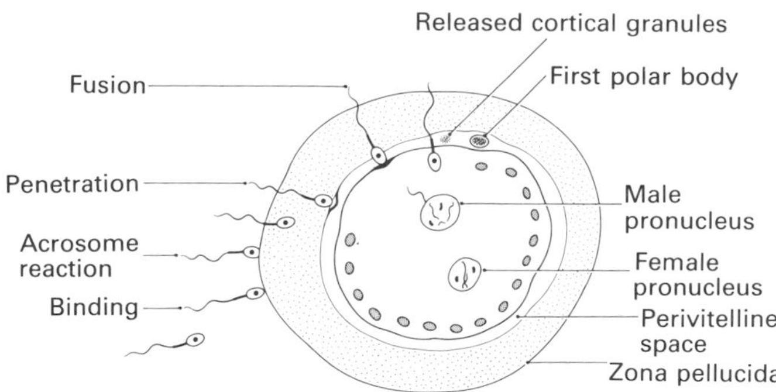

Fig. 11.8 Schematic respresentation of fertilization.

matozoa come in contact with the ovum and its cellular coverings. Before a spermatazoon can do this it must first penetrate the cellular covering of the oocyte, the cumulus oophorus, the corona radiata and the zona pellucida (Fig. 11.7). The cumulus cells are embedded in a matrix rich in hyaluronic acid and the acrosome located at the end of the spermatozoon contains the enzyme hyaluronidase. This may well be important in the dispersion of the cumulus cells. This process of dispersion is further completed by the action of the cilia of the fallopian tube.

The zona pellucida

The zona pellucida is a dense translucent protein layer immediately surrounding the oocyte. It has been suggested that penetration of the zona occurs as a result of release of acrosin — a trypsin-like enzyme-released from the inner acrosome membrane of the spermatozoon. The spermatozoon attaches itself to specific glycoprotein receptors on the outer surface of the zona pellucida (Fig. 11.8). During this process, a proteolytic proenzyme appears on the exposed acrosomal membrane and is activated to yield acrosin to digest a path through the zona.

Penetration of the egg

Once through the zona pellucida, the spermatozoon enters the perivitelline space. The microvilli on the surface of the egg envelope the sperm head and the sperm membrane in the equatorial region of the head fuses with the surface or vitelline membrane of the oocyte. When this has happened there is a cessation of movement by the spermatozoon. Once attachment has occurred, rapid electrical changes occur on the membrane surface which prevent penetration of additional spermatozoa (polyspermia). After the spermatozoon penetrates, corticle granules are released — these are peripherally located particles in the cytoplasm of the oocyte — which contain proteolytic enzymes. The spermatozoon — both its head and tail — is then incorporated in the cytoplasm of the oocyte, completing the penetration process. The first phase of fertilization, from entry of the cumulus mass to fusion, lasts between 10 and 20 min. Ensuing phases of fertilization last some 20 h or so and will result in the return of the diploid genetic constitution of the embryo and the initiation of the developmental programme of the embryo.

Conception

Within 2 or 3 h of oocyte–sperm fusion, the second polar body has been expelled and the remaining haploid set of female chromosomes lies in the ooplasm. When the sperm head enters the ooplasm its chromosome material is tightly packed. During the next 2–3 h these chromosomes uncoil under the influence of cytoplasm of the oocyte, and the sperm head is transformed into the male pronucleus. The male and female pronuclei increase somewhat in size and then migrate towards the centre of the egg; with the formation of the metaphase spindle, the chromosomes assume their position at its equator. This occurs 18–21 h after gamete fusion. The coming together of the gametic chromosomes, syngamy, is the final phase of fertilization. Immediately anaphase and telophase are completed, the cleavage furrow forms and the one-cell zygote becames a two-cell embryo.

Endometrial development

The endometrium has undergone extensive proliferation under the influence of oestrogen in the days prior to ovulation. Its cells exhibit marked mitotic activity. Under the combined influence of oestrogen and progesterone following ovulation, with the increasing quantities of these hormones secreted by the corpus luteum, the endometrial stroma and glands change rapidly. The glands displace a secretory pattern and the products of their secretion are discharged into the uterine lumen (for further details see Ch. 14).

The embryo remains in the fallopian tube in the site of fertilization for approximately 3–4 days. It is suspended in the tubal fluid and continues to develop into the morula. It is then transferred through the isthmus of the tube into the uterine cavity. This transfer is facilitated by the changing endocrine environment of the early luteal phase. There are rapid increasing levels of progesterone in the circulation altering the ratio of progesterone to oestrogen. This affects the oviduct and uterine musculature, inducing relaxation of the sphincter. However it seems more likely that the cilia rather than the musculature of the fallopian tube are the primary active transporters of the embryo.

Within the uterine cavity the embryo establishes nutritional and physical contact with the maternal tissue at the site of implantation (Fig. 11.9). Secondly, it begins to create its own substances which make its presence felt and primarily affect the maternal pituitary–ovarian axis, which ceases to go through its normal cyclical pattern of oscil-

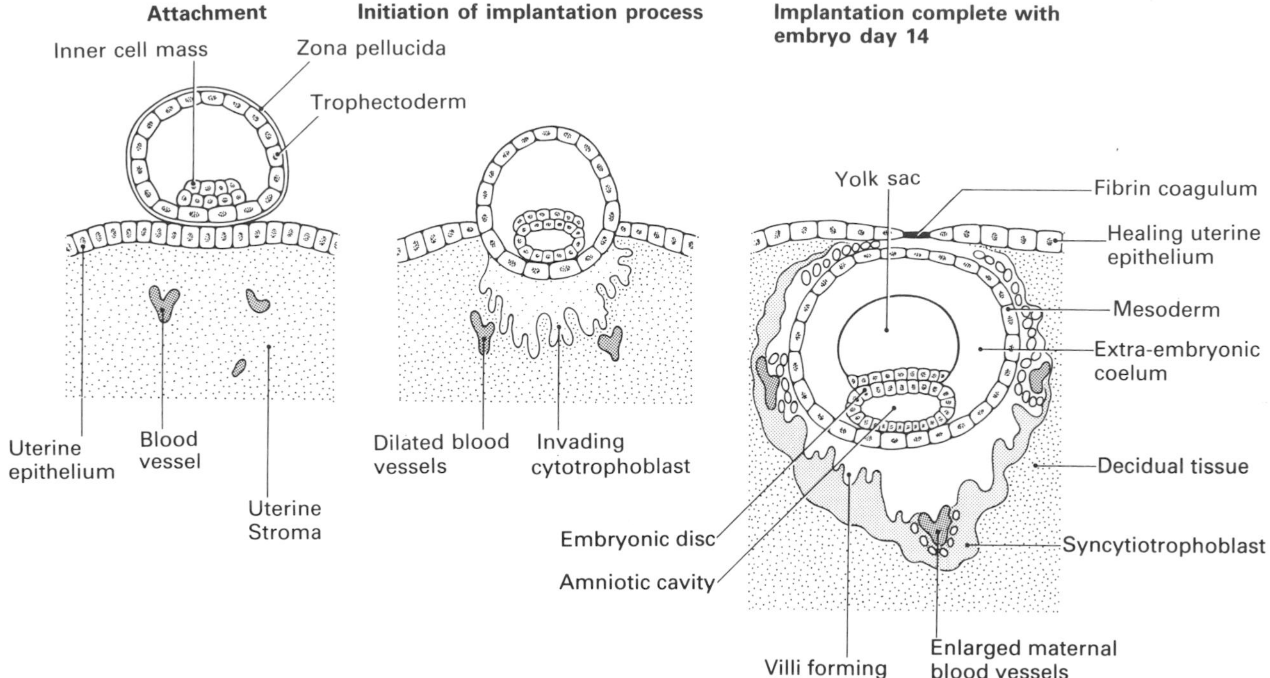

Fig. 11.9 Stages of implantation.

lating oestrogen/progesterone dominance and convert it to a non-cyclic pattern with progesterone dominance throughout.

Growth of the preimplantation embryo

Development of the embryo into the blastocyst continues within the uterine fluid in which it is suspended for 3–4 days. Each cell or blastomere of the two-cell embryo undergoes a series of divisions. Although the actual size of the embryo remains much the same, at the eight-cell stage the cleaving embryo changes its morphology by undergoing a process of compaction to yield the morula. At the same time there is a marked quantitative increase in its biosynthetic capacity and the net synthesis of RNA and protein increases, and there are changes in the synthetic patterns of phospholipase and cholesterol. Between the 32- and 64-cell stage it undergoes morphological changes during transition into the blastocyst. The blastocyst is composed of a fluid-filled cavity surrounded by one layer of trophoblastic cells. An aggregate of cells appears in the periphery, called the inner cell mass. It is from these cells that the fetus will eventually develop; the trophoblast at periphery gives rise to the placental tissue. At this point the blastocyst is still surrounded by the zona pellucida. However, during this time the process of hatching occurs whereby an opening forms in the zona and the blastocyst is freed.

Implantation

The free living morula and then blastocyst is bathed in the secretions in the fallopian tube and uterus respectively and draws from them the oxygen and metabolic substrates it requires for its continued growth. There is a limit to the size the embryo can grow as this process alone cannot satisfy all its nutritional requirements by simple diffusion or active ion exchange.

The site of implantation is perhaps determined by the activity of the uterine musculature which dictates where the blastocyst makes contact with the uterine tissue. The process of implantation involves the adherence of the trophoblast tissue, adjacent to the inner cell mass, to the epithelium of the endometrium. It is at this point that the dissolution of the zona pellucida occurs, thus exposing the trophectoderm to the luminal epithelium of the endometrium. Initial contact between the trophectoderm and the uterine epithelium induces vascularization and then eventual differentiation in the underlying endometrial stromal tissue. In addition, at the point of contact with the maternal epithelium trophectoderm cells, through a process of erosion of the surface epithelium, begins the invasion of the underlying decidualized tissue. During the process of invasion some trophectodermal cells fuse together forming a syncytium (syncytiotrophoblast). Some of those remaining retain their cellularity (cytotrophoblast). These may serve as a proliferative source for generating more trophoblastic cells. Rapid invasion of the trophoblastic tissue causes local disruption of the maternal capillaries, forming venous pools of blood within the decidual tissue. Within 3–5 days of attachment, the whole embryo is completely embedded under the uterine epithelium in the endometrial stroma. By 14–21 days after fertilization the trophoblastic structure at the periphery of the blast cells resembles the villi of the mature placenta and the area of the inner cell mass has started to organize itself into the embryo proper.

SUMMARY

Details of further development go beyond the scope of this book, and readers are referred to relevant chapters in textbooks of obstetrics. The whole process of maturation of the gametes, fertilization, early embryonic development and implantation are highly complex and at many steps problems may arise. Approximately one-third of post-implantation embryos exhibit abnormalities which suggest that they were destined to fail to achieve successful implantation even before the missed period. Embryonic defects may occur as a result of faulty implantation but many are caused by failures at an earlier stage of development. In addition, factors of delayed fertilization when penetration of an oocyte is over-ridden, or genetically induced defects in the oocyte and spermatozoa, together go to explain the high rate of pregnancy wastage in the human.

KEY POINTS

1. Final differentiation of spermatozoa occurs during spermatogenesis.
2. Activation of acrosome reaction in the spermatozoa is calcium dependent.
3. Primordial follicles contain oocytes arrested in the diplotene stage of the first meiotic field.
4. Maturation of ovarian follicles involves a progressive increase in follicular diameter.
5. Oestrogen and FSH play a crucial role during the second phase of growth.
6. The fallopian tube provides the ideal environment where fertilization can take place.
7. Fertilization is a multiple process, in the first step of which sperm attach to glycoprotein receptors on the zona pellucida.
8. Polyspermia is prevented by release of cortical granules and the second polar body is expelled after oocyte and sperm fusion.
9. Implantation occurs after hatching of the blastocyst and the fetus develops from the differentiating inner cell mass.

FURTHER READING

Coutinho E M, Mala H S 1971 The contractile response of the human uterus, fallopian tubes and ovary to prostaglandins in vivo. Fertility and Sterility 22: 539–543

Denker H W 1983 Basic aspects of ova implantation. Obstetrical and Gynaecological Annual Reviews 12: 15–42

Diaz S, Ortiz M-E, Crozatto H B 1980 Studies on the duration of ovum transport by the human oviduct. The time interval between the luteinizing hormone peak and recovery of ova by transcervical flushing of the uterus in normal women. Amcrican Journal of Obstetrics and Gynecology 137: 116

Di Zerega G S, Hodgen G D 1981 Folliculogenesis in the primate ovarian cycle. Endocrine Reviews 2: 27

Erickson G F 1986 An analysis of follicle development in ovum maturation. Seminars in Reproductive Endocrinology 4: 233–254

Glasser S R 1986 Current concepts of implantation and decidualization. In: Hoszar G (ed) The physiology and biochemistry of the uterus in pregnancy and labor. CRC Press, Boca Raton, Florida.

Harper N J K 1988 Gamete and zygote transport. In: Knobil E, Neill J (eds) The physiology of reproduction. Raven Press, New York, pp 103–134

Johnson M, Everitt B 1982 Essential reproduction. Blackwell Scientific Publications, Oxford

Lippes J, Enders R G, Pragay D A, Bartholomew W R 1973 The collection and analysis of human fallopian tube fluid. Contraception 5: 85–93

Mastroianni L, Coutifaris C (eds) 1989 Reproductive physiology, vol 1. Parthenon Publishing, Carnforth

12. Sexual differentiation — normal and abnormal

D. K. Edmonds

INTRODUCTION

Sexual differentiation and its control is fundamental to the continuation of most species. The understanding of this process has advanced greatly in recent years and before abnormalities of intersex can be discussed, an understanding of normal sexual development is important. At fertilization, the haploid gametes unite and the conceptus contains 46 chromosomes, 22 autosomes derived from each of the sperm and ovum, the ovum donating one X chromosome and the sperm either one X or a Y. The axiom of mammalian reproduction is that 46XX embryo will differentiate into a female whereas a 46XY embryo becomes a male. However, it is the presence or absence of the Y chromosome which determines whether the undifferentiated gonad becomes a testis or an ovary.

Genetic control of testicular differentiation

A factor must exist on the Y chromosome which is responsible for testicular differentiation. Localization of the testicular-determining factor (TDF) was finally discovered when individuals with 46X,i(Yq) were found to be phenotypically female with streak gonads. The lack of the short arm of the Y chromosome (Yp) in those individuals localised TDF to this area.

Recent work (Page et al 1987), using DNA probes for the gene copies in XX males, has localized a segment of the short arm of the Y chromosome that contains the gene for TDF, confirming that the position of DXYS5 is the most likely sequence.

The mechanism by which differentiation occurs seems to depend on a cell surface antigen (histocompatibility antigen Y or H-Y antigen). The evidence for this is based on the work summarized by Wachtel (1983):

1. H-Y antigen is present in all individuals containing the Y chromosomes.
2. H-Y antigen is found in XY females.
3. Sex-reversed males (46XX) and true hermaphrodites have H-Y antigen.
4. H-Y antigen is present in the testicular portion of ovotestes but not the ovarian part.

Wachtel also suggests that the locus for the H-Y antigen is near that of TDF, and it may be that TDF regulates H-Y antigen expression (Wolf 1981).

Although H-Y antigen plays an integral part in testicular development, other autosomally located genes must also be involved, as evidenced by the hereditary disorder of testicular regression syndrome. Here, the testes atrophy in late gestation — although normally functional during differentiation — and the familial nature of the condition makes autosomal genetic control most likely. Cryptorchidism is also hereditary and is associated with other genetically determined syndromes.

Genetic control of ovarian differentiation

The presence of two X chromosomes results in ovarian development, but some females with deletions of either the short or long arms of the X chromosome have variable ovarian development, or even streak ovaries alone. With regard to the short arm of X, ovarian determinants seem to be located in the region p11.2 to p21 as loss of this region results in ovarian agenesis (Simpson 1987). Deletions of the long arm in the region of Xq13 are usually associated with ovarian failure, but distal deletions may be of less importance, although X926 deletion seems to be as-

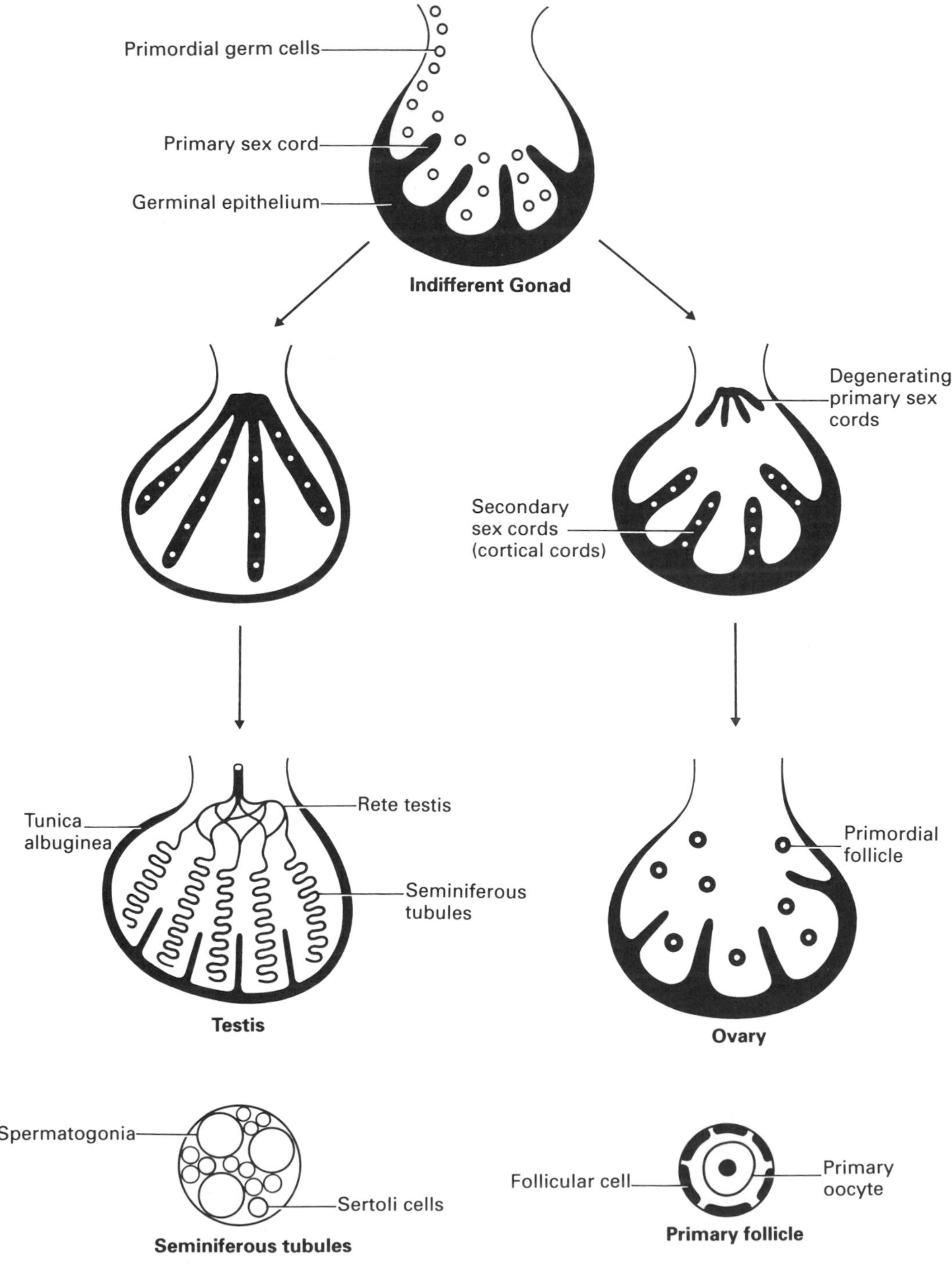

Fig. 12.1 Normal gonadal differentiation.

sociated with premature menopause (Fitch et al 1982). Autosomal loci are certainly involved in ovarian maintenance as gonadal dysgenesis in 46XX females is often a familial autosomal recessive disorder (Simpson 1979).

The development of müllerian and wolffian structures must also be under genetic control. The inheritance is probably polygenic multifactorial although autosomal recessive genes may be involved.

Normal embryological development of the reproductive system (Fig. 12.1)

Although the chromosomal sex is determined at the time of fertilization, gonadal sex results from differentiation of the indifferent gonad to become either a testis or an ovary. This begins during the fifth week of development. At this time, an area of coelemic epithelium develops on the medial aspect of the urogenital ridge and proliferation leads to the establishment of the gonadal ridge. Epithelial cords then grow into the mesenchyme (primary sex cords) and the gonad now possesses an outer cortex and inner medulla. In XY individuals, the medulla becomes the testis and the cortex regresses, and in embryos with an XX complement, the cortex differentiates to become the ovary and the medulla regresses. The primordial germ cells develop by the fourth week in the endodermal cells of the yolk sac and during the fifth week they migrate along the dorsal mesentery of the hindgut to the gonadal ridges, eventually becoming incorporated into the mesenchyme and the primary sex cords by the end of the sixth week.

Development of the testis

The primary sex cords become concentrated on the medulla of the gonad and proliferate and their ends anastomose to form the rete testis. The sex cords become isolated by the development of a capsule called the tunica albuginea, and the developing sex cords become the seminiferous tubules; mesenchyme grows between the tubules to separate them (Leydig cells). The seminiferous tubules are composed of two layers of cells, supporting cells (Sertoli cells) derived from the germinal epithelium and spermatogonia derived from the primordial germ cells.

Development of the ovary

The development of the ovary is much slower than that of the testis, and the ovary is not evident until the 10th week. Now the primary sex cords regress and finally disappear. Around 12 weeks, secondary sex cords arise from the germinal epithelium and the primordial germ cells become incorporated into these cortical cords. At 16 weeks, these cortical cords break up to form isolated groups of cells called primordial follicles; each cell contains an oogonium derived from a primordial germ cell, surrounded by follicular cells arising from the cortical cords. These oogonia undergo rapid mitosis to increase the numbers to thousands of germ cells called primary oocytes. Each oocyte is surrounded by a layer of follicular cells, the whole structure being called a primary follicle. The surrounding mesenchyme becomes the stroma.

Development of the genitalia

Both sexes develop two pairs of genital ducts, known as wolffian ducts (mesonephric ducts) and the müllerian ducts (paramesonephric ducts; Fig. 12.2). The wolffian ducts arise in the mesonephros on either side and run caudally to enter the urogenital sinus near the müllerian tubercle. The müllerian duct develops laterally to the wolffian duct and has an open upper end into the peritoneal cavity. It runs inferiorly and parallel to the wolffian duct, but as it reaches the caudal region, it crosses the wolffian duct anteriorly and meets it opposite, to fuse in the midline and enter the urogenital sinus, forming the müllerian tubercle.

Male development

Development of the male internal structures requires regression of the müllerian ducts by müllerian inhibitor secreted by the testis, primarily by Sertoli cells. This seems to be mediated through the release of hyaluronidase by the müllerian duct cells and thus local destruction, and also inhibition of growth factor stimulation, presumably through a specific cell membrane-associated receptor as the regression is tissue-specific. The wolffian ducts develop under the stimulation of testosterone and result in the epididymis and vas deferens, and the seminal vesicles. The urogenital sinus undergoes masculinization; the penis forms from the müllerian tubercle, and the urethra forms as a result of elongation of the urogenital folds which fuse with each other along the ventral surface. The scrotum forms from fusion of the labioscrotal swellings.

Female development

The open cranial ends of the müllerian ducts become the fallopian tubes and the fused portion gives rise to the epithelium and glands of the uterus; the myometrium is derived from surrounding mesenchyme. At the point of fusion, a uterine septum is present for a short time before regressing to form a single cavity. The fusion of the müllerian ducts brings two peritoneal folds towards the midline, forming the broad ligaments. The vagina develops from two sources — the vaginal plate which arises from the sinovaginal bulbs, in the urogenital sinus, and the uterovaginal canal. As the uterovaginal canal reaches the pelvic portion of the urogenital sinus, there is stimulation of two endodermal autogrowths which are called the sinovaginal bulbs. These fuse to form a solid vaginal plate

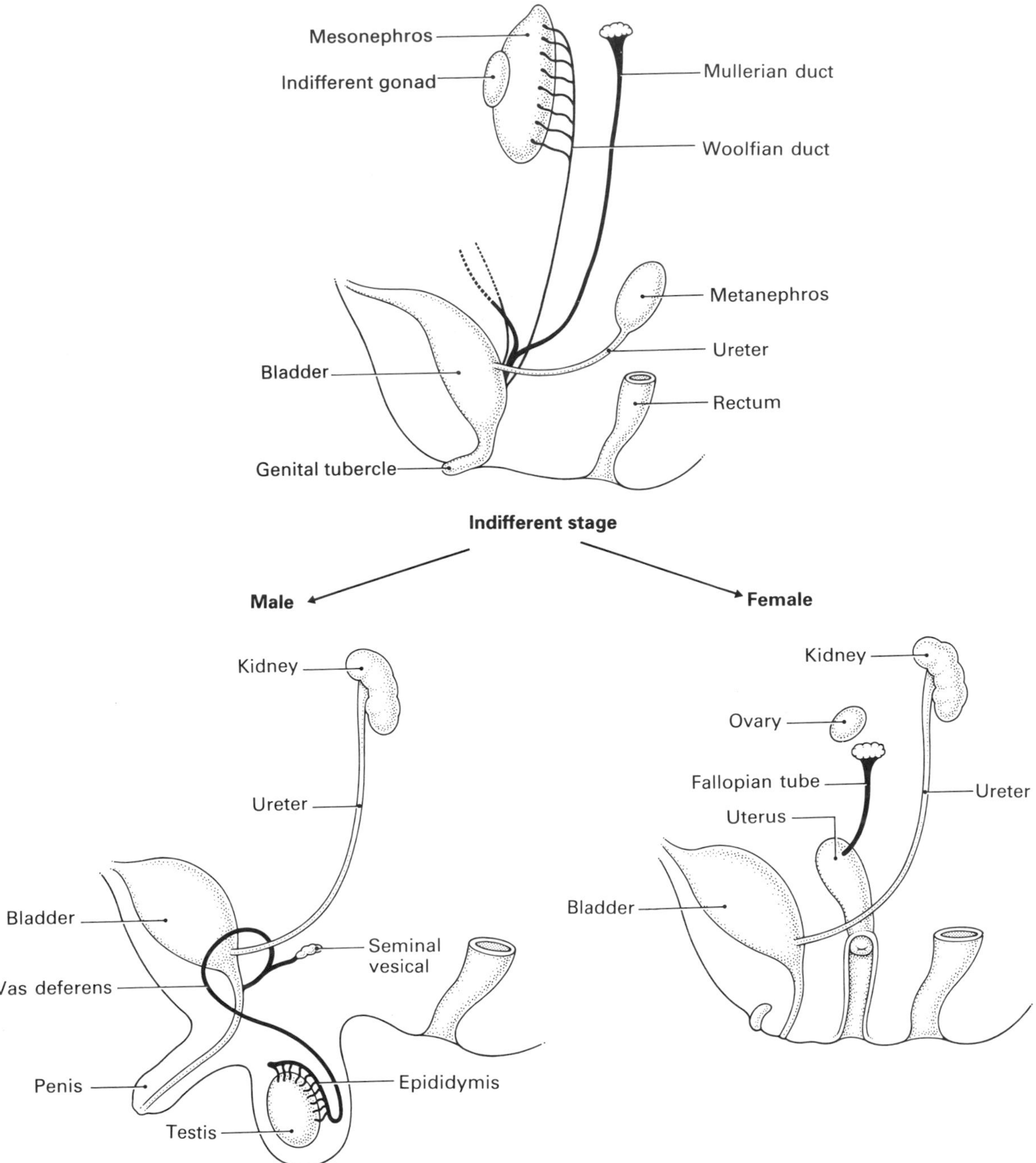

Fig. 12.2 Development of internal genitalia.

and this grows rapidly in a cranial direction giving the vaginal plate length. It eventually cavitates, beginning caudally, and by 20 weeks the vagina is fully formed (Fig. 12.3). The hymen represents the remains of the müllerian tubercle. The wolffian structures regress due to lack of testosterone stimulation, although occasional remnants may persist, i.e. hydatid cyst of Morgagni, Gartner's duct cysts.

The external genitalia in the female result from feminization of the urogenital sinus. The müllerian tubercle grows initially before ceasing and becoming the clitoris. The unfused urogenital folds form the labia minora; the labioscrotal folds form the labia majora.

FEMALE INTERSEX DISORDERS

Definition

This group of disorders comprises conditions in which masculinization of the external genitalia occurs in patients

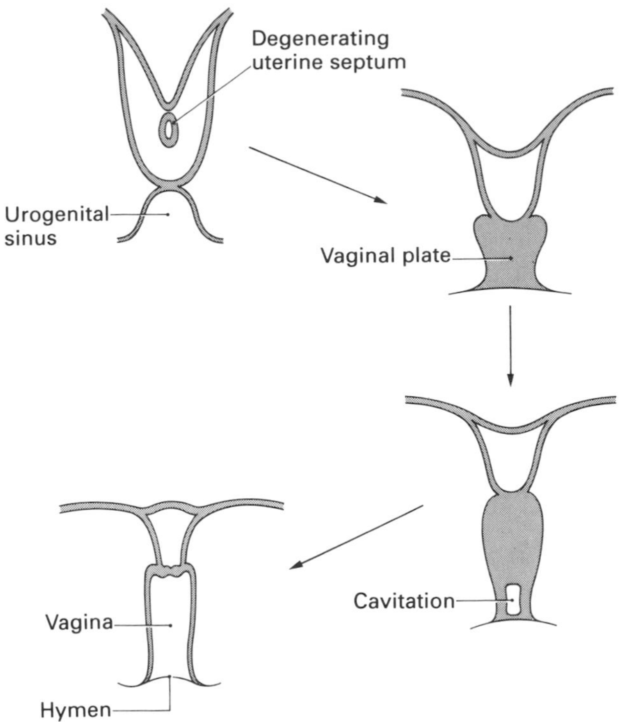

Fig. 12.3 Development of uterus and vagina.

with a normal 46XX karyotype. The degree of masculinization is variable, ranging from mild cliteromegaly to complete fusion of the labial folds with a penile urethra.

Pathophysiology

The abnormalities occur when a female fetus is exposed to elevated levels of androgens. As the differentiation of the external genitalia to male or female depends on the conversion of testosterone to dihydrotestosterone (DHT) in the tissues of the cloaca, the presence of DHT leads to male-type development. If the female fetus is exposed to low levels of androgen, partial masculinization may occur, leading to ambiguous genitalia, but if the levels are high enough, then complete male external genital development may occur, although the testes are naturally absent. If androgen exposure is delayed until after 12 weeks, then virilization is limited to clitoral enlargement with no effect on the already differentiated labia. Androgens have no effect on internal sexual development and therefore the ovaries, uterus and upper vagina are normally formed and functional.

Aetiology

The causes of the androgenization are due to excessive androgens either:

1. arising in a fetus, e.g. congenital adrenal hyperplasia;
2. arising in the mother, e.g. androgen-secreting tumour;
3. ingested by the mother, e.g. progestogens, danazol.

There are also cases which are associated with other congenital abnormalities or idiopathic.

Congenital adrenal hyperplasia

Pathophysiology

This is the most common cause of female pseudohermaphroditism and is an autosomal recessive disorder

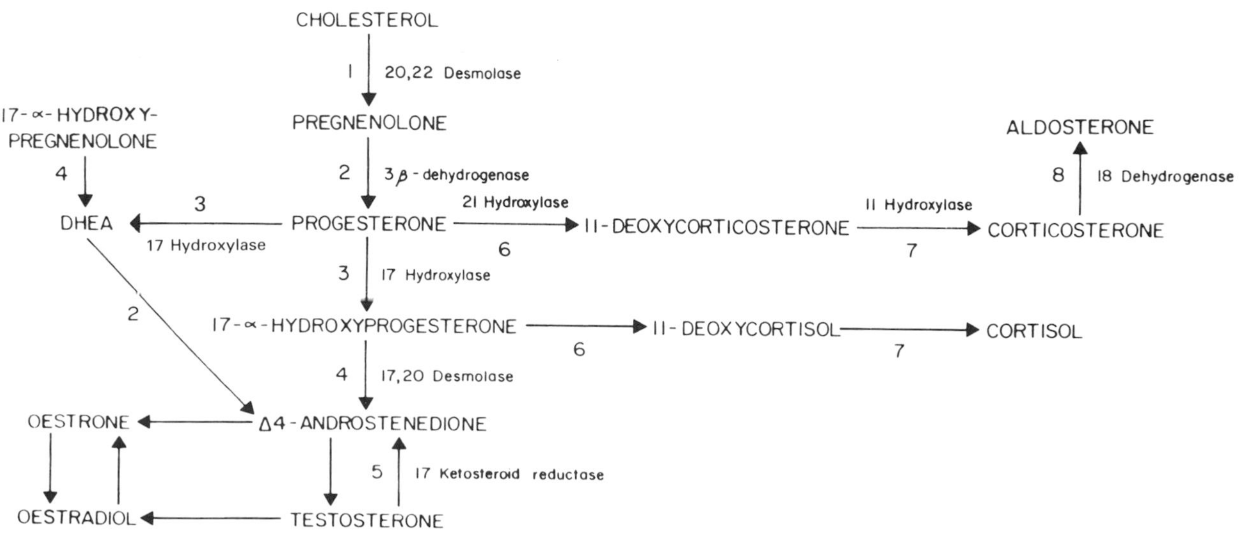

Fig. 12.4 Adrenal synthesis of steroids.

resulting in enzyme deficiency in the biosynthesis of cortisol in the adrenal. Cortisol production occurs in the zona fasciculata and zona reticularis (Fig. 12.4) and is controlled by adrenocorticotrophic hormone (ACTH) secreted by the pituitary gland. Adrenal androgen production occurs in the same area and is influenced by ACTH. A deficiency in any enzyme in the pathway results in decreased production of cortisol with resultant elevated levels of ACTH. This leads to increased steroid production by the adrenal reticularis and consequent hyperplasia. The stimulation by ACTH elevates the levels of circulating androgens and this results in the virilization of the female fetus.

There are three adrenal enzyme deficiencies which result in masculinization — 21-hydroxylase, 11-hydroxylase and 3β-dehydrogenase deficiency.

21-Hydroxylase deficiency

This accounts for 90% of all cases of congenital adrenal hyperplasia. The deficiency results in an increase in progesterone and 17α-hydroxyprogesterone and this substrate is therefore converted to androstenedione and subsequently to testosterone.

Failure of 21-hydroxylase to convert progesterone to 11-deoxycorticosterone may result in aldosterone deficiency; this occurs in about two-thirds of cases. This is the so-called 'salt-losing' type of CAH.

Aetiology. Deficiency of 21-hydroxylase is an autosomal recessive disorder. The link between human leukocyte antigen (HLA) type and 21-hydroxylase deficiency was established by Dupont et al (1977) and this allowed mapping of the gene which was located on the short arm of chromosome 6. It is located between the HLA-B and HLA-DR loci, and subgroups of HLA-B have been closely linked to congenital adrenal hyperplasia types; HLA-BW47 is linked to salt-losing congenital adrenal hyperplasia, and HLA-BW51 to the simple virilizing form. Studies by Donohoue et al (1986) have shown that there are two 21-hydroxylase genes — 21-OHA and 21-OHB. Only one is active (21-OHB) and they both lie between the fourth components of complement C4A and C4B. A variety of mutations have been reported, including gene deletions of 21-OHB, gene conversions and point mutations.

Epidemiology. The incidence of 21-hydroxylase deficiency is between 1/5000 and 1/15 000, based on neonatal screening programmes (Cacciari et al 1983), although a higher incidence (1/700) has been reported in specific populations of Eskimos (Pang et al 1982). The incidence of the non-classic form of the disease, when androgenization fails to appear before late childhood or puberty, is much more common, about 1/300 in the white population, and 1/30 in European Jews (Spencer et al 1985).

Presentation. Affected females are born with an enlarged clitoris, fused labioscrotal folds and a urogenital sinus which may become a phallic urethra. There is often a great variation of the degree of masculinization of the external genitalia; this is classified according to Prader (1958).

The internal genitalia develop normally as they are not influenced by androgens.

In the salt-losing form, the infants develop dehydration, hypotension and hyponatraemia between 7 and 28 days of age, known as a salt-losing crisis. The non-salt-losing form tends to cause less severe masculinization than the salt-losing type. In general, all children born with ambiguous genitalia, including cryptorchidism and hypospadias, should be screened for congenital adrenal hyperplasia. Without treatment, severe salt-losing disease is fatal.

When an infant is born with ambiguous genitalia, the management of the parents is very important. It is helpful to reassure them that the infant is healthy and that there is a developmental anomaly of the genitalia. If the initial examination of the child fails to identify palpable gonads, it is most likely that the child is female, and the parents should be informed as such and the likelihood of congenital adrenal hyperplasia may be raised. The diagnosis must then be made with as much haste as possible to alleviate parental anxiety.

Investigation. The initial investigations are karyotyping, pelvic ultrasound and then endocrine studies. The karyotype maybe performed on a sample of cord blood or on a venous sample and rapid results obtained. Pelvic ultrasound to discover the presence of a uterus and vagina will confirm the diagnosis. The specific diagnosis is made by measuring 17α-hydroxyprogesterone in serum, although a 24-hour urinary estimate of 17-ketosteroids will also confirm the diagnosis.

Treatment. This is divided into four parts:

1. *Acute salt-losing crisis*: This involves correcting the electrolyte imbalance and replacing the cortisol deficiency with desoxycorticosterone acetate (DOCA), 1 mg/24 h. For the majority of cases (9α-fludrocortisol is used in a dose of 0.1–0.2 mg/day added to the oral feed, and the dosage of DOCA or fludrocortisol adjusted against the electrolyte levels.
2. *Long-term cortisol replacement therapy*: Although previous reports suggested that mineralocorticoid therapy could be discontinued after infancy (Newns 1974), more recent data suggest that it is essential to continue therapy for life (Hughes et al 1979).
3. *Surgical correction*: Once the sex of rearing has been established as female, some attempt to feminize the genitalia may be made, usually within the first 18 months of life. If the clitoris is enlarged, a reduction clitoridectomy can be performed, and the perineal region modified (Edmonds 1989). There are major surgical problems associated with severe virilization in congenital adrenal hyperplasia. The urogenital sinus has been formed by labial fold fusion and the folds

are usually thin, but may be thick with associated narrowing of the lower vagina, especially in salt-losers. If the labial folds are thin, division by a simple posterior incision may be performed around age 3 or 4 years. However, thick perineal tissue should be left until after puberty and no attempt at surgery should be made until the girl is physically and mentally sexually mature. The operation, when it is performed, involves a flap vaginoplasty with a pedicle graft of labia used to recreate the vagina. Alternatively, a William's vaginoplasty may be used.

Mulaikal et al (1987) reviewed the fertility rates in 80 women with 21-hydroxylase deficiency: of 25 with the simple form who attempted pregnancy, 15 were successful, whereas of the salt-losers who tried to become pregnant, only one succeeded. There is no doubt that a major reason for the failure of the salt-loser group is the disappointing results of surgery and subsequent lack of adequate sexual function.

4. *Psychological support*: As the child grows, long-term psychological guidance and support will be required for the parents initially, and then the child.

Prenatal diagnosis. If the parents are heterozygous carriers of 21-hydroxylase deficiency, the fetus has a 1 in 4 chance of being affected. Thus, prenatal diagnosis is important, either by amniocentesis to measure amniotic fluid 17-hydroxyprogesterone levels or by HLA typing of amniotic cells, or chorionic villus sampling and the use of specific DNA probes. Once the diagnosis has been made, the option is available to treat the pregnant woman with oral dexamethasone, which crosses the placenta and suppresses the secretion of ACTH and thus the circulating androgen levels.

11-Hydroxylase deficiency

This is the hypertensive form of congenital adrenal hyperplasia which accounts for about 5–8% of all cases (Zachmann et al 1983). The absence of 11-hydroxylase leads to elevated levels of 11-deoxycorticosterone (DOC) and although this means a decreased amount of aldosterone, DOC has salt-retaining properties, leading to hypertension. Androstenedione levels are also elevated and this can result in ambiguous genitalia.

The diagnosis is made by measuring elevated levels of urinary 17-hydroxycorticosteroids, and raised serum androstenedione. Treatment is similar to 21-hydroxylase deficiency, with glucocorticoid replacement therapy.

The genetics, however, are rather different. There is no HLA association with 11-hydroxylase deficiency, but the use of a DNA probe has located the gene on the long arm of chromosome 8 (White et al 1985).

3β-Dehydrogenase deficiency

This rare form of congenital adrenal hyperplasia results in a block of steroidogenesis very early in the pathway, giving rise to a severe salt-losing adrenal hyperplasia. The androgen most elevated is dehydroepiandrosterone, an androgen which causes mild virilization. The diagnosis rests on the measurement of elevated dehydroepiandrosterone. The gene encoding 3β-dehydrogenase has not yet been cloned but it is not linked to HLA.

Androgen-secreting tumours

Androgen-secreting tumours are rare in pregnancy, but may arise in the ovary or the adrenal. They cause fetal virilization. When they occur in the non-pregnant woman, anovulation is induced.

Ovary

A number of androgen-secreting tumours have been reported including luteoma (Hensleigh & Woodruff 1978; Cohen et al 1982), polycystic ovaries (Fayez et al 1974), mucinous cystadenoma (Novak et al 1970; Post et al 1978), arrhenoblastoma (Coignet et al 1966) and Krukenberg tumours (Connor et al 1968; Forest et al 1978). Not all female fetuses will be affected and there is no association with gestation and exposure. The fetus may be partly protected by the conversion of the maternally derived androgen to oestrogen in the placenta, and thus the degree of virilization is variable.

Adrenal

There are only two reports of adrenal adenomas causing fetal masculinization (Murset et al 1970; Fuller et al 1983). These tumours may be human chorionic gonadotrophin-responsive, and thus levels of androgen may be higher in pregnancy than in the non-pregnant state, leading to androgenization of the fetus.

Drugs

The association between the use of progestogens and masculinization of the female fetus has received much publicity, but the only progestogen proven to have such an effect is 17-ethinyl testosterone (Ishizuka et al 1962). These infants had cliteromegaly and in some cases labioscrotal fusion, but the risk is very small (1/50). Gestogens which are derived from testosterone should be avoided in the pregnant woman. There have been two case reports of androgenization of female fetuses from exposure to danazol during pregnancy (Castro-Magana et al 1981; Duck & Katamaya 1981) and both babies were born with external genitalia similar to those with adrenogenital syndrome.

Associated multiple congenital abnormalities

Female intersex has been described in association with a number of multiple abnormality states, most commonly those associated with the urinary and gastrointestinal tracts. It has also been described in association with VATER syndrome (Say & Carpentier 1979).

The management of these children with masculinized genitalia is to ensure the assignation of a sex of rearing and modify the genitalia appropriately. In all of these rare cases, the female role has been chosen and reduction clitoroplasty performed.

XY FEMALE

The normal differentiation of the gonad to become a testis has been described above, and its subsequent secretion of testosterone leads to development of the wolffian duct and the urogenital sinus to produce the normal male internal and external genitalia. Testosterone is the predominant male sex hormone secreted by the testis but two other processes are necessary for normal development: the conversion of testosterone to DHT by 5α-reductase, and the presence of androgen receptors in the target cell which bind with the DHT or testosterone and produce appropriate nuclear function. Thus, normal male genotype — i.e. XY — with a female phenotype will occur if there is:

1. Failure of testicular development.
2. Error(s) in testosterone biosynthesis.
3. Androgen insensitivity at the target site.

Failure of testicular development

This group of disorders includes true gonadal dysgenesis, Leydig cell hypoplasia and the persistent müllerian duct syndrome.

True gonadal agenesis

True gonadal agenesis is characterized by the complete absence of any gonadal tissue and therefore the development of female internal and external genitalia. The karyotype can be either 46XY or 46XX. These patients present in the teenage years with failure of pubertal development (Chapter 13).

Leydig cell hypoplasia

Leydig cell hypoplasia is an uncommon condition, of which the aetiology remains speculative. The role of fetal luteinizing hormone in normal testicular development is unknown, but it may be necessary for maturation of the interstitial cells into Leydig cells. Failure of luteinizing hormone production in the first trimester will result in Leydig cell hypoplasia and male pseudohermaphroditism (or an autosomal recessive disorder resulting in absent luteinizing hormone receptors will cause absence of Leydig cells). This manifests as ambiguous genitalia, in both circumstances due to some androgen production by Sertoli cells. Clinically, Leydig cell hypoplasia usually presents as a phenotypical female with primary amenorrhoea and sexual infantilism (see Chapter 1) but ambiguity at birth may result in the diagnosis in infancy.

Errors in testosterone biosynthesis

This type of disorder accounts for only 4% of XY females, and results from deficiency of an enzyme involved in testosterone synthesis (see Fig. 12.4).

20–22 Desmolase deficiency

Absence of this enzyme results in failure to convert cholesterol to pregnenolone and a failure of subsequent steroid production. Most of the reported cases have died in early life due to adrenal insufficiency, but the XY individuals are all partially virilized with a small blind vaginal pouch. It is considered to be an autosomal recessive disorder.

3β-Hydroxysteroid dehydrogenase deficiency

This is a rare disorder which affects both adrenal and gonadal function, and is again autosomally recessive. The deficiency may be complete or incomplete and thus the degree of virilization is variable, to various degrees of hypospadias, or a small blind vagina with normal internal male genitalia and absent müllerian structures. Those individuals who have survived and reached puberty have developed gynaecomastia, presumably because the absence of testosterone during fetal life has allowed breast bud development. The diagnosis is made by elevated levels of pregnenolone and 17-hydroxy-pregnenolone and low levels of corticosteroids and testosterone.

17α-Hydroxylase deficiency

This syndrome produces a phenotype in XY individuals, varying from normal female external genitalia and a blind vaginal pouch to hypospadias with a small phallus. The diagnosis is usually only made in adulthood with failure to develop secondary sexual characteristics. The impaired adrenal production of cortisol is not associated with clinical symptoms as the elevated levels of corticosterone compensate. The gonads should be removed if the patient is assigned a female gender and hormone replacement therapy instituted.

17–20 Desmolase deficiency

This enzyme defect primarily affects testosterone production and there is no adrenal insufficiency. The clinical findings range from normal female to undervirilized male genitalia, and the endocrine findings are of very low serum levels of testosterone with normal corticosteroids. Again, diagnosis may not be made until failure of pubertal development.

17-Ketosteroid reductase deficiency

This enzyme is responsible for the reversible conversion of androstenedione to testosterone and oestrone to oestradiol. These patients almost always present at birth with female external genitalia and testes in the inguinal canal, and undergo masculinization at puberty. Those individuals to be raised as females should have their gonads removed before puberty, and oestrogen therapy begun at puberty.

Androgen insensitivity at the target site (Table 12.1)

In this group of patients testicular function is normal and circulating levels of androgen are consistent with normal male development. The majority of patients present at puberty with primary amenorrhoea, but some will present with ambiguous genitalia. The defect may be 5α-reductase deficiency, complete or partial androgen insensitivity.

Table 12.1 Types of androgen insensitivity and their abnormalities

Defect	External genitalia	Internal genitalia	Gonad	Phenotype at puberty
5α-Reductase deficiency	Female or ambiguous	Male	Testis	Masculine
Complete androgen insensitivity	Female	Male	Testis	Infantile and breast growth
Partial androgen insensitivity	Ambiguous	Male	Testis	Partial masculine and breast growth

5α-Reductase deficiency

This results in the failure of the conversion of testosterone to DHT in target tissues and thus a failure of masculinization of the site. In infancy, there is usually a small phallus, some degree of hypospadias, a bifid scrotum and a blind vaginal pouch. The testes are found either in the inguinal canal or in the labioscrotal folds, and müllerian structures are absent. At puberty, elevated levels of androgen lead to masculinization, including an increase in phallic growth, although this remains smaller than normal. Seminal production has been reported (Petersen et al 1977).

It is an autosomal recessive trait, and the resulting enzyme defect gives predictable hormone profiles with normal levels of testosterone, but low levels of DHT. The diagnosis is important in individuals born with ambiguous genitalia in order to assign the sex of rearing, and this should be based on the potential for normal sexual function in adult life. The gonads should be removed if the sex of rearing is to be female, and at puberty oestrogen replacement therapy instituted.

Complete androgen insensitivity

This is an X-linked recessive disorder characterized by the clinical features of normal female external genitalia, a blind vaginal pouch and absent müllerian and wolffian structures. The testes are found either in the labial folds or inguinal canal or they may be intra-abdominal.

These patients may lack the presence of the androgen receptor, and may be shown to lack the gene located on the X chromosome between Xp11 and Xq13. Work by Brown et al (1982) however suggests that there may be a variety of defects, ranging from absence of receptors to presence of a normal number of receptors which are inactive. The exact mechanism of the defects in patients with androgen receptors awaits definition.

The hormonal levels of testosterone which are elevated above normal due to increased luteinizing hormone production and the associated increase in testicular oestradiol and peripheral conversion of androgens to oestradiol promotes some breast development. Pubic hair growth depends on the degree of insensitivity but is usually rather scanty.

Patients either present with a hernial mass or with primary amenorrhoea despite secondary sexual characteristics; karyotyping makes the diagnosis. The gonads should be removed because of the malignant potential. The vagina may be of variable length and may be adequate, but those with a short vaginal pouch may need manual dilatation.

Partial androgen insensitivity

This is a complex condition which has been found to be due to a reduced binding affinity of DHT to the receptor, or because the receptor binds the DHT but there are defects in the transcription to the nucleus. It is an X-linked recessive disorder and the partial expression means inevitable ambiguous genitalia with a blind vaginal pouch and phallic enlargement. The penis can be normal. The wolffian ducts can be rudimentary or normal, but the testes are azoospermic. The most common presentation in infancy is hypospadias with the urethra opening at the base of the phallus, and there may be cryptorchidism. At puberty, male secondary sexual characteristics develop poorly, but there is usually gynaecomastia. The management is dependent on the degree of ambiguity and subsequent choice of sex of rearing, with gonadectomy and hormone replacement therapy for those assigned the female role.

ANOMALOUS VAGINAL DEVELOPMENT

When the vagina does not develop normally, a number of abnormalities have been described. The vagina may be partially maldeveloped, leading to a vaginal obstruction which may be complete or incomplete, or there may be total maldevelopment of the müllerian ducts leading to various disorders.

Classification

Vaginal anomalies may be categorized as follows:

1. Congenital absence of the müllerian ducts (the Mayer–Rokitansky–Kuster–Hauser syndrome).
2. Disorders of a vertical fusion.
3. Failure of lateral fusion.

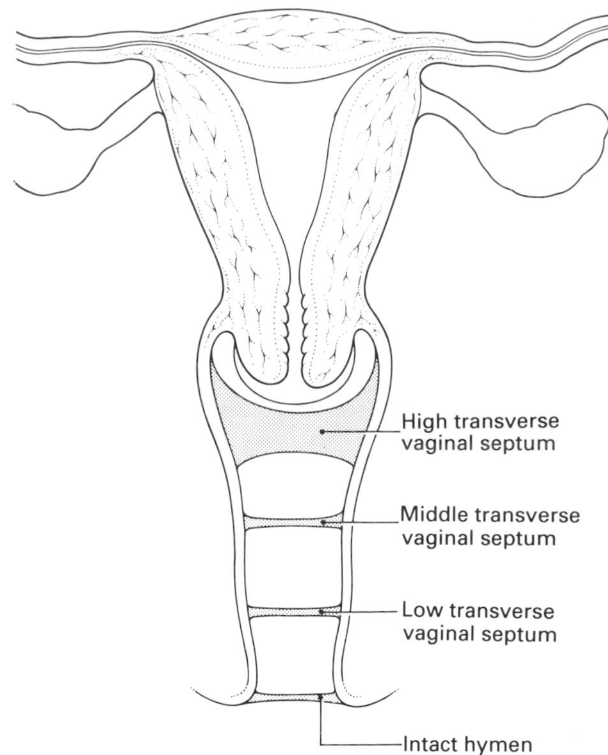

Fig. 12.5 Disorders of vertical fusion.

Aetiology

There are three mechanisms which may explain most vaginal anomalies. They may be familial, for example XY females who have a hereditary disorder as described previously. Congenital absence of the vagina has been very rarely reported in XX siblings (Jones & Murmut 1974) and also in monozygotic twins with only one child affected (Lischke et al 1973).

The case of a female limited autosomal dominant trait was first reported by Shokeir (1978) who studied 16 Saskatchewan families in which there was a proband with vaginal agenesis. However Carson et al (1983), in a study of 23 probands, disputed the Shokeir theory. The previous evidence with regard to monozygotic twins also makes this mode of inheritance unlikely. Polygenic or multifactorial inheritance does, however, offer some explanation that families may exhibit the trait as reported. The recurrence risk of a polygenic multifactorial trait in first-degree relatives is reported to be between 1 and 5%.

Finally, it is possible that müllerian duct defects could be secondary to teratogens or other environmental factors but no definite association has been demonstrated.

Epidemiology

The incidence of vaginal malformations has been variously estimated between 1/4000 and 1/10 000 female births (Evans et al 1981). The infrequency of this anomaly makes accurate estimates of the true incidence very difficult to obtain but when considered as a cause of primary amenorrhoea, vaginal malformation ranks second to gonadal dysgenesis.

Pathophysiology

The pathophysiology of vaginal absence may be either as a result of failure of the vaginal plate to form, or failure of cavitation. Absence of the uterus and fallopian tubes indicates total failure of müllerian duct development but in the Rokitansky syndrome, the uterus is often present although rudimentary, and therefore it must be failure of vaginal plate formation and subsequent vaginal development which leads to the absent vagina. Vertical fusion defects (Fig. 12.5) may result from failure of fusion of the müllerian system with the urogenital sinus, or it may be due to incomplete canalization of the vagina. Disorders of lateral fusion are due to the failure of the müllerian ducts to unite and may create a duplicated uterovaginal septum which may be obstructive or non-obstructive, depending on the mode of development (Fig. 12.6).

Presentation

Vaginal atresia

Vaginal atresia presents at puberty with complicated or uncomplicated primary amenorrhoea. In the majority who have an absent or rudimentary uterus, uncomplicated primary amenorrhoea is the presenting symptom, but those women who have a functional uterus may develop an associated haematometra and present with cyclical abdominal

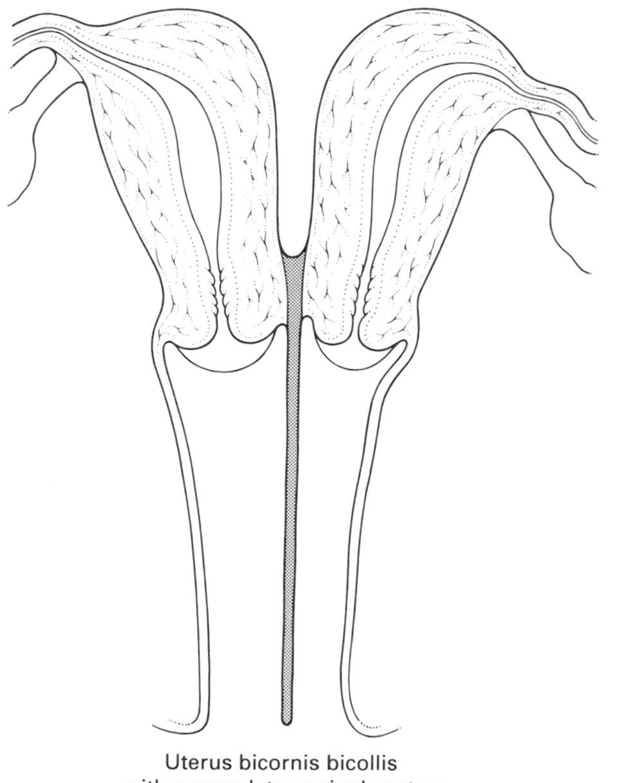

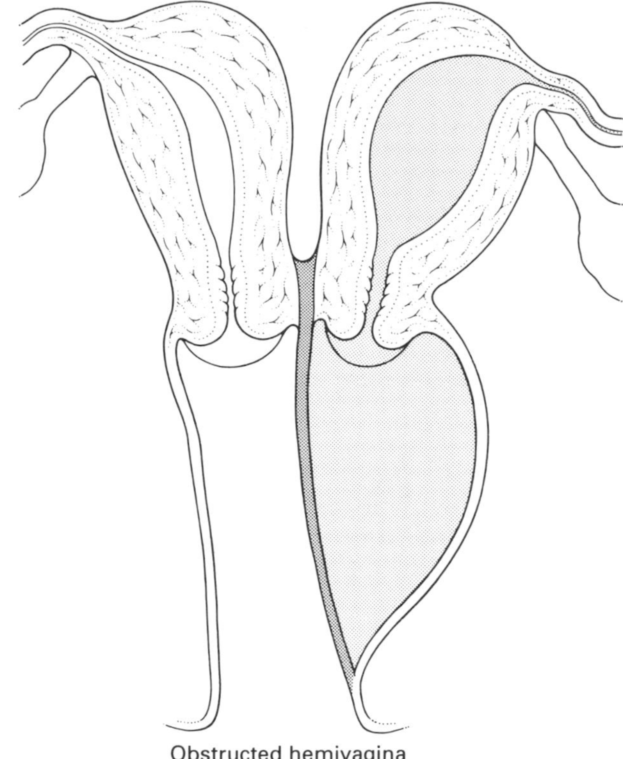

Fig. 12.6 Lateral fusion defects.

pain. If a haematometra does develop, there will be uterine distension and an abdominal mass may be palpable but more commonly is felt on rectal examination.

Vertical fusion defects

Here, the transverse vaginal septum prevents loss of menstrual blood and therefore cryptomenorrhoea results. Most patients present as teenagers with cyclical abdominal pain and a haematocolpos will be palpable within the pelvis on rectal examination. The patient may also present from associated pressure symptoms of urinary frequency and/or retention. The incidence of vertical fusion defects is reported as 46% high, 35% mid, and 19% low septae in the vagina (Rock et al 1982).

Disorders of lateral fusion

These patients usually present with the incidental finding of a vaginal septum which is usually asymptomatic. It may well first be diagnosed during pregnancy at which time excision will be necessary to ensure a vaginal delivery. However, these patients may present with dyspareunia caused by the septum and in most cases one vagina is larger than the other and intercourse may have occurred partially successfully in the larger side. In the unilateral vaginal obstruction group, presentation is usually with abdominal pain and the associated symptoms of a haematometra and haematocolpos. The confusing clinical sign is the associated menstruation from the other side and the diagnosis may be missed if careful examination is not performed in these teenagers.

Investigation

Vaginal atresia

A patient presenting with a clinically absent vagina and no cyclical abdominal pain requires an ultrasound examination of the pelvis to determine the presence or absence of a uterus and/or a haematometra. Laparoscopy in these patients is unnecessary. Some 15% of patients with the Rokitansky syndrome suffer major defects of the urinary system, including congenital absence of a kidney: 40% of patients also have trivial urinary abnormalities (D'Alberton et al 1981). It is therefore important to perform an intravenous urogram in order to establish any abnormalities in the renal system or the presence of a pelvic kidney which may alert the surgeon to take extra care if abdominal operation becomes necessary.

Anomalies of the bony skeleton occur in about 12% of patients. These include abnormalities of the lumbar spine, the cervical vertebrae and also limb abnormalities. However, it may be that the incidence of bony abnormalities is higher than this as investigation of the skeletal system is rarely performed.

Transverse vaginal septum

Investigations in these patients is limited to ultrasound assessment of the uterus for the detection of a haematometra and haematocolpos, and this may also be used to assess the level of the septal defect. Again, investigation of the urinary tract is pertinent.

Lateral fusion defects

Investigations in this group are only important if there is an obstructed outflow problem and should follow those outlined for vertical fusion defects.

Treatment

Vaginal atresia

The patient with müllerian agenesis requires careful psychological counselling and associated therapy. The psychological impact of being informed that there is an absent vagina comes as an immense shock to both patient and parents. It is almost always followed by a period of depression in which many patients question their femininity and look upon themselves as abnormal females. They very much doubt their ability to enter a heterosexual relationship which will be lasting, and feel worthless both sexually and certainly as regards being a reproductive partner. In some patients the depression can be very profound and suicide may be threatened. There is also great maternal anxiety over the aetiology as most mothers feel that they are responsible for the abnormality. Reassurance of the mother is equally as important that of the daughter in the management of the patient.

Occasionally cultural problems arise which make management much more difficult, especially in ethnic groups where the ability to procreate is fundamental to marriage and social acceptance. These patients and their parents can be very difficult to console and often refuse to accept the situation, questioning the diagnosis of their sterility over a number of years. The immediate reaction of most patients is to request surgical correction of the abnormality to return them to 'normal'. Unfortunately, opting for surgical treatment without adequate psychological and physical preparation inevitably leads to disaster. We recommend a minimum of 6 months of preparation before any surgical procedure is performed, and during this time psychological support can be implemented for the patient and her parents. There are two major areas of support required: firstly, the correction of the loss of esteem and inevitable depression, and repeated counselling sessions by trained personnel are required if these symptoms are to be overcome. The second problem involves the psychological aspect, and again prolonged counselling sessions will be required if an adequate and fulfilling sex life is going to be possible in the future. The sexual life achieved by well managed patients can be excellent and has been reported as comparable to that of the normal population (Raboch & Horejsi 1982; Poland & Evans 1984).

Management of the absent vagina with a non-functioning uterus

In a patient with an absent or rudimentary uterus, the creation of a vaginal passage may be non-surgical or surgical. The non-surgical technique involves the repeated use of graduated vaginal dilators over a period of 6–12 months. A minimum of 1 cm of vaginal dimple is necessary for this technique to succeed and patients require support and encouragement during this time. Patients are instructed to begin with a small vaginal dilator which is pressed firmly against the vaginal dimple for a period of some 20 minutes twice a day. Pressure is exerted but pain should be avoided and repeated use of these vaginal dilators will be met with success in about 90% of cases with appropriate selection (Broadbent & et al 1984). This technique was first described by Frank in 1938 and in view of the undoubted success of this technique with no complications, this method must be attempted in all girls with an absent vagina and a 1 cm dimple before any surgical procedure be considered.

In those girls with a vagina of less than 1 cm or those in whom Frank's procedure fails, vaginoplasty will be required. There are currently three techniques in popular usage: the McIndoe–Reed operation, the amnion vaginoplasty and the William's vulvovaginoplasty.

The *McIndoe–Reed* procedure was first described in 1938 (Mc Indoe & Banister 1938) and involved the use of a split-thickness skin graft over a solid mould; this mould is placed in a surgically created space between the urethra and the rectum. This space is created digitally following a transverse incision in the vaginal dimple. Digital exploration of the space must be performed with great care as damage to the bladder or the rectum may occur. The space created must reach the peritoneum of the pouch of Douglas if an adequate length of vagina is to be created. A split-thickness skin graft is then taken from a donor site and an appropriately sized mould is chosen. The skin graft is then fashioned over the mould with the external skin surface in apposition to the mould. The skin-covered mould is then placed in the neovaginal space and the labia are sutured together to hold the mould in situ. McIndoe reported his own series of 105 patients in 1959 and had a satisfactory outcome in 80% of patients. Cali & Pratt (1968) reported on their series of 123 patients; 90% had good sexual function. However, 6% had major complications which were primarily fistulae; subsequent reconstructive surgery was necessary in 8%. These complications resulted in modifications of the technique and the use of a soft material for the mould to prevent fistula formation due to pressure necrosis.

The search for an alternative material to line the neovagina and avoid the scarring of the donor skin site led to the use of *amnion* for the vaginoplasty procedure (Ashworth et al 1986). The technique involves the creation of a neovaginal space in the same way as described for the McIndoe–Reed procedure but amnion obtained at the time of elective caesarean section is used to line the neovagina. The mesenchymal surface of the amnion is placed against the new vaginal surface to promote epithelialization and the mould is kept in situ for 7 days and then replaced with a new amnion graft for a further 7 days. Subsequently patients are encouraged in the frequent use of dilators to maintain the vaginal passage. Again, reported success of around 90% has been achieved by these authors.

The *Williams' vulvovaginoplasty* (Williams 1976) still has an important place in the management of these disorders, but is much less frequently used than in the past. In patients in whom dissection of a neovagina is impossible but the labia majora are normal, this technique is invaluable. The principle of the operation is to create a vaginal pouch from the full-thickness skin flaps created from the labia majora, which are united in the midline. Following surgery and adequate healing, the patient is taught to use vaginal dilators in the same way as described in the Frank technique. There is no doubt that this does allow the patient and her partner to enjoy a sex life with mutual orgasm but the angle of the vagina is unnatural and unsatisfactory for some patients. Although the operation is simple to perform, the psychological problems of the distorted external genitalia can be considerable.

The absent vagina with a coexistent functional uterus

This situation presents major problems as the release of menstrual blood and the relief of associated pain are the primary aims; the creation of a normal vagina is an equally important yet secondary role. The functional uterus may be normal and a cervix may be present or absent. This situation is very rare; an operation to create a neovagina in an attempt to reanastomose a uterus which has been drained of its haematometra is highly specialized and will not be discussed further.

Complications

Some 25% of women will have some degree of dyspareunia following a vaginoplasty (Smith 1983). This is most commonly due to scarring at the upper margin of the vagina, involving the peritoneum. Similar incidences of dyspareunia occur in nearly all series and it is difficult to know how best to avoid this. It seems to occur regardless of technique but contraction of the upper part of the vagina is difficult to avoid. The artificial vagina created in these ways acquires all the characteristics of normal vaginal epithelium and the exposure of the grafted epithelium to a new environment means that care has to be taken to ensure it remains healthy. Four cases of intraepithelial neoplasia in neovaginas have been reported (Jackson 1959; Duckler 1972; Rotmensch et al 1983; Imrie et al 1986).

Management of disorders of vertical fusion

In these abnormalities, the type of procedure is governed by the type of abnormality. In the obstructed hymen the procedure is extremely simple and a cruciate incision through the hymen will release the accumulated menstrual blood and resolve the problem. In obstructing transverse vaginal septae in the lower and middle thirds, surgical removal of the septum can almost always be performed transvaginally and a reanastomosis of the upper and lower vaginal segments may be performed. Great care must be taken to ensure that the excision is adequate or a vaginal stenosis at the site of the septum will remain a problem. The high vaginal septum is the most difficult abnormality to manage and it is almost always necessary to perform a laparotomy in order to expose the haematometra. The passage of a probe through the uterine cavity and cervix into the short upper vagina allows a second vaginal surgeon to explore the vagina from below and excise the septum. It is usual that the absent portion of vagina is so great that reanastomosis of the vaginal mucosa cannot be achieved and either a soft mould is inserted and granulation allowed to occur, or an amnion-covered soft mould should be inserted to promote epithelialization. Vaginal dilatation following removal of the mould must be encouraged in order to prevent constriction of the new vaginal area.

Results. The results of surgery are extremely good when judged by sexual satisfaction. However, Rock et al (1982) reported pregnancy success following surgical correction of transverse vaginal septa and noted that patients with a transverse vaginal septum had only a 47% pregnancy rate when the site of the septum was taken into account. If the obstruction was in the lower third, then all patients achieved a pregnancy; in the middle third 43% and in the upper third 25% of patients became pregnant. It is suggested that the difficulties in conceiving may be secondary to the development of endometriosis and the higher the site of the septum, the more likely the development of this disorder may be. Thus prompt diagnosis and surgical correction is important in an attempt to preserve the maximum reproductive capacity in these patients.

Complications. Complications are primarily those of dyspareunia and failure of pregnancy, as described above.

Disorders of lateral fusion

The treatment of this condition depends on the abnormality. In patients with a midline septum and no other abnormality, excision of the septum should be performed and care must be taken as these septa can be very thick and removal can be rather difficult. When resecting the septum, generous pedicles should be taken to ensure haemostasis and the results are extremely good as the remaining tissue usually retracts and causes no problem. In patients in whom there is an incomplete vaginal obstruction, again the septum needs to be removed and care must be taken to remove as much of it as possible. Failure to do this will result in healing of an ostium and repeat obstruction of the hemivagina. The results and outlook for these patients are extremely good.

MALFORMATIONS OF THE UTERUS

Classification and pathophysiology

There have been numerous classification systems for uterine malformations varying between those based on embryological development to those based on obstetric performance. However, the most widely used classification in current use is that of Buttram & Gibbons (1979) which is based upon the degree of failure of normal development. There are six categories described.

Class I: Müllerian agenesis or hypoplasia.
Class II: Unicornuate uterus.
Class III: Uterus didelphis.
Class IV: Uterus bicornuate.
Class V: Septate uterus.
Class VI: Diethylstilboestrol (DES) anomalies.

A separate class of uterine malformations has been identified in the presence of communication between two separate uterocervical cavities.

The pathophysiology of failure of normal union of the müllerian ducts is not clear. As proposed in the section on vaginal agenesis, the hypothesis of teratogens has been been suggested but again evidence is unsupported. It is most likely that this is a polygenic or multifactorial inheritance which slightly increases the risk of a uterovaginal abnormality arising in a family with no anomalies.

Incidence

The incidence of uterine anomalies is difficult to define as it depends entirely upon the interest of the investigator and the diligence to which investigation will be pursued. Obstetric series show an incidence of uterine abnormalities ranging from 1/100 to 1/1000 (Semmens 1962). In an infertile population, the incidence increases to around 3% (Sanfillippo et al 1978). It is likely that the incidence of uterine malformations is greatly underestimated as in the vast majority of patients no gynaecological or reproductive problems are ever experienced.

Presentation

Abnormal uterine development may be symptomatic or asymptomatic. The most common clinical situations that will lead to a diagnosis of malformation of the uterus are recurrent pregnancy loss, primary infertility, urological abnormalities, menstrual disorders and DES exposure.

Recurrent pregnancy loss

Recurrent pregnancy wastage in the form of abortion or premature labour is a common way in which uterine anomalies will be discovered. The role of uterine anomalies in pregnancy wastage is discussed in Chapter 15.

Primary infertility

Uterine abnormalities may be discovered during investigation of an infertile woman. However, the relationship between infertility and uterine abnormalities remains controversial.

Urological abnormalities

Not uncommonly, urologists who discover malformations of the urinary system investigate the genital system and find abnormalities. Thompson & Lynn (1966) reported that 66% of patients with a maldevelopment of the renal tract had an associated müllerian duct abnormality. However only 13.5% of women with anomalous renal development had anomalous uterine development. In patients with a single kidney, the most common uterine abnormality is uterus didelphus with a vaginal septum which is associated with unilateral occlusion.

Menstrual disorders

Uterine abnormalities may be responsible for a number of menstrual disorders including oligomenorrhoea, dysmenorrhoea and menorrhagia. The specific menstrual symptoms will depend on the anomaly. In an interesting study by Sorensen (1981), investigating infertile women with oligomenorrhoea, 56% of patients were found to have mild uterine abnormalities. The author suggested that this oligomenorrhoea might be due to poor vascularization or steroid receptor development in the malformed uterus. With regard to dysmenorrhoea, uterine abnormalities seem to be associated with a higher incidence of primary dysmenorrhoea, although this may also be associated with obstructed outflow problems. Rudimentary hemiuteri may be also the cause of dysmenorrhoea in some women.

DES exposure

The malformations associated with DES exposure have been well described (Kaufman et al 1980). These abnormalities include the classic T-shaped uterus with a widening of the interstitial and isthmic portions of the fallopian tubes and narrowing of the lower two-thirds of the uterus, as well as non-specific uterine abnormalities with changes of cavity seen on hysterosalpingography. These patients may present with impaired reproductive function and pregnancy wastage may be as high as 50–60%.

Investigations

It is obvious that investigation of patients with suspected uterine abnormalities must be done with the aid of hysterosalpingography. This radiographic demonstration of the intrauterine shape is the most appropriate procedure, although care must be taken to ensure that if a double cervix is present, both cervical canals are cannulated and contrast medium is injected. A wide range of uterine abnormalities has been described and this has led to the classification system of Buttram & Gibbons (1979).

Treatment

A number of uterine malformations are suitable for surgical repair and the types of treatment and results are seen in Chapter 15.

KEY POINTS

1. Gonadal differentiation into a testicle or ovary depends on the presence or absence of a Y chromosome.
2. The testis develops from the medulla whereas the ovary originates from the cortex of the primitive gonad.
3. Development of normal ovaries depends on the presence of two X chromosomes.
4. Deletion of either the short or long arms of the X chromosome may result in variable ovarian development or dysgenesis.
5. Development of the testis depends on the testicular determining factor which controls the expression of the H-Y antigen, but other autosomally located genes are also involved.
6. Female intersex disorders denote external genitalia masculinization in patients with 46 XX karyotype.
7. Differentiation of internal female sexual organs is not androgen dependent and unlike the clitoris, the labia are adversely affected only if exposed to androgens before the 12th week of intrauterine life.
8. 21-Hydroxylase deficiency is an autosomal recessive disorder and accounts for 90% of cases of congenital adrenal hyperplasia (CAH).
9. 21-Hydroxylase deficiency is the only adrenal enzymatic deficiency associated to the HLA gene located in chromosome 6.
10. Female fetus defeminization may follow maternal use of testosterone related progestogens.
11. Prenatal diagnosis of CAH in heterozygous carriers is necessary and treatment with dexamethasone prevents fetal infliction.
12. Successful pregnancy following resection of vaginal septa is inversely related to the level of the septa in the vagina.
13. Intrauterine diethylstilboestrol (DES) exposure may lead to T-shaped uterus with impaired reproductive function.

REFERENCES

Ashworth M F, Morton K E, Dewhurst C J et al 1986 Vaginoplasty using amnion. Obstetrics and Gynecology 67: 443–444

Broadbent R T, Woolf R M, Herbertson R 1984 Non-operative construction of the vagina. Plastic and Reconstructive Surgery 73: 117–122

Brown T R, Maes M, Rothwell S W, Migeon C J 1982 Human complete androgen insensitivity with normal dihydrotestosterone receptor binding capacity in cultured genital skin biopsies. Journal of Clinical Endocrinology and Metabolism 55: 61–69

Buttram V S, Gibbons W E 1979 Mullerian anomalies — a proposed classification. Fertility and Sterility 32: 40–48

Cacciari E, Balsamo A, Cassio A et al 1983 Neonatal screening for congenital adrenal hyperplasia. Archives of Disease in Childhood 58: 803–806

Cali R W, Pratt J H 1968 Congenital absence of the vagina. American Journal of Obstetrics and Gynecology 100: 752–754

Carson S A, Simpson J L, Malinak L R et al 1983 Heritable aspects of uterine anomalies II. Genetic analysis of mullerian aplasia. Fertility and Sterility 40: 86–91

Castro-Magana M, Chervanky T, Collipp P J, Ghavami-Maibadi Z, Angulo M, Stewart C 1981 Transient adrenogenital syndrome due to exposure to danazol in utero. American Journal of Archives of Diseases of Childhood 135: 1032–1034

Cohen V A, Daughaday W H, Weldon V 1982 Fetal and maternal virilization association with pregnancy. American Journal of Diseases of Childhood 136: 353–356

Connor T B, Ganis F M, Levin H S, Migeon C J, Martin L G 1968 Gonadotrophin dependent Krukenberg tumour causing virilization during pregnancy. Journal of Clinical Endocrinology and Metabolism 28: 198–201

D'Alberton A, Reschini E, Ferrari N, Candiani P 1981 Prevalence of urinary tract abnormalities in a large series of patients with uterovaginal atresia. Journal of Urology 126: 623–627

Donohoue P A, Van Dop C, McLean R H et al 1986 Gene conversion in salt-losing congenital adrenal hyperplasia with absent complement C4B protein. Journal of Clinical Endocrinology and Metabolism 62: 995–1002

Duck S C, Katamaya K P 1981 Danazol may cause female pseudohermaphroditism. Fertility and Sterility 35: 230–231

Duckler L 1972 Squamous cell carcinoma developing in an artificial vagina. Obstetrics and Gynecology 40:35

Dupont B, Oberfield S E, Smithwick E M et al 1977 Close genetic

linkage between HLA and congenital adrenal hyperplasia. Lancet ii: 1309–1312
Edmonds D K 1989 Intersexuality. In Dewhurst's practical paediatric and adolescent gynaecology, 2nd ed. Butterworths, London, pp 6–26
Evans T N, Poland M L, Boving R L 1981 Vaginal malformations. American journal of Obstetrics and Gynecology 141: 910–916
Fayez J A, Bunch T R, Miller G L 1974 Virilization in pregnancy associated with polycystic ovary disease. Obstetrics and Gynecology 44: 511–521
Fitch N, de Saint Victor J, Richer C L et al 1982 Premature menopause due to a small deletion in the long arm of the X chromosome. American Journal of Obstetrics and Gynecology 142: 968–971
Forest M G, Orgiazzi J, Tranchant D, Mornex R, Bertrand J 1978 Approach to the mechanism of androgen production in a case of Krukenberg tumor responsible for virilization during pregnancy. Journal of Clinical Endocrinology and Metabolism 47: 428–434
Frank R T 1938 The formation of an artifical vagina without operation. American Journal of Obstetrics and Gynecology 35: 1053–1055
Fuller P J, Pettigrew I G, Pike J W, Stockigt J R 1983 An adrenal adenoma causing virilization of mother and infant. Clinical Endocrinology 18: 143–153
Hensleigh P A, Woodruff D A 1978 Differential maternal fetal response to androgenizing luteoma or hyperreactio luteinalis. Obstetrical and Gynecological Surgery 33: 262–271
Hughes I A, Wilton A, Lole C A, Gray O P 1979 Continuing need for mineralocorticoid therapy in salt-losing congenital adrenal hyerplasia. Archives of Disease in Childhood 54: 350–358
Imrie J E A, Kennedy J H, Holmes J D et al 1986 Intraepithelial neoplasia arising in an artificial vagina. British Journal of Obstetrics and Gynaecology 93: 886–887
Ishizuka S C, Kawashima Y, Nakanishi T et al 1962 Statistical observations on genital anomalies of newborns following the administration of progestins to their mothers. Journal of the Japanese Obstetrical and Gynaecological Society 9: 271–282
Jackson G W 1959 Primary carcinoma of an artifical vagina. Obstetrics and Gynaecology 14: 534
Jones H W, Mermut S 1974 Familial occurrence of congenital absence of the vagina. Obstetrics and Gynecology 42: 38–40
Kaufman R H, Adam E, Binder G L, Gerthoffer E 1980 Upper genital tract changes and pregnancy outcome in offspring exposed in utero to DES. American Journal of Obstetrics and Gynecology 137: 299–306
Lischke J H, Curtis C H, Lamb E J 1973 Discordance of vaginal agenesis in monozygotic twins. Obstetrics and Gynecology 41: 920–922
McIndoe A H 1959 Discussion on treatment of congenital absence of the vagina with emphasis on long term results. Proceedings of the Royal Society of Medicine 52: 952–953
McIndoe A H, Banister J B 1938 An operation for the cure of congenital absence of the vagina. Journal of Obstetrics and Gynaecology of British Commonwealth 45: 490–495
Mulaikal R M, Migeon C J, Rock J A 1987 Fertility rates in female patients with congenital adrenal hyperplasia due to 21-hydroxylase deficiency. New England Journal of Medicine 316: 178–181
Murset G, Zachmann M, Prader A, Fischer J, Labhart A 1970 Male external genitalia of a girl caused by a virilizing adrenal tumour in the mother. Acta Endocrinologica 65: 627–638
Newns G H 1974 Congenital adrenal hyperplasia. Archives of the Diseases of Childhood 49: 716–724
Novak D J, Lauchlan S C, McCauley J C 1970 Virilization during pregnancy: case report and review of literature. American Journal of Medicine 49: 281–286
Page D C, Mosher R, Simpson E M et al 1987 The sex determining region of the human Y chromosome. Cell 51: 1091–1104
Pang S, Murphey W, Levine L S et al 1982 A pilot newborn screening for congenital adrenal hyperplasia in Alaska. Journal of Clinical Endocrinology and Metabolism 55: 413–420
Petersen R E, Imperato-McGinley J, Gautier T, Sturla E 1977 Male pseudohermaphroditism due to 5αreductase deficiency. American Journal of Medicine 62: 170–191
Poland M L, Evans T N 1985 Psychologic aspects of vaginal agenesis. Journal of Reproductive Medicine 30: 340–348
Post W D, Steele H D, Gorwill H 1978 Mucinous cystadenoma and virilization during pregnancy. Canadian Medical Association Journal 118: 948–953
Prader A 1958 Vollkommen männlichie aussere Genitalentwicklung und Salzverlustsyndrom bei Mädchen mit kongenitalem adrenogenitalem Syndrom. Helvitica Paediatrica Acta 13: 5–14
Raboch J, Horejsi J 1982 Sexual life of women with Kuster–Rokitansky sydrome. Archives of Sexual Behavior 11: 215–219
Rock J A, Zacur H A, Dlugi A M et al 1982 Pregnancy success following surgical correction of imperforate hymen and complete transverse vaginal septum. Obstetrics and Gynaecology 59: 448–454
Rotmensch J, Rosenheim N, Dillon M et al 1983 Carcinoma arising in a neovagina. Obstetrics and Gynecology 61: 534
Sanfillippo J S, Yussman M A, Smith O 1978 Hysterosalpingography in the evaluation of infertility. Fertility and Sterility 30: 636–639
Say B, Carpentier N J 1979 Genital malformations in a child with VATER association. American Journal of Diseases of Childhood 133: 438–439
Semmens J P 1962 Congenital anomalies of the female genital tract. Obstretrics and Gynecology 19: 328–333
Shokeir M H K 1978 Aplasia of the mullerian system. Evidence of probable sex limited autosomal dominant inheritance. Birth Defects 14: 147–151
Simpson J L 1979 Gonadal dysgenesis and sex chromosome abnormalities. In: Vallet H L, Porter I H (eds) Genetic mechanism of sexual development. Academic Press, New York p 365
Simpson J L 1987 Genetic control of sex determination. Seminars in Reproductive Medicine 5: 209–220
Smith M R 1983 Vaginal aplasia: therapeutic options. American Journal of Obstetrics and Gynecology 146: 534–538
Sorensen S S 1981 Minor mullerian anomalies and oligomenorrhoea in infertile women. American Journal of Obstetrics and Gynecology 140: 636–640
Thompson D P, Lynn H B 1966 Genital abnormalities associated with solitary kidney. Mayo Clinic Proceedings 41: 438–442
Wachtel S S 1983 H-Y antigen and the biology of sexual differentiation. Grune & Stratton, New York
White R, Leppert M, Bishop D T et al 1985 Construction of linkage maps with DNA markers for human chromosomes. Nature 313: 101–105
Wolf U 1981 Genetic aspects of H-Y antigen. Human Genetics 58: 25–34
Zachmann M, Tassinari D, Prader A 1983 Clinical and biochemical variability of congenital adrenal hyperplasia due to 11-hydroxylase deficiency. Journal of Clinical Endocrinology and Metabolism 56: 222–229

13. Disorders of puberty

S. Duncan

INTRODUCTION

Puberty in girls is the first phase of transition from child to mature woman. Normally, it is a coherent process involving oestrogen production, increased somatic growth and the development of secondary sexual characteristics. Most of the changes occur gradually, though menarche can be dated. Normal puberty involves a fairly regular sequence of events between the age of 10 and 16 years and abnormal puberty can be defined as any disturbance in this. However, the range of normality is wide and the overlap can tax clinical acumen and ability to interpret laboratory data.

In this chapter, puberty is defined as the first phase of the changes which incorporate the development of secondary sex characteristics and the onset of menstruation. Full sexual maturity, which involves completion of breast development, the occurrence of regular ovulation and especially psychological maturity related to sexuality, takes longer and occupies the mid and later teens.

There are some gynaecological conditions liable to arise for the first time in the early teenage girl. These include vaginitis, genital warts, problems of menstrual hygiene (e.g. retained tampon). In the early teenage girl they acquire special importance in diagnosis and management but are outside the scope of this chapter. Likewise, causes of secondary amenorrhoea will not be considered. However, pubertal menorrhagia and dysmenorrhoea, when associated with the first menstrual year, have important implications and will be referred to.

PATHOPHYSIOLOGY AND CLASSIFICATION

Normal puberty

The key events of puberty development are well described (Huffman et al 1981; Dewhurst 1984) and the normal sequence of events should be understood by all doctors and by all nurses and health care personnel who deal with this very sensitive age group.

Longitudinal studies of pubertal girls have been conducted as part of more comprehensive studies of human growth (auxology) and our understanding of this area owes much to the pioneering work of Marshall and Tanner (for references see Tanner 1981; Brook 1982). The first external sign is increased growth (the onset of the growth spurt) then breast budding, and almost simultaneously, the appearance of pubic hair — all being consequences of oestrogen production (Figs 13.1–13.3; Marshall & Tanner 1969).

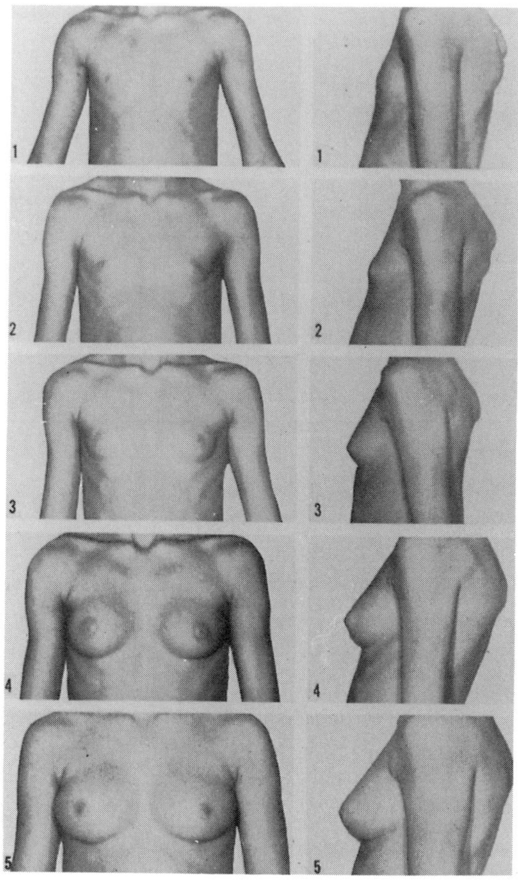

Fig. 13.1 Stages of breast development at puberty. **Stage 1**: This is the infantile stage which persists from the time the effect of maternal oestrogen on the breasts disappears, shortly after birth, until the changes of puberty begin. **Stage 2**: The bud stage. The breasts and papillae are elevated as a small mound and there is an increase in the diameter of the areola. This stage represents the first indication of pubertal change in the breast. **Stage 3**: The breasts and areola are further enlarged to create an appearance similar to that of a small adult breast, with a continuous rounded contour. **Stage 4**: The areola and papilla enlarge further to form a secondary mound projecting above the contour of the remainder of the breast. **Stage 5**: The typical adult breast with smooth rounded contour. The secondary mound present in stage 4 has disappeared.

Hormonal events

The hormonal secretions are an essential feature. They involve the hypothalamus, the pituitary and the ovaries and are a co-ordinated evolution of the behaviour of the relevant endocrine glands. These glands are all capable of promoting ovarian function very much earlier — even in utero — and the events of puberty result from a maturation of dynamic processes rather than the acquisition of new functions. Much study has gone into understanding these inter-relationships from early childhood to teens (for a discussion see Huffman et al 1981 or Reindollar & McDonough 1987) and with progressive refinement of measurement of hormones our concepts have required constant fine-tuning. Only a brief summary is given here.

Essentially, the hypothalamus receives stimuli from the

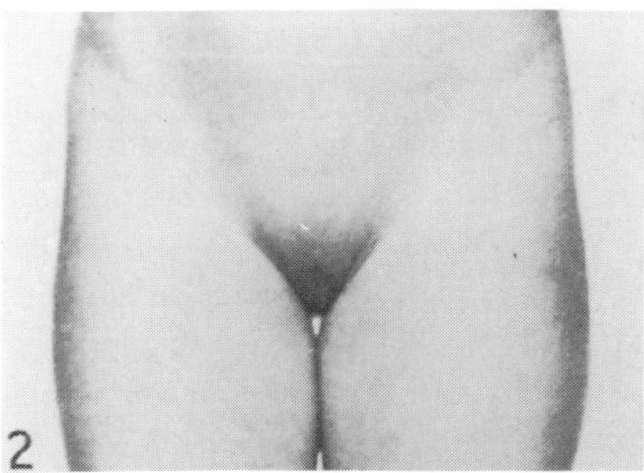

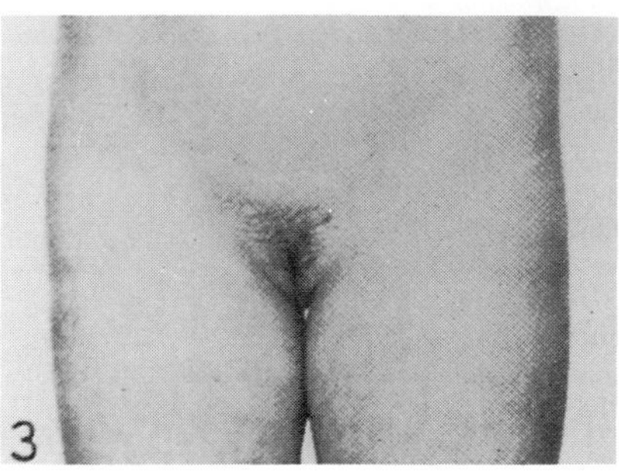

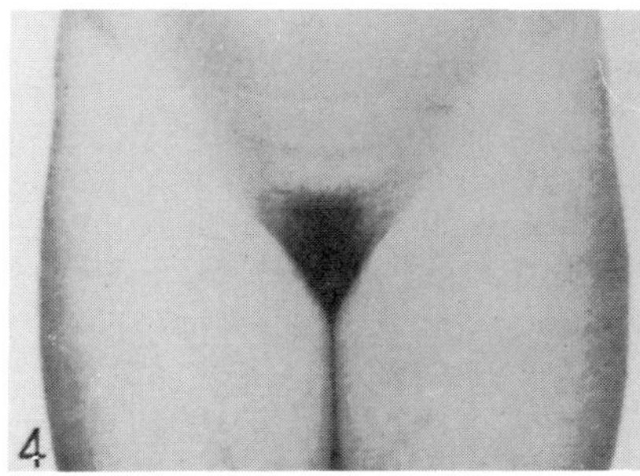

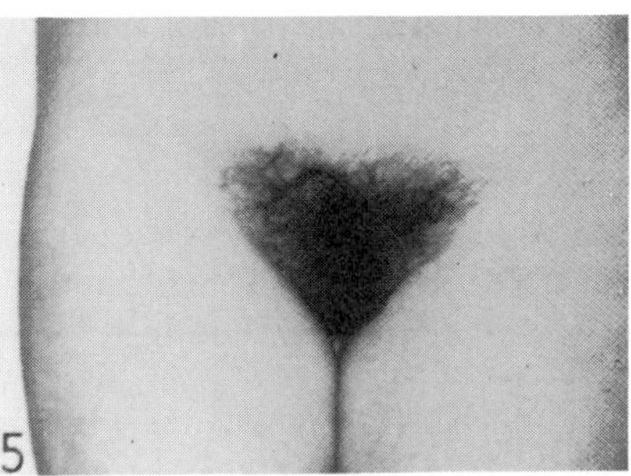

Fig. 13.2 Stages of pubic hair development at puberty. **Stage 2**: Sparse growth of slightly pigmented hairs on either the labia or the mons pubis. **Stage 3**: The hair is darker and coarser and spreads sparsely over and on either side of the midline of the mons pubis. **Stage 4**: The hair is adult in character but covers a smaller area than in most adults and has not spread to the medial surface of the thighs. **Stage 5**: Hair distributed as an inverse triangle and spreading to the medial surfaces of the thighs. It does not spread to the linea alba or elsewhere above the base of the triangle.

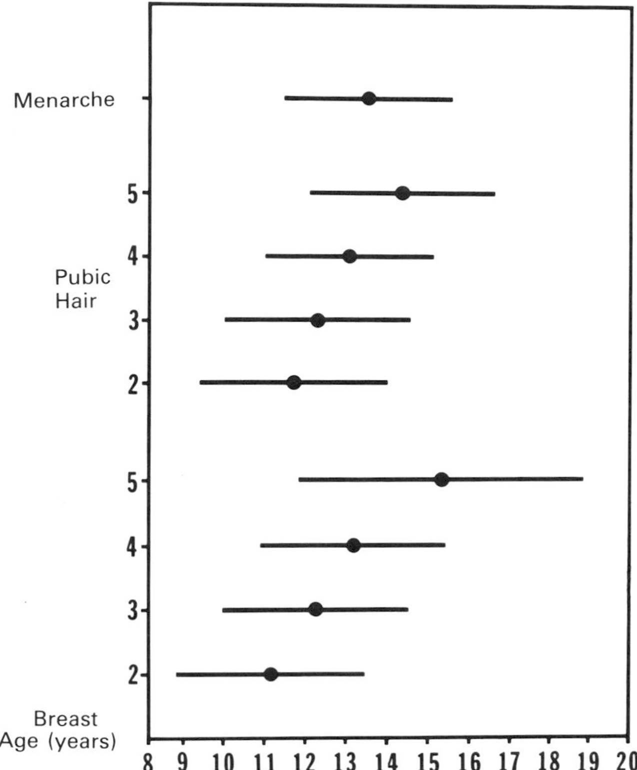

Fig. 13.3 Timing of pubic hair and breast changes and menarche. Horizontal line represents mean ± 2 s.d.

central nervous system and other endocrine organs. The hypothalamus both stores and releases gonadotrophic (as well as other)-releasing hormones, which pass to the anterior pituitary via the portal vessels. Both follicle-stimulating hormone and luteinizing hormone (LH) are released from the pituitary during late childhood (i.e. from about 5–10 years onwards). The circulation of these two hormones, as judged by either serum or urinary levels is neither equal nor synchronous. LH tends to be released in spurts, especially nocturnally, and levels measured on different days may vary widely. The net effect, however, is of intermittent bursts of hormonal stimuli to the ovaries and uterus, and ovarian activity in response to these can be detected from about 7–8 years of age. Small amounts of oestrogen are secreted throughout childhood, possibly from the adrenals as well as the ovaries, but differences in measured levels are detected between boys and girls only after about 8 years. Thereafter, in the girl, increased oestrogen levels occur gradually and the negative feedback mechanism, which has apparently operated very closely during the childhood years, appears to become less sensitive. This means that more oestrogen is required to suppress gonadotrophin activity, or rather that gonadotrophin effects are greater despite increasing oestrogen levels. Whether the negative feedback mechanism is the primary one in childhood is currently being challenged (Reindollar & McDonough 1987) as there is increasing evidence of the importance of central nervous system influence on arcuate activity. The final event of pubertal maturation of this system is the development of the positive feedback system which requires pulsatile secretion and eventually leads to regular LH surges and ovulation.

This hypothalamus–pituitary–ovarian process is not occurring in isolation. The thyroid gland plays an interactive though ill defined role. The adrenal glands also increase their activity of sex steroids from about 7 years of age in girls. Increased sebum formation, pubic and axillary hair, erectility of the clitoris and change in voice timbre are attributed primarily to the production of adrenal androgens but these differential roles are not clear-cut and both adrenal and ovarian hormone levels are rising at the same time.

The role, if any, of the pineal gland in influencing gonadal function in the human is obscure. In sub-primates, it appears to exert a suppressive role on gonadotrophin release and this effect is influenced by exposure to light. Such a regulatory mechanism is of importance in seasonal mating behaviour but has no exact parallel in the human. Nevertheless, it is of interest that girls who are blind to light perception (as well as vision) tend to have an earlier menarche (Zacharis & Wurtman 1964). Without some light there may be release of the inhibitory effect.

Ovarian development

Development of primordial follicles and secretion of oestrogens may be regarded as the final common path in all this hormonal activity and there is a close correlation between oestrogen levels and sexual maturation. Blood oestrogen levels rise before and during puberty and continue to do so for about 3 years after menarche before the normal adult follicular levels of oestrogen are seen. This gradual maturation is a reflection of the finding that many of the early cycles are not ovulatory, and of the observation that the early postmenarchial years are relatively infertile, even in populations where sexual activity without contraception is usual in these years.

Menarche. The first period occurs because there has been sufficient endometrial stimulation to result in a withdrawal bleed when there is a temporary fall in the oestrogen level. It is not usually, although it can be, associated with the first ovulatory/corpus luteum sequence. Although it really just indicates that a particular threshold has been reached in an already oscillating system, its objectivity enhances its significance. In so far as it denotes an intact hypothalamic–pituitary–ovarian axis, functioning ovaries, presence of a uterus and patency of the genital tract it is indeed a notable event. It may occur anywhere between 10 and 16 years (peak time is 13 years). The exact age is of less importance in diagnosis than its place in a girl's developmental process. Menarche generally occurs within 1 year of peak growth velocity and within 2 years of the earliest pubic hair and breast changes and it tends to occur earlier in girls who are taller and heavier for their age. Bone age is generally about 13 years.

Disorders of timing of puberty

The gynaecologist is most likely to be involved in delay or arrest of puberty or of anomalous development.

Delay and arrest

Delay and arrest can overlap but include:

1. No thelarche by age 13.
2. Abnormalities in the sequence and tempo of puberty development.
3. Amenorrhoea.

Any classification of delay in the onset of puberty depends on the diagnostic techniques available and these have evolved over recent years. A useful aetiological classification is given in Table 13.1. Girls with ovarian failure — more than half of whom have chromosome anomalies — constitute the largest single group. Arrest of development involves initial changes, with incomplete development of secondary sex characters and/or failure of menarche.

Table 13.1 Causes of delayed onset of puberty

With little or no evidence of gonadal function		
Hypergonadotrophic		
Chromosomal, e.g. 45X, mosaic cell lines	27%	43%
Normal chromosomes but ovarian failure (includes 46XY, gonadal failure)	16%	
Hypogonadotrophic		
Reversible causes — constitutional delay, weight loss, adrenal disease, thyroid disorder	19%	31%
Irreversible causes — pituitary deficiency, cerebral tumours, congenital central nervous system defects	12%	
With definite evidence of gonadal function		
Anatomical causes, e.g. müllerian agenesis, genital tract obstruction	18%	26%
Inappropriate feedback anovulation		
Androgen insensitivity	8%	

From Reindollar et al 1981.

Precocious puberty

Breast development before 8 years of age or menarche before 10 years is regarded as sexual precocity (Kulin 1987). There may or may not be accompanying presence of pubic hair and sebaceous secretion (adrenarche). Basic reasons are central — gonadotrophin production driving the ovaries — or peripheral — autonomous adrenal or ovary production. The commonest cause is constitutional early development (Table 13.2).

Table 13.2 Causes of precocious puberty

Basic drive	Origin	Example
Central	Constitutional	More likely when approaching the time of normal onset, i.e. 6 years upwards.
	Hypothyroidism	Autoimmune thyroiditis
	Specific central nervous system lesion	Craniopharyngioma Hydrocephaly Postinfective encephalitis Neurofibromatosis Congenital brain defects Cysts of third ventricle Hamartomas McCune Albright syndrome
Peripheral	Ovary	Tumour
	Adrenal	Tumour
	Rare tumour	Chorion epithelioma
Extraneous	Exogenous oestrogens	

When precocious puberty occurs, there is disturbance of the normal sequence of changes and evidence of dissociation between adrenarche and gonadarche (Sklar et al 1980). Thus, where precocious puberty is evident under the age of 6 years some important disturbance driving ovarian development is usually operating and (except in primary adrenal disorders) the adrenal status is not affected and is in accordance with chronological age. However, when precocious features occur closer to the normal time of puberty onset, it is more likely that the problem is one of general advance of maturational processes and the adrenal status is more likely to be part of this and be advanced for age. Bone maturation is accelerated in precocious puberty, leading to premature epiphyseal closure and curtailed stature. If menstrual cycles occur, they may be ovulatory.

If a girl has primary hypothyroidism, there is elevation of thyroid-stimulating hormone, maintained by production and release of thyrobropin-releasing hormone and this also causes some release of follicle-stimulating hormone.

Anomalous puberty

This arises when there is inappropriate hormonal secretion with virilization. Causes include:

1. Partial androgen insensitivity.
2. 5α-reductase deficiency.
3. Gonadal dysgenesis with formation of functioning tumour.
4. Congenital adrenal hyperplasia.
5. Adrenal tumours.

Pubertal menorrhagia

This is usually due to anovulation with cystic glandular hyperplasia

Pubertal dysmenorrhoea

This can be caused by:

1. Early ovulatory cycles.
2. Congenital anomaly of genital tract causing obstruction (can be partial or unilateral).
3. Endometriosis.
4. Other pelvic disease.

AETIOLOGY

Delay

Essentially, delay or arrest of puberty development is due to the following reasons:

1. The ovary is not stimulated.
2. The ovary cannot respond.
3. The hormones produced are inappropriate.
4. There is no uterus to respond to hormonal stimulation.
5. There is obstruction.

These causes are set out in Table 13.1; differentiation between them depends on the outcome of investigation. Precocious or anomalous puberty may be due to tumour or inappropriate hormonal release. Menorrhagia is usually due to unopposed oestrogen action; dysmenorrhoea may be obstructive or due to adnexal disease.

EPIDEMIOLOGY

Earlier menarche

Much interest has been shown in recent years in the tendency for menarche to occur at progressively earlier ages, thus tending to shorten childhood and prolong the interval between physiological and psychosocial maturity. There are many reviews of this trend (Tanner 1978; Dewhurst 1984). The essential conclusion from the study of many facets is that this change has coincided with a period of dramatic improvement in social conditions and nutrition. Children progress through childhood with comparatively accelerated growth, with fewer impediments and are, on average, taller and heavier than children of comparable age in previous generations. This trend has not been limited to those previously recognized to be deprived. In the past, even the well born were subject to debilitating illnesses and, sometimes, poor nutrition. It is not, therefore, so much that all girls are maturing earlier but rather that more are reaching their genetic potential and physiological maturity unimpeded by malnutrition and illness. Within a population, age of menarche is mainly correlated with socioeconomic factors including education, nutrition and urbanization. Adverse factors include poor nutrition and increasing size of family. Climate, season and race are not, of themselves, important. There is a strong genetic component and a correlation in the time of menarche between uniovular twins, binovular twins, sisters and mother–daughter pairs (Huffman et al 1981).

The concept of a critical weight or at least, a critical weight-for-height in determining the onset of menarche has been much debated in recent years (Frisch 1985). In well nourished girls, genetic influences seem to matter more (for discussion and references see Stark et al 1989).

Incidence of puberty disorders

The incidence of many of the conditions affecting puberty is not known because systematic surveys have not been carried out on a firm geographic base. Many valuable series (Reindollar et al 1981) have been from tertiary centres where there has been high selectivity for referral and treatment. Thus, a girl with Turner's syndrome or an imperforate hymen is more likely to be treated locally whereas a girl with precocious puberty or anomalous development is more likely to be referred to an expert in a more limited field. Although some very important conditions are quite rare, there is a large number of them and the combined clinical effect is of significance. Most early teenage girls have normal pubertal development and the few with a significant underlying anomaly are easily overlooked among many comparatively minor problems. Thus, most girls with an unusual problem of development are likely to be seen first by a doctor who has never encountered that problem before.

For example, if an average practice cares for 2000 people

= 1000 females of all ages
= about 70 girls between 10–15 years at any one time.

This number will obviously vary with the age distribution of the practice. Even if one allows for 30 years of practice with 15 girls/year growing up, a general practitioner would deal primarily with about 500 girls in a professional lifetime. Conditions rarer than 1 in 500 are quite likely never to be seen and even for commoner conditions random chance will affect the number. A consultant gynaecologist might be expected (and there are wide variations) to be seeing referred problems from about 350 girls of any one age at a time (assuming one gynaecologist per 50 000 total population). In a professional lifetime this represents the problems of about 10 000 girls passing through puberty. On average, a family doctor may see a fair selection of commoner anomalies, e.g. uterine abnormalities, but only about 4 girls with Turner's syndrome (incidence about 1 in 2500) and only 2 or 3 girls with an imperforate hymen (incidence about 1 in 4000).

PRESENTATION

Initial consultation

The manner of handling the initial approach is crucial to the doctor's future relationship with the girl. The exact circumstances and age will determine the best way to proceed. Extreme sensitivity about burgeoning sexuality or its failure can be assumed even if not overtly expressed. The occasional important deviation from normal puberty development has to be distinguished from the much commoner minor variations within the normal but it is better to err on the side of excessive rather than too little concern. However, apart from a few urgent conditions, study of the problem can be stepwise and based on observations of dynamic changes. When a mother brings a girl (or she comes of her own accord) there is a problem, no matter how trivial it may appear to be. A dismissive approach may be disastrous and inhibit correct diagnosis for years. Acceptance of the presenting feature in an open-minded and interested way is most likely to lead to diagnosis or exclusion of any disorder.

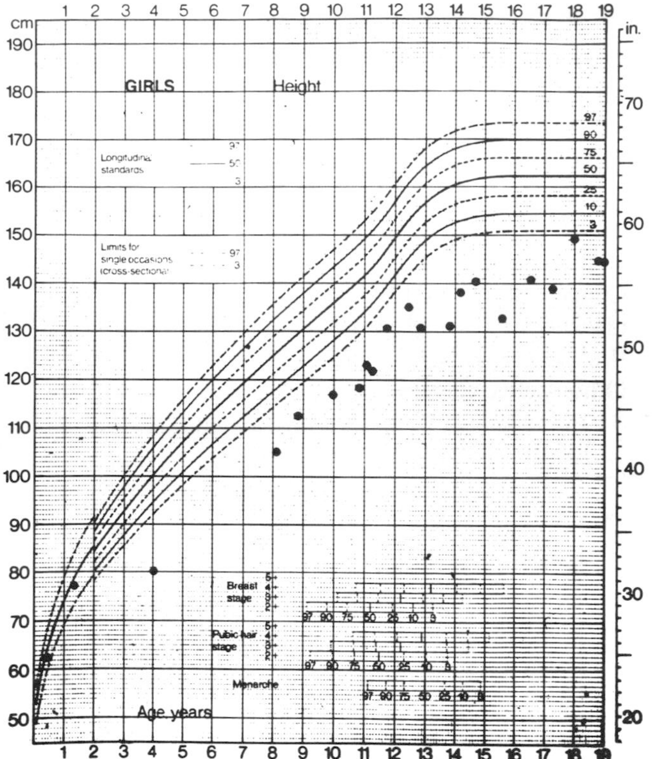

Fig. 13.4 Height of 21 girls with Turner's syndrome at the time of first diagnosis. Several were over 14 years of age before the diagnosis was made, despite the short stature which was a feature in all.

The prepubertal girl

Some puberty problems will have been foreseen since infancy, e.g. imperforate vagina or congenital adrenal hyperplasia. Problems of genital anatomy may come to notice at any stage of childhood. Differentiation will be that appropriate to age. In the prepubertal child an unusual appearance may be associated with:

1. Labial adhesions.
2. Vaginal agenesis.
3. Vaginal cyst.
4. Unusual anomalies.
5. Uterovaginal prolapse.

Any bleeding prior to secondary sexual development should be investigated further.

Precocious puberty will present with the untimely appearance of breast development together with pubic hair or vaginal bleeding.

Around the time of puberty

The main presenting features include:

1. Lack of breast development.
2. Amenorrhoea.
3. An unusual genital feature, e.g. enlarged clitoris or enlarged labia.
4. Abdominal swelling.
5. Inability to insert a tampon.
6. Abdominal pain.
7. Heavy or irregular bleeding.
8. Dysmenorrhoea.

An important aspect of presentation is the combination of features. Short stature has not been included in the above list, but it is a very important accompanying feature and is sometimes present, yet has often been overlooked when a girl presents with puberty delay (Fig. 13.4). It is easy to screen for but if it is the primary presenting feature it is more likely to be noted in childhood and referred to a paediatric endocrinology clinic (Fig. 13.5).

In considering the history at the presenting consultation it should be appreciated that a girl this age (10–16 years) will often seem to have little awareness of the timescale of her body development and of previous events. Her mother may be helpful over early childhood illnesses but may have limited awareness of puberty changes to date.

Particular attention should be paid to some associations:

1. Heart disorders or operations — chromosome anomalies.
2. Bowel or urinary investigations — anatomical anomalies of the genital tract.
3. Hernia repair — gonadal disorder.
4. Hip or leg problems — apt to be blamed for short stature.
5. Slow general development — hypothyroidism, hypothalamic disorder.
6. Anorexia — hypothalamic delay.

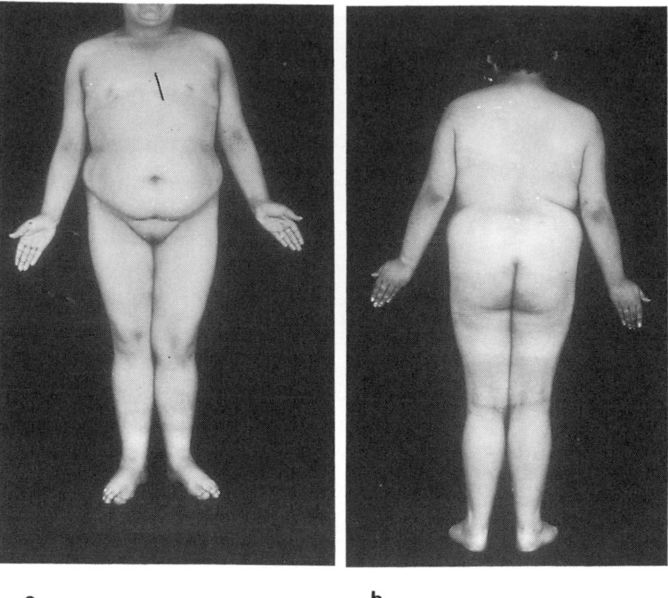

a b

Fig. 13.5 Characteristic phenotype of Turner's syndrome.

Where the presenting features include abdominal swelling with or without a history of amenorrhoea, pregnancy as well as ovarian swellings and menstrual obstruction should be remembered.

If primary amenorrhoea is the presenting feature the following differential approach can streamline the possibilities. If secondary sex characteristics are:

1. Good
   a. Haematocolpos.
   b. No vagina or uterus.
   c. Polycystic ovary disorder.
   d. (Pregnancy.)
2. Poor or absent
   a. Constitutional delay.
   b. Primary gonadal failure.
   c. Hypothalamic or pituitary failure (includes weight-related arrest of development).

Heavy, prolonged bleeding may be a feature of early cycles. There may be dramatic exsanguination.

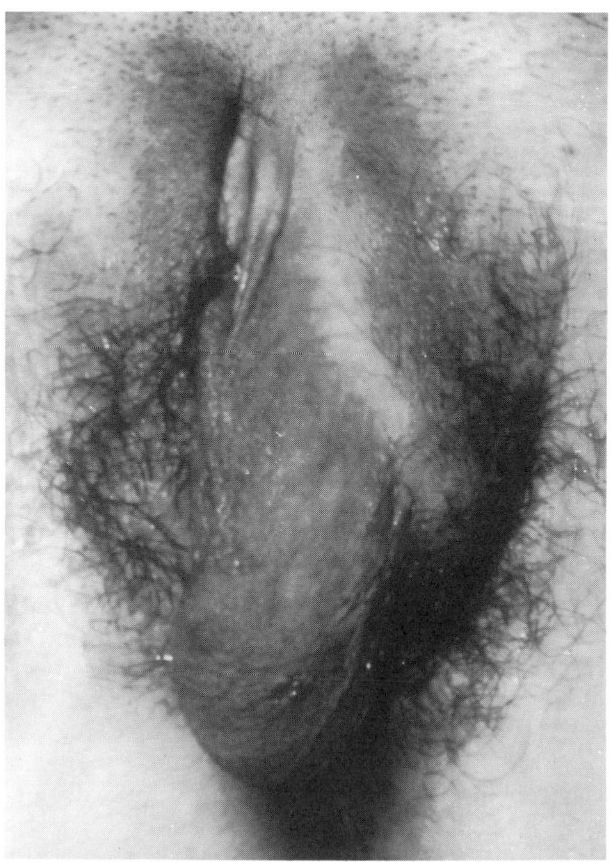

Fig. 13.6 Swelling within left labia majora occurring soon after puberty. Although alarming to a teenage girl, this proved to be a simple cyst.

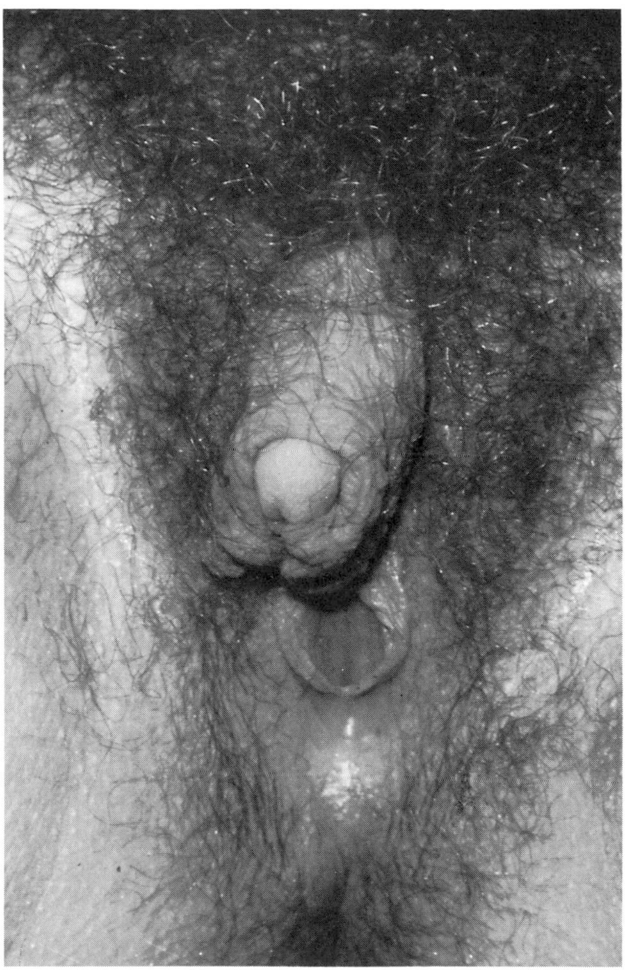

Fig. 13.7 Clitoral enlargement occurring at puberty due to tumour in an abdominal testis.

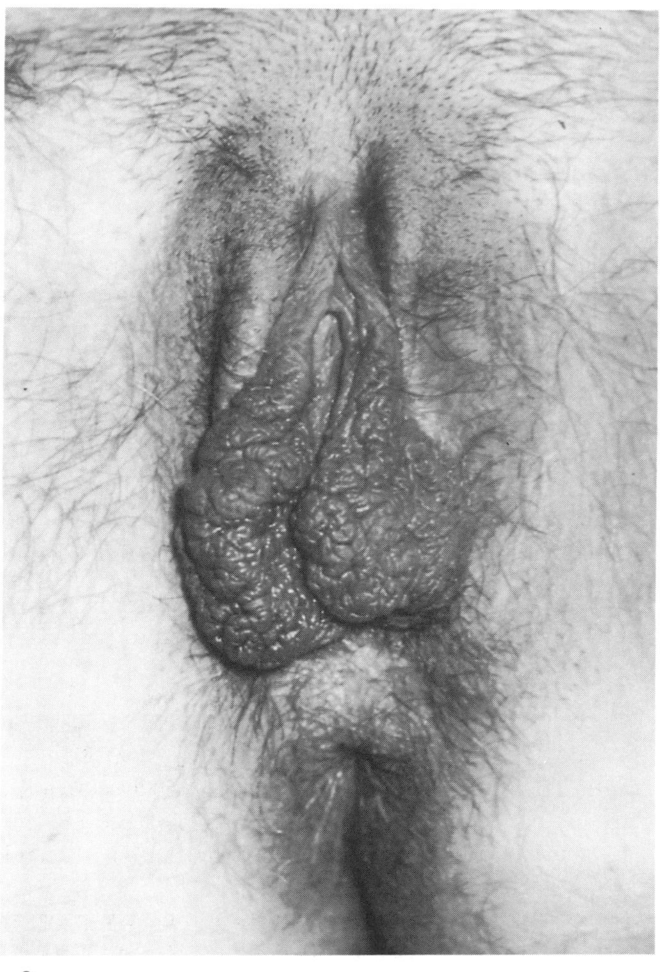

a

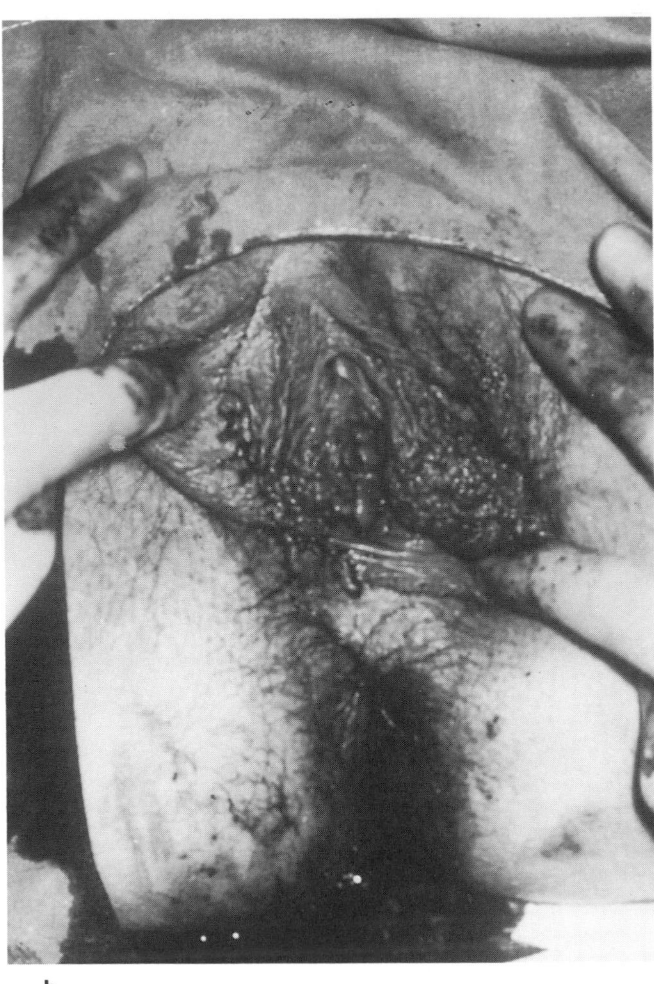

b

Fig. 13.8 (**a**) Unduly large pigmented labia causing discomfort. (**b**) Reduction in progress: right side completed; left intact.

Awareness of genital anomaly by the girl or her mother is an unusual presentation and is likely to be associated with secondary sex characteristics since it is the gonadal function that has probably caused the change (Fig. 13.6). Clitoral enlargement (Fig. 13.7), unduly large labia (Fig. 13.8) or awareness of a septum or blockage may be the presenting event.

INVESTIGATION AND DIAGNOSIS

The history, clinical examination, assessment of stature and stage of puberty development are fundamental and will often lead to identification of the category of problem if not the exact diagnosis.

The range and sophistication of investigations have developed in recent years. Some are basic and others are best reserved for interpretation at specialized centres.

Karyotype

This is particularly relevant where there is short stature and/or suspicion of ovarian failure. A buccal smear for Barr bodies is of very limited value since some of the girls with a mosaic pattern will be positive (see Chapter 1).

Banding techniques will clarify some of the more complex X chromosome patterns. Where there is deletion of X material, cardiac screening should be performed.

Endocrine

Measurement of gonadotrophin levels (follicle-stimulating hormone and LH) is an important starting point where there is amenorrhoea and lack of secondary sex development. This distinguishes hyper-from hypogonadotrophic causes and enables rationalization of further testing. Where levels are low, then testing of the pituitary response to gonadotrophin-releasing hormone will help to distinguish primary pituitary from hypothalamic causes.

Measurement of thyroxine and prolactin levels is useful in amenorrhoea.

Measurement of oestrogen levels is of little value if there is no clinical evidence of ovarian activity but it is useful where there is apparent arrest of early development or where there are secondary sex characteristics and when menstrual obstruction has been excluded. In the latter event, normal or even above normal levels may be associated with polycystic ovarian disorder or congenital adrenal hyperplasia, even with primary amenorrhoea.

Testosterone blood level is essential where there is suspicion of testicular or Leydig cell tissue.

17-αOH-progesterone will be raised where congenital adrenal hyperplasia is due to 21-hydroxylase deficiency.

X-rays

Bone age is extremely useful where there is delay or acceleration of puberty development. It permits a biological rather than chronological age to frame other observations.

Where there are anatomical abnormalities of the genital tract the renal tract should be investigated by intravenous pyelography (unless ultrasound has provided or excluded a diagnosis).

Ultrasound

Pelvic ultrasound scanning has extended diagnostic possibilities in recent years. It is particularly useful where there is menstrual obstruction (see Chapter 1, Fig. 1.16) and polycystic ovaries (e.g. in pubertal menorrhagia), abdominal swelling and for identification of kidneys. It is of some use in clarifying the anatomy in girls with delayed puberty in that the presence of ovaries and uterus can generally be established. However, there are some pitfalls. The prepubertal ovary is not usually identifiable. The gonad without a müllerian system may be very high and lateral and is easily missed. Recognition of an unstimulated uterus (e.g. in primary ovarian failure) may be difficult and presence of a rudimentary, but uncanalized uterus may deceive. Awareness and better technical resolution will hopefully reduce these misinterpretations. Scanning of the premenarchial pelvis has proved particularly useful in surveillance of ovarian or uterine development during spontaneous or therapeutic progress towards menarche. Thus, in infancy after postnatal regression of the uterine and ovarian enlargement due to maternal hormones, the uterus remains very small (about 2.5 × 1.0 cm) until nearly puberty. Thereafter there is increase in size, amenable to measurement, with a steep curve from 10–13 years (Ivarsson et al 1983). It is hard to see the ovaries in a girl less than 7 years in age but thereafter there is a rapid increase in size by menarche when there is a mean volume of 3.30 cm^3. The growth correlates with the stage of puberty. Girls with precocious puberty tend to have ovaries greater than 2 s.d. for age while girls with Turner's syndrome are less than 2 s.d. (Ivarsson et al 1983).

Normally, as menarche approaches, there is a 'megalocystic' appearance indicative of multiple follicular development without ovulation (Stanhope et al 1985).

Where hypogonadotrophic hypopituitarism is diagnosed studies of the pituitary fossa by X-ray or computerized tomography scan are indicated. Anosmia (Kallman's syndrome) is an unusual accompaniment.

Similarly, where precocious puberty is being investigated, abdominal ultrasound and hormonal investigation are basic. If peripheral causes are excluded, cerebral investigation by computerized tomography scan and nuclear magnetic resonance investigation will require specialized referral.

Where pubertal menorrhagia is the problem, a balance has to be struck between reluctance to interfere and concern lest there is a pathological cause. An ultrasound scan may reveal unusual intrauterine contents — the possibility of an incomplete abortion should be remembered. The multicystic ovaries associated with anovulation and endometrial hyperplasia are an exaggeration of the normal findings and the condition is self-limiting but may require treatment.

Laparoscopy

Where there is doubt about the internal anatomy, obstruction that cannot be drained effectively vaginally or severe dysmenorrhoea in the early cycles, this is a useful investigation.

It is of very limited value if there is primary gonadal failure. If there are raised gonadotrophins it is possible to establish whether there are streak gonads or ovaries with unstimulatable primordial follicles (resistant ovary syndrome). However, elucidation of the precise status of the ovaries can be deferred since there appear, at present, to be very limited therapeutic options (Ledger et al 1989).

Special situations

In general, the assessment of overall growth and development and identification of discrepancies provide the important diagnostic clues. If a girl is well grown, has had a growth spurt but no menarche, there is likely to be a significant cause and investigation must be pursued. Precocious puberty may be accepted to be constitutional once important pathological causes have been excluded. However, there are times when a systematic sequence of investigation does not enable diagnosis, and observation over a period of weeks or months may be helpful.

A particular difficulty is to distinguish between constitutional delay, hypothalamic causes and weight-related delay.

Where there is hypogonadotrophic hypogonadism, normal chromosomes, normal anatomy and delayed bone age, an increase in weight, increased growth velocity and onset

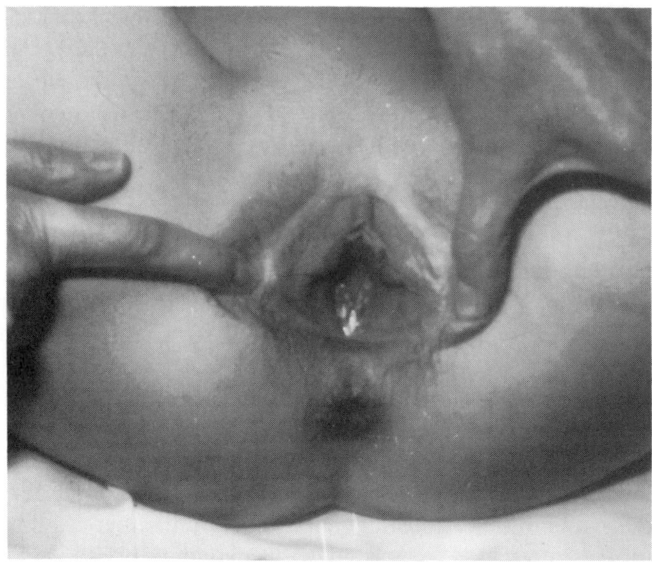

Fig. 13.9 Imperforate hymen, presenting with amenorrhoea and requiring excision and drainage.

of breast development on successive examinations would be important clues.

TREATMENT

This follows from the cause. Therapeutically, there may be several possible outcomes.

Cure

Surgical

1. Imperforate hymen: incision only may suffice (Fig. 13.9).
2. Vaginal atresia with a functioning uterus: this may be difficult and prolonged but the aim is the restoration of normal function (where there is cervical atresia this would still be the primary objective; see Chapter 1 for discussion and references).
3. Unduly enlarged labia.
4. Removal of ovarian or adrenal cyst or tumour.
5. Some cerebral tumours.

Medical

1. Hypothyroidism: treatment of this may normalize the puberty development.
2. Hyperprolactinaemia.
3. Constitutional delay: self-limiting but puberty development can be expedited.

Management with irremediable cause

1. Primary ovarian failure, e.g. Turner's: replacement therapy if Y chromosome material plus gonadectomy.
2. Androgen insensitivity: gonadectomy advisable; oestrogen replacement.
3. Müllerian agenesis: need for and timing of vaginal enlargement.
4. Pituitary deficiency (± cerebral tumour): replacement treatment.
5. Hypothalamic deficiency: LH-releasing hormone may enable puberty development.

Treatment of cause

When treatment is possible but may not cure the puberty problem:

1. Polycystic ovarian disorder: treatment may suppress the condition and the problem may be self-limiting.
2. Congenital adrenal hyperplasia: steroid treatment may enable the menarche to occur.
3. Weight-related amenorrhoea: this is apt to persist or recur.
4. Some pituitary/hypothalamic disorders may be treatable.

Primary ovarian failure

Replacement oestrogen is the basis of treatment. In most circumstances of primary ovarian failure there is a uterus and vagina and in the long term oestrogen/progestagen in an oral contraceptive type of pill is advisable for endometrial protection. Initial replacement with oestrogen alone is reasonable, especially if the girl is young, as this simulates nature. The starting dose in girls of average stature is not critical and 0.02 mg ethinyloestradiol or equivalent is reasonable. This will usually produce a growth spurt and then hasten epiphyseal closure as well as encourage breast and pubic hair development. If the girl is eunuchoid and considerably above average height, increased dosage may be used to accelerate the growth spurt and close the epiphyses quickly.

Where gonadal failure accompanies short stature (Turner's syndrome and its variants) special considerations apply and treatment depends on age. Hopefully the diagnosis will increasingly be made before the age of puberty and treatment started in a paediatric clinic. Without treatment there is no growth spurt (Ranke et al 1983) and although oestrogen and oxymetholone have been used for many years to achieve one, there is doubt about the best timing and regime. The growth spurt tends to be short-lived and of limited magnitude (Fig. 13.10). In normal puberty, peak height velocity occurs before menarche and at very low oestrogen levels. Bone growth is better at lower oestrogen doses and if epiphyseal closure can be delayed by lower doses there may be greater final height (Ross et al 1986). Oestrogen administration is therefore best started

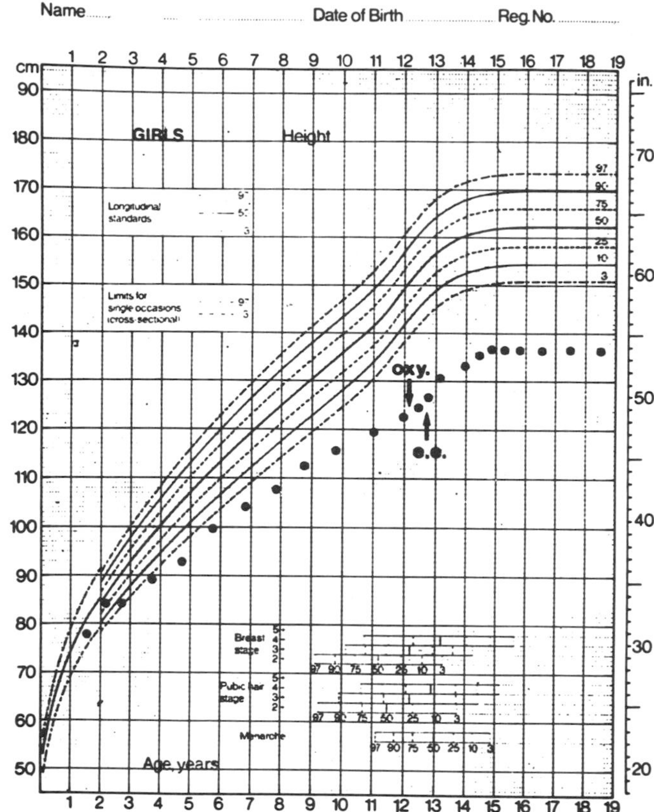

Fig. 13.10 Growth spurt in a girl with Turner's syndrome, following oxymetholone and later oestrogen administration.

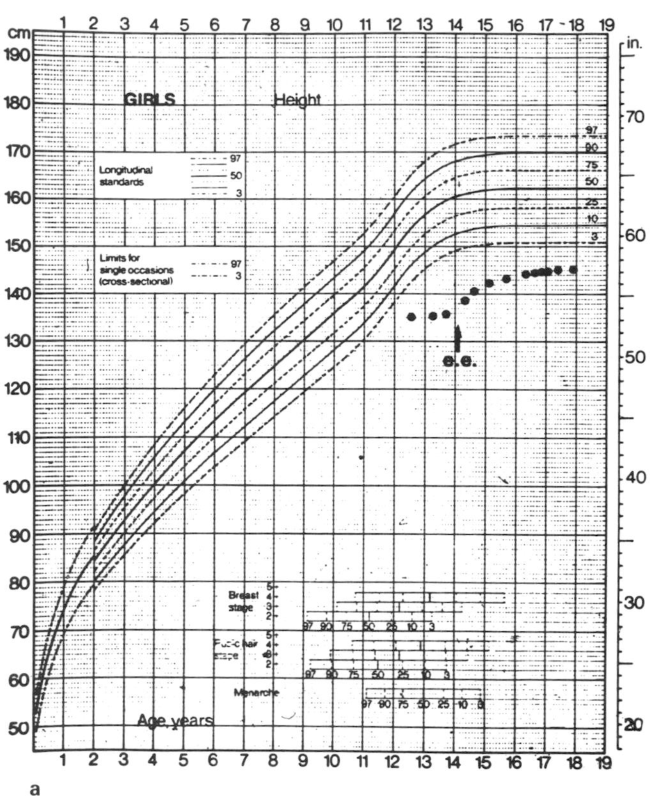

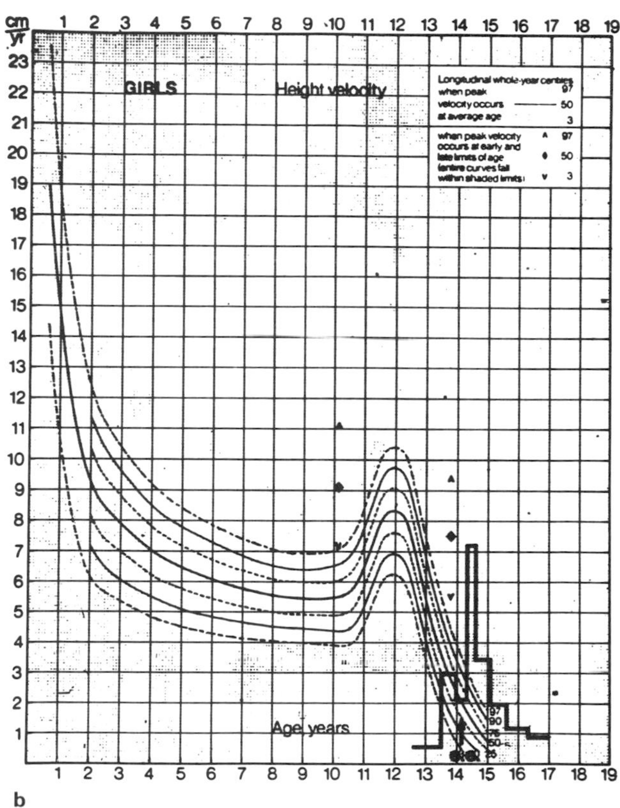

Fig. 13.11 Growth spurt in a girl with Turner's syndrome following oestrogen administration (**a**). Although there is a clear growth spurt with increased height velocity (**b**), the spurt is short-lived and makes little impact on the deficit in stature.

at about 10 years of age — the physiological time — with a dose (100 ng/kg/day) calculated to achieve physiological blood levels for age. This is 2–5 μg/day, increasing to 10–20 μg once a growth spurt is achieved. Continuous administration with less than 10 μg/day will not usually result in withdrawal bleeding, but at an appropriate age (e.g. 13 years), when taking 10–20 μg/day, a girl will usually have a 'period' if administration is cyclical. Alternative or additional strategies for increased height are under trial.

Oxymetholone (or similar steroids) and human growth hormone also produce a temporary growth spurt (Rosenfeld et al 1986). Trial of human growth hormone was halted because of Creutzfeldt–Jakob disease (Buchanan et al 1987). Synthetic growth hormone looks promising (Rongen-Westerlaken et al 1988) but it is unclear yet whether any of these regimes influence final height (which is on average 150 cm). The basic problem is that prepubertal growth has been slow and by 10 years of age girls are substantially short. A growth spurt which is short-lived achieves little or no 'catch-up' (Fig. 13.11 and 13.12). To make progress it will be essential to decrease the deficit before the peak velocity or greatly prolong the growth spurt. Nevertheless, early treatment prevents the girl falling even further behind her peer group and the development of secondary sex characteristics and 'periods'

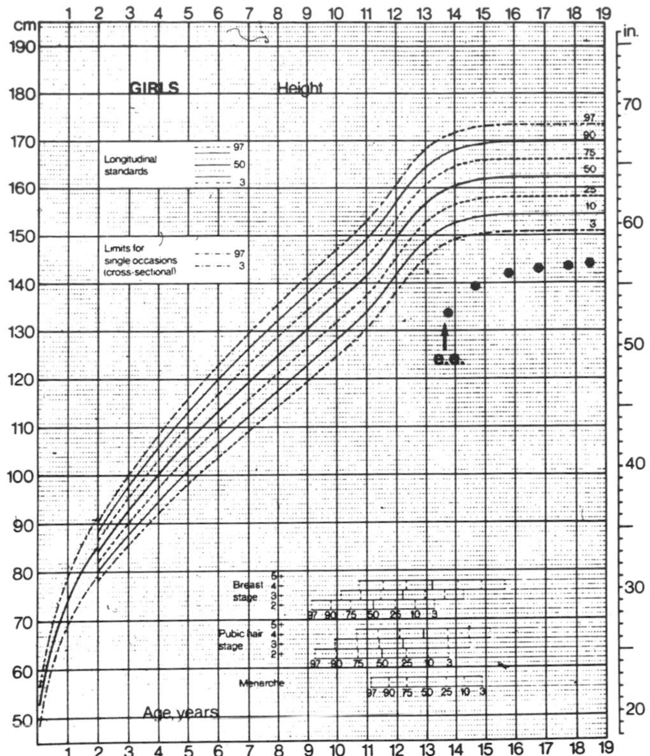

Fig. 13.12 Mean growth spurt in 7 girls with Turner's syndrome treated with oestrogens at a mean age of just under 14 years and followed annually for 5 years. There was continuing slow growth.

provides an important psychological boost. The quality of breast development appears to be very variable and it is uncertain whether dosage or turning of oestrogens affects this critically (Figs 13.13 and 13.14).

Girls who look younger than their years tend to be treated accordingly and advice should be offered to counteract this. Ensuring that the girl and her mother understand about infertility despite apparent puberty development requires tact with clarity. Long-term considerations include the addition of progestagens to the oestrogen replacement, advice concerning the value of continuing replacement treatment throughout the reproductive years and the possibility of donor egg pregnancies. Where there is a Y chromosome (e.g. 45X/46XY) the streak gonads should be removed (see below).

Androgen insensitivity

Once the diagnosis has been made, management must include advice concerning removal of gonads and then replacement oestrogens. Because the growth spurt is at the mean age for boys, there is longer than usual prepubertal growth and final stature therefore is usually above the female mean. Breast development varies but tends to be less than usual and there is poor vulvar development with almost no pubic hair. The build is generally slim and boyish. Once growth is completed there is no advantage in retaining the gonads. The exact incidence of gonadoblastoma or dysgerminoma formation in XY individuals is uncertain since there may be biased reporting from positive cases, but it is estimated at about 30% (for discussion see Verp & Simpson 1987). Girls are often reluctant to have their gonads removed in this condition as it seems unphysiological and the miracles of modern reproductive technology appear to them to offer hope. It remains to be seen whether regular ultrasound scanning (e.g. at 6-monthly intervals) offers sufficient reliability in this situation at least to defer gonadectomy.

After gonadectomy, long-term oestrogens should be prescribed for their effect on vaginal epithelium, osteoporosis and cardiovascular system. There seems no point in recommending progestagens as well unless there is shown to

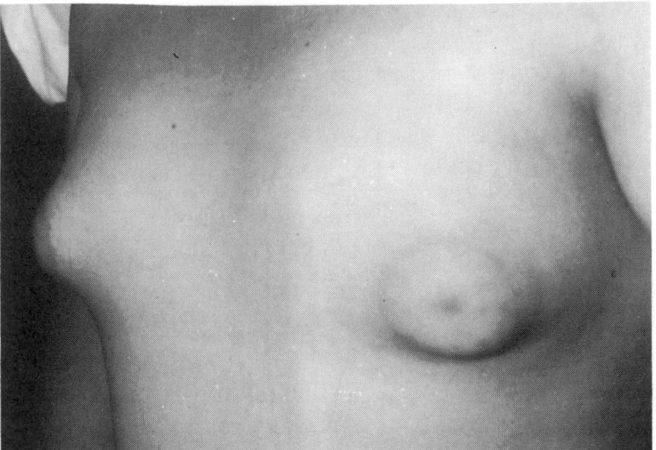

Fig. 13.13 Breast development in Turner's syndrome following oestrogen administration. There is good areolar development but little breast tissue after several years of hormone replacement.

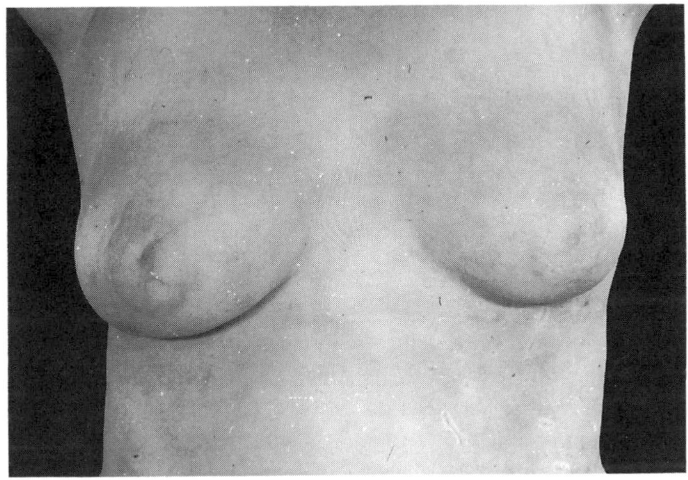

Fig. 13.14 In this girl with Turner's syndrome, hormone replacement resulted in good breast but poor nipple development.

be a protective effect on breast disease. Where incomplete androgen insensitivity or 5α-reductase deficiency is diagnosed, there is concomitant virilization and, assuming reinforcement of the female gender, gonadectomy becomes a matter of greater urgency. Clitoral reduction or recession may be required.

Hypogonadotrophic hypogonadism

Where the cause is treatable, this should be effected first.

Where the basic cause is hypogonadotrophic there are options. Replacement oestrogens (later, with progestagens) can be offered and the effect should be similar to that in girls with ovarian failure. Gonadotrophin therapy should be reserved for induction of ovulation and prior achievement of secondary sex characteristics is preferable. A more physiological approach is the use of pulsatile LH-releasing hormone (Stanhope et al 1987).

Anorexia nervosa and weight-related amenorrhoea

The management of these girls is notoriously difficult and essentially similar whether there is delay in onset of puberty, arrest of development or secondary amenorrhoea. Use of oestrogens to promote puberty development may also be associated with slight weight gain and may help over a difficult patch.

Precocious puberty

Treatment depends on the cause which should, where possible, remove the gonadotrophic or oestrogen stimulus. This may require neurosurgery for intrinsic reasons. Where the diagnosis is that of constitutional early development treatment options include:

1. Down-regulation with LH-releasing hormone analogues (Comite et al 1981; Pescovitz et al 1985).
2. Cyproterone acetate, which suppresses gonadotrophin secretion (Lorini et al 1981).
3. Medroxyprogesterone acetate (Grumbach 1985).
4. Danazol.

Psychological aspects of treatment are important. Management should usually be according to age, despite the physical appearance.

Pubertal menorrhagia

If rare pathological causes are excluded, anovulation is present and treatment is required, then use of oestrogen/progestagen as in the combined pill will usually permit acceptable withdrawal bleeds. If not, then continuous administration to achieve complete amenorrhoea may be more acceptable. Treatment should be discontinued after, say, 6 months and the natural cycle reviewed. Alternative hormonal treatment includes dihydrogesterone, which is less likely to inhibit ovulation, or depot injections of a progestogen.

Dysmenorrhoea

If this is due to a rudimentary horn which may be obstructed, then removal may be indicated. Occasionally endometriosis may be present, apparently from menarche, and if diagnosed should be appropriately treated.

RESULTS

Where the cause of the puberty problem is reversible the outcome is good and sometimes normal.

Continuing problems are described below.

Following obstruction

Vaginal or cervical atresia. Maintenance of patency for menstrual function may be difficult or impossible (see Chapter 1). Endometriosis may be a severe problem resulting from obstruction.

Müllerian agenesis

Available techniques usually enable a good vaginal result.

Gonadal failure or removal

Results in terms of maintenance of secondary sex characteristics are usually good. Long-term replacement treatment, especially the addition of progestagens, where indicated, may be difficult to sustain. Sexual function is usually good.

Weight-related amenorrhoea

Despite achievement of normal weight for height, amenorrhoea may persist or recur.

Congenital adrenal hyperplasia

Good adrenal control may not necessarily result in normal ovarian function. Inappropriate feedback with hypergonadotrophin and polycystic ovarian disorder may occur. Fertility is reduced and early ovarian failure appears to be common.

Precocious puberty

It is of some encouragement gynaecologically that the long-term outlook for girls with precocious puberty in terms of menstrual function and subsequent fertility is good, provided there was no serious pathology in the first instance (Murram et al 1984).

Pubertal menorrhagia

The condition is generally self-limiting and results are excellent.

Dysmenorrhoea

Teenage endometriosis, arising either spontaneously or as a result of premenarchial obstruction, may have a very variable outcome. Treatment should aim for eradication.

COMPLICATIONS

The main complication is failure to achieve a physiological result with fertility. Only conditions resulting in positive complications are referred to here.

Cervical or vaginal atresia

Despite surgical endeavours there may be severe pelvic infection with pyosalpinx or peritonitis. Hysterectomy may be necessary.

Vaginal agenesis

Despite surgery, apareunia may result.

CONCLUSIONS

There is overlap between normal and abnormal pubertal development. Anatomical abnormalities of the genitalia are often multiple. Short stature or the presence of other disorders may provide important diagnostic clues when pubertal development seems to be disordered.

It is important to avoid false reassurance of abnormal features such as short stature, unexpected bleeding, failure to develop secondary sex characteristics or failure to menstruate. It is wise to seek another opinion if there are unresolved or unusual features.

It is extremely important to avoid undermining a girl's confidence in her own observations or her sexuality. A poor prognosis with respect to fertility must be conveyed tactfully.

KEY POINTS

1. Puberty is a coherent process involving oestrogen, increased somatic growth and the development of secondary sexual characteristics.
2. Menarche: the first period occurs because there has been sufficient endometrial stimulation to result in a withdrawal bleed when there is a temporary fall in the oestrogen level.
3. Ovarian failure constitutes the largest single cause of delayed puberty.
4. The commonest cause of precocious puberty in the female is central constitutional early development.
5. Measurement of gonadotrophin levels is important in distinguishing hyper- from hypogonadotrophic causes of delayed puberty.
6. Pelvic ultrasound scanning has extended diagnostic possibilities in recent years.
7. Oestrogen replacement (later, with progestogens) is the basis of treatment in primary ovarian failure to induce pubertal growth and secondary sexual development.
8. It is extremely important to avoid undermining a girl's confidence in her own observations or her sexuality and false reassurance of abnormal features.

REFERENCES

Brook C G D 1982 Growth assessment in childhood and adolescence. Blackwell Scientific Publications, Oxford

Brook C G D 1986 Turner syndrome. Archives of Disease in Childhood 61: 305–309

Buchanan C R, Law C M, Milner R D G 1987 Growth hormone in short, slowly growing children and those with Turner's syndrome. Archives of Disease in Childhood 62: 912–916

Comite F, Cutler G B, Rivier J et al 1981 Short-term treatment of idiopathic precocious puberty with a long-activating analogue of luteinizing hormone releasing hormone. New England Journal of Medicine 305: 1546

Dewhurst C J 1984 Female puberty and its abnormalities. Churchill Livingstone, Edinburgh, pp 57–81

Frisch R E 1985 Body fat, menarche and reproductive ability. Seminars in Reproductive Endocrinology 3: 45

Grumbach M M 1985 True or central precocious puberty. In: Krieger D T, Bardin C W (eds) Current therapy in endocrinology and metabolism. Dekker, Toronto

Huffman J W, Dewhurst C J, Capraro V D 1981 The gynaecology of childhood and adolescence. W B Saunders, Philadelphia

Ivarsson S A, Nilsson K O, Persson P-H 1983 Ultrasonography of the pelvic organs in prepubertal and post pubertal girls. Archives of Disease in Childhood 58: 352–354

Kulin H E 1987 Precocious puberty. Clinical Obstetrics and Gynecology 30: 714

Ledger W L, Thomas E J, Browning D, Lenton E A, Cooke I D 1989 Suppression of gonadotrophin secretion does not reverse premature ovarian failure. British Journal of Obstetrics and Gynaecology 96: 196

Lorini R, Colombo A, Ugazio A G et al 1981 Cyproterone acetate in precocious puberty. Journal of Endocrinological Investigation 4: 263

Marshall W A, Tanner J M 1969 Variations in the pattern of pubertal changes in girls. Archives of Disease in Childhood 44: 291–303

Murram D, Dewhurst J, Grant D B 1984 Precocious puberty: a follow up study. Archives of Disease in Childhood 59: 77–78

Pescovitz O H, Cutler G B, Loriaux D L 1985 Management of

precocious puberty. Journal of Pediatric Endocrinology 1: 85
Ranke M B, Pfluger H, Rosendahl W et al 1983 Turner syndrome: spontaneous growth in 150 cases and review of the literature. European Journal of Pediatrics 141: 81
Reindollar R H, McDonough P G 1987 Neuroendocrine processes relevant to the childhood years. Clinical Obstetrics and Gynecology 30: 633
Reindollar R H, Byrd J R, McDonough P G 1981 Delayed sexual development: a study of 252 patients. American Journal of Obstetrics and Gynecology 140: 371–380
Rongen-Westerlaken C, Wit J M, Drop S L S et al 1988 Methionyl human growth hormone in Turner's syndrome. Archives of Disease in Childhood 63: 1211–1217
Rosenfeld R G, Hintz R L, Johanson A J et al 1986 Methionyl human growth hormone and oxandrolone in Turner's syndrome. Preliminary results of a prospective randomised trial. Journal of Pediatrics 109: 936–943
Ross J L, Long L M, Skerda M et al 1986 Effects of low doses of oestradiol on 6-month growth rates and predicted height in patients with Turner syndrome. Journal of Pediatrics 109: 950–953
Sklar C A, Kaplan S L, Grumbach M M 1980 Evidence for dissociation between adrenarche and gonadarche. Journal of Clinical Endocrinology and Metabolism 51: 548–556
Stanhope R, Adams J, Jacobs H S, Brook C G D 1985 Ovarian ultrasound assessment in normal children, idiopathic precocious puberty, and during low dose pulsatile gonadotrophin releasing hormone treatment of hypogonadotrophic hypogonadism. Archives of Disease in Childhood 60: 116–119
Stanhope R, Brook C G D, Pringle P J, Adams J, Jacobs H S 1987 Induction of puberty by pulsatile gonadotropin releasing hormone. Lancet ii: 552–555
Stark O, Peckham C S, Moynihan C 1989 Weight and age at menarche. Archives of Disease in Childhood 64: 383–387
Tanner J M 1981 A history of the study of human growth. Cambridge University Press, Cambridge
Verp M S, Simpson J L 1987 Abnormal sexual differentiation and neoplasia. Cancer Genetics and Cytogenetics 25: 191–218
Zacharis L, Wurtman R 1964 Blindness: its relation to age of menarche. Science 144: 1154

14. Menstruation and menstrual abnormality

M. Lumsden S. Smith

INTRODUCTION

Menstrual abnormality is a frequent cause for presentation of women to gynaecological clinics and menorrhagia is one of the commonest causes of iron deficiency anaemia in western women (Cohen & Gibor 1980). However before discussing the aetiology of menstrual abnormality, the mechanism of normal menstruation will be reviewed.

MENSTRUATION

At the end of the ovarian cycle, a major portion of the endometrium in primates undergoes periodic necrosis and sloughing associated with blood loss. This is at a time when the gonadal steroids reach their lowest levels. The nature of the supportive effect on the endometrium is unknown, although possible mechanisms will be discussed later.

The mechanism of menstruation

The uterine wall consists of three layers: the serous coat, the myometrium and the endometrium. The serous coat is firmly adherent to the myometrium which consists of smooth muscle fibres, the main branches of the blood vessels and the nerves of the uterus and connective tissue. The endometrium consists principally of glandular and stromal cells although its structure does vary with the position in the uterus and the stage of the menstrual cycle.

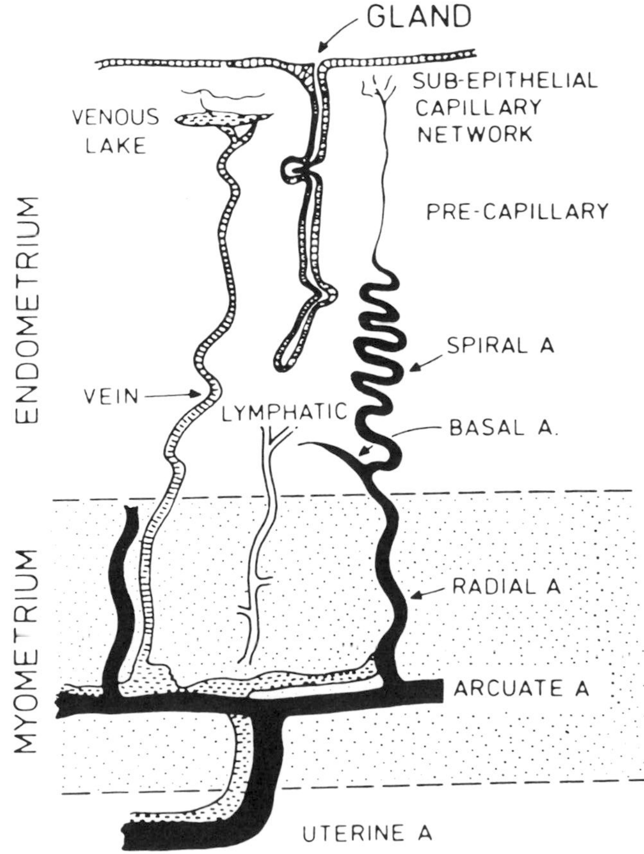

Fig. 14.1 Schematic representation of the blood supply of the uterus. A = artery.

The blood supply of the uterus

This is illustrated in Figure 14.1. The arcuate and radial arteries which supply the myometrium and basal endometrium have vascular fields which overlap. On approaching the surface epithelium, the radial arteries develop a corkscrew appearance and are known as spiral arterioles. These are present only in species which menstruate and are end arterioles, each supplying an area of 4–7 mm^2. They are sensitive to changes in gonadal steroid levels and the capillaries are lost with the glands and stroma at menstruation. There is an irregular network of venous vessels with the veins frequently intersecting, forming venous lakes. The radial and arcuate veins drain via the uterine vein into the iliac vein.

The histology of the uterus

The histology of the uterus is illustrated in Figure 14.2a. The zona compacta, which is adjacent to the uterine cavity, and the zona functionalis (spongy layer) are sensitive to

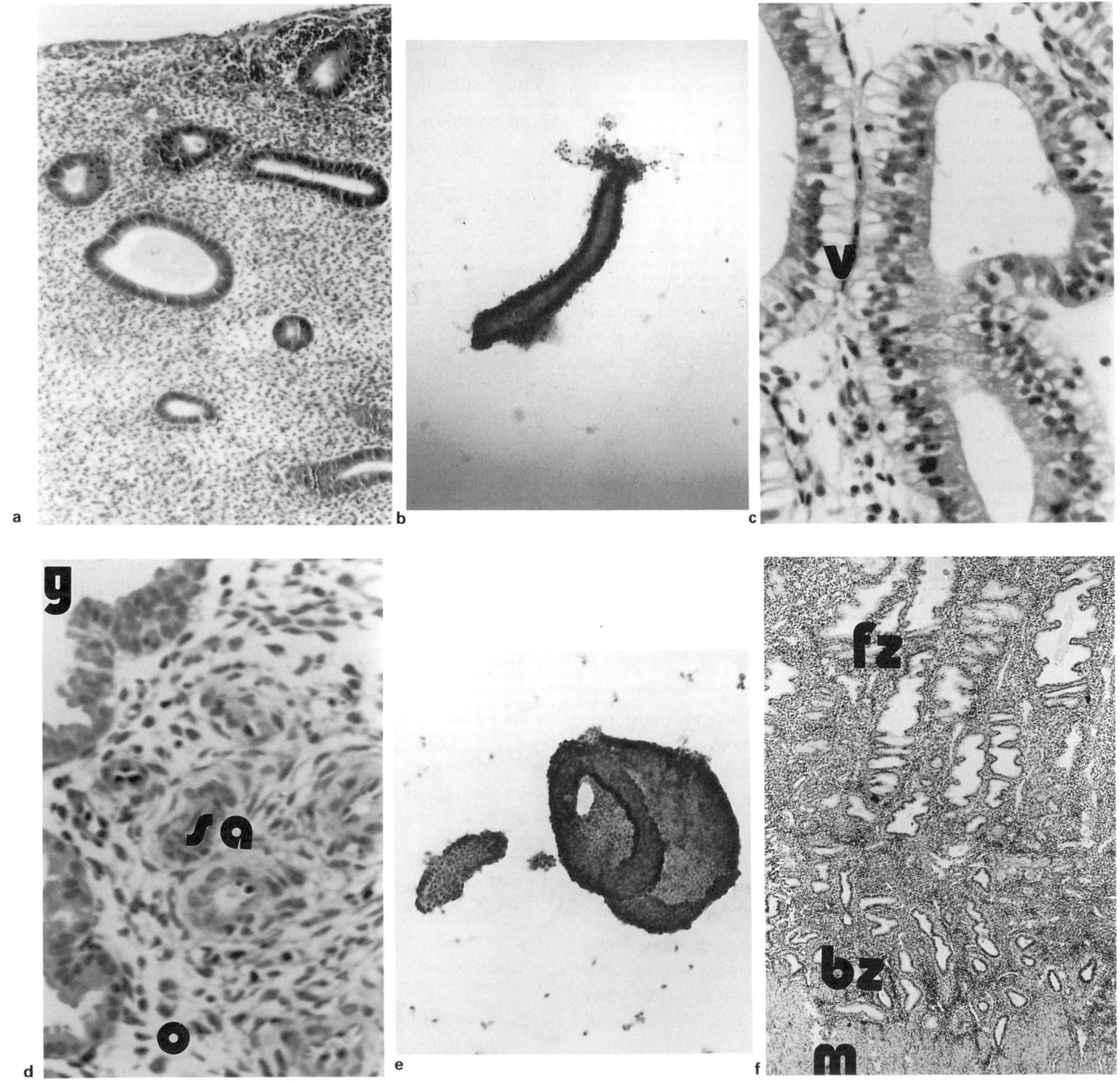

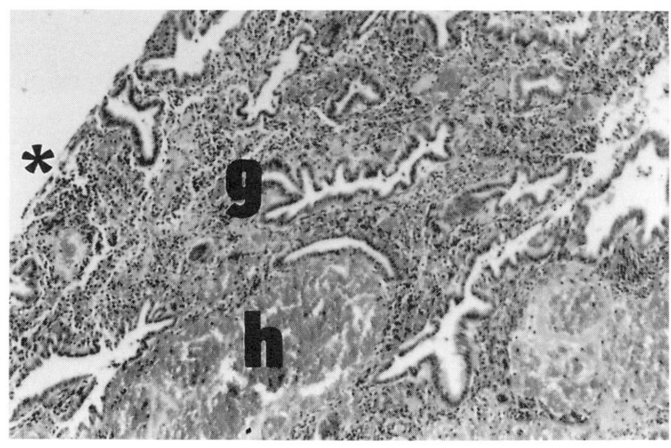

g

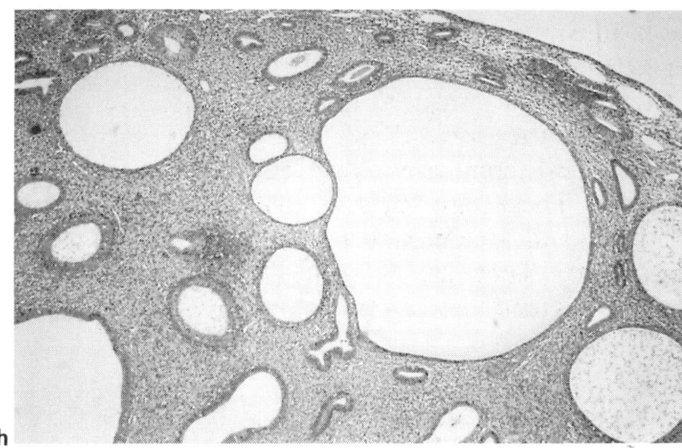

h

Fig. 14.2a Proliferative endometrium showing tubular glands. Mitoses are present in glands and stroma (× 10). **b** A proliferative gland (× 63) separated from endometrium by collagenase digestion. **c** Early secretory endometrium showing sub-nuclear vacuolation (v) and the presence of secretions. There are now few mitoses (× 40). **d** Mid-secretory endometrium (day 23) characterized by 'saw-toothed' glands (g), convoluted spiral arterioles (sa) and stromal oedema (o) (× 40). **e** Mid secretory gland illustrating the coiled shape (compare with Fig. 14.2b) (× 40). **f** Late secretory endometrium showing the functional zone (fz), basal zone (bz) and myometrium (m). **g** Menstruating endometrium. The glands (g) are now thin and show little secretory activity. There are lakes of haemorrhage (h) and the endometrium is beginning to break up (*). There is infiltration with white blood cells (× 10). **h** Cystic glandular hyperplasia (× 4).

changes in gonadal steroids whereas the basal layer, which joins the myometrium, is not. The myometrium, which consists principally of smooth muscle cells, is connected by gap junctions allowing free movement of ions; it offers low electrical resistance. There is functional resemblance to cardiac muscle although there is no conclusive evidence for a pacemaker within the uterus. The endometrium responds to the cyclical changes in the gonadal steroid levels described elsewhere (see Chapter 10); these changes are probably in preparation for blastocyst implantation, as menstruation only happens when this fails to occur.

The first half of the cycle involves tissue growth and proliferation and the second, epithelial and stromal differentiation. During the proliferative phase, the short, straight, epithelial glands elongate and become tortuous (Fig. 14.2a). Changes occur in the position of the nuclei and the number of mitoses (Fig. 14.2a). During the secretory phase, the glands increase in diameter and tortuosity and vacuoles appear in the cellular cytoplasm (Fig. 14.2c). The tissue also becomes markedly more oedematous.

The spiral arterioles also undergo cyclical change. Following the cessation of menstruation they are simple in form, extending just into the endometrium. The secretory phase is characterized by growth of arterioles. In the late secretory phase coiling occurs due to proliferation and extension of the arterioles as well as the resorption of the stromal oedema (Fig. 14.2d). With the fall in steroid concentrations menstrual shedding of the endometrium occurs (Fig. 14.2g). Cell injury becomes increasingly evident and infiltration of macrophages occurs.

Endometrial shedding varies remarkably from one woman to another and from one area of the uterus to another in the same woman.

Dramatic changes occur in the spiral arterioles at menstruation. These changes were described by Markee (1948) after experiments involving the transplantation of endometrium into the anterior chamber of the eye of the rhesus monkey. This work is the cornerstone of the current-day concepts of the menstrual process. On observing the bleeding process, Markee suggested that the arteriolar coiling caused constriction of the vessel lumen with vascular stasis and leukocytic infiltration. About 24 hours premenstrually intense vasoconstriction led to ischaemic damage which was then followed by vasodilatation with haemorrhages from both arterial and venous vessels: 75% of the loss was arteriolar, 15% venous and 10% diapedesis of erythrocytes. This work has never been repeated although some support comes from experiments where endometrium was implanted into the hamster cheek pouch (an immunologically privileged site) and changes observed through a plastic window. Bleeding was observed although no hormonally induced changes in the blood vessels occurred.

The myometrium

There is no evidence for a structural change in the myometrium during the menstrual cycle. However, it is well known that changes occur in the pattern of contractility. This can be assessed by measuring intrauterine pressure, which demonstrates maximum activity during the first days of the menses, when a labour-like activity is observed which may or may not lead to pain (Fig. 14.3).

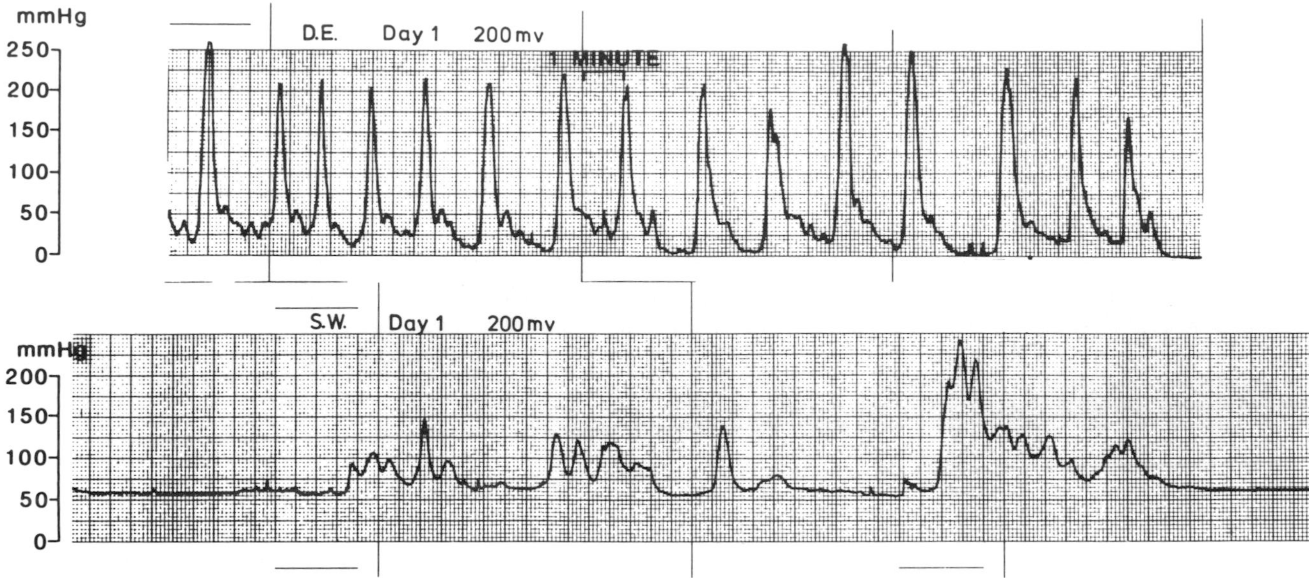

Fig. 14.3 Uterine contractility on day 1 of the menses as assessed by measuring the intrauterine pressure using a microtransducer catheter. Subject DE suffered from dysmenorrhoea whereas subject SW did not.

CONTROL OF MENSTRUAL BLOOD LOSS

The endometrial surface area is large (10–45 mm^2), indicating that haemostasis during menstruation is usually very efficient. Possible factors in the control of blood loss are:

1. Myometrial contractility.
2. Haemostatic plug formation.
3. Vasoconstriction.

Drugs which inhibit uterine contraction, such as prostaglandin synthetase inhibitors (see p. 200), and which are used to treat dysmenorrhoea do not increase menstrual blood loss whereas ergot alkaloids which cause muscle contractions are of no use in treating menorrhagia. Myometrial activity is therefore not considered to be the principal mechanism.

Menstrual blood was thought not to clot and to be free of platelets and fibrin. However more recent work suggests that menstruation is initiated by tissue alterations involving vascular disintegration and extravasation of blood with a general lack of haemostatic reaction. Once clinical bleeding and tissue shedding has started, haemostatic plug formation occurs, but less rapidly and less completely than is observed in human skin wounds (Christiaens et al 1982). Menstrual fluid and endometrium have marked fibrinolytic activity. Anti-fibrinolytic agents decrease the menstrual blood loss significantly and certain haemorrhagic conditions (e.g. thrombocytopenic purpura) are associated with an increased incidence of menorrhagia. Thus menorrhagia may occur in the presence of abnormalities of platelet structure or function and in clotting disorders, as described later. Lack of clotting makes physiological sense since clotting would lead to fibrosis which would impair fertility and cyclical uterine function.

Vasoconstriction is currently considered to be the most important mechanism controlling menstrual blood loss, although studies measuring endometrial blood flow have failed to confirm premenstrual vasoconstriction (Fraser et al 1987). Much work has recently centred on the role of prostaglandins since as a group, they have many properties, which makes it likely that they play a vital part.

Prostaglandins and menstruation

The evidence for a role for prostaglandins in menstruation is summarized below:

1. Prostaglandins of the 2 series, which are synthesized from arachidonic acid (Fig. 14.4), are present in endometrium and menstrual fluid in high concentrations.
2. Their synthesis by endometrium is influenced by steroid hormones and highest levels are found during the menses. This is particularly true for prostaglandin $F_{2\alpha}$, the synthesis of which rises significantly during the secretory phase of the menstrual cycle under the influence of progesterone.
3. They are vasoactive. Prostaglandin $F_{2\alpha}$ is a potent vasoconstrictor whereas others, e.g. prostaglandin E_2 and prostacyclin lead to vasodilatation.
4. Prostacyclin is a potent inhibitor of platelet aggregation.
5. Inhibitors of their synthesis decrease menstrual blood loss and myometrial contractility.

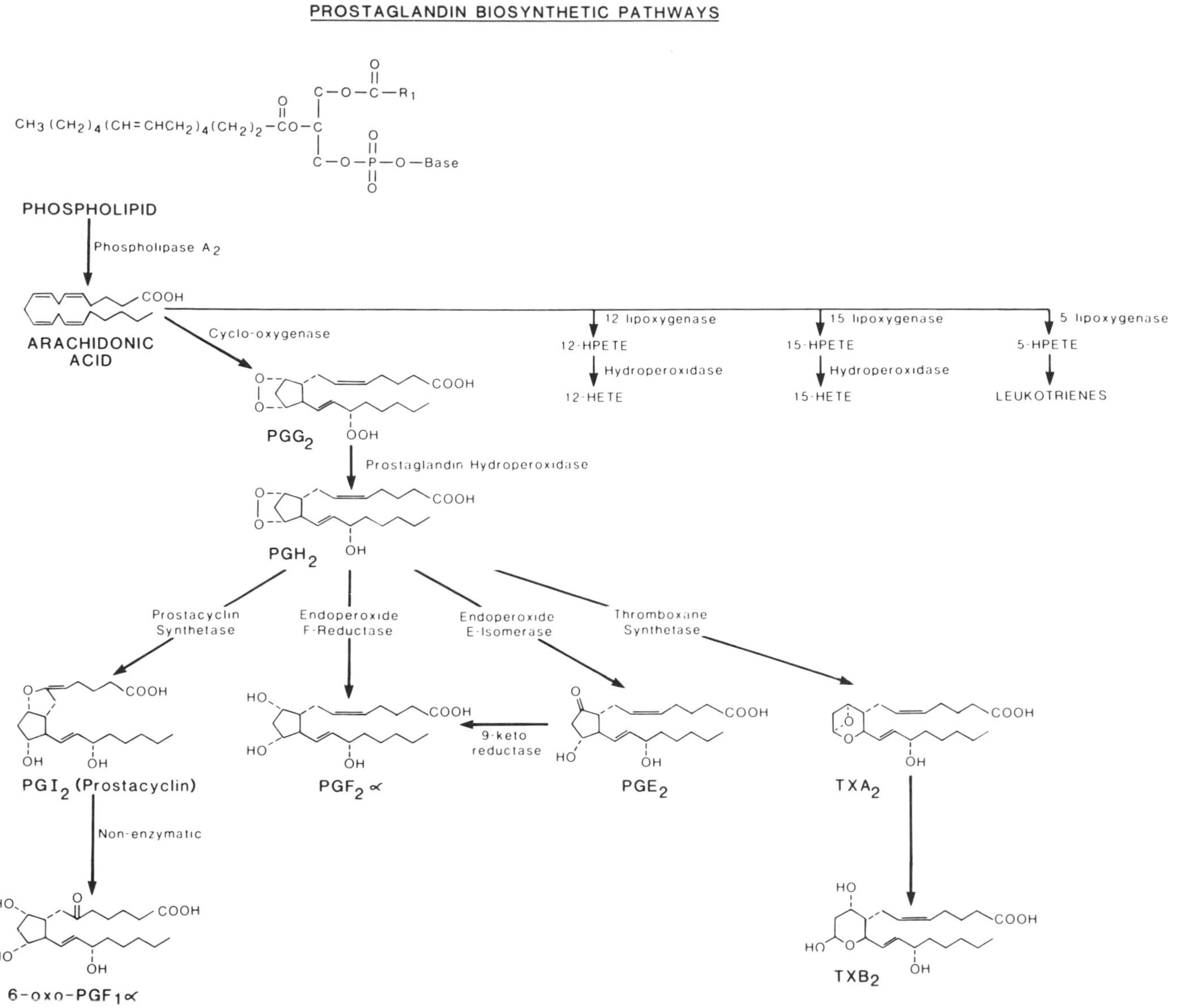

PROSTAGLANDIN BIOSYNTHETIC PATHWAYS

Fig. 14.4 The synthesis of prostaglandins from arachidonic acid. The most important products of endometrium are PGE_2, $PGF_{2\alpha}$ and PGI_2.

6. Exogenous prostaglandins affect uterine contractility and can induce menstrual-type bleeding.

A possible mechanism for menstruation is illustrated in Figure 14.5.

Phospholipase A2 controls the release of arachidonic acid from cell membranes and stimulates arachidonic acid and prostaglandin release. Production of the latter is also enhanced by tissue death and ischaemia. The factors controlling the differential production of the prostaglandins are unknown, although this is important when considering abnormal menstruation, for reasons which will be discussed later.

Arachidonic acid is also converted by another mechanism to leukotrienes. These are present in endometrium and their receptors have also been identified in the uterus.

The normal menstrual cycle

A majority of cycles are between 24 and 32 days and a normal cycle is considered to be 28 days. Menstrual cycle length varies during reproductive life, being most regular between the ages of 20 and 40 years. It tends to be longer after the menarche and shorter as the menopause approaches. The mean menstrual blood loss per menstruation in a healthy west European population ranges between 37 and 43 ml; 70% of the loss occurs in the first 48 hours. Despite the large interpatient variability, loss between consecutive menses in the same woman does not vary to a great extent (Fig. 14.6). Only 9–14% of women lose more than 80 ml/period and 60% of these women are actually anaemic. The upper limit of normal menstruation is thus taken as 80 ml/menses (Rybo 1966). However, actual fluid

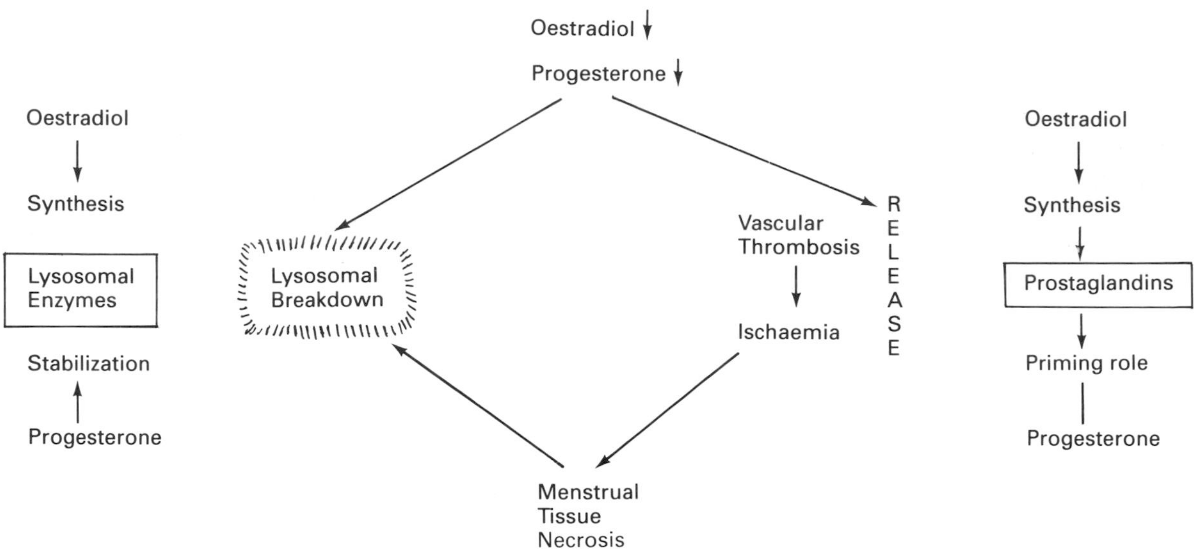

Fig. 14.5 Schematic representation of the events leading to endometrial breakdown and menstruation.

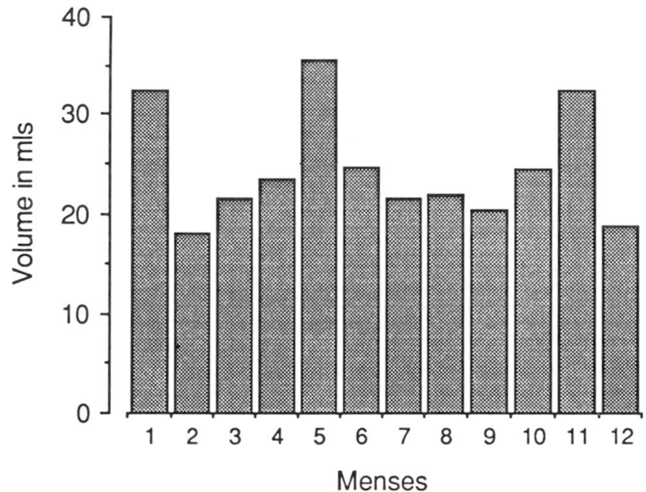

Fig. 14.6 The variability in menstrual blood loss in a single individual: values for 12 consecutive periods (adapted from Hallberg & Nilsson 1964).

loss (mucus, tissue etc.) may be considerably more than the blood loss alone and amounts vary considerably.

During the first day or two of the menses uterine contractility is at its greatest. This may possibly aid expulsion of the degenerating endometrium from the uterus. Activity is extremely variable between women although it is remarkably constant between menses in the same women. There is no objective method of separating normal and abnormal contractility; normal contractility is considered to be that which causes no debility to a woman although mild discomfort may occur.

ABNORMAL MENSTRUATION

During this century, widespread use of contraception and sterilization with reduction in family size has resulted in a significant increase in the number of menstrual periods experienced by women. As a result, menstrual problems have became increasingly important. The defects considered here will be menorrhagia with particular reference to dysfunctional uterine bleeding (DUB) and dysmenorrhoea. Those defects particularly associated with infertility, e.g. oligo- or amenorrhoea, will not be discussed further.

Menorrhagia

The causes of menorrhagia fall into four categories:

1. Clotting defects.
2. DUB.
3. Pelvic pathology.
4. Medical disorders.

Clotting defects

Certain haemorrhagic conditions, e.g. thrombocytopenic purpura and Von Willebrand's disease, are associated with an increased incidence of menorrhagia. However there is no impairment of blood coagulation in those with excess menstrual loss, nor are fibrin degradation products elevated in the menstrual fluid of those with heavy menstrual loss (Bonnar et al 1983). Patients with platelet and coagulation disorders frequently suffer from excessive menstrual blood loss, necessitating hormonal or surgical therapy and sometimes multiple transfusions. In women with thrombocytopenia, menstrual blood loss correlates broadly with platelet count at the time of the menses. Splenectomy has been known dramatically to reduce the menstrual blood loss in these patients.

DUB

Disturbances in the pattern of menstruation are a common clinical presentation for abnormalities of the hypophyseal–pituitary–ovarian axis. DUB is defined as heavy and/or irregular menses in the absence of recognizable pelvic pathology, pregnancy or general bleeding disorder. It commonly occurs at the extremes of reproductive life (adolescence and perimenopausally). The abnormalities of ovarian activity may be classified as follows:

1. *Anovulatory*
   a. Inadequate signal, e.g. in polycystic ovarian disease or premenopausally.
   b. Impaired positive feedback, e.g. in adolescence.
2. *Ovulatory*
   a. Inadequate luteal phase.
   b. Idiopathic.

Anovulatory DUB. Occasionally anovulatory cycles occur in all women. Chronic anovulation, however, is associated with an irregular and unpredictable pattern of bleeding ranging from short cycles with scanty bleeding to prolonged periods of irregular heavy loss. Normal bleeding occurs in response to withdrawal of both progesterone and oestradiol. If anovulation does not occur then the absence of progesterone results in no secretory changes in the endometrium accompanied by abnormalities in the production of steroid receptors, prostaglandins and other locally active endometrial products. Unopposed oestrogen gives rise to persistent proliferative or hyperplastic endometrium and oestrogen withdrawal bleeding is characteristically painless and irregular. It tends to occur at the extremes of reproductive life but is rare at other times. Only 20% of those cycles with excessive menstrual blood loss are anovulatory (Haynes et al 1979); this same study fails to demonstrate any abnormalities in gonadotrophin or circulating steroid concentrations. In anovulatory cycles, the endometrium appears to be unable to produce prostaglandin $F_{2\alpha}$ (Smith et al 1982). This may account for the painless nature of the bleeds.

Ovulation occurs in response to the mid-cycle surge of luteinizing hormone. If this fails to occur due to insufficient oestradiol secretion or impaired positive feedback, ovulation will not occur.

Failure of follicular development. This occurs perimenopausally and in the polycystic ovarian syndrome (the aetiology and treatment of the latter are dealt with elsewhere; Ch. 22). Follicular development insufficient to produce an oestrogen signal sufficient to induce a luteinizing hormone surge is one of the common reasons for the irregularities in menstrual cycle pattern in premenopausal women. Decreased ovarian activity due to diminished oocyte population may last weeks.

Gonadotrophin secretion rises, since feedback with the ovarian steroids is minimal, and then declines as follicles develop. The level of oestradiol may never be sufficient to induce endometrial development. Stimulation by the oestrogen may be unopposed by progesterone for long periods and cause irregular and unpredictable bleeding. The mechanism of this bleeding is unknown although it may result from the lack of secretory change in the endometrium (already described).

Failure of positive feedback. Anovulatory bleeding may be associated with cystic glandular hyperplasia of the endometrium (Fig. 14.2h). This occurs in some older women and also in prepubertal girls where the positive feedback mechanism is absent. It is normal for the first few cycles after the menarche to be anovulatory, scanty and painless. However, if anovulation persists, a long period of amenorrhoea is accompanied by endometrial hyperplasia. This is probably a result of multiple follicular development (multicystic ovaries) with failure of antral follicle formation. Levels of oestradiol fluctuate, but levels of follicle-stimulating hormone are more resistant than normal to the negative feedback effects of oestradiol due to a defect in either the hypothalamus or pituitary. Thus the mechanism by which a single follicle is selected for development each month is disturbed with a higher than normal level of oestrogen secretion. The resulting endometrial hyperplasia may cause excessive bleeding, anaemia, infertility and even cancer of the endometrium.

Ovulatory DUB.

Inadequate luteal phase. The luteal phase is usually over 10 days with a serum progesterone peak on at least 1 day in excess of 20 nmol/l. Anything less is inadequate. The short luteal phase arises from inadequate follicular development, possibly due to a lower than normal secretion of follicle-stimulating hormone. This syndrome may be associated with irregular bleeding and infertility.

Idiopathic bleeding. A relationship between prostaglandin production and menorrhagia was suggested in the mid 1970s by work showing a relationship between total endometrial prostaglandin content and the degree of menstrual loss — work which has received support in recent publications (Cameron et al 1987). The total amount of prostaglandin E_2 and $F_{2\alpha}$ in menstrual fluid is elevated during the first 2 days of the menses in women with menorrhagia, as is the endometrial content of prostaglandins. In patients experiencing regular ovulatory cycles there is an association between the menstrual blood loss and the ratio of prostaglandin. $E_2{:}F_{2\alpha}$. This suggests that excessive bleeding results from a shift in endometrial conversion of endoperoxide from the vasoconstrictor prostaglandin $F_{2\alpha}$ to the vasodilator prostaglandin E_2. This work was substantiated by later in vitro work which showed that secretory endometrium taken from women with menorrhagia in the presence of added precursor (arachidonic acid) has a greater capacity to produce prostaglandin E_2 and D_2 (vasodilatory prostaglandins) at the expense of prostaglandin $F_{2\alpha}$ (a vasoconstrictor) than endometrium from women with light periods, and may also enhance the synthesis of prostacyclin (vasodilator and inhibitor of platelet aggregation) from myometrium (Smith et al 1981a, b).

The differential action of the endometrium would seem to arise from an increased availability of precursor. The basic concept that there is an alteration in prostaglandin synthesis resulting in increased vasodilation rather than vasoconstriction is also supported by the finding that there are a greater number of prostaglandin E_2 receptors in the myometrium of menorrhagic women. However, the cause of the abnormal prostaglandin production is unknown since there is no evidence of an endocrine abnormality in those with DUB.

Menorrhagia in the presence of pathology

Menorrhagia is thought to be associated with uterine fibroids, adenomyosis, pelvic infection, endometrial polyps and the presence of a foreign body such as an intrauterine contraceptive device (IUCD). Also the rare conditions of myometrial hypertrophy and vascular abnormality may be associated with severe — even life-threatening — menorrhagia. However, objective evidence of menorrhagia in most of these situations is remarkably limited. In women with menstrual blood loss greater than 200 ml, over half will have fibroids, although only 40% of those with adenomyosis actually have menstrual blood loss in excess of 80 ml/menses. Whether chronic pelvic inflammatory disease or endometrial polyps are associated with above average loss is unclear.

Menorrhagia is well documented in the presence of an IUCD and morphological studies of IUCD-influenced endometrium have shown an impaired haemostatic reaction during menstruation, as compared with the normal situation. Only a small proportion of the vessels in the menstrual endometrium contain intravascular platelets and fibrin.

There is evidence for a role for prostaglandins in the menorrhagia associated with adenomyosis, uterine leiomyomata and the presence of an IUCD (Fraser et al 1986). Endometrial production of prostaglandin $F_{2\alpha}$, E_2 and 6-oxo-prostaglandin F_1 (the stable metabolite of prostacyclin) is raised in the presence of adenomyosis, although the increase in the vasodilators prostaglandin E_2 and 6-oxo-prostaglandin F_1 is greater than that of prostaglandin $F_{2\alpha}$. Prostaglandin production is also increased in the presence of an IUCD. However, the non-steroidal anti-inflammatory agents are less effective in menorrhagia associated with IUCD presence that in DUB, making it likely that other factors are also important.

Medical problems

Menorrhagia is associated with various endocrine disorders such as thyrotoxicosis and Cushing's disease, although the mechanism is unknown.

DYSMENORRHOEA

Dysmenorrhoea comes from the Greek and means difficult monthly flow, but is now taken to mean painful menstruation. It is a symptom complex with cramping lower abdominal pain radiating to the back and legs, often accompanied by gastrointestinal and neurological symptoms as well as general malaise. As with menorrhagia, it may be associated with pathology or may be idiopathic in origin.

Idiopathic (primary) dysmenorrhoea

There are many different theories as to why women suffer from dysmenorrhoea. The following factors may be of importance:

1. Prostaglandins (leukotrienes).
2. Increased myometrial contractility.
3. Decreased uterine blood flow.
4. Vasopressin.
5. Cervical sympathetic innervation.
6. Cervical stenosis.
7. Psychological.

Hysterosalpingographic studies performed during the menses failed to show any increase in the tightness of the cervical canal in those with dysmenorrhoea; therefore cervical stenosis is of doubtful importance. Patients often describe the pain as 'labour-like' and an increase in uterine contractility can be demonstrated by measuring the intrauterine pressure in those with dysmenorrhoea compared with controls (Lumsden & Baird 1985). This may be associated with a decrease in endometrial blood flow. The

Table 14.1 Drugs commonly used in the treatment of menorrhagia as a percentage of the total number of prescriptions written for menorrhagia in the UK during 1988

Drug	Proportion of prescriptions
Non-steroidal anti-inflammatory agents	13.8%
Gestogens, e.g. norethisterone	31.6%
Antigonadotrophins, e.g. danazol	9.8%
Antifibrinolytics, e.g. tranexamic acid	Unknown
Ethamsylate	10.8%
Anti-anaemics	13.0%
Other	21%

Total number of patients with primary indication of menorrhagia = 646 000.

evidence that prostaglandins are involved in the aetiology of primary dysmenorrhoea is good. Both prostaglandin $F_{2\alpha}$ and E_2 are found in higher concentrations in the menstrual fluid of those with dysmenorrhoea. Prostaglandin $F_{2\alpha}$ is a potent oxytocic and vasoconstrictor. When administered into the uterus it will give rise to dysmenorrhoea-like pain and occasionally menstrual bleeding. Menstrual fluid prostaglandin $F_{2\alpha}$ concentrations also correlate with uterine work during the menses in those with dysmenorrhoea (Lumsden et al 1983). These properties of prostaglandin $F_{2\alpha}$ could thus lead to 'angina' of the myometrium (Fig. 14.7). The role of prostaglandin E_2 is less clear although its administration may increase the sensitivity of nerve endings. The reason for the abnormal prostaglandin levels is unknown. Primary dysmenorrhoea occurs almost exclusively in ovulatory cycles and steroid hormones affect

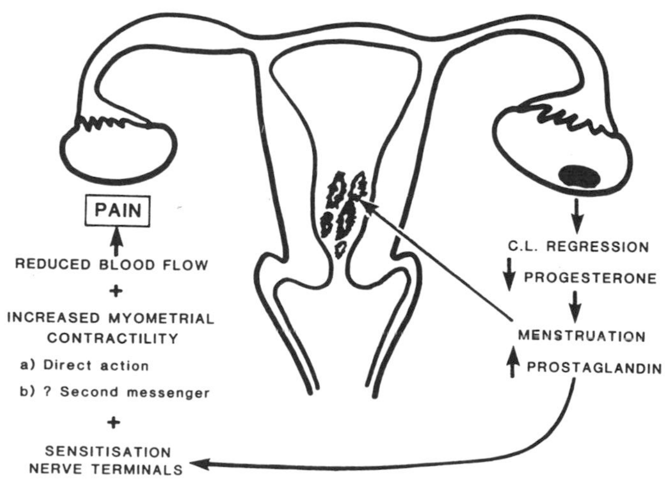

Fig. 14.7 A possible mechanism whereby the prostaglandins could produce dysmenorrhoea.

both uterine prostaglandin concentration and myometrial contractility. However, no consistent abnormality of the hormone levels has been demonstrated in those with dysmenorrhoea.

Leukotrienes are also produced by the endometrium; increased myometrial contractility and receptor sites are present in myometrium, although evidence for a role in dysmenorrhoea is still preliminary (Rees et al 1987). There are also other stimulants of the non-pregnant uterus such as vasopressin, which is particularly active at the onset of menstruation. On day 1 of the menses, plasma concentrations are higher in those with dysmenorrhoea than those without although there is no good evidence that it acts via stimulation of prostaglandin release and its mechanism of action is not clear. Preliminary studies also indicate that vasopressin analogues may have a place in treating dysmenorrhoea. Other factors of importance may be that there are nerve endings in the myometrium and cervix which are destroyed during pregnancy and fail to regenerate. This may explain the observation that primary dysmenorrhoea is relieved by the birth of a baby. The literature suggests that a psychological and physical cause for dysmenorrhoea is mutually exclusive. The evidence for physical factors is strong, treatment is very effective and it is unlikely that psychological problems would be removed simply by tablet-taking. However, a recurring, debilitating pain may well cause depression and anxiety in women of any age.

Secondary dysmenorrhoea

As with menorrhagia, this may be associated with uterine and pelvic pathology such as fibroids, the presence of an IUCD, pelvic inflammatory disease, adenomyosis, endometriosis or cervical stenosis. The cause of the pain is not always clear. Abnormal uterine contractility has been observed in those with fibroids and prostaglandins may be involved when dysmenorrhoea is associated with an IUCD, pelvic inflammatory disease, adenomyosis and possibly endometriosis. However, the use of prostaglandin synthetase inhibitors is not very effective in the presence of pathology, making it likely that there are also other factors.

THE EPIDEMIOLOGY OF MENSTRUAL ABNORMALITY

The distribution of blood loss for a normal population shows a positively skewed distribution, as mentioned above (Cole et al 1971). Age per se does not influence the menstrual blood loss until the sixth decade. This may be due to an increased incidence of pathology (e.g. fibroids or premenopausal endocrine abnormalities). A hereditary influence has been demonstrated following twin studies and parity is also thought to be an important factor; parous women have a greater menstrual blood loss than nulliparous women. Uterine pathology is a well documented cause for menorrhagia, particularly fibroids, although endometrial pathology is rather uncommon in menorrhagic women; it is found as a reasonable cause for menorrhagia in only about 6%.

The variation between menses for an individual (intramenses) is between 20 and 40% (Fig. 14.6). The reason for this variation is unknown. About 90% of blood is lost during the first 3 days of the menses in both normal and menorrhagic women. These studies are based on objective measurement of menstrual blood loss, which is rarely done except for research purposes. The measurement of menstrual blood loss is very straightforward and perfectly safe for the patient. The most commonly used is the alkaline haematin technique in which used menstrual pads are soaked in sodium hydroxide and haemoglobin is converted to alkaline haematin, causing a characteristic change in the colour of the solution. Blood loss is calculated after spectrophotometry (Hallberg & Nilsson 1964).

There is a poor correlation between subjective and objective assessment of loss (Chimbira et al 1980), which means that most gynaecologists treat patients with no objective tests — apart from a haemoglobin test. This is important as medical treatment for menorrhagia is unlikely to be effective in those with normal loss and surgical treatment carries a risk. Only about 50% of women presenting with menorrhagia actually have a loss outside the normal range (> 80 ml), which indicates that the changes which occur in the cycle are often perceived erroneously as abnormal.

The results of epidemiological studies performed over the last 50 years give a variable incidence for dysmenorrhoea. This is due to the fact that pain is a subjective symptom and cannot be assessed accurately by an outsider. Different women will react to the same pain in different ways and how each women perceives the pain will vary with altered circumstances. Also, the definition and diagnosis allow different interpretations by different workers. Severe dysmenorrhoea which causes disruption of daily routine with time off work or study occurs in 3–10% of 19-year-olds (Andersch & Milsom 1982), while mild discomfort occurs in a majority of women. Dysmenorrhoea frequently starts within 1 year of the menarche and is accompanied by premenstrual symptoms in 40%. Girls whose mothers have dysmenorrhoea are more likely to suffer; lifestyle and occupation are also important. Although primary dysmenorrhoea is frequently cured by parturition, the fact that many women delay starting their families means that the consequences of the high incidence of this disorder are important both socially and economically.

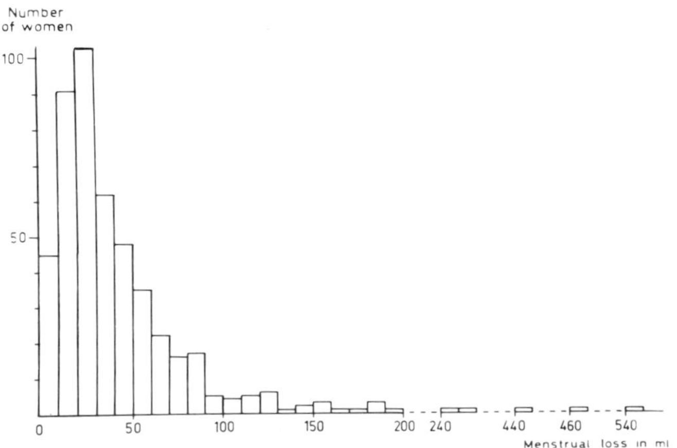

Fig. 14.8 The distribution of menstrual blood loss for a population of women who did not consider they had any menstrual abnormality (from Hallberg et al with permission).

PRESENTATION

Menstrual problems are a common cause for presentation to both the general practitioner and the gynaecological outpatients clinic. The bleeding pattern may be cyclical or irregular and may be accompanied by dysmenorrhoea. The latter symptom is less often the major complaint. Patients often complain of 'clots' and 'flooding' and the severity is often assessed only by asking the degree of disability experienced, e.g. the time lost from work. As stated above, the amount of protection used does not correlate with blood loss. Other gynaecological problems may also be present, such as intermenstrual bleeding, vaginal discharge or premenstrual syndrome.

Clinical examination seldom reveals significant observation. An enlarged uterus may suggest uterine leiomyomata or a cervical polyp may cause intermenstrual bleeding. Anaemia may also be present since menorrhagia is the commonest cause of iron deficiency anaemia in the western world. Menorrhagia may arise as a consequence of disorders of the haemopoietic system, as described above.

INVESTIGATION

The measurement of menstrual blood loss should be the cornerstone of the diagnosis of menorrhagia, since 50% of those complaining of heavy loss are within the normal range. In fact this measurement is rarely performed. The investigation thus depends on whether the cycle is regular or irregular since 80% of those with three or more consecutive regular cycles are ovulating.

Anovulatory menorrhagia

In the younger patient (< 40 years of age) assessment of the hypothalamic–pituitary–ovarian axis is indicated. The diagnosis of polycystic ovarian disease has increased over recent years with the finding of altered luteinizing hormone: follicle-stimulating hormone ratios in the follicular phase of the cycle and the identification of micro-

and macrocystic disease by vaginal ultrasound. The presence of hirsutism requires the investigation of the hypothalamo–pituitary–adrenal system; this should include measurement of dehydroepiandrosterone sulphate levels which reflect adrenal androgen synthesis, and testosterone which reflects primarily ovarian synthesis. Anovulatory menorrhagia is commoner in the older women since failure of ovulation frequently precedes the menopause. Anovulation may be associated with intermittent ovulatory cycles characterized by a short follicular phase and raised follicle-stimulating hormone levels (Van Look et al 1977).

Dilatation and curettage

Dilatation and curettage (D&C) is advocated to exclude the diagnosis of endometrial malignancy. The incidence of this diagnosis in women under the age of 40 is of the order of one in 10 000–100 000 and is probably not indicated in women below this age (Grimes 1982). Towards the menopause the incidence increases to around 1%. Recently thin plastic cell samplers have been developed which provide a histological sample without the need for dilation and anaesthetic. Several makes are now available. If the initial analyses are substantiated by larger-scale studies, these techniques are likely to supersede D&C as the main means of endometrial sampling. The Vabra aspirator usually provides a greater amount of tissue for analysis and is probably no less efficient in diagnosing endometrial malignancy than D&C, but may not be tolerated by some patients as an outpatient procedure.

Hysteroscopy

The hysteroscope is an important aid to diagnosis. The rate of detection in women with abnormal bleeding ranges between 43 and 85% (Valle & Sciarra 1979). The frequent findings of endometrial polyps and submucus fibroids are often missed by a 'blind' D&C. Hysteroscopic examination with tissue biopsy gives as accurate a histopathological diagnosis as D&C and the use of a microhysteroscope allows this to be performed as a day-case procedure.

Ovulatory menorrhagia

This requires no endocrinological investigation and in women under the age of 35 years a tissue biopsy is no longer considered mandatory. However, those with abnormal findings on examination may require further investigation, such as pelvic ultrasound or D&C. A clotting screen may need to be performed as suggested by the history.

Dysmenorrhoea

Those with normal pelvic examination require no further investigation initially. Laparoscopy is indicated for those with a provisional diagnosis of endometriosis or pelvic inflammatory disease. D&C and examination under anaesthetic are required only if uterine abnormality is suspected. The standard treatment for dysmenorrhoea (prostaglandin synthetase inhibitors and the oral contraceptive pill) is so effective that laparoscopy in treatment failures will often demonstrate previously unsuspected abnormalities such as mild endometriosis, even in teenage girls.

TREATMENT

Women require rapid, safe and effective treatment for their menstrual problems. There are three main categories of treatment — surgical, medical and the newer hysteroscopic techniques. In Scotland during 1987, 2300 women had a hysterectomy and 30 000 'bed days' were occupied by women presenting primarily with heavy menses, giving some indication of the extent of the problem (data from the Common Services Agency, Scottish Home and Health Department).

Surgical treatment

Hysterectomy is certainly an effective treatment for menstrual problems. However, it is a major operation and is not without risk in terms of both mortality and morbidity. The incidence of hysterectomy is gradually increasing in the western world. The number performed in Scotland over the last 15 years is shown in Figure 14.9. The incidence varies considerably from one country to another (Fig. 14.10), reflecting differences in the attitude of both patients and gynaecologists rather than a variation in pathology. Women in Scotland have a 20% chance of losing their uterus before the age of 60 years whereas in California this figure is 50% (Bunker & Brown 1974). It appears that a decrease in the incidence of hysterectomy may be achieved by influencing the attitudes of patients and doctors as a result of mass media campaigns. This sug-

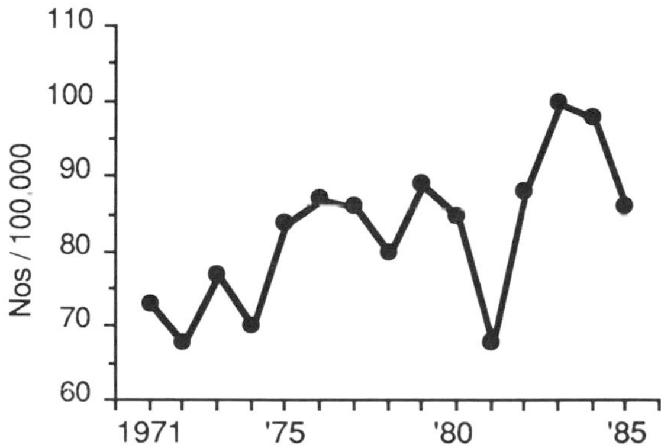

Fig. 14.9 Graph depicting the number of hysterectomies performed in Scotland between the years 1971 and 1985.

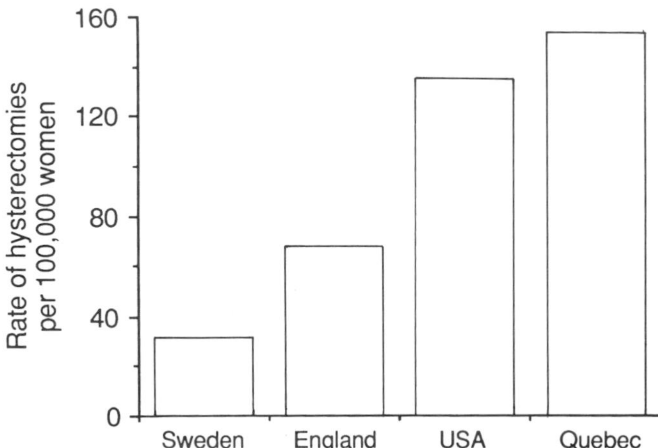

Fig. 14.10 The incidence of hysterectomy/100 000 women for Sweden, England, the USA and Quebec (from Domenighetti et al 1989, with permission).

gests that we are performing more hysterectomies than are necessary.

Both abdominal and vaginal hysterectomy are accompanied by considerable morbidity; the mortality rate in non-pregnant women under 54 years of age without cancer is 6/10 000. Morbidity, which is frequently caused by infection or haemorrhage, causes prolonged stay in hospital and weeks or months off work. The cost to both the women and the National Health Service is thus considerable.

Drug treatment

Drugs are now commonly prescribed by general practitioners for the treatment of menorrhagia and dysmenorrhoea. About 1 200 000 prescriptions were written in the UK during 1988 for menorrhagia and dysmenorrhoea. The commonly prescribed drugs for menorrhagia are shown in Table 14.1 together with the proportion of the market controlled by each drug. The acceptability of each treatment depends on the balance between effectiveness and side-effects. Menorrhagia is very rarely life-threatening and the aim of treatment is to improve the quality of life. Side-effects may therefore make an effective drug unacceptable.

Prostaglandin synthetase inhibitors

The role of prostaglandins in abnormal menstruation has already been discussed. Prostaglandin synthetase inhibitors, of which the different types are shown in Table 14.2, are thus a logical mode of treatment (Anderson 1981). The fenamates not only inhibit the synthesis of prostaglandins but also interfere with the binding of prostaglandin E_2 to its receptor. The mean decrease in blood loss varies between 20 and 44.5% and there is a suggestion that there is a correlation between the pretreatment menstrual blood loss and the volume reduction in menstrual blood loss during therapy. A decrease in the number of days of bleeding has also been reported.

Table 14.2 The non-steroidal anti-inflammatory agents

Parent compound	Example
Salicylate	Aspirin Aloxiprin
Indole	Indomethacin
* Propionic acid	Ketoprofen Ibuprofen
* Fenamates	Mefenamic acid
Pyrazone	Phenylbutazone
Indene	Sulindac
Alkanone	Nabumetone
Benzotriazine	Azapropazone
Phenylacetic acid	Diclofenac sodium

* Most commonly used for menstrual problems.

The percentage decrease in menstrual blood loss in 13 women taking mefenamic acid is shown in Figure 14.11 and illustrates the variable results obtained with this treatment. IUCD-associated menorrhagia also responds well to prostaglandin synthetase inhibitors although there is little evidence that they are as effective in the presence of

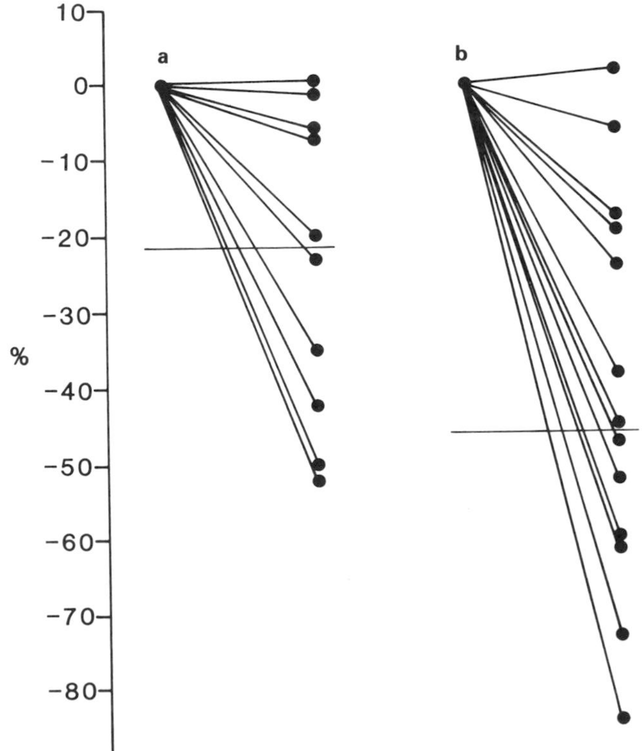

Fig. 14.11 Percentage change in menstrual blood loss (mean of two cycles) of women receiving (**a**) norethisterone (5 mg b.d. days 19–25) and (**b**) mefenamic acid (250 mg t.d.s. days 1–5).

pathology such as fibroids. About 80% of women with primary dysmenorrhoea can be successfully treated with this group of drugs although, once again, they are less effective in the presence of pathology.

Side-effects. Gastrointestinal symptoms occur in up to 50% of those taking these drugs although they are often very mild and may be decreased by taking the drug with food. Patient response may be idiosyncratic, making the testing of different members of the group worthwhile if symptoms occur. Central nervous system symptoms such as dizziness and headache occur in around 20%. Although significant changes in liver function have been reported, the indices have remained within the normal range. Potential serious side-effects such as blood dyscrasias and nephropathy have not been reported in any study, possibly because of the intermittent nature of drug administration.

Hormonal treatment

Gestagen therapy

Synthetic progestins have been employed for at least 25 years in the treatment of menorrhagia with few objective studies to validate their use. There is histological evidence that in women with metropathia haemorrhagica, progestin administration will cause secretory change in the endometrium accompanied by a subjective decrease in blood loss. However, in those with ovulatory DUB, the effect is unpredictable and the overall median decreased menstrual blood loss is less than 25% (Fig. 14.11a). The progestin-impregnated IUCD has proved successful in reducing menstrual blood loss, possibly by inducing extreme endometrial atrophy. Some advocate the use of depot medroxyprogesterone acetate as a therapy for DUB since it induces amenorrhoea in 50% after 1 year of use, but the 15–20% incidence of episodes of frequent or prolonged bleeding make this treatment unacceptable to many.

Side-effects. Blood lipid profiles are altered in patients on gestagen therapy with an increase in low-density lipoprotein and an decrease in high-density lipoprotein, thus increasing the potential risk of vascular disease. This is an androgenic effect common to both C19 (e.g. norethisterone) and C20 (e.g. medroxyprogesterone) analogues and is due to active metabolites. However the risk is dose-dependent and is reduced by the intermittent nature of administration. Minor side-effects such as nausea, headache, a bloated feeling, weight gain and skin rashes are common but rarely significant.

Combined oestrogen/progesterone formulations

The combined oral contraceptive pill gives a significant decrease in menstrual blood loss although their use is often accompanied by oestrogen-related side-effects. The use of low-dose oestrogen pills in the management of menorrhagia is affected by the adverse publicity associated with their use in women over the age of 35 who are obese, smoke and have a family history of heart disease. However in the younger patient with irregular bleeding they not only reduce the menstrual blood loss but provide a regular menstrual loss. Dysmenorrhoea is also reduced by oral contraceptive therapy which enhances their acceptability.

The mechanism by which exogenous steroids reduce menstrual blood loss is unknown, though the induction of atrophy and the reduction of prostaglandin release from endometrium may play a part.

Antifibrinolytic drugs

Fibrinolytic inhibitors act by inhibiting plasminogen activator, reducing the accelerated fibrinolytic activity found in menorrhagic women. Tranexamic acid is of value in the treatment of excessive menstrual bleeding, giving around a 50% decrease in those with DUB- as well as IUCD-associated menorrhagia. They are very widely used in Scandinavia although they have achieved less acceptance in the UK.

Side-effects. The commonest side-effects reported include nausea, dizziness, tinnitus, rash and abdominal cramps. Oral administration does give rise to low systemic levels of tranexanic acid and case reports of serious thromboembolic disorders following administration have been reported, although the underlying incidence of these disorders in women of reproductive age must always be borne in mind.

Danazol

Danazol is the isoxazole derivative of 17α ethinyl testosterone. Its mechanism of action is not clear but it is thought to act both directly by inhibiting endometrial proliferation causing endometrial atrophy, and by displacement of endometrial oestrogen receptors. It also has an indirect action, reducing pituitary gonadotrophin secretion and inhibiting the enzymes involved in ovarian steroidogenesis. It is an effective treatment for menorrhagia even at low doses although it must be given continuously, as it is ineffective when administered cyclically. At moderate or high doses (400 mg daily), danazol induces amenorrhoea in a majority of women, but at low doses (200 mg daily), although it reduces loss, it has no effect on cycle length. Dosage of 100 mg daily has no effect on the duration of bleeding and the mean cycle length is significantly shorter.

Side-effects. The side-effects of danazol have been extensively documented and include weight gain, acne, hirsutism, muscle cramps, headaches and in severe cases, breast atrophy.

Ethamsylate

Ethamsylate is thought to act by inhibiting the increase in capillary fragility measurable in premenopausal women by reducing the rate of breakdown in mucopolysaccharide ground substance in the capillary wall. Its effectiveness has not been well documented by objective study but a significant decrease in menstrual loss in women with DUB- and IUCD-associated menorrhagia is reported. Side-effects appear to be minor.

Luteinizing hormone-releasing hormone (LHRH) agonists

LHRH agonists are derived from the LHRH decapeptide with a 140-fold more potent action then endogenous LHRH. They induce down-regulation of the pituitary with an initial agonist phase followed by exhaustion of the pituitary and hypogonadotrophic hypogonadism. This results in either amenorrhoea or oligomenorrhoea, depending on the route of administration. Intranasal administration reduces menstrual blood loss by about 50% (Shaw & Fraser 1984) although it tends to increase cycle irregularity. It can also be administered subcutaneously using implants; this results in more consistent suppression of oestrogen production and amenorrhoea is the norm. However, side-effects due to hypo-oestrogenism occur which could lead to bone mineral loss in the long term. Either they must be used only for short periods or they must be used in combination with bone-sparing agents, e.g. progestogens. The acceptability and suitability of these regimes are under investigation at the present time.

Endometrial ablation techniques

Attempts at endometrial destruction with the aim of producing a therapeutic Asherman's syndrome in cases of abnormal menstruation have been made by a variety of techniques. Early trials involved the intrauterine application of cytotoxic chemicals, intracavity radium, steam and cryosurgery. However these were either ineffective or had unacceptable side-effects. They were also carried out blindly and since the endometrium has remarkable powers of regeneration, any missed areas resulted in failure.

More recently, hysteroscopic techniques of laser ablation and endometrial diathermy or resection have been described. Visualization allows complete endometrial destruction which produces amenorrhoea in as many as 50% of cases. As with hysterectomy, it is only suitable for women who have completed their families as the uterine cavity is frequently completely obliterated.

Laser ablation

Laser beams may be produced from a variety of sources although currently neodymium:ytrium-aluminium-garnet (Nd:YAG) is optimal for intrauterine surgery since it can be delivered along a flexible fibre, can be transmitted through a liquid medium, and the depth of tissue penetration can be controlled. The beam produces warming, coagulation, evaporation and carbonization. Tissue destruction typically occurs to a depth of 4–5 mm. Heat transmission through the myometrium is minimized by the continuous flow of cold irrigation fluid. Results from a large study with 6 years' follow-up indicate improvement in up to 98% of women with only 3% coming to hysterectomy (Loffer 1987).

Endometrial diathermy/resection

The technique of transcervical resection of the endometrium is essentially similar to that of transurethral prostatectomy in men and can be performed through an unmodified continuous flow resectoscope. The endometrium is systematically excised down to the superficial myometrium either over the entire cavity (total resection) or to within 1 cm of the internal os (partial resection). It appears to be quicker than laser ablation and can also be performed as an outpatient procedure under intravenous sedation or analgesia. Long-term follow-up is not available as yet, but in the short term, results look promising (Goldrath et al 1981).

Risks of intrauterine surgery

This technique requires a basic knowledge of hysteroscopy. Risks include haemorrhage, infection and in particular uterine perforation. The use of large volumes of irrigating fluid is associated with the risk of excessive absorption resulting in fluid overload, hypertension, hyponatraemia, neurological symptoms, haemolysis and death.

Other treatments for dysmenorrhoea

In young women dysmenorrhoea is frequently the only menstrual abnormality. Prostaglandin synthetase inhibitors and the oral contraceptive pill are very effective, but in some women even in the absense of disease these measures are insufficient. Calcium channel blockers (e.g. nifedipine) have been used in Scandinavia and are effective, although their use is limited by cardiovascular side-effects. In the past presacral neurectomy was performed but this involved major abdominal surgery and was effective in only about 50%. Recently neurectomy has been performed using intra-abdominal lasers. The long-term effect of this treatment has not been reported and it is only available in a few centres in the UK. In the older women where childbearing is completed, hysterectomy is often the solution since dysmenorrhoea in this group is frequently associated with other menstrual problems.

RESULTS

The results of the treatment of menstrual problems are difficult to determine. Hysterectomy is undoubtedly effective in curing menstrual problems but its effect on the quality of life of the woman is largely unknown. This is a difficult parameter to measure but the information is vital when considering patient acceptability.

Drug treatments are very effective in some women although the response tends to be variable. In the main they are safe and reported serious side-effects are unusual. However acceptability must be questioned since it has been demonstrated that side-effects may make a very effective drug (in terms of reduction in menstrual blood loss) unacceptable (Dockeray et al 1989). Many women also find the prospect of long-term drug therapy unappealing. Endometrial destruction by laser or electrocautery is an attractive alternative to both long-term drug therapy and hysterectomy for the common gynaecological complaint of abnormal menstruation. It is associated with a shorter hospital stay and a faster recovery. Clinical improvement occurs in a vast majority of women, although its long-term efficacy is not yet proven.

CONCLUSIONS

Menstrual dysfunction remains one of the commonest causes for women to seek medical advice yet the process of menstruation is poorly understood. Strategies to improve the investigation and management of this problem are likely to arise from two directions. Firstly, a thorough investigation of the medicosociological factors is required. Secondly, the role of vasoactive substances in the endometrium needs to be further investigated as well as determining the factors which control endometrial proliferation. At present, the diagnosis of menorrhagia is inadequate and medical treatment is disappointing. Gynaecologists need to address these problems before significant improvements in management will arise.

KEY POINTS

1. The smooth muscle of the myometrium shows functional resemblance to cardiac muscle although there is no conclusive evidence for a pacemaker within the uterus.
2. The mean menstrual blood loss per menstruation in a healthy West European population ranges between 37 and 43 ml; 70% of the loss occurs within the first 48 hours.
3. Vasoconstriction is currently considered to be the most important mechanism controlling menstrual blood loss.
4. Patients with platelet and coagulation disorders frequently suffer from excessive menstrual blood loss.
5. There is evidence for a role for PGs in the menorrhagia associated with adenomyosis, uterine leiomyomata and the presence of an IUCD.
6. The incidence of endometrial malignancy in women with menorrhagia under the age of 40 is of the order of 1:10 000–1:100 000, rising to 1% perimenopausally.
7. Hysteroscopy is more helpful in identifying intrauterine pathology than dilatation and curettage.
8. Antifibrinolytic drugs and prostaglandin synthetase inhibitors are of value in the treatment of menorrhagia, in those with DUB as well as IUCD associated menorrhagia.
9. The effect of danazol on reducing menstrual blood loss, length of period and length of cycle is dose dependent.
10. The production of a therapeutic Asherman's syndrome in cases of abnormal menstruation is an attractive alternative to both longterm drug therapy or hysterectomy.

REFERENCES

Andersch B, Milsom I 1982 An epidemiologic study of young women with dysmenorrhoea. American Journal of Obstetrics and Gynecology 144: 655–660

Anderson A 1981 The role of prostaglandin synthetase inhibitors in gynaecology. Practitioner 225: 1460–1470

Bonnar J, Sheppard B L, Dockeray C J 1983 The haemostatic system and dysfunctional uterine bleeding. Research and Clinical Forums 5: 27–36

Bunker J P, Brown B W 1974 The physician–patient as an informed consumer of surgical services. New England Journal of Medicine 290: 1051–1055

Cameron I T, Leask R, Kelly R W, Baird D T 1987 Endometrial prostaglandins in women with abnormal menstrual bleeding. Prostaglandins, Leukotrienes and Medicine 29: 249–257

Chimbira T H, Anderson A B M, Turnbull A C 1980 Relation between measured menstrual blood loss and patients' subjective assessment of loss, duration of bleeding, number of sanitary towels used, uterine weight and endometrial surface area. British Journal of Obstetrics and Gynaecology 87: 603–609

Christiaens G C, Sixma J J, Haspels A A 1982 Haemostasis in menstrual endometrium: a review. Obstetrical and Gynecological Survey 37: 281–303

Cohen B J B, Gibor Y 1980 Anaemia and menstrual blood loss. Obstetrical and Gynecological Survey 35: 597–618

Cole S K, Billewicz W Z, Thomson A M 1971 Sources of variation in menstrual blood loss. Journal of Obstetrics and Gynaecology of the British Commonwealth 78: 933–939

Dockeray C J, Sheppard B L, Bonnar J 1989 Comparison between mefenamic acid and danazol in the treatment of established menorrhagia. British Journal of Obstetrics and Gynaecology 96: 840–844

Domenighetti G, Luraschi P, Gutzwiller F et al 1989 Effect of information campaign by the mass media on hysterectomy rates. Lancet ii: 1470–1473

Fraser I S, McCarron G, Markham R, Resta T, Watts A 1986 Measured menstrual blood loss in women with menorrhagia associated with pelvic disease or coagulation disorder. Obstetrics and Gynecology 68: 630–633

Goldrath M H, Fuller T A, Segal S 1981 Laser photovaporisation of endometrium for treatment of menorrhagia. American Journal of Obstetrics and Gynecology 140: 14–19

Grimes D A 1982 Diagnostic dilatation and curettage: a reappraisal. American Journal of Obstetrics and Gynecology 142: 1–6

Hallberg L, Nilsson L 1964 Consistency of individual menstrual blood loss. Acta Obstetricia et Gynecologica Scandinavica 43: 352–359

Hallberg L, Högdahl A, Nilsson L, Rybo G Menstrual blood loss and iron deficiency. Acta Medica Scandinavica 180: 639–655

Haynes P J, Anderson A B M, Turnbull A C 1979 Patterns of menstrual blood loss in menorrhagia. Research and Clinical Forums 1: 73–78

Loffer F D 1987 Hysteroscopic endometrial ablation with the Nd:YAG laser using a nontouch technique. Obstetrics and Gynecology 69: 679–682

Lumsden M A, Baird D T 1985 Intrauterine pressure in dysmenorrhoea. Acta Obstetricia et Gynecologica Scandinavica 64: 183–186

Lumsden M A, Kelly R W, Baird D T 1983 Is prostaglandin $F_{2\alpha}$ involved in the increased myometrial contractility of primary dysmenorrhoea? Prostaglandins 25: 683–692

Markee J E 1948 Morphological basis for menstrual bleeding. Relation of regression to the initiation of bleeding. Bulletin of the New York Academy of Medicine 24: 253–270

Rees M C, DiMarzo V, Tippins J R, Morris H R, Turnbull A C 1987 Leukotriene release by endometrium and myometrium throughout the menstrual cycle in dysmenorrhoea and menorrhagia. Journal of Endocrinology 113: 291–295

Rybo G 1966 Clinical and experimental studies on menstrual blood loss. Acta Obstetricia et Gynecologica Scandinavica 45(suppl): 1–23

Shaw R W, Fraser H M 1984 Use of a superactive luteinizing hormone-releasing hormone (LHRH) agonist in the treatment of menorrhagia. British Journal of Obstetrics and Gynaecology 91: 913–916

Smith S K, Abel M H, Kelly R W, Baird D T 1981a Prostaglandin synthesis in the endometrium of women with ovular dysfunctional uterine bleeding. British Journal of Obstetrics and Gynaecology 88: 434–442

Smith S K, Kelly R W, Abel M H, Baird D T 1981b A role for prostacyclin (PGI_2) in excessive menstrual bleeding. Lancet i: 522–524

Smith S K, Abel M H, Kelly R W, Baird D T 1982 The synthesis of prostaglandins from persistent proliferative endometrium. Journal of Clinical Endocrinology and Metabolism 55: 284–289

Valle R F, Sciarra J J 1979 Current status of hysteroscopy in gynecological practice. Fertility and Sterility 32: 619–625

Van Look P F A, Lothian H, Hunter W M, Michie E A, Baird D T 1977 Hypothalamic-pituitary-ovarian function in perimenopausal women. Clinical Endocrinology 7: 13–31

FURTHER READING

Baird D T, Michie E A (eds) 1985 Mechanism of menstrual bleeding. Serono symposia publications no 25. Raven Press, New York

Drife J O (ed) 1989 Dysfunctional uterine bleeding and menorrhagia. Clinical obstetrics and gynaecology, vol 3. Baillière Tindall, London, p 2

Lumsden M A 1985 Dysmenorrhoea. In: Studd J (ed) Progress in obstetrics and gynaecology, vol 5. Churchill Livingstone, Edinburgh

Shaw S T, Roche P C 1980 Menstruation. In: Finn C A (ed) Oxford reviews of reproductive biology, vol II. Clarendon Press, Oxford, pp 41–96

Smith S K 1985 Menorrhagia. In: Studd J (ed) Progress in obstetrics and gynaecology, vol 5. Churchill Livingstone, Edinburgh

15. Spontaneous and recurrent abortion

D. K. Edmonds

INTRODUCTION AND DEFINITION

In the UK, a spontaneous abortion is defined as a pregnancy loss occurring before 28 completed weeks of gestation. In 1977, the World Health Organization defined an abortion as 'the expulsion or extraction from its mother of a fetus or an embryo weighing 500 gms or less' (WHO Recommended Definitions 1977). A woman who has three or more spontaneous abortions is generally accepted to be a recurrent aborter although the definition is complicated by the interspersion of successful pregnancies.

SPONTANEOUS ABORTION

This is a hugely traumatic emotional event in any woman's reproductive career, and greatly underestimated by medical practitioners in its impact. Great care and compassion are required in order to manage these women efficiently and sympathetically so that they return to physical and mental health as soon as possible.

Pathophysiology and classification

It is evident that the process of abortion is the major route by which natural selection operates in humans. It may be considered that the abortion results either from an inherent abnormality in the conceptus or is related to outside influences leading to elimination of the pregnancy from the uterus. The pathophysiological processes will depend upon the aetiology and will be considered in this regard in the next section. The causes of spontaneous abortion may be classified depending on the aetiological defect, which may relate to the fetus, placenta or uterus:

1. Genetic factors.
2. Developmental problems.
3. Placental problems.
4. Infection.
5. Undetermined cause.

A number of these causes may result in recurrent miscarriage.

Aetiology

Fetal problems may be divided into chromosomal problems and developmental abnormalities.

Chromosomal anomalies

It is generally accepted that 50% of all clinically recognized first-trimester losses are chromosomally abnormal. In the second trimester the incidence falls but is still significant. Table 15.1 gives the combined data from nine cytogenetic surveys of spontaneous abortuses, showing an overall rate of 49% chromosomal abnormalities. However, the prevalence of chromosomal abnormalities is gestation-dependent (Table 15.2) and the variation in prevalence shown in Table 15.1 is explained by the greater proportion of abortuses in the second trimester in the studies of Dhadial et al (1970), Creasy et al (1976), Geisler & Kleinebrecht (1978) and Warburton et al (1980). Some concern has been expressed with regard to the culture techniques used to derive these figures, as evidenced by Simoni et al (1985), who showed that 15% of abnormalities seen in chorionic villus sampling were not subsequently confirmed when

Table 15.1 Frequency of chromosomal abnormalities from nine major studies of spontaneous abortion

Authors	No. of abortuses	No. abnormal	% abnormal
Dhadial et al 1970	547	128	23
Boue et al 1975	1498	921	61
Creasy et al 1976	986	290	29
Takahara et al 1977	505	237	47
Therkelsen et al 1977	254	139	54
Geisler & Kleinebrecht 1978	166	65	39
Hassold et al 1980	1000	463	46
Kajii et al 1980	402	215	54
Warburton et al 1980	967	312	32
	6325	3069	49

Table 15.2 Chromosomal abnormalities related to gestational age

Gestation	Chromosomal abnormalities
8–11 weeks	50%
12–15 weeks	40%
16–19 weeks	19%
20–23 weeks	12%
24–28 weeks	8%

From Warburton et al (1980).

fetal tissue was cultured. Thus, a slight overestimate may result in the studied series.

About 30% of abortuses have an extra chromosome (trisomy) which is usually an autosome, and only 0.6% have a sex chromosome polysomy. The other major abnormalities are monosomy X and triploidy (Table 15.3). However, over 54% of all abortuses are euploid.

Table 15.3 Types of chromosomal abnormalities in abortions

Abnormality	%
Normal	54.5
Monosomy X	8.6
Triploidy	7.0
Tetraploidy	2.6
Trisomy	30.4
Sex chromosomal polysomy	0.6
Structural abnormalities	1.5

Trisomy has been described for all chromosomes except number 1 and the Y chromosome, although the frequency is vastly different (Fig. 15.2). Some 32% of cases are trisomy 16, whilst chromosomes 2, 13, 15, 18, 21 and 22 account for the majority of the remainder. Increasing maternal age increases the risk of trisomic conception, although there is no age effect on trisomy 16. Most trisomies are believed to be a consequence of non-disjunction during maternal meiosis. Trisomic pregnancies result in empty sacs ('blighted ova' or 'anembryonic pregnancies') or very stunted fetal growth, although trisomies 13–15 show cyclopia and facial abnormalities. Trisomy 16 gives rise to only the most rudimentary embryonic growth with an empty sac.

Monosomy X is usually associated with the presence of a fetus, although focal abnormalities may occur, e.g. encephaloceles, hygromata. It results from paternal sex chromosome loss, which can probably be X or Y.

Polyploidy (triploidy or tetraploidy) results from the addition of complete haploid sets of chromosomes. Triploid abortions are usually 69 XXY or 69 XXX and usually result from dispermy. The mean duration of survival is around 5 weeks of embryonic life, and polyploidy is characterized by neural tube defects and omphaloceles and

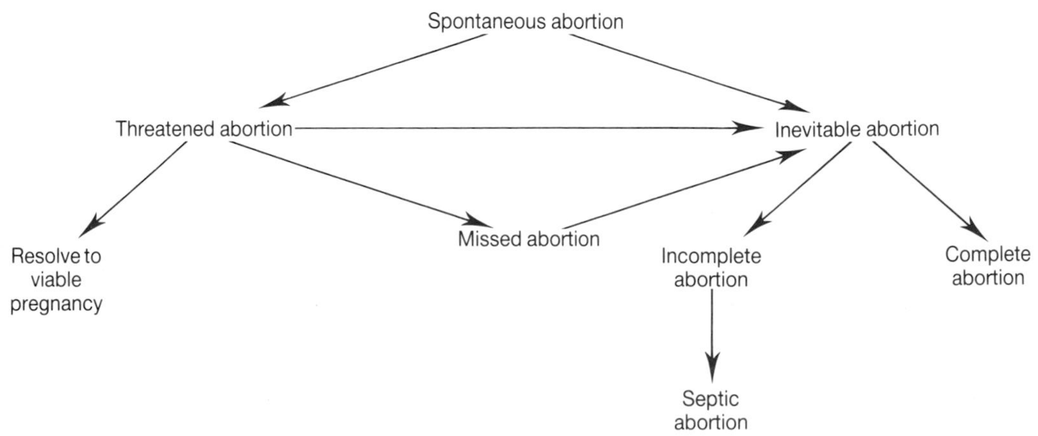

Fig. 15.1 Clinical classification of spontaneous abortion.

Table 15.4 Defect rate per 1000 cases.

Structural abnormality	Spontaneous abortuses	Liveborn
Neural tube defect	1.38	0.6
Cleft palate	1.3	1.8
Cleft lip or palate	6.9	0
Cyclopia	2.7	0
Polydactyly	2.7	0.95
Sirenomelia and caudal regression	4.2	0
Amniotic bands	4.2	0.03

Modified from Fantel & Shepard (1987).

Table 15.5 Placental abnormalities associated with macerated abortions

Placental abnormality	%
Maternal floor infarction	22.1
Malformation	11.2
Uteroplacental ischaemia	10.0
Chorioamnionitis	8.5
Hydrops	8.5
Retroplacental clot	5.6
Cord abnormalities	3.0
Non-specific	31.1

Adapted from Rushton (1988).

Table 15.6 Placental pathology in association with a fresh fetus

Placental abnormality	%
Chorioamnionitis	30.1
Retroplacental haemorrhage	12.6
Uteroplacental ischaemia	5.8
Malformations	5.3
Non-specific	46.2

Adapted from Rushton (1988).

placental changes including a large sac, hydropic villi and intrachorial haemorrhage. Tetraploidic pregnancies (92 chromosomes) are rare and the majority are empty sacs or grossly abnormal stunted fetuses which rarely progress beyond 3 weeks of embryonic life.

Sex chromosome polysomy 47XXX, 47XXY or 47XYY occurs infrequently in abortuses, and is more commonly seen in liveborn infants. It is not considered a lethal gene constitution.

Structural chromosomal rearrangements may arise de novo, or may be inherited. They are rarely the cause of spontaneous abortion per se but are associated with recurrent abortion.

In a large series by Fantel & Shephard (1987) reporting the morphological abnormalities in 1441 specimens, a wide variety of structural defects were discovered. Many were related to chromosomal defects, but it is interesting to compare the defect rate in abortions and in liveborns (Table 15.4). The major abnormalities are more frequently seen in the abortuses, and there is little difference in the more minor abnormalities.

Placental abnormalities

There have been scant data published on placental findings in spontaneous abortions, in comparison with the information with regard to the fetus. However, the role of the placenta must be paramount in the maintenance of pregnancy and the continued growth of the fetus. Rushton (1988) has reported the largest study of placentae, considering 1426 specimens. The pregnancies were grouped into those with blighted ova, those with macerated fetuses and those with fresh fetuses.

The blighted ova group showed a mixed histological pattern with fibrotic avascular villi as well as microscopic hydropic villi. The macerated group showed a much greater variety of changes (Table 15.5). The maternal floor infarction probably reflects cessation of blood flow following fetal demise, but the uteroplacental ischaemia and retroplacental haemorrhage group also showed evidence of placental bed fibrinoid necrosis and spiral artery atherosis, as is seen in pre-eclampsia and intrauterine growth retardation. Perhaps these cases are the early end of this disease spectrum.

In the third group associated with a fresh fetus, the placental changes were as seen in Table 15.6. In 30% of cases, chorioamnionitis was present although no specific infections were identified. As in the macerated group, the presence of ischaemia and haemorrhage were associated with vascular lesions.

Thus the role of the process of abnormal placentation may have greater importance in the aetiology of chromosomally normal and some chromosomally abnormal spontaneous abortions than previously realized; some may be amenable to treatment.

Infection and spontaneous abortion

A number of organisms have been associated with spontaneous abortion (Table 15.7) and although anecdotal evidence exists for sporadic abortion, no evidence exists for a role in recurrent abortion.

Listeria monocytogenes is a notorious pregnancy-associated pathogen and spontaneous abortion clearly may result from maternal bacteraemia during early pregnancy. Cases of abortion associated with *Campylobacter* spp. have been reported although they are scant. *Brucella* spp. are well known as a cause of abortion in animals and human infec-

Table 15.7 Organisms associated with spontaneous abortion

Bacteria	*Parasites*
Listeria monocytogenes	Toxoplasma gondii
Campylobacter spp.	*Viruses*
Brucella spp.	Cytomegalovirus
Mycoplasma hominis	Rubella Herpes
Ureaplasma urealyticum	Coxsackie
Spirochaetes	
Treponema pallidum	

Adapted from Watts & Eschenbach (1988).

tion can occur, but rarely cause abortion. Both *Ureaplasma urealyticum* and *Mycoplasma hominis* have been associated with spontaneous abortion. However, much emphasis has been laid on these organisms as a cause of recurrent abortion but no evidence exists for this. The confusion arises as *Ureaplasma* and *Mycoplasma* can be isolated from 40–90% of pregnant women where no evidence of chorioamnionitis exists, and a successful pregnancy results.

Syphilis is more commonly the cause of late second-trimester abortion and stillbirth but cases have been reported in the first trimester and of course this is a treatable cause of miscarriage. *Toxoplasma gondii* has also been linked to spontaneous abortion, although there are no studies to corroborate the relationship.

Cytomegalovirus (CMV) is a common infection and known to affect the neonate prenatally but reports of CMV causing abortion are scant (Kriel et al 1970) and inconclusive. Rubella, however, has been alleged to increase the risk of spontaneous abortion and congenital abnormalities (Charles & Larsen 1987) and herpes simplex may increase the risk of abortion by threefold (Gronroos et al 1983).

It is evident, therefore, that whilst spontaneous abortion may result from isolated placental and fetal infection with various organisms, no evidence exists for their involvement in a recurrent problem.

Undetermined causes

A percentage of spontaneous abortions — perhaps around 25% — remain undetermined in their aetiology, but it is most likely that a lack of ability to investigate these cases is the reason. A greater diligence amongst clinicians and pathologists is necessary if a greater understanding of these tragic cases is to be gained.

Epidemiology

It is very difficult to estimate the frequency of early pregnancy loss since the advent of sophisticated biochemical assays which detect the presence of human chorionic gonadotrophin (hCG) in women. There have been five studies considering early pregnancy loss prior to 6 weeks' gestation (Table 15.8). There is considerable variation in the results, which may well be explained by the sensitivity and specificity of the methods used to detect β-hCG. It is of note, however, that the data from Walker et al (1988) is unique in not detecting any evidence of β-hCG, which differs from all other studies. Whilst the figure of 58% by Edmonds et al (1982) is probably an overestimate, the results of Wilcox et al (1988) using a highly specific β-hCG assay are probably the best estimate at 22%. All these studies are based on the detection of postimplantation hCG and thus any losses of pre-embryos or blastocysts which failed to implant are undetected. In a mathematical consideration of the total loss rate, Roberts & Lowe (1975) calculated the total loss to be around 78%. The risk of spontaneous abortion of a clinically recognized pregnancy is around 15% (Warburton & Fraser 1964) and this is borne out by the longtitudinal studies quoted in Table 15.8.

Presentation

Spontaneous abortion may present clinically as either a threatened or inevitable abortion (Fig. 15.1).

Threatened abortion

This is said to occur when a woman bleeds from the uterus prior to 28 weeks of gestation. The bleeding is not associated with pain although there may be some backache. It is assumed that the bleeding is placental in origin, from some placental disruption or as a result of vascular disturbance at the site of implantation or the union of the decidua capsularis and the decidua vera. The bleeding is initially

Table 15.8 Preclinical and clinical pregnancy loss rates

Authors	Positive hCG	Clinical pregnancies	Preclinical loss rate	Clinical loss rate
Miller et al (1980)	152	102	50/152 (33%)	14/102 (14%)
Edmonds et al (1982)	118	51	67/118 (58%)	6/51 (12%)
Whittaker et al (1983)	92	85	7/92 (8%)	11/85 (13%)
Walker et al (1988)	25	25	0/0 (0%)	4/25 (16%)
Wilcox et al (1988)	198	155	44/198 (22%)	18/155 (12%)

hCG = human chorionic gonadotrophin.

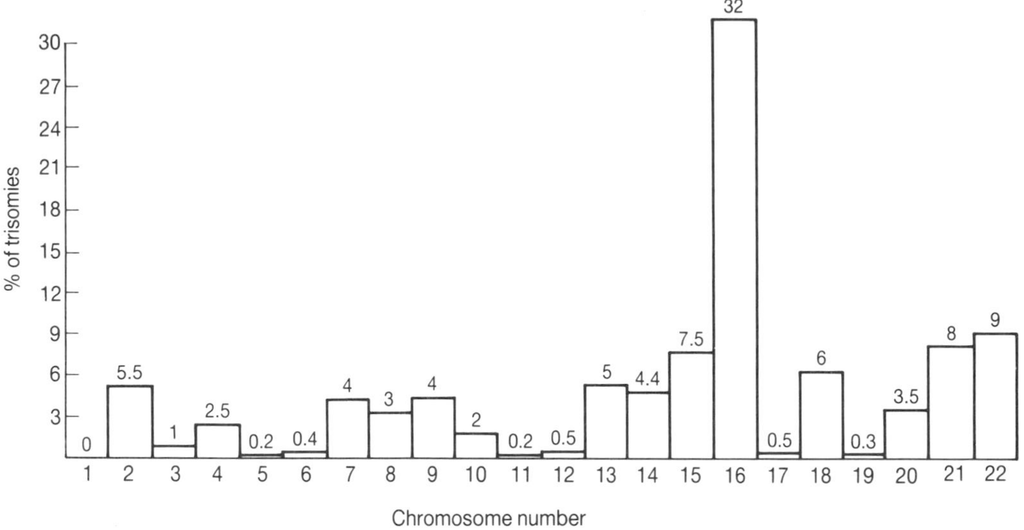

Fig. 15.2 Distribution of differing trisomies (based on Kajii et al 1973, Boué et al 1975, Hassold et al 1980, Warburton et al 1980).

bright red and then becomes brown, presumably as the primary vessel ceases bleeding and any surrounding clot breaks down. Clinical examination reveals a soft, non-tender uterus of appropriate size for gestation with a closed cervix. Whilst there may be considerable anxiety shown by the mother at the thought of being examined per vaginam, there is no evidence that this procedure precipitates miscarriage. If the mother is reluctant or refuses examination, then one should not persist but rather assess the pregnancy using ultrasound. The course of the pregnancy may proceed in three ways from here — resolution, becoming a missed or an inevitable abortion.

Missed abortion

In this condition there is either failure of embryonic growth in spite of placental viability or a viable fetus dies. In the first instance, an empty amniotic sac develops and this is known as a missed abortion (i.e. there is maternal failure to recognize the non-viable pregnancy) or, incorrectly, an anembryonic pregnancy (all pregnancies develop from an embryo) or blighted ovum (the pregnancy cannot result from an ovum alone). The situation of fetal demise usually occurs before 8 weeks' gestation, although the uterus does not expel the products. In both instances, the question of dependence of the placenta on fetal circulation for viability is undermined; much more research in this area needs to be performed to delineate the mechanisms of placental growth in the early weeks in order to define the causes of demise. The mother usually reports a disappearance of the symptoms and signs of pregnancy and a brown vaginal loss may ensue which may result from increasingly non-viable placental tissue. When the non-viable pregnancy becomes surrounded by clot in utero, it is termed a carneous mole.

Examination of the patient reveals a uterus which is smaller than the gestation would suggest but the cervical os is closed. Further assessment of the pregnancy involves an ultrasound examination which will either confirm a missed abortion, or the possibility of a viable pregnancy at a lesser gestational age than expected. A missed abortion may proceed in time to an inevitable abortion.

Inevitable abortion

If a woman presents with vaginal bleeding in association with crampy lower abdominal pain, the abortion is said to be inevitable. The pain is due to cervical dilatation secondary to uterine contractions and this results from prostaglandin release as the placenta and membranes separate from the uterine site. Once the internal os is open, the products will be expelled, either completely or, as in the vast majority, incompletely. Thus, the patient may give a history of passing products of conception. Blood loss may be considerable and care must be taken not to underestimate this fact. Examination reveals a tender, firm uterus which may be smaller than the gestational age expected and the internal cervical os is open. Products of conception may be felt through the os.

Occasionally, the woman may present with shock, either secondary to haemorrhage which will require appropriate measures, or out of proportion to the blood loss. This is due to products of conception being held in the cervix with a resultant sympathetic stimulation, known as cervical shock syndrome. Removal of the products results in relief of the shock.

Complete and incomplete abortion

If the pregnancy is expelled intact, the abortion is said to be complete, but this is a rare event in the first trimester;

in the majority of cases products of conception remain behind, and liable to cause bleeding or become infected if untreated. Examination reveals the os to be open and products may be palpated or discovered in the vagina.

Septic abortion

Failure of the patient to present with an incomplete abortion, or failure to diagnose the condition means that non-viable tissue remains in the uterus and may become infected. Whilst this is an unlikely event following spontaneous abortion, the risk is considerably higher following therapeutic abortion — around 3.6% (Frank 1985). The most common organisms are *Escherichia coli*, *Bacteroides* spp., streptococci (both anaerobic and, less commonly, aerobic) and *Clostridium welchii*.

The patient usually complains of abdominal suprapubic pain, malaise, some mild vaginal bleeding and pyrexia. Examination reveals abdominal rigidity and the bimanual examination reveals a tender uterus and adnexae, with the cervical os closed. Rarely, a septicaemia may ensue — bacteraemic endotoxic shock — which may result in maternal death.

Investigations

In threatened abortion or in patients suspected of having a missed abortion, an ultrasound scan for fetal viability is vital. The presence of a fetal heart can be reliably identified by 7 weeks' gestation and its presence or absence governs subsequent management. If a gestation sac is seen on a scan and there is no fetus visible, the diagnosis rests between a missed abortion or a pregnancy of earlier gestation than expected. Management at this stage depends on the clinical assessment, but frequently repeat ultrasound examination in 7–10 days is suggested, and failure to demonstrate the appearance of a fetus or diminution of the size of the gestation sac confirms the diagnosis of a missed abortion.

In some cases of threatened abortion, with a viable pregnancy, a second sac may be seen, indicating a non-viable twin gestation which is the cause of the symptoms and signs. These sacs usually reabsorb and the viable pregnancy proceeds unaffected. A low placental site is not a reliable ultrasound diagnosis to the aetiology of a threatened abortion in early pregnancy, although this may be the case.

The diagnosis of a *hydatidiform* mole on ultrasound is particularly obvious and the 'snowstorm' appearance of earlier technologies is now superseded by the appearance of the vesicles.

Patients with an inevitable complete or incomplete abortion require no further investigations in order to manage their situation. The management is entirely based on the clinical findings unless the patient refuses vaginal examination and then ultrasound may be performed to confirm the diagnosis. Care must be taken in managing these patients as there is an expectation amongst them that a scan is the ultimate diagnostic test. The role of the scan is very important in that the patient is able to visualize the viability or non-viability of the pregnancy, and if the latter is the case, she is able to accept the demise more readily. Thus *any* patient who requests a scan should be allowed to have that investigation.

All women who present with any degree of spontaneous abortion should have their blood group investigated so that any Rhesus-negative mothers may receive anti-D immunoglobulin.

Treatment

This depends on the clinical presentation and the results of the ultrasound investigations performed.

Threatened abortion

The traditional management for this condition is bedrest and forbidden intercourse. However, there are no studies to suggest that such management has any bearing on the outcome of the pregnancy. Having considered the aetiologies, bedrest will have no influence on a chromosomally or developmentally abnormal fetus, and neither will there be any change in abnormal placentation. If there is an infective cause, the difficulty of diagnosing the organism until the products have been expelled negates the efficacy of bedrest, although if a specific agent is identified the appropriate antibiotic can be administered.

Whilst most women may express the desire for and necessity of bedrest, the medical support of this wish merely surrounds the problem of miscarriage with a sense of desperation. Patients should be reassured and not made to feel that the threatened loss of a pregnancy is their fault by doing something they ought not to have done, or not doing something they should have done. When ultrasound has demonstrated a viable pregnancy, the chances of a spontaneous abortion occurring subsequently are only 2–3% (Christiaens & Stoutenbeck 1984) and thus reassurance and support will suffice in the vast majority.

Inevitable abortion and missed abortion

Having established the diagnosis, the primary aim of treatment is evacuation of the retained products of conception (ERPC) from the uterus, as the only way of being certain that the abortion is complete is the demonstration of no products of conception at ERPC. All cases, whether thought to be complete or incomplete, ought to have an ERPC. If bleeding has been sufficient to result in compromise of the maternal condition, then appropriate resuscitative measures should be taken prior to surgery. Bleeding may be arrested with the aid of Syntocinon

(20 i.v.) or ergometrine malleate (0.5 mg i.v.) if the situation requires this.

Evacuation should be performed under general anaesthesia and a suction curettage should be performed. The use of sharp curettes in the uterus should be avoided in view of the risk of surgical removal of the basal endometrium by over-vigorous curettage, leading to Ascherman's syndrome and subsequent fertility problems. Whilst it is ideal to arrange histological and chromosomal analysis of the products to help reach a possible diagnosis, this service is rarely available in the UK.

In the case of missed abortion, evacuation is again required, but the cervix should be prepared preoperatively using a gemeprost 1 mg pessary inserted high in the vagina. This synthetic prostaglandin acts by softening the cervix and inducing uterine contractions to cause cervical dilatation and allow easy access to the uterine cavity with the suction curette. Attempts to dilate the cervix forcibly with Hegar dilators should be avoided so that traumatic damage does not occur to the internal cervical os, with a subsequent risk of cervical incompetence.

Septic abortion

These cases present in two ways, either with a localized infection in the uterus and fallopian tubes, or with bacteraemic endotoxic shock. The management of the latter problem is outside the remit of this chapter (see Wright & Trott 1988), but the initial problem requires prompt action. If the patient is not bleeding heavily, which is usually the case, systemic antibiotics should be given for 24 hours before the ERPC because the action of curettage exposes arterioles into which bacteria enter and a bacteraemia results. Great care must be taken at the time of the ERPC as the risk of Ascherman's syndrome is highest in these patients. The most appropriate antibiotic regimen would be ampicillin 500 mg 6-hourly combined with metronidazole 200 mg 8-hourly.

Complications

Spontaneous abortion is such a common phenomenon that scant attention is paid to the associated risks. There is a mortality rate of 12.5 per million pregnancies; death occurs primarily as a result of haemorrhage and/or sepsis (Reports on confidential enquiries into maternal deaths in England and Wales 1986).

There is always blood loss associated with abortion and this is often impossible to assess from the patient's history. Thus, careful attention to physical signs of acute anaemia and anticipation of a problem by cross-matching blood, prompt use of antibiotics when appropriate, and the use of oxytocics can avoid the chance of severe problems. Rarely, a coagulopathy may develop, particularly in association with septic cases; management, with the aid of a haematologist, needs to be swift and effective. The use of fresh whole blood and fresh frozen plasma may be life-saving. Acute, prolonged hypovolaemia may result in renal cortical necrosis or renal tubular necrosis, and careful management of fluid balance is required to avoid this.

Patients who suffer a threatened abortion during the first trimester, and in whom the situation resolves, are prone to late pregnancy complications. These include an increased incidence of preterm labour, small-for-dates infants and retained placentae, and therefore a patient reporting bleeding in the first trimester must be identified as being in a higher-risk group.

Psychological aspects

The emotional effect of an abortion varies greatly. Some women report frank happiness or had positive feelings at the loss of an 'abnormal' pregnancy, whilst almost 60% had feelings of depression and hostility (Seibel & Graves 1980). There is always associated fear and anxiety caused by the pain and bleeding and the uncertainty with regard to the cause. Bereavement is the typical reaction to abortion. Around 30% of women begin to regard the fetus as a 'real person' by the 8th to 12th week of pregnancy and a miscarriage at this stage is seen as the loss of a child. There is often a loss of self-esteem with the view of a failure of womanhood and a loss of social identity — the 'mother-to-be'. Often the intensity of the emotions is not appreciated by those who care for the patient, or by her friends and relatives. Interaction with other people is very important and unfortunately, many people try to avoid discussing the loss, thereby further isolating the woman and prolonging the grief. Thus, all health workers should aim to help the woman express her grief and then reinforce her self-esteem.

The giving of the news to the patient that the pregnancy is lost should be done in the best possible surroundings so that the parents may express emotion without embarrassment, but patients should not be isolated. The use of sedatives is inappropriate in these circumstances. It is important to understand that these women have a deep desire for an explanation of what happened and why, and this information helps greatly in their acceptance of the tragedy of their pregnancy loss. Women who have experienced a loss will require considerable reassurance and support in a subsequent pregnancy if they are to have the confidence necessary to enjoy the — hopefully successful — outcome.

RECURRENT SPONTANEOUS ABORTION

There must be few conditions encountered by reproductive gynaecologists which are as distressing for the patient or frustrating to the doctor as recurrent miscarriage. The very large deficiency in our knowledge of fertilization, embryo development, implantation and the maintenance of pregnancy means that our understanding of repetitive pregnancy wastage is also limited.

Aetiology

The causes of recurrent spontaneous abortion are summarized below.

1. Genetic factors
   a. Parental chromosomes.
   b. Recurrent aneuploidy.
   c. Multifactorial.
   d. Recurrent euploidy.
2. Anatomical factors
   a. Uterine problems.
   b. Cervical problems.
3. Endocrine factors
   Corpus luteum problems.
4. Immunological factors
5. Maternal chronic disease

Chromosomal anomalies

Recurrent genetically abnormal pregnancy may result from parental chromosomal anomalies or the parents may be euploid. The incidence of chromosome abnormalities in couples who experience recurrent pregnancy loss is 6.14%, as opposed to a 1/500 rate in the normal population. When the couples are divided into recurrent aborters or multiple reproductive losses (i.e. recurrent aborters with live or stillborn offspring), there is still an equally high incidence of parental chromosome anomaly (Warburton & Strobino 1987) and the incidence of anomalies is threefold higher in women than men (Lippman-Hand & Vekemans 1983).

Robertsonian translocations. This is a condition in which two chromosomes adhere to each other, at either the centromere or the short arms. The total chromosome number is then 45, although one chromosome represents two. The frequency in the normal population is around 1/1000 and in recurrent aborters this is 10/1000 individuals (or 2% of couples). The risk of an abnormal conceptus is 100% if the translocation involves homologous chromosomes; only those involving chromosomes 13 and 21 result in live birth (i.e. trisomy 13 and trisomy 21). Thus chromosomal analysis resulting in the recognition of a robertsonian translocation is important for the counselling of these couples.

Reciprocal translocations. Here, a portion of one chromosome is exchanged with a portion of another, resulting in two abnormal chromosomes, but a total complement of 46. This occurs in around 3% of recurrent aborters and here the female to male ratio is 2:1. Translocations are reported for all the chromosomes and in all combinations and therefore estimating risk factors is very difficult. The risk of an unbalanced fetus is 11% in a subsequent pregnancy at amniocentesis, although 40% of chorionic villus samples demonstrate the translocation (Mikkelson 1985).

Inversions. This involves the reversal of order of genes, usually as a result of two chromosomal breaks, followed by reinsertion in reverse order of the free segment. Inversions in which the breakpoints are on either side of the centromere are known as pericentric inversions, and those on the same side are known as paracentric inversions. Inversions increase the risk of fetal loss due to abnormal combinations during cross-over of the meiotic loop. The result is fetal wastage, although if a balanced situation exists the fetus may be normal. Interestingly, inversions of chromosome 9 are relatively common and are generally considered of no clinical consequence (for review, see Simpson & Bombard 1987).

X chromosome mosaicism. This has been reported on a number of occasions, associated with recurrent miscarriage. Recurrent abortion seems to depend on the ratio of 45X:46XX cells, with the greater risk associated with a larger percentage of 45X.

Recurrent aneuploidy

The risk of a chromosomal abnormality in a second abortus depends on the chromosomal complement of the first (Table 15.9). If the complement of the first abortus is normal, the likelihood of the second being normal is 80%, whereas a repeated trisomy chance is 70%. This implies that some couples are predisposed to production of chromosomally abnormal conceptions. There are several suggested mechanisms for this phenomenon. If there is an

Table 15.9 Risks of karyotypes in successive abortuses

First abortus	Second abortus			
	Normal	Trisomy	Monosomy	Polyploidy
Normal	80%	9%	4%	7%
Trisomy	24%	70%	3%	3%
Monosomy	45%	36%	9%	9%
Polyloidy	40%	40%	10%	10%

From Hassold (1980).

error in gametogenesis in the oocyte, abnormal embryos may result and increased maternal age may be associated with an increased incidence of such oocytes being selected. Ageing of the oocyte following ovulation and prior to fertilization has also been suggested as increasing the abnormalities of the embryo. Human trisomy is almost always maternal in origin whereas triploidy is male in origin — fertilization by diploid sperm in 30% of cases or dispermy in 70%.

Multifactorial problems

These situations are most commonly neural tube defects, although other syndromes, e.g. Potter's syndrome, are described. There seems to be an increased risk of subsequent abortion if a pregnancy is diagnosed as having a neural tube defect, especially anencephaly, although the exact risks are difficult to estimate.

Genetic factors in recurrent euploid abortion

Many abortuses which are examined cytogenetically turn out to be euploid (46XY or 46XX) — even missed abortions — and the possibility of the presence of lethal genes seems highly likely. Much work on transgenic mice has indicated that DNA fragments can be inserted to cause lethal mutations in recessive or dominant offspring. In the mouse, a lethal gene called the complex can be found on chromosome 17, but no equivalent has been found in the human although the hypothesis that certain homologues exist on human chromosome 6 and 19 suggests that lethal mutations could exist in these sites. Abnormal development may occur as a result of another mutation. Homeobox genes control the expression of groups of genes through transcription regulation; they regulate the development of groups of cells which become morphologically recognized. Mutation of a homeobox sequence results in inappropriate or abnormal development and their importance is proven in mice and *Drosophila*. Whether the early findings of homeobox genes in humans on chromosome 17 (Rabin et al 1985) will lead to further discovery of homeobox genes and their mutations remains to be seen, but the potential for discovering the control of development is immense.

Another genetic possibility in normal and abnormal development is the role of oncogenes. Oncogenes are established as involved in unregulated neoplastic growth and may be the origin of growth factors which are involved in embryo growth. An abnormality or absence of an oncogene may lead to failure of embryonic growth or perhaps selective failure. Thus, whilst routine karyotyping may fail to identify a chromosomal cause for recurrent abortion, the possibility of gene mutations and deletions remains a very likely aetiology for euploid abortion.

Anatomical factors

Uterine problems

The origin of congenital uterine anomalies is not straightforward and requires an understanding of normal development. The müllerian ducts give rise to the fallopian tubes, uterus and upper two-thirds of the vagina. Each duct grows in a cephalocaudal direction, canalizing as they do so, and eventually uniting in the midline to form the uterus and müllerian tubercle. This forms the vaginal plate which grows inferiorly to reach the urogenital sinus, canalization of this downgrowth results in the vagina. It seems that the uterus is distinguishable by 11 weeks' gestation and the vagina complete by weeks 20–22. Defects in the process of fusion or canalization can produce numerous anomalies, from complete failure of fusion and duplication of the system (uterus didelphys), partial fusion (uterus bicornus), failure of reabsorption (septate uteri) and failure of canalization (vaginal agenesis).

The incidence of uterine anomalies is unknown, but patients with recurrent pregnancy loss have a 10–15% incidence of uterine anomalies (Sandler 1977). The aetiology of the recurrent reproductive failure is not clear although implantation on a septum may lead to decreased placental vascularization. Uterine anomalies also arise secondary to intrauterine exposure to diethylstilboestrol, which results in abnormal development of the uterus and cervix, and reproductive failure is high. The existence of Ascherman's syndrome is associated with recurrent abortion, presumably due to inadequate placentation. Finally, the role of fibroids in recurrent abortion is somewhat contentious, although Buttram & Reiter (1981) suggested a reduction in recurrent abortion following myomectomy.

Cervical factors

Pregnancy loss from cervical incompetence is due to weakness in the sphincteric mechanism of the internal os. This may be congenital (rare) or acquired and the aetiology is primarily a previous pregnancy. The history of a therapeutic abortion or a dilatation and curettage prior to pregnancy are risk factors, as is a previous cone biopsy. Finally diethylstilboestrol exposure results in an incompetent cervix in about 20% of patients.

Endocrine factors

The functional corpus luteum is essential for the implantation and maintenance of early pregnancy, through the production of progesterone. A normally functional corpus luteum follows the adequate growth and maturation of the follicle, without which the corpus luteum will be inadequate. Hence, progesterone production is reduced, endometrial maturation is retarded and menstruation may occur prematurely.

Whilst measurement of luteal phase parameters, e.g. progesterone levels, may be valuable in the non-conceptual cycle, there is no method of assessing luteal phase function in a pregnant patient. In fact, the corpus luteum of pregnancy and that in the non-conceptual cycle are entirely different, both morphologically and endocrinologically. The idea, however, that 'inadequate' production of progesterone is associated with recurrent abortion seems to have persisted without any evidence to support the theory. Attempts to improve pregnancy outcome using clomiphene citrate have failed, as has the use of luteal phase progesterone. Similarly, the use of hCG in the luteal phase and early pregnancy remains unsubstantiated, although studies are in progress (Harrison 1988). It would seem unlikely that inadequate luteal function is a cause of recurrent abortion.

Immunological factors

The risk of a recurrent abortion following three consecutive spontaneous miscarriages is variously reported as between 26 and 47% (Warburton & Strobino 1987). The percentage of aneuploidy in this population is small (6%) and thus another explanation for recurrent euploid losses may be immunological.

The major histocompatibility complex is located on chromosome 6 and is encoded for two classes of antigens. Class I antigens are glycoproteins, coded by the genes human leukocyte antigen (HLA) A, B and C, and are the cell surface antigens which are responsible for cytotoxic reactions and allograft responses. Class II antigens are also glycoproteins and are products of the gene HLA D, and are responsible for presenting antigens to immunocompetent cells, thereby regulating the immune response. The continuous layers of syncytiotrophoblast and underlying cytotrophoblast that surround the conceptus are HLA class I and II antigen-negative.

Class I antigen production seems to be inhibited at the stage of transcription. The cytotrophoblast attaching the trophoblast to the decidua certainly does express class I antigens; however the expression is incomplete. The lack of class II antigens, especially HLA DR, implies an inability to mount a cytotoxic immune response at this level, which may be important in pregnancy maintenance.

Another antigen has been found to bind to both trophoblast and leukocytes, referred to as trophoblast-leukocyte cross-reacting (TLX) antigen. A positive response to this antigen is considered necessary in the establishment of fetomaternal immunological coexistence. Why there is no graft–host rejection response at the site of placentation has concerned a number of investigators. It seems that local production of suppressor cells within the decidua may play a role in this phenomenon. Two types of suppressor cell have been described, one which is non-antigen-specific and suppresses all cytotoxic immune responses, and a second type which is immunosuppressive through its ability to produce prostaglandin E_2, which indirectly inactivates uterine T helper cells. Macrophages also accumulate in the uterus during pregnancy and they too suppress T helper cells.

Thus a major modification of the normal immune mechanism is necessary in the establishment of a successful pregnancy, and failure to achieve this may result in recurrent abortion. Why some women fail to mount this response is uncertain, although some suggest that HLA compatibility between couples, especially HLA B and DR, and perhaps the TLX antigens, means a failure to generate an immune response. However, if this theory were correct, couples with recurrent abortion would not benefit from immunotherapy; the HLA theory has few advocates.

Unsuccessful pregnancies may arise because of:

1. Failure to mount a protective maternal immune response.
2. Failure of the cytotrophoblast to express a local non-cytotoxic immune response.
3. Failure of T lymphocytes to produce lymphokines which induce trophoblastic growth.

These deficiences will result in an immune response mounted by the mother against the pregnancy, and its subsequent demise.

Maternal chronic disease

Diabetes mellitus

There is general agreement that there is an increased risk of spontaneous abortion in uncontrolled diabetics who may become recurrent aborters. The rate of spontaneous abortion is 26–30% overall (Wright et al 1983) although the series by Crane & Wahl (1981) failed to demonstrate that the risk was increased above the normal population.

Systemic lupus erythematosus (SLE)

There is no doubt that pregnancies in patients with SLE have a very poor prognosis. Patients who are positive for lupus anticoagulant prior to the clinical onset of the disease have a high spontaneous abortion rate, and those with the clinical disease almost always result in fetal death. Lupus anticoagulant is an antiphospholipid antibody which interferes with coagulation by excluding the phospholipid surface of platelets from the generation of thrombin. The most appropriate test for the presence of lupus anticoagulant is the kaolin clotting time, although other autoantibodies are also often present, e.g. anticardiolipin antibody (100% of cases), antinuclear antibody (90% of cases).

Chronic systemic diseases

Conditions such as chronic essential hypertension and chronic renal diseases may be associated with recurrent abortion. This may be as a result of reduction of uterine blood flow due to small vessel damage.

Smoking and alcohol consumption

These have been implicated by some investigators as associated with recurrent abortion (Kline et al 1980). The risk of abortion seems to be increased by 1.5–2 times that of normal.

Investigations

History-taking is very important in cases of recurrent abortion and must include:

1. History of the abortions and the histological/karyotype findings.
2. Family history of neural tube defects or other malformations.
3. History of chronic disease states.

The patient should be examined, but there are rarely any physical signs. Investigations must include a full blood count and a kaolin clotting time (or lupus anticoagulant level) karyotyping of both partners and a hysterosalpingogram. Further investigations are probably of little value in managing the patient.

Treatment

This must be tailored towards the identified cause, although in the majority of cases the investigations will reveal no apparent abnormality.

One of the problems faced in advising patients is an understanding of the risks of recurrence. Only four prospective studies address this problem (Table 15.10); and the risk of repeated abortion rises with increasing recurrence. However, it is important to note that even after three miscarriages, without any treatment, a couple may expect a 71% chance that the next pregnancy will be successful, and when evaluating treatments this must be used as the standard rate upon which improvement is based. Patients may therefore be given positive advice if the investigations discover no obvious cause.

Table 15.10 Probability of a spontaneous abortion given the previous abortion history

Authors	No. of previous abortions 0	1	2	3+
Warburton & Fraser (1964)	12.3%			
Boue et al (1975)		13.8%		24.9%
Lauritsen (1976)		13.2%		32.5%
Harger et al (1983)			17.4%	29.2%
Total	12.3%	13.5%	17.4%	28.9%

Chromosomal problems

Genetic counselling is of paramount importance for couples who have either a chromosomal disorder themselves, or in whom there is a history of recurrent chromosomal abortions. Couples with balanced translocations can be positively advised with regard to further pregnancies and the availability of prenatal diagnosis by either chorionic villus sampling or amniocentesis. In reciprocal translocation, again counselling should be against further pregnancies in view of the absolute nature of the problem. In certain circumstances, when the abnormal chromosome complement is traced to the male partner, artificial insemination with donor sperm may be suggested as a possible solution, but great care must be taken when introducing this concept. Gynaecologists must be certain of the genetic basis of the disease process for which they are counselling and if any uncertainty exists, referral to a clinical geneticist is strongly advised.

Anatomical problems

Uterine anomalies. Patients with a unicornuate uterus have a high abortion rate, but if there is evidence of cervical incompetence (which may occur in about 25% of cases), cervical cerclage should be inserted in the first trimester. If a rudimentary horn also exists, serious consideration should be given to its removal as a pregnancy in a rudimentary horn has a 90% chance of rupturing the uterus (O'Leary & O'Leary 1963). It is probably adequate to rely on ultrasound to identify the pregnancy in the rudimentary horn and remove the horn if this occurs. In uterus didelphys, there is no proven therapy to improve the obstetric performance.

Bicornuate uteri have been treated primarily by Strassman's procedure (Strassman 1966); he reported an 85% fetal survival out of 289 women. The use of cervical cerclage has also been used to improve the reproductive outcome of bicornuate uteri with similar success, but no trials to compare these two methods have been reported.

Patients with the septate uterus may be managed by abdominal (Tompkin's metroplasty) or hysteroscopic metroplasty with dramatic improvement of fetal survival, from around 6 to 80%. However, there is infertility following abdominal surgery due to adhesion formation; this may be as high as 30%. The use of the hysteroscope may improve this rate, and DeCherney et al (1986) report a 7% rate of failure to conceive, and hysteroscopic resection of a septum is the preferred operative choice.

In patients who have uterine anomalies secondary to

diethylstilboestrol exposure, the obstetric outlook is poor and there are no surgical procedures which improve the uterus. Patients who have had second trimester abortions may benefit from cervical cerclage in a subsequent pregnancy (for review, see Kaufman & Irwin 1987).

Fibroids. Women whose uterine cavity is distorted by fibroids may be advised to undergo myomectomy but again great care must be taken as the adhesion rate postoperatively is high and a significant infertility rate will ensue. However, fetal loss rate may be reduced from around 40 to 20% (Buttram & Reiter 1981).

Incompetent cervix. The incompetent cervix and its management is controversial. The role of cervical cerclage and the effect on outcome remains unresolved as there are no truly randomized trials. Two studies which have attempted this have unfortunately a patient select bias (Papiernik et al 1984; Rush et al 1984) but neither of these studies was able to support the concept that cervical cerclage is valuable in prolonging pregnancy. In view of the exclusion of patients with proven cervical incompetence by HSG, the data for these patients must be based on uncontrolled series. If a cerclage is inserted prophylactically, one can expect an 80% successful outcome, and 60% if inserted after cervical dilatation has commenced.

Whilst cervical incompetence is usually associated with mid-trimester abortion, Ayers et al (1982) and Edmonds (1988) have attempted its use to prevent recurrent first trimester losses. Both studies showed an equal improvement to other therapies with successful outcome in excess of 80%. However, the series were not randomized and the results must be interpreted with caution. There may well be a major effect of psychotherapy which is influencing the outcome.

Immunological therapy

Blood transfusions containing leukocytes have been demonstrated to have a number of effects on the immune system, primarily the concept of increased allograft survival. This led to the idea of using leukocyte transfusions in women with idiopathic recurrent abortion in an attempt to modify the immune response within the uterus. The leukocytes have been given by various routes — intravenously, subcutaneously and intradermally — and the doses have varied also. The results of success overall seem very consistent, around 77%, although there is an obvious lack of control data. The only randomized study was that of Mowbray et al (1985) which demonstrated a significant advantage of immunotherapy. The risk of recurrent abortion in the control groups seems unexpectedly high in comparison with previous published estimates. It would seem that a group of patients are suitable for immunotherapy as a treatment to improve their obstetric outcome, but the numbers of patients who need treatment is undetermined. Attempts to identify a suitable population have as yet been unsuccessful. Mowbray et al (1985) have suggested using antipaternal cytotoxic antibody, but studies on the normal population have found this insensitive and invalid (Regan & Braude 1987). Beer (1988) has suggested the use of a maternal serum mixed lymphocyte culture blocking assay as an index of immune response and thus an indicator for patients who are suitable for immunization. However, although the preliminary results are encouraging, much work needs to be done before immunotherapy can be used routinely.

Psychotherapy

Whether psychological factors affect the outcome of pregnancy has perplexed clinicians and patients for many years. A spontaneous abortion has, until recently, been considered a less serious emotional event than other types of bereavement, but these beliefs are changing. The eventual effect on subsequent reproductive performance is difficult to quantify but could be significant, and this belief has led to the use of psychotherapy in the management of recurrent abortion. The largest study was published by Stray-Pedersen & Stray-Pedersen (1988) in which 205 patients with idiopathic recurrent abortion received psychotherapy and 42 did not, and the success rate was 85 and 36% respectively. Thus, although these studies are not randomized, there is a suggestion that psychological factors may adversely affect pregnancy outcome and therapy may improve the reproductive performance.

CONCLUSIONS

The aetiology of repetitive fetal wastage is diverse and ill understood. Whilst we await further advances in our knowledge, we must rely on good clinical skills and resist the temptation to treat unnecessarily. The results of Stray-Pedersen & Stray-Pedersen (1988) must make us aware of the fact that intervention is not necessarily the answer and conservative management may be just as successful.

KEY POINTS

1. A woman who has three or more successive spontaneous abortions is generally accepted to be a recurrent aborter.
2. The process of abortion is the major route by which natural selection operates in humans with 50% of all clinically recognized first trimester losses being chromosomally abnormal.
3. Trisomic pregnancies result in blighted ova or very stunted fetal growth.
4. Structural chromosomal rearrangements are rarely the cause of spontaneous abortion.
5. Abnormal placentation may be important in the

aetiology of chromosomally normal spontaneous abortions: some may be amenable to treatment.
6. Spontaneous abortion may result from isolated placental and fetal infections but no evidence exists for their involvement in recurrent spontaneous abortions.
7. The risk of spontaneous abortion in a clinically recognized pregnancy is around 15%.
8. Patients who suffer a threatened abortion are prone to late pregnancy complications and must be identified as a high risk group.
9. The incidence of chromosome abnormalities in couples with recurrent pregnancy loss is 6.14%.
10. 10–15% of women who suffer recurrent pregnancy loss have a uterine anomaly.
11. Failure to achieve the major modification of the normal immune mechanism necessary to establish a successful pregnancy may result in recurrent abortion.
12. Psychological factors may adversely affect pregnancy outcome and therapy may improve reproductive performance.

REFERENCES

Ayers J W, Petersen E P, Ansbacher R 1982 Early therapy for the incompetent cervix in patients with habitual abortion. Fertility and Sterility 38: 177–181

Beer A E 1988 Pregnancy outcome in couples with recurrent abortions following immunological evaluation and therapy. In: Beard R W, Sharp F (eds) Early pregnancy loss: mechanisms and treatment. Royal College of Obstetricians and Gynaecologists, London, pp 337–349

Buttram V C, Reiter R 1981 Uterine leiomyomata: etiology, symptomatology and management. Fertility and Sterility 30: 644–652

Charles D, Larsen B 1987 Infectious agents as a cause of spontaneous abortion. In: Bennett M J, Edmonds D K (eds) Spontaneous and recurrent abortion. Blackwell Scientific Publications, Oxford, pp 149–167

Christiaens G C M L, Stoutenbeck P H 1984 Spontaneous abortions in proven intact pregnancies. Lancet ii: 572–574

Crane J P, Wahl N 1981 The role of maternal diabetes in repetitive spontaneous abortion. Fertility and Sterility 36: 477–479

Creasy M R, Crolla J A, Alberman E D 1976 A cytogenetic study of human spontaneous abortions using banding techniques. Human Genetics 31: 177–196

DeCherney A H, Russell J B, Graebe R A, Polen M L 1986 Resectoscopic management of mullerian fusion defects. Fertility and Sterility 45: 726–728

Dhadial R K, Machin A M, Tait S M 1970 Chromosomal anomalies in spontaneously aborted human fetuses. Lancet ii: 20–21

Edmonds D K, 1988 Use of cervical cerclage in patients with recurrent first trimester abortion. In: Beard, R W, Sharp F (eds) Early pregnancy loss: mechanisms of treatment. Royal College of Obstetricians and Gynaecologists, London, pp 411–415

Edmonds D K, Lindsay K S, Miller J F, Williamson E, Wood P J 1982 Early embryonic mortality in women. Fertility and Sterility 38: 447–453

Fantel A G, Shepard T H 1987 Morphological analysis of spontaneous abortuses. In: Bennett M J, Edmonds D K (eds) Spontaneous and recurrent abortion. Blackwell Scientific Publications, Oxford, pp 8–28

Frank P 1985 Sequelae of induced abortion. In: Abortion: medical progress and social implications. Pitman, London, pp 67–82

Geisler M, Kleinebrecht J 1978 Cytogenetic and histological analysis of spontaneous abortions. Human Genetics 45: 239–251

Gronroos M, Honkonen E, Punnonen R 1983 Cervical and serum IgA and serum IgG antibodies to *Chlamydia trachomatis* and herpes simplex virus in threatened abortion. British Journal of Obstetrics and Gynaecology 90: 167–170

Harrison R F 1988 Early recurrent pregnancy failure treatment with human chorionic gonadotrophin. In: Beard R W, Sharp F (eds) Early pregnancy loss: mechanisms and treatment. Royal College of Obstetricians and Gynaecologists, London, pp 421–431

Hassold T 1980 A cytogenetic study of repeated spontaneous abortions. American Journal of Human Genetics 32: 723–731

Hassold T, Chen N, Funkhouser J et al 1980 A cytogenetic study of 1000 spontaneous abortions. Annals of Human Genetics 44: 151–178

Kajii T, Ferrier A, Niikawa N, Takahara H, Ohama K, Aviroachan S 1980 Anatomic and chromosomal anomalies in 639 spontaneous abortuses. Human Genetics 55: 87–98

Kaufman R H, Irwin J F 1987 Diethylstilboestrol exposure and reproductive performance. In: Bennett M J, Edmonds D K (eds) Spontaneous and recurrent abortion. Blackwell Scientific Publications, Oxford, pp 130–148

Kline J, Stein Z, Susser M, Warburton D 1980 Environmental influences on early reproductive loss. In: Porter I H, Hook E B (eds) Embryonic and fetal death. Academic Press, New York, pp 225–240

Kriel R L, Gates G A, Wulff H 1970 Cytomegalovirus isolations associated with pregnancy wastage. American Journal of Obstetrics and Gynecology 106: 885–890

Lauritsen J G 1976 Aetiology of spontaneous abortion. Acta Obstetrica Gynaecologica Scandinavica 52: 1–9

Lippman-Hand A, Vekemans 1983 Balanced translocations among couples with two or more spontaneous abortions. Human Genetics 63: 252–257

Mikkelson M 1985 Cytogenetic findings in first trimester chorionic villus sampling. In: Fraccaro G, Simoni G, Brambati B (eds) First trimester fetal diagnosis. Springer-Verlag, Berlin, p 108

Miller J F, Williamson E, Glue J, Gordon Y B, Grudzinskas J G, Sykes A 1980 Fetal loss after implantation: a prospective study. Lancet ii: 554–556

Mowbray J F, Gibblings C, Liddel H, Reginald P W, Underwood J L, Beard R W 1985 Controlled trial of treatment of recurrent abortion by immunization with paternal cells. Lancet i: 941–943

O'Leary J L, O'Leary J A 1963 Rudimentary horn pregnancy. Obstetrics and Gynaecology 22: 371–375

Rabin M, Hart C P, Ferguson-Smith A et al 1985 Two homeobox loci mapped in evolutionary related mouse and human chromosome. Nature 314: 175–178

Regan L, Braude P R 1987 Is antipaternal cytotoxic antibody a valid marker in the management of recurrent abortion. Lancet ii: 1280

Reports on confidential enquiries into maternal deaths in England and Wales 1979–1981 1986 HMSO, London

Roberts C J, Lowe D B 1975 Where have all the conceptions gone? Lancet i: 498

Rushton D I 1988 Placental pathology in spontaneous miscarriage. In: Beard R W, Sharp F (eds) Early pregnancy loss: mechanisms and treatment. Royal College of Obstetricians and Gynaecologists, London, pp 149–157

Sandler S W 1977 Spontaneous abortion in perspective. South Africa Medical Journal 52: 1115–1124

Seibel M, Graves W L 1980 The psychological implications of spontaneous abortion. Journal of Reproductive Medicine 25: 161–172

Simoni G, Gimelli G, Cuoco C 1985 Discordance between prenatal cytogenetic diagnosis after chorionic villus sampling and chromosomal constitution of the fetus. In: Fraccaro M, Simoni G, Brambati B (eds) First trimester fetal losses. Springer-Verlag, Berlin, pp 108–119

Simpson J L, Bombard A 1987 Chromosomal abnormalities in spontaneous abortion. In: Bennett M J, Edmonds D K (eds)

Spontaneous and recurrent abortion. Blackwell Scientific Publications, Oxford, pp 51–76

Strassman E O 1966 Fertility and unification of the double uterus. Fertility and Sterility 17: 165–171

Stray-Pedersen B, Stray-Pedersen S 1988 Recurrent abortion: the role of psychotherapy. In: Beard R W, Sharp F (eds) Early pregnancy loss: mechanisms and treatment. Royal College of Obstetricians and Gynaecologists, London, pp 433–440

Takahara H, Ohama K, Fukiwara A 1977 Cytogenetic study in early spontaneous abortion. Hiroshima Journal of Medical Science 26: 291–296

Therkelsen A J, Grunnet N, Hjort T, Myre Jansen O, Jonasson J, Lauritsen J G 1977 Studies in spontaneous abortion. In: Boue A, Thibault C (eds) Chromosomal errors in relation to reproductive failure. INSERM, Paris, pp 81–83

Walker E M, Lewis M, Cooper W, Marnie M, Howie P W 1988 Occult biochemical pregnancy: fact or fiction? British Journal of Obstetrics and Gynaecology 95: 659–663

Warburton D, Fraser F C 1964 Spontaneous abortion risks in man: data from reproductive histories collected in a medical genetics unit. Human Genetics 16: 1–25

Warburton D A, Strobino B 1987 Recurrent spontaneous abortion. In: Bennett M J, Edmonds D K (eds) Spontaneous and recurrent abortion. Blackwell Scientific Publications, Oxford, pp 193–213

Warburton D, Stein Z, Kline J, Susser M 1980 Chromosome abnormalities in spontaneous abortions. In: Porter I H, Hook E B (eds) Human embryonic and fetal deaths. Academic Press, New York, pp 261–287

Watts D H, Eschenbach D A 1988 Reproductive tract infections as a cause of abortion and preterm birth. Seminars in Reproductive Medicine 6: 203–215

Whittaker P G, Taylor A, Lind T 1983 Unsuspected pregnancy loss in healthy women. Lancet i: 1126–1127

WHO recommended definitions, terminology and format for statistical tables related to the perinatal period. 1977 Acta Obstetrica Gynecologica Scandinavica 56: 247–253

Wilcox A J, Weinberg C R, O'Connor J F et al 1988 Incidence of early pregnancy loss. New England Journal of Medicine 319: 189–194

Wright S W, Trott A T 1988 Toxic shock syndrome: a review. Annals of Emergency Medicine 17: 268–273

16. Investigation of the infertile couple

W. Thompson R. N. Heasley

INTRODUCTION

This chapter aims to present a simple account of the investigation of the infertile couple, emphasis being placed on clinical practice and an ordered scheme of basic tests. This is supported by descriptions of more complex procedures which may be required in some situations and of which the practising gynaecologist should be aware. In our opinion, it is more important to perform relevant tests in their proper order and at the correct time than to subject the couple to a large range of investigations, many of which bear little relevance to the day-to-day management of their problem.

Using life table analysis it has been calculated that the chances of conception for a given couple having regular unprotected intercourse are 80 and 90% after 12 and 18 months respectively (Cooke et al 1981). Based on this it is usual to begin investigations after 1 year when there will be a reasonable chance that one or more problems may exist. Once a programme of basic tests is initiated it is important that it is completed within a defined period of time, usually 6 months, so that the couple can be offered a realistic prognosis and an appropriate treatment schedule. Prompt recognition of the factors which may cause infertility leads to ordered and logical attempts at treatment and this is particularly important in view of the availability of new technologies which now offer real hope to couples whose prognosis would have been hopeless just a few years ago. It is also important that a clear explanation of each of the tests, and the reasons for doing them, is given to both partners. It goes without saying that the couple must always be seen in parallel, a condition best achieved in dedicated infertility clinics. Here adequate time is available for counselling and facilities exist to permit a proper assessment of the situation. In many instances however, the female partner is simply referred to a routine gynaecology clinic by her family doctor. In this situation the general gynaecologist should always encourage the husband to attend, perhaps setting aside time at the end of the clinic to deal with such infertile couples.

The causes of infertility and their relative frequency are shown in Figure 16.1. Unexplained infertility is an ill defined entity. Its frequency will depend on the extent and complexity of investigations available to a particular clinic, consequently the reported incidence varies between 6 and 60% (Templeton & Penney 1982).

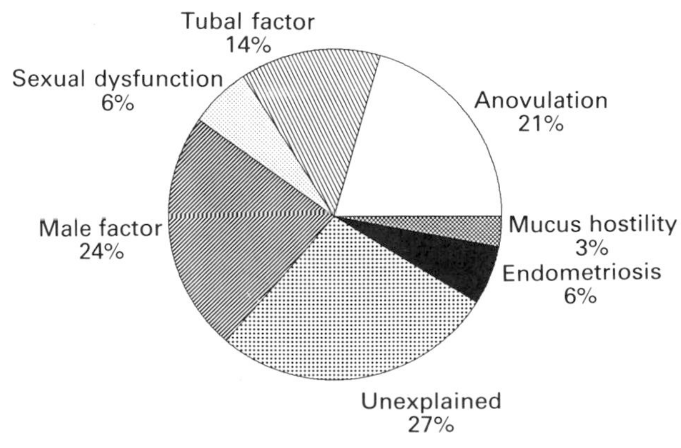

Fig. 16.1 The causes of infertility.

Investigation of infertility can conveniently be divided into two phases. At the beginning a number of tests aimed at confirming normal ovulation, sperm production and gamete transport are undertaken. Depending upon the results and also the duration of infertility, more complex investigations may be pursued, although the value of many of these is debatable (see below).

The approach to the infertile couple should begin with a detailed medical, sexual and social history followed by physical examination of both partners. The sequence of investigations should be ordered so that the simplest, least invasive and most productive tests are completed first. Therefore at the initial clinic visit semen analysis and a simple test to confirm ovulation are arranged. If these are normal, tubal patency is assessed and the cervical factor investigated by means of a properly timed postcoital test.

HISTORY AND EXAMINATION

In the female partner the presence of previous significant illnesses should be sought, particularly a history of pelvic infection or sexually transmitted diseases; previous abdominal surgery may also be relevant (Table 16.1). When obtaining details of the medical history it is important to ascertain whether or not infertility investigations have been undertaken elsewhere. Infertile couples often move from clinic to clinic in the hope that something new or different can be offered. In such a situation, needless repetition of tests is wasteful of time and resources, prolongs the investigative process and often falsely raises the patients' hopes.

Details of menstruation should include the regularity and duration of bleeding and the presence of associated symptoms suggestive of ovulation, e.g. mittelschmerz. A history of irregular cycles is suggestive of ovulatory dysfunction, most commonly due to polycystic ovary disease.

Table 16.1 Investigation of infertility — the female history

Sexual dysfunction	Dyspareunia Vaginismus
Cervical factor	Mucus secretion Conization/cautery Incompetence
Uterine and tubal	Pelvic/abdominal surgery Pelvic infection Pelvic pain Dysmenorrhoea
Endocrine	Hirsutism Weight changes Menstrual pattern Galactorrhoea
Previous obstetric history	Pregnancy loss Puerperal sepsis
Contraception	Hormonal Intrauterine contraceptive device

In the case of secondary infertility, the obstetric history is important. For instance, prolonged rupture of membranes associated with chorioamnionitis, or puerperal sepsis, may have led to ascending infection and tubal damage.

A clear history should also be obtained from the male; points of particular importance are the occurrences of testicular pain, swelling, or trauma. Surgical operations such as orchidopexy or herniorrhaphy may also be relevant. The social history includes reference to drug intake, occupation, tobacco and alcohol consumption and occupation (Table 16.2).

Table 16.2 Investigation of infertility — the male history

Occupation	Sedentary Toxin/irradiation
Illnesses/operations	Febrile conditions Bladder neck surgery Cryptorchidism
Infection	Venereal Orchitis/epididymitis Tuberculosis
Drugs	Sulphasalazine Chemotherapy Antimicrobials Antihypertensives Alcohol/nicotine
Sexual function	Coital frequency Erection/orgasm Ejaculation
Trauma/stress	

A careful physical examination of both partners is also mandatory. In the female, general assessment must include the height and weight, breasts and secondary sexual characteristics. Abdominal palpation is performed prior to a full pelvic examination. In the male, weight and general appearance are recorded, the abdomen palpated, hernial orifices checked and the external genitalia examined. The latter is best performed with the subject standing. The penis is inspected and the testes assessed for size with reference to an orchidometer; testicular consistency is also important. An attempt should be made to palpate the vasa deferentia which characteristically feel like a 'whipcord' and to check for the presence of varicoceles. This is best achieved by asking the patient to perform a Valsalva manoeuvre.

MALE FACTORS

It is accepted that a substantial proportion of infertility is due to deficiencies in semen; nevertheless, controversy still surrounds the question of what constitutes a normal semen analysis. Consequently, many men who were previously categorized as sterile are now classified as subfertile. It is unwise to state that a man is infertile if any number of motile sperm are found on semen analysis — conceptions have been reported with counts as low as 1 million per ml — with values below 20 million per ml the overall pregnancy rate without therapy is approximately 20–25% (MacLeod & Gold 1951). The dissatisfaction with traditional methods of assessing male fertility potential (i.e. the routine semen analysis) has led to the introduction of more elaborate diagnostic tests. These include computer-assisted analysis of sperm motility patterns, sperm penetration of mid-cycle cervical mucus in vitro and the ability of sperm to penetrate zona-free hamster eggs.

Routine semen analysis

Despite the recognized limitations, a careful examination of the ejaculate is an essential part of an infertility investigation. For detailed technical information on methods the reader is referred to the World Health Organization laboratory manual for the examination of human semen and semen–cervical mucus interaction (World Health Organization 1987). There follows a brief description of the minimum information which should be obtained from the routine semen analysis (Table 16.3) and a discussion of the further investigations which might be undertaken if the results prove to be outside the widely accepted normal limits.

Table 16.3 Routine semen analysis

Volume	2–6 ml
Liquefaction	Complete in 30 min
Count	20 million/ml or more
Motility	60% (forward progressive)
Morphology	70% or more normal forms
Mixed antibody reaction test	Negative

Collection of semen samples

The collection of semen specimens must be organized by experienced staff and only after full discussion with the male partner as to the details of the arrangements. A clearly written instruction sheet concerning the collection and transport of the specimen is useful.

The patient must be allowed, within reason, to choose where he wishes to produce the sample. If he lives a long distance from the clinic and is willing to produce the specimen in hospital then a room should be provided which is quiet and secluded and which will guarantee total privacy. The production of semen by masturbation usually results in a specimen that is complete and otherwise uncontaminated and hence it is the preferred method. The specimen is collected in a clean, wide-mouthed non-toxic plastic container which must be protected from the cold and delivered to the laboratory within 1–2 hours.

However, there are some who find this method difficult or offensive and others who have religious objections. In these cases a specimen can be obtained following coitus provided a sheath designed for this purpose has been used; contraceptive condoms are unsuitable since the majority contain spermicidal agents which rapidly obliterate all sperm motility. Collection of semen samples by coitus interruptus is not recommended because the first part of the ejaculate may be lost; it is this portion which contains the highest concentration of sperm.

The length of abstinence prior to the production of semen alters to some extent both the sperm numbers and their motility. Nevertheless, if the specimen is not produced within 24 hours of a previous ejaculation and the length of abstinence is known, a proper assessment can be made. It would be more logical to obtain a history of the couple's sexual practice and then collect semen samples in keeping with the intervals between coitus since this would reflect the semen quality to which the cervical mucus is regularly exposed. Because of the known variability in semen quality from the same individual, at least two specimens should be examined during the course of the infertility investigations.

Semen liquefaction and viscosity

Human semen forms a gel-like clot soon after ejaculation. Liquefaction of this coagulum normally occurs within 30 minutes and is a necessary prerequisite to undertaking microscopic examination of the specimen. Coagulation is dependent on the presence of a fibrinogen-like substrate derived from the seminal vesicles, whereas the liquefying enzyme, vesiculase, is produced by the prostate gland. A complete absence of the coagulum indicates an obstruction of the ejaculatory duct or congenital absence of the seminal vesicles.

On the other hand a prolonged liquefaction time (more than 1–2 hours) or complete absence of liquefaction can be caused by a deficiency of vesiculase from reduced prostatic secretion. This situation, particularly if found in association with a negative postcoital test, may be a cause of infertility. Several methods can be used to liquefy the ejaculate prior to microscopic examination; these include addition of 5% alpha-amylase or proteolytic enzymes such as trypsin.

Increased viscosity may also lead to difficulties with the laboratory assessment of the specimen but there is some doubt whether it is associated with infertility, since sperm from hyperviscid semen usually show no difficulty in entering cervical mucus at microscopy. The viscosity of the ejaculate may vary considerably between different patients and also between samples from the same individual. If the specimen of semen is excessively viscid it should be repeatedly forced through a narrow gauge hypodermic needle (no. 19) prior to microscopic examination.

Volume

The volume of the ejaculate should be measured either with a graduated cylinder or by aspirating the whole sample into a pipette; the average range is 2–5 ml. A low volume may indicate that the complete specimen was not collected into the container or that spillage had occurred before it reached the laboratory. This should be ascertained by questioning the patient and the test repeated.

A persistently low semen volume (less than 0.5 ml) may be due to an obstruction of the ejaculatory ducts or the congenital absence of the seminal vesicles. In both cases, the low volumes are associated with reduced fructose levels in the seminal plasma. Absence of ejaculatory fluid in the presence of a normal orgasm may suggest a diagnosis of retrograde ejaculation and such men will sometimes have noted a 'cloudy' urine after coitus. To confirm this diagnosis a urine sample is obtained as soon as possible after masturbation and the voided specimen centrifuged for 10 minutes at 3000 r.p.m. The residue is then resuspended in a small volume of a physiological solution (Ringer's lactate) and examined for the presence of motile sperms.

An abnormally large semen volume (greater than 6 ml) is usually associated with a reduced sperm concentration and this could theoretically interfere with sperm transport in the female. Furthermore, leakage of semen from the vagina is more likely to occur. When a large volume of semen is considered to be a possible factor for the infertility the sperm can be concentrated by centrifugation at 3000 rpm for 5 minutes and resuspended in a small volume of Ringer's lactate; this is then used for artificial insemination. It is generally accepted that the volume of the ejaculate has little effect on fertility if the sperm concentration is not significantly reduced.

Sperm count and concentration

Several methods are available to determine the number of sperm per ml in the ejaculate (sperm concentration). These provide a good estimate but variations of 10–20% from true concentrations can be expected; this should be borne in mind when interpreting reports.

The haemocytometer (improved Neubauer) counting chamber is most frequently used to estimate the sperm concentration. The ejaculate must be diluted (usually 20-fold) with a spermicidal solution and after counting, the number of sperm in a fixed volume is calculated by correcting for the dilution factor. Other techniques to count sperm include the Makler chamber (Makler 1980) or a similar device such as the Howell fertility counting chamber. These chambers have a depth of 10 μm and permit direct estimation of the sperm concentration without dilution.

Sperm can also be counted with an electronic particle analyser such as the Coulter counter. However aberrant results are not infrequent as the ejaculate can contain agglutinated sperm or cell debris of similar size and it is doubtful if this method is useful in clinical practice. It should be emphasized that these methods may give different results for the same semen sample.

Oligozoospermia

A patient should be considered oligozoospermic and the ejaculate abnormal if his sperm concentration is less than 10 million per ml, although some laboratories now set the limit at 5 million per ml. It must be emphasized that it is extremely difficult to state definitively when the sperm count is so low that the patient is completely infertile. Not only is the concentration of sperm important but the total number (sperm count) is significant as well. A good concentration but poor volume will produce a low overall sperm count (less than 20 million) which may cause fertility problems. The use of the motile sperm concentration rather than the total sperm concentration is perhaps a better index for fertility assessment in that it takes two variables into consideration.

Azoospermia

If two semen analyses show azoospermia blood should be taken for follicle-stimulating hormone (FSH) and testosterone estimation. A high FSH with a normal or low testosterone confirms testicular failure and is not remediable. Azoospermia in the presence of testes of normal size and consistency with a normal FSH level can be regarded as an indication for an exploration of the scrotal contents and evaluation for a possible obstructive lesion by vasography. A testicular biopsy may also be performed but in practice it is unlikely that a situation which can be corrected surgically will be encountered. In the majority of patients (95%) with azoospermia it will be a question of accepting the situation and providing realistic counselling as to donor insemination or adoption. In a few cases, where FSH levels are low (hypogonadotrophic hypogonadism), the situation is more optimistic and fertility can be restored in more than 50% of cases by the use of exogenous gonadotrophins.

Azoospermia in association with eunuchoid features suggests a diagnosis of Klinefelter's syndrome and this can be confirmed by chromosomal analysis following examination of a peripheral blood sample.

Sperm morphology

To assess the morphology of sperm, a semen smear is prepared on a slide and air-dried or the sperm may be fixed before the smear is prepared. The Giemsa or other sample stains are often used for this purpose but the Papanicolaou stain is preferred as it produces excellent cytological and nuclear detail, including identification of the acrosome cap. Abnormalities are noted in the head, mid-piece and tail and reported as such; the diagnostic use of further subdivisions is questionable, although certain clinical conditions are associated with well defined sperm abnormalities, e.g. amorphous and tapered sperm with variocele. Human semen samples usually contain a high percentage of abnormal sperm forms and up to 30% are reported in otherwise 'fertile' ejaculates. However, the presence of more than 60% of abnormal sperm cells, particularly if the lesion is well defined and constant, are likely to be significant and related to infertility.

Debilitating illnesses, including viral and bacterial infections, will produce an increase in the number of abnormal sperms as well as certain drugs, such as nitroferans. In a long-term follow-up of patients, Bostofte et al (1982) have shown a clear relationship between a high number of abnormal sperm and reduced fertility. The increase in abnormal sperm cells usually starts occurring within 30 days of an acute illness and may be present for up to 2–3 months, even though the clinical condition of the patient has markedly improved. The presence of a large number of sperm containing cytoplasmic droplets may suggest incomplete maturation and thus epididymal pathology. Scanning and transmission electron microscopy may also be employed to identify specific structural abnormalities of the sperm, but routine evaluation of the ultrastructure is neither practical nor necessary.

Sperm motility

The motility is expressed as the percentage of moving sperm in the sample; the accepted normal value is at least 60% after 1 hour. It is particularly important to assess the number of sperm exhibiting progressive forward motility across the field of view; at least 50% should show this quality. Poor motility, particularly in the presence of normal sperm numbers, suggests that the sample may simply have become cold and a repeat specimen should be analysed. Other causes of reduced motility per se include seminal infection and sperm autoantibodies but most often it is merely one aspect of poor semen quality, together with reduced count and increased numbers of abnormal sperm.

Recently, objective measurement of human sperm movement characteristics using computerized image analysis have been developed (Cellsoft, Cryo Resources, New York). This method can provide information on sperm velocity, linearity of sperm progression and amplitude of lateral head displacement — parameters that cannot be obtained by routine semen analysis. The amplitude of lateral head displacement correlates with in vitro fertilizing capacity as evaluated by the hamster egg penetration assay in both normal fertile men and in the male partners of couples with unexplained infertility (Aitken et al 1985).

In samples of semen exhibiting no sperm motility further investigation can be undertaken using the supravital staining technique. Semen is mixed 1:1 with 0.5% eosin Y and after 1–2 min a smear is prepared (World Health Organization 1987). Sperm with physically intact membranes appear bluish-white, whereas dead sperm are coloured reddish-yellow. A sample is considered abnormal if more than 50% of the sperm stain 'dead'.

The recently introduced hypo-osmotic swelling test not only evaluates whether the sperm head membrane is intact but also if it is biochemically active. For this test 0.1 ml semen is mixed with 1 ml of hypo-osmotic medium (2.7 g fructose and 1.47 g sodium citrate:$2H_2O$ in 200 water); after 30 min at 37°C the percentage of sperm with coiled or bent tails is evaluated microscopically. If less then 50% of sperm fail to show these changes the test is positive. In human in vitro fertilization programmes the hypo-osmotic swelling test has been shown to be a much better predictor of fertilizing capacity than conventional semen analysis (Van der Ven et al 1986).

The zona-free hamster egg penetration test

This test of sperm function is based on the property of zona-free golden hamster eggs to be able to be penetrated by sperm of other species, including the human. Eggs are collected from golden hamsters that have been superovulated with gonadotrophins. The zonae are removed by enzymatic treatment and the eggs are then cultured with human sperm that has been washed, resuspended in a physiological solution and incubated for 6 hours. This incubation allows the acrosome reaction to occur, a prerequisite for sperm penetration. Sperm which have penetrated the zona-free eggs will show swollen heads with decondensation of the chromatic material. The results of the test are reported as the percentage of eggs penetrated or the average number of sperm penetrations per egg.

Unfortunately the variability of the test conditions between laboratories makes comparisons of normal values difficult, but an abnormal test is defined as less than 10% of eggs penetrated. Despite this attempt at standardization, there are reports of conceptions with male partners who have consistently negative penetration tests. In a routine laboratory this test is expensive to establish and good quality control is difficult to maintain. This, associated with lack of correlation with human egg fertilization as reported from in vitro fertilization programmes, means that the technique is probably best confined to specialized units for research studies.

OVULATION DETECTION

Symptoms and signs

Ovulation pain (mittelschmerz) and mid-cycle staining occur regularly in a small percentage of women and may be a useful adjunct to coital timing, indicating that ovulation is likely to be taking place. In clinical practice, no definite conclusions regarding ovulatory status should be drawn from their occurrence. Observation of mid-cycle mucus is the best clinical marker of ovulation and is useful in the timing of procedures such as donor insemination. It is important to note that these changes do not provide proof of ovulation since an increase in cervical mucus can occur in anovulatory cycles where there is good endogenous oestrogen production.

Basal body temperature recording

This is a widely used technique which has been employed for ovulation detection in infertility, as a method of natural family planning and as a means of diagnosing luteal phase deficiency. The mid-cycle rise of 0.5–1°C due to the thermogenic effect of progesterone can be detected using a fertility thermometer; the body temperature is recorded at the same time each day, usually first thing in the morning. Vaginal or rectal readings approximate better to core temperature than oral recordings, although this is aesthetically unacceptable to many women. Because basal body temperature recording is still frequently used as a method of ovulation detection it is important to reappraise its value in the light of more scientific methods such as hormone assays and ultrasonography. Such critical review suggests that this method is unreliable as a marker of ovulation (Heasley & Thompson 1986); in addition, it can be confusing, stressful and inconvenient for the patient. However, from a practical point of view, it may be of some value for timing luteal phase progesterone estimation or as an adjunct to monitoring the response to clomiphene in anovulatory women.

Hormone assays

In women with regular periods the simplest and most reliable method of detecting ovulation is to measure a single mid luteal serum progesterone whereas those with oligomenorrhoea or amenorrhoea warrant a full hormonal profile. It is important to measure serum progesterone in at least two consecutive cycles and to ensure that blood sampling is performed approximately 1 week prior to the onset of subsequent menstruation. The minimum level of serum progesterone taken to indicate ovulation to within 95% confidence limits is usually accepted as 30 nmol/l. This is in keeping with the data of Hull et al (1982) although higher values have been suggested. Some flexibility in sample timing is possible but suboptimal values interpreted without reference to the subsequent menstrual period are meaningless.

It has been suggested that a single progesterone estimation is not sufficient and that four samples should be taken in the mid luteal phase on consecutive days. This is obviously less convenient for the patient but the use of such a 'progesterone index' eliminates errors which may arise due to episodic fluctuations in daily progesterone levels. Daily estimations of progesterone in serum or alternatively in saliva have also been used but are impractical for everyday use. They may however be employed in an effort to detect luteal phase deficiency (see p. 227).

Detection of the preovulatory oestradiol peak and the mid-cycle surge of luteinizing hormone (LH) may also be used to predict ovulation. The LH peak is of most value, occurring between 8 and 20 hours prior to ovulation, but its accurate delineation requires at least daily blood or urine sampling. It is not usual to perform these investigations as a routine but when accurate ovulation timing is required, for instance in procedures like donor insemination, such methods are helpful. There are several commercially available kits allowing women to undertake daily urine testing for the LH peak with minimal supervision.

Ovarian ultrasonography

Ultrasonographic visualization of developing follicles has become an established method for studying ovulation; increases in follicular diameter and observation of follicular rupture correlate well with cyclical hormonal changes during the ovarian cycle. The recent introduction of vaginal ultrasonography has added an even greater degree of sophistication to the technique. Ovulation is presumed to have occurred when there is a sudden reduction in size or complete disappearance of the dominant follicle, which measures 18–25 mm prior to its rupture.

This method is rarely necessary during the basic investigations but is of great value in monitoring ovulation induction. It has also been employed to assess follicular growth in cases of unexplained infertility.

Endometrial biopsy

Formal dilatation and curettage is rarely indicated in modern practice. It is expensive and potentially harmful since it can (rarely) cause intrauterine adhesions and lead to pelvic inflammatory disease. It is therefore indicated only if significant endometrial pathology, such as tuberculosis, is suspected. Endometrial tissue adequate for ovulation detection may be readily obtained as a simple outpatient procedure using instruments such as the Vabra or Sharman curettes, dispensing with the need for cervical dilatation. The presence of secretory change in the premenstrual biopsy implies a normal response to progesterone in a properly primed endometrium.

Using the criteria of Noyes et al (1950), the endometrium in the luteal phase can also be histologically dated, providing a detailed assessment of the response to oestrogen and progesterone. Biopsies should be obtained from high in the uterus and close to the onset of subsequent menstruation for maximum accuracy. If endometrial development lags by 2 or more days in two consecutive cycles a diagnosis of luteal phase deficiency is made.

This method is widely regarded by many as the best way of assessing luteal function; it should be noted however that the original baseline criteria for endometrial dating employed rather inaccurate methods of ovulation timing (cycle length and basal body temperature charts). When the LH peak is used as a reference point the method has been shown to be rather imprecise (Tredway et al 1973).

Endometrial biopsy and dating are not essential during the routine investigation of infertility. If detailed ovulation studies are thought to be necessary, for instance in cases of unexplained infertility, then a combination of serum progesterone measurements and endometrial dating seems the most logical approach to the assessment of luteal function.

Tubal, uterine and pelvic factors

Traditionally, three methods have been employed to assess the patency of the fallopian tubes in infertile women. However, only two of these, hysterosalpingography and laparoscopy, merit serious consideration in modern practice. The third, tubal insufflation (Rubin's test) is very imprecise and carries a risk of carbon dioxide embolism; its use should therefore be abandoned.

Hysterosalpingography

In this investigation a radiopaque dye is injected into the uterus by means of a Leech–Wilkinson cannula inserted into the cervical canal. During injection of dye fluoroscopic screening is performed permitting visualization of the uterine cavity, the fallopian tubes and the presence of free spill into the peritoneal cavity.

The method suffers from several disadvantages, not least that it can be a painful and unpleasant experience for the patient. Consequently, it is usual to give sedation (such as Omnopon) prior to the procedure. Tubal spasm may occur in some women, creating a false positive result and suggesting cornual blockage, and there is also a risk of reactivation of previous salpingitis. However, hysterosalpingography remains a helpful investigation which is widely used in clinical practice.

Laparoscopy

Whether or not laparoscopic examination is used as the sole method of investigating tubal patency, it is widely agreed that this method is essential for a full assessment of the infertile couple. Excellent accounts of the technique are described elsewhere (Steptoe 1967; Gordon & Lewis 1988). However, it is important to emphasize two practical points regarding laparoscopy in cases of infertility. Firstly, a thorough examination of the pelvic organs cannot be obtained unless a double-puncture technique is employed. This permits the introduction of a probe which can be used to ensure that the operator has clearly visualized the whole length of the fallopian tubes, in particular the fimbriated ends and their apposition to the ovaries. Additionally, the ovaries may be elevated to allow inspection of their undersurface and of the broad ligaments and pelvic side walls in a careful search for endometriotic deposits. A second puncture can also be used for the introduction of scissors to divide adhesions and bipolar coagulation or laser for the local treatment of endometriosis.

Secondly, when the laparoscopic examination has been completed a detailed description of all the findings (including negative ones) should be made with the aid of simple diagrams. This ensures that others gain an accurate impression of the problems that may be present and of the prognosis for fertility.

Several retrospective studies have compared the reliability of the results obtained by laparoscopy and hysterosalpingography. The general conclusions are that both should be performed for maximum accuracy (Moghissi & Sim 1975). In a prospective study Okonofua et al (1989) suggest that laparoscopy should be the primary procedure and, if normal, precludes the need for hysterosalpingography since no additional information will be gained.

There is widespread agreement that laparoscopy is superior for the detection of peritubal adhesions and for the accurate diagnosis of cornual blockage, where hysterosalpingography gives a significant number of false positives. In addition, laparoscopy is much better for the detection of pelvic pathology such as endometriosis or ovarian cysts. If performed at the appropriate time of the cycle it also provides evidence that recent ovulation has occurred. While hysterosalpingography is of undoubted value for the detection of intrauterine pathology such as polyps, myomas and synechiae, the increasing use of hysteroscopy may further reduce its value in infertility investigations (Leeton 1988).

The modern approach is to regard laparoscopy as the primary procedure because of its much higher diagnostic yield. However, there are undoubtedly some situations where hysterosalpingography is more appropriate. These include patients in whom laparoscopy would be technically difficult or when it is necessary to define accurately the shape of the uterine cavity.

Cervical factor

The postcoital test

During the immediate preovulatory period sperm rapidly reach the endocervical canal where they are distributed and stored in the cervical mucus (Moghissi 1976). The number of sperm remains fairly constant between 10 and 150 min after intercourse, following which there is a progressive reduction. The only practical way of testing the integrity of this physiological process is by performing a postcoital test (PCT). A negative PCT may be due to poor semen quality, coital difficulty, failure to produce adequate cervical mucus or immunological factors in either partner. There is controversy regarding the value of the PCT which has undoubtedly arisen because of poor standardization of the technique and differences in interpretation of the results.

The PCT is not of value unless performed in the immediate preovulatory phase when the cervical mucus is profuse, virtually acellular and exhibits ferning and Spinnbarkeit. These changes may be limited to 2 or 3 days in each cycle, making timing difficult, and a negative test in the presence of poor cervical mucus should be repeated in a subsequent cycle. Even apparently 'good' cervical mucus may be found to be unreceptive to sperm and if any doubt exists then a fern test should be performed. If there is difficulty in pinpointing the correct time it is important to ensure that ovulation is occurring, since the production of good mucus is dependent on a normal preovulatory oestradiol surge. It may also be necessary either to perform the test on alternate days near mid-cycle or to see the patient daily until adequate cervical mucus is observed; the PCT should then be performed the next day.

It is widely accepted that a period of abstinence of 2 or 3 days before the test is sufficient although there are no firm rules. There has also been disagreement about the optimum timing of the PCT in relation to coitus; intervals of 2–24 hours have been reported. A 2-hour interval usually means having intercourse in the early morning and can often lead to practical difficulties including temporary impotence as a result of having to adhere to a strict time schedule. A more reliable approach is to perform the test 8–12 hours after coitus so the couple can have intercourse the previous evening; this also has theoretical advantages when it comes to interpreting the results.

For the test, mucus is collected using either a tuberculin syringe or a fine plastic tube (Rocket UK) and its amount, viscosity and cellularity are recorded. In the standard PCT the cervical mucus is placed on a slide, a coverslip applied and microscopic examination performed at high power (× 400).

A more complex capillary tube method has been devised but is only employed for research purpose. Various scoring systems have been proposed for the interpretation of results but the scores obtained do not correlate well with future fertility. A simpler classification, based on the presence or absence of progressively motile sperm, is easier to use and correlates better with the final outcome in terms of pregnancy rates (Kroeks & Kremer 1987).

If sperm are not present in repeated PCTs despite a normal semen analysis a coital problem should be suspected. Gross asthenospermia or a very low semen volume may also give a negative test; the presence of sperm which are immotile or which exhibit the 'shaking phenomenon' (non-progressive motility) suggests the presence of anti-sperm antibodies. In a few instances non-progressive motility may simply be due to thick sticky cervical mucus, despite proper timing of the test.

The PCT is best considered as a prognostic index for future fertility; those with a positive test have a significantly better outlook. A negative test should lead to more specific investigations such as those for anti-sperm antibodies.

In vitro mucus penetration tests

A negative PCT is most often due to inappropriate timing and should be repeated. If, however, the test is negative despite good cervical mucus, some form of in vitro mucus penetration test should be performed. This permits a more detailed assessment of sperm–mucus interaction and allows cross-over tests with donor sperm and donor mucus to be undertaken. The two commonly used techniques are the sperm penetration test (SPT) and the sperm–cervical mucus contact test (SCMCT).

The former is usually performed on a microscope slide although tube methods have also been described. A drop of semen is placed adjacent to an equivalent amount of preovulatory mucus and a coverslip applied so that an interface is formed (Fig. 16.2). Penetration of the mucus by sperm is assessed by microscopic examination over the course of the next hour. A negative test is indicated by complete failure of penetration or immobilization of those sperm which have penetrated; the shaking phenomenon (see below) may also be observed. This test is simple to perform but is less specific for the presence of sperm

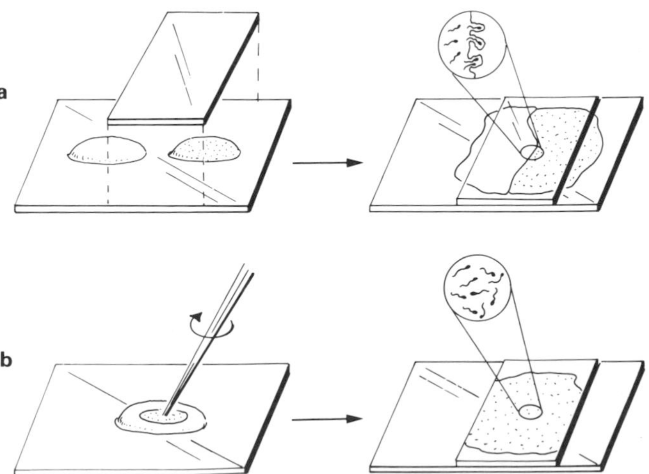

Fig. 16.2 The sperm penetration test and the sperm–cervical mucus contact test. In the former (**a**) an interface is produced; in the latter (**b**) there is mixing of the components.

antibodies than the SCMCT, since non-immunological factors may lead to a negative test.

The SCMCT, devised by Kremer & Jager (1976), is reported to correlate well with the presence of anti-sperm antibodies in either semen or cervical mucus. It can therefore be used as the primary diagnostic method for local immunological factors if more complex antibody tests are not available. The test is performed by mixing a drop of cervical mucus with a similar volume of semen on a slide and observing after 30 min (Fig. 16.2). If more than 25% of the sperm are exhibiting jerking or shaking movements rather than forward motility the presence of antibodies is presumed and in strongly positive tests the proportion of such sperm equates to the antibody titre. Cross-over testing with donor sperm or mucus permits an accurate assessment of whether the antibodies are present in the semen or the mucus.

Unexplained infertility

If the basic investigations are normal yet there is a persistent failure to conceive, couples are said to have unexplained (idiopathic) infertility. This poorly defined entity is usually reported in 20–30% of cases although a range of 6 to 60% has been cited (Templeton & Penney 1982). It has been clearly demonstrated that the chance of conception in such couples is most closely related to the duration of their infertility; the age of the female partner and the type of infertility (either primary or secondary) are also relevant (Lenton et al 1977; Hull et al 1985). These authors all basically agree that an eventual pregnancy rate of 60–70% will be achieved after 3 years of follow-up with no specific treatment being offered. In view of this, counselling forms the basis of management in a situation which is frustrating for both patient and doctor.

Despite the presence of these solid epidemiological data, in some clinics couples with unexplained infertility may undergo a range of more detailed investigations in an effort to find a cause for their failure to conceive. There is no evidence that this approach is superior to simply waiting for spontaneous conception to occur. Furthermore, if treatment is undertaken on the basis of results of these tests its apparent success may be wrongfully attributed to the therapy, rather than to natural conception. The major investigations which are sometimes performed in unexplained infertility are briefly described below. For more detailed accounts the reader is referred to Moghissi & Wallach (1983) and McBain and Pepperell (1987).

Hysteroscopy

This technique is increasingly performed in infertile women and is complementary to laparoscopy and hysterosalpingography. It provides an accurate clinical evaluation of the uterine cavity leading to the diagnosis of uterine malformations, endometrial polyps and intrauterine adhesions. Unfortunately, the importance of such pathology in the aetiology of infertility remains unclear at the present time and there is no convincing evidence that treatment improves the prognosis. However such conditions are likely to be associated with recurrent loss of early pregnancy.

Ovarian ultrasonography

This has been employed in an effort to detect subtle abnormalities of follicular growth and rupture. Accelerated follicular growth has been demonstrated in women with unexplained infertility and there are several reports of the 'luteinized unruptured follicle' syndrome (Daly et al 1985; Haxton et al 1987). It is not known whether such anomalies occur in repeated cycles or if they are seen only in unexplained infertility. Furthermore, there is no proven treatment, apart from in vitro fertilization; their diagnosis is therefore of academic interest since in vitro fertilization is increasingly offered to couples with idiopathic infertility.

Investigation of corpus luteum function

Luteal deficiency is a poorly defined entity which has been implicated as a cause of unexplained infertility. Unfortunately there has been a lack of standardization of diagnostic methods and treatment, leading to confusion about its aetiological role. There is no doubt that defective luteal function can occur and is probably the end-result of a disordered follicular phase. However, it can only be implicated as a cause of infertility if it is more common in infertile women and seen to occur repetitively. This would entail studying a large number of consecutive cycles in each patient, a condition which is difficult to meet in practice.

Luteal deficiency has been diagnosed on the basis of suboptimal serum progesterone (or urinary pregnanediol) levels or by histological dating of the endometrium (Noyes et al 1950); basal body temperature records are too imprecise to be of value. Serum progesterone can be measured daily throughout the cycle, three times at the mid luteal phase or simply once at the mid luteal peak. Daily salivary progesterone estimations provide an alternative method of assessing luteal function. Histological evidence of luteal deficiency is based on retarded maturation of the endometrium, the accepted diagnostic criterion being a lag of 2 days or more in endometrial development in two consecutive cycles.

There is no clear answer at present to the question: 'Does luteal phase deficiency cause infertility?' Our approach is to perform a well timed mid luteal progesterone estimation in two or three consecutive cycles, and if suboptimal values are found, to prescribe clomiphene citrate. Although this simple approach is acceptable in clinical practice at the present time, more prospective controlled studies are required in this whole area in order to clarify the role of luteal deficiency in infertility.

Sperm antibodies

The precise role of immunological factors in the aetiology of infertility remains controversial. It is accepted that sperm are highly antigenic and antibodies to them have been detected in both male and female serum, cervical mucus and seminal fluid. During the routine investigation of the male partner a simple screening test such as the mixed antiglobulin reaction (MAR) or the immunobead test is worthwhile (Figs 16.3 and 16.4). However when such tests are positive the semen analysis is usually abnormal and a diagnosis of unexplained infertility is therefore not entertained. Similarly the presence of sperm antibodies in cervical mucus will lead to negative postcoital and sperm penetration test.

MAR Test

R.B.C coated with Anti D

R.B.C coated with Anti D and IgG or IgA

Mixed agglutinate of RBC and Speratozoa

Sperm coated with antisperm antibodies

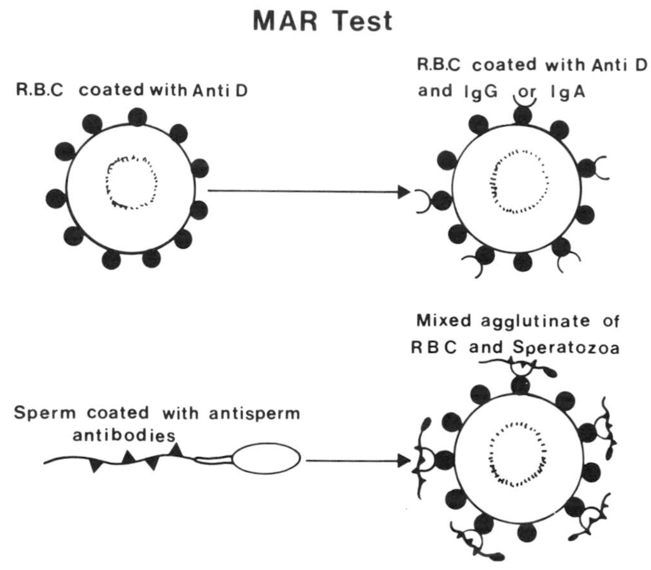

Fig. 16.3 The mixed antiglobulin reaction (MAR) test. Red blood cells, coated with IgA or sensitized with IgG, are mixed with a non-specific anti-IgA or an anti-IgG and then incubated with sperm under test. Sperm with anti-sperm antibodies will adhere to the treated red blood cells (RBC).

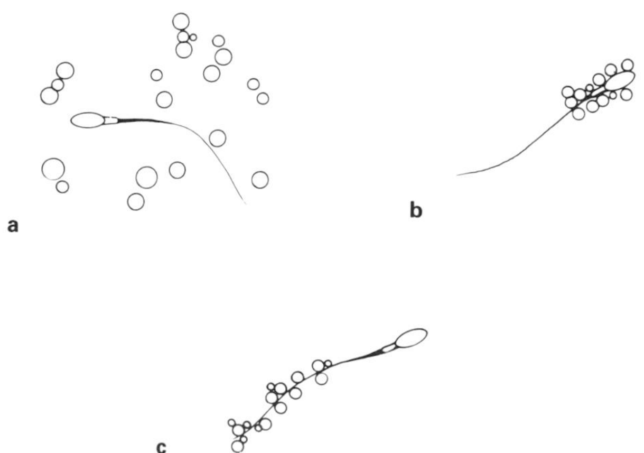

Fig. 16.4 The immunobead test. (**a**) Negative test; (**b**) and (**c**) positive tests showing beads attached to sperm head and tail respectively.

This leads to the question of whether additional screening for sperm antibodies using elaborate techniques is justified in couples with unexplained infertility or whether it should be limited to those with abnormal semen samples or negative mucus penetration tests. Serum antisperm antibodies may be detected by a number of methods (Kibrick et al 1952; Isojima et al 1968) and are reported to be present in 10–20% of couples with unexplained infertility. However it remains to be proven whether or not such antibodies are a cause of infertility and their detection is therefore of little value during the routine investigation of the infertile couple. It is our practice to use the postcoital and sperm penetration tests as screening procedures for antibodies in cervical mucus. In addition, the presence of a positive MAR test, particularly in combination with sperm agglutination and poor motility, is regarded as being indicative of autoantibodies in semen. Consequently we do not see the need to employ tests for serum agglutinating or immobilizing antibodies in unexplained infertility.

KEY POINTS

1. It is more important to perform relevant tests in their proper order, and at the correct time, than to subject the couple to a large range of investigations.
2. Once investigation is initiated it is important that it is completed within a defined period of time so that a realistic prognosis and an appropriate treatment schedule can be offered.
3. The sequence of investigations should be performed so that the simplest, least invasive and most productive tests are completed first.
4. A history of irregular cycles is suggestive of ovulatory dysfunction, most commonly due to polycystic ovarian disease.
5. In couples where the man has a sperm count of less than 20 million per ml, there is an overall pregnancy rate of about 25%, so it is extremely difficult to state definitively that a count is so low that the patient is completely infertile.
6. The first part of the ejaculate contains the highest concentration of sperm.
7. Azoospermia coupled with a high FSH and normal or low testosterone indicates testicular failure and is not remediable.
8. In human IVF programmes, the hypo-osmotic swelling test has been shown to be a much better predictor of fertilizing capacity than conventional semenanalysis.

9. At least two semen specimens should be examined due to the known variability in each individual.
10. Observation of mid-cycle mucus is the best clinical marker suggestive of ovulation, while basal body temperature charts are unreliable and sometimes stressful for the patient.
11. Detection of the mid-cycle surge of LH, 8–20 hours before ovulation, is not routinely necessary but is useful when accurate timing of ovulation is required.
12. Formal D & C for endometrial biopsy is only indicated if significant endometrial pathology, such as tuberculosis, is suspected.
13. Laparoscopy has the highest diagnostic yield, and should be regarded as the primary procedure for the investigation of tubal patency.
14. A negative PCT may be due to poor semen quality, coital difficulty, failure to produce adequate cervical mucus or immunological factors in either partner, though is most often due to inappropriate timing.
15. 60–70% of couples with unexplained infertility will conceive within 3 years with no treatment.
16. Intrauterine pathology is more likely to be associated with recurrent early pregnancy loss than infertility.
17. The role of luteal phase deficiency in infertility is not clear.

REFERENCES

Aitken R J, Sutton M, Warner P, Richardson D W 1985 The relationship between the movement characteristics of human spermatozoa and their ability to penetrate cervical mucus and zona-free oocytes. Journal of Reproduction and Fertility 73: 411–449

Bostofte E, Serup J, Rebbe H 1982 Relation between morphologically abnormal spermatozoa and pregnancies obtained during a 20-year follow-up period. International Journal of Andrology 5: 379–386

Daly D C, Soto-Albors C, Walters C, Ying Y, Riddick D H 1985 Ultrasonic evidence of luteinised unruptured follicle syndrome in unexplained infertility. Fertility and Sterility 43: 62–67

Haxton M J, Fleming R, Hamilton M P R, Yates R W, Black W P, Coutts J R T 1987 Unexplained infertility — results of secondary investigations in 95 couples. British Journal of Obstetrics and Gynaecology 94: 539–542

Heasley R N, Thompson W 1986 The prediction and detection of ovulation in artificial insemination. In: Andrology. Male fertility and sterility. Academic Press, Florida pp 491–509

Isojima S, Li T S, Ashitake Y 1968 Immunologic analysis of sperm immobilizing factor found in sera of women with unexplained infertility. American Journal of Obstetrics and Gynecology 101: 677–683

Kibrick S, Belding D, Merrill B 1952 Method for the detection of antibodies against mammalian spermatozoa. II. A gelatin agglutination test. Fertility and Sterility 3: 430–438

Kremer J, Jager S 1976 The sperm–cervical mucus contact test: a preliminary report. Fertility and Sterility 27: 335–340

Leeton J 1988 The investigation of pelvic lesions in infertility. Australian and New Zealand Journal of Obstetrics and Gynaecology 28: 126–127

Lenton E A, Weston G A, Coke I D 1977 Long term follow-up of the apparently normal couple with a complaint of infertility. Fertility and Sterility 28: 913–919

Makler A 1980 The improved 10-micrometer chamber for rapid sperm count and motility evaluation. Fertility and Sterility 33: 337–338

Moghissi K S 1976 Postcoital test: physiological basis, technique and interpretation. Fertility and Sterility 27: 117–129

Moghissi K S, Sim G S 1975 Correlation between hysterosalpingography and pelvic endoscopy for the evaluation of tubal factor. Fertility and Sterility 28: 1178–1183

Moghissi K S, Wallach E E 1983 Unexplained Infertility. Fertility and Sterility 39: 5–21

Okonofua F E, Essen U I, Nimalaraj T 1989 Hysterosalpingography versus laparoscopy in tubal infertility: comparison based on findings at laparotomy. International Journal of Gynaecology and Obstetrics 28: 143–147

Steptoe P C 1967 Laparoscopy in gynaecology. Churchill Livingstone, Edinburgh

Templeton A A, Penney G C 1982 The incidence, characteristics and prognosis of patients whose infertility is unexplained. Fertility and Sterility 37: 175–181

Tredway D R, Misschell D R Jr, Moyer D 1973. Correlation of endometrial dating with luteinizing hormone peak. American Journal of Obstetrics and Gynecology 117: 1030–1033

Van der Ven H H, Jeyendran R S, A I Hasani S et al 1986 Correlation between human sperm swelling in hypoosmotic medium (hypoosmotic swelling test) and in vitro fertilization. Journal of Andrology 7: 190–196

17. New frontiers in assisted reproduction

N. N. Amso R. W. Shaw

INTRODUCTION

Perhaps no other breakthrough in the field of reproductive medicine has generated such hope for thousands of subfertile women as the development of in vitro fertilization (IVF).

The past decade has witnessed dramatic changes in patient expectations, the attitudes of clinicians and the public towards the problems and needs of the subfertile couple, and the provision of highly complicated and expensive treatments. The natural cycle was quickly replaced with the use of superovulation protocols to increase the number of oocytes obtained, and hence optimize the number of embryos replaced. Similarly, laparoscopic egg collection was replaced by less invasive ultrasound-guided techniques, thus transforming an inpatient treatment into an outpatient day-case approach. New methods of sperm preparations, embryo culture and freezing have resulted in improved fertilization and pregnancy rates. These exciting advances, often magnified by the popular press, unjustly raised patient expectations and placed enormous pressure and demand for such treatment on the underfunded health service. Pregnancy rates unfortunately remain low, and couples are subjected to great stress and trauma before, during, and after their treatment. This necessitated the establishment of counselling as an integral part of any assisted reproduction programme. Finally, the need for continued research and increase in knowledge has generated widespread debate, nationally and internationally, especially on the emotive subject of embryo research. Many countries have already introduced legislation controlling or banning embryo research (the UK, Australia, Germany) and many others are in the process of doing so.

This chapter will address the developments in patient management, laboratory techniques, and the outcome of these treatments. It will also try to outline the controversies that are presently being hotly debated.

SELECTION AND PREPARATION OF PATIENTS

Although IVF was initially instituted to bypass tubal blockage, it is now utilized in the treatment of various causes of infertility. The current indications are listed below:

1. Tubal disease.
2. Unexplained infertility.
3. Treated endometriosis.
4. Male factor infertility.
5. Failed artificial insemination by donor (AID).
6. Cervical hostility.
7. Failed ovulation induction.
8. Absent or inappropriate ovaries.
9. Therapy for female cancer.

Many units have evolved specific criteria for inclusion of patients on their programmes. Each couple should be assessed carefully prior to their enrolment on the waiting list. Factors like female age, antisperm antibodies, sperm dysfunction and severe endometriosis affect the success rate considerably. Women with mild and treated endometriosis or unexplained infertility have a better prognosis. Some assisted reproduction programmes may be selective in entering patients on their programmes. Prior to initiation of therapy, it is important to evaluate the couple's suitability for IVF treatment. Additionally, information-giving and decision-making aspects of counselling should be made available by a specially trained counsellor as a matter of routine to all couples. These couples have frequently undergone extensive investigations, are under considerable stress, and their marriage is often under strain. IVF treatment should not be used as a panacea for marital or psychosexual disorders, but to fulfil the wishes of a well adjusted couple to have a baby.

The male and female partner are interviewed together and an appropriate history and clinical examination are undertaken for both. A number of tests are carried out prior to initiation of the treatment (Table 17.1). Hepatitis B and human immunodeficiency virus (HIV) III screening is carried out to ensure safety of the staff, to prevent spread of infection should the patient's serum be used for culture media, or when oocytes are being donated. Laparoscopy should be carried out to confirm a normal pelvis if gamete intrafallopian transfer (GIFT) is to be the treatment of choice. Similarly, the male partner undergoes various tests. Semen assessment should be repeated more than once before initiation of the treatment cycle and all semen parameters (total count, density, motility, progression, morphology and presence of white cells) should be recorded.

Table 17.1 Tests indicated for female and male partners

Female
Baseline hormone profile
Luteal-phase progesterone
Assessment of tubal patency
Serum antisperm antibodies
Rubella status
HIV III and hepatitis B screening
Male
Semen analysis and microbiology
Hamster egg penetration test*
Serum antisperm antibodies
HIV III, and hepatitis B screening

* Where indicated in unexplained infertility and male sperm dysfunction.
HIV III = human immunodeficiency virus III.

The couple must be well informed about the details of their treatment, the techniques involved, and the indications for the tests they have to undergo. Assisted reproduction involves four principal steps;

1. The induction and timing of ovulation.
2. Egg collection.
3. Fertilisation (IVF).
4. The replacement of gamete/embryos.

CLINICAL MANAGEMENT OF THE TREATMENT CYCLE

The first successful birth from IVF-embryo transfer (ET) in 1978 resulted from a single oocyte obtained from the dominant follicle in a natural ovarian cycle. Success rates were found to be improved when multiple embryos were transferred thus at present, the majority of assisted reproduction programmes undertake ovarian stimulation to induce multiple follicular development.

Normal folliculogenesis

This involves several important and inter-related steps:

1. Follicular recruitment: this occupies the first few days of the ovarian cycle and allows the follicle to continue

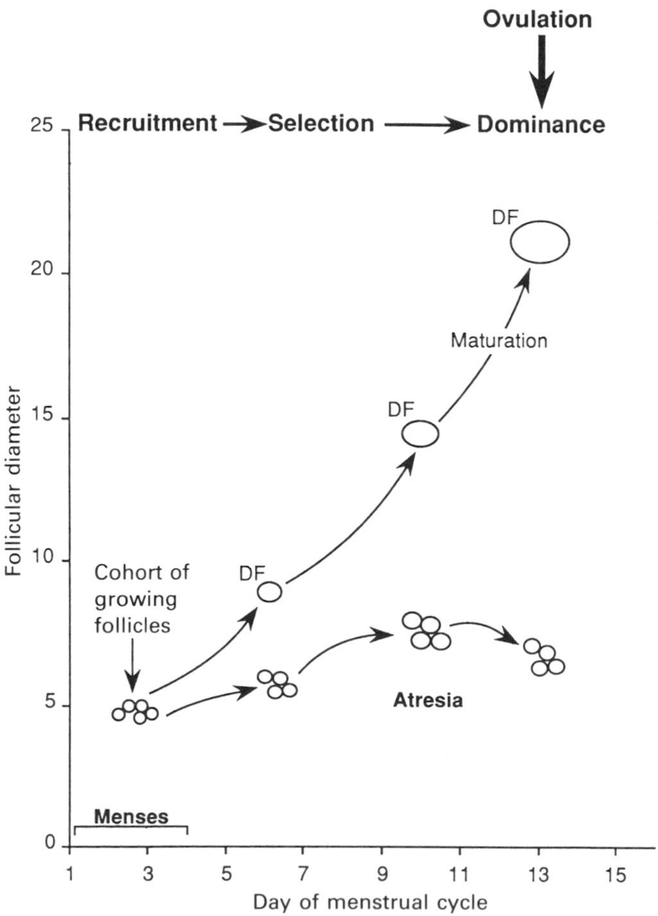

Fig. 17.1a Selection and maturation of the dominant follicle (DF) during a natural cycle.

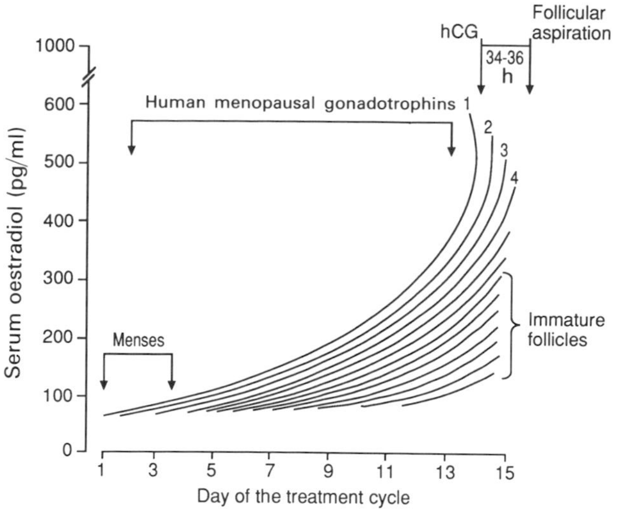

Fig. 17.1b Induced follicular maturation with gonadotrophin therapy over-riding selection of a single dominant follicle, as in the natural cycle.

to mature in the correct gonadotrophic environment and to progress towards ovulation.

2. Selection: this is the mechanism whereby a single follicle is chosen and ultimately achieves ovulation.
3. Dominance: the selected follicle maintains its pre-eminence over all other follicles and occupies days 8–12 of the primate ovarian cycle.

Follicular development beyond the antral stage depends on the concentration of follicle-stimulating hormone (FSH) in the circulation. Once a threshold level has been attained, follicular growth beyond 4 mm occurs. The interval during which FSH remains elevated above threshold level can be regarded as a gate through which a follicle must pass to avoid atresia. The width of the gate will therefore determine the number of follicles which can be selected for ovulation (Fig. 17.1). The preovulatory luteinizing hormone (LH) surge is triggered by the positive feedback of oestradiol (E_2) from the dominant follicle as well as other follicular contributory factors. Ovulation occurs between 24 and 36 h after the onset of the LH surge.

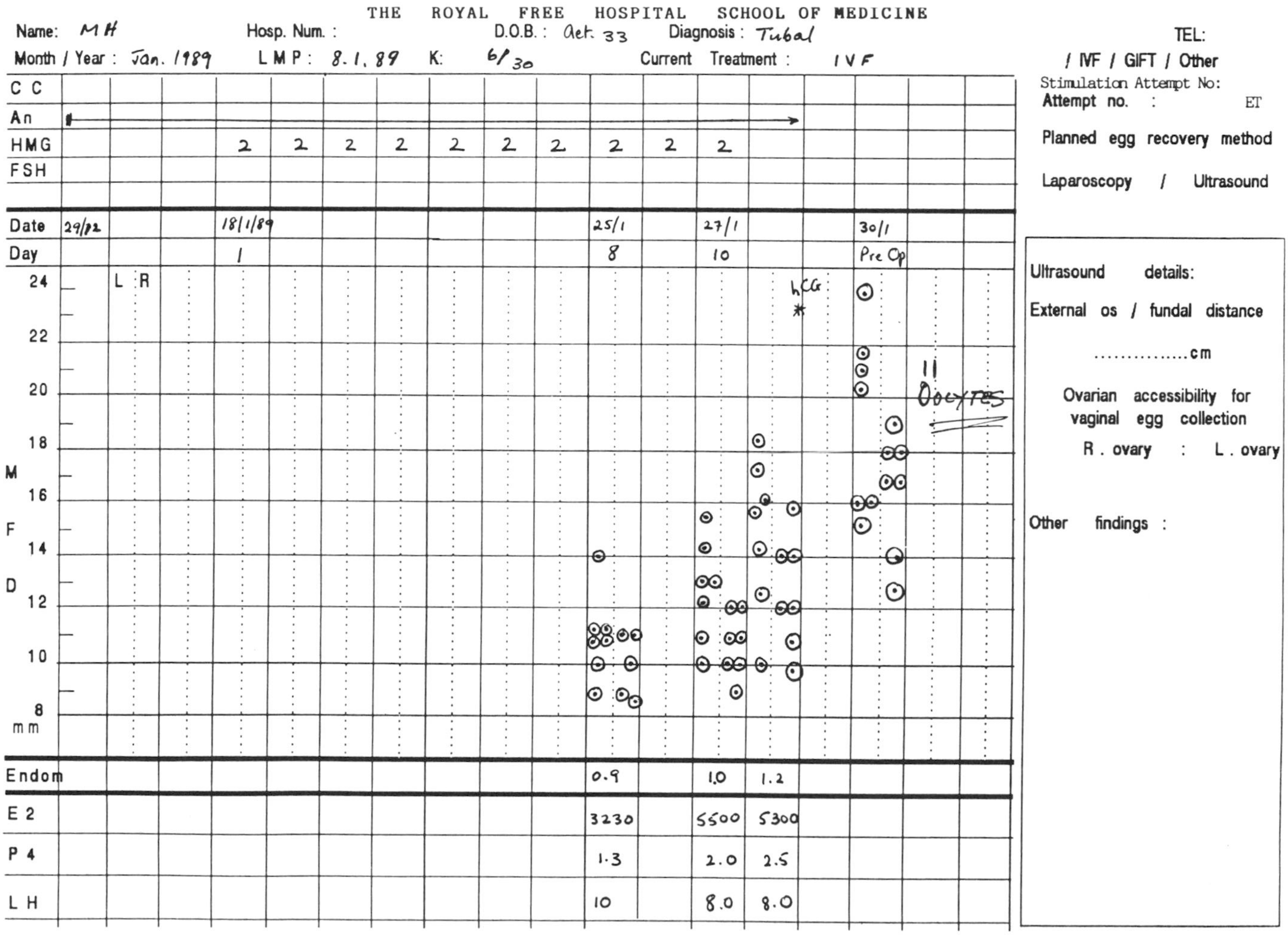

THE ROYAL FREE HOSPITAL SCHOOL OF MEDICINE

Name: MH Hosp. Num.: D.O.B.: Aet. 33 Diagnosis: Tubal TEL:

Month / Year: Jan. 1989 LMP: 8.1.89 K: 6/30 Current Treatment: IVF / IVF / GIFT / Other

CC															
An															
HMG			2	2	2	2	2	2	2	2	2	2			
FSH															
Date	29/12		18/1/89							25/1		27/1		30/1	
Day			1							8		10		Pre Op	

Stimulation Attempt No:
Attempt no. : ET
Planned egg recovery method
Laparoscopy / Ultrasound

24, 22, 20, 18, 16, 14, 12, 10, 8 mm — MFD — L R — hCG * — 11 Oocytes

Ultrasound details:
External os / fundal distance
...............cm
Ovarian accessibility for vaginal egg collection
R. ovary : L. ovary
Other findings :

	25/1	27/1	
Endom	0.9	1.0	1.2
E 2	3230	5500	5300
P 4	1.3	2.0	2.5
L H	10	8.0	8.0

Fig. 17.2 Folliculogram showing satisfactory ovarian response after 10 days of gonadotrophin therapy.

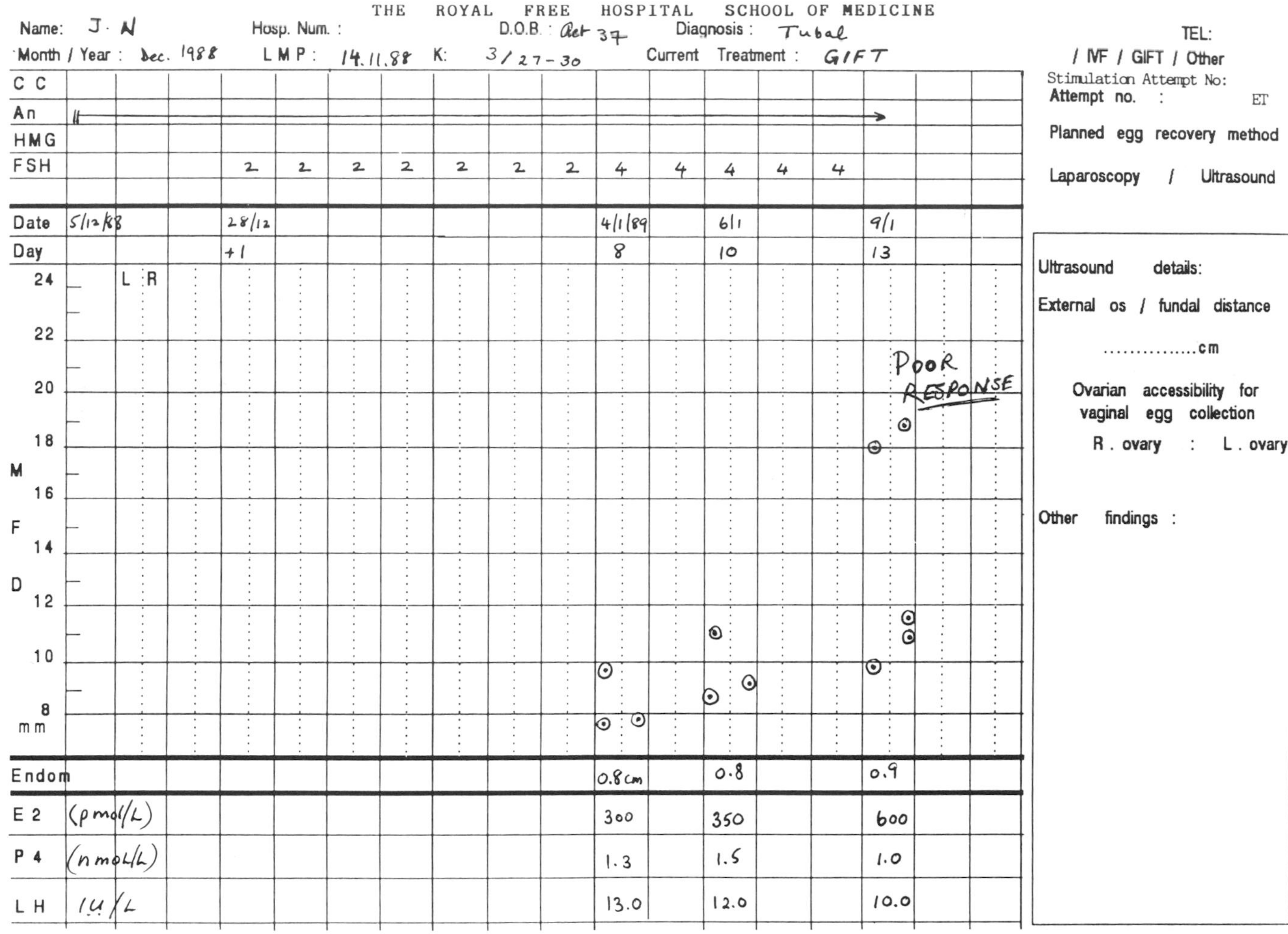

THE ROYAL FREE HOSPITAL SCHOOL OF MEDICINE

Name: J. N   Hosp. Num. :   D.O.B. : Aet 37   Diagnosis : Tubal   TEL:

Month / Year : Dec. 1988   LMP : 14.11.88   K: 3/27–30   Current Treatment : GIFT   / IVF / GIFT / Other

Stimulation Attempt No:
Attempt no. : ET

Planned egg recovery method

Laparoscopy / Ultrasound

CC																	
An	→	→	→	→	→	→	→	→	→	→	→	→	→	→	→		
HMG																	
FSH				2	2	2	2	2	2	2	4	4	4	4	4		
Date	5/12/88			28/12							4/1/89		6/1			9/1		
Day				+1							8		10			13		

Endom											0.8cm		0.8			0.9		
E 2	(pmol/L)										300		350			600		
P 4	(nmol/L)										1.3		1.5			1.0		
LH	IU/L										13.0		12.0			10.0		

Ultrasound details:

External os / fundal distance

..............cm

Ovarian accessibility for vaginal egg collection

R. ovary : L. ovary

Other findings :

Fig. 17.3 Poor follicular response in a patient aged 37 years.

The aims of superovulation regimens in assisted reproduction are to maximize the number of follicles which mature; to minimize the degree of asychrony amongst developing follicles and to minimize the deleterious effects of the abnormal follicular environment on luteal function and endometrial receptivity. Multiple follicular development and ovulation can be achieved by widening the FSH gate. Several drug combinations have been used to achieve this, and are listed below:

1. Clomiphene citrate + human menopausal gonadotrophin (hMG) and/or pure FSH.
2. hMG and/or pure FSH alone.
3. Gonadotrophin-releasing hormone (GnRH) analogue + hMG and/or pure FSH.

Clomiphene citrate, alone or in combination with gonadotrophins, has been very popular. More recently, GnRH analogues have been increasingly used in superovulation protocols in conjunction with gonadotrophins. The GnRH analogue is commenced either in the mid luteal phase and continued until complete down-regulation is achieved (long protocol), or started on the first day of the menstrual cycle (short protocol).

Many programmes commence ovarian stimulation with the onset of the menstrual cycle. This will lead to oocyte recoveries taking place at random according to follicular development and maturation. Consequently, such units are obliged to work 7 days a week, which streches human resources. Alternatively, oocyte retrieval may be programmed to coincide with a working day by manipulating the onset of the menstrual cycle using norethisterone tablets or utilizing the hypogonadotrophic effect of GnRH analogues prior to commencing gonadotrophins on a predetermined day of the week. The down-regulatory phase may be prolonged to allow a fixed number of patients to be treated each week. Follicular response is monitored by ultrasound scans and serum hormone assays for oestrogen, LH, and progesterone commencing on the 8th day of the treatment cycle. The gonadotrophin dosage is adjusted according to ovarian response. When three or

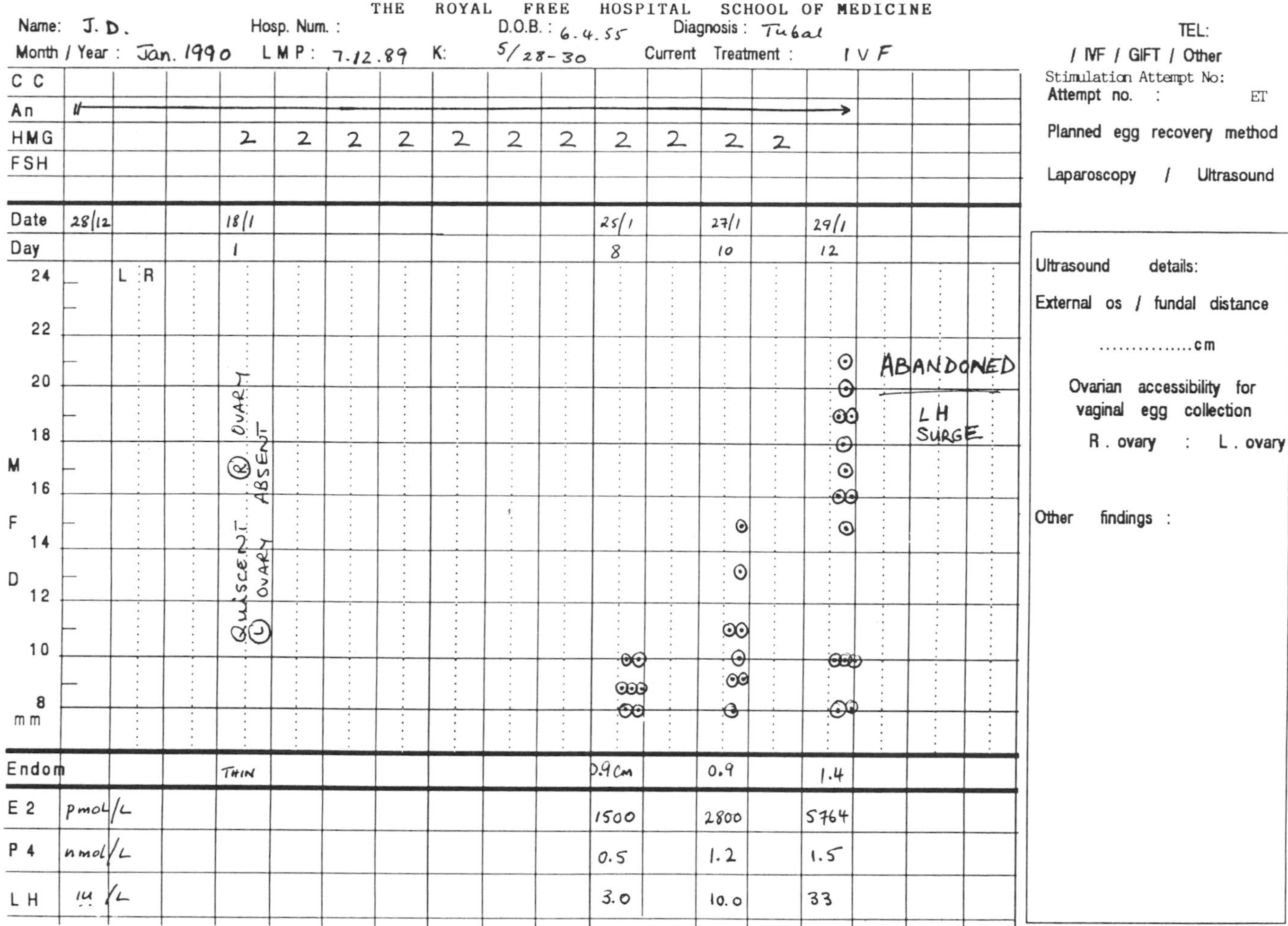

Fig. 17.4 Premature LH surge prior to the hCG injection. The treatment cycle was abandoned.

more follicles are greater than 18 mm in diameter, 5000 u of human chorionic gonadotrophin (hCG) is given intramuscularly 34–36 hours prior to oocyte collection. Oocyte retrieval takes place on a weekday, 13 days or more after commencing gonadotrophin stimulation.

Figure 17.2 depicts a typical ovarian response, where follicles are noted to grow at rate of 2–3 mm/day accompanied by a steady increase in serum E_2 levels. Unfortunately, not all stimulation cycles progress in this typical pattern, and many may have to be abandoned before oocyte collection for a variety of reasons. In a retrospective analysis of 314 stimulation cycles commenced in 1988, we found that 30.9% of cycles were abandoned before oocyte collection (Table 17.2). While premature LH surge and preoperative ovulation have been largely eliminated by the introduction of GnRH analogue, other problems such as poor ovarian response or the development of ovarian hyperstimulation remain unresolved.

Table 17.2 Causes of abandoned stimulation cycles in IVF/GIFT

Total number of IVF/GIFT cycles	314
Number of abandoned cycles	97 (30.9%)
Poor/no response	56 (57.7%)
Premature LH surge	15 (15.5%)
Preoperative ovulation	12 (12.4%)
Risk of hyperstimulation	11 (11.3%)
Other	3 (3.1%)
Number proceeded to oocyte collection	217 (69.1%)

Poor ovarian response

When no or fewer than three follicles develop after 14 days of gonadotrophin treatment, the stimulation cycle is aborted (Fig. 17.3). This problem is frequently encountered in women over the age of 37 years and those with severe ovarian endometriosis. Often, few oocytes of low quality are obtained and pregnancy rates are usually poor. Increasing the starting dose of gonadotrophins may somctimes improve the response and enable recruitment of a larger number of oocytes. The use of GnRH analogues in patients with moderate or severe endometriosis has resulted in a better response, an increase in the number of oocytes retrieved and fertilized and an improved outcome.

Premature LH surge/preoperative ovulation

These constitute a high proportion of abandoned cycles, especially when facilities to carry out oocyte retrieval, once the surge is detected, are not available; when endocrine monitoring is not performed, and when oocyte retrievals are programmed to take place on determined days of the week only. The introduction of GnRH analogues in superovulation protocols has largely eliminated these problems and enabled a better control of the stimulation cycle (Fig. 17.4).

Risk of hyperstimulation

Women with polycystic ovarian disease are at a particular risk of developing hyperstimulation, may have high tonic LH levels or suffer premature ovulation (Fig. 17.5). Their ovarian response is often unpredictable (Shaw & Amso 1991). When there is a risk of hyperstimulation developing, withholding the hCG injection will almost completely eliminate that risk (Fig. 17.6). However, when clinical symptoms and signs develop after the hCG injection, operation or before the embryo transfer, then an alternative approach may be adopted. The follicles are aspirated, the oocytes fertilized, but embryo replacement is postponed, and the developing embryos are cryopreserved. If the patient is on GnRH analogues, then treatment is continued throughout the luteal phase to induce luteolysis. The embryos are transferred in subsequent cycles, resulting in pregnancies (Amso et al 1990).

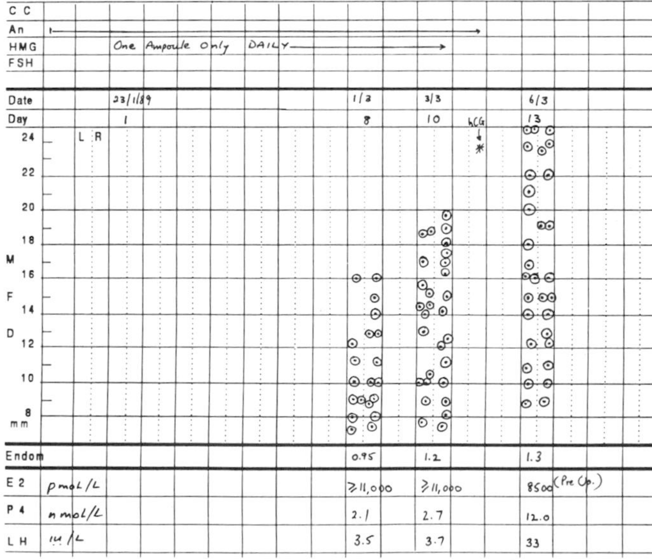

Fig. 17.5 Excessive follicular response in a patient with polycystic ovaries in spite of receiving only one ampoule of Pergonal daily. A total of 23 oocytes were retrieved at vaginal egg collection. The patient, however, did not develop symptoms and signs of ovarian hyperstimulation syndrome.

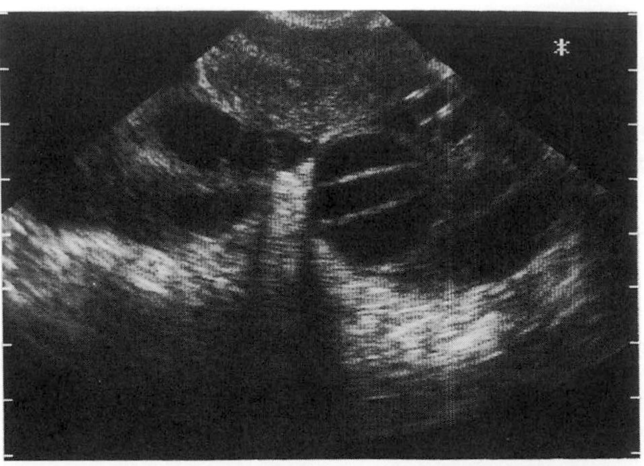

Fig. 17.6a Vaginal ultrasound appearance of the hyperstimulated ovaries. The enlarged ovaries almost completely occupy the pelvis and contain an excessive number of large, intermediate and small follicles.

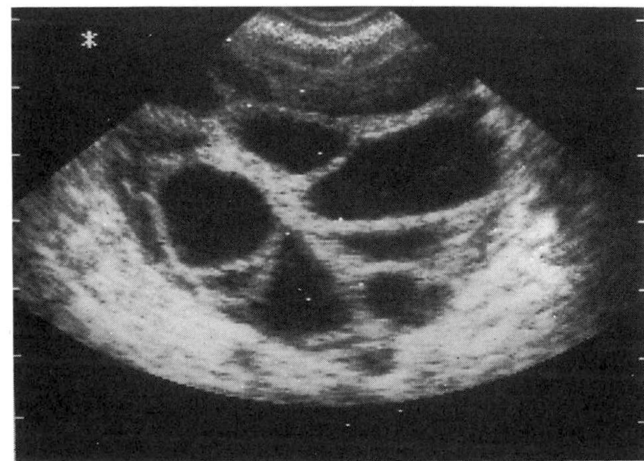

Fig. 17.6b Vaginal ultrasound appearance of the mature follicles in a normal ovary prior to vaginal egg collection.

OOCYTE COLLECTION

Methods of egg collection have improved considerably over the past few years. The main motivation for these technical advances is to limit the high cost of IVF treatment which is largely due to time spent in hospital, the type of anaesthesia, and the degree of invasiveness of the procedure and its morbidity.

Laparoscopic egg collection

At first, all egg collections were laparoscopic. Presently, laparoscopic egg collection is reserved for patients being treated with GIFT. The need for general anaesthesia and the frequently encountered limited access to adherent or covered ovaries have meant that simpler ultrasound-guided techniques have replaced laparoscopy as the principal method for egg collection in IVF.

Ultrasound-guided egg collection

Transvesical/transurethral techniques

Abdominal transducers with frequencies between 3.5 and 5.0 MHz are used to visualize the follicles through the full bladder. Both techniques are easy to learn, quick and do not require hospitalization for a long period. However, local anaesthesia is often insufficient for adequate pain relief, in addition to the discomfort experienced by filling the bladder. The transurethral approach may also be complicated by haematuria.

Vaginal egg collection

A specially designed vaginal ultrasound transducer is used to visualize the follicles and along its side the aspirating needle is passed. This method is generally well tolerated when carried out under light intravenous sedation, can be learnt very quickly and is associated with minimal morbidity. It has almost completely replaced all previously described ultrasound methods. Ideally, both laparoscopy and ultrasound-guided techniques should be available to accommodate the anatomical needs of all patients.

Equipment and preparation. Several ultrasound machines are now equipped with slim-line vaginal probes with frequency of between 6 and 7.5 MHz. The probes may have a diameter of 1.5 cm only and together with the needle guide occupy minimum space in the vagina, causing least discomfort.

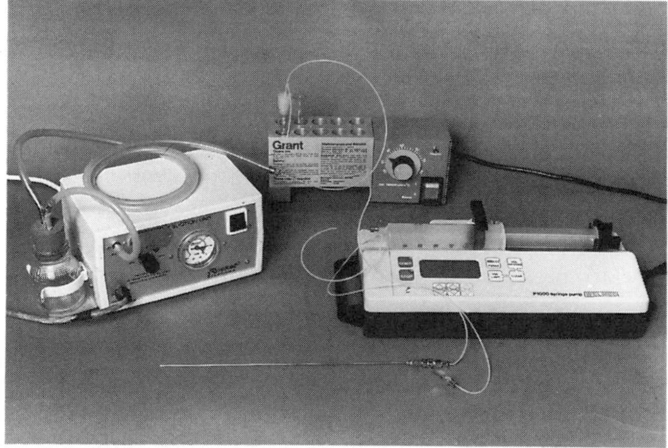

Fig. 17.7 An assembled follicle aspiration needle connected to a test-tube and a flushing syringe pump. The test-tube is in turn connected to a suction pump.

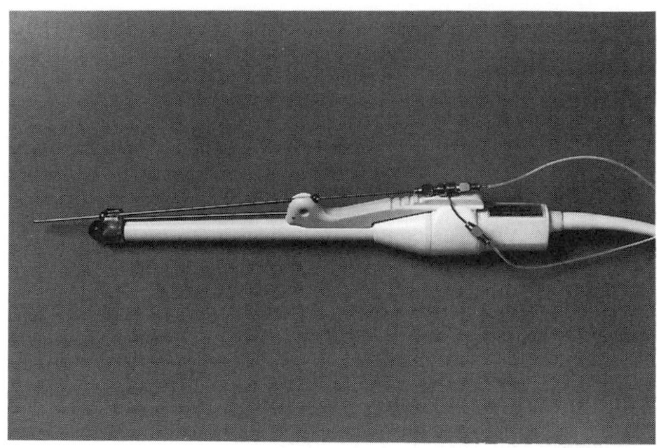

Fig. 17.8 Vaginal ultrasound transducer with needle bracket and guide. The needle tip is protruding from the proximal end of the probe.

Several designs of aspiration needles are available. They may have a single or double lumen to enable aspiration and flushing through different routes. The needle must have a very sharp tip to enable easy puncture of mobile ovaries and its distal 2 cm should be roughened to enhance ultrasound visualization. The needle is connected by tubing to a test-tube to which suction is applied from a foot-operated pump (Fig. 17.7).

The ultrasound transducer (Fig. 17.8) is enclosed in a special sterile condom and plastic sleeve prior to insertion into the vagina and should be thoroughly cleaned with a damp cloth after each procedure.

Anaesthesia. Vaginal egg collections may be performed under general anaesthesia or intravenous sedation with diazepam (5–12.5 mg) and pethidine (75–125 mg). The dose given varies according to the patient's tolerance and the time taken to complete the operation.

Technique. The patient is placed in the lithotomy position and the vagina is cleaned carefully. Prior to puncture of the lateral vaginal vault, the ovaries should be carefully scanned to determine the plane which will enable the best access to the largest follicles. The needle is pushed through the vaginal wall and into the first follicle by a single, firm thrusting movement. Suction is applied as soon as the needle tip is seen to be within the follicle which will be seen to collapse as the follicular fluid is aspirated (Fig. 17.9). During aspiration, the needle is rotated and moved gently in all directions within the follicle to increase the chance of oocyte retrieval. If the oocyte is not recovered in the first aspirate, the follicle is flushed several times. We use a footpedal-controlled pump to facilitate delivery of flushing media at a steady rate. Once the egg is obtained, the needle is lined against a neighbouring follicle without

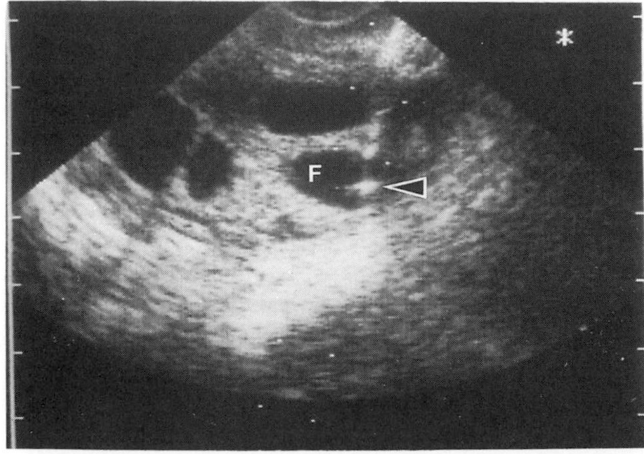

Fig. 17.9 Ultrasound picture during vaginal egg recovery. The tip of the needle (arrow) is seen within the follicle (F). The two parallel dotted lines demarcate the path of the needle. The dots are 1 cm apart.

removing it from the ovarian surface. Unanaesthetized patients will experience pain when the external follicular surface is entered. However, the procedure is well tolerated and usually completed in about 30 min. At the end, the vaginal vault should be inspected to exclude bleeding from puncture sites. The patient recovers quickly, and will be able to leave the hospital after a few hours.

Complications. In our experience, very few difficulties have been encountered during vaginal egg collections:

1. Mobile ovaries may be stabilized with gentle suprapubic or iliac fossa pressure; the use of sharp needles usually overcome this difficulty.
2. If the uterus lies between the vaginal vault and the ovary, manual suprapubic pressure or redirection of the transducer will often bring the ovary in direct line with the needle. Occasionally, the ovary will need to be accessed by passing the needle through the uterus. This is rather painful for the unanaesthetized patient but appears to have minimal risk of damage or bleeding.
3. Pelvic vessel puncture has been reported but appears to be without sequelae.
4. Severe pelvic sepsis may develop, most commonly in patients with a history of chronic pelvic inflammatory disease or following inadvertent bowel injury. Prophylactic antibacterial cover may be given preoperatively either routinely or for certain high-risk patients. In over 250 vaginal procedures we have carried out so far, only 1 patient developed clinical pelvic infection postoperatively.

GAMETE/EMBRYO REPLACEMENT

Embryo replacement into the uterine cavity is a relatively simple procedure, but must be carried out very meticulously to ensure appropriate placement of the embryos approximately 1 cm from the uterine fundus (Fig. 17.10).

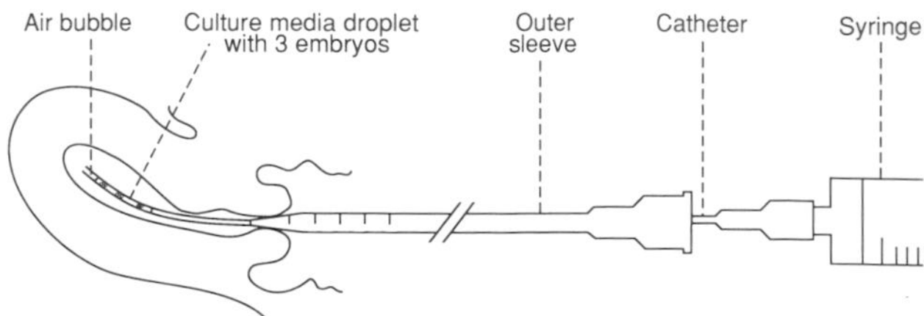

Fig. 17.10 Loaded ET catheter. Three embryos are ready to be deposited within 1 cm of the uterine fundus.

Intrafallopian replacement, at present, is carried out mainly laparoscopically. The gametes or embryos are loaded into a specially designed catheter which is passed through the fimbrial end and manipulated 3–6 cm into the ampulla. Catheterization of the fallopian tube may sometimes be difficult and a Palmer grasping forceps may be used to secure the fallopian tube by pinching a small amount of serosa close to the fimbrial end. Recently, ultrasound-guided transvaginal cannulation of the fallopian tube has been tried for intratubal insemination/embryo transfer.

LABORATORY PROCEDURES IN ASSISTED REPRODUCTION

General principles

The laboratory procedures involved include:

1. Sperm preparation and separation from the seminal plasma.
2. The identification of oocytes at the time of operation.
3. The addition of washed sperm to human eggs in culture media resulting in the dissociation of the cumulus oophorus, binding of sperm to, and penetration of the zona pellucida.
4. Embryo assessment at 20 and 48 h after insemination.

Although the above steps appear relatively simple, it is considered that this part of the IVF procedure is the one most likely to cause difficulty. It is certainly the part most likely to be considered at fault when a programme suffers a low success rate (Trounson 1989). However, it is often difficult to identify a specific problem because of our inability to measure embryo quality. In this section, the general principles of laboratory procedures will be described and emphasis will be placed on those aspects which require careful attention.

Quality control

It is very important to institute strict quality control measures in the human reproduction laboratory to ensure high fertilization rates, embryo quality and consequently to maintain consistent pregnancy rates. Unfortunately, there is no simple quality control test that will guarantee optimal laboratory procedures. Mouse embryo cultures have been widely used as a quality control model to identify sub-optimal culture media conditions or toxic effects in culture components. Incubators must be cleaned and sterilized on a regular basis, and measures taken to ensure that temperature, carbon dioxide and humidity controls are functioning properly. Heating blocks and warm plates must be constantly checked to prevent overheating as temperatures $\geqslant$ 40°C will irreversibly damage cells in mitosis. All glassware and items which come into contact with culture media, gametes or embryos should be thoroughly cleaned, adequately rinsed with ultrapure water and sterilized before use. Contamination of culture ware and incubators with micro-organisms, yeast and fungi has occurred in laboratories from presumed sterile sources, resulting in the loss of all the eggs and embryos in culture at the time.

Media for insemination and culture of embryos

There are no specific guidelines for the choice of an ideal culture medium. However, a wide range of culture media has been used. They can be divided into complex and simple balanced salt solutions. Complex tissue culture media contain many substances and are made commercially. Simple balanced salt solutions are used by the majority of assisted reproduction laboratories for egg handling, insemination and culture of embryos. Several formulae are available but probably Earle's solution and Whittingham's T6 are the most commonly used media. Human serum is routinely added to culture media as proteins allow easier handling of embryos and prevent their adherence to plastic or glass surfaces. Embryos in vitro appear to develop more slowly than in vivo and their viability is reduced with increasing time in culture. It is of interest to note that, at present, results of GIFT/ZIFT (zygote intrafallopian transfer) are better than IVF, thus highlighting the influence of in vitro conditions.

Evaluation of eggs

Determination of egg quality is a subjective and difficult task. Oocytes from atretic follicles can be identified by their dark and gritty granulosa, and oocytes from immature follicles by their poorly dispersed cumulus cells and tightly packed granulosa cells. However, these parameters are non-specific and it has been shown that 29% of eggs with completely expanded cumuli are mitotically immature.

Sperm preparation

The sperm used for insemination in vitro or for GIFT is prepared by the wash and swim-up technique. Briefly, culture media is added to the semen sample, centrifuged for 10 min at 600 g and the supernatant is then discarded. The semen pellet is then resuspended in a small volume (0.5 ml) of medium, gently layered with fresh medium and incubated for 45–60 min. The uppermost portion containing the actively motile sperm is removed and approximately 50 000 sperm (10 000–500 000) are added to the egg in tissue culture dishes. Increasing sperm concentration is likely to increase the rate of polyspermic fertilization. Semen samples from patients with male factor infertility require different methods of preparation to obtain a high proportion of actively motile sperm.

Embryo assessment

The eggs may demonstrate signs of fertilization when examined 12–24 h after insemination. The presence of two distinct pronuclei is an indication of successful fertilization (Fig. 17.11). This is important for several reasons: it has been shown that delayed fertilization is associated with severely reduced embryo viability. Moreover, 87% of eggs which formed pronuclei later than 17–20 h after insemination had chromosomal anomalies, compared with 29% of those which had developed two pronuclei at the 17–20 h stage. The latter group obviously have priority for transfer. Polyspermy (fertilization by more than one sperm) as manifested by the presence of more than two pronuclei results in embryos with variable potential for cleavage. Triploidy usually causes the death of the embryo or fetus, and triploid or androgenetic embryos contribute to trophoblastic disease, e.g. *hydatidiform* mole and chorionic tumours, thus these embryos should not be replaced.

At present, the evaluation of embryo viability is subjective. However, it is generally agreed that embryos which divide evenly, regularly and rapidly have the highest viability or the capacity for development to term when

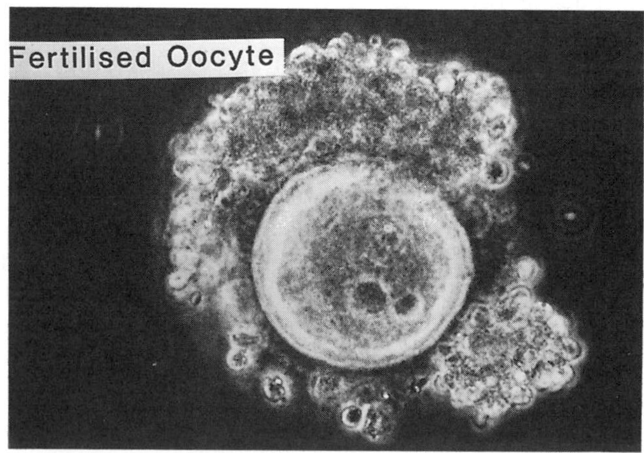

Fig. 17.11 Pronuclear embryo 18 h post insemination. The two pronuclei are clearly visible.

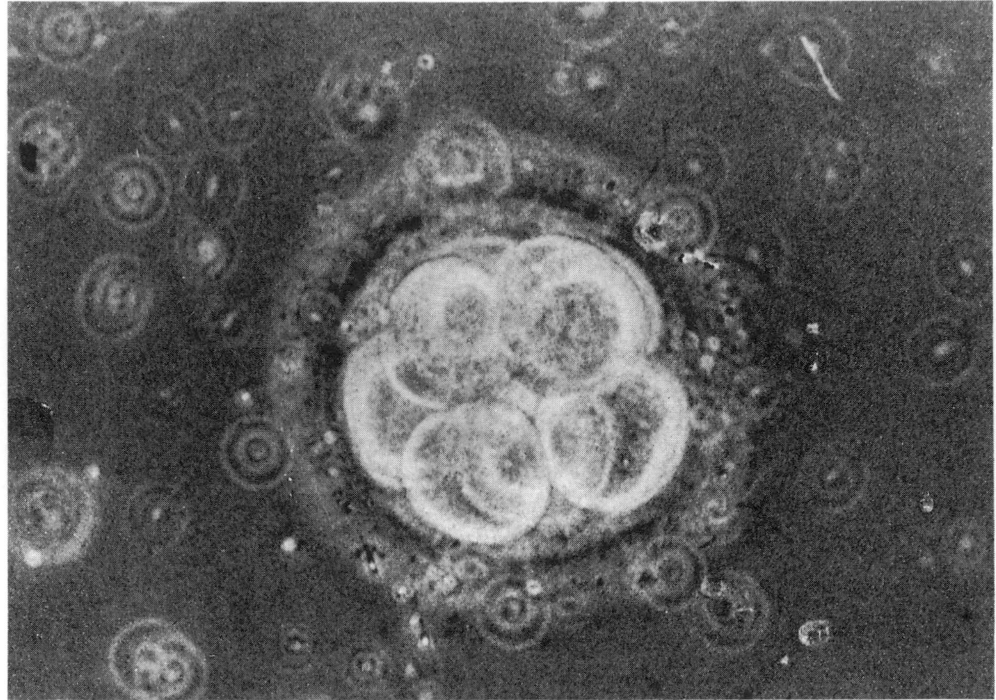

Fig. 17.12 An 8-cell stage pre-embryo. The blastomeres are evenly divided.

replaced in utero (Fig. 17.12). Scoring systems of embryo quality have been devised and are based on the symmetry and rate of cleavage, evenness of cytoplasm, and the presence or absence of anucleate fragments. These indices give a good guide to the prospects of pregnancy, but while they may be helpful, there is an urgent need to develop other tests (invasive or non-invasive) of embryonic normality. These may be biochemical assays (pyruvate and glucose uptake); biophysical (quantitative fluorescence microscopy) or microsurgical (embryo biopsy) techniques to detect chromosomal anomalies (Handyside 1990).

Embryo cryopreservation

Human embryos were successfully cryopreserved as early as 1983 using techniques adapted from methods initially introduced for cattle embryos. Since then, cryopreservation has been introduced into clinical IVF as a way of dealing with excess embryos resulting from superovulation protocols. Current methods of cryopreservation involve slow cooling of embryos to temperatures around −30 to −40°C in the presence of cryoprotectant to avoid intracellular ice formation. The embryos are then rapidly cooled to −196°C by transfer into liquid nitrogen. Thawing of embryos may be either a rapid or a slow process depending on initial freezing protocols. The aim in either case is to avoid growth of intracellular ice crystals and prevent damaging osmotic effects on the dehydrated cells. The main cryoprotectants in use are dimethyl sulphoxide (DMSO), glycerol, and 1,2-propanediol. There is no general agreement as to which slow cooling method or cryoprotectant is the best, but it is probable that success rates of a cryopreservation programme may depend more on the quality and viability of the embryos produced than the individual programme. It also depends on the critical training of the embryologist in freezing techniques, the quality of equipment used and the timing of embryo replacement. Survival rates of thawed embryos are variable but figures up to 88% (Testart et al 1986) have been achieved for pronuclear stage embryos frozen in 1,2-propanediol, decreasing progressively with increasing numbers of blastomeres. Furthermore, addition of 0.1 mol/l sucrose to propanediol in the freezing medium significantly improves the survival of embryos after thawing and pregnancy rates, irrespective of the cleavage stage.

Recently, interest has developed in rapid freezing techniques such as vitrification (where concentrated solutions of cryoprotectant solidify or form glass instead of crystals), vapour freezing and ultrafreezing. These techniques have not yet been used in human cryopreservation programmes on a large scale. Results from experiments on mouse embryos are encouraging and early reports from human work suggest that survival rates after thawing can approach those following slow cooling methods, and that a high proportion of embryos continue to cleave after thawing (Trounson 1989). These methods are simple, quick and inexpensive and may change the currently complex processes significantly. The successful introduction of embryo cryopreservation has helped to increase success rates, simplified the treatment of women on oocyte donation programmes and given hope to others suffering from malignant disease as embryos can be stored before chemotherapy or radiotherapy is begun.

Male factor infertility and IVF

When one or more sperm parameters are below what is regarded as normal (according to World Health Organization criteria), then chances of fertilization and pregnancy are greatly reduced. Sperm density and motility are the two most important criteria for successful IVF. Several studies have reported the successful use of IVF for male factor infertility, achieving good pregnancy rates (Cohen et al 1985; Mahadevan et al 1985, Yovich et al 1985). Attempts have been made to improve sperm quality used for insemination by utilizing newer methods of sperm preparation. These include the Percoll gradient, Ficoll entrapment, glass bead column, and glass wool filtration method. The Percoll gradient is the most popular and its use significantly decreases the amount of debris present and increases the percentage of motile sperm.

Difficulties encountered in treating male factor infertility have prompted the development of a new technique called microsurgical fertilization. This may be achieved by microinjection of a single sperm into the egg cytoplasm — a technique not successful in humans — or subzonal insertion of sperm, or zona drilling. The latter two techniques are still being evaluated. However, several problems remain unresolved: there is a higher incidence of polyspermy; fertilization rates are low; special equipment and training are needed, and the risk of inducing chromosomal anomalies is high. Improvements in these procedures indicate that IVF will be of major use in the future treatment of male infertility.

Table 17.3 Fecundibility and mean time to conception in different groups of women

Fecundibility	Example	Mean time to conception
0.4	Age 25, fertile, first pregnancy	2–3 months
0.158	All ages, attempting first pregnancy	6 months
0.11	AID frozen semen, age <25 years	9 months
0.07	Treated endometriosis	16 months
0.065	AID frozen semen, age ≥35 years	15 months
0.011	Treated endometriosis + AID, age ≥35	7.3 years
0.0083	Unexplained primary infertility ≥2 years	10 years
0	Tubal obstruction or azoospermia	—

EFFICACY OF ASSISTED REPRODUCTION TECHNIQUES

Conception is a matter of chance. It is a complex process in which all 'normal' couples do not have equal potential for fertility, as manifest by a substantial biological variation in the length of time required to conceive. Several factors influence the couple's chance of conception (fecundibility) and the mean time required to achieve pregnancy (Jansen 1987; Table 17.3).

Therefore, it is important when evaluating the efficacy of assisted reproduction techniques to bear in mind the duration of infertility, the age of the female partner, the multiplicity of factors responsible for the couple's subfertility, and the number of treatment cycles they have undergone. Similarly, it is essential to conduct properly designed randomized clinical trials, including the use of appropriate control groups, to ascertain the efficacy of these therapeutic modalities in a specific clinical setting (Haney 1987). At present, the most common indicators for successful treatment are biochemical, clinical or live birth pregnancy.

Successful outcome after IVF/GIFT depends on:

1. Attention to techniques for sterilization of equipment, gamete preparation and the technique of tubal catheterization and embryo transfer.
2. The number of pre-embryos/oocytes transferred (Table 17.4).
3. The number of treatment cycles carried out yearly in the institution.
4. The age, length of previous infertility, and diagnosis of the woman being treated.

Table 17.4 Pregnancy and multiple pregnancy rates per pre-embryo or gamete transfer

No of pre-embryos or eggs transferred	IVF		GIFT	
	Pregnancy rate (%)	Multiple pregnancy rate (%)	Pregnancy rate (%)	Multiple pregnancy rate (%)
One	9.6	1.0	10.0	—
Two	14.2	13.1	12.6	9.3
Three	25.2	29.2	23.1	19.1
Four	23.4	24.2	26.9	21.0
Five or more	—	—	25.8	31.2

From Interim Licensing Authority (1990).

Table 17.5 Efficacy of IVF/ET treatment as reported by various registers

Study	Efficacy per 100 cycles		Efficacy per 100 ET cycles	
	Clinical pregnancy	Live birth	Clinical pregnancy	Live birth
ANZ	11.6*	8.3	15.5	11.1
USA	16.0†	12.0	19.0	14.0
UK	12.5*	10.1	16.4	13.6

* Efficacy per 100 stimulation cycles; † Efficacy per 100 retrieval cycles.
ANZ = National Perinatal Statistics Unit and Fertility Society of Australia (1988).
USA = Medical Research International, and the Society for Assisted Reproductive Technology, American Fertility Society (1990).
UK = Interim Licensing Authority (1990).

Pregnancy rates vary inversely with duration of infertility and the age of the patient. Increasing the number of pre-embryos/oocytes transferred to above 3/4 respectively will need to be balanced by the empirically quantifiable risk of multiple pregnancy, but also the qualitative hazard of high multiple pregnancy in which no embryo may reach viability. Currently, assisted reproduction techniques contribute significantly to the aetiology of triplets and higher multiples, and strain the capacities of medical care for premature neonates. Efficacy rates are then calculated by using one of these outcomes as the numerator over a denominator of all stimulation cycles reaching the oocyte retrieval or pre-embryo transfer stage. However, it should be acknowledged that apart from a live birth outcome, all other pregnancies may result in preclinical spontaneous abortion, early or late spontaneous abortion, blighted ova, ectopic pregnancies and fetal death. When success is defined as biochemical pregnancy related to embryo transfer cycles, efficacy rates may be as high as 35–55%. If instead the numerator is the number of clinical pregnancies or live births, efficacy rates are more modest.

Efficacy is even lower when outcome is related to all stimulation cycles, since the ET stage is often never reached. It is estimated that the number of healthy babies per stimulation cycle amounts to about 4–5% only. Different centres vary considerably in their reported success rates and several countries have reported overall results from their assisted reproduction units (Table 17.5). The results are disappointing and rather discouraging, especially when it has been reported that a treatment-independent pregnancy rate of 12–25% occurs in women (with non-tubal factor infertility) either on the waiting list or within 2 years of discontinuation of therapy. Indeed, in some centres patients wait 1–2 years before undergoing IVF treatment to allow for spontaneous conception to occur. However, such a policy does not appreciate the psychological impact of infertility on the couples, their advancing age, social pressures and their willingness to pursue almost any reasonable effort towards achieving their goal of parenthood. More importantly, the chances of any woman conceiving are higher at a younger age and delay of treatment in many instances will be disadvantageous to the couple.

The prognosis for pregnancy also depends on the number of attempts undergone by the couples (cumulative pregnancy rate). Clinical pregnancy rate does not appear to differ after multiple attempts as long as embryo transfer occurs and the increase in calculated cumulative pregnancy rate for cycles 1–6 ranges from 13–59% in one study to 25–88% in another (Padilla & Garcia 1989). The message is that with careful evaluation, persistence in IVF-ET can lead to a successful outcome for a large proportion of couples.

Efficacy of GIFT and other assisted reproduction techniques

Since the first report which indicated consistent success with GIFT in 1984, the technique has gained wide acceptance for the treatment of unexplained infertility. Results of an international co-operative study (Asch 1987) indicated an overall pregnancy rate of 28.7% per treatment cycle (Table 17.6). It should be noted however that some studies could not detect a significant difference between the success rate of IVF-ET and GIFT in a specified group of patients.

Table 17.6 Pregnancy rate per oocyte/embryo transfer by aetiology in women treated with GIFT/ZIFT

	Asch (1987)		USA*
GIFT			
Endometriosis	32%		27%
Unexplained infertility	31%		24%
Cervical factor	28%		
Male factor	15%		24%
Immunological (male and female)	10%		30%
ZIFT			
Unexplained infertility (Deveroy et al 1989)		48%	
Male factor (Yovich et al 1988)		31%	
All categories*		35%	

*Medical Research International, and the Society for Assisted Reproductive Technology, American Fertility Society (1990).

The results also show that poor sperm parameters are not readily overcome by GIFT, thus it is essential to confirm fertilization in vitro when male factor disorders are present or suspected. The fallopian tubes should provide a more physiological environment for early embryonic development: transfer of the zygote or early cleaved embryo (ZIFT) or tubal embryo transfer (TET) into the fallopian tube has been carried out with a view to improving the outcome for such couples; a pregnancy rate of 31% per transfer has been obtained in couples with male factor infertility (Yovich et al 1988). More recently, a pregnancy rate of 48.1% per ZIFT replacement was reported in women with unexplained infertility (Deveroy et al 1989). These reports are preliminary and more definitive assessment is required.

PREGNANCIES AND THEIR OUTCOME

In the past decade, several thousand babies have been born following assisted reproduction techniques worldwide. However, large studies answering the many questions related to these pregnancies and their outcome have only recently been published. The issues which need clarification are:

1. Do these pregnancies and their outcome differ from those occurring spontaneously in normal women?
2. Are there increased risks for the mother or fetus? If so, are these risks attributed to the women, to the procedures involved, or to the management of the pregnancies?
3. Is the fetus affected in any way, either in the long or short term?

National registers obtaining results from all assisted reproduction units in the countries concerned have provided some answers to the above questions. Other advantages of these registers are:

1. The results are for the total population.
2. The data relate to a much larger number of pregnancies than is available from a single programme.
3. They enable more detailed analysis of outcomes.
4. They avoid the tendency to publish only optimal results.

The reproductive potential of subfertile women (as a cohort) appears to be different from that of normal women. Substantial and consistent differences exist in the incidence of spontaneous clinical abortion in different women: it increases with age, with previous history of abortion and perhaps with increasing gravidity. First-pregnancy abortion incidence in normal young women under the age of 30 years is low and varies between 8.3 and 11% of all intrauterine pregnancies, increasing to between 15.3 and 22.4% in women over 35 years. Most forms of infertility treatment are accompanied by an increased risk of spontaneous abortion (Table 17.7). This increased risk is not explained merely by heightened surveillance for early pregnancy losses but may be a residue of incompletely treated reproductive abnormality, or may be introduced by therapy, or both. Therefore, spontaneous abortion deserves attention and recognition equal to that of refractory infertility (persistent infertility despite technically adequate therapy) and ectopic pregnancy as a specific reproductive difficulty that may accompany treatment of infertility. Whenever controversy surrounds the relative effectiveness of different therapeutic modalities for the treatment of a particular type of infertility, the spontaneous abortion incidence may be a sensitive and objective way of assessing therapeutic efficacy. The reader is referred to a comprehensive review on the subject by Jansen (1982).

Table 17.7 Spontaneous clinical abortion and ectopic pregnancy rates among different groups of subfertile women

Cause of infertility and/or treatment	Spontaneous abortion rate (%)	Ectopic rate (%)
Primary infertility — no treatment	21.7	1.6
Anovulatory infertility treated with		
gonadotrophins	22.7	1.4
clomiphene	19.3	1.2
bromocriptine	11.8	0.9
Insemination		
Donor sperm	14.0	0.3
Husband sperm	24.3	1.9
Previous tubal surgery		
Salpingostomy	26.7	15.5
Uterotubal implantation	22.4	12.5
Macrotubal anastomosis	2–13	14.7
Microsurgical anastomosis	5–18	2.5
Salpingolysis	16.6	9.0
IVF-ET		
ANZ	23.0	5.2
ILA	20.5	5.1
USA	24.0	5.0
GIFT		
Craft et al (1988)	25.0	6.9
USA	20.0	5.0
Frozen embryo replacement		
Frydman et al (1989)	12.2	4.7
USA	23.0	5.0

ANZ = National Perinatal Statistics Unit and Fertility Society of Australia (1988).
ILA = Interim Licensing Authority (1990).
USA = Medical Research International, and the Society for Assisted Reproductive Technology, American Fertility Society (1990).

Early pregnancy loss

Sub/preclinical abortion

The diagnosis of pregnancy loss in this instance is based on embryological and endocrinological evidence of pregnancy prior to reaching the clinical stage. This seems to be a distinct problem in a number of fertility populations.

Table 17.8 Effect of maternal age on the rate of clinical spontaneous abortion

	≤25 years	25–29 years	30–34 years	35–39 years	40+ years	Overall abortion rate (%)	Total
IVF-ET							
ANZ	14.8	21.8	21.0	33.8	44.4	24.3%	(290/1194)
USA		(32.0)	22.0	24.0	60.0	25.3%	(107/422)
GIFT							
Craft et al (1988)	N/A	23.4	19.5	24.6	48.6	25%	(90/360)
USA		(13%)	14.0	29.0	38.0	20%	(42/215)

ANZ = National Perinatal Statistics Unit and Fertility Society of Australia (1988).
USA = Medical Research International, and the Society for Assisted Reproductive Technology, American Fertility Society (1990).

However, its prevalence in normal women of low age and parity may have been exaggerated. In contrast to the pattern seen in spontaneous abortion, there is no clear-cut association between preclinical abortion and maternal age, possibly indicating that embryo quality may be a more important factor in the failure of pregnancy.

Spontaneous abortion

Clinical spontaneous abortion of less than 20 weeks' gestation occurs in about 25–33% of pregnancies. It is considerably more common in IVF than in spontaneous pregnancies among young normal women. Maternal age at conception appears to be the most important factor determining continuation of pregnancy (Table 17.8). There is no evidence that an increase in the number of embryos replaced increases the abortion rate.

Ectopic pregnancy

Ectopic pregnancy occurs in about 1/200 of natural conceptions and several studies have shown it to be increasing. Its incidence is higher following most assisted reproduction techniques and especially in women <25 and >35 years. It is more likely to occur with tubal causes and frequently following tubal surgery. The results of a multicentre study covering 1163 IVF pregnancies observed a 5% ectopic pregnancy rate (Schoen & Novak 1975; Rubin et al 1983; Cohen et al 1986). Two factors were found to have a specific influence: the therapeutic use of clomiphene, which increased the rate from 3 to 6%, and the number of patent fallopian tubes with an increase from 3% (no or two patent tubes) to 13% with one patent tube. The incidence of ectopic pregnancy in different groups of subfertile women is depicted in Table 17.7. Heterotopic pregnancy (combined intra- and extrauterine pregnancy), usually a rare phenomenon, is much commoner following assisted reproduction techniques. It must be suspected in patients who present with symptoms and signs of acute abdomen with intrauterine pregnancy(ies) apparently progressing satisfactorily. Live births have been reported after surgical and conservative treatment of the ectopic pregnancy.

Anembryonic pregnancy

The final diagnosis of anembryonic pregnancy is based on the absence of sonographic or histological evidence of fetal or embryonic parts independent of the menstrual cycle or clinical data. Anembryonic pregnancy occurs in 14.4% of women presenting with threatened miscarriage, and 45.5% of those whose pregnancy has failed at the time of clinical presentation. The proportion of women with anembryonic pregnancy varies from 12% at 8 weeks to 37% at 10 weeks. Its incidence following IVF-ET or GIFT is approximately 16% of all clinical pregnancies (Riddle et al 1988).

Antenatal complications and outcome of viable pregnancies

A higher frequency of adverse outcome is encountered among these pregnancies, in part due to the increased occurrence of multiple implantations secondary to the transfer of three or more embryos. There is an increase in first-trimester bleeding in IVF as compared to spontaneous pregnancies. Also, women present more often with pregnancy-induced hypertension requiring treatment in the third trimester. This is possibly due to a greater number of primigravidae and older maternal age among these mothers. There is also a significantly higher incidence of breech presentations.

Multiple pregnancy

There is a threefold increase in the risk of multiple pregnancy when three or more pre-embryos are transferred. In recent years more pre-embryos have become available for transfer. In the UK, the Interim Licensing Authority (1986) has recommended limiting the number of eggs/pre-embryos transferred to three, or four in exceptional circumstances, in order to lower the risk of multiple pregnancy. Approximately 19% of IVF-ET live birth pregnancies in the USA were multiple in 1988. In the UK, 24% of IVF and 19.9 of GIFT pregnancies in 1988 were multiple, and consequently contributed significantly to the number of higher-order multiple births (Medical Research 1990).

Preterm delivery and low birth weight

There is a high incidence of preterm delivery in pregnancies resulting from assisted conception. Recently, the report by the Medical Research Council working party (1990) on births in Great Britain resulting from assisted conception between 1978 and 1987 found that overall, 24% of deliveries were preterm (<37 completed weeks). Although multiple pregnancy is an important factor, preterm birth among singleton pregnancies is approximately twice that in spontaneous conceptions (13 compared with 6%).

There is a more than fourfold increase in the incidence of low birth weight (<2500 g) in IVF/GIFT pregnancies, comprising 12% of singletons, 55% of twins and 94% of triplet births. Birth weights of singletons were significantly lower than those of all singletons born in England and Wales.

The reason for this unduly high frequency of preterm delivery and low birth weight babies is unclear. Maternal age, cause of infertility and high incidence of induced labour do not seem to be contributory factors. Similarly, fetal growth retardation does not appear to be significantly increased in these pregnancies. However, the average gestational age and birth weight declined with the number of embryos replaced and were also lower for babies of women admitted to hospital for bleeding and hypertension during pregnancy.

Rates of perinatal and infant mortality were about twice the national average. This was accounted for entirely once allowance had been made for multiple births and maternal age.

Mode of delivery

More babies are born by caesarean section than in natural conceptions. The overall rate ranges between 43.9 and 58% and is higher in multiple pregnancies. Many factors may contribute to this increased rate:

1. Advanced maternal age.
2. History of prolonged infertility.
3. Multiple pregnancy.
4. Breech presentation in preterm labour.
5. Low clinician threshold for operative delivery.

Congenital malformations

Many factors may contribute to a greater risk of congenital abnormalities following assisted reproduction. Several studies could not detect a significantly higher incidence of major congenital malformations or chromosomal abnormalities in these pregnancies (Frydman et al 1986). Similarly, although the numbers are still small, there is no evidence to suggest that births resulting from frozen embryo replacements are associated with an increase in these abnormalities (Frydman et al 1989). Although there is no conclusive evidence that these techniques are not associated with an increased risk of congenital malformation, the risk, if any, appears small and maternal age remains the main indication for carrying out routine tests for the detection of pregnancy abnormalities.

The long-term developmental and psychological assessment of these children in comparison with a suitable control group has not yet been thoroughly evaluated. The high incidence of preterm delivery and low birth weight emphasizes the importance of selecting appropriate controls in follow-up studies. It is known that major and minor neurological and sensory disability occurs more frequently in low birth weight infants. Information on the long-term morbidity of these babies should become available in the near future.

EMBRYO/OOCYTE DONATION

The introduction of IVF techniques and oocyte/pre-embryo donation has allowed certain categories of women now to achieve pregnancy (Table 17.9). Candidates for these procedures fall into two main groups: those with normal ovarian function and those with ovarian failure. Oocyte donors may be women undergoing IVF treatment themselves where excess oocytes may be donated, or women undergoing laparoscopic tubal sterilization. Donated embryos may be obtained from paid volunteers who are artificially inseminated with the recipient's husband's sperm and the resulting embryos are obtained by non-surgical flushing of the donor's uterine cavity.

In all instances, the most critical component is the synchronization between the donor and recipient for appropriate timing of embryo replacement (Cameron et al 1989). In recipients with normal ovarian function, the

Table 17.9 Indications for oocyte/embryo donation

Normal ovarian function
Abnormal, unfertilized or degenerate oocytes
Inadequate response to ovarian stimulation
Hereditary genetic disease
No ovarian function
Primary gonadal failure
Gonadal dysgenesis
Resistant ovary syndrome
Autoimmunity
Secondary ovarian failure
Premature menopause
Surgically absent ovaries
Failure induced by chemotherapy or radiotherapy

surge of LH can be monitored easily, in addition to determining serum levels of *oestradiol* (E_2) and progesterone (P_4). Recipients with ovarian failure must have oestrogen and progesterone therapy to prime the endometrium prior to embryo replacement. Hormonal replacement regimens may be either a fixed cyclical regimen, with E_2 administered in an incrementally increasing fashion in the follicular phase to mimic a natural cycle, followed by the introduction of progesterone$_4$ on day 15 of E_2 replacement in a 28-day cycle. Alternatively, a constant low-dose, variable-length E_2 regimen may be employed. This approach will overcome the problem of donor–recipient asynchrony by extending the follicular phase of the latter. Progesterone is commenced the day before or the day of oocyte retrieval. Embryos at 4–8-cell stage should be available for transfer on days 17–19 of the recipient's menstrual cycle. In agonadal women, exogenous steroids must be continued for at least 10 weeks until it is certain that the placenta will provide adequate endogenous support.

Results of oocyte donation and fresh gamete/embryo transfer have been very encouraging. Success rates of 14–36% per embryo transfer have been reported for natural or low-dose E_2 replacement cycles respectively. Furthermore, the integration of oocyte donation with embryo freeze-thawing has overcome many problems of cycle synchronization.

COST-EFFECTIVENESS

Assisted reproduction techniques are complex procedures usually requiring frequent hospital attendance, repeated tests and at least one operative procedure (Wagner & St Clair 1989). Hence the cost of one treatment cycle, irrespective of the outcome, may vary considerably depending on the particular set-up in which it is carried out. It has been estimated that a treatment cycle costs approximately £1500. Understandably, the cost of a live birth is considerably higher in view of the low success rate and the high incidence of early pregnancy failure. Valid estimates should also include the cost of all subsequent procedures that occur more often with these pregnancies (e.g. high-risk obstetric care, caesarean section and neonatal intensive care).

EMOTIONAL ASPECTS OF ASSISTED REPRODUCTION AND COUNSELLING

A diagnosis of infertility is profoundly distressing and represents a major life crisis for many couples. All staff working in assisted reproduction centres must recognize the emotional reactions experienced by these couples and be able to distinguish between those who are coping with their anxieties and those who need more specialized counselling services. Reactions to infertility are varied and have been likened to those associated with grief. They include initial shock, disbelief, frustration, anger and depression as well as feelings of guilt. Dealing with these reactions may lead to marital discord, sexual problems, and withdrawal from social situations which involve children. Additional emotional trauma is generated by the strains of infertility treatment. Couples require information about the demands of the stage-by-stage nature of the treatment, coping strategies and sources of emotional support available to them. Counselling referrals should be made such that couples feel that they will be helped by discussion rather than be punished for an inability to cope effectively.

Counselling is not synonymous with accepting or rejecting the couple for treatment, but is to help the couple to determine their own needs, recognize the source and nature of pressures on them, and make decisions appropriate to them. Although all medical and nursing staff in contact with the patients have a counselling component to their work, a specially trained and qualified person should provide a more specialized and intensive service. Programmes vary in their approach, from those offering it to all couples on an individual basis or in group sessions to those availing it on an as-needed basis.

Timing of counselling will vary according to the couple's — or even each partner's — needs. Certain phases are more stressful than others and require additional attention. At the time of initial diagnosis, couples often wish to discuss the medical options and alternatives available to them as well as the implications of each option. The first treatment cycle is often reported as the most emotionally demanding, combining a mixture of high hopes and apprehension. An unsuccessful treatment attempt may be associated with severe emotional reactions and couples will need to adjust to the idea that medical technology does not yet have all the answers in this area. Couples may need help to determine the number and timing of treatment cycles. Similarly, deciding to finish treatment can represent a dilemma for many. Such a decision is often traumatic although it may be accompanied by a sense of relief. Occasionally the partners may not be in agreement to stop treatment and it is helpful for them to use counselling sessions to time their final treatment course rather than after-the-event counselling.

The use of donor gametes poses additional emotional, social, legal and ethical concerns for the couple. The counsellor will discuss the implications resulting from such treatments and help couples to deal with their fears in a supportive environment.

Counselling may also be necessary to deal with pregnancy-related anxieties, and sometimes needs to be extended into the neonatal period.

ETHICAL AND LEGAL CONSIDERATIONS

The expanding indications for IVF and the introduction of new techniques such as GIFT, embryo freezing and, oocyte/embryo donation have posed ethical, moral and legal dilemmas for all workers in the field. IVF and the use of donor gametes are morally unacceptable to certain religious groups.

Advances in superovulation protocols have meant that more oocytes are generated per treatment cycle than are needed for replacement. This surplus of oocytes/embryos has allowed cryopreservation of embryos, donation of gamete/embryos to other couples, and for embryo research to be practised on a large scale.

The use of cryopreserved embryos could increase pregnancy rates by an extra 10% per cycle, avoid the need for an additional oocyte retrieval procedure, reduce the overall cost of treatment, and lessen the stress for the couple. The main legal issues concern the authority to dispose of the embryos, length of storage, posthumous use, inheritance rights and family relations after embryo donation. Ethical concerns include whether the embryo has any rights before implantation and whether dissociation of fertilization from reproduction represents an unacceptable intrusion into the natural process of reproduction.

There are many ethical and as yet unresolved legal problems associated with gamete (sperm/egg) donation. Anonymity, the source and logistics of obtaining sperm/eggs, reimbursement, and the screening of donors are constant sources of debate in the profession. The legal status of the offspring and their rights are still unsettled. Embryo donation represents a prenatal adoption for couples suffering from female and male sterility and those at risk of transmitting a serious hereditary anomaly. At present, embryo donation is not widely practised but no doubt patient demand will bring an enormous pressure on clinicians and scientists to offer this service within a strictly defined legal and ethical framework.

The issue of embryo research represents a major challenge for clinicians, scientists and society. The main reasons why such research is required are:

1. To improve the success rate in present clinical assisted reproduction programmes (Editorial 1989).
2. To continue research into genetic disorders and prevent the transmission of such disorders in couples at risk.
3. To develop better methods of contraception.

On the other hand, those opposed to research believe that life begins from the moment of conception and are concerned that uncontrolled research, or that not carried out for the benefit of the embryo, or research involving genetic selection and gene manipulation in vitro will further infringe on the rights of the embryo as a potential human being and endanger the future of the human species.

Other practical ethical considerations should address the question of who should be involved in assisted reproduction. All these concerns have led to the introduction of the Bill on human fertilization and embryology in Parliament with a view to constructing an ethically acceptable and legal framework in which to practise assisted reproduction and embryo research within specific confines and timescales.

CONCLUSION

The development of new methods for the treatment of male infertility would assist a high proportion of couples currently with bleak prospects. Embryo research may enable the identification of embryos with greater potential for implantation and development. This would be a major advance in our efforts to improve success rates. Innovations in ultrasound technology and the ability to study blood flow in the uterus and pelvis may help to identify causes of failed or poor implantation of embryos and early pregnancy loss.

All these advances will no doubt raise more ethical and legal concerns. It is our duty to reassure the public by maintaining conscientious and honest control of our practice for the benefit of humanity.

KEY POINTS

1. In vitro fertilization treatment should not be used as a panacea for marital or psychosexual disorders, but to fulfil the wishes of a well adjusted couple to have a baby.
2. The aims of superovulation regimens in assisted reproduction are to maximize the number of follicles which mature, minimize the degree of asychrony amongst developing follicles, and minimize the deleterious effects of the abnormal follicular environment on luteal function and endometrial receptivity.
3. While premature LH surge and preoperative ovulation have been largely eliminated by the introduction of GnRH-analogues, other problems such as poor ovarian response or the development of ovarian hyperstimulation remain unresolved.
4. The couple must be well informed about the details of their treatment, the techniques involved, and the indications for the tests they have to undergo.
5. The use of GnRH-analogues in patients with moderate/severe endometriosis has resulted in a better response, increase in the number of oocytes retrieved and fertilized and an improved outcome.
6. Vaginal egg collection has almost completely replaced all other ultrasound guided methods.
7. It is very important to institute strict quality control measures in the human reproduction laboratory to ensure high fertilization rates, embryo quality and consequently to maintain consistent pregnancy rates.
8. There is an urgent need to develop new tests

(invasive or non-invasive) to determine embryonic normality.

9. It is probable that success rates of an embryo cryopreservation programme may depend more on the quality and viability of the embryos produced; on the critical training of the embryologist in freezing techniques; on the quality of equipment used, and timing of embryo replacement than any individual programme.
10. Conception is a matter of chance.
11. It is important when evaluating the efficacy of assisted reproduction techniques to bear in mind the duration of infertility, age of the female partner, the multiplicity of factors responsible for the couple's subfertility, and the number of treatment cycles which they have undergone.
12. The reproductive potential of subfertile women (as a cohort) appears to be different from that of normal women.'
13. A higher frequency of adverse outcome is encountered among pregnancies resulting from assisted reproduction techniques.
14. All staff working in assisted reproduction centres must recognize the emotional reactions experienced by these couples and be able to distinguish between those who are coping with their anxieties and those who need more specialized counselling services.
15. It is our duty to reassure the public by maintaining conscientious and honest control of our practice for the benefit of humanity.

REFERENCES

Asch R H, Ellsworth L R, Balmaceda J P, Wong P C 1984 Pregnancy after translaparoscopic gamete intrafallopian transfer. Lancet ii: 1034

Amso N, Ahuja K, Morris N, Shaw R 1990 The management of ovarian hyperstimulation involving gonadotropin-releasing hormone analogue with elective cryopreservation of all pre-embryos. Fertility and Sterility 53: 1087–1090

Asch R 1987 GIFT: a multicentric international study In: Proceedings of the VIth world congress on human reproduction, Tokyo

Cameron I, Rogers P, Caro C, Harman J, Healy D, Leeton J 1989 Oocyte donation: a review. British Journal of Obstetrics and Gynaecology 96: 893–899

Cohen J, Edwards R, Fehilly C B et al 1985 In vitro fertilization: a treatment for male infertility. Fertility and Sterility 43: 422

Cohen J, Mayaux M-J, Guihard-Moscato M-L, Schwartz D 1986 In vitro fertilization and embryo transfer: a collaborative study of 1163 pregnancies on the incidence and risk factors of ectopic pregnancies. Human Reproduction 1: 255–258

Craft I, Al-Shawaf T, Lewis P et al 1988 Analysis of 1071 GIFT procedures — The case for a flexible approach to treatment. Lancet i: 1094–1097

Deveroy P, Staessen C, Camus M, De Grauwe E, Wisanto A, Van Steirtegham A 1989 Zygote intrafallopian transfer as a successful treatment for unexplained infertility. Fertility and Sterility 52: 246–249

Editorial 1989 Embryo research: yes or no? British Medical Journal 299: 1349–1350

Frydman R, Belaissch-Allart J, Fries N, Hazout A, Glissant A, Testart J 1986 An obstetric assessment of the first 100 births from in vitro fertilisation programme at Clamart, France. American Journal of Obstetrics and Gynecology 154: 550–555

Frydman R, Forman R, Belaissch-Allart, Hazout A, Fernandez H, Testart J 1989 An obstetric analysis of 50 consecutive pregnancies after transfer of cryopreserved human embryos. American Journal of Obstetrics and Gynecology 160: 209–213

Handyside A 1990 Sex and the single cell. New Scientist 126: 34–35

Haney A 1987 What is efficacious infertility therapy? Fertility and Sterility 48: 543–545

Interim Licensing Authority 1986 The first report of the Interim Licensing Authority for human in vitro fertilisation and embryology. Interim Licensing Authority, London

Jansen R 1982 Spontaneous abortion incidence in the treatment of infertility. American Journal of Obstetrics and Gynecology 143: 451–473

Jansen R 1987 The clinical impact of in-vitro fertilization. Part 1. Results and limitations of conventional reproductive medicine. Medical Journal of Australia 146: 342–253

Mahadevan M M, Leeton J F, Trounson A O, Wood C 1985 Successful use of in vitro fertilization for patients with persisting low quality semen. Annals of the New York Academy of Sciences 442: 293–300

Medical Research Council working party on children conceived by in vitro fertilisation 1990 Births in Great Britain resulting from assisted conception, 1978–1987. British Medical Journal; 300: 1229–1233

Medical research international, and the society for assisted reproductive technology, American Fertility Society 1990 In vitro-fertilization embryo transfer in the United States: 1988 results from IVF-ET registry. Fertility and Sterility 53: 13–20

National perinatal statistics unit and fertility society of Australia 1988 IVF and GIFT pregnancies: Australia and New Zealand, 1987. National perinatal statistics unit, Sydney

Padilla S, Garcia J 1989 Effect of maternal age and number of in vitro fertilization procedures on pregnancy outcome. Fertility and Sterility 52: 270–273

Riddle A, Stabile I, Sharma V, Campbell S, Mason B, Grudzinskas J 1988 Early pregnancy and its failure after assisted conception: diagnosis by ultrasonic and biochemical techniques. In: Chapman M, Grudzinskas J, Chard T (eds) Implantation. Biological and clinical aspects. Springer-Verlag, Berlin pp 207–215

Rubin G L, Peterson H B, Dorfman S F et al 1983 Ectopic pregnancy in the United States: 1970 through 1978. Journal of the American Medical Association 249: 1725–1729

Schoen J A, Novak R J 1975 Repeat ectopic pregnancy. A 16 year clinical survey. Obstetrics and Gynecology 45: 542–546

Shaw R, Amso N 1991 New concepts in GnRH-a associated superovulation for polycystic ovarian disease in assisted reproduction programmes. In: Coelingh Bennink H J T, Vemer H M, Van Keep P A (eds) Proceedings of the symposium on chronic hyper-androgenic anovulation pp 121–129. Parthenon Press, Carnforth, Lancs

Testart J, Lassall B, Belaisch-Allart J 1986 High pregnancy rate after early human embryo freezing. Fertility and Sterility 46: 268–272

Trounson A 1989 Fertilization and embryo culture. In: Wood C, Trounson A (eds) Clinical in vitro fertilization, 2nd edn. Springer-Verlag, London, pp 33, 127

Wagner M, St Clair P 1989 Are in-vitro fertilisation and embryo transfer of benefit to all? Lancet ii: 1027–1029

Yovich J L, Stanger J D, Yovich J M 1985 The management of oligospermic infertility by in vitro fertilization. Annals of the New York Academy of Sciences 442: 276–286

Yovich J M, Yovich J M, Edivisinghe W 1988 The relative chance of pregnancy following tubal or uterine transfer procedures. Fertility and Sterility 49: 858

World Health Organization 1987 WHO Laboratory manual for the examination of human semen and semen–cervical mucus interaction. Cambridge University Press, Cambridge

18. Amenorrhoea and oligomenorrhoea, and hypothalamic–pituitary dysfunction

M. G. R. Hull M. I. M. Abuzeid

INTRODUCTION

This chapter focuses attention on the understanding and practical management of amenorrhoea and oligomenorrhoea due to endocrine disorders involving the hypothalamus and anterior pituitary as they usually present to a gynaecologist, i.e. because of consequent ovarian endocrine and reproductive failure. Therefore discussion will be limited in the case of, for example, disorders of the thyroid or adrenal axis, and of primary ovarian failure, to what is needed for essential awareness and basic diagnosis. Some aspects are only touched on here because they are detailed in other chapters in this book.

Amenorrhoea and oligomenorrhoea are of course not diagnoses but the common presenting symptoms of a wide range of different causes. Each cause will therefore be separately discussed as a whole.

DEFINITIONS AND CLASSIFICATION OF CAUSES

Pathological amenorrhoea

Pathological amenorrhoea is usually defined as the absence of menstruation for at least 6 months, not due to pregnancy, in a woman of child-bearing age. The usual age limits are 16 and 40 years, the normal limits for menarche and menopause respectively. On the other hand, amenorrhoea may be recognized and specific treatment required before 16 years of age in a girl who has previously menstruated, or after 40 years if a cause is established other than primary ovarian failure.

Primary amenorrhoea

Primary amenorrhoea is defined as failure even to have menstruated by the age of 16 years, as the normal upper age limit for menarche is 15 years. It therefore means the same as delayed menarche, but may or may not be associated with delayed puberty. Puberty strictly means procreative ability but is generally used to mean secondary sexual development. Secondary sexual development begins before menarche with the onset of breast development (thelarche), normally by 13 years of age. Delayed puberty can therefore be recognized at 14 years, and its definition need not wait to include delayed menarche at 16 years.

Oligomenorrhoea

Oligomenorrhoea is usually defined by menstrual intervals between 6 weeks and 6 months. Those definitions are, however, arbitrary and do not necessarily reflect important distinctions; indeed they can be misleading. Oligomenorrhoea is so defined because the upper normal limit of the menstrual cycle length is 5 weeks. On the other hand, cycles of around 6 weeks' length are usually indistinguishable from normal in terms of follicular growth and hormonal development apart from the delay in onset (Aksel 1981). Therefore oligomenorrhoea is likely to include a spectrum of conditions ranging from virtual normality at one end to the same causes as of amenorrhoea at the other. The main difference appears to be in the frequency of polycystic ovaries, which ultrasound and endocrine studies show account for about 90% of cases of oligomenorrhoea and 33% of amenorrhoea (although often without the classical syndrome, including hirsutism and obesity; Adams et al 1986; Hull 1987; Hull 1989).

Some authors take 4 or 12 months as the criterion for amenorrhoea. Absence of menstruation for only 4 months after sudden cessation of previously normal cycles is undoubtedly appropriate to treat as amenorrhoea; oligomenorrhoea implies repeated occurrence of prolonged menstrual intervals.

The distinction between primary and secondary amenorrhoea can also be misleading. Menstrual periods are sometimes described as having occurred once or twice at the expected age by patients who could not possibly have menstruated, for example with male pseudohermaphroditism and vaginal atresia, presumably from self-examination and wishful thinking! Primary and secondary amenorrhoea cannot be distinguished by any tests of endocrine function. The only endocrine disorder presenting specifically in either way is congenital hypothalamic failure (it presents of course with primary amenorrhoea and lack of pubertal development). By contrast, ovarian dysgenesis if partial can present with secondary amenorrhoea, whilst anorexia nervosa or hyperprolactinaemia can occur before puberty.

For all those reasons, primary and secondary amenorrhoea and oligomenorrhoea should be considered in the same way clinically and within a unified classification of causes as described later.

The definitions of individual conditions accounting for oligomenorrhoea will be considered where they are described. The reader first needs to appreciate that different authors employ inconsistent or ill defined terminologies, for example hypothalamic–pituitary failure versus disorder, and polycystic ovarian syndrome, polycystic ovarian disease, and polycystic ovaries. These distinctions must be made within the context of a particular classification.

Physiological amenorrhoea

Physiological amenorrhoea occurs, of course, as normal before menarche and after the menopause. It is important never to overlook the possibility of pregnancy as the cause, even after years of amenorrhoea. Some conditions can resolve spontaneously, such as weight loss-related hypothalamic disorder, whilst in others like polycystic ovarian disease ovulation may occur sporadically at long intervals; when ovulation occurs it does so unheralded by any warning menstruation.

CLASSIFICATION OF CAUSES

Anatomical abnormalities of the genital tract account for only about 1% of cases of amenorrhoea. The usual causes, affecting endocrine function, used to be classified nosologically (e.g. psychological, tumour, autoimmune disease) but this has given way to a systematic endocrinological approach:

1. Disorders of the hypothalamic (anterior)–pituitary–ovarian (H–P–O) axis
   a. hypothalamic.
   b. pituitary.
   c. ovarian.
2. Disorders of other endocrine systems, e.g. thyroid, adrenal.

Disorders of the H–P–O axis

The disorders of the H–P–O axis can be further classified into primary failures and functional disorders. We now run into difficulties due to inconsistent use of such terms by different authors. Some use the term 'hypothalamic–pituitary failure' to mean any condition affecting the hypothalamus or pituitary resulting in impaired gonadotrophin secretion (hypogonadotrophism), whilst others simply use 'hypothalamic amenorrhoea'. Another common term is 'functional amenorrhoea', which is generally used to mean disorders not due to any evident lesion such as a tumour. We do not hold with the use of these terms and must make our own views clear.

We use primary failure to mean inherent failure of an endocrine organ, or at least of a specific cellular component, e.g. the gonadotrophin-releasing hormone (GnRH) neurons of the hypothalamus, or gonadotrophs of the pituitary, which may be affected selectively. This could result for example from a congenital malformation, compression by a tumour, or surgical destruction. This will lead to secondary (or tertiary) failure further down the axis; for example, a tumour compressing the hypothalamus can cause secondary pituitary failure and consequent (tertiary) ovarian failure.

By contrast, we use the term *functional disorder* to imply a reversible functional failure in which the affected functional elements are structurally undamaged. Thus psychological disturbance can lead to *hypothalamic disorder*. An interesting example is a prolactin-secreting adenoma of the pituitary (prolactinoma). It is the commonest tumour disturbing reproductive function, but it rarely compresses the pituitary sufficiently to cause primary pituitary failure. It acts by short-loop feedback of the excess prolactin on hypothalamic GnRH secretion, i.e. causing secondary hypothalamic disorder and consequent (tertiary) pituitary hypogonadotrophism and (quaternary) ovarian failure.

There are anomalies in any classification. Pubertal failure, for example, may be due to primary hypothalamic failure, which can be permanent (e.g. Kallman's syndrome) or temporary (delayed puberty). It is often not possible, however, to predict whether puberty will merely be delayed, and all cases are treated in the same way.

Another odd example is polycystic ovarian disease, which is difficult to classify. Its aetiology is unclear, but it now appears to be an inherent primary abnormality of the ovary affecting structure and function, although subject also to extraneous hormonal influences, notably insulin. Associated disorders of the hypothalamus and pituitary affecting luteinizing hormone (LH) secretion now appear to be secondary features. We therefore classify polycystic ovarian disease as an ovarian functional disorder in the following system concerning the H–P–O axis (Table 18.1).

Table 18.1 Disorders of the H–P–O axis

Hypothalamic
Primary failures
Compression by tumours
Kallman's syndrome
Functional disorders
Psychological disturbances
Weight loss
Extreme exercise
Pituitary
Primary failures
Compression by tumours
Damage by surgery, radiotherapy
Infarction (e.g. Sheehan's syndrome)
Hyperprolactinaemia
Functional failure secondary to hypothalamic failure or disorder
Ovarian
Primary failures
Dysgenesis
Damage by surgery, radiotherapy, chemotherapy
Autoimmune disease
Premature menopause
Resistant ovary syndrome
Functional failure secondary to hypothalamic–pituitary failure or disorder
Polycystic ovarian disease

Unclassified disorders

Conditions are commonly described, such as 'post-pill amenorrhoea' and 'pseudocyesis', which are not proven entities. The particular historical features have been taken as distinctive, but the conditions appear to be no more than one or other of the functional disorders mentioned above.

Anatomical causes of amenorrhoea

These are detailed in Chapter 14 but will be summarized here for systematic completeness (Table 18.2). Note that incomplete endometrial fibrosis will present with hypomenorrhoea, not oligomenorrhoea.

Table 18.2 Anatomical causes of amenorrhoea

Simple developmental defects
Absent ovaries (extremely rare)
Absent uterus
With or without absent vagina
'Imperforate hymen' (lower vaginal aplasia)
Developmental defects of endocrine origin
Androgen-resistant syndrome (testicular feminization) in male pseudohermaphrodites (genetic and gonadal males) including inhibition of uterovaginal development
Acquired conditions
Endometrial fibrosis
Traumatic (Asherman's syndrome)
Infective (tuberculosis)
Cervical stenosis (extremely rare)
Surgical trauma
Infective
Vaginal stenosis (extremely rare)
Chemical inflammation

INDIVIDUAL CAUSES OF ENDOCRINE DISORDER

Kallman's syndrome

Absent or impaired olfactory sensation (anosmia or hyposmia, respectively) is the characteristic feature of the syndrome described by Kallman and colleagues in 1944 associated with delayed pubertal development, occurring much less frequently in girls than boys. The impairment of olfactory sensation is often subtle. The classic test is to distinguish between the smell — not the taste — of coffee and tea. Failure is diagnostic in a girl with delayed pubertal development and serum follicle-stimulating hormone (FSH) and prolactin levels are not raised.

Failure is permanent and treatment is needed without delay. The theoretical choice is pulsed GnRH but this is unnecessarily complicated and oestrogen therapy is employed until ovulation induction is eventually required to achieve pregnancy. Oestrogen dosage and combination with progestagen will depend primarily on skeletal development as discussed later.

Idiopathic delayed puberty

As discussed earlier, delayed puberty can be recognized by the age of 14 years in girls if breast development has still not started. Idiopathic hypothalamic failure, which usually resolves spontaneously, accounts for most cases of delayed puberty in boys but a minority in girls. There is often a family history of delayed puberty. If there is no history of hyposmia, obsessive dieting or ill health, other causes of amenorrhoea with oestrogen deficiency must be excluded by lateral skull X-ray (non-endocrine tumours, e.g. craniopharyngioma) and serum prolactin (prolactinoma) and FSH measurement (ovarian dysgenesis).

It is not reliably possible to distinguish between primary hypothalamic and primary pituitary failure by measuring the gonadotrophin response to an acute stimulus with GnRH, because that only tests the releasable pool of LH and FSH; in either condition positive or negative results can be obtained. The secretory capacity of the pituitary can be properly tested only by prolonged repeated stimulation, preferably using relatively physiological pulses about every 90 minutes.

Thus, a diagnosis of idiopathic delayed puberty due to hypothalamic failure can be made after relatively simple exclusion of other causes. It only remains to distinguish whether the failure is permanent or whether puberty will only be delayed. The distinction is impossible, however, although suggested by a familial association. Treatment should begin anyway without delay as for Kallman's syndrome. The only difference is that when secondary sexual maturation is complete, treatment might be interrupted from time to time in order to test for spontaneous H–P–O activity.

Hypothalamic lesions

Congenital aplasia

Congenital aplasia can occur in association with other rare midline malformations of the head and central nervous system, including pituitary aplasia and cleft palate.

Traumatic lesions

Traumatic lesions include accidental injury, surgical damage and post-radiotherapy fibrosis. Forward whiplash injuries are more likely to transect the pituitary stalk than damage the hypothalamus, however. Hypothalamic infarction can occur in association with hypophyseal portal vein thrombosis after prolonged hypovolaemia, hypotension and coma.

Inflammatory lesions

Inflammatory lesions include, particularly, tuberculous meningitis, granulomas and abscess; also sarcoidosis, giant cell granulomas in middle-aged women, and hystiocytosis-X in children causing delayed growth and puberty (Hand–Schüller–Christian disease).

Tumours

The most likely cause to present to a gynaecologist is a tumour, particularly a craniopharyngioma, compressing the hypothalamus and suppressing GnRH secretion or interrupting portal flow of GnRH in the pituitary stalk. Craniophyaryngiomas arise from remnants of Rathke's pouch and commonly present clinically around the age of onset of puberty. They are usually cystic and calcification is common and is readily recognizable on a lateral skull radiograph. Other tumours of the hypothalamus include gliomas (which may arise in the optic tract), meningiomas, endodermal sinus tumour (or yolk sac carcinoma) which secretes alpha-fetoprotein, and congenital hamartomas composed of GnRH neurosecretory cells which can lead to precocious puberty.

Pineal tumours can affect hypothalamic function in different ways. Melatonin secretion by the pineal, which is increased during darkness, suppresses reproductive function. Non-parenchymal pineal tumours (gliomas, teratomas) thus tend to cause sexual infantilism presumably by secreting excessive melatonin. By contrast, parenchymal tumours (e.g. germinomas, which are similar to ovarian dysgerminomas and testicular seminomas, and were previously called pinealomas) can cause sexual precocity, presumably by suppressing pineal function; however, this is rare in girls compared with boys.

Psychoneuroendocrine disorders

The modulatory influence of extrahypothalamic brain centres on hypothalamic pulsatile secretion of GnRH was discussed in Chapter 9 to explain the possible mechanisms whereby psychological disorders cause amenorrhoea. They are the commonest cause, accounting for about a third of all cases of amenorrhoea.

Weight loss by associated dietary restriction is a common accompaniment of psychological disorder, and weight loss alone may contribute to neuroendocrine disturbance. Fat tissue is an important extragonadal source of oestrogens by conversion from adrenal androgen precursors. Lack of oestrogen appears to withdraw the normal oestrogenic inhibition of endogenous opioid peptide production; opioids normally inhibit pulsatile GnRH secretion (Bhanot & Wilkinson 1983). Another effect of weight loss is disturbance of the metabolism of oestrogens both in the liver and brain in favour of catechol oestrogens (e.g. 2-alpha-hydroxy- and 4-hydroxy- metabolites of oestrone, oestradiol and oestriol). Catechol oestrogens appear to have contrasting effects to the classical oestrogens in the hypothalamus and pituitary on gonadotrophin secretion, amplifying the negative rather than positive effects (Fishman 1980).

Psychological and weight disturbances take various forms, which may explain the variety of neuroendocrine and clinical features. Weight loss may result from true anorexia (loss of appetite) in response to stress, or from obsessional starvation as a primary psychological feature of anorexia nervosa. Extreme exercise is obviously stressful in other ways, but amenorrhoea is common only in competitive long-distance runners, unlike swimmers (Sanborn et al 1982), and in ballet dancers.

The hypothalamus is the focus of neuroendocrine

disturbance; in particular there is functional impairment of the GnRH pulse generator in the arcuate nucleus. Excessive hypothalamic beta-endorphin and dopamine have been implicated as a cause in some but not all cases (Quigley et al 1980), and naloxone infusion has been shown to increase pulsatile secretion of LH (Laatikainen et al 1986). It is also possible that augmentation of opioid secretion is the mechanism whereby corticotrophin-releasing factor (CRF) has been shown to inhibit gonadotrophin secretion experimentally in monkeys. Stress-induced stimulation of CRF secretion is suggested by the unique pattern of hypersecretion of cortisol, characterized by increased amplitude of secretory episodes during the daytime in women with functional amenorrhoea (Suh et al 1988).

The pineal may also play a part in suppressing hypothalamic GnRH secretion, as suggested by raised plasma melatonin levels in women with hypothalamic amenorrhoea (Berga et al 1988; Brzezinski et al 1988). This may be associated with disturbance of sleep patterns as occurs in chronic anorexia, or with acute effects of exercise, as discussed later.

Indirect evidence of hypothalamic impairment is provided by the normal pituitary responsiveness to administration of exogenous releasing hormones, in particular by restoration of normal pituitary–ovarian cyclicity and ovulation in response to prolonged physiological pulsed treatment with GnRH. Direct evidence of other specific hypothalamic disturbances is provided by abnormal body heat production in response to changes in environmental temperature, demonstrable at least in women with weight loss-related amenorrhoea (Vigersky 1981).

Weight loss-related amenorrhoea

According to the critical weight hypothesis of Frisch & McArthur the onset of female puberty and the maintenance of regular menstrual cycles depend on reaching a critical body weight (47 kg) and ratio of fat to lean mass. It is estimated that body fat should reach at least 17% to achieve menarche, and at least 22% to sustain the adult menstrual pattern (Frisch 1984). Loss of 10–15% of body weight, equivalent to a loss of about one-third of body fat, commonly results in amenorrhoea. There is, however, marked individual variation. The rate of loss of weight seems to be important, and rapid loss is frequently associated with psychological disturbance.

There are different patterns of dieting to lose weight, as originally emphasized by Fries et al (1974). There is dieting for straightforward cosmetic reason; loss of appetite (true anorexia) in response to stress, as often occurs when young women are taking examinations, or leave home for the first time to travel abroad or take up institutional training; and anorexia nervosa, a specific psychiatric disorder which, after the obvious acute phase, commonly persists in a partly recovered chronic phase that is easily overlooked. A more subtle variation of anorexia nervosa, or at least related to it, is bulimia nervosa ('bulimia' means self-induced vomiting). These conditions will be discussed in more detail later.

Dieting in adolescence. It is important to appreciate how widespread dieting is in adolescent girls and that simple cosmetic dieting can lead directly to anorexia nervosa. In Sweden, where the prevalence of anorexia nervosa seems to be the same as in the UK (about 0.5–1.0% of teenage girls), it has been found that about half of all teenage girls feel fat and most diet to lose weight. It is clear that such weight loss due to cosmetic dieting in adolescence is a warning of serious danger. Other particular warning signs are faddishness about the preparation and eating of food (often in isolation) combined with one or more of the following: signs of anxiety, depression, feeling cold, constipation, mental sluggishness, loss of interest in previous activities, and of course amenorrhoea.

Anorexia nervosa

Anorexia nervosa is a misnomer. 'Nervous' the patients may be, but there is no loss of appetite. The starvation is self-imposed; hunger could not be admitted when refusing to eat. The condition is more readily recognized in its acute phase than its chronic phase when some of the lost weight has been regained, as when a woman commonly presents to the gynaecologist some years later with a complaint only of amenorrhoea. Amenorrhoea is an invariable feature of anorexia, not only in its acute phase but also if it continues chronically.

Then, as the patient walks into the consulting room, she seems unremarkable — perhaps only modishly slim and a little reserved in her manner. She will usually admit on direct questioning to an episode of rapid weight loss associated with the onset of amenorrhoea. It can require skilful questioning, however, and usually only at subsequent visits, to uncover the typical, bizarre features of chronic anorexia nervosa: whilst at first claiming to eat normally, she takes irregular and often lonely meals, carefully avoiding carbohydrate; so faddish that she may have ostracized herself rather than dine socially; sometimes giving in to her appetite by gargantuan but secret binges, immediately followed by self-induced vomiting so as to enjoy feeling empty again, or purging habitually to achieve the same end.

At the first consultation few clues are likely to be revealed apart from the history of the original acute weight loss. Constipation is commonly admitted, and often used to explain the need for purgatives. While claiming unconcern about weight, when encouraged to increase her weight she could not bear to do so as she would feel too fat. Yet such patients are usually markedly underweight, and to demonstrate that, it is particularly useful to have a weight/height charge available for reference, as shown in

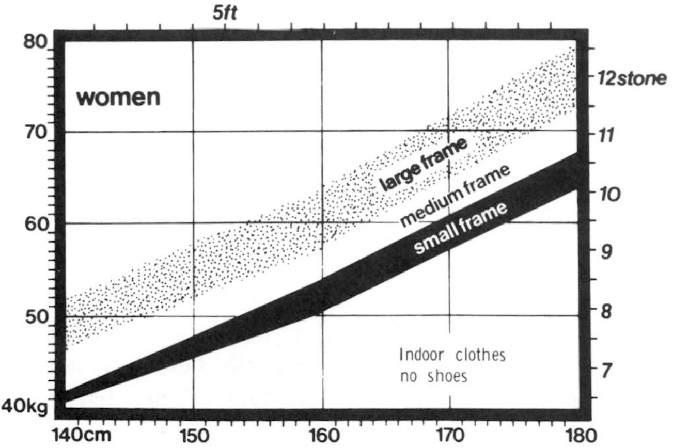

Fig. 18.1 Normal weight of women for height and frame size. Modified From Fletcher (1974).

Figure 18.1. That is more effective than calculating the body mass index (weight (kg)/height $(m)^2$), which should be greater than about 19.

Anorexia nervosa does not seem to be a specific psychological disease as once believed. The self-imposed starvation is now thought to be a response to the psychosexual pressures of adolescence, the response in these particular individuals being conditioned by their constitution and family environment, in which there is often marked weight consciousness including obesity and sometimes anorexia nervosa in other members. There are usually greater family problems than weight consciousness, however, and the parents' own anxieties are easily conveyed to their daughter.

One particular characteristic is the patient's illusion of her body size and shape, which is grossly overestimated and distorted in her mind, particularly after meals. Although this may be part of her strategy of denying her abnormality, it is probably a genuine distortion effected by the memory of her premorbid obesity as this same phenomenon is observed in previously obese but otherwise normal women.

Management of weight loss-related amenorrhoea

Weight loss accounts for about a third of all cases of amenorrhoea presenting to gynaecologists, and chronic anorexia nervosa accounts for half of those. Anorexia nervosa tends to be a lifelong condition and acute exacerbations can be life-threatening. Chronic anorexia nervosa is difficult to treat because patients deny their problem, an attitude that hardens with time, and they reject formal psychiatry. Gynaecologists can be faced with an ethical dilemma when very disturbed patients want help to become pregnant because the risk of psychological disturbance in their children is high. That may be difficult to argue, but the physical risks for the fetus associated with an underweight mother are clearly defined and the patients should be encouraged to restore themselves to normal reproductive function by dietary measures to increase their weight rather than resort to pharmacological stimulation of ovulation.

Increasing their weight can be too difficult for some patients with anorexia nervosa, however. It is essential strategy to set a target weight, which usually needs to be the premorbid weight. If reached, ovulation induction should be promised then if necessary. The patient can often be helped to accept the importance of weight by appreciating the serious endocrinological and other physical consequences of her being underweight.

Endocrinopathy of weight loss-related amenorrhoea

The distinct effects of weight loss and psychological disorder on central neuroendocrine processes have been discussed. In the acute phase of anorexia nervosa there is almost complete suppression of gonadotrophin secretion and pulsatility evident peripherally, as shown in Figure 18.2. As weight is restored FSH secretion returns ahead of LH as in prepuberty, and LH pulsatility returns in association with sleep (or improved sleep in the case of anorexia nervosa) as initially occurs through the stages of puberty (Fig. 18.3). LH pulsatility is entrained particularly with rapid eye movement sleep, which is only restored when weight has returned to within 15% below the normal mean for height and age (Lacey et al 1975).

As weight is gradually restored there is gradual restoration of pituitary LH production even before normal pulsatility is achieved, as indicated by the differential basal levels and responses to acute stimulation with GnRH shown in Figure 18.4 of patients remaining amenorrhoeic. This partial but still incomplete return of LH secretion may explain the ultrasound evidence of early ovarian follicular development described as 'multicystic ovaries'. These are the typical appearances of prepubertal ovaries, with a few small or medium-sized follicles in ovaries that are not enlarged (distinct from polycystic ovaries) representing at most feeble activity associated with infrequent LH pulses (Mason et al 1988). The patients are still demonstrably oestrogen-deficient.

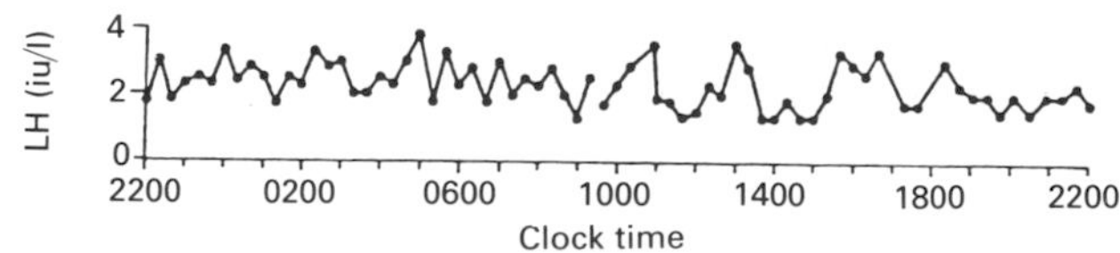

Fig. 18.2 Plasma luteinizing hormone (LH) concentration every 20 min for 24 h in a case of acute anorexia nervosa. Modified from Boyar et al (1974).

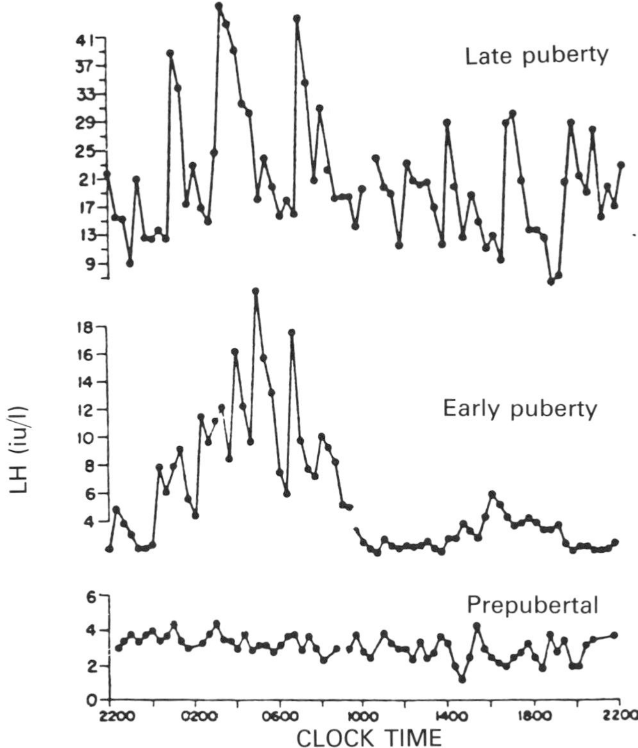

Fig. 18.3 Plasma luteinizing hormone (LH) concentration every 20 min for 24 h in individual girls at different stages around the onset of puberty. Modified from Boyar et al (1974).

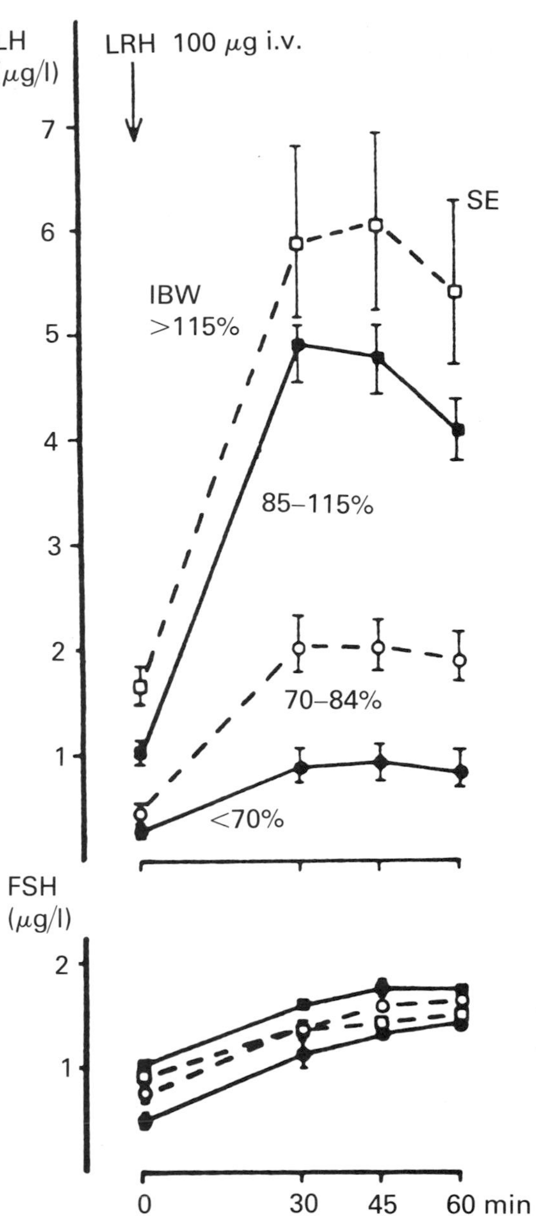

Fig. 18.4 Plasma luteinizing hormone (LH) and follicle-stimulating hormone (FSH) responses to intravenous luteinizing hormone-releasing hormone (LRH = GnRH) in women with amenorrhoea related to their ideal (normal mean) body weight (IBW). (Modified from Bergh et al 1978).

There is also continuing evidence of impaired negative and positive feedback by oestrogen on the hypothalamus and pituitary. There is lack of gonadotrophin and consequent ovulatory response to clomiphene, and lack of differential LH response to acute GnRH stimulation after priming with oestrogen. Responsiveness to clomiphene may return in the final stage of weight recovery before menstrual cycles are restored, however, and if the target weight has been reached but amenorrhoea continues clomiphene therapy is worth trying again before resorting to pulsed GnRH or gonadotrophin therapy to achieve pregnancy.

Serum oestradiol levels are reduced on average, and the menstrual response to a progestogen challenge is almost invariably lacking or at least impaired.

One consequence of oestrogen deficiency — the importance of which is becoming increasingly recognized — is osteoporosis. Loss of bone mineral content particularly affects weight-bearing vertebral trabecular bone (Cann et al 1984), and crush fractures sometimes occur without specific injury.

Another effect of oestrogen deficiency, of minor diagnostic importance, is reduction in certain hormone-binding proteins in plasma, notably thyroxine-binding protein. This leads to misleadingly reduced thyroxine levels but the free thyroxine index is normal, like thyroid-stimulating hormone.

In clinical practice, to define the endocrinopathy of weight loss-related amenorrhoea it is sufficient to detect normal or low basal FSH and LH levels, oestrogen deficiency by a progestogen challenge test, and if pregnancy is desired, failure to ovulate normally or usually even to menstruate in response to a single course of clomiphene. The history of weight fluctuation and psychological disturbance is the critical diagnostic feature.

Other causes of weight loss

Physical illness, famine and chronic undernutrition can all cause amenorrhoea, but are of little relevance to gynaecologists. It is of passing interest, however, that chronic undernutrition may be an important regulator of general fertility: the onset of puberty is delayed; skeletal growth although delayed is protected until reproductive maturity is reached, and the effects of physiological (lactational) hyperprolactinaemia may be accentuated, so extending birth intervals.

Other psychological disorders

In the absence of a distinct history of weight loss related to the onset of amenorrhoea, the cause can be ascribed confidently to psychological disorder only if there is an obvious condition like chronic depression or if there had been unusual emotional disturbance or anxiety such as commonly leads to amenorrhoea when young women commence institutional life. The latter should not be taken as a simple explanation and consequently dismissed as unimportant.

Patients with serious psychiatric disorders are unlikely to present to a gynaecologist. It should be remembered, however, that psychotropic drug therapy could be the direct cause of amenorrhoea by inducing hyperprolactinaemia (see later).

Bulimia nervosa

Bulimia nervosa is becoming increasingly recognized as a common psychological disorder characterized by covert self-induced vomiting to achieve weight control while overeating in response to normal appetite, associated with morbid fear of fatness (Fairburn & Cooper 1982). It is difficult to diagnose because weight is usually normal and bulimia is not readily admitted. The psychological disorder seems to be related to anorexia nervosa and is therefore interesting, demonstrating that it can lead to amenorrhoea independent of weight loss. Only a minority of bulimic women develop amenorrhoea but many have menstrual irregularity.

Exercise-related amenorrhoea

An uncommon cause of amenorrhoea is extreme exercise involving endurance, as occurs in up to half of top-class competitive long-distance runners and professional ballet dancers. World-class gymnasts also seem to be at their best during the early teenage years and their pubertal development is commonly delayed. The exact aetiology and endocrine mechanisms are, however, unclear.

There appear to be anomalies, such as swimmers, in whom amenorrhoea is relatively infrequent and unrelated to distance training (Sanborn et al 1982). This is likely to be related to greater redistribution of fat to lean weight in the runners combined with general loss of weight. Psychological factors associated with extreme competitiveness are important determinants (Gadpaille et al 1987), and ballet dancers are also specially concerned by their weight. Physical stress is, however, a key factor as indicated by the rapid return of menstruation when rest is enforced by injury without any increase in weight.

Acute exercise is known to lead to rapid increases in stress hormones including adrenocorticotrophic hormone, cortisol, beta-endorphin, beta-lipoprotein, growth hormone, prolactin and catecholamines; it is also known to cause an increase in melatonin. Acute exercise in already amenorrhoeic runners, however, does not increase prolactin levels, which suggests that it is not the mechanism by which GnRH secretion is suppressed.

The endocrine effects of chronic exercise are not well defined, but in patients who develop amenorrhoea the clinical endocrine picture is that of hypothalamic disorder and secondary ovarian failure, as already described for psychogenic and weight loss-related amenorrhoea. The secretion and control of prolactin are normal (Chang et al 1984). It is perhaps specially important to appreciate that even in such physically fit athletes there is reduction in mineral density of weight-bearing (vertebral) bones associated with oestrogen deficiency (Drinkwater et al 1984).

Obesity

In contrast to weight loss-related amenorrhoea, from which recovery can be confidently predicted if weight is restored, there is no clear relationship to obesity or therapeutic certainty from shedding excess weight.

Obesity may be associated with polycystic ovarian disease and Cushing's syndromes but those conditions involve specific endocrine disorders that can cause oligo- or amenorrhoea. Otherwise obesity, even when gross, is associated with menstrual disturbance in only about one-third of cases, and there are no endocrine features to distinguish those from non-obese patients with similar menstrual disturbances. Only in the massively obese is there any convincing evidence that weight reduction (when massive) leads to improvement in endocrine state and menstrual function (Kopelman et al 1981).

Congenital pituitary endocrine failures

Congenital absence of the anterior pituitary in association with other midline structural developmental defects is extremely rare and in the presence of the gland, primary deficiencies of pituitary hormone secretion are very uncommon. Growth hormone deficiency is the commonest, in isolation or with panhypopituitary dwarfism. Reproductive capacity is potentially intact, usually together with lactation. Isolated deficiencies of prolactin and thyroid-stimulating hormone have been reported, but not of adrenocorticotrophic hormone, as this is incompatible with life.

Gonadotrophin deficiency is usually secondary — rarely primary — to hypothalamic failure of GnRH secretion as previously described. Isolated LH deficiency in a man gives rise to a 'fertile eunuch'. Isolated FSH deficiency has been reported in men and in one case in a woman; it was successfully treated using exogenous gonadotrophins.

Other genetic syndromes involving hypogonadotrophic hypogonadism and various congenital defects include the Laurence–Moon–Biedl syndrome (with obesity, retinitis pigmentosa, mental retardation and polydactyly) and various syndromes with cerebellar ataxia that are thought to be inherited as X-linked recessive conditions.

A not uncommon congenital defect that may present in adult life is the (presumably gradual) herniation of the arachnoid through the dura roofing the pituitary fossa. The fossa becomes filled with cerebrospinal fluid within the hernia which can compress the pituitary stalk and gland. The fossa may be enlarged, giving the appearance of an intrasellar tumour on ordinary radiography, and giving rise to the so-called empty sella syndrome including hyperprolactinaemia (see below).

Pituitary lesions

Congenital absence in association with other midline structural developmental defects has been mentioned as an extremely rare occurrence. Haemochromatosis of the pituitary is the consequence of a hereditary disorder of iron metabolism but functional damage from the iron deposition presents relatively late in life.

Traumatic lesions include accidental injury such as whiplash transection of the pituitary stalk, surgical damage and post-radiotherapy fibrosis. Infarction can occur as a result of hypovolaemic shock, notably as a result of massive postpartum haemorrhage (Sheehan's syndrome), presumably because of increased vascularity and growth of the pituitary (specifically of the lactotrophes) that occur in pregnancy in response to the massive increase in oestrogens from the placenta. Tuberculous and other granulomas can affect the pituitary as well as the hypothalamus (see above).

Tumours arising in the hypothalamic area or from the integuments of the pituitary fossa can compress the pituitary stalk or the gland itself, as in the case of the hypothalamus (see above). Tumours arising in the anterior pituitary gland are common, usually benign and small in women, and often of no functional relevance. Macroadenomas are more common in men. Amongst normal women about one-third can be found to have a tumour on radiological or subsequent post-mortem examination. Some may be trophic tumours representing nodal hypertrophy of the secretory cells in response to their respective hypothalamic stimulatory hormones (although classically only when the stimulation is excessive, as for example in primary hypothyroidism).

About a quarter of all pituitary adenomas appear to be non-secretory and present a clinical problem only by compression of the normal pituitary tissue or the pituitary stalk. FSH- and/or LH-secreting tumours are extremely rare, and then usually occur in men rather than women. Prolactin secretion is commonest, but is sometimes combined with growth hormone or adrenocorticotrophic hormone secretion, which may not be clinically evident at first. Non-secretory tumours can present with hyperprolactinaemia, usually of only modest degree, by compressing the pituitary stalk and interrupting hypothalamic dopamine inhibition of normal pituitary secretion of prolactin.

Hyperprolactinaemia

Unlike the other trophic hormones secreted by the anterior pituitary, prolactin is controlled primarily by inhibition from the hypothalamus (by dopamine, and to a minor extent, gamma-amino butyric acid), and in common only with growth hormone is not subject directly or indirectly to negative feedback by peripheral hormones. It exercises inhibitory self-regulation via short-loop feedback on hypothalamic dopamine by means of counter-current flow in the hypophyseal portal system (as well as inhibition of GnRH pulsatile secretion). Hypothalamic stimulatory factors appear to be of minor importance normally; they include serotonin, opioids and notably thyrotropin-releasing hormone (TRH). Prolactin secretion is stimulated by peripheral oestrogen, particularly in pregnancy from the placenta, and by a thoracic sensory nerve pathway from the nipple in reflex response to suckling.

Thus pathological hyperprolactinaemia can be caused by drugs that inhibit dopamine production or action; primary hypothyroidism via excessive TRH; tumours or granulomas compressing the pituitary stalk or hypothalamus, and rarely, traumatic or neoplastic lesions of the thorax or spine affecting the suckling sensory nerve pathway. An additional rare cause is ectopic production of prolactin by a tumour. Chronic renal failure is also often associated with hyperprolactinaemia, both due to reduced excretion of the hormone and probably by central mechanisms affecting dopamine action. By far the commonest causes of hyperprolactinaemia, however, are a pituitary prolactinoma and idiopathic hypersecretion. Amongst patients presenting to a gynaecologist the key diagnostic considerations are a tumour (found in 40–50% of cases), primary hypothyroidism (3–5%) and pharmacological causes (1–2%). First, however, it is necessary to confirm hyperprolactinaemia as the cause of oligo- or amenorrhoea.

Diagnosis of hyperprolactinaemia. Galactorrhoea, the typical symptom of hyperprolactinaemia, is not a reliable index. It occurs in less than half the patients with hyperprolactinaemic amenorrhoea. Conversely, only about half the patients with galactorrhoea and normal menstrual cycles have hyperprolactinaemia.

Serum prolactin measurement is therefore critical and always needs to be undertaken in cases of ovulatory failure. Spurious hyperprolactinaemia was commonly attributed to the stress of clinical procedures, examination of the breasts, or normal episodic secretion of prolactin, but these explanations are now generally discounted. It now seems necessary to repeat prolactin measurement in a second blood sample only if the first is raised, and again if the second is discrepant, accepting normal values and excluding an isolated raised value.

The commonest problem has been simple misinterpretation of the upper normal limit by assuming arithmetic instead of the actual geometric (skewed) distribution of normal. The upper limit should be taken at about 800 mu/l. There is of course overlap between normal and abnormal ranges, and there are anomalies to mislead the unwary diagnostician. Unfortunately there is no endocrine test to distinguish the functional relevance of borderline hyperprolactinaemia. What really matters, it seems, is how well distinguished the ovulatory disorder is for which hyperprolactinaemia is being considered as a possible cause — true hyperprolactinaemia nearly always causes amenorrhoea or severe oligomenorrhoea.

One anomaly is the association of mild hyperprolactinaemia with some cases of polycystic ovarian disease (see Chapter 22). Although there is some evidence that excessive prolactin might stimulate adrenal androgen precursor secretion, it appears more likely to be the consequence rather than the cause of polycystic ovarian disease, due to stimulation by oestrogen which is produced in substantial amounts both by the polycystic ovaries and by peripheral conversion in fat tissue from androgens. By contrast, prolactin levels tend to be subnormal in amenorrhoea due to hypothalamic disorder, presumably because of lack of oestrogenic stimulation.

Another uncommon anomaly is the occurrence of molecular forms (notably 'big, big' prolactin) that are biologically inactive but detected by radioimmunoassay for prolactin. This may explain many of the cases of very high prolactin levels sometimes found in normally ovulating women. It is worth repeating: it is the distinctiveness of ovulatory disorder that determines the pathological relevance of raised prolactin levels.

Endocrine effects of hyperprolactinaemia. Hyperprolactinaemia interferes with ovarian function by indirectly suppressing gonadotrophin secretion, by means of short-loop feedback via the hypophyseal portal system on hypothalamic GnRH pulsatile release. Whilst basal gonadotrophin levels and release remain normal there is suppression of LH pulsatility (Moult et al 1982) and loss of positive and negative feedback by oestrogen.

Early in vitro studies suggesting a direct inhibitory effect of excess prolactin on human granulosa cell function were clearly misleading and there is now much indirect evidence to disprove that idea. Both the pituitary and ovary respond as normal to pulsed GnRH therapy in arcuate-lesioned and pituitary stalk-sectioned monkeys despite accompanying hyperprolactinaemia (Knobil 1980), and in women with pathological hyperprolactinaemic amenorrhoea (Polson et al 1986).

There appears to be a relationship between the degree of hyperprolactinaemia and that of secondary ovarian dysfunction, but there is usually progression to amenorrhoea or severe oligomenorrhoea and associated oestrogen deficiency. Hyperprolactinaemia accounts for about 20% of patients with amenorrhoea and 2% with oligomenorrhoea. It is very unconvincing as a cause of persistent follicular/luteal dysfunction and infertility in normally menstruating women. The only convincing association with such dysfunction is in temporary situations as after stopping bromocriptine therapy before amenorrhoea supervenes again; or after incomplete surgical excision of a prolactinoma; or in women during prolonged lactation. Generally in normally menstruating women there is no relation between prolactin levels and mid luteal progesterone levels or pregnancy rates (Glazener et al 1987).

In women with hyperprolactinaemic amenorrhoea one important consequence of oestrogen deficiency is osteoporosis, which deserves specific therapeutic consideration (Klibanski & Greenspan 1986; Schlecte et al 1987). Some women may also be troubled by atrophic changes in the vulva and vagina.

Pharmacological causes of hyperprolactinaemia

Drugs are an uncommon but easily identified cause of hyperprolactinaemia. They are all dopamine antagonists

Table 18.3 Pharmacological agents associated with hyperprolactinaemia

Phenothiazines
Perphenazine (Fentazin)
Chlorpromazine (Largactil)
Thioridazine (Melleril)
Trifluoperazine (Stelazine)
Prochlorperazine (Stemetil)
Butyrophenones
Haloperidol (Haldol, Serenace)
Pimozide (Orap)
Benzamides
Metoclopramide (Maxolon)
Clebopride (Cleboril)
Cimetidine (Tagamet)
Rauwolfia alkaloids
Reserpine (Serpasil)
Methyldopa (Aldomet)

but have a wide range of therapeutic uses, as shown in Table 18.3. Oestrogens, as in contraceptive pills, also increase prolactin levels but only slightly — within the normal range. The usual drug to cause hyperprolactinaemia in a young women is a phenothiazine or metoclopramide.

Prolactinomas

Prolactinomas are benign prolactin-secreting adenomas that arise in the lower lateral wings of the anterior pituitary from lactotrophes (the prolactin-secreting cells), which are normally sited there and make up about one-third of the functioning cells of the pituitary gland. The tumours are usually soft and discrete, sometimes partly degenerated and cystic, surrounded by a pseudocapsule of compressed pituitary tissue. Infrequently, the tumour may be diffuse and locally invasive, but rarely malignant. The bony fossa of the pituitary often becomes remodelled in response to a large tumour but is seldom eroded by it. Extension mostly occurs upwards and can compress the optic tracts. Compression of the hypothalamus and pituitary stalk can lead to panhypopituitarism. When the tumour is less than 10 mm in diameter it is called a microadenoma; otherwise it is a macroadenoma.

Diagnosis. Diagnostic confirmation requires special immunohistochemical staining of the tissue, but surgical extirpation is seldom undertaken except in the case of particularly large tumours with suprasellar extension. Most prolactinomas (in women) are microadenomas. Unfortunately the radiological appearances of a microprolactinoma are unreliable. Standard radiology may show downward distortion of one side of the fossa floor (reflecting the usual site of origin of a prolactinoma) but is easily misinterpreted. Computerized tomographic (CT) scanning shows a rounded area of inhomogeneity in the pituitary gland, which is usually taken as diagnostic in combination with hyperprolactinaemia, That is an unreliable conclusion, however, given the high frequency of adenomas to be found in women without endocrine disease. Therefore the main diagnostic value of a CT scan is to detect a macroadenoma, whether prolactin-secreting or not, and not to make a diagnosis of a microprolactinoma. Magnetic resonance imaging offers even better resolution to detect very small microprolactinomas, but in the light of the previous discussion there is little practical relevance in that.

Non-secreting macroadenomas can lead to hyperprolactinaemia by compressing the pituitary stalk, but the prolactin levels are usually much lower than with a prolactinoma of the same size. Prolactin levels correlate roughly with the size of prolactin-secreting adenomas, and a macroprolactinoma is to be expected when serum prolactin levels are greater than 2500–3000 mu/l. However, because lower levels may be due to a non-secreting macroadenoma, or occasionally a subarachnoid hernia expanding the fossa (empty sella syndrome; see earlier), CT scanning of the pituitary region is always advisable in addition to a lateral radiograph, which is mainly intended as a simple crude screening method for gross abnormality of the pituitary fossa or calcification in a craniopharyngioma. Radiology is of no value in oligomenorrhoeic patients who are not hyperprolactinaemic and do not have clinical evidence of other distinct endocrine disorders.

Pathogenesis and natural history. The aetiology and pathogenesis of prolactinomas are unknown; indeed it is arguable whether a microprolactinoma is a true neoplasm. Adenoma cells behave like normal lactotrophes and are normally receptive to dopamine.

Studies over the course of several years have shown that microprolactinomas generally show little or no enlargement (Sisam et al 1987; Schlecte et al 1989). However, because enlargement can occur annual monitoring by prolactin measurement is advisable. Prolactin levels reflect the functional size of a tumour. Up to a third of patients with apparent prolactinomas experience spontaneous resolution (Schlecte et al 1989), which may be encouraged by pregnancy possibly by inducing infarction of the tumour (Crosignani et al 1989).

Treatment. Transnasal–trans-sphenoidal microsurgical excision of a microadenoma is a fairly straightforward safe procedure. Unfortunately excision is often incomplete, therefore fails to cure the condition although prolactin levels are lower than before. Furthermore, even after apparent cure later relapse often occurs. Interestingly, when hyperprolactinaemia then recurs it is usually not associated with any evidence of tumour, suggesting there may be an inherent functional disturbance of the pituitary or hypothalamus–pituitary affecting prolactin secretion and underlying the pathogenesis of prolactinomas (Ciccarelli et al 1990). Surgery and radiotherapy are therefore usually reserved for very large tumours with suprasellar and frontal extension.

The treatment of choice is a dopamine agonist like bromocriptine. Shrinkage of tumour usually occurs rapidly, with concomitant improvement of any associated visual field defects. Although prolactin levels may not be fully suppressed at first, steady improvement can be achieved by prolonged treatment, which can often be reduced gradually to quite low maintenance doses but should be continued indefinitely. Tumour re-growth usually occurs again quickly after stopping treatment.

In pregnancy, after bromocriptine has been used to induce ovulation but then discontinued, the possibility of serious enlargement of a tumour can be monitored by visual field perimetry every 2 months, and bromocriptine therapy can be effectively reintroduced if necessary. Alternative urgent treatment including surgery needs specialist consideration. The reader is referred to a review of the management of prolactinomas by Molitch (1989).

Idiopathic hyperprolactinaemia

This diagnosis is made by exclusion of identifiable causes and will apply to about half the cases of hyperprolactinaemic amenorrhoea or oligomenorrhoea. The aetiology and pathogenesis are unknown, as for prolactinomas. Serum prolactin levels are usually only modestly raised (to less than 2500 mu/l) and some authors consider, although speculatively, that idiopathic hyperprolactinaemia may be an entity distinct from a prolactinoma, partly because there appears to be a greater chance (about 20%) of eventual spontaneous recovery (Schlecte et al 1989).

Treatment. Spontaneous recovery is unlikely and unpredictable, therefore treatment is specifically needed to achieve pregnancy, suppress galactorrhoea, or relieve symptoms associated with vulvovaginal atrophy. Furthermore, greater liveliness and libido, previously forgotten, are often distinct benefits, to be gained from restoration of ovarian function. In the long term, however, the main considerations are choice of contraceptive method and protection from osteoporosis, and these apply along with specific management of a prolactinoma as described above.

Dopamine receptor agonists like bromocriptine are very effective inhibitors of prolactin secretion by the normal pituitary, and in cases of idiopathic hyperprolactinaemia. Fertility is not restored in cases of (apparent) hyperprolactinaemia without associated ovulatory failure.

Bromocriptine is also very effective in suppressing galactorrhoea, although that is not of inherent concern, only in so far as it is a nuisance. Oestrogen deficiency symptoms are overcome by restoration of normal ovarian hormone production. Fertility is of course also restored, and contraceptive measures need to be taken if required. The choice can be made from the full range, including oral oestrogenic preparations, which have no adverse effect on prolactin secretion during bromocriptine therapy.

Osteoporosis. Perhaps most important of all, oestrogen therapy can be used to protect against osteoporosis which results from the lack of ovarian oestrogen production (Klibanski & Greenspan 1986; Schlecte et al 1987). The use of a simple contraceptive preparation is therefore particularly attractive for that purpose in the long term. It needs to be used with special caution if there is a macroadenoma because of the limited experience with it. On the other hand, the risk of osteoporosis is also of serious concern and deserves effective treatment.

A reasonable compromise with oestrogen therapy, particularly when there is intolerance of bromocriptine, might be to combine it with only a small dose of bromocriptine, sufficient to be protective without aiming to suppress prolactin levels substantially.

Control of bromocriptine therapy. The aim should be to suppress serum prolactin levels to around mid normal values (200–300 mu/l), not to very low levels. The dose should therefore be titrated accordingly. When attempting to induce ovulation there is usually scarcely time to optimize the dose before pregnancy is achieved. A daily dose of 5.0 mg is effective in about two-thirds of cases, but to save time we usually commence with 7.5 mg. Only about 10% of patients will need a higher dose than that but it is usually ineffective to raise the dose above 20–30 mg/day if prolactin levels are still not adequately suppressed. Side-effects are discussed in Chapter 10.

Alternative drug treatments. The search continues for dopamine receptor agonists with fewer side-effects and longer action. Many have been reported but none have proved superior to bromocriptine, although they may be of occasional benefit in cases of apparent idiosyncratic intolerance of bromocriptine. Lysuride is available in the UK but other effective agents include pergolide, terguride, metergoline and cabergoline, all ergot/ergoline derivatives.

Other hypothalamic–pituitary disorders

The hypothalamic–pituitary failures and disorders described so far, which are mostly related to weight loss and psychological disorders, and hyperprolactinaemia, account for about 50% of cases of amenorrhoea and 10% of oligomenorrhoea. In addition, primary ovarian failure accounts for about 10 and 2% respectively. What about the remainder?

It is notable that the foregoing disorders are all associated with secondary ovarian failure, and consequent oestrogen deficiency is evident in nearly all cases. By contrast, the remainder are nearly all oestrogenized. Polycystic ovarian syndrome, typified by hirsutism, accounts for about 8% of the amenorrhoea cases and 20% of oligomenorrhoea. The few cases of polycystic ovarian syndrome that appear to be oestrogen-deficient do not so much have low serum oestrogen levels as exceptionally high androgen levels, often with specific evidence of adrenal origin (because of raised dehydroepiandrosterone sulphate levels).

The rest, about a quarter of all patients with amenorrhoea and two-thirds of those with oligomenorrhoea, are oestrogenized and present no unusual features in their histories or physical make-up. For want of an explanation these patients are sometimes said to have 'euestrogenic oligo- or amenorrhoea'. Some authors have assumed a diagnosis of hypothalamic disorder, to distinguish the condition from hypothalamic failure which they use to describe the patients with oestrogen deficiency, inferring more profound disturbance (failure) of the H–P–O axis. However, patients with euestrogenic oligo- or amenorrhoea nearly all respond fully to treatment with clomiphene, which clearly indicates intact responsiveness of the hypothalamus–pituitary to negative and positive feedback signals. For that reason the condition has also been called 'cycle initiation defect', implying a simple but unexplained inability to trigger a H–P–O cycle in response to the usual decline in luteal hormone levels, although otherwise normal.

Some patients with euestrogenic oligo- or amenorrhoea have raised serum LH levels, but normal FSH, which has led some authors for many years to assume a diagnosis of polycystic ovarian disease even in the absence of hirsutism or obesity. It is now becoming clear by the use of refined vaginal ultrasonography that the ovaries are in fact polycystic in nearly all the oestrogenized patients (Hull 1989; Shulman et al 1989; Fox et al 1991a,b). The specific ultrasound features are at least 15 follicles of 2–10 mm diameter per ovary, usually but not invariably arranged around the cortex, and in particular a prominent expanded, echogenic stroma. These ultrasound appearances of polycystic ovarian disease have been confirmed histologically (Saxton et al 1990).

Thus it is now clear that polycystic ovarian disease, with or without hirsutism, accounts for about a third of all cases of amenorrhoea and nearly 90% of oligomenorrhoea (Adams et al 1986; Hull 1987), and the most consistent endocrine feature is oestrogenized state. The reader should appreciate that this view of polycystic ovarian disease as the essential cause of euestrogenic oligo amenorrhoea or cycle initiation defect is new and not universally accepted yet.

Feedback mechanisms in the hypothalamus–pituitary are intact, and the primary disorder appears to be usually in the ovary, although other factors such as hyperinsulinism and adrenal hyperandrogenism in a few cases are commonly involved (see Chapter 22). We therefore classify polycystic ovarian disease as an ovarian, not a hypothalamic–pituitary disorder.

Unclassified causes of oligo/amenorrhoea

Post-pill amenorrhoea and pseudocyesis are two conditions in particular that need discussion here because they are reported as though specific entities, usually along with the assumption that the underlying mechanism is hypothalamic–pituitary dysfunction in response to a particular pharmacological or psychological stimulus. It seems clear to us, however, that they are not specific entities, bearing only coincidental not causal relations to the factors suggested by their names; they encompass any and many of the conditions discussed earlier in this chapter.

Post-pill amenorrhoea

A causal relation to combined oestrogen–progestogen oral contraception was assumed for several reasons: the coincidental timing of onset with cessation of treatment; the common association with previous menstrual disorder, which is presumed to represent special susceptibility; the common delay in first menstruation after cessation of oral contraceptive treatment, and apparent reduced fertility subsequently.

Post-pill amenorrhoea occurs in about 0.5% of oral contraceptive users, not significantly more than the incidence in non-users as suggested by the prospective study (at least up to 3 months' duration) by Berger et al (1977). Also, previous menstrual disturbance was as common in women whose amenorrhoea is unrelated to oral contraceptive usage as in those with post-pill amenorrhoea (Hull et al 1981; Sherman et al 1984). Endocrine studies have revealed no consistent mechanism. Prospective and case-controlled studies have specifically shown no relationship of hyperprolactinaemia and prolactinomas to oral contraceptive usage, which had once been of particular concern (Sherman et al 1984). It seems that the coincidental timing of post-pill amenorrhoea is to be expected, the underlying cause having been masked by oral contraceptive-induced menstruation.

The usually brief initial impairment of fertility after oral contraceptive use may not be entirely due to biological effects, but may be at least partly behavioural. Spira et al (1985) noted that amongst women in Paris giving up contraception to conceive, 60% delayed their attempts after using oral contraceptives by nearly 4 months on average, and 30% did so after an intrauterine contraceptive device (IUCD) by nearly 3 months. After correction for these delayed attempts the differences in observed conception rates disappeared completely (Fig. 18.5).

Conclusions. The H–P–O system is remarkably robust, predictable in its response to contraceptive steroids, and in its return to normal function and fertility. There is no

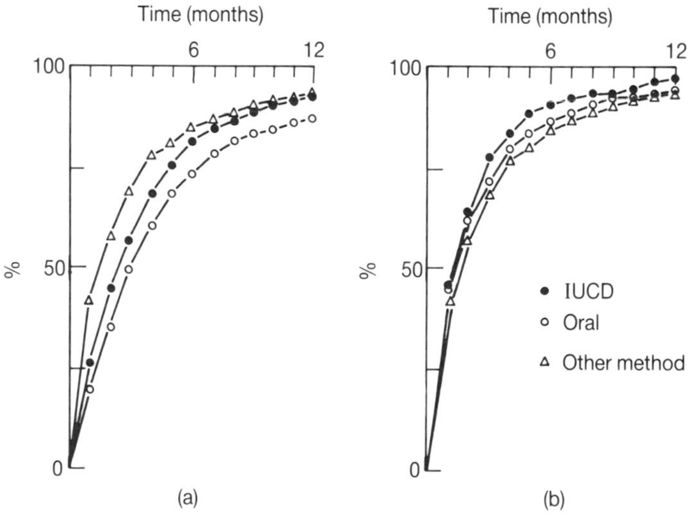

Fig. 18.5 Cumulative conception rates in fertile women after discontinuing contraception related to the method used. (**a**) From the time of discontinuing contraception; (**b**) after correcting for those who delayed their attempts to conceive. IUCD = intrauterine contraceptive device; Oral = oral contraceptive. Modified from Spira et al (1985).

evidence that oral contraceptives cause subsequent amenorrhoea. Therefore in practice post-pill amenorrhoea should not be treated as an entity. It should not be dismissed, but investigated and treated as any case of amenorrhoea. If reliable contraception is required again, standard oestrogen/progestogen preparations can be safely recommended. Hyperprolactinaemia is a possible exception because of oestrogenic stimulation, as discussed earlier.

Pseudocyesis

Phantom pregnancy and its psychological origin have been recognised since ancient times but the condition is now rare. It is still relatively common in some parts of the world, probably because of the overwhelming importance attached to fecundity in certain cultures, even amongst older women. The menopause accounts for many cases reported from West Africa, for example (Osotimehin et al 1981). Although a persistent corpus luteum occurs in some non-primates it does not explain human pseudocyesis. A wide range of disparate endocrinopathies have been reported (e.g. Osotimehin et al 1981; Tulandi et al 1983; DeVane et al 1985; Starkman et al 1985) including primary ovarian failure, hyperprolactinaemia, polycystic ovarian disease and psychogenic hypothalamic disorders.

The only sensible conclusion is that pseudocyesis is usually nothing more than an exaggerated emotional misinterpretation of amenorrhoea of different origin as being due to pregnancy; whilst in some cases the overwhelming desire for pregnancy can lead to typical psychogenic hypothalamic disorder. Pseudocyesis is not an entity and should be managed as any case of amenorrhoea, of course attending to the particular emotional problems of each patient.

Primary ovarian failure

There is space here for only an outline of the subject to fit into the context of management of oligo/amenorrhoea. There are numerous possible causes, briefly listed in the introductory classification given at the beginning of this chapter, and reviewed by Friedman et al (1983). The essential questions are whether primary ovarian failure can resolve, whether resolution is predictable, and whether any treatment can help recovery. In fact recovery is very uncommon and unpredictable, and treatment seems ineffective.

The key diagnostic feature is postmenopausal levels of FSH. Laparoscopic visualization alone is sufficient in the case of 'streak' ovaries, but in other cases laparoscopic and even laparotomy ovarian biopsy is unreliable. The typical inflammatory cell infiltration of autoimmune disease in the presence of plentiful follicles provides a little more optimism for recovery, but the diagnosis could be made equally by serology and other autoimmune endocrine disorders should be considered.

Immunosuppressive therapy for autoimmune ovarian failure even with high dosage of glucocorticoids is ineffective, but spontaneous recovery occurs occasionally and then sometimes intermittently. In the general type of case, claims for successful treatment with exogenous oestrogen, sometimes followed by gonadotrophins, are unconvincing. Any chance of recovery seems to be entirely fortuitous, the only optimistic hints being in those women with some menstrual activity, without extremely low oestrogen or extremely high FSH values, and with histological evidence of primordial follicles. None of those features discriminate between outcome completely, however. Up to 10% of women with primary ovarian failure recover and conceive. What is clear is that recovery is impossible while FSH levels remain raised.

Advice to individual patients is a matter of practical philosophy. Those who do not want to conceive need to be aware of the small chance of recovery and consider contraception if reliability is essential. Oestrogen replacement therapy will usually be necessary and a contraceptive preparation would do well. Those who want to conceive should interrupt the replacement therapy from time to time to reassess symptoms and FSH levels. Egg donation in vitro fertilization is an alternative.

Resistant ovary syndrome

This diagnosis implies the presence of ovarian follicles that are temporarily unresponsive to the usual gonadotrophic stimuli. The reasons for that are not clear except in the case of autoimmune disease. Also, the diagnosis and prognosis are unreliable because recovery can occur even when there were insufficient follicles to have been found on biopsy, as already discussed. The diagnosis can only be made in retrospect, when recovery has occurred, and is of no practical importance.

Endocrine disorders arising outside the H–P–O axis

It is beyond the scope of this chapter to review in detail other specific endocrine disorders. They seldom present simply with oligo/amenorrhoea to a gynaecologist. Routine attention in the history to involuntary weight changes, true anorexia, weakness, or heat or cold intolerance should point to Cushing's or Addison's adrenal disorder or thyroid disorder. The latter can also be easily screened by serum thyroid-stimulating hormone measurement (using the new assays with improved sensitivity to detect reduced levels or the free thyroxine index). Routine testing for glycosuria is sufficient for diabetes mellitus, although it is not clear whether that can cause oligo/amenorrhoea. Acromegaly should be recognized by the typical clinical features, particularly if hyperprolactinaemia is found by routine assay,

Table 18.4 Basic diagnostic classification and frequencies of endocrine disorders causing amenorrhoea or oligomenorrhoea

Class	Percentage of cases of		Criterion	Oestrogen state
	Amenorrhoea	Oligomenorrhoea		
Primary failures (H–P–O axis)				
Hypothalamic	2	0	History	Deficient
Pituitary	<1	0	History	Deficient
Ovarian	12	2	Raised FSH	Deficient
Functional disorders (H–P–O axis)				
Hypothalamic	30	5	History	Deficient
Hyperprolactinaemia	20	2	Raised PRL	Deficient
Polycystic ovaries	33	88	(Hirsutism if present)	Oestrogenized
Other endocrine disorders				
Thyroid	1	2	TSH (or FTI)	Variable
Adrenal	<1	<1	History (cortisol if indicated)	Variable

FSH = Follicle-stimulating hormone; PRL = prolactin; TSH = thyroid-stimulating hormone
FTI = free thyroxine index.

being commonly associated with excessive growth hormone secretion.

A common effect of these disorders on the H–P–O axis is by modulating circulating levels of sex hormone-binding globulin which is increased in thyrotoxicosis and reduced in hypothyroidism, hyperadrenalism and acromegaly. Other specific mechanisms also occur. In hyperadrenalism excess cortisol may directly suppress gonadotrophin secretion. Addison's disease does not seem to interfere with ovarian function except by association with polyendocrine autoimmune disease. Most notably, primary hypothyroidism often leads to hyperprolactinaemia essentially by excess TRH stimulation of prolactin secretion. A prolactinoma may be induced, which may explain why the degree of hyperprolactinaemia is usually related to the duration of hypothyroidism. Otherwise there is plentiful evidence that appropriate treatment of specific underlying endocrine disorders restores normal reproductive function.

GENERAL MANAGEMENT OF OLIGO/AMENORRHOEA

The prevalence of pathological amenorrhoea in young women is 1–2% and oligomenorrhoea about the same. They are common conditions with a wide range of causes. Specific diagnosis and treatment may in some cases need referral to other specialists by a gynaecologist but most can be managed along common lines within a simplified diagnostic framework as follows.

Apart from wanting a diagnosis, patients have different requirements which include advice about future fertility and its possible protection, contraception, hirsutism (see Chapter 22), secondary sexual development, protection against osteoporosis, and protection against endometrial cancer.

Basic diagnosis of endocrine disorder

After simply excluding an unlikely anatomical cause of amenorrhoea, the first step in diagnosis is to classify the type of endocrine disorder in a systematic way as shown in Table 18.4. Then more detailed investigations can be undertaken to define the specific underlying cause if necessary. The diagnosis of hypothalamic–pituitary failure or disorder requires routine exclusion of primary ovarian failure (raised serum FSH), hyperprolactinaemia (raised serum prolactin) and thyroid disorder (raised or low thyroid-stimulating hormone or free thyroxine index). Distinction between hypothalamic failure and hypothalamic disorder then depends primarily on the history because dynamic gonadotrophin-releasing tests are unhelpful, e.g. history of hyposmia, a known treated pituitary tumour, or weight fluctuation or psychological disorder.

In the diagnosis of polycystic ovarian disease hirsutism is specific but occurs in only about 25% of cases. The remainder, usually identifiable by high-resolution vaginal ultrasonography, are distinguished endocrinologically by their oestrogenized state, in contrast to the oestrogen deficiency which characterizes ovarian failure both primary and secondary to hypothalamic–pituitary failure or disorder. LH and androgen measurements are less reliable. Ultrasound diagnosis is also limited in some ways: it is not always possible to define the ovaries well enough, or to use a vaginal probe; on the other hand, polycystic ovaries can be found misleadingly (because of their common occurrence in apparently normal women; Polson et al 1988) in some women with amenorrhoea due to some other overriding cause.

From an ovarian viewpoint the classification of oligomenorrhoea can be simply reduced to the following: whether failure is primary or secondary there is consequent oestrogen deficiency.

1. Primary ovarian failure.
2. Secondary ovarian failure — due to hypothalamic or pituitary failure or disorders, including hyperprolactinaemia which acts by hypothalamic disorder of GnRH secretion.
3. Polycystic ovarian disease — essentially a primary ovarian disorder although modulated by extraneous influences like hyperinsulinaemia.

Assessment of oestrogen state

Assessment of oestrogen state provides 90% diagnostic reliability in distinguishing between polycystic ovarian disease and other causes of oligo/amenorrhoea (Hull 1989, Fox et al 1991a,b). It also provides a reliable index of responsiveness to clomiphene when ovulation induction is needed. In addition, it indicates the need for long-term therapy to protect the endometrium from overstimulation with endogenous oestrogen, or the bones from lack of it.

Assessment of oestrogen state is therefore of central importance in the management of oligo/menorrhoea. Some use oestrogen measurements in blood or urine, whilst others favour biological methods, including simple examination of the lower genital tract, particularly the cervix, vaginal cytology, and ultrasound measurement of uterine size and endometrial thickness (Shulman et al 1989), and the menstrual (endometrial) response to administered progestogen (the progestogen challenge test). Various progestogen regimens are used, by injection or tablet, but the one that has been systematically studied is a 5-day oral course of medroxyprogesterone acetate, in a daily dose of 5 mg (Hull et al 1979) or 15 mg (Shulman et al 1989).

The menstrual response to a progestogen challenge test is assessed in the following week: a normal menstrual loss indicates oestrogenized state (of the endometrium) and failure to menstruate indicates oestrogen deficiency. In only a small proportion of cases an impaired response occurs, defined by only scanty menstrual bleeding for no more than 2 days, and this also indicates oestrogen deficiency by correlation with other indices of oestrogen state (Hull et al 1979) including ultrasound measurement of double endometrial thickness of 4 mm or less (Shulman et al 1989).

By contrast, serum oestradiol levels range too widely, overlapping to a large extent between oestrogenized and oestrogen-deficient groups of patients, to be diagnostically useful (Shulman et al 1989) except when the level is distinctly low, below 100 pmol/l (Hull et al 1979) as illustrated in Figure 18.6.

Summary of primary investigations

1. History
   a. Previous weight loss.
   b. Psychological disorder.

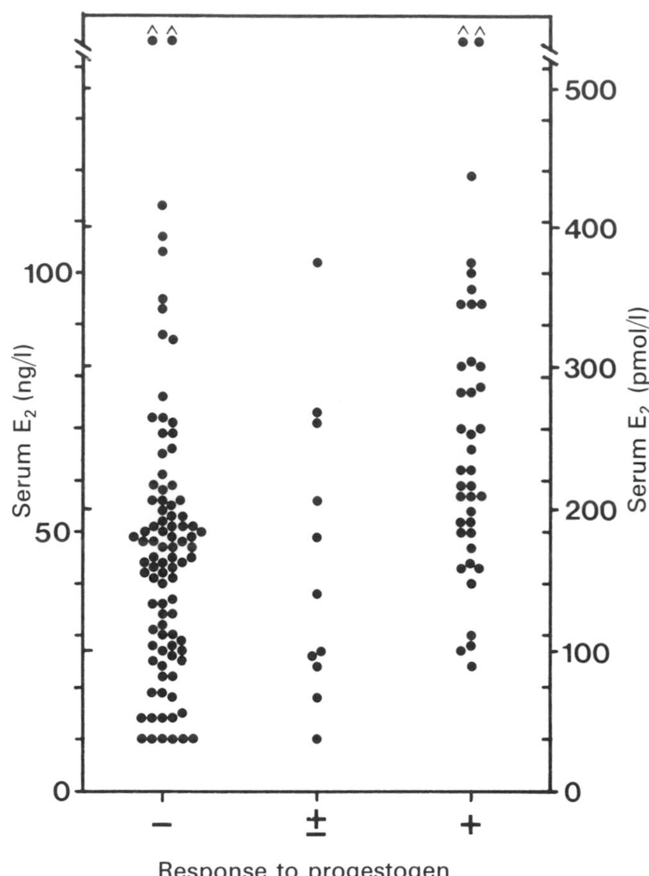

Fig. 18.6 Serum oestradiol (E_2) concentrations in women with amenorrhoea related to their menstrual response to a progestogen challenge: menstrual bleeding (+); positive — normal, impaired — scantly loss (±); negative — nil loss (−); From Hull et al (1979) with permission.

   c. Prolactinergic drugs.
   d. Thyroid symptoms.
   e. Hirsutism.
2. Examination
   a. Hirsutism.
   b. Vaginal atresia.
3. Serum
   a. FSH.
   b. Prolactin.
   Thyroid-stimulating hormone (or free thyroxine index).
4. Progestogen challenge test (oestrogen state).
5. Clomiphene test (only if pregnancy is desired).

Future fertility

Patients can be reassured about their future fertility. Given appropriate treatment, those with amenorrhoea have been shown to have a completely normal chance of conceiving and delivering a baby, excluding those with primary ovarian failure, while those with oligomenorrhoea have only a slightly reduced chance overall (Hull et al 1982). In fact the majority have a better chance than average because the overall success rates are reduced by the subgroup with overt polycystic ovarian syndrome (Hull 1987).

Patients with clinically 'occult' polycystic ovarian disease, i.e. as indicated only by evident oestrogen production and ultrasound appearance of the ovaries, are mostly successfully responsive to clomiphene treatment (Hull 1987). Those with overt polycystic ovarian syndrome have a more severe disorder as indicated for example by higher levels of androgens and insulin; they are much less likely to respond adequately to clomiphene, whilst their response to gonadotrophin therapy is particularly difficult to control.

Contraceptive advice

Nulliparous patients with oligo/amenorrhoea may be concerned about contraceptive need while protecting their future fertility. Others need advice having had a baby after successful ovulation induction therapy. An unexpected pregnancy is likely to be as unwelcome to such a woman as any other new mother. Advice will depend on knowing their chance of spontaneous ovulation and the possible effect of oral contraception generally on future fertility.

Oligomenorrhoeic women may ovulate normally in association with menstruation, albeit infrequently, and even amenorrhoea can resolve spontaneously and unpredictably. Virtually only Kallman's syndrome and ovarian failure with streak ovaries are certain not to resolve. The chance of conception is reduced, however — sometimes severely so — and this must be balanced against the degree of contraceptive reliability required. A married amenorrhoeic patient may be happy to do without any contraceptive protection.

The usual range of contraceptives can be considered, but with certain limitations. An IUCD should of course be avoided if possible in nulliparous women as usual. It should also be avoided, however, in all oligo/amenorrhoeic patients who are oestrogen-deficient because of uterine atrophy, which occurs even in parous women to such a degree as to prevent proper containment of the IUCD.

The choice of oestrogen/progestogen oral contraception depends partly on the evidence for any possible association with subsequent amenorrhoea or subfertility following its use generally. Those fears are unfounded, as discussed earlier, therefore such contraception can be safely considered. It may also carry other advantages (see below). In women with polycystic ovarian disease androgenic progestogens should be avoided. A preparation containing an antiandrogenic progestogen like cyproterone acetate would seem particularly appropriate.

One concern about oestrogenic contraceptives is possible worsening of hyperprolactinaemia and in particular critical enlargement of a prolactinoma. Protective combination with low-dose bromocriptine could be considered but needs studying, and progestogen-only therapy may be a reasonable compromise.

Endometrial protection

Cystic hyperplasia of the endometrium is a well recognized association with prolonged anovulatory intervals between menstruation, as typically occurs with polycystic ovarian disease, and polycystic ovarian syndrome has been clearly linked with an increased risk of endometrial carcinoma in relatively young women, under 40 years of age (Lucas 1974; Nisker et al 1978). It therefore seems important to offer protective therapy to oligo/amenorrhoeic patients who are oestrogenized. Progestogen courses of at least 12 days are required, although in low dose — sufficient to induce menstrual bleeding only in young oligo/amenorrhoeic women. How often such cyclical therapy needs to be given is unclear, but every 1–2 months would seem appropriate and timing will depend partly on the personal wishes of each patient. An alternative form combining menstrual cycle control with reliable contraception would of course be a standard combined oestrogen/progestogen contraceptive preparation.

Oestrogen deficiency

Oestrogen deficiency is a consequence of all the hypothalamic–pituitary disorders leading to secondary ovarian failure associated with oligo- or usually amenorrhoea, as well as primary ovarian failure. This may result in acute symptoms, or chronic but often unrecognized impairment of well-being, and osteoporosis. Osteoporotic fractures including vertebral crush fractures can occur in young women. Oestrogen replacement therapy is therefore a major prophylactic requirement, particularly because of the young age of the patients. Points of practical concern are possible risks of adverse stimulation in cases of hyperprolactinaemia; unwelcome return of menstruation in some patients with particular psychological disorders, and the dosage required.

Delayed puberty

The particular therapeutic needs of young patients with primary amenorrhoea and lack of secondary sexual development are early recognition of their need, low-dose oestrogen therapy to stimulate skeletal growth, and warning that full secondary development requires patience. Delayed pubertal development should be recognized and treatment started for its psychological benefit by the age of 14 years if breast development has not started by then. Full breast development takes 4–5 years to complete and cannot be hurried by increasing the dose of oestrogen; indeed the shape of the breasts, in particular the areolae, can become distorted.

In general, without allowing for variation in body weight, it requires a dose of ethinyl oestradiol of only 5 μg daily to stimulate bone growth maximally, and any stimulant effect is lost at about 20 μg/day. Breast development, by contrast, is less sensitive to oestrogen and needs about 10 μg/day (Ross et al 1983). Continuous oestrogen alone seems appropriate at first, combining later with progestogen only if any irregular vaginal bleeding occurs or when breast development is well advanced.

KEY POINTS

1. Delayed puberty is diagnosed if breast development does not start by 14 years of age. It should not be delayed to include menarche.
2. Primary and secondary amenorrhoea and oligomenorrhoea should be considered in the same way clinically as distinction may be misleading. In addition oligomenorrhoea is likely to include a spectrum of conditions ranging from virtual normality at one end to the same causes as those of amenorrhoea at the other.
3. It is not possible to distinguish between primary hypothalamic or pituitary failure by measuring the gonadotrophins response to an acute GnRH stimulus. The secretory capacity of the pituitary gland can be tested by prolonged repeated GnRH pulses.
4. Psychological causes account for about one-third of all causes of amenorrhoea. This affirms the modulatory influence of extra hypothalamic brain centres on pulsatile GnRH secretion.
5. Cosmetic weight loss in adolescent girls may be a warning sign of future anorexia. This is especially so if it is associated with faddishness about the preparation and eating of food (often in isolation) and combined with anxiety, depression, feeling cold, constipation and behavioural changes.
6. Weight loss accounts for about one-third of all cases of amenorrhoea presenting to the gynaecologist and anorexia nervosa accounts for half of those.
7. Anorexia nervosa may not be a specific psychological disease as once believed. Starvation may be a response to the psychosexual pressure of adolescence conditioned by the individual's constitutional and family environment (parents' own anxieties).
8. In anorexia nervosa there is increased hypothalamo-adrenocorticotrophic activity coupled with failure of the hypothalamo-pituitary-ovarian axis. This is reflected by high cortisol levels and low gonadotrophins and oestrogen values coupled with failure of the pituitary gland to respond to an acute GnRH stress.
9. Women with weight-related amenorrhoea should not be encouraged to get pregnant by using drugs. They should rather be encouraged to gain weight first as a low BMI is associated with an adverse fetal outcome.
10. The most common causes of hypoprolactinaemia are pituitary adenomas (40–50%) and idiopathic hypersecretion (50%). Primary hypothyroidism and pharmacological causes account for 3–5% and 1–2% respectively.
11. Amongst normal women, one-third can be found to have a pituitary tumour on radiological or subsequent post-mortem examination.
12. True hypoprolactinaemia nearly always causes amenorrhoea or severe oligomenorrhoea with no convincing evidence of causing persistent follicular or luteal dysfunction and infertility in normally menstruating women.
13. Treatment of hyperprolactinaemia is necessary, even if pregnancy is not desired, to reduce tumour size and relieve symptoms of oestrogen deficiency and galactorrhoea.
14. Polycystic ovarian disease with or without hirsutism accounts for about one-third of all cases of amenorrhoea and nearly 90% of oligomenorrhoea.
15. Amenorrhoeic women with oestrogen deficiency should receive HRT to guard against oestrogen deficiency related symptoms. On the other hand, well oestrogenized amenorrhoeic women should receive cyclic progestogen treatment to guard against endometrial hyperplasia and atypia.
16. Menstrual dysfunction associated with obesity may be a reflection of an associated endocrine dysfunction (e.g. PCO) rather than being due to obesity itself. Only in massive obesity is there any convincing evidence that weight reduction may lead to improvement in the endocrine state and menstrual function.

REFERENCES

Adams J, Polson D W, Franks S 1986 Prevalence of polycystic ovaries in women with anovulation and idiopathic hirsutism. British Medical Journal 292: 355–359

Aksel S 1981 Hormonal characteristics of long cycles in fertile women. Fertility and Sterility 36: 521–523

Berga S L, Mortola J F, Yen S S 1988 Amplification of nocturnal melatonin secretion in women with functional hypothalamic amenorrhea. Journal of Clinical Endocrinology and Metabolism 66: 242–244

Berger G S, Taylor R N, Treloar A E 1977 The risk of post-pill amenorrhea: a preliminary report from the menstruation and reproduction history research program. International Journal of

Gynaecology and Obstetrics 15: 125–127
Bergh T, Nillius S J, Wide L 1978 Serum prolactin and gonadotrophin levels before and after luteinizing hormone-releasing hormone in the investigation of amenorrhoea. British Journal of Obstetrics and Gynaecology 85: 945–956
Bhanot R, Wilkinson M 1983 Opiatergic control of gonadotrophin secretion during puberty in the rat: a neurochemical basis for the hypothalamic 'gonadostat'? Endocrinology 113: 596–603
Boyar R M, Katz J, Finkelstein J W et al 1974 Anorexia nervosa. New England Journal of Medicine 291: 861–865
Brzezinski A, Lynch H J, Seibel M M, Deng M H, Nader T M, Wurtman R J 1988 The circadian rhythm of plasma melatonin during the normal menstrual cycle and in amenorrheic women. Journal of Clinical Endocrinology and Metabolism 66: 891–895
Cann C E, Martin M C, Genant H K, Jaffe R B 1984 Decreased spinal mineral content in amenorrhoeic women. Journal of the American Medical Association 251: 626–629
Chang F E, Richards S R, Kim M H, Malarkey W B 1984 Twenty four-hour prolactin profiles and prolactin responses to dopamine in long distance running women. Journal of Clinical Endocrinology and Metabolism 59: 631–635
Ciccarelli E, Ghigo E, Miola C, Gandini G, Muller E E, Camanni F 1990 Long-term follow-up of 'cured' prolactinoma patients after successful adenomectomy. Clinical Endocrinology 32: 583–592
Crosignani P G, Mattei A M, Scarduelli C, Cavioni V, Boracchi P 1989 Is pregnancy the best treatment for hyperprolactinaemia? Human Reproduction 4: 910–912
DeVane G W, Vera M I, Buhi W C, Kalra P S 1985 Opioid peptides in pseudocyesis. Obstetrics and Gynecology 65: 183–188
Drinkwater B L, Nilson K, Chesnut C H, Bremner W J, Shainholtz S, Southworth M B 1984 Bone mineral content of amenorrheic and eumenorrheic athletes. New England Journal of Medicine 311: 277–281
Fairburn C G, Cooper P J 1982 Self induced vomiting and bulimia nervosa: an undetected problem. British Medical Journal 284: 1153–1155
Fishman J 1980 Fatness, puberty and ovulation. New England Journal of Medicine 303: 42–43
Fletcher R 1974 Assessment of nutritional status. Medicine Series 1 28: 1650–1666
Fox R, Corrigan E, Thomas P, Hull M G R 1991a Oestrogen and androgen states in oligo-amenorrhoeic women with polycystic ovaries. British Journal of Obstetrics and Gynaecology 98: 294–299
Fox R, Corrigan E, Thomas P, Hull M G R 1991b The diagnosis of polycystic ovaries in women with oligo-amenorrhoea: predictive power of endocrine tests. Clinical Endocrinology 34: 127–131
Friedman C I, Barrows H, Kim M H 1983 Hypergonadotropic hypogonadism. American Journal of Obstetrics and Gynecology 145: 360–372
Fries H, Nillius S J, Petterson F 1974 Epidemiology of secondary amenorrhea. II. A retrospective evaluation of etiology with special regard to psychogenic factors and weight loss. American Journal of Obstetrics and Gynecology 118: 473–479
Frisch R E 1984 Body fat, puberty and fertility. Biological Reviews 59: 161–188
Gadpaille W J, Sanborn C F, Wagner W W 1987 Athletic amenorrhoea, major affective disorders, and eating disorders. American Journal of Psychiatry 144: 939–942
Glazener C M A, Kelly N J, Hull M G R 1987 Prolactin measurement in the investigation of infertility in women with a normal menstrual cycle. British Journal of Obstetrics and Gynaecology 94: 535–538
Hull M G R 1987 Epidemiology of infertility and polycystic ovarian disease: endocrinological and demographic studies. Gynecological Endocrinology 1: 235–245
Hull M G R 1989 Polycystic ovarian disease: clinical aspects and prevalence. Research and Clinical Forums 11: 21–30
Hull M G R, Knuth U A, Murray M A F, Jacobs H S 1979 The practical value of the progestogen challenge test, serum oestradiol estimation or clinical examination in assessment of the oestrogen state and response to clomiphene in amenorrhoea. British Journal of Obstetrics and Gynaecology 86: 799–805
Hull M G R, Bromham D R, Savage P E, Barlow T M, Hughes A O, Jacobs H S 1981 Post-pill amenorrhoea: a causal study. Fertility and Sterility 36: 472–476
Hull M G R, Savage P E, Bromham D R 1982 Anovulatory and ovulatory infertility: results with simplified management. British Medical Journal 284: 1681–1685
Klibanski A, Greenspan S L 1986 Increase in bone mass after treatment of hyperprolactinemic amenorrhea. New England Journal of Medicine 315: 542–546
Knobil E 1980 The neuroendocrine control of the menstrual cycle. Recent Progress in Hormone Research 36: 53–88
Kopelman P G, White N, Pilkington T R E, Jeffcoate S L 1981 The effect of weight loss on sex steroid secretion and binding in massively obese women. Clinical Endocrinology 15: 113–116
Laatikainen T, Virtanen T, Apter D 1986 Plasma immunoreactive beta-endorphin in exercise-associated amenorrhea. American Journal of Obstetrics and Gynecology 154: 94–97
Lacey J H, Crisp A H, Kalucy R S, Hartmann M K, Chen C N 1975 Weight gain and the sleeping electroencephalogram: study of 10 patients with anorexia nervosa. British Medical Journal iv: 556–558
Lucas W E 1974 Causal relationships between endocrine-metabolic variables in patients with endometrial carcinoma. Obstetrics and Gynecology Survey 29: 507–528
Mason H D, Sagle M, Polson D W et al 1988 Reduced frequency of luteinizing hormone pulses in women with weight loss-related amenorrhoea and multifollicular ovaries. Clinical Endocrinology 28: 611–618
Molitch M E 1989 Management of prolactinomas. Annual Reviews of Medicine 40: 225–232
Moult P J A, Rees L H, Besser G M 1982 Pulsatile gonadotrophin secretion in hyperprolactinaemic amenorrhoea and the response to bromocriptine therapy. Clinical Endocrinology 16: 153–162
Nisker J A, Ramzy I, Collins J A 1978 Adenocarcinoma of the endometrium and abnormal ovarian function in young women. American Journal of Obstetrics and Gynecology 130: 546–550
Osotimehin B O, Ladipo O A, Adejuwon C A, Otolorin E O 1981 Pituitary and placental hormone levels in pseudocyesis. International Journal of Gynaecology and Obstetrics 19: 399–402
Polson D W, Sagle M, Mason H D, Adams J, Jacobs H S, Franks S 1986 Ovulation and normal luteal function during LHRH treatment of women with hyperprolactinaemic amenorrhoea. Clinical Endocrinology 24: 531–537
Polson D W, Adams J, Wadsworth J, Franks S 1988 Polycystic ovaries — a normal variant? Lancet i: 870–872
Quigley M E, Sheehan K L, Casper R F, Yen S S 1980 Evidence for increased dopaminergic and opioid activity in patients with hypothalamic hypogonadotropic amenorrhea. Journal of Clinical Endocrinology and Metabolism 50: 949–954
Ross J L, Cassorla F G, Skerda M C, Valk I M, Loriaux D L, Cutler G B 1983 A preliminary study of the effect of estrogen dose on growth in Turner's syndrome. New England Journal of Medicine 309: 1104–1106
Sanborn C F, Martin B J, Wagner W W 1982 Is athletic amenorrhea specific to runners? American Journal of Obstetrics and Gynecology 143: 859–861
Saxton D W, Farquhar M, Rae T, Beard R W, Anderson M C, Wadsworth J 1990 Accuracy of ultrasound measurements of female pelvic organs. British Journal of Obstetrics and Gynaecology; 95–699
Schlecte J, El-Khoury G, Kathol M, Walkner L 1987 Forearm and vertebral bone mineral in treated and untreated hyperprolactinemic amenorrhea. Journal of Clinical Endocrinology and Metabolism 64: 1021–1026
Schlecte J, Dolan K, Sherman B, Chapler F, Luciano A 1989 The natural history of untreated hyperprolactinemia: a prospective analysis. Journal of Clinical Endocrinology and Metabolism 68: 412–418
Sherman B M, Wallace R B, Chapler F K, Luciano A A, Bean J A 1984 Prolactin-secreting pituitary tumors: an epidemiologic approach. In: Cammani F, Muller E E (eds) Pituitary hyperfunction: physiopathology and clinical aspects. Raven Press, New York, pp 167–174
Shulman A, Shulman N, Weissenglass L, Bahary C 1989 Ultrasonic assessment of the endometrium as a predictor of oestrogen status in amenorrhoeic patients. Human Reproduction 4: 616–619
Sisam D A, Sheehan J P, Sheeler L R 1987 The natural history of untreated microprolactinomas. Fertility and Sterility 48: 67–71

Spira N, Spira A, Schwartz D 1985 Fertility of couples following cessation of contraception. Journal of Biosocial Science 17: 281–290
Starkman M N, Marshall J C, La Ferla J, Kelch R P 1985 Pseudocyesis: psychologic and neuroendocrine interrelationships. Psychosomatic Medicine 47: 46–57
Suh B Y, Liu J H, Berga S L, Quigley M E, Laughlin G A, Yen S S 1988 Hypercortisolism in patients with functional hypothalamic amenorrhea. Journal of Clinical Endocrinology and Metabolism 66: 733–739
Tulandi T, McInnes R A, Lal S 1983 Altered pituitary hormone secretion in patients with pseudocyesis. Fertility and Sterility 40: 637–641
Vigersky R A 1981 Functional disorders of the hypothalamic–pituitary axis. In: Beardwell C, Robertson G L (eds) The pituitary. Butterworths, London, pp 1–46

19. Tubal disease

R. A. Margara

INTRODUCTION

Tubal disease can be defined as tubal damage caused by pelvic infection such as pelvic inflammatory disease, tuberculosis, salpingitis isthmica nodosa or iatrogenic disease with varying degrees of tubal damage or obstruction, sometimes involving the surrounding ovary or pelvic peritoneum, and adhesion formation. As a result patients with tubal damage suffer from infertility and/or pelvic pain. Tubal disease is accountable for 30–40% of cases of female infertility.

AETIOLOGY OF TUBAL DISEASE

Salpingitis

Most salpingitis is the result of an ascending infection from the lower genital tract (Fig. 19.1). The mechanisms whereby the infection ascends through the cervical canal and reaches the tubes is still unknown. It is possible that cervical resistance diminishes, allowing the bacteria to pass through, and is at its lowest during ovulation and menstruation. This theory fits with observations that in cases of cervical gonorrhoea the symptoms of salpingitis appear after menstruation, and patients on oral contraception appear to be 'protected', due to anovulation.

Salpingitis is not in general seen in women who are not sexually active and, it is possible that coitus produces uterine contractions, facilitating the spread of infection into the uterus and tubes. In other cases, iatrogenic manoeuvres such as insertion of an intrauterine device, termination of pregnancy, hysterosalpingography or curettage can spread a cervical infection into the uterus and tubes.

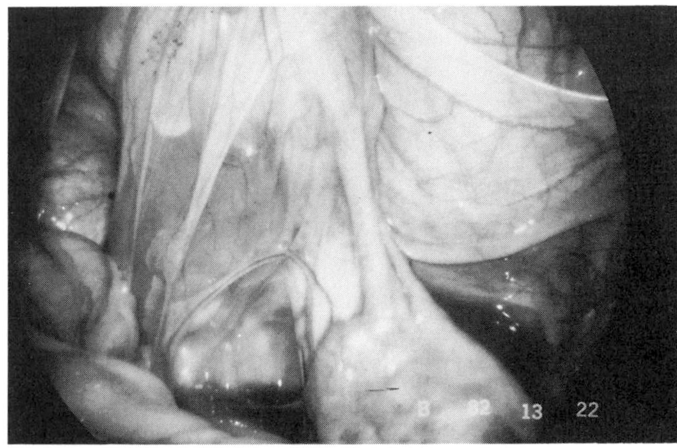

Fig. 19.1 Laparoscopic view of a pelvis after pelvic inflammatory disease. There is a 'curtain' of adhesions covering the pelvic organs.

Iatrogenic tubal disease is tubal damage caused by surgical procedures carried out in a manner damaging the peritoneum and tubes, rendering young women infertile.

Pelvic inflammatory disease has by tradition been associated with gonorrhoea. Improvement of microbiological techniques has allowed the identification of numerous other organisms capable of producing salpingitis, including *Chlamydia trachomatis*, *Mycoplasma hominis* and anaerobic bacteria.

Neisserial gonorrhoeae

Neisseriae gonorrhoeae has been isolated from cervical mucus in women with salpingitis in between 10 and 70% of cases, but among those that have positive cervical cultures not all have positive peritoneal cultures. What are the

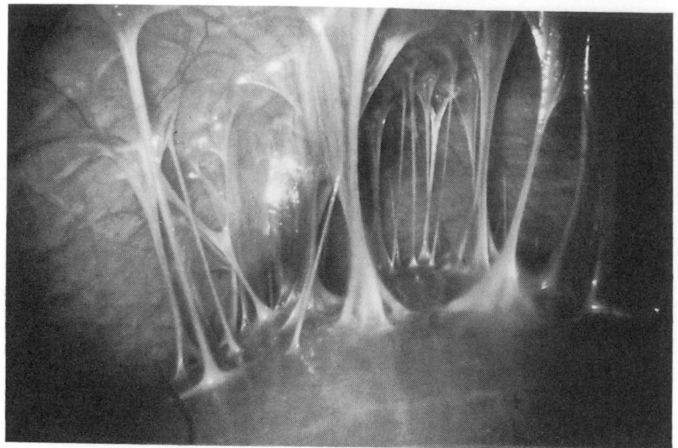

Fig. 19.2 Laparoscopic photograph of perihepatic adhesions: Fitz–Hugh–Curtis syndrome.

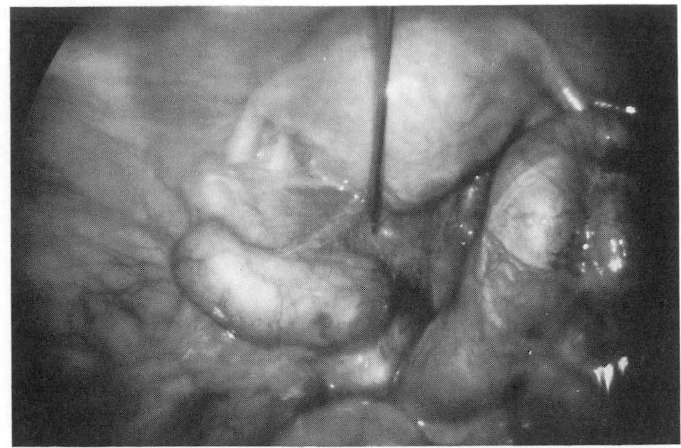

Fig. 19.3 Laparoscopic appearance of bilateral hydrosalpinges as a result of previous pelvic inflammatory disease.

reasons for the variation? There may be differences in host resistance to the organisms; the non-white population seems to be more at risk of having salpingitis with gonococcal cervicitis than others. The use of oral contraception may increase resistance towards the gonococcus and it is probably because of this that in the USA, where since 1974 the use of oral contraception has decreased, the risk of women having salpingitis has increased.

Certain auxotypes of gonococcus are more sensitive to antibiotics; when they are localized in the cervix they are easily treated, thus preventing the organism spreading to the tubes.

Chlamydia trachomatis

Chlamydia trachomatis was isolated for the first time in Sweden by Eilard et al (1976) from women with salpingitis. Positive cultures from cervices have been found in up to 36% of patients, but only 6% of them have positive cultures from the tubes. There is no doubt, that *Chlamydia* is responsible for a significant amount of salpingitis but it is not possible to determine how much. There is a discordance between identification of *Chlamydia*-positive cultures and the titre of immunoglobulin gamma M; this titre does not correlate with the severity of salpingitis found at the time of laparoscopy.

There is evidence that *Chlamydia* is also responsible for causing postpartum endometritis with perihepatic adhesions (Fig. 19.2). Infertile women on average have higher *Chlamydia* antibody titres than pregnant women. Peritonitis following salpingitis may be the result of an immunological mechanism and it has been suggested that the perihepatic adhesions are not caused by *C. trachomatis* directly, but more likely to be caused by a heterologous infection.

Other organisms

In the general female population there are many organisms capable of producing salpingitis. Most of them are part of the vaginal flora or from the perianal region and are called polymicrobial salpingitis.

Gonococcal infection seems to pave the way for other micro-organisms to cross the cervical mucus and affect the uterus or the tubes; there may be a relation between the intensity of the symptoms, the duration of a gonococcus salpingitis and superinfection with other micro-organisms (Fig. 19.3). Gonococcal salpingitis may increase tubal susceptibility to a subsequent infection, and one attack of salpingitis may protect against the same strain of gonococcus, the subsequent salpingitis being non-gonococcal.

Mycoplasma hominis

Mycoplasma hominis has been isolated from peritoneal fluid from patients with salpingitis. Animal experiments suggest that *M. hominis* produces parametritis as well salpingitis, implying a source of infection other than canalicular.

Mycobacterium tuberculosis

Tubal damage of tuberculous origin is still seen in developed countries, although rarely. *Mycobacterium tuberculosis* reaches the pelvic organs from a primary focus of entry — lung or intestine — and then spreads to the genital organs. The most common organs affected are the endometrial cavity and the tubes. Primary genital tuberculosis has been described as a result of infection from semen of an affected partner, this being the most common source of entry to the cervix.

The aetiology, trends, incidence and epidemiology of pelvic inflamatory disease are discussed in other chapters.

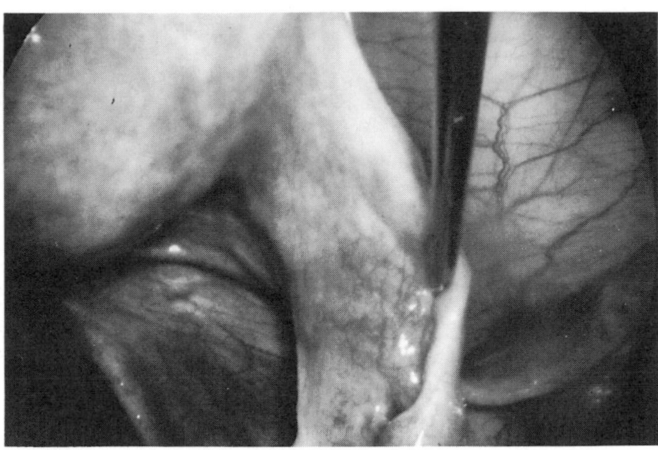

Fig. 19.4 Laparoscopic photograph of the same patient as in Figure 19.3 with salpingitis isthmica nodosa. There is extravasation of dye through the tubal wall.

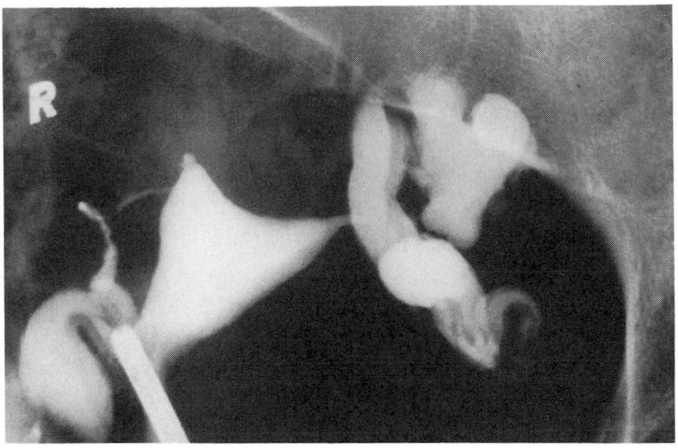

Fig. 19.5 Hysterosalpingogram of a patient with bilateral hydrosalpinges.

Salpingitis isthmica nodosa

Salpingitis isthmica nodosa was described Chiari (1887) as nodular thickening of the proximal part of the fallopian tube. The aetiology of this entity is unknown but it is probably due to a non-inflammatory process similar to adenomyosis (Benjamin & Beaver 1951) or related to diverticulosis in other organs (Burne 1973); infection may always be a secondary process (Fig. 19.4).

Salpingitis isthmica nodosa can be defined as the microscopic presence of tubal epithelium within a hypertrophied and hyperplastic myosalpinx or beneath the tubal serosa and characterized radiologically by a small diverticulum. It has been classified into grades I–III according to the degree of invasion or depth of the tubal epithelium in the myosalpinx.

The real incidence of salpingitis isthmica nodosa is very difficult to determine. Honore (1978) reported an incidence of 0.6% in a control population who had undergone salpingectomy for sterilization. He also noted a frequency of 2.86% in patients with ectopic pregnancy. Creasy et al (1985) reported in a large series of hysterosalpingograms of infertile women that 3.9% had changes of salpingitis isthmica nodosa on their hysterosalpingograms and half of them had bilateral involvement.

Other causes

Endometriosis, endosalpingiosis and cornual polyps can be the cause of cornual obstruction or tubal damage. Endometriosis has been reviewed in Chapter 30.

Cornual polyps

Cornual polyps have been described by Lisa et al (1954); they can cause infertility if they are bilateral. The exact aetiology is not known, but they seem to have two origins — infection and endometriosis.

Previous tubal/pelvic surgery

In a survey done at Hammersmith Hospital in 1980, in 100 consecutive patients referred to the unit for a mechanical cause of their infertility, no less than 24 had had previous pelvic surgery which appeared to be the reason for the tubal damage (Winston, unpublished results). The operations that had been performed were ovarian cystectomy, wedge resection, myomectomy, salpingectomy, and shortening of round ligament.

Tubal sterilization procedures

Tubal sterilization can be done by laparotomy, culdoscopy and laparoscopy; probably the latter is the most widely used. The laparoscopic methods can be diathermy (monopolar or bipolar); tubal clips (Hulka–Clemens or Filshie) and Yoong's tubal rings. Laparotomy is most used in general at the time of a caesarean section. Methods of sterilization are reviewed in Chapter 21.

DIAGNOSIS AND TREATMENT

The diagnosis of tubal disease is made by laparoscopy and hysterosalpingography. Laparoscopy does not replace the hysterosalpingogram and vice versa. The two are complementary investigations, both offering very important information (Figs 19.5 and 19.6).

Laparoscopy

Laparoscopy should be performed by the surgeon or a member of the team who will eventually operate on the

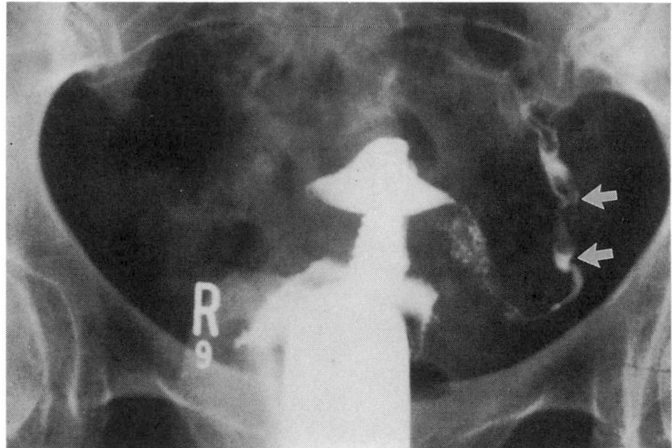

Fig. 19.6 Hysterosalpingogram of a patient with salpingitis isthmica nodosa. Arrows indicate the diverticula filed with contrast medium.

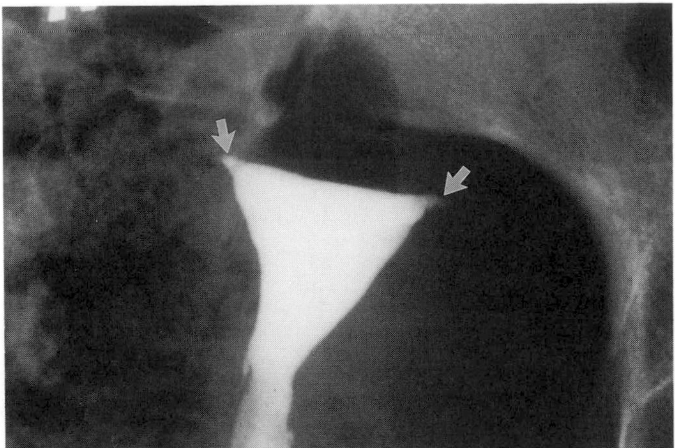

Fig. 19.8 Hysterosalpingogram of a patient with bilateral tubal block (arrows).

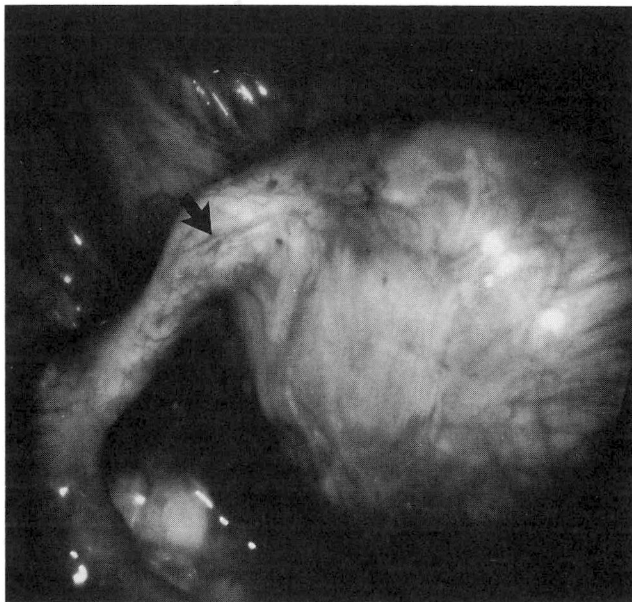

Fig. 19.7 Tubal cornual block: there are irregular vessels on the peritoneum surface as a result of previous inflammation (arrow).

patient if surgery is the treatment of choice. The reason is the variation between units in experience and approaches to varying tubal diseases.

The criteria of patient selection for treatment depend very much on the surgeon's experience and the possibility of being able to offer alternative treatment. Other points to be considered at the time of making the decision regarding treatment are the patient's wishes of the type of treatment that she and her husband prefer, and the problem of pain. Large numbers of patients with tubal disease have pelvic pain due to adhesions. In some of them the freeing of the ovaries and tubes of adhesions surgically can give symptomatic relief.

The treatment of tubal disease in the infertile patient is surgical and based on the principles of microsurgery, but microsurgery is not merely the use of a microscope and involves gentle tissue handling, reperitonealization of raw areas, the use of fine non-absorbable suture material and irrigation of the tissues using Ringer's lactate tend to prevent adhesion formation. Repair of the ovarian capsule, if it has been damaged, is a basic step in surgical treatment in the infertile patient.

Microsurgery

The microscope was used for tubal surgery for the first time by Walz (1959). Whilst others used delicate electrosurgery and magnification (loupes) in the treatment of hydrosalpinges. Paterson & Wood (1974) in Australia and Winston & McClure-Browne (1974) in England adapted their laboratory techniques to the human and operated on infertile women under high magnification using an operating microscope. There were heated arguments about how useful the microscope was and how much its use improved pregnancy rates. Now microsurgery is well established and is a routine procedure for tubal infertility.

Coadjuvants

The use of coadjuvants can sometimes help to avoid adhesion formation, but remember no coadjuvant will replace a lack of surgery. If a coadjuvant is used probably the best choice is the use of steroids (Winston 1982).

Cornual occlusion (Figs 19.7, 19.8)

Cornual occlusion due to inflammatory causes was treated by uterotubal implantation with very poor results. Ehrler

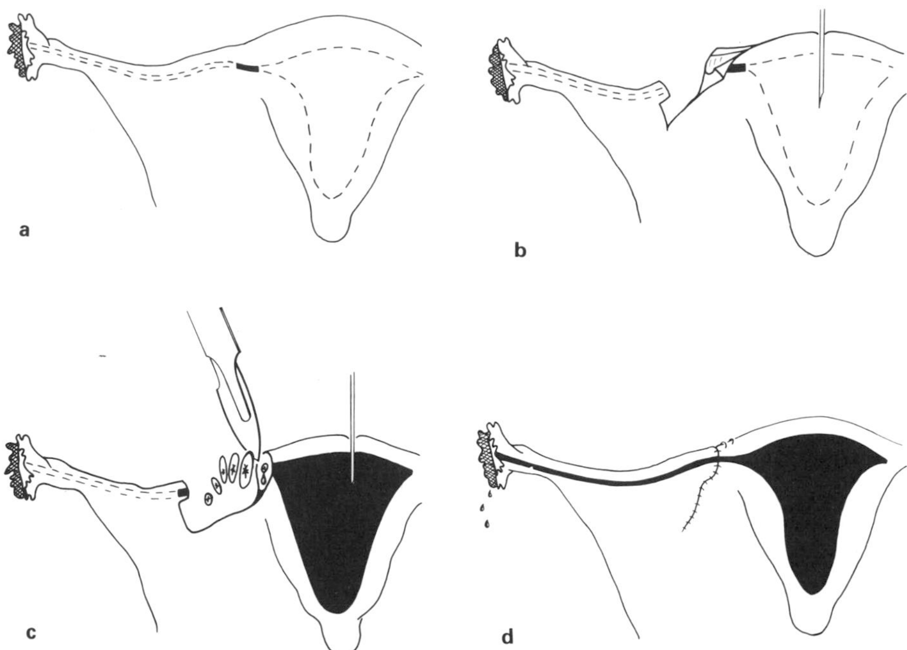

Fig. 19.9 Cornual block diagram showing a cornual anastomosis. (**a**) Superficial cornual block; (**b**) opening of the cornua to expose the intramural part of the tube); (**c**) shaving of the tube to find healthy mucosa of anastomosis; (**d**) cornual anastomosis completed.

(1963) describes his technique and suggested that in most patients the intramural portion of the tube could be spared. Since Winston (1977) and Gomel (1977) described their methods based on the use of the microscope it has become the surgical technique of choice. Cornual implantation is now rarely used in our department except in cases of severe damage of the intramural portion of the tubes, and is reserved for cases where there is a severe degree of adenomyosis or tubal damage. We avoid tubocornual implantation whenever possible. Destroying a possible sphincter at the utero tubal junction is associated with excessive bleeding and damage to the tubal blood supply; it shortens the tube and may increase the risk of rupture of the uterus in the event of subsequent pregnancy, thus patients must be delivered by caesarean section.

The use of magnification allows the surgeon better identification of the intramural portion of the tube by careful shaving of the cornua until healthy tissue is found, permitting a more accurate tissue apposition with a watertight anastomosis between healthy tubal tissues. Once the ends are well defined the anastomosis is done in two layers, using 8/0 nylon as a suture. The suture material should not penetrate the mucosa, only the muscularis (Seki et al 1977). In some cases the use of a temporary splint gives considerable help, especially in deep cornual tubal anastomosis (Fig. 19.9), but it should be removed at the end of the surgical procedure, and if left in situ should not remain more than 48 h. Longer periods of time cause mucosal damage. Tension between the anastomosed ends must be avoided. A stitch of 6/0 prolene between both ends of the mesosalpinx should be applied as a stay suture. More details about the technique have been given elsewhere (Winston 1977; Margara 1982).

Cornual polyps

Removal of cornual polyps is still a matter of controversy. Glazener et al (1987) stated that the removal of cornual polyps does not improve fertility, and they are not a cause of infertility. We believe that large polyps present in the intramural or isthmic portion of the tube should be removed depending on the location and size of the polyp. This can involve salpingotomy and resection of the polyp without tubal resection or the opening of the cornu and removal of the affected portion of the tube followed by cornual–isthmic anastomosis in two layers. In some cases when a large polyp is implanted deep in the intramural portion of the tube the anastomosis can be difficult due to disparity of the lumen of the tubal ends. The portion where the polyp was present is wider than the isthmic portion of the tube and it is not always easy to achieve a watertight anastomosis. For this reason some surgeons prefer salpingotomy whenever possible.

Tubal anastomosis

Tubal anastomosis for reversal of sterilization is the most successful technique in microsurgery for two reasons: healthy tissues are anastomosed and the localised damage is removed completely (Fig. 19.10). These patients are in

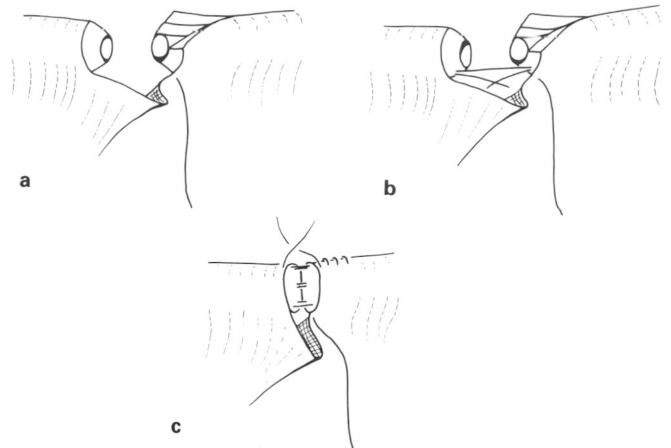

Fig. 19.10 Anastomotic procedure (**a**) Both tubal lumens are exposed (healthy mucosa); (**b**) the first stitch is at 6 o'clock and must be extra mucosa; (**c**) the anastomosis is completed in two layers. The suture material used is 8/0 nylon.

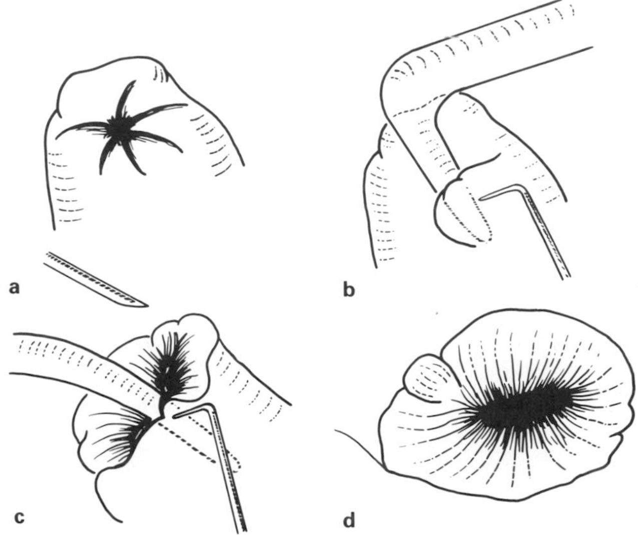

Fig. 19.11 Salpingostomy: (**a**) Identification of the terminal part of the hydrosalpinge where the incision must be made. (**b**) An incision is made using diathermy and the tip of the glass is inserted into the hole in the tube. (**c**) The salpingostomy is enlarged using the diathermy needle and glass rods. (**d**) The salpingostomy is completed.

general fertile. Success depends on the length of the remaining tube. The minimum length of tube necessary to maintain fertility in women is not known. Winston & Boeckx (unpublished data), studied its importance in rabbits. Fertility diminished in a linear fashion depending on the length of the ampulla resected; when more than 70% was missing, none of the animals became pregnant. Resection of the ampullary isthmic junction did not appear to alter fertility (Winston et al 1977). The rabbit is far from an ideal model for human tubal physiology, but these results emphasize the fact that the ampulla seems to be important to maintain fertility. We have found that women with very short tubes occasionally conceive, but patients with very short ampullary segments are less fertile, and when the total length of the tube following anastomosis is shorter than 4 cm the pregnancy rate decreases markedly.

The length of time between sterilization and reversal is important and has a prognostic value. Vasquez et al (1980), demonstrated that after 5 years of sterilization the proximal portion of the tube has a severely damaged mucosa with flattening of the epithelium and polyp formation. The surgical technique of reversal of sterilization has been described elsewhere (Winston 1977; Margara 1982).

Hydrosalpinges

The value of microsurgery varies in the treatment of hydrosalpinges. In some cases where the tube is completely free of adhesions the use of loupes suffices. Where complex adhesions are present the use of the microscope is mandatory. When performing a salpingostomy the following points should be borne in mind. Before starting the salpingostomy mobilization of the tube must be completed. Division of adhesions between tube and ovary or other pelvic organs is very important in order to leave the tube fully mobile, with the possibility of the new ostium being able to cover the whole ovarian surface and make egg pick-up more likely.

While dividing adhesions special care must be taken to avoid damage to the fimbrial blood supply. These vessels are in the area of the connecting ligament between the ovary and the tube at the outer margin of the mesosalpinx. The hydrosalpinge must be open at the most terminal part, the 'pucker point'. This is where the fimbrial end has closed; it is clearly seen under the microscope as a thin fibrous line, often with an H-shaped configuration and is not always the thinnest part of the tube. Linear salpingostomy has a high chance of healing over. Using fine diathermy, the tube is then opened and a glass probe introduced, following the fibrous tracts parallel to the blood vessels and ensuring that the mucosal folds are not cut. Using small incisions the new tubal ostium is completed and then the mucosa can be everted (Fig. 19.11).

Two or three stitches of 8/0 nylon are used to secure the mucosal eversion. If the ovarian surface is damaged during the division of adhesions, the raw area should be repaired using fine non-absorbable suture material to avoid recurrence of adhesions.

Adhesions

Omental adhesions are not infrequent and where more than minimal, a partial omentectomy is performed. It is best done at the beginning of the operation. Fine 2/0 linen is

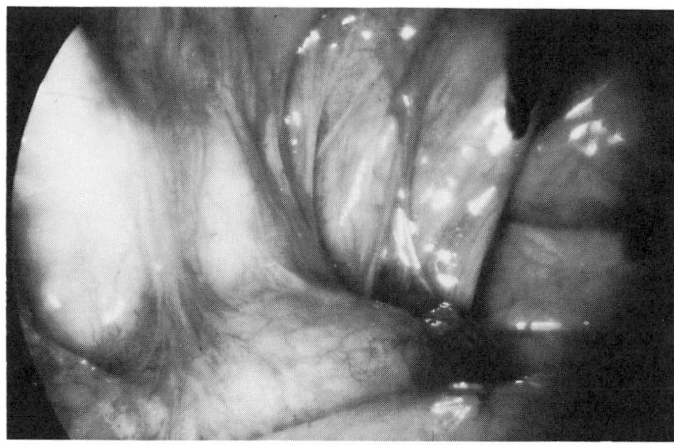

Fig. 19.12 Laparoscopic appearance in a patient with severe periovarian adhesions after pelvic inflammatory disease.

used to secure the pedicles. We do not use this as a routine precedure, but it seems to be a very effective way of avoiding recurrent adhesion in the pelvis (Fig. 19.12).

The most frequent adhesions are between the ampulla, the ovary and the mesosalpinx. It is easy to work from the isthmus towards the fimbrial end. Using a glass probe the adhesions are hooked and with monopolar diathermy they are incised. Care should be taken not to damage the tubal peritoneum. The use of the microscope simplifies the process because the peritoneal edges can be easily seen. If the tubal peritoneum is incised it must be repaired using 8/0 nylon as suture material.

Ovarian adhesions should be removed from the ovarian capsule using diathermy or scissors, leaving the ovarian capsule as free as possible. Ovulation and egg release seem to improve after careful ovariolysis and may depend on the amount of the ovarian surface left free.

Special attention must be paid to raw areas. The uterine surface and the surrounding peritoneum must be carefully inspected. Peritonealization is very important and must be done using fine suture material. If the ovarian fossa has been damaged in order to free or liberate a firmly adherent ovary, the raw area should be closed using a linear suture of 4/0 prolene. If the raw area cannot be peritonealized using the surrounding peritoneum, a peritoneal graft can be applied. The peritoneum should be thin and without fatty tissue. It is attached to the raw area using 8/0 nylon or 6/0 prolene. The donor areas can be the peritoneum layer of the anterior abdominal wall, the peritoneal space between the round ligament and the bladder, and in some cases the peritoneum of the mesentery of the small or large bowel. This technique has proved very effective in experimental animals and the results with humans are very encouraging.

Special mention should be made of the treatment of tubal damage due to tuberculosis. The treatment is always medical and the tubal damage cannot be repaired by surgery. In this group of patients if the uterine cavity remains unaffected or without damage, in vitro fertilization is the only option.

RESULTS

Cornual anastomosis

Cornual anastomosis offers very good results in selected groups of patients; 50% of our patients with inflammatory cornual block have conceived, providing the isthmic portion resected was 1 cm or less. With greater degrees of damage the results are not so good. The miscarriage rate was high (5 among 14 patients) but all of them managed to deliver one full-term pregnancy (Table 19.1). In all, 85% of the patients who conceived did so during the first 6 months after surgery.

Table 19.1 Cornual anastomosis after inflammatory damage

	Patients	Pregnancies	Miscarriages	Ectopic pregnancies
Isolated cornual block	29	14	5	1
Salpingitis isthmica nodosa	15	4	1	0
Total	44	18	6	1

Data from Hammersmith Hospital.

Postoperative laparoscopies show a high patency rate among those patients who have not conceived. The major limiting factors seem to be the recrudescence of the disease or extension of the original inflammation into the anastomotic site rather than luck of patency. Gomel (1980) has reported similar results: 53% of his patients conceived and had at least one term pregnancy. Only 9% of his patients had abortions. At Hammersmith Hospital we have found abortion to be very common after cornual anastomosis, but ectopic pregnancy has not been a major problem.

Salpingitis isthmica nodosa

The surgical treatment of salpingitis isthmica nodosa in the infertile patient is similar to that of cornual block. In nearly half of the patients the tubes are open and the diagnosis is made on the basis of the typical images of diverticula on the hysterosalpingogram and at laparoscopy. The anastomotic procedure is in general much easier but the length of isthmic portion that must be removed can be difficult to assess. The prognosis depends on the length of tube removed, but if we do not remove enough tissue the surgical procedure will probably fail.

The use of the microscope and the experience of the surgeon are very important in the evaluation of the amount or

Table 19.2 Reversal of sterilization according to the site of the anastomosis

Site of anastomosis	Number of patients	Number of pregnant patients	Number of ectopic pregnancies	Percentage of pregnancies
Cornu–isthmus	17	12	0	71%
Cornu–ampulla	26	14	1	54%
Isthmus–isthmus	16	12	0	75%
Isthmus–ampulla	27	17	2	63%
Ampulla–ampulla	19	8	0	42%
Others	21	10	0	48%
Total	126	73	3	58%

Data from Hammersmith Hospital.

length of tissue that must be resected. In general we must accept that this condition involves most of the isthmic portion of the tube, so the anastomosis is between the cornu and the ampullary–isthmic junction.

When the intramural portion of the tube is extensively involved in the process this patient probably should not be treated surgically. The surgical procedure itself does not vary from that of tubocornual anastomosis. When the whole of the isthmus is removed the problem of tension at the anastomotic level can be solved using stay sutures of 6/0 prolene between the uterus and the mesosalpinx in order to approximate the tubal ends. Conception rates in this group of patients are approximately 35%.

Reversal of sterilization

Reversal of tubal sterilization is the most successful procedure in tubal microsurgery. At Hammersmith Hospital in a series of 126 patients 58% conceived; the pregnancy rates varied according to the site of the anastomosis (Table 19.2). Results with reversal of sterilization are very much influenced by the length of tube remaining (Table 19.3).

Table 19.3 Reversal of sterilization in 95 patients: pregnancy rates according to the length of the longer tube

Length of tube	Patients	Number of pregnancies	Percentage
<2.5 cm	7	2	28
2.5–4 cm	15	4	30
4.1–6 cm	30	14	46
6.1–8 cm	25	16	64
>8 cm	20	18	90

Data from Hammersmith Hospital.

Salpingostomy

It is in general difficult to assess results of salpingostomy because a very heterogeneous group of patients is involved. Patient selection varies widely between different units and there is no agreement regarding classification, especially where salpingostomy and fimbrioplasty are concerned.

Salpingostomy is a surgical procedure that many gynaecologists think is obsolete, because in vitro fertilization techniques offer comparable or better results in some cases. As in any other surgical procedure, if we select the patients well, good results will be achieved.

Boer-Meisel et al (1986) in a prospective study classified hydrosalpinges as grades I, II and III, based on the nature and extent of the adhesions, the microscopic aspect of the endosalpinx, the thickness of the tubal wall and the diameter of the hydrosalpinx. In their series 77% of patients with grade I hydrosalpinx have the possibility of conception, 21% with grade II, and only 3% with grade III. Thus surgery is the obvious treatment for patients with grade I hydrosalpinges. Patients with grade III should avoid surgery and be treated using in vitro fertilization techniques. The difficult group is the grade II hydrosalpinx, where treatment with in vitro fertilization or tubal surgery has the same prognosis. Age, social and religious background, possibility of alternative treatment, and the patients' wishes must be considered very carefully.

In a series of 323 patients from Hammersmith Hospital, 81 (25%) of the patients conceived, most of them during the first 8 months following surgery, or after the second year. After the second year the ectopic pregnancy rate seemed to be higher. Twenty of these patients have more than one child, and one has already had four (Table 19.4).

Table 19.4 Results of salpingostomies (1971–1985)

Patients	Pregnancies	Miscarriages	Ectopic pregnancies
323	81 (25%)	54 (16.7%)	32 (10%)

Data from Hammersmith Hospital.

CONCLUSIONS

There is no doubt that we can treat a large group of patients with tubal disease using in vitro fertilization techniques, but in a well selected group of infertile patients with tubal damage microsurgery offers a very good prognosis, and with only one treatment many of them can conceive more than once. In a highly specialized unit both methods should be available and the choice adapted to each individual case.

KEY POINTS

1. Tubal disease is tubal damage caused by pelvic infection or iatrogenic disease with varying degrees of damage, and sometimes involving surrounding structures.
2. Tubal disease is accountable for 30–40% of cases of female infertility.
3. Salpingitis most commonly results from ascending infection from the lower genital tract.
4. Cervical resistance diminishes during ovulation and menstruation, possibly then allowing bacteria to ascend.
5. Salpingitis is not in generally seen in women who are not sexually active.
6. The non-white population seems to be more at risk of salpingitis with gonococci cervicitis. Host resistance is important and may be increased to gonococcus by use of the oral contraceptive pill.
7. *Chlamydia trachomatis* is responsible for a significant amount of salpingitis, postpartum endometriosis and perihepatic adhesions.
8. Many organisms are capable of producing salpingitis. Gonococcal infection seems to pave the way for other micro-organisms to cross the cervical mucus and affect the uterus or tubes.
9. Tubal damage of tuberculus origin is rare in developed countries. *Mycobacterium tuberculosis* reaches pelvic organs either by spread from a primary focus or occasionally occurs as the primary disease resulting from infection with infected semen.
10. The treatment of tubal disease in the infertile patient is surgical and based on the principles of microsurgery: gentle tissue handling; reperitonealization of raw areas; use of fine non-absorbable sutures; irrigation with Ringers' solution.
11. Tubocornual implantation is avoided if possible since destroying a possible sphincter at the uterotubal junction is associated with excessive bleeding and may increase the risk of rupture.
12. Tubal anastomosis for reversal of sterilization is the most successful technique of microsurgery and the success depends upon the length of the remaining tube and the time elapsed since the sterilization.

REFERENCES

Benjamin C L, Beaver D C 1951 The pathogenesis of salpingitis isthmica nodosa. American Journal of Clinical Pathology 21: 212–222

Boer-Meisel M E, te Velde E R, Habbena J D F, Kardaun J W P F 1986 Predicting the pregnancy outcome in patients treated for hydrosalpinx: a prospective study. Fertility and Sterility 45: 23–29

Burne J C 1973 Salpingitis isthmica nodosa. In: Fox H, Langley F A (eds) Postgraduate obstetrical and gynaecological pathology. Pergamon Press, Oxford, p 269

Chiari H 1887 Zur pathologischen Anatomie des Eileiter-Catrrhs. Zeitschrift für Heilkunde 8: 457–473

Creasy J L, Clark R L, Cuttino J T, Groff T R 1985 Salpingitis isthmica nodosa: radiologic and clinical correlates. Radiology 154: 597–600

Eilard T, Brorsson J E, Hamark B, Forssman L 1976 Isolation of *Chlamydia* in acute salpingitis. Scandinavian Journal of Infectious Diseases a (suppl): 82–84

Ehrler P 1963 Die intramurale Tubenanastomoze (ein Beitrag zur Uberwindung der tubaren Sterität). Zentralblatt für Gynaekologie 85: 393–400

Eschenbach D A, Holmes K K, 1979. The ethiology of acute pelvic inflmamtory disease. Sexually Transmitted Diseases 6: 224–227

Glazener C M A, Loveden L M, Richardson S J, Jeans W D, Hull M G R 1987 Tubocornual polyps: their revelance in subfertility. Human Reproduction 2: 59–65

Gomel V 1977 Tubal reanastomosis by microsurgery. Fertility and Sterility 28: 59

Gomel V 1980 Clinical results of infertility microsurgery. In: Crosignany P G, Rubin B L (eds) Microsurgery in female infertility. Academic Press, New York, pp 77–94

Honore L H 1978 Salpingitis isthmica nodosa in female infertility and ectopic tubal pregnancy. Fertility and Sterility 29: 164–168

Lisa J R, Gioia J D, Rubin I C 1954 Observations on interstitial portion of the fallopian tube. Surgery, Gynecology and Obstetrics 99: 159–169

Margara R A 1982 Tubal reanastomosis. In: Chamberlain G, Winston R L M (eds) Tubal infertility. Blackwell Scientific, Oxford, pp 106–119

Paterson P, Wood C 1974 The use of microsurgery in the reanastomosis of the rabbit fallopian tube. Fertility and Sterility 25: 757–761

Seki K, Eddy C A, Smith N K, Pauerstein C J 1977 Comparison of two techniques of suturing in microsurgical anastomosis of the rabbit oviduct. Fertility and Sterility 28: 1215–1219

Vasquez G, Winston R L M, Boeckx W, Brosens I 1980 Tubal lesions subsequent to sterilisation and their relation to fertility after attempts at reversal. American Journal of Obstetrics and Gynecology 138: 86–92

Walz W 1959 Fertilitäts Operationen mit Hilfe eines Operationenmikroscopes. Geburtshilfe und Gynaecologie 153: 49–53

Winston R L M 1977 Microsurgical tubocornual anastomosis for reversal of sterilisation. Lancet i: 284–285

Winston R L M 1982 Reconstructive microsurgery at the lateral end of the fallopian tube. In: Chamberlain G, Winston R L M (eds) Tubal infertility. Blackwell Scientific, Oxford; pp 79–104

Winston R L M, McClure-Browne J C 1974 Pregnancy following autograph transplantation of the fallopian tube and ovary in the rabbit. Lancet ii: 494–497

Winston R L M, Frantzen C, Oberti C 1977 Oviduct function following resection of the ampullary–isthmic junction. Fertility and Sterility 28: 284

20. Ectopic pregnancy

R. A. Margara

INTRODUCTION

Ectopic pregnancy can be defined as the implantation of a fertilized ovum outside the uterine cavity. It was first described in the literature in 936 AD by Abulcasis. Parry & Lea in 1876 reported a mortality of nearly 70%, and it was Tait who in 1884 published the first cases of surgical management of ectopic pregnancy.

PATHOPHYSIOLOGY

The reason why a fertilized ovum can implant in an apparently normal fallopian tube is still unknown but abnormalities of the mechanisms involved in ovum transport may be a predisposing factor. Ovum transport from when the ovum is released by the ovary until it reaches the uterine cavity takes 3–4 days with the ovum being retained in the ampulla for most of that time. Passage through the isthmus is very rapid.

Innervation

The adrenergic innervation of the myosalpinx is important; the nerve fibres are concentrated in the isthmus. This suggests that a sphincter mechanism might influence ovum transport but adrenergic or anti-adrenergic drugs do not seem to disrupt transport to any great extent in primates.

Muscular contractions

The contribution of contractions of the tubal muscle to tubal transport varies according to the portion of the tube and the time from when the ovum was released. Measurement of tubal contractility without interference with tubal function is practically impossible. One of the methods used for assessment is electrical activity: electrical stimuli to the circular muscle of the ampulla increase intraluminal pressure and movement of the ovum. In rabbits this mechanism is complicated by the flow of fluid in the tubal lumen.

The muscle has longitudinal and circular layers, making the interpretation of measurements difficult as they may have functional independence between layers.

Ovarian hormones

Tubal transport is influenced by hormone levels; oestrogens stimulate tubal contractility but progesterone causes decreased activity. Progesterone also decreases local prostaglandin secretion and causes relaxation of the isthmic portion of the tube, which may allow the fertilized ovum to progress into the uterus.

Cilial action

Beating of the cilia is also involved in transporting the egg towards the uterus. At the ampulla the cilia beat towards the isthmus, assisting transport. In animals, tubal contractions can be stopped pharmacologically but the egg still progresses. Surgical reversal of 1 cm of the isthmus in rabbits does not prevent pregnancy but if the segment reversed is from the ampulla no pregnancy occurs (Eddy et al 1977). Cilia beating continues, but after the reversal it is in the opposite direction to that in the remaining portion of the ampulla. If ova are placed in the fimbrial end of these tubes they are transported until they reach the reversed segment; if they are placed on the surface of the reversed segments, transport is back towards the ovary. In contrast, in oviducts in which 1 cm segments were transected but not reversed, ovum transport was normal. These observations suggest an important role for the cilia in transporting the ova through the ampulla but not through the isthmus.

Loss of ciliated cells due to pelvic inflammatory disease may decrease the quality of ovum transport and delay the ovum reaching the isthmus and the uterine cavity (Brosens & Vasquez 1976). Cilia do not seem to be strictly necessary for ovum transport as patients with Kartagener's syndrome, where the cilia are immobile, are able to conceive and have intrauterine pregnancies.

Changes at site of implantation

Exactly where the blastocyst implants in the tube is still a matter of speculation, as it is difficult to observe very early tubal implantation. It seems likely that the blastocyst implants on the tips of the papillary fronds.

It has been assumed that when an ectopic pregnancy implants and grows in the tubal lumen, placentation involves the endosalpinx with obliteration of the tubal epithelium without trophoblastic invasion into the muscularis. The trophoblast does not differ histologically from that normally formed in the uterus; as it penetrates the tubal wall and invades the muscularis it becomes extraluminal although retroperitoneal. When blood vessels are involved bleeding occurs and a retroperitoneal haematoma is formed with tubal dilatation. The haematoma, with dilation of the retroperitoneal space, may explain the pain that patients observe well before the occurrence of tubal rupture and complications of ectopic pregnancy.

CLASSIFICATION

Tubal ectopic pregnancy can be classified in order of frequency according to the site of implantation. It can be ampullary, isthmic, fimbrial or in the interstitial portion of the tube (Fig. 20.1). These sites account for 95% of ectopic pregnancies.

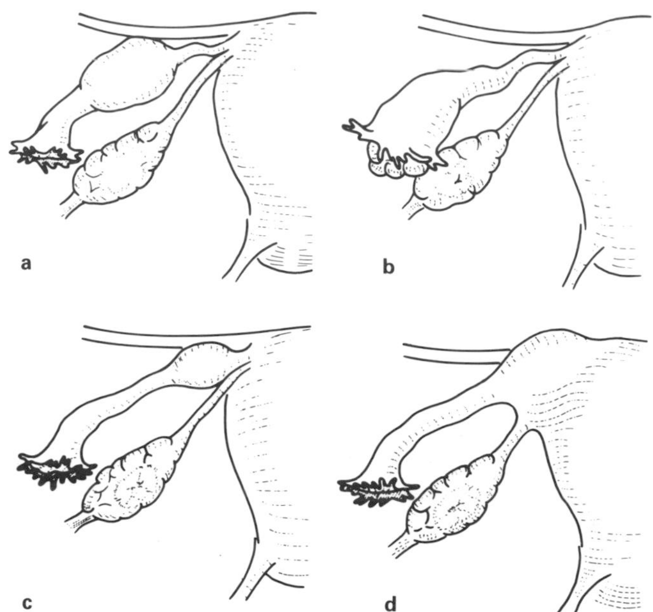

Fig. 20.1 Appearance of ectopic pregnancy implanted in different parts of the tube. (**a**) Ampulla; (**b**) infundibulum/fimbria; (**c**) isthmus; (**d**) cornual or interstitial.

Douglas, in 1963, reviewed 438 ectopic pregnancies; 417 were tubal and the implantation sites were as shown in Table 20.1.

Table 20.1 Implantation sites of 417 tubal ectopic pregnancies

Site	*n*	%
Fimbrial	29	7.0
Ampullary	176	42.0
Isthmic	117	28.0
Interstitial	54	13.0
In stump of tube	9	2.0
Unrecorded	32	8.0

From Douglas (1963).

Ovarian ectopic

Ovarian ectopic pregnancies can be primary or secondary, depending upon whether the implantation was directly on the ovary or the result of a tubal abortion and re-implantation on the ovary. The incidence is reported as being in between 1/2000 to 1/8500 deliveries. The identification of this type of ectopic pregnancy can be difficult. To classify an ectopic pregnancy as a primary ovarian implantation the fallopian tube should be normal and the gestational sac has ovarian tissue in its wall.

Abdominal ectopic

Similarly, abdominal implantation of an ectopic pregnancy can be primary or secondary, depending on the pregnancy implanting directly in the abdominal cavity or implantation occurring as a result of a tubal abortion or ruptured tubal ectopic pregnancy without major clinical symptoms. In primary implantation the tubes and ovaries are intact and the pregnancy is associated with peritoneal tissue only. The frequency of abdominal pregnancies varies between 1/3400 and 1/8000 deliveries.

Cervical ectopic

Cervical ectopic pregnancy is a rare event with a frequency varying between 1/10 000 and 1/16 000 deliveries. To identify a cervical ectopic pregnancy, cervical glands must be attached to the placenta, the placenta must be implanted below the place where the uterine vessels reach the uterus, and the attachment between the placenta and the cervix should be intimate.

Other sites

A case of vaginal ectopic pregnancy presented as a sub-urethral cyst has been described by Duckman et al (1984). After removal of the cyst the presence of trophoblastic tissue was confirmed histopathologically.

Intraligamentous ectopic pregnancy has been defined by Kobak et al (1955) as a pregnancy below the tube bordered by the broad ligament, the levator ani muscle, laterally by the pelvic side wall, and medially by the uterus. It is extremely uncommon.

Ectopic pregnancy in a rudimentary uterine horn has also been reported and live births have been confirmed as resulting from such an implantation site.

Heterotopic pregnancy is the combination of an intrauterine and an ectopic pregnancy, generally tubal. Heterotopic pregnancy used to be a very rare eventuality with an incidence of 1/30 000 deliveries. Since in vitro fertilization and multiple embryo transfers have become common practice, the incidence of heterotopic pregnancy has increased, but at the moment it is not possible to confirm by how much.

AETIOLOGY

Many factors are known to contribute to the cause of ectopic pregnancy or can put patients at risk of having an ectopic pregnancy. Any mechanism — infectious, surgical or hormonal — that can alter tubal transport or the quality of the egg may contribute directly or indirectly to the aetiology of ectopic pregnancy.

Causes related to tubal function

Pelvic inflammatory disease

Ectopic pregnancies associated with pelvic inflammatory disease have increased dramatically in the last 15 or 20 years. Endosalpingitis may damage the tubal endothelium and cause adhesion formation, creating gland-like spaces and pockets where the fertilized ovum may be trapped and implant. Westrom et al (1981) found that in Sweden the likelihood of ectopic pregnancy is correlated with the age of the woman. The incidence was 4.1/1000 in teenagers, 6.9/1000 in women 20–29 years old and 12.9/1000 in the age group of 30–39 years. The risk of an ectopic pregnancy increased sevenfold after acute salpingitis and was associated with the use of intrauterine contraceptive divices.

Clark & Baranyai (1987) found a 38% increase in ectopic pregnancy in New Zealand over 15 years (1970–1984) and histological evidence of tubal infection in patients with ectopic pregnancy increased from 40% in 1970 to 61% in 1984.

There is an association between ectopic pregnancy and *Chlamydia trachomatis* infection and in general the infection was subclinical. Brunham et al (1986) reported that only 10% of women with ectopic pregnancy and 6% with serology positive for *Chlamydia trachomatis* had a history of clinical pelvic inflammatory disease.

Salpingitis isthmica nodosa

Salpingitis isthmica nodosa was first described by Chiari in 1887 and its incidence, aetiology and clinical significance are still a matter of controversy. It seems to have an effect on the reproductive performance of the infertile woman and is often associated with ectopic pregnancy — to what degree is very difficult to establish. Persaud (1970) found diverticula which occur in salpingitis isthmica nodosa in 49% of specimens of ectopic pregnancies and Majmudar et al (1983) found that 57% of specimens of their cases of ectopic pregnancies had signs of salpingitis isthmica nodosa. A possible reason why ectopic pregnancy occurs in the tubes damaged by this condition is that the embryo is trapped in extensions of the tubal mucosa into the myosalpinx, with subsequent nidation. One of the major problems in accepting this mechanical theory is that in the majority of patients ectopic pregnancies are implanted on the distal part of the tube, where salpingitis isthmica nodosa is less common. It might be that, due to the thickness of the muscular layer of the tube in patients with the condition, the women may have spasmodic contractions of the tubes and obstruction or dysfunction of the mechanism of tubal transport without a real mechanical obstruction.

Tubal reconstruction

Tubal reconstruction is associated with an increased incidence of ectopic pregnancy. The success of tubal surgery is measured by a high intrauterine and low extrauterine pregnancy rate. The fact that microsurgery can achieve tubal patency in severely damaged tubes with abnormal function may predispose to or increase the risk of ectopic pregnancy.

In a large series of 653 patients from 14 different centres, 54% of patients had ectopic pregnancies when the microsurgical approach was used (Winston 1981). In his first series after the magnification and electrocautery were introduced for tubal surgery, Swolin (1975) had 18% of ectopic pregnancies after salpingostomy.

The ectopic pregnancy rate is less among patients who have had tubal anastomosis due to tubal damage. Reversal of sterilization is the most successful of the anastomotic surgical procedures and carries a lower risk of ectopic pregnancy.

Conservative surgery for ectopics

Conservative surgery in ectopic pregnancies may increase the chances of having another ectopic pregnancy, but it will depend very much on any pre-existing conditions in the tube where the first ectopic originated, the localization of the ectopic and whether the contralateral tube is healthy or damaged.

Intrauterine contraceptive devices

The use of intrauterine contraceptive devices has been associated with an increase in ectopic pregnancy. Although Ory (1981) in a multicentre study concluded that women who had never had an intrauterine device had the same chances of having an ectopic pregnancy as those who had, Erkkola & Liukko (1977) found that in Finland there is an increase with time in the number of ectopic pregnancies in patients who have had a device; 59% of their patients with ectopic pregnancy had had devices inserted. Contraceptive users of any kind have less chance of having an ectopic pregnancy than non-users, but long-term device users were 2.5 times more likely to have an ectopic pregnancy than those who had the device for a shorter period of time (less than 25 months).

Ovarian pregnancy appears to have an increased incidence amongst intrauterine device users and it has been postulated that deciliation of the endosalpinx might be the cause or that increased secretion of prostaglandins by mast cells of the mesosalpinx can alter tubal transport.

Tubal sterilization procedures

A high risk of ectopic pregnancy has been reported in patients who conceive after sterilization, as there has been major destruction of tube. When a tuboperitoneal fistula results there is a higher chance of pregnancy and also a higher chance that it will be an ectopic. Patients who are sterilised and have had a previous illegal abortion are at higher risk of having an ectopic pregnancy than those who have had an induced abortion, but previous intrauterine device usage is not a factor. No differences were found in cases of old pelvic infection or device users before sterilization.

The chances of conceiving after sterilization are very low — approximately 1/1000 — and the chances of that pregnancy being an ectopic range between 15.6 and 63.3%.

Exposure to diethylstilboestrol

Women who were exposed to diethylstilboestrol in utero have an increased chance of ectopic pregnancy. DeCherney et al (1981) reported that 16 such patients had unique findings at laparoscopy with 'withered' tubes, described as a 'foreshortened, sacculated, convoluted tube with a pinpoint os and constricted fimbria' and all had the classic T-shaped uterus. There were no significant findings with respect to the tubal lumen or any other pathology in the hysterosalpingogram. The effect of diethylstilboestrol was said to be related to the dose used but no specific evidence was given.

Previous termination of pregnancy

Controversy still exists regarding the incidence of ectopic pregnancy related to termination of pregnancy. In 1948 Sawar & Roth suggested a relationship between the increase in ectopic pregnancy and termination of pregnancy.

Induced abortion may be one of the factors that increases the risk of having an ectopic pregnancy; the risk increases among those who have had two or more terminations of pregnancy.

Causes related to the embryo

Ovulation induction

Gemzell et al in 1982 showed that in women who have had ovarian stimulation with gonadotrophins there is an increased chance of having an ectopic pregnancy. The theory is that hyperstimulation produces higher oestrogen levels, affecting tubal transport and that oocytes of different degrees of maturity are released at the same time, with possible delay of fertilization. High level of oestrogen before human chorionic gonadotrophin (hCG) is released might increase this risk.

In vitro fertilization

In vitro fertilization has been associated with increased chances of ectopic pregnancy. The reasons are not very clear but the possible explanations are that the embryo might be injected directly into the tube; that it migrates spontaneously, or that is moved by uterine contractions. It is possible that some such embryos are expelled back into the uterine cavity by the tube but the largest group of

Table 20.2 Ectopic pregnancies deaths and rates per million estimated pregnancies from 1970 to 1984

Trienna	Total estimated pregnancies (in thousands)	Ectopic pregnancies in HIPE*	Ectopic pregnancies per 10 000 estimated pregnancies	Number of deaths	Death rate per 1000 ectopic pregnancies
1970–1972	2890.7	11.6	40	34	2.9
1973–1975	2578.4	11.7	45	21	1.6
1976–1978	2323.0	11.6	50	21	1.8
1979–1981	2543.0	12.1	48	20	1.7
1982–1984	2507.0	14.4	57	10	0.7

*Hospital inpatient enquiry.
*From Report on confidential enquiries into maternal deaths in England and Wales 1979–1984.

patients in an in vitro fertilization programme have tubal disease. Tubal function is impaired so that re-expulsion of embryos may not always be possible. In vitro fertilization patients have high oestrogen levels and this could contribute to altered tubal transport by affecting the beating of the cilia.

Direct placement of gametes as in gamete intrafallopian transfer (GIFT) or zygote intrafallopian transfer (ZIFT) may well increase the risk further.

Gamete transmigration

Many series have reported the finding of the corpus luteum in the contralateral ovary to the side of the ectopic, suggesting ovum transmigration.

In theory the fimbria may aspirate the oocyte or a fertilized egg from the pouch of Douglas. If an embryo has been aspirated it can then implant in the ampulla, or because of its size cannot go through the intramural portion of the tube-ending as in an interstitial implantation. The hormonal background with high levels of progesterone may influence tubal transport.

Transmigration of spermatozoa has been described as a possible cause of ectopic pregnancy. There are cases where the tubal lumen has been interrupted by sterilization, or conservative surgery in a previous ectopic pregnancy. It has also been suggested that in cases of reversal of sterilization where only one oviduct could be repaired, the remaining portion of the other tube should be removed, especially the fimbrial end.

EPIDEMIOLOGY

The increased number of ectopic pregnancies is well documented but it is in some way related to the fact that an early diagnosis of pregnancy can be made with the use of beta-hCG and the ability to locate the site of implantation at an early stage. The gynaecologist feels it is urgent to confirm the diagnosis, which always involves in one way or another a surgical procedure. Possibly a proportion of ectopic pregnancies with abnormal implantation or abnormal embryos would resolve on their own without any consequences.

Race and socioeconomic factors influence the risk of ectopic pregnancy. In the USA ectopic pregnancy is twice as high in non-white than in white populations (Lehfeldt et al 1970; Erkkola & Liukko 1977). In England and Wales, there was little change in the incidence of ectopic pregnancy or death due to ectopic pregnancy between 1970 and 1981, but from 1982 to 1985 the number of ectopic pregnancies increased by 19% (Table 20.2).

Until 1981 ectopic pregnancy had been the leading cause of maternal mortality in the first trimester. The decrease in the subsequent 3 years may be due to chance, but the incidence of non-fatal cases has increased, so the decrease of mortality is due to earlier diagnosis and better treatment. Similar trends have been seen in the USA.

The availability of early diagnosis and treatment, and the degree of awareness of doctors and patients of the possibility of ectopic pregnancy are very important factors which contribute to the decrease of maternal deaths.

PRESENTATION

Ectopic pregnancy can present in different ways. Probably the most important factor in detection and making an early diagnosis is always to think about that possibility in patients at high risk, such as infertile patients or those who have had previous tubal surgery; those with a history of pelvic inflammatory disease, and those who have been sterilized or are using intrauterine contraceptive devices.

The signs and symptoms of ectopic pregnancy vary according to their presentation, whether acute or subacute.

Acute presentation

Acute presentation is associated with rupture of the ectopic pregnancy and massive intraperitoneal bleeding, with acute abdominal pain and cardiovascular collapse. Some patients have a history of menstrual irregularity, local pain and shoulder pain. Abdominal rigidity and rebound tenderness are in general present. Vaginal examination is not necessary: it does not add any specific information except that there may be some localized tenderness in one of the fornices and it can be dangerous, producing the total rupture of the ectopic gestation and increasing intraperitoneal bleeding.

Subacute presentation

Subacute presentation occurs in the majority of cases. The patient complains of abdominal pain which may be localized to one iliac fossa, vaginal bleeding and a delayed menstrual period. She may report shoulder pain if free blood is in the peritoneal cavity, due to the irritation of the peritoneum. On bimanual examination there may be localized tenderness in one of the fornices, cervical excitation pain, and sometimes a very tender posterior fornix, due to the presence of the affected tube in the pouch of Douglas. This examination has to be very gentle due to the possibility of rupture of an unruptured ectopic pregnancy with severe intraperitoneal bleeding and collapse. In some cases the patients are referred by the family doctor due to the symptoms of pregnancy and a positive urine pregnancy test.

Since the availability of beta-hCG subunit assay, the early diagnosis of ectopic pregnancy can be made in most cases, and with the help of ultrasound to exclude intrauterine pregnancy the diagnosis is often made even before the patient has symptoms. With other than tubal ectopic pregnancies, the diagnosis is sometimes made late due to lack of symptoms.

Non-tubal ectopics

The diagnosis of abdominal pregnancy can be very difficult. Abdominal tenderness in a pregnant woman with a mass separated from the uterus and cervical displacement can be present. Some patients have bowel or urinary symptoms related to the implantation of the ectopic placenta. Beta-hCG and ultrasound scan can confirm the absence of an intrauterine pregnancy, but routine diagnostic ultrasound scans are usually done in patients who are between 12 and 14 weeks pregnant.

The symptoms of an ovarian ectopic pregnancy do not differ from those of a tubal pregnancy, which in general are abdominal pain, vaginal bleeding and menstrual irregularity.

Cervical pregnancy in general has the manifestations of a threatened or incomplete abortion. Uterine bleeding in a pregnant women with a partially open cervix which is enlarged and sometimes bigger than the uterus are suggestive of a cervical pregnancy. The products of conception are attached to and confined to the cervix.

Implantation of pregnancies in a rudimentary horn, whether connected to the main uterine cavity or vagina or not, is very infrequent and does not have specific signs. Pregnant women with a known uterine abnormality, where the pregnancy has been identified by ultrasound outside the main uterine cavity but still surrounded by myometrium, should suggest the presence of the anomalous implantation.

Patients with an intrauterine pregnancy and an ectopic pregnancy — heterotopic pregnancies — have often had multiple embryos transferred during an in vitro fertilization–embryo transfer (IVF–ET) treatment cycle. They do not have special signs or symptoms except of abdominal pain and if complicated, those of the ectopic pregnancy as well as those of a normal pregnancy. The in vitro fertilization practitioner must bear the possibility of heterotopic pregnancy in mind and arrange careful ultrasound scans on patients with pain until he or she is completely certain that a heterotopic pregnancy has not been missed.

INVESTIGATION AND DIAGNOSIS

Laparoscopy

The early diagnosis of ectopic pregnancy depends very much on the environment in which the practitioner is working and the facilities available. Years ago a patient with the symptoms of early pregnancy complaining of irregular bleeding, abdominal pain or adnexal mass with excitation pain would have proceeded directly to emergency laparotomy. Laparoscopy as a method of diagnosis of ectopic pregnancy has been used since 1937, when Hope reported the first 10 cases. The development of laparoscopy and its wide use have facilitated the diagnosis and treatment of ectopic pregnancy, thereby decreasing its mortality. When laparoscopy became a routine procedure, up to 40% of laparotomies were avoided and definitive diagnosis was possible early, with less morbidity and mortality. The development of a very sensitive radioimmunoassay capable of detecting beta-hCG subunits at an early stage of pregnancy, together with the use of ultrasound, has again changed the diagnosis and management of suspected ectopic pregnancy.

Measurement of beta-hCG

Detection of beta-hCG in serum confirms the presence of trophoblastic tissue in 99–100% of cases. In normal pregnancy, gonadotrophins have a pattern of regular increase in the first weeks of pregnancy. Variation or abnormalities in the rate of increase can indicate the presence of an abnormal implantation.

When fertilization and implantation occur hCG can be detected in serum as early as 7–10 days after ovulation or embryo transfer and it increases exponentially, following the development of trophoblastic tissue, but with daily spasmodic variations. The increase in hCG level in a normal pregnancy has a doubling time of 48 h and can be predicted using a formula or nomogram. The normal range of the doubling time is from 1.2 to 3.5 days, depending on the age of the pregnancy. In a normal pregnancy the doubling time is 1.2–1.4 days during the first week after conception, before menstruation, and 3.3–3.5 days 6–8 weeks after conception.

Abnormal hCG rises can be compatible with both normal and abnormal pregnancies. In general, when doubling time is less than 85% or the level starts reaching a plateau or decreasing, it is most likely is that there is an abnormal pregnancy of undermined site of implantation which needs to be confirmed by ultrasound or laparoscopy.

Ultrasound

Ultrasound has been widely used in the diagnosis of ectopic pregnancy since the times of Donald (1965), but to rely on ultrasound scans to diagnose the presence of an ectopic pregnancy can be dangerous because a tubal pregnancy can be missed. The role of ultrasound scanning is to exclude an intrauterine pregnancy (Figs 20.2 and 20.3). The presence of an intrauterine gestational sac in general excludes an ectopic pregnancy, but is possible in the presence of a heterotopic pregnancy.

The use of beta-hCG and ultrasound in combination is the safe way of making a really early diagnosis, although serum beta-hCG is detected very early in pregnancy whereas an intrauterine gestational sac cannot be visualized by ultrasound until 28 days after conception.

Confirmation of the presence of an ectopic pregnancy in the tube can eventually be made by ultrasound but this may be too late. An intrauterine sac can be detected in normally ovulating women at 5½ weeks after the last menstrual period, when the beta-hCG titre is above 6.500 miu/ml. Kadar et al (1981) demonstrated that the presence of an intrauterine sac and beta-hCG below 6.500 miu/ml carry a poor prognosis and it is very probable that it is an ectopic pregnancy or a pregnancy that will miscarry. The visualization by ultrasound of an image like a gestational sac has been observed in suspected ectopic pregnancies, but it may be the endometrial cavity with a decidualized endometrium.

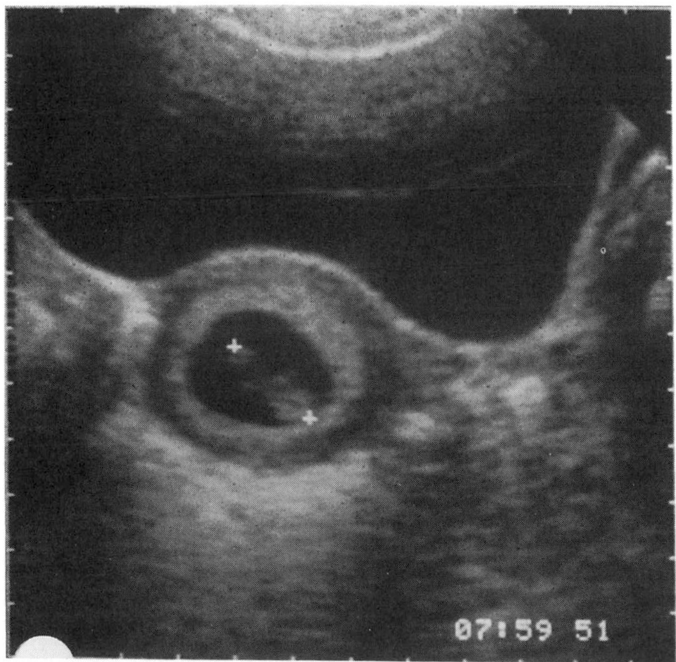

Fig. 20.2 Abdominal scan of pelvis. Transverse section of uterus showing a normal intra-uterine pregnancy (fetal pole 1.77 cm).

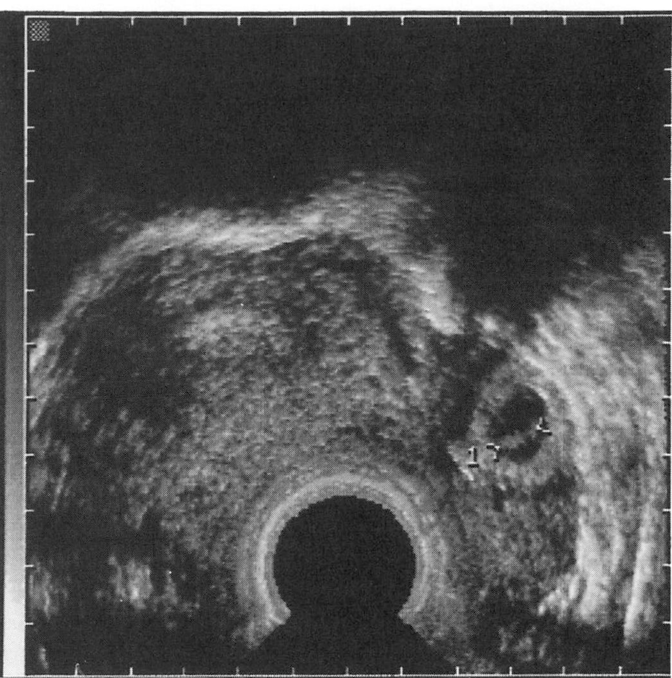

Fig. 20.3 Vaginal scan of pelvis. Transverse view of the pelvis. Arrow shows an empty uterine cavity. Dots show an ectopic pregnancy of the left tube lying on the ovary.

The presence of a 'double ring' image has been proposed to differentiate between a healthy intrauterine sac and a pseudouterine sac with an ectopic pregnancy. These images are produced by the presence of decidua capsularis and parietalis, with a double ring in a normal pregnancy and only a single ring in a sac of an abnormal one.

Ultrasound diagnosis of abdominal pregnancy can sometimes be made at an early stage with an empty cavity, fetal parts outside of the uterine cavity, and the identification of an ectopic placenta. In some patients it can be very difficult to identify the uterus or the placenta due to their displacement in the abdominal cavity.

Arias–Stella phenomenon

The Arias–Stella phenomenon consists of marked secretory and proliferative activity, often on the same endometrial gland lumen, forming syncytial masses with very tall and vacuolated cells which have hypertrophic and hyperchromatic nuclei with different shapes and bizarre forms. The phenomenon has been said to be important in the diagnosis of ectopic pregnancy but its incidence in ectopic pregnancies varies from 3 to 100%. The exact nature of the Arias–Stella phenomenon is still obscure: it may be due to the response of the stimulation produced by oestrogens and chorionic gonadotrophins. This process is not typical of ectopic pregnancy but can be associated with normal pregnancy, abortion, chorioepithelioma, endometritis and patients treated with oestrogens and progestogens for a long time.

Abdominal X-rays

In advanced abdominal pregnancies X-ray of the abdominal and pelvic cavities can be very useful. A lateral view can show fetal parts lying on the maternal spine and this is a sign of abdominal pregnancy. Hysterosalpingography can be of use as a diagnostic tool but carries the risk of irradiation of a viable pregnancy.

The wide use of ultrasound has practically displaced the use of X-rays in the diagnosis of abdominal pregnancy.

TREATMENT

Ectopic pregnancy still presents problems of choice of the best treatment in spite of the advances in diagnosis and surgical or medical treatment. There are very important considerations to be taken into account at the time of the surgical procedure in order to decide on the type of operation. These include the site of the ectopic pregnancy, the past history of the patient, the desire for further pregnancies, and future options for treatment, such as in vitro fertilization. In principle the attitude should be as conservative as possible, according to the circumstances.

Salpingectomy

Salpingectomy, as first described by Tait (1884), is still the method mostly used as a treatment for ectopic pregnancy, with or without an ipsilateral oophorectomy. For a large number of authors salpingectomy is still an orthodox management of ectopic pregnancy in patients with a normal contralateral tube. Salpingectomy is particularly indicated in patients with a second ectopic pregnancy in a tube already treated conservatively; patients who have been sterilized and do not desire further pregnancy; ruptured ectopic pregnancy with severe destruction of tubal tissue or severe haemorrhage, and patients with a frozen pelvis, in whom the severity of the tubal damage is pre-existing and does not justify conservative treatment. For many clinicians salpingectomy would still be the orthodox management of ectopic pregnancy in patients with a normal contralateral tube, although this should be questioned.

The removal of the ipsilateral ovary is very rarely indicated these days. The one indication is when the ectopic pregnancy has involved the ovarian tissue to a great extent and the remaining ovarian tissue is badly damaged by a previous disease such as endometriosis, severe pelvic inflammatory disease or previous ovarian surgery.

Conservative procedures

Conservative procedures for ectopic pregnancies were probably attempted at the end of the last century, but it was Stromme (1953) who published the first case of salpingotomy in an unruptured ectopic pregnancy. Partial salpingectomy with removal of the site of implantation is performed in cases of early isthmic ectopic implantation, followed by reanastomosis of the remaining segments, allowing the patient to conceive again spontaneously (Figs 20.4 and 20.5). The anastomosis can be done immediately after the removal of the ectopic pregnancy during the same procedure or at a later stage in a separate or second procedure.

Based on the fact that the ectopic trophoblast invades the muscularis leaving the tubal lumen undamaged, conservative procedures such as salpingotomy without removing the segment of the tube have become widely used by many authors with good results.

At the time of the laparotomy or laparoscopy the tube is opened in the anti-mesenteric border on the site of the tubal implantation using scalpel or electrobistoury, and once the embryonic sac has been exposed and removed

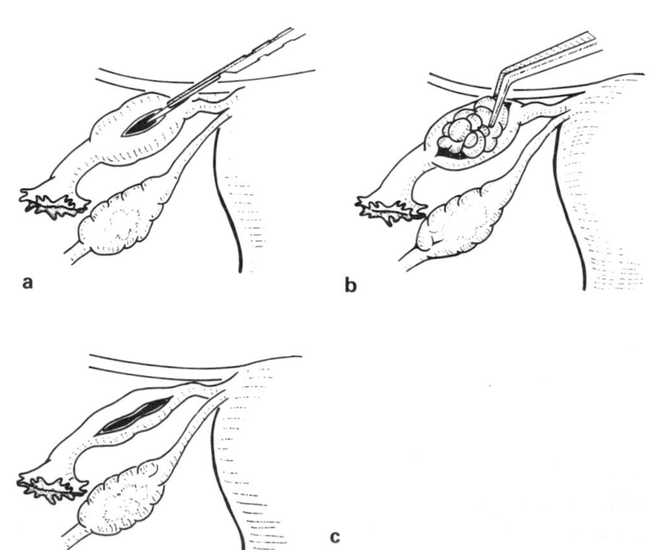

Fig 20.4 Conservative surgical management of an ampullary ectopic pregnancy. (**a**) Linear salpingotomy; (**b**) removal of the gestational sac; (**c**) Salpingotomy left open to heal without closure.

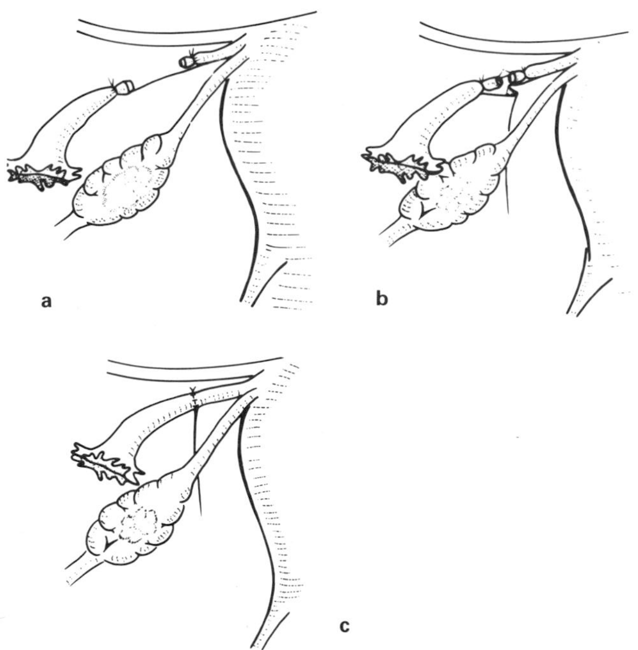

Fig 20.5 Conservative surgical management of an isthmic ectopic pregnancy. (**a**) Resection of the gestational sac; (**b**) Blind ends left tied in order to perform a reanastomosis as a second procedure; (**c**) reanastomosis done on the same surgical procedure.

using gentle pressure, or by aspiration if done by laparoscopy, haemostasis is completed using electrocoagulation. The salpingotomy can then be closed or not. If the salpingotomy is closed a fine non-absorbable suture material such as 6/0 prolene should be used. If the bleeding does not stop some sutures can be placed in the mesosalpinx in the base of the tube in the area where the ectopic pregnancy implanted, and good haemostasis will be accomplished. In cases where the ectopic pregnancy is situated in the ampulla very close to the fimbrial end or on the fimbria, 'milking' of the ectopic pregnancy can be the method of choice. Once the pregnancy has been milked out, gentle pressure on the site of implantation is necessary to complete haemostasis.

Whatever the surgical procedure, radical or conservative, it must always be based on microsurgical principles — gentle handling of the tissues, avoidance of peritoneal damage, peritonealization of the raw areas, and the use of fine and non-resorbable suture material (prolene 5/0 or 6/0) which will prevent further damage and adhesion formation. If the tube is to be removed, it should be done so that the ovary is not displaced from its anatomical position, leaving it available for egg retrieval should the patient wish to be included in an in vitro fertilization programme. The use of drugs in order to diminish adhesion formation is debatable, but always remember that no drug or coadjuvant will compensate for a lack of surgical technique, and if the decision is made to use one, probably the best choice is steroids with local effect.

Laparoscopic techniques

The early diagnosis of ectopic pregnancy and the improvement of laparoscopic surgical methods and instruments, allowing the surgeon to perform laparoscopic surgery, have opened a new chapter in the treatment of ectopic pregnancy. Semm was the pioneer of laparoscopic surgery for ectopic pregnancy, and his first series of cases was published in 1980. The same principles of conservation should be applied with laparoscopic surgery as with open operations. For successful laparoscopic surgery, selection of patients is important. They should be haemodynamically stable. The ectopic pregnancy should be small, less than 6 cm in diameter, and the hCG level less than 6000 miu/ml; the pelvis should have only a minor amount of adhesions, and the pregnancy should be implanted in the tube.

For a very experienced laparoscopist, cornual or interstitial implantation is not an absolute contraindication to laparoscopic surgery at an early stage. It might even be reasonable to attempt laparoscopic surgery in cases with pelvic adhesions or a haemoperitoneum. In this type of procedure multiple punctures are needed. The use of dilute vasopressin 5 iu in 20 ml of saline, injected in the mesosalpinx, seems to have an important role in controlling bleeding.

Ovarian ectopic surgery

Ovarian ectopic pregnancy is a rare event and in general treatment depends on how early the diagnosis is made and how much the ovary and the tube, bowel or other pelvic organs are involved. The experience of the surgeon and the circumstances determine the type of operation necessary, but in general oophorectomy or salpingo-oophorectomy are the most common options.

Abdominal pregnancy

Abdominal pregnancy is a completely different problem, and fortunately a very rare one. The mortality is not negligible. The fetus can be removed or delivered without major problem. The main difficulty is presented by the ectopic placenta, sometimes inserted in the bowel or over-large vessels. In these cases the removal of the placenta should not be attempted because it can cause major bleeding, and sometimes even ligation of the internal iliac artery may not save the patient's life. In general placental function disappears over several weeks. Resorption of the placenta can be a very slow process and in some cases can last years. Methotrexate has been used to manage residual placenta, but can accelerate necrosis of the tissue causing severe infections and adding another morbidity factor.

Cytotoxic agents

Methotrexate may be useful in the treatment of ectopic pregnancy. In cases of interstitial ectopic pregnancy, Tanaka et al (1982) obtained good results without surgery and without major complications. Other uses are in cases where there is residual trophoblastic tissue after conservative surgery, or in cases of cornual or interstitial pregnancies where the surgeon was not able to remove the trophoblastic tissue totally and the follow-up beta-hCG remained high.

RESULTS

Analysis of long-term results of treatment of ectopic pregnancy is rather difficult due to the diversity of surgeons and procedures involved. It is even more difficult to compare or draw conclusions when treatment has been conservative. Due to the frequency of ampullary ectopic pregnancy the major published series are related to this site of ectopic implantation.

There does not seems to be a great difference in long-term results whether radical or conservative methods are used in the treatment of ectopic pregnancy in patients in whom both fallopian tubes are present. Oelsner (1987) collected a series of 1630 patients from the literature, and found that 40.9% had intrauterine and 14.2% repeated ectopic pregnancy when radical surgery (salpingectomy) was the treatment of choice; with a conservative approach 45.5% had an intrauterine and 11.5% repeated extra-uterine pregnancy. When analysing their results of salpingostomy DeCherney et al (1982) reported that among 15 patients with only one functional tube, 53% subsequently had an intrauterine pregnancy and 20% a recurrent extrauterine pregnancy.

Results of treatment of isthmic ectopic pregnancy are very few due to the low frequency of implantation of the pregnancy in this site. Stangel & Gomel (1980) reported on 7 patients: only 2 desired further pregnancies and both achieved intrauterine pregnancy. Gomel (1983) in another series of 9 patients with delayed reanastomosis found that 6 subsequently conceived with only 1 repeat ectopic pregnancy. DeCherney & Boyers (1985) found that among 6 patients with segmental resection and delayed reanastomosis, 4 conceived and only 1 had a recurrent ectopic pregnancy.

Since the wider application of laparoscopic treatment of ectopic pregnancies larger series have been published, but most have been concentrated on the success of the technique rather than the reproductive outcome for the patient. Pouly et al (1986) in their series of 321 ectopic pregnancies performed conservative surgery, using laparoscopic linear salpingostomy only. Of these 321, 5.9% needed a laparotomy after laparoscopic surgery due to bleeding, and 4.8% a secondary procedure for retention of trophoblastic tissue.

COMPLICATIONS

The major complication of ectopic pregnancy is death and ectopic pregnancy is still an important cause of maternal mortality in the first trimester of pregnancy.

One of the complications of treatment of ectopic pregnancy is iatrogenic disease. It is quite common and very disappointing to laparoscope patients complaining of infertility to find the pelvis covered by adhesions following ectopic pregnancy although the remaining fallopian tube is reasonably healthy. The fact that ectopic pregnancies are in general operated on in emergencies is no justification not to take maximum precautions and so avoid this common problem. Gentle handling of the tissues and the use of wet swabs and fine sutures, aspiration of the free blood in the abdominal cavity, and washing the peritoneal cavity using Ringer's lactate are all that is required.

Since early diagnosis of pregnancy has become possible with the use of beta-hCG and ultrasound, doctors can perform a laparoscopy on a patient too early and miss seeing an ectopic gestation, especially in a patient with distorted anatomy due to pelvic adhesions. In these cases a close follow-up with beta-hCG measurements and ultrasound are mandatory in order to avoid fatal consequences.

Persistent ectopic trophoblast can remain in the implantation site after conservative surgery. In some cases this is asymptomatic, the only finding being a persistent beta-hCG which slowly resolves. In other patients persistent trophoblast can cause intra-abdominal haemorrhage requiring an emergency laparotomy.

Severe intra-abdominal bleeding can be a complication after conservative laparoscopy, but with the injection of vasopressin in the mesosalpinge of the affected tube this eventuality has decreased greatly.

A new problem occurs in those patients who have successfully been through an IVF–ET programme when multiple embryo transfer has been performed. An intrauterine pregnancy may be confirmed by ultrasound without follow-up in later weeks to exclude the possibility of a heterotopic pregnancy. This used to be a rare event, but is not so now and the doctor should always be aware of it as a possibility.

KEY POINTS

1. Ectopic pregnancy occurs when there is implantation of the fertilized ovum outside the uterine cavity.
2. Abnormalities of the mechanisms involved in ovum transport may be a predisposing factor.
3. Tubal transport is influenced by hormone levels. Oestrogens stimulate tubal contractility but progesterone decreased the activity. Progesterone also decreases local prostaglandin secretion, causes relaxation of the isthmic portion of the tube which

may allow the fertilized ovum to progress into the uterus.
4. Cilia are important in transporting the ovum through the ampulla but not through the isthmus.
5. The most common site for tubal implantation is the ampulla.
6. Ovarian or abdominal ectopics may be primary or secondary depending on whether the pregnancy implants directly or as a result of tubal abortion.
7. A cervical ectopic is rare. To identify it, cervical glands must be attached to the placenta, the placenta must be implanted below where the uterine vessels reach the uterus.
8. Heterotopic pregnancy is the combination of an intrauterine pregnancy and an ectopic (generally tubal) pregnancy. It occurs in 1:30 000 pregnancies although this has risen with IVF techniques.
9. The risk of an ectopic increases 7-fold following an attack of salpingitis and is associated with the use of the IUCD.
10. Tubal reconstruction is associated with an increased incidence of ectopic.
11. The likelihood of conceiving after a sterilization procedure is 1:1000.
12. Race and socioeconomic factors influence the risk of ectopic pregnancy. In the USA, ectopic pregnancy is twice as high in non-white than in white populations.
13. The decrease in mortality rate is due to earlier diagnosis and better and earlier treatment.
14. When laparoscopies became a routine procedure, up to 40% of laparotomies were avoided and an early diagnosis was possible with less morbidity and mortality.
15. Serum B hCG is detectable 7–10 days after ovulation. The role of ultrasound scanning is to exclude an intrauterine sac after 5½ weeks.
16. For laparoscopic treatment, patient selection is important. The ectopic pregnancy should be small, less than 6 cm in diameter, and the hCG levels less than 6000 miu/ml.

REFERENCES

Abulcasis [Abul Qasim] 936–1013. De chirrugia, Arabice et Latine cura Johannis Channing, vol 3. Oxonii, e typ. Clarendoniano, 1778. M S Spink & G L Lewis, London: Wellcome Institute for the History of Medicine 1973

Brosens I A, Vasquez G 1976 Fimbrial microbiopsy. Journal of Reproductive Medicine 16: 171–178

Brunham R C, Binns B, McDowell J, Paraskevas M 1986 Chlamydia trachomatis infection in women with ectopic pregnancy. Obstetrics and Gynecology 67: 722–726

Clark K, Baranyai J 1987 Pelvic infection and the pathogenesis of tubal ectopic pregnancy. Australian and New Zealand Journal of Obstetrics and Gynaecology 27: 57–60

DeCherney A H, Maheux R, Naftolin F 1982 Salpingostomy for ectopic pregnancy in the sole patent oviduct: reproductive outcome. Fertility and Sterility 37: 619–622

DeCherney A H, Boyers S P 1985 Isthmic ectopic pregnancy: segmental resection as the treatment of choice. Fertility and Sterility 44: 307–312

DeCherney A H, Cholst I, Naftolin F 1981 Structure and function of the fallopian tubes following exposure to diethylstilbestrol (DES) during gestation. Fertility and Sterility 36: 741–745

Douglas C P 1963 Tubal ectopic pregnancy. British Medical Journal 2: 838–841

Donald I 1965 Diagnostic uses of sonar in obstetrics and gynaecology. Journal of Obstetrics and Gynaecology of the British Commonwealth 72: 907–919

Duckman S, Suarez J, Spitaleri J 1984 Vaginal pregnancy presenting as a suburethral cyst. American Journal of Obstetrics and Gynecology 149: 572–573

Eddy C A, Antonini R Jr, Pauertein C L 1977 Fertility following microsurgical removal of the ampullary–isthmic junction in rabbits. Fertility and Sterility 28: 1090–1093

Erkkola R, Liukko P 1977 Intrauterine devices and ectopic pregnancy. Contraception 16: 569–580

Gemzell L, Guillome J, Wang F C 1982 Ectopic pregnancy following treatment with human gonadotropins. American Journal of Obstetrics and Gynecology 143: 761–765

Gomel V 1983 Conservative surgical treatment of tubal pregnancy. In: Gomel V (ed) Microsurgery in female infertility. Little, Brown, Boston, p. 53

Hope R B 1937 The differential diagnosis of ectopic gestation by peritoneoscopy. Surgery, Gynecology and Obstetrics 64: 229–233

Kadar N, DeVore G, Romero R 1981 Discriminatory hCG zone: its use in the sonographic evaluation for ectopic pregnancy. Obstetrics and Gynecology 58: 156–161

Kobak A J, Fields C, Pollack S L 1955 Intraligamentary pregnancy: the extraperitoneal type of abdominal pregnancy. American Journal of Obstetrics and Gynecology 70: 175–184

Lehfelft H, Tietze C, Gorstein F 1970 Ovarian pregnancy and the intrauterine device. American Journal of Obstetrics and Gynecology 108: 1005–1009

Majmudar B, Henderson PH III, Semple E 1983 Salpingitis isthmica nodosa: a high risk factor for tubal pregnancy. Obstetrics and Gynecology 62: 73–78

Oelsner G, Morad J, Carp H, Mashiach S, Serr D M 1987 Reproductive performance following conservative microsurgical management of tubal pregnancy. British Journal of Obstetrics and Gynaecology 94: 1078–1083

Ory H W and The Women's Health Study 1981 Ectopic pregnancy and intrauterine contraception devices: new perspectives. Obstetrics and Gynecology 57: 137—144

Parry J S, Lea H C 1876 Extrauterine pregnancy. American Journal of Obstetrics and Gynecology 9: 169–170

Persaud V 1970 Etiology of tubal ectopic pregnancy. Obstetrics and Gynecology 36: 257–163

Pouly J L, Manhes H, Mage G, Canis M, Bruhat M A 1986 Conservative laparoscopic treatment of 321 ectopic pregnancies. Fertility and Sterility 46: 1093–1097

Semm K, Mettlesr L 1980 Technical progress in pelvic surgery via operative laparoscopy. American Journal of Obstetrics and Gynecology 138: 121–127

Stangel J J, Gomel V 1980 Techniques in conservative surgery for tubal gestation. Clinical Obstetrics and Gynecology 23: 1221–1228

Stromme W B 1953 Salpingotomy for tubal pregnancy. Obstetrics and Gynecology 1: 472–476

Swolin K 1975 Electromicrosurgery and salpingostomy long term results. American Journal of Obstetrics and Gynecology 121: 418–419

Tait T 1884 Five cases of extrauterine pregnancy operated upon at the time of rupture. British Medical Journal 1: 1250–1251

Tanaka T, Hayashi H, Kutsuzawa T, Fujimoto S, Ichinoe K 1982

Treatment of interstitial ectopic pregnancy with methotrexate: report of a successful case. Fertility and Sterility 37: 851–852
Westrom L, Bengtsson L P H, Mardh P A 1981 Incidence, trends and risks of ectopic pregnancy in a population of women. British Medical Journal 282: 15–18
Winston R L M 1981 Is microsurgery necessary for salpingostomy? The evaluation of results. Australian and New Zealand Journal of Obstetrics and Gynaecology 21: 143–152

21. Contraception, sterilization and abortion

John Newton

WORLD POPULATION GROWTH AND CONTRACEPTIVE PREVALENCE

Despite the decline in fertility rate seen in some countries, there is still a massive increase predicted for world population within the next 20 years. This population explosion is best seen in the years needed to double the world's population; from the time of the first settlements the years required to double the population have been 5000, 2500, 1500, 75 and 50 years. In 1975, the world population was 4000 million, by 1980 it was 4400 million and a massive total of 5900 million is predicted for the year 2000. Because of current size China and Asia will increase by 63% but growth will be most rapid in sub-Saharan Africa (76% of the projected total). Population growth in developed countries will be less.

There are major differences in contraceptive use by geographical regions. These are due in part to history, religious, cultural and social factors, government policies and the availability of family planning services and methods. Approximately 51% of the world's population (females at risk of pregnancy and male partners) will use some method of contraception — 70% in the more developed regions and 45% or less in the less developed regions (United Nations 1989). The method used and percentage by region are summarized in Figures 21.1 and 21.2 and Table 21.1.

'No contraception used' is another category worthy of scrutiny. Rates as high as 94% in Pakistan, 66% in Mexico, and 23% in the UK are the current range. In many cases this leads to unwanted and unplanned pregnancy.

Given these figures it is clear that we need all the available low-failure-rate methods plus new developments to prevent a further population explosion. Contraceptive use will have to increase by 150% within the next 10–15 years if we are to keep pace with increases in population growth, due to the number of women reaching 15 years and beyond in this time. This goal is attainable as, when compared with total fertility rates and population growth, the rate of increase of contraceptive use since 1960 has shown that contraceptive use can contain excessive growth.

INTRAUTERINE DEVICES (IUDs)

The IUD is now probably the second most commonly used reliable reversible method of preventing pregnancy; only

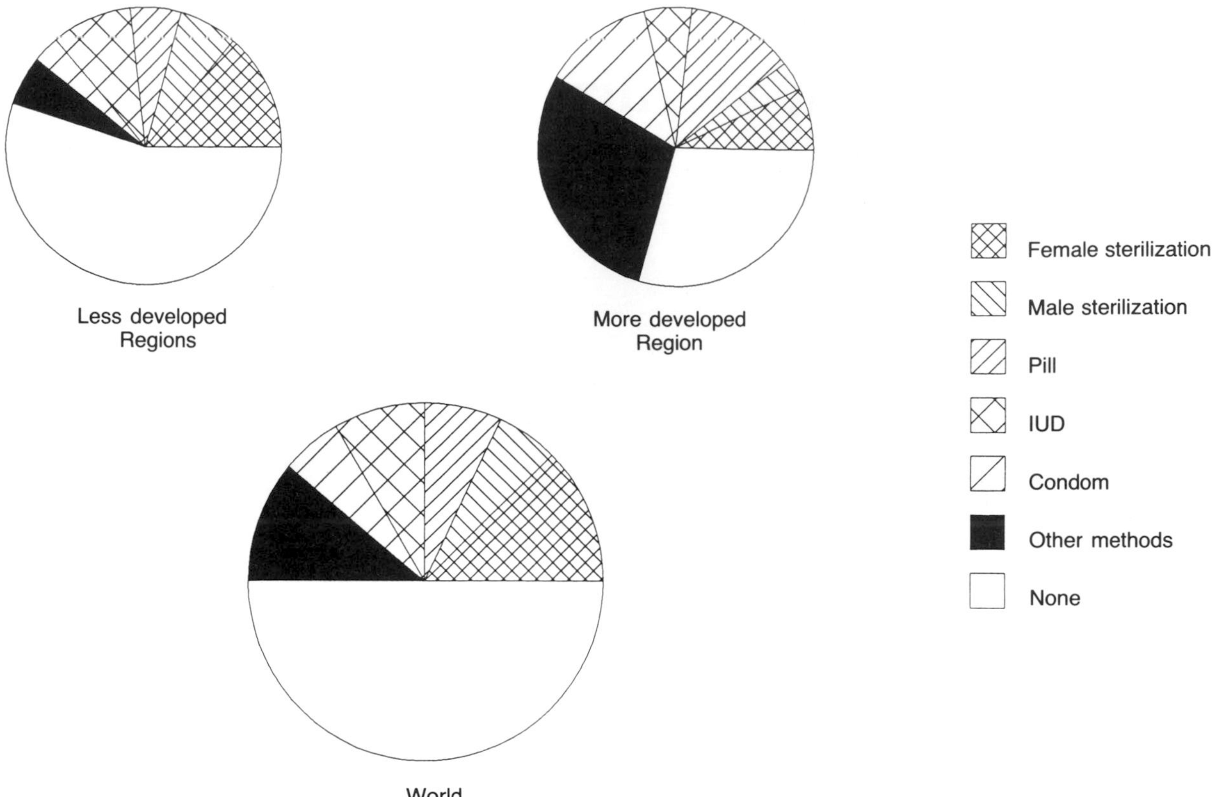

Fig. 21.1 Diagrammatic representation of form of contraception usage worldwide.

Table 21.1 WHO data 1989: percentage of current contraceptive use

Area	Sterilization		'Pill'*	IUD	Condom	Other methods†	Total
	Female	Male					
World	13	5	8	9	5	11	51%
More developed regions	7	4	13	6	13	27	70%
Less developed regions	15	5	6	10	3	6	45%
Africa	1	–	5	2	0.5	5	13.5%
Latin America	19	0.5	17	4	2	11	53.5%
East Asia	27	9	5	29	3	1.5	74.5%
South Asia	10	6	4	2	3	8	33%

IUD = Intrauterine device.
* Pill equivalent to all normal methods.
† Includes other supply and non-supply methods.

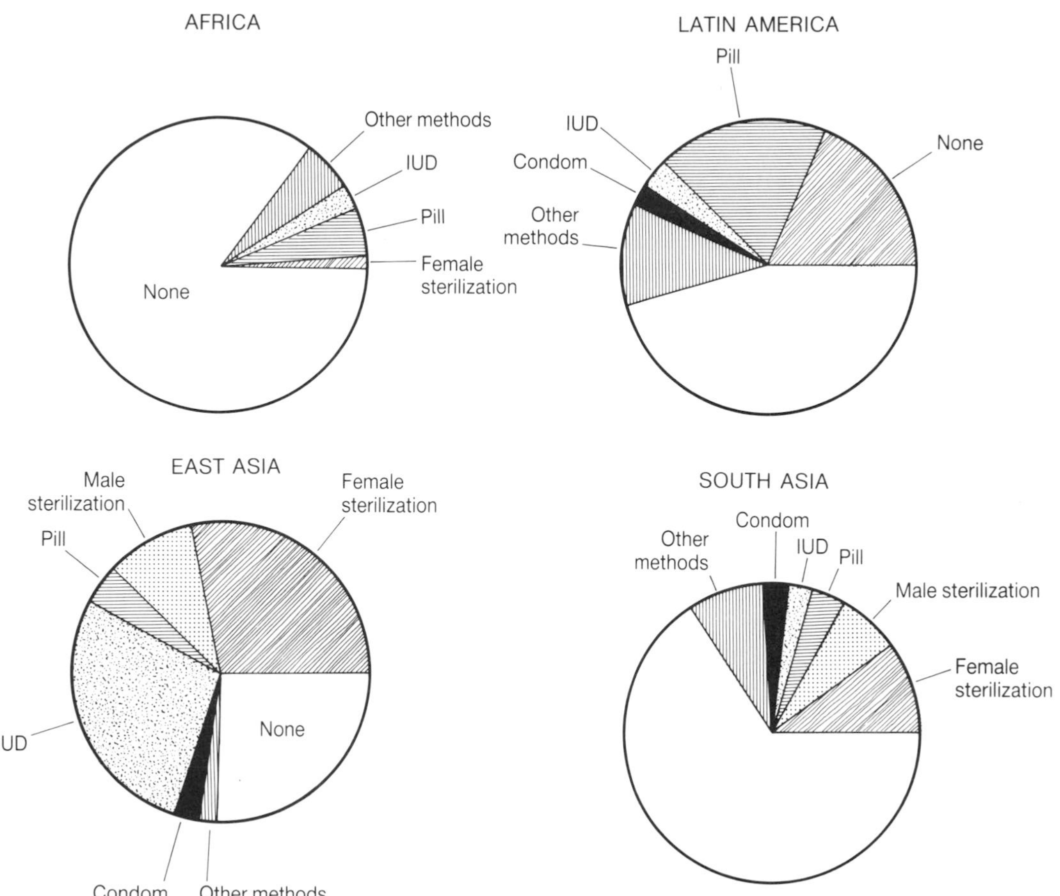

Fig. 21.2 More detailed breakdown of contraceptive usage in various continents.

oral hormonal contraceptives are used more frequently. It is estimated that more than 60 million women are using IUDs, of whom at least 80% are in China where, in some areas, more than 50% of women of child-bearing age have had an IUD inserted. IUD use in other areas of the world is very much less, ranging from about 6% in developed countries to 0.5% in sub-Saharan Africa (Table 21.2).

Table 21.2 IUD use worldwide

Region	Estimated number of IUD users	Percentage of married women reproductive of age
Africa (sub-Saharan)	0.3 million	0.5
Asia (excluding Japan)	49.5 million*	13.0
Developed countries	11.7 million	6.0
Latin America/Caribbean	1.8 million	2.2
South-west Asia/North Africa	0.8 million	2.0
World	60.5 million	23.7

* Includes 42.3 million in China.
After Newton et al (1987).

Types of IUD in common use

Lippes loop (size C) non-medicated

This serpentine (double-S)-shaped device is made of Silastic impregnated with barium sulphate to render it radio-opaque. It is 27 × 5 mm long and 30 mm wide and it has two threads attached to the lower end. It is inserted by straightening it inside an introducer tube; it is then inserted through the cervix into the uterine cavity. Due to its size, it is larger than most uterine cavities, even in multiparous women. Its use has been superseded by modern copper-containing and hormone-releasing devices.

First-generation copper devices

Copper Seven (Gravigard). The polypropylene carrier is shaped like a 7 and copper wire is wound round the vertical stem (200 mm^2 surface area). It is 36 mm long and 26 mm wide. It is also available in a smaller size — the mini-gravigard (28 × 22 mm).

Copper T 200 (Gynae T). This is T-shaped. The carrier

is made of polyethylene containing 200 mm^2 of copper wire on the vertical stem. It measures 36 × 32 mm.

Second-generation copper devices

Multiload 250. This polyethylene carrier has a vertical stem with two wings containing protrusions. Copper wire (250 mm^2) is on the vertical stem; wire thickness is increased to 0.3 mm to give longer efficacy. The overall dimensions are 26 × 18 mm. It is also available in a short form measuring 25 × 18 mm.

Nova T (Novagard). This T-shaped polyethylene device has a silver-cored copper wire wound round the stem of 200 mm^2. The dimensions are 32 × 32 mm.

Third-generation copper devices

Multiload 375. Of similar construction to the Multiload 250, it has copper wire of 0.4 mm thickness with a surface area of 375 mm^2 and hence a longer life and lower pregnancy rate. The overall dimensions are 26 × 18 mm.

Copper T 380S, 380A and 380 Ag. This family of copper devices is similar to the T-shaped device, 36 mm × 32 mm, using a polyethylene carrier where copper wire is wound round the vertical stem. The copper T380 Ag has a silver core similar to the Nova T. All three devices have in addition two copper collars or sleeves, one on each of the transverse arms. In the copper T 380A and Ag, these sleeves are mid-way along each horizontal arm. In the copper T 380S the sleeves are crimped on to the ends of the arms and hence are nearer to the tubal opening into the uterine cavity.

Hormone-releasing devices

Progestasert. This T-shaped device (36 × 32 mm) is made of a semi-permeable membrane of ethylene/vinyl acetate releasing progesterone at a rate of 65 mg/day for 1 year.

Levonorgestrel IUD. The frame of this IUD is identical to the Nova T without the copper. The levonorgestrel is released at 20 mg/day from a reservoir in the polymethylsiloxane collar around the vertical stem.

All these copper-containing and hormone-releasing devices have removal threads attached to the lower end of the device. This comes down through the cervix (see section on removal). They all also contain barium sulphate to render them radio-opaque.

Method of action

It is clear that the mechanism of action is multi-functional. Whenever a foreign body is inserted into the uterine cavity, specific changes occur: leukocyte infiltration, increased vascular permeability and oedema. This foreign body reaction takes place in the absence of bacteria and should not be confused with endometritis.

Biochemical changes seen with copper-bearing IUDs include changes in endometrial enzyme DNA cellular content, glycogen metabolism and oestrogen uptake by the uterine mucosa. The copper ions released by the device also inhibit sperm transport and affect tubal fluid and oocytes.

Hormone-releasing IUDs produce endometrial changes similar to hormonal contraception with a thinned atrophic endometrium and cervical mucus changes.

Insertion

Intermenstrual

It is wise to insert an IUD when a patient is menstruating, or immediately after. This has two benefits: the doctor can be certain the patient is not pregnant and insertion is easier due to the natural dilatation of the cervix at menstruation. Insertion at other times during the cycle may be necessary due to need, the type of patient and the time of referral. Pregnancy should be excluded before insertion.

Postnatal

Higher expulsion rates with certain devices are seen with early insertion during the first week of the puerperium. However immediate postplacental insertion is possible provided fundal insertion is achieved with a special long introducer. There is no benefit in waiting until 6 weeks after delivery; side-effects, perforation and expulsion are no higher of the device if inserted earlier, e.g. 3–4 weeks after delivery. There is no increased risk to the patient if she is breast-feeding, or if she has had a caesarean section.

Post-termination of pregnancy or miscarriage

There is no increased risk of perforation, side-effects, bleeding or infection, nor later side-effects e.g. medical removals. Expulsion is no higher for first-trimester miscarriage but is increased if insertion takes place after a second-trimester miscarriage or termination of pregnancy; however, this slightly increased risk has to be weighed against the benefits of IUD insertion (WHO 1983a,b).

Method of insertion

Proper IUD insertion reduces the risk of pregnancy and all the major risks. Each IUD has its own specific method of insertion but the object is the same: to achieve correct fundal placement allowing the IUD to open to its preinsertion shape and to do this without pain or discomfort to the patient. Successful insertion requires:

1. Careful explanation of the procedure to the patient.
2. Careful bimanual pelvic examination of the uterus with sounding of the cavity to determine its length and direction.
3. Careful technique — this reduces discomfort.
4. Aseptic technique — this prevents infection.
5. Fundal placement of the IUD high in the uterus — this reduces pregnancy and expulsion.

IUD efficacy

The modern copper-bearing IUD is one of the most effective methods of contraception, with pregnancy rates below 1 per 100 women at the end of 1 year of use. Recent WHO studies indicate that after 72 months — 6 years — of use the copper T 380A has a cumulative pregnancy rate of 1.4 per 100 women years (Newton et al 1987; Population Reports 1988).

In general terms non-medicated devices have higher pregnancy rates than copper- or hormone-releasing devices and therefore should not be used as routine IUDs of choice. The copper devices can be divided into three distinct groups according to pregnancy rates:

Group 1: pregnancy rates in excess of 2 per 100 women; the copper 7 and the copper T 200.

Group 2: pregnancy rates less than 1.5 but not better than 1 per 100; the Nova T and Multiload 250.

Group 3: the preferred IUDs on the basis of pregnancy rates alone are the Copper T 380A or 380S, the Multiload 375 and the levonorgestrel-releasing device.

Continued use of IUDs

It is already clear from the clinical data that all copper-releasing IUDs can be used for longer than the initial recommended period of time. Copper release rates are low and effective and pregnancy rate data show that even the Copper 7 and Copper T200 can be left in place for up to 5 years without lowering of efficacy. The newer second and third generation devices can be left for at least 6 years and probably 8 years without significant increase in the pregnancy rates.

Pregnancy with the IUD in place

The IUD is a very effective contraceptive. However, if pregnancy does occur there are potential complications. It is important that the patient is seen as early in the pregnancy as possible.

Spontaneous abortion is the most common complication if the IUD is not removed (Population Reports 1988); it is up to 5 times more common than if the IUD were not in place. In the USA with certain devices, septic mid-trimester abortion occurred (Foreman et al 1981); however, this was not seen in other countries.

About 3–9% of pregnancies with the IUD in place are ectopic. Therefore if pregnancy is suspected, an ectopic should be excluded.

Because of risks later in pregnancy, especially that of intrauterine infection and abortion, the IUD should always be removed as soon as pregnancy is confirmed. If the threads are not visible then careful counselling about the risks of continuing with the pregnancy is necessary.

IUD use and side-effects

The majority of women who use an IUD do so without side-effects. However, certain well recognized conditions do occur; these are described below.

Bleeding and pain

This is still the commonest medical reason for removal of an IUD. Usually it is increased menstrual bleeding or a longer period loss, though with some hormone-releasing IUDs intermenstrual spotting or bleeding may be more common in the first few months of use. Removal rates range from 4 to 13 per 100 women for copper devices at the end of 1 year of use. Higher rates of removal are seen for the larger non-medicated devices, e.g. Lippes loop.

The average increase in monthly blood loss with copper devices appears to be about 40–50% when compared with preinsertion levels. In contrast, hormone-releasing devices reduce monthly blood loss by 40–50% at the expense of an increase in intermenstrual spotting and bleeding in 50–80% of patients. The aetiology of this increased loss is due to endometrial lesions which predispose to this bleeding. Superficial microscopical ulceration of the endometrium may be caused by pressure from the IUD; the endometrial capillaries are eroded, leading to interstitial haemorrhage.

Expulsion

Uterine contraction can push the IUD downwards and either partially or completely expel the device. Again the rates vary from 1 to more than 10 per 100 women in the first year of use. The design of the IUD, the method of insertion, the skill of the person inserting the device and the size and shape of the uterine cavity all influence expulsion. Women of younger age — below 30 — and nulliparous women have higher expulsion rates than older and multiparous women.

Ectopic pregnancy

It is clear that the rate of ectopic pregnancy has increased in some western societies and that this increase is related to the rapid rise in the rate of sexually transmitted infections. If a patient becomes pregnant with an IUD in place then the risk of ectopic pregnancy is estimated at 1 in 30 or 3–4% whereas in the non-IUD user it is 1 in 125 or 0.8%.

However recent studies (WHO 1985) have shown that the copper-releasing devices have a definitive protective effect against the occurrence of an ectopic pregnancy: the relative risk is less than 1. Duration of IUD does not seem to effect the incidence of ectopic pregnancy (WHO 1987).

Any pregnancy with an IUD is uncommon, thus ectopic pregnancy with an IUD in situ is fortunately rare. The rate for modern IUDs is less than 1.5 per 1000 women years of IUD use (WHO 1987, Population Reports 1988).

Pelvic inflammatory disease

Many epidemiological studies in the 1970s tended to overestimate the incidence of pelvic inflammatory disease due to the methodology used, i.e. inappropriate control groups, ascertainment and diagnostic bias. Recent studies reviewed in a WHO technical report (WHO 1987) and Population Reports (1988) confirm that the risk of developing infection following IUD insertion is much less than at first thought — probably 1.5–2 times the background rate of pelvic inflammatory disease in the population, and then only for the first few weeks of IUD use. After that time the rate of pelvic inflammatory disease with an IUD is no greater than the rate within a population. Stable monogamous relationships reduce the incidence of pelvic inflammatory disease significantly and copper-releasing IUDs have the lowest rate. Correct selection of patients and screening of 'at-risk' cases before IUD insertion will reduce the risk of infection to a minimum.

Uterine perforation

Occasionally, in less than 1.2 per 1000 insertions, the uterus will be perforated by the introducer tube and the IUD placed partially or wholly outside the uterus. The IUD may come to lie intra- or extraperitoneally. Once identified the IUD should be removed as soon as is practical as copper-containing devices can cause an intense inflammatory reaction with structures such as omentum or bowel becoming adherent to the IUD. Usually laparoscopic retrieval is possible but occasionally — in 1 in 10 cases — a laparotomy may be needed to retrieve the device.

Correct identification of the position and angulation of the body of the uterus will allow proper intrauterine placement of the IUD; force should never be used during insertion as this may lead to perforation.

Management of missing IUD threads

Sometimes the thread of the IUD gets drawn up into the cervical canal or uterine cavity. In this situation the cervical canal should be gently sounded and sometimes the thread will be visualized. If ultrasound is not available and there is no chance of pregnancy, gentle cavity sounding using a plastic thread retrievial device, e.g. M-one spiral, will often bring down the thread. Alternatively, a small biopsy forceps can be used. Ideally an ultrasonic examination should be done before this as it will localize the IUD. A lateral X-ray with uterine sound can be used if necessary or if perforation is suspected.

If the patient is asymptomatic and wishes to continue with the IUD then it should be left in place. The thread does not have to be brought down. On the other hand if removal is required this can usually be achieved with biopsy forceps as an outpatient procedure.

Removal of an IUD

A request for removal or medical reason for removal should lead to an easy withdrawal of the IUD from the uterine cavity by gentle traction on the threads which are visible in the cervical canal. It is best to grip the threads firmly with a pair of forceps, e.g. long Spencer Wells; stabilize the cervix with a pair of tissue forceps and then apply traction downwards in the line of the uterine cavity. Occasionally the threads break and if they do the forceps can be used to explore the cervical canal. Often the lower part of the IUD stem is resting in the canal and the IUD can be retrieved. If it cannot be felt then a retrieval hook or uretheral biopsy forceps can be inserted into the uterine cavity. Local anaesthesia (1% Xylocaine) may be needed in some cases.

Return to fertility following removal

There is no evidence of impaired fertility in women who discontinue the use of an IUD to become pregnant. Conception rates vary between the various services published but with all modern copper- and hormone-releasing IUDs fertility rates vary between 75.8 and 96.4% pregnant at the end of 1 year and 93.3–96.8% at the end of 2 years (WHO 1987).

Selection of patients for an IUD

The critical factor in successful IUD use without unnecessary side-effects is careful selection of appropriate patients, together with pre-IUD screening when necessary.

Table 21.3 summarizes the absolute and relative contraindications to IUD use. A case history must be obtained with special reference to any pregnancies, menstrual cycle, past or present genital infection, number of sexual partners and previous attempts at contraception. A careful abdominal pelvic examination must follow; the size, shape, and position of the uterus must be verified and

Table 21.3 Contraindications to IUD insertion and use

Event	Types of contraindication Nulliparous women	Parous women	Remarks
Pregnancy	Absolute	Absolute	Suspected or confirmed
Genital infection	Absolute	Absolute	Active, with the exception of candidiasis
Sexually transmitted disease during the past 12 months	Absolute	Absolute	Does not apply to bacterial vaginosis, candidiasis, recurrent herpes virus infection, hepatitis B or cytomegalovirus
Serious pregnancy-related pelvic infection during the past 12 months	Absolute	Relative	
Previous ectopic pregnancy	Absolute	Relative	
Previous pelvic inflammatory disease	Absolute	Relative	
Multiple sexual partners	Relative	Relative	Absolute for nulliparae in areas of high prevalence of sexually transmitted disease
Anaemia	Relative	Relative	
Pathology of the uterine corpus	Relative	Relative	
Immunosuppressive therapy	Relative	Relative	
Wilson's disease	Relative	Relative	Copper IUDs

gynaecological infection excluded. Due to the recent increase in *Chlamydia* infection with little or nothing in the way of symptoms, consideration should be given to screening high-risk patients.

Absolute contraindications to IUD insertion include malignant disease of the uterus, cervical or vaginal bleeding of undiagnosed aetiology, suspected pregnancy and active pelvic inflammatory disease.

The following points may help in the selection of an appropriate IUD.

Nulliparity

Provided the patient understands the slight risk of tubal infection and is in a stable monogamous relationship then an appropriate small copper IUD can be inserted. These include a Copper 7 (if still available), a Nova T or a Multiload Short.

There is always a group of nulliparous women who cannot or will not use other methods of contraception and in whom the IUD is an appropriate choice.

Previous pelvic sepsis

So often when a careful history is taken, suspected pelvic sepsis turns out to be nothing more than undiagnosed abdominal pain. Nevertheless, lifestyle, sexual partners and vaginal discharge may make the use of an IUD inappropriate. If an IUD is needed then a copper or levonorgestrel-releasing IUD is the most appropriate.

Previous ectopic pregnancy

The incidence of repeat ectopic pregnancy is as high as 15%. While IUDs do not cause ectopics, ectopics do occur and it is usually preferable to use another form of contraception.

COMBINED ORAL CONTRACEPTION

Introduction

It is now more than 30 years since combined oestrogen and progestogen oral contraception was developed. The first paper was presented at the 13th Annual Laurentian Hormone Conference in 1956 under the title 'Synthetic progestins in the normal human menstrual cycle'. At that time there were debates and considerable disagreement as to the likely impact of contraception on population growth. However, the 'pill', as it is now universally known, is widely accepted and more than 60 million women were using it by 1989.

Monophasic oral contraceptives

The first types of oral contraception contained the same

Table 21.4 Combined oral contraception: selected examples of monophasic preparations (daily dose of steroids)

Oestrogen dose	Name	Progestogen	Dose
Ethinyloestradiol 50 μg (selected preparations)	Anovlar	NET-Ac	4.0 mg
	Gynovlar 21	NET-Ac	3.0 mg
	Minovlar	NET-Ac	1.0 mg
	Eugynon 50	Norg	500 μg (contains 250 μg LNg)
Ethinyloestradiol 35 μg	Norimin	NET	1.0 mg
	Ovysmen	NET	500 μg
Ethinyloestradiol 30 μg	Eugynon 30	LNg	250 μg
	Microgynon 30	LNg	150 μg
	Marvelon	DES	150 μg
	Femodene	GE	75 μg
	Loestrin	NET-Ac	1.5 mg
Ethinyloestradiol 20 μg	Mercilon	DES	150 μg
	Loestrin 20	NET-Ac	1.0 mg

Progestogens: NET = norethisterone; NET-Ac = norethisterone acetate; LNg = levonorgestrel; Norg = norgestrel; DES = desogestrel; GE = gestodene.

dose of oestrogen and progestogen each day for 21 (or 22) days. This approach is still used and called monophasic preparations (Table 21.4). Initial doses of oestrogen were often 75 or 100 μg (high-dose) and were either mestranol or ethinyloestradiol. Now only ethinyloestradiol is used and the dose has been progressively reduced in response to the findings that oestrogen side-effects were dose-related. The dose was reduced initially to 50 μg (medium-dose) and then to 30 μg (low-dose). The range of low-dose monophasic pills usually includes a range of oestrogen dose from 20 to 35 μg.

The progestogens commonly used in oral contraceptive pills are shown in Table 21.4. The first-generation progestogens used in early oral contraceptives included norethynodrel and norethisterone and due to relative low potency the dose used tended to be high (4–5 mg). Then in the 1960s the second generation of more potent progestogens were introduced — levonorgestrel. Initial oral contraceptives used norgestrel, a mixture of active and inactive isomers, hence the reduced dosage when the active isomer levonorgestrel was purified. These potent compounds allowed the dose to be reduced to 150 μg; however, some undesirable metabolic side-effects occurred despite good cycle control.

The third generation of highly discriminatory progestogens were introduced in the 1970s — desogestrel, and in the 1980s gestodene. These two potent compounds have few or no metabolic effects in the doses used in oral contraceptives (Table 21.4).

Phasic preparations

In an effort to reduce total steroid intake per month, the manufacturers prepared formulations with low doses of progestogen for the first part of the cycle, increasing it slightly for the last part. This increase was needed to maintain cycle control. If only one change in dose occurs, a biphasic preparation results; if there are two dose changes then the oral contraceptive is called a triphasic preparation. In some cases the oestrogen had to be increased slightly at mid-cycle to maintain cycle control (see Table 21.5 for examples of phasic preparations). These phasic preparations are now being replaced by the modern third-generation progestogen monophasic pills.

Progestogen-only pill

Alternatively, oral contraceptives can contain a small dose of progestogen without oestrogen; this type is useful in certain clinical situations and for certain patients (Table 21.6).

Table 21.5 Combined oral contraception: selected examples of phasic preparations (daily dose of steroids)

Type of pill	Name	Progestogen dose		Oestrogen dose		Regime
Biphasic	BiNovum	NET	0.5 mg	EE	35 μg	7 days followed by
			1.0 mg	EE	35 μg	14 days
Triphasic	Trinordial (also known as Logynon)	LNg	50 μg	EE	30 μg	6 days then
			75 μg	EE	40 μg	5 days then
			125 μg	EE	30 μg	10 days

NET = Norethisterone; LNg = levonorgestrel; EE = ethinyloestradiol

Table 21.6 Progestogen-only preparations

Progestogen	Dose/day (μg)	Name	Supplied as packs of
Ethynodiol diacetate	500	Femulen	28 pills
Norethisterone	350	Noriday (or Micronor)	28 pills
Norgestrel	75*	Neogest	35 pills
Levonorgestrel	30	Microval (or Norgeston)	35 pills

* Only contains 37.5 μg of the active isomer levonorgestrel.

The progestogens are those used in combined oral contraceptives but at a much reduced dose.

Clinical studies of combined oral contraception

Data on cycle control, the incidence of breakthrough bleeding and side-effects are obtained from large-scale clinical trials (stage III) and past marketing surveillance studies. These have been widely reported and include single-drug studies in a multicentre setting or, in a few cases, random allocation studies of different combined oral contraceptives, and also in a multicentre study (WHO 1982a). These show that for the first 3–4 months there is a slightly higher incidence of breakthrough spotting or bleeding for a few days per cycle, but that by the sixth cycle of use the pattern is no different from pretreatment cycles, i.e. there is a spotting incidence of 1 or more days in about 6% of women.

Epidemiological studies have been ongoing since the late 1960s and are usually of two types: case control studies to investigate a particular problem or large cohort studies to observe the beneficial and adverse long-term effects in a given population of women. Three that are worth mentioning are the Oxford Family Planning Study (for review see Vessey 1984) of 17 032 women; 57% were oral contraceptive users and for entry to the study they had to be married and have been using the method for 6 months. The Royal College of General Practitioners' (RCGP) study (for review see Kay 1984) recruited 23 000 pill users and 23 000 'never' users by 1400 general practitioners and was conducted by Dr Clifford Kay. These two studies started in 1968; they are ongoing and provide relative risks for both beneficial and adverse effects in their population. Most of these women started with what we would now term medium-dose first- and second-generation oral contraceptives. The third major study is the Walnut Creek study from the USA (Rinehart & Piotrow 1979) which recruited some 18 000 women. It is these three major studies and some other smaller studies that give us most of the data on long-term adverse and beneficial effects. They also allow us to look at some aspects of association of these effects, e.g. length of taking the pill versus effect.

Beneficial effects

Combined oral contraceptives reduce blood loss by at least 50% and therefore it is not surprising that the incidence of anaemia, dysmenorrhoea and menorrhagia is significantly reduced. Fibroids causing significant problems were also reduced in the RCGP study (by 30% by 10 years of use) and functional ovarian cysts were also reduced by more than 50%. This is to be expected, due to the suppression of ovulation seen with combined oral contraceptives.

The cervical mucus is also altered by combined oral contraceptives to the progestogenic 'thick' mucus plug. Pelvic inflammatory disease was reduced in pill users by at least 50%, partly due to this action, and the pill provides some protection against ascending infection (Kay 1984; Vessey 1984; Grimes 1979). The risk of ectopic pregnancy is also reduced due to the ovulation suppressive effect: no ectopics were seen in the oral contraceptive group of the Oxford study (Vessey 1984) when compared with barrier methods (0.6%).

Subsequent fertility is not affected by pill use — no delay in return to ovulation is seen in the majority of women. In a small number of women having oligomenorrhoea or a tendency to secondary amenorrhoea, a delay in return to regular ovulatory cycles has been seen. However, this responds to correct treatment.

Adverse effects

Minor or nuisance side-effects are now uncommon with low-dose combined oral contraceptives. Side-effects range from breast tenderness, nausea and vomiting to weight gain and mood change. There is a pronounced 'placebo effect' in relation to these side-effects and adequate counselling often prevents problems. These side-effects can also 'come and go' with different cycles and are often related to non-medical events. Weight gain, common with levonorgestrel pills, is not a problem with desogestrel- and gestodene-containing pills. Weight increase will be seen with adolescents due to their continued development and body area increase during teenage years. Inappropriate weight distribution, e.g. on the hips, is a sign of progestogen-related weight increase and needs to be checked.

Major side-effects are fortunately rare and can largely be avoided by risk assessment before starting oral contraception (see section on prescribing oral contraception). The major effects can be usefully grouped under cardiovascular, gastrointestinal and cancer.

Cardiovascular side-effects

These were among the first side-effects to be reported in the 1960s. Confounding factors such as family history of cardiovascular disease and smoking made the interpretation of early data difficult. It is best to subdivide cardiovascular disease into the following groups:

1. *Venous thrombosis*: Early reports with high-dose oestrogen-containing pills suggested a relative risk (RR) of 2:1 up to 11:1. However when the dose was reduced the RR went down and now with low-dose combined oral contraceptives the RR ratio is less than 2.

   There is little or no association with superficial venous thrombosis. No link appears to exist between progestogens and venous thromboembolism or to duration of pill use. Smoking and blood group A are confounding factors.
2. *Arterial and venous cerebral haemorrhage ('Stroke')*: Subarachnoid haemorrhage is the commonest type of stroke. The UK epidemiological studies (Kay 1984; Vessey 1984) indicate that there is an increased risk with combined oral contraceptive use, probably in the order of 1.5 to 2 (RR). However, smoking again significantly increases the risk, and pre-existing raised blood pressure also increases the risk.
3. *Thrombotic stroke*: This is rare and in about 1 in 10 000 women years results in a fatal stroke, whereas for non-fatal stroke the risk is between 2 and 4 per 10 000 women years. From the RCGP study (Kay 1984) the risk was shown to be less with reduced oestrogen and reduced progestogen dose. At present there is no conclusive evidence of an effect due to duration of use.
4. *Hypertension*: Modern low-dose combined oral contraceptives cause little change in diastolic or systolic blood pressure. Blood pressure returns to normal when oral contraceptives are stopped.
5. *Myocardial infarction and ischaemic heart disease*: In early reports, again with higher-dose pills, RR appeared to be raised between 1 and 14. However, most studies indicate an RR of between 3 and 5. Fatal infarction occurs in about 1 in 10 000 women years. There also appeared to be evidence linking both the oestrogen and progestogen dose to this increased risk. Confounding bias again occurs with other risk factors such as smoking, age, hypertension, diabetes mellitus and hyperlipidaemia. Again from the RCGP study (Kay 1984) excess deaths due to pill use in non-smokers never reach a significant level but in those who smoke the rate becomes significant by the age of 35.

Gastrointestinal disorders

The incidence of gallstones and cholecystitis is increased in some of the cohort studies in earlier reports. Recent reports (Hennekens et al 1984) do not confirm this early increased risk. The rate appears to be associated with oestrogen dose (RCGP study) (Kay 1984) and therefore with the new low-dose combined oral contraceptives the RR is not significant. Other chronic bowel disease such as ulcerative colitis and Crohn's disease has also been seen in some studies to have a slightly increased risk. However the confounding influence of smoking may be responsible for this.

Cancer and combined oral contraceptive use

Several factors need to be taken into consideration. The first is the latent interval between exposure to oral contraceptive use and the onset of cancer several years later — (more than 10 years in some cases). The time of exposure before first full-term pregnancy can affect some cancers, as can the known high-risk groups, e.g. multiple sexual partners and cervical neoplasia, and a family history of breast cancer in oral contraceptive users. These factors need to be taken into account together with the changes that have occurred both in the dose of oestrogen and progestogen and the potency of the progestogen used.

Ovarian cancer. Most epidemiological studies show a significant (more than 50%) reduction in the incidence of ovarian cancer and studies (Kay 1984) indicate that this protective effect persists for many years after stopping oral contraceptives.

Endometrial cancer. This is rare before 45 years of age. However most of the epidemiological data supports the observation of a significant reduction in the incidence of endometrial cancer by at least 50%.

Cervical neoplasia. Data presented on cervical carcinoma sometimes confuse invasive carcinoma with preinvasive disease, e.g. cervical intraepithelial neoplasia (CIN) I, II and III. Pick-up rates of cervical lesions are bound to be higher in combined oral contraceptive users due to more frequent screening, cervical assessment and cytology. An increase in number of sexual partners also predisposes to cervical neoplasia and there is the confounding influence of smoking and wart virus infection. Many of the earlier studies did not control for sexual partners and other variables and therefore the early reports of an increase in risk need to take into account this bias. Nevertheless, reports (Kay 1984) indicate that the increased risk is very slight and early detection is possible, together with adequate treatment. It is also the view of one leading authority (Vessey 1989) that it is impossible to be sure that this slight increase is not due to the confounding sexual factors.

Breast cancer. This is still a complex issue and more than any other cancer is affected by latent time to disease and time of exposure. Use of combined oral contraceptives is associated with a protective effect against clinically detectable benign breast disease (Kay 1984; Vessey 1984). Most of the recent data comes from case control studies and from the three major cohort studies (Vessey 1989). The majority of the data is reassuring and does not show an increased risk of developing breast cancer; therefore there does not seem at this time to be any need to change prescribing habits. However, there may be certain groups of patients who will possibly be more at risk in the future and warrant the continued collection of data. The older woman (over 30 years) appears not to be at risk and sufficient long-term data exist (Vessey 1989). However, data on young women and those who use combined oral contraceptives before first full-term pregnancy are conflicting and often confusing, due to small numbers of women included in the surveys. The question of a possible relationship between early oral contraceptive use and breast cancer remains unresolved at present. For a recent review see Vessey (1989).

Efficacy

Failure can be due to failure of the pill (method failure) or poor patient compliance with missed pills (patient failure). With older medium-dose combined pills in clinical trials the total failure rate was less than 1 per 100 women years. However, the margin for error is less with modern low-dose pills and recent studies by the WHO indicate failure rates in the order of 3.0 per 100 women years, which equates with rates seen in routine use and post-marketing surveillance studies (WHO 1982a).

Failure can be reduced by adequate counselling and teaching patients to use the schemes described for missed pills.

Starting the pill, follow-up and review

It is wise to start the first packet of combined oral contraceptives on day 1 of the cycle. If this is not possible, then it should be no later than day 5. After spontaneous abortion or therapeutic termination of pregnancy the pill should be started immediately rather than waiting for the first period. After pregnancy in non-breast-feeding women the combined oral contraceptives can be started immediately; for breast-feeding women a progestogen-only formulation is preferred; combined oral contraceptives can be started when partial breast-feeding is in progress or when breast-feeding ceases. Steroid contraceptives cross into the breast milk and while they do not appear to affect development adversely, it is wise to choose a pill with the lowest dose, hence the progestogen-only pill recommendation.

Once combined oral contraceptives have been started the patient should be seen regularly for interview, reinforcement of 'pill rules' and examination. At each visit weight and blood pressure are recorded together with menstrual cycle details and details of any abnormal bleeding. At least once a year a pelvic examination should be carried out and cervical smears taken at appropriate intervals. These visits can be used for other health screening, e.g. self breast examination and health education on diet and prevention of smoking. Follow-up should be within 6 weeks of the initial visit or when switching from one brand to another type of pill; thereafter for the first year follow-up is advisable at 3–4 monthly intervals and then twice a year. There is no need for patients to have a 'rest' from the pill. Some doctors still recommend this but it is unnecessary with modern low-dose pills.

Prescribing oral contraception

This section reviews the essential factors relating to prescribing of oral contraception. For more detailed information the reader should consult the data sheets and *The Handbook of Family Planning* (Loudon 1991).

The objective is always to use the lowest suitable dose of combined pill which is safe and effective. Modern progestogens, being very potent, can be used in very low doses. These low-dose combined oral contraceptives, containing either desogestrel or gestodene, are highly discriminatory and have little effect on the biochemical parameters that have been measured. Thus insulin, carbohydrate and plasma lipids remain within the normal range for the population who are likely to take oral contraceptives.

Selection

To select a user for a combined oral contraceptive it is necessary to have a checklist of absolute and relative contraindications (Tables 21.7 and 21.8). Women will often come to an initial counselling session knowing which pill they want due to discussions with family, or previous reading.

Table 21.7 *Absolute contraindications to use of combined oral contraceptives*

Present or past circulatory disease
- Arterial or venous thrombosis
- Angina or ischaemic heart disease
- Hyperlipidaemia
- Known abnormalities of coagulation/fibrinolysis
- Focal migraine, transient ischaemic attacks
- Past cerebral haemorrhage
- Most types of valvular disease
- Combination of risk factors (see text)

Liver disease
- Active liver disease, cholestatic jaundice of pregnancy, recurrent jaundice
- Gallstones (see text)
- Porphyrias
- Liver adenomas

Previous serious conditions affected by combined oral contraceptives
- Herpes gestationis
- Trophobastic disease (see text)
- Haemolytic uraemic syndrome

Undiagnosed genital tract bleeding

Oestrogen-dependent neoplasms

Pregnancy

Table 21.8 Relative contraindications to combined oral contraceptive use (after counselling appropriate oral contraceptives can be used)

Risk factors for cardiovascular disease, e.g. smoking (see text)
Migraine (excluding focal migraine — see Table 21.7)
Past sex steroid-dependent cancer (see text)
Family history of breast cancer (first-degree relative)
Preinvasive cervical disease (see text)
Long-term immobilization
Homozygous sickle cell disease
Long-term treatment with drugs which are likely to interact with oral contraceptives

In the counselling session a full medical, reproductive, social and family history is taken. It is necessary in the family history to enquire about cardiovascular disease, age of onset of disease, smoking, and breast cancer in addition to other factors. These risk factors can be graded from relative to absolute contraindications, thus for smoking: less than 40 cigarettes/day = relative; more than 40/day = absolute.

For cardiovascular disease, if a first-degree relative under the age of 45 has had a major event, e.g. stroke or ischaemic heart disease, then this plus a normal blood biochemical profile would be a relative contraindication, whereas the presence of an abnormal profile would be an absolute contraindication. Diabetes mellitus, hypertension and obesity can be treated in the same way.

It is clear from the epidemiological data mentioned earlier that women who do not smoke and have no risk factors can continue to take low-dose combined oral contraceptives up to the menopause. Women with risk factors will need to change either to progestogen-only pills or to another method at an earlier age. Discussions on method changes in this group need to start between 30 and 35 years.

Missing pills

Patient compliance is essential to prevent 'pill failure' and unintended pregnancy. If a patient misses one pill then that pill should be taken as soon as she remembers or within 24 h. Missing two pills, especially with modern low-dose combined oral contraceptives, will often cause breakthrough bleeding and leave the patient at risk of pregnancy. Extra precautions need to be taken, e.g. barrier contraception for at least 7 days. Missing pills at times when the 7-day pill-free interval can be extended by these missed pills, e.g. the last week or first week of pill-taking, is also a risk factor. Missing pills in the last week should be treated by abolishing the pill-free interval and starting the next packet immediately after the current one. Missing pills in the first or second week should be covered by barrier contraception for at least 7 days. The patient should continue with her oral contraceptives and disregard any breakthrough bleeding.

Drug interaction

Drugs that increase the breakdown of oral contraceptives by liver enzyme induction or prevent absorption of the drug, e.g. in gastroenteritis, can affect the efficacy of the pill. The two well known situations are enzyme indication due to drugs used to treat epilepsy, e.g. phenytoin: here a stronger combined oral contraceptive (medium-dose) will be needed to maintain bioavailability. Certain antibiotics are also known to affect combined oral contraceptives, e.g. long-term treatment for tuberculosis and, in certain cases, ampicillin. For a full list of drug interactions please see the review article by Back et al (1982) and Loudon (1991).

Surgery

Minor and intermediate surgery, e.g. laparoscopic sterilization, is not a contraindication to pill continuation. For major surgery, e.g. cholecystectomy or hysterectomy, then oral contraceptives should be stopped at least 4 weeks before surgery to allow the changes in the fibrinolytic system and the clotting cascade to return to normal.

Pregnancy

If pregnancy is suspected then the pill should be stopped and appropriate tests used to confirm the pregnancy. The data with modern low-dose contraceptives and continuing pregnancy are reassuring as it is suggested that there is little if any effect on the fetus in terms of abnormality.

ORAL PROGESTOGEN-ONLY CONTRACEPTION — 'THE MINI PILL'

Several progestogens have been used for this type of oral contraception (see Table 21.6). The dose is considerably less than with combined oral contraceptives — 30 μg levonorgestrel compared with 150 μg in the combined oral contraceptives. The progestogen-only pill (POP) works by affecting cervical mucus, altering it so that it becomes thick and progestogenic and prevents sperm penetration. In addition up to 40 or 50% of cycles will have disordered luteal phases; recent ultrasound studies (Jackson & Newton 1989) have shown that persistent follicles (small cysts) are formed in the ovary in up to 50% of treated cycles. This explains why the major side-effects of this type of contraception are irregular and unpredictable bleeding. The pills are taken one every day, continuously without a break.

The blood levels of the synthetic steroid are directly related to time of ingestion and reach low levels between 20 and 24 h after ingestion. Timing of intake is critical and should relate to the patient's lifestyle. Pills should be taken at a time related to the usual time of intercourse and not 20 h later. This will reduce failure rates.

Clinical side-effects

Non-menstrual side-effects are minor and less than with combined oral contraceptives. Menstrual side-effects include irregular cycles, unpredictable bleeding, amenorrhoea and spotting. When properly counselled, women can usually accept this pattern.

Cycle lengths of 25–35 days occur in 55–65% of women (Fotherby 1982; WHO 1982b). As use is continuous then the incidence of cycle disruption decreases; after 6 months of use most women have predictable bleeding patterns.

Efficacy

Table 21.9 lists published studies and failure rates.

Table 21.9 Efficacy of progestogen-only pills

Drug	Dose (μg)	Women months of use	Pregnancy rate (pearl index)*
Femulen (ethynodiol diacetate)	500	24534	2.1
Micronor (Noriday) (norethisterone)	350	26173	2.3
Microval (Norgeston) (levonorgestrel)	30	36118	3.0

* Pearl index (pregnancy rate) = $\frac{\text{Number of pregnancies}}{\text{Number of months of use}} \times 1200$

Return to fertility

There is no delay in return to fertility, and cycle delay which is sometimes seen with combined oral contraceptives is not seen with the mini pill.

Use in special groups

Due to its low dose, absence of systemic side-effects and no significant risk of cardiovascular disease, the mini pill is often the method of choice for those who cannot take the combined oral contraceptive. It is therefore useful in the 'at-risk' older woman, e.g. one who smokes, is obese and over 35 years; those with severe side-effects of combined oral contraceptives or a family history that prohibits the use of oestrogen-containing pills.

The mini pill is useful in lactating women, as only a small amount of the progestogen crosses into the breast milk. Follow-up studies have shown no harmful effect on the infant nor on the quality of the milk.

Metabolic effects

These are few in number and minor in nature.

POSTCOITAL CONTRACEPTION

Oestrogens have been used successfully as a postcoital contraceptive for a number of years, usually after unprotected intercourse or following an accident with barrier contraception. However, ethinyloestradiol given for 5 days in this way had a high — 30% or more — incidence of nausea and vomiting. More recently a combined progestogen–oestrogen regime (the Yuzpe method) has been used with success. Ethinyloestradiol 100 μg and levonorgestrel 300 μg are given stat and then 12 h later. This medication, PCC4, is in the form of a standard combined 50 μg oestrogen-containing oral contraceptive, so 2 tablets are taken and then a further 2 12 h later. To be effective this must be used within 48 h of intercourse. If the patient presents later than this then an IUD, either copper-containing or inert, can be inserted up to 5 days after intercourse.

When this method has been used as a 'first aid' contraceptive method it is important to see the patient at the time of the next period to establish a suitable long-term method.

Table 21.10 Injectable preparations
Progestogen-only preparations

Name	Progestogen	Dose	Frequency of injections	Type of preparation
Depo-Provera	Depot medroxyprogesterone acetate	150 mg	Every 90 days (12 weeks)	Aqueous micro-crystalline suspension
Noristerat	Norethisterone acetate	200 mg	Every 8 weeks for 6 months then 8 or 12 weeks (see text)	In vehicle of benzyl benzoate and caster oil

Combined preparations given every 30 days ('once a month')

Name	Progestogen	Dose	Oestrogen	Dose
Cyclofem (HRP 102)	Medroxyprogesterone acetate	50 mg	Oestradiol valerate	5 mg
HRP 112*	Norethisterone acetate	50 mg	Oestradiol cyprionate	5 mg

* Under development by World Health Organization and used extensively in clinical trials.

INJECTABLE CONTRACEPTION

Two long-acting progestogen-only contraceptive agents have been available for some years and in excess of 6 million women worldwide use this method. The first to be introduced was Depo-Provera DMPA (medroxyprogesterone acetate: a microcrystalline suspension of the drug in an oily solution), usually given in the dose of 150 mg every 12 weeks by deep intramuscular injection. The second and more recent is Noristerat (norethisterone oenanthate — NET-EN: a micronized suspension of the drug); 200 mg is given by injection every 8 weeks (Table 21.10). Some of the early studies repeated use of this injectable every 60 days for 6 months and then every 84 days, with acceptable pregnancy rates. However, pharmacokinetic data support injections every 8 weeks (see Table 21.10).

These methods offer several advantages: a low failure rate, good patient compliance, especially in women who forget to take tablets, and infrequent visits (every 2–3 months) for medical attention. As with all progestogen-only agents the main disadvantage is irregular, often unpredictable bleeding which is worse in the first few months of use. However, with reassurance and forewarning it can be only a minor nuisance for the majority. Depo-Provera also has an increased incidence of amenorrhoea (absent withdrawal bleeds) but this is often welcomed by patients when they realize they are not pregnant.

Although animal data have raised concern about the safety and long-term side-effects of DMPA and NET-EN, certain animal models and the doses used appear not to be appropriate for studying human effects of these steroids. Extensive clinical and epidemiological studies among women using these drugs have thus far demonstrated no life-threatening events and no increased incidence of cancer. These studies over the last 15 years have shown that injectables may well have fewer adverse effects than are found with other hormonal agents.

In an effort to improve cycle control and reduce irregular menstrual bleeding, WHO and other agencies have developed one-a-month combination injectables which contain both oestrogen and a progestogen. These are now used by more than 1 million women. They have highly predictable bleeding patterns; the first bleed occurs a few days after the first injection and thereafter bleeding occurs every 28–30 days. The injections need to be given regularly every 28 days, i.e. the same day each fourth week. Contrary to expectations, women do not find it difficult to return for injections every month and any inconvenience is offset by the better cycle control. The incidence of irregular bleeding compared with the progestogen-only injectable is half that seen with Depo-Provera.

It is important for the first injection of either progestogen-only or combined injectables to be given within 5 days of the start of a normal period or within 5 days of a miscarriage.

Pregnancy rates with these methods are very low — 0–0.4 per 100 women.

Implants

Now being used or introduced in 15 countries of the world, a slow-release subcutaneous implant of a silactic tube containing levonorgestrel (Norplant), is the most recent new contraceptive method to be introduced. It has been developed by the Population Council. Six small implants are placed under the skin using a local anaesthetic infiltration and an introducer. Pregnancy rates remain low for at least 5 years. The side-effects are similar to other progestogen-only systems, i.e. bleeding irregularities. Removal is easy, either when the patient wishes it removed or at the end of its useful life, which is about 5 years.

Other implants using 3-ketodesorgesterel (Implanon) are being developed while other delivery systems are also being tried, e.g. microspheres containing norethisterone and biodegradable systems also containing norethisterone.

Vaginal rings

Soft torodial silastic rings, approximately 55 mm in diameter, have been developed as drug delivery systems for hormones. Progestogen-only rings using either levonorgestrel or 3-ketodesorgesterel and combined rings using an oestrogen plus a progestogen have been developed. The steroid is released at a zero-order rate using either a rate-limiting membrane or another system. The progestogen-only rings are changed every 3 months; the combined rings are used like combined pills (left in for 3 weeks and taken out for 7 days). The vaginal route of administration avoids the first-pass liver effect and therefore the dose of the steroid can be significantly reduced, e.g. oestrogen reduced by 50% from 30 to 15 μg.

With the progestogen-only system, menstrual irregularity is still a nuisance but tolerable. With the combined system cycle, control is similar to oral contraceptive. The rings are well tolerated, highly acceptable in the studies so far completed and expulsion rates are low provided constipation and straining are avoided. Pregnancy rates are low and acceptable.

STERILIZATION

Sterilization of either partner has become one of the most widely used methods of contraception in the world with over 90 million couples choosing this option. Over the years it has become a simple reliable procedure with low morbidity. Female sterilization methods have been simplified and improved, with the change from methods requiring laparotomy up to the 1960s and then the change to laparoscopic methods. It is usual for general anaesthesia to be used but local anaesthesia can be used for some methods.

Female sterilization methods

Current methods of female sterilization use a laparoscopic or mini-laparotomy technique. Before the 1960s, some form of tubal occlusion was usually performed through a laparotomy incision. For review see Newton (1984).

Laparoscopic techniques

Laparoscopic sterilization was introduced in England in 1967 by Steptoe and this technique has revolutionized the procedure of female sterilization. Methods which initially used diathermy to destroy the tubes have now been replaced by mechanical methods, of which the most common are the Filshie clip and the Fallope ring.

Unipolar diathermy. A minimum of 3 cm of tube is diathermized from the cornu of the uterus. Morbidity has been found to be higher than in other diathermy techniques. Bowel and abdominal burns have also been reported. Reversal is usually impossible due to postoperative ischaemic necrosis destroying up to seven-eighths of the tube.

Bipolar diathermy. This method has allowed a smaller segment of the tube to be destroyed. The tube is grasped several times beginning at the cornu to achieve a confluent coagulated zone of 1.5 cm.

Thermal coagulation. Low voltage and low temperature produce coagulation. Semm and Wolf techniques of thermal coagulation have been described.

Fallope ring. This was introduced in 1972. The ring is made of silicone rubber with 5% barium sulphate. The dimensions are: outer diameter 3.6 mm, inner diameter 1 mm and thickness 2.2 mm. The ring (or rings) is loaded on to the applicator. A loop of tube is then drawn into the applicator with forceps and the ring is forced off to occlude the piece of tube.

Hulka Clemens clip. This was developed in 1972. It is made of the plastic plexine and has teeth which interlock when the clip is closed. When closed it is locked in place by a gold-plated stainless steel spring.

Filshie clip. This is the latest clip to be designed and was introduced in 1975. Its main advantages are minimal destruction of tube (4 mm), complete occlusion, no possibility of migration once the clip is locked, and complete tubal ischaemia due to the constant pressure of the silicone rubber insert until tubal necrosis and separation of the two portions of the tube on either side of the clip are complete. Failure rates are also reported to be low, in the region of 1 per 1000 cases.

As with any surgical procedure there is a learning curve for the operation and strict attention to detail minimizes failure rates.

Mini-laparotomy

This provides an alternative method of sterilization as not all cases are suitable for laparoscopy. Morbidity associated with a laparotomy can be reduced by a mini-laparotomy incision (3–5 cm) with an appropriate tubal occlusion technique. It is usually used in conjunction with a uterine manipulator to allow the fallopian tubes to be presented in turn beneath the mini-laparotomy incision for easier application of the clip or ring.

Culdotomy

This is an alternative method used not infrequently in some countries, e.g India, where an incision in the posterior fornix allows access for vaginal tubal sterilization. Culdotomy has higher complication rates than laparoscopy or laparotomy.

Hysteroscopic techniques

Modern hysteroscopes developed in the 1970s allowed further study on transcervical tubal sterilization. Techniques included diathermy, ceramic tubal plugs, chemical agents and silicone splints formed in place in the tube. Unfortunately all these methods have high ectopic rates and an inability to guarantee bilateral occlusion following a single application. This method still remains a research technique, requiring further development.

Morbidity following sterilization

Several studies have sought to identify the morbidity associated with sterilization. This can be classified as *early*, including difficulties encountered at the time of operation and in the immediate postoperative period, and *late*, including long-term possible ill effects.

Early morbidity

Several large studies have shown current laparoscopic techniques to be safe, with low overall morbidity rates (Chamberlain & Brown 1978, Phillips et al 1977, 1981). Early morbidity should be considered under surgical difficulty and surgical complications.

Surgical difficulty. Here a problem interferes with the procedure and may result in a change in method or abandonment of the sterilization. Two problems were identified by Mumford & Bhiwandiwala (1981): firstly those particular to the patient (thick tubes, obesity, previous abdominal surgery), and secondly those relating to the instrument (e.g. slipping of a ring).

Surgical complications. This includes problems such as bleeding during the procedure or torn tubes. Technical failure results when the planned technique could not be carried out and the method was changed or abandoned.

Bhiwandiwala et al (1982) found variations from 0.6 to 1% for different laparoscopic techniques.

Technical failure shows a strong association with a history of pelvic inflammatory disease, recent use of IUD and a history of spontaneous abortion, obesity and previous abdominal and pelvic surgery.

Long-term morbidity

Long-term morbidity associated with sterilization is more difficult to quantify, due to the fact that few long-term follow-up studies exist. The most currently suggested sequelae include abdominal pain, dyspareunia, menstrual disturbance and possibly an increased incidence of gynaecological surgery. These require critical review as often no inappropriate or control groups of patients are included.

Abdominal pain and dyspareunia. These are well known sequelae but reports vary on their incidence. Stock (1978) reported that up to 31% of patients experience some lower abdominal pain following sterilization; he noted that ring application was associated with a lower incidence (24%) compared with cautery (31%). Dueholm et al (1986, 1987) reported that up to 13% of women complained of abdominal pain and 6.6% of dyspareunia following sterilization. He again confirmed reduced rates with the ring procedure (8.6% pain and 1.9% dyspareunia respectively).

Menstrual disturbance. The incidence of post-sterilization dysfunctional bleeding varies more than any other sterilization-attributed sequelae. Studies rely on subjective assessment and therefore may be inaccurate. In an objective evaluation of pre- and postmenstrual loss Kasonde & Bonnar (1976) reported no significant changes.

Contraceptive use prior to sterilization is the most important component in subsequent menstrual disturbance — thus those taking hormone contraception need to be warned that period loss may increase after sterilization, while those using an IUD may notice a decrease.

Gynaecological surgery. It has been debated whether sterilization predisposes to an increased incidence of subsequent gynaecological surgery. Letchworth & Noble (1977) noted a higher incidence of hysterectomy in post-sterilization women (up to 9%) compared with women whose husbands had had a vasectomy. Whitelaw (1979) reported an incidence of 11.8% of patients requiring a further gynaecological operation following sterilization. Vessey et al (1983) in contrast found little evidence of any excess of gynaecological disorders, especially dilatation and curettage and hysterectomy, when comparing tubal sterilization patients and vasectomy wives. Newton & Gillman (1980) also confirmed in a large follow-up study no increase in gynaecological surgery following sterilization.

Psychological morbidity

Several recent papers have tried to assess any possible psychological ill effects associated with sterilization (Clarkson & Wayne 1975; WHO 1982; Cooper et al 1982, 1985). In Philliber's review (1985) many studies reported a better mental state following sterilization. Cooper (1982) confirmed that postoperative mental status was dependent upon preoperative mental health.

Studies have shown no difference in frequency of intercourse (Philliber 1985) and no change in the sexual relationship (Cooper et al 1982).

In some studies up to 16% of women have noted a worsening of the marital relationship but Philliber & Philliber (1985) reported only a few respondents who made a causal connection between marital difficulties and sterilization.

Since psychological state, sexual desire, frequency of intercourse and other patterns of behaviour change with age, it is important to separate life cycle changes from those resulting from sterilization.

Regret following sterilization (requests for reversal)

Sterilization is essentially a permanent procedure and therefore any measure of regret after the decision is of serious consequence. Cooper et al (1982) noted that 10.9% of patients expressed some dissatisfaction at 18 months and 38% of these wished they had not had the operation. The common reasons for regret were change of partner, desire for another child, menstrual problems, loss of sense of fertility, and sexual problems.

A more appropriate interpretation of regret may be those patients who actually seek reversal. Cooper et al (1982) found 9% of those expressing regret sought reversal by 18 months after the operation.

Identification of factors associated with regret. Several studies have tried to identify factors to help predict the patient who might regret her decision and seek reversal at a later date. Taylor et al (1986) compared women requesting reversal and those undergoing sterilization and found the most discriminatory characteristics were youth at first birth, lack of spousal support and failure to choose 'completed family' as a reason for sterilization. At the time of counselling it is important to confirm that both partners agree with the decision for sterilization.

Failure rates

Pregnancy can follow sterilization as a result of failure (true method failure), surgical error (misidentification of tubes) or because of a luteal phase pregnancy (the woman was pregnant at the time of sterilization). Pregnancy rates differ according to the method, surgical approach, operator skill and type of patient.

Söderstrom (1985) reviewed repeat sterilization cases to assess the cause of failure, and highlighted interesting findings in relation to modern methods of sterilization: fimbriectomy — a remnant of the fimbriae ovarica and spontaneous reanastomosis; Pomeroy method — fistula formations; bipolar coagulation — an intact serosa coagulated muscularis and a viable though constricted endosalpinx; unipolar diathermy — fistula formation. With mechanical methods the following reasons for failure were found: Weck, Blier and Hulka Clemmens clips — tubal patency despite clip application across the tube. All these are probably due to the inherent design fault in these clips. Once the clip is applied, further pressure to cause necrosis is not possible, and with thick tubes the clip can be left in place but not completely closed. However in the design of the Filshie locking clip, a silicone rubber insert causes complete tubal blockage. With the Fallope ring failures, the knuckle of the tube had atrophied but the viable ends had not separated and fistula formation had occurred.

To minimize failure correct training of surgeons and surgical procedure on the correct structure — namely the fallopian tube — is important. If diathermy is used a minimum length of 2 cm of each tube from the cornu needs to be coagulated. Tubal division post-sterilization is to be avoided as this may predispose to fistula formation.

Sterilization in the luteal phase of the cycle when no contraception has been used should be avoided. If contraception is continued oral contraception should not be stopped until after the sterilization.

Male sterilization (vasectomy)

The exact incidence rates for vasectomy are unknown; however, like female sterilization, it has become popular over the last 10–15 years.

Vasectomy has always been an easy operation to perform, owing to the accessibility of the vas deferens beneath the scrotal skin. Many operations are under local anaesthesia as an outpatient or 'office' procedure and the approach to the vas is through a single midline scrotal incision or, more commonly, through small bilateral scrotal incisions located over each vas on the anterior surface of the scrotum (McEwan et al 1974). Various methods of occluding the vas have been tried, including cutting followed by ligation, diathermy of the cuttings or cautery of the cuttings and on occasions chemical sclerosing agents.

Failure of vasectomy

It has become common practice to ask for two sperm samples at 3 and 4 months after vasectomy and provided both of these are negative, i.e. azoospermic, then the vasectomy is considered complete. If sperm are present in small numbers then further samples are taken at 5 and 6 months and reanalysed. If sperm are still present then re-exploration under general anaesthesia is desirable.

Persistent sperm may indicate an immediate or early vasectomy failure or a low rate of ejaculation and non-clearance of the sperm down the stream of the vasectomy site. The failure rate, i.e. the recanalization rate, is low and comparable to female sterilization, being of the order of 1–4 per 1000 procedures.

Early morbidity of vasectomy

Severe complications of vasectomy are exceedingly rare. The usual postoperative complications of infection and haematuria are fortunately very low (less than 3% — McEwan et al 1974).

Later changes

Here several areas need to be mentioned:

1. *Morphology of the testis*: There appears to be little histological change in the testis or on spermatogenesis.
2. *Antibody production*: After vasectomy sperm production continues, and there is also increased phagocytosis. Antisperm antibodies can be demonstrated; 50–60% develop sperm-agglutinating antibodies while up to 30% may develop sperm-immobilizing antibodies. These can persist and may affect the success of reversal operations.
3. *Other late changes*: There is no evidence from long-term studies of an increase in any major general disease, nor is there an increase in atherosclerosis or ischaemic heart diseases.

Reversibility

Surgically it is technically easy to reverse a vasectomy if the vas has a thick muscular wall and is easily accessible. The rates of reversal appear to be similar to those seen for women; tubal and successful patency as judged by sperm in the ejaculate can be as high as in 90% of cases. However, the time after vasectomy affects the reversal. Reversal occurring after less than 10 years is associated with high sperm counts postoperatively, whereas those more than 10 years after vasectomy achieve positive sperm count in only half of the cases operated on. The overall pregnancy rate is lower, partly due to the often unproven fertility on the part of the new partner and perhaps because of some sperm antibodies.

Acceptability

Adequate counselling must take place as for female sterilization. Men who are not psychologically adjusted to vasectomy and those with psychosexual problems prior to operation are unsuitable for male sterilization. It is important therefore to take a full sexual history at counselling. The majority of studies confirm that vasectomized men and their spouses report improvements in sexual relationships and marital harmony following vasectomy.

INDUCED ABORTION (termination of pregnancy)

The abortion Act 1967

Therapeutic termination of pregnancy or induced abortion is the term used to describe medical or surgical intervention to terminate pregnancy. While abortion has been practised by many societies since early history, modern law in the UK stems from the 1803 Act and then the 1967 Abortion Bill. This modern bill permits abortion under the following clauses:

1. '. . . continuing the pregnancy would involve risk to the life of the pregnant woman greater than if the pregnancy were terminated'.
2. '. . . continuing the pregnancy would involve risk of injury to the mental and physical health of the woman greater than if the pregnancy were terminated'.
3. '. . . continuing the pregnancy would involve risk of injury to the mental and physical health of the woman and also the mental and physical health of the child (children) greater than if the pregnancy were terminated'.
4. '. . . a substantial risk of the baby being born suffering from a mental or physical abnormality or to be seriously handicapped'.

Following the introduction of this bill those working in family planning, general practice and gynaecology have with the general public reached a consensus on the interpretation of the Act and this was supported by the Lane Commission Inquiry into the Abortion Act in 1972. The majority of abortions fall into clause 2 or 3 and the interpretation here is mental stress, too many children too frequently, unwanted unplanned pregnancy, failed contraceptive methods and socioeconomic factors.

With modern genetic counselling and prenatal testing, e.g. chorionic villus sampling, amniocentesis, chromosome culture, alpha-fetoprotein screening and ultrasound scanning for fetal abnormalities, clause 4 can be interpreted with ease. Only rarely is clause 1 invoked.

Statistics

In 1963 some 23 000 abortions (RCOG 1982) were reported and this figure has risen to 198 000 in 1987. This is not due to an increasing rate of abortions per 1000 women but rather to an increase in the number of women aged 15 to 44.

Table 21.11 shows the figures reported to the Department of Health for 1989. Regional services vary according to the facilities available. The table also shows the distribution by age and gestation, indicating the need to provide facilities for second-trimester termination of pregnancy either because of late diagnosis of pregnancy or fetal abnormality diagnosis, which may not be before 18–20 weeks of pregnancy. An RCOG report (RCOG 1982) highlighted the need to provide adequate services for those who were disadvantaged and often did not know of available services and hence presented late.

Table 21.11 Termination of pregnancy in England and Wales (1989) (Resident Women)

	Number	Percentage
Total number 147 619		
Single	93 041	63
Married	38 203	26
Widowed/divorced/separated	14 827	
Unknown	1548	
Category of premises		
NHS	67 529	44
Non-NHS	80 168	52
Agency	6839	4
Gestation at termination of pregnancy		
Under 9 weeks	49 287	33
9–12 weeks	79 371	54
13–18 weeks	15 981	11
19–24 weeks	2945	2

Counselling

This is a process of discussions between the woman, sometimes her partner or family member and a professional group. This may include the general practitioner, the practice nurse, the family planning clinic staff (nurse plus doctor) and the gynaecologist. Non-directional counselling is essential so that in what is a potentially negative situation positive and constructive advice is given. In the UK it is necessary for two doctors to agree that termination is indicated and to sign the Schedule A form (the Blue form). To do this an adequate counselling session needs to be available. The objectives are:

1. To take a full medical, social, family and contraceptive history.
2. To give information on methods of termination of pregnancy, their risks and benefits.
3. To discuss alternative courses of action, e.g. adoption, fostering and continuation with the pregnancy.
4. To give factual advice and determine what the woman's real wishes are.
5. To allow her to reach a decision.

High-risk groups require special counselling. These are:

1. *Teenagers*: lack of parental support or parental interference, the inability in the very young to comprehend what is really needed and post-termination contraceptive needs.
2. *Repeat terminations*: problems with contraception, reason for repeat request, contraceptive compliance post-termination.

3. *Patients with genetic risk factors*: adequate genetic and prepregnancy screening is needed.
4. *Sexual abuse*: these women need extra counselling and support.
5. *Late terminations* (e.g. 18–20 weeks): These women need extra counselling, support and to be helped to understand the method to be used.

Methods

These are best described by the time in pregnancy when termination is carried out — first trimester, second trimester and very early termination of pregnancy.

First-trimester surgical termination of pregnancy

This is the most common method and accounts for more than 70% of all cases. While local anaesthesia can be used in certain patients, it is not commonly used in the UK. A short general anaesthetic is all that is required and patients often only have to stay in hospital a few hours (day-care). In many hospitals due to administrative arrangements or due to the gestation (i.e. at 12 weeks) or a 'high-risk' factor (see above) the patients will stay in hospital overnight.

The procedure consists of dilation of the cervix followed by evacuation of the products of contraception. Dilation of the cervix is most commonly carried out using mechanical dilatation stretching the cervical muscle to an appropriate point to allow easy evacuation, e.g. 8 mm = 8 weeks; 10 mm = 10 weeks. However medical priming to dilate the cervix with prostaglandin, e.g. prostaglandin E_2, is also used, as is a water-absorbing sponge or plastic placed in the cervical canal, this sponge then swells over a period of a few hours, e.g. Lamicel.

Following dilatation the contents of the uterus are then evacuated, usually using a suction curette, e.g. Karman curette, which decreases blood loss and is more efficient than simple surgical forceps evacuation. It is wise to check that the uterine cavity is empty using a curette and to examine the products of gestation to check that they are complete in terms of volume and weight.

Second-trimester termination of pregnancy

Dilatation and surgical evacuation of a pregnancy up to 17 weeks are practised in certain specialized centres, e.g. Holland (Van Lith et al 1984). However, in the UK it is more usual to use a medical method — commonly prostaglandin instillation into the space between the membranes and myometrium via the cervix: the extraovular method. A Foley catheter is inserted transcervically and then a solution of a prostaglandin E or $F_{2\alpha}$ analogue, e.g. 15 methyl prostaglandin F_2 (Bygdeman 1984). The action is prolonged and the induction–abortion interval is usually of the order of 14 h. Intravenous Syntocinon is often used to potentiate the action of the prostaglandin and reduce the induction–abortion interval.

Alternative delivery routes for prostaglandins are the use of vaginal tablets and intramuscular injections.

Hysterotomy

The removal of the uterine contents via laparotomy and a vertical or transverse uterine incision was common in the late 1960s (Newton 1984) but is now rarely used due to the lower morbidity seen with the other methods described above.

Complications of first- and second-trimester TOP

Generally speaking, termination of pregnancy is a safe and relatively easy operation to complete. Complications arise with the increase in gestation but mortality is rare (Table 21.12).

Table 21.12 Complications of termination of pregnancy

	Number	Percentage
Vacuum aspiration only		
Procedures	113 568	
Total complications	542	0.48
Sepsis	60	0.05
Haemorrhage	219	0.19
Perforation	151	0.13
Other	143	0.12
Prostaglandins only		
Procedures	3584	
Total complications	70*	1.9
Sepsis	6	0.16
Haemorrhage	40	1.1
Perforation	1	0.03
Other	25	0.7

* This does not include routine curettage for retained products.

Early complications

These include retained products of conception — 0.1–2.9%, depending on the series reviewed. After a second-trimester termination it is often routine to carry out a curettage to prevent retained products.

Haemorrhage. Blood loss increases with gestation at termination — 50 ml at 8 weeks, 100 ml at 12 weeks. Loss in excess of 500 ml is considered significant and may be due to uterine atony, retained products, trauma to the cervix or uterus or uterine perforation. Re-evacuation, egbolic drugs, intravenous fluid balance and if necessary transfusion is all that is usually required. Hysterectomy is only needed rarely.

Uterine perforation. This is a rare occurrence and often requires no further treatment as the small perforation caused by the sound or dilator closes as the uterus retracts when the termination is complete. Rarely, however, a large perforation is mistaken by the operator and bowel can then be brought down into the uterus, requiring abdominal surgery to repair the damage. If the surgeon is in doubt, then a laparoscopy should be performed to ascertain the site of perforation and its severity.

Cervical trauma. This rarely occurs and is due to splitting of the cervix with dilatation, trauma with cervical traction or tears due to a false passage being made with the dilators. Observation and suture when necessary are all that is required.

Sepsis. This is also rare and is most usually caused by retained products; antibiotics and re-evacuation are then required.

Table 21.13 Very early termination of pregnancy with prostaglandin analogues

Prostaglandin analogue	Gestation	Route	Success — complete abortion
16 Phenoxy prostaglandin E_2 methyl sulphonylamide	< 7 weeks	Vaginal suppository Intramuscular injection	95% 94%
16.16 Dimethyl prostaglandin E_2	< 4 weeks	Vaginal suppository	100%
16.16 Methylester	< 7 weeks	Vaginal suppository	92%
9 Methylene prostaglandin E_2	< 7 weeks	Vaginal suppository	92%

Later complications of termination of pregnancy

Psychiatric sequelae. Most women at some time following a termination will develop feelings of guilt and minor depression. Serious psychiatric disturbance is rare however, and these sequelae can be minimized by adequate pre-termination counselling, postoperative support and follow-up.

Infertility. Studies indicate that abortion is rarely associated with subsequent infertility (Franks & Kay 1981). If a woman presents with infertility following a termination of pregnancy, tubal status and confirmation of male fertility need to be assessed early in the investigation cycle.

Rhesus isoimmunization. This can be prevented by routinely giving anti-D to rhesus-negative patients.

Cervical incompetence. Cervical incompetence requiring treatment in subsequent pregnancy has been reported by the RCOG/RCGP study (Franks & Kay 1981). Cervical softening agents listed above, e.g. prostaglandins, rather than forceful mechanical dilatation will reduce the incidence of this complication.

Very early termination of pregnancy

Prior to the eighth week of pregnancy both surgical and medical methods have been used to terminate pregnancy (see Table 21.13).

Menstrual extraction (surgical). This consists of a small plastic catheter 2–3 mm wide attached to a vacuum source-syringe or pump. A suction curettage is then carried out with either no anaesthesia or a cervical local anaesthetic block. The problems with this method are a continuing pregnancy in 2.6% and retained products in a further 2.6% (Table 21.14).

Prostaglandins. Since the report by Karim et al in 1977, prostaglandin research has continued to find a safe and effective method for early pregnancy termination without side-effects (Table 21.13). Unfortunately all prostaglandins given in the doses needed to effect complete abortion produce gastrointestinal side-effects; vomiting and diarrhoea in fewer than 30% and uterine pain in up to 30% of cases (Table 21.14). Table 21.14 shows a selection of analogues that have been used and their success rates; efficacy is however less than 90% and the future lies with these analogues when used in combination with antiprogestins.

Antiprogestogens (medical). these are compounds which block the receptor sites for progesterone or block its synthesis. They are effective in achieving complete abortion in up to 61% of cases when used alone. Several compounds are available e.g. Epostane, Mifepristone (RU486). Various dose levels have been investigated however, an acceptable complete abortion rate has not been

Table 21.14 Comparison of side-effects and complete abortion with different methods for early termination of pregnancy

	Complete abortion (%)	Gastrointestinal side-effects (%)	Uterine pain (%)	Excessive bleeding (%)
Surgical evacuation	95–100			<0.5
Mifepristone	61	0	0	5.6
16 Phenoxy prostaglandin E_2	94	55	56	0
Day 1 Mifepristone plus prostaglandin day 3 (see text)	96	0	13	0

After Swahn & Bygdman (1987).

Table 21.15 Antiprogestins for early termination of pregnancy

	Mifepristone		Epostane
Drug dose	25 mg × 2	50 mg × 2	200 mg × 4
Number of patients	26	26	26
Complete abortions	16 (61%)	16 (61%)	19 (73%)
Incomplete abortions	2	2	0
Vaginal bleeding	8	8	4
No response	0	0	3

After Odlind & Birgenson (1987).

achieved with these compounds alone (see Table 21.13).

Combinations of prostaglandin plus antiprogestogens. This combination therapy has achieved complete abortion rates similar to surgical evacuation (Table 21.15). Data now exist on 1 year's experience of the method in clinical trials from France (Silvestre et al 1990). The regime is 600 mg of Mifepristone taken orally on Day 1 followed on day 3 by prostaglandins either as an injection 0.5 ml intramuscularly or a 1 mg pessary. The patient then stays in hospital and abortion usually occurs within a few hours.

A very small number of women have a serious blood loss requiring treatment. These cases cannot be identified prior to the haemorrhage.

With this combination therapy there was a 95.7% success rate in 2115 cases. Incomplete miscarriage occurred in 2.1% of cases and 1.0% continued, requiring surgical evacuation. With this method pregnancy loss needs to be monitored by decreasing human chorionic gonadotrophin titres and/or ultrasound scans.

CONCLUSIONS

This chapter has reviewed the reversible methods of contraception, sterilization and abortion that are currently available. The risks and benefits are presented together with information on counselling, choice of method and the ranking of methods by failure rate (Table 21.16).

In any choice of method the patient's wishes, medical history and her attitude to various methods will determine the choice. It is unfortunate that still much of the information that patients obtain about contraceptive methods is second-hand, with the client often seeking advice from a friend or article in the popular press. While lay press articles have improved tremendously over the last few years, education of both the general public and professionals of all groups is still needed to provide up-to-date information and eradicate old-fashioned ideas.

It is essential to increase family planning services and family planning use worldwide if we are to contain the population explosion. The uptake of family planning over the last 15 years suggests that this is possible. The World Health Organization has a goal for the year 2000: 'health for all'; this includes adequate family planning services and methods for all.

KEY POINTS

1. Insertion of an IUD at time of termination of pregnancy does not increase infection rates.
2. Pregnancy with an IUD in situ increases the risk of miscarriage by a factor of 5.
3. 3–4% of pregnancies with an IUD in place are ectopic.
4. Copper-releasing IUDs reduce ectopic pregnancy rates.
5. IUDs should not be used in women who have had a previous ectopic pregnancy.
6. The oral contraceptive pill reduces incidence of menorrhagia, functional ovarian cysts, fibroids, PID and ectopic pregnancy.

Table 21.16 Range of failure rates with common methods of contraception

Group	Failure rate	Range of failure (%)	Method of contraception
I	15	0.1–1.0	Male sterilization (vasectomy) Female sterilization (Filshie clips) Progestogen-only implants Injectable contraception — progestogen-only or monthly combined; Third-Generation copper IUDs e.g. Multiload 375, T 380S
II	Up to 2%	0.5–2.0	Combined oral contraception; second-generation medicated IUDs, e.g. Nova T, Multiload 250
III	Up to 6%	0.5–5.4 0.5–6.0 2.0–6.0	Progestogen-only contraception Some combined oral contraception (see text) Non-medicated IUDs, e.g. Lippes loop
IV	Above 6%	3.0–15.0 4.0–25.0 10.0–25.0 10.0–30.0	Condoms Diaphragms Spermicides alone Periodic abstinence

Sources: Contemporary published papers (see References list); WHO Reports 1985–1988; United Nations 1989

7. The oral contraceptive pill does not affect subsequent fertility.
8. The oral contraceptive pill reduces the incidence of ovarian and endometrial carcinoma by 50%.
9. An association between the oral contraceptive pill use and cervical and breast carcinoma is as yet unproven.
10. Women with no risk factors can take the oral contraceptive pill until their menopause.
11. PC4 can be given for 48 hours and an IUD inserted up to 5 days after intercourse is post-coital contraception.
12. Failure rates of laparoscopic sterilization are approximately 1:1000.

REFERENCES

Back D J et al 1982 The effects of ampicillin on OCs in women. British Journal of Clinical Pharmacology 14; 43

Bhiwandiwala P P et al 1982 A comparison of different laparoscopic sterilization occlusion techniques in 24,439 procedures. American Journal of Obstetrics and Gynecology 144: 319–331

Bygdeman M 1984 The use of prostaglandins and their analogues for abortion. Clinics in Obstetrics and Gynaecology 11: 573–584

Chamberlain G, Brown J C (eds) 1978 Gynaecological laparoscopy — the report of the working party of the confidential inquiry into gynaecological laparoscopy. Royal College of Obstetricians and Gynaecologists, London

Clarkson S E, Wayne R G 1985 Psychological aspects of female sterilization. New Zealand Medical Journal 98: 748–750

Cooper P et al 1982 Psychological sequelae to elective sterilization. British Medical Journal 284: 461–464

Cooper P et al 1985 Effects of female sterilization; a 1 year follow up. Journal of Psychosomatic Research 29: 13–22

Dueholm S et al 1986 Late sequelae following laparoscopy sterilization employing electrocautery and tubal ring techniques. Annales Chirurgiae et Gynaecologiae 75: 285–289

Dueholm S et al 1987 Late sequelae after laparoscopic sterilization in pregnant and non-pregnant women. Acta Obstetricia et Gynaecologica Scandinavica 66: 227–231

Foreman H et al 1981 Intrauterine device usage and fetal loss. Obstetrics and Gynaecology 58: 669–677

Fotherby K 1982 Progestogen only contraceptives. British Journal of Family Planning 8: 7–10

Franks S, Kay C R 1981 Characteristics of women recruited into a long term study of the sequelae of induced abortion. Journal of the Royal College of General Practitioners 31: 473–477

Grimes J 1979 Reversible contraception for the 1980s. Journal of the American Medical Association 255: 69–75

Jackson R, Newton J R 1989 The in vivo release characteristics of a multicompartment vaginal ring releasing 3 keto desogestrel. Contraception 40: 615–621

Karim S M M, Ratnam S S 1977 Termination of pregnancy with vaginal administration of 16,16-dimethylprostaglandin E_2. British Journal of Obstetrics and Gynaecology 84: 135–137

Kay C R 1984 The RCGP oral contraception Study. Clinics in Obstetrics and Gynaecology 11(3): 759–786

Kasonde J M, Bonnar J 1976 Effect of sterilization on menstrual blood loss. British Journal of Obstetrics and Gynaecology 83: 572–575

Lane Commission Inquiry into the Working of the Abortion Act 1972 Chairman: The hon. Mrs Justice Lane DBE. HMSO, London

Letchworth A T, Noble A D 1977 Late effects of female sterilization. Lancet ii: 768

Loudon N B (ed) 1985 Handbook of Family Planning. Churchill Livingstone, Edinburgh

McEwan J et al 1974 Hospital family planning: a vasectomy service. Contraception 9: 177–192

Mumford S D, Bhiwandiwala P P 1981 Tubal ring sterilization experiences with 10,086 cases. Obstetrics and Gynaecology 57: 150–157

Newton J R 1984 Sterilization. Clinics in Obstetrics and Gynaecology 11(3): 603–640

Newton J R, Gillman S 1980 Retrospective survey of female sterilization. Contraception 22: 295–312

Odlind V, Birgenson L 1987 Interruption of early pregnancy with antiprogestins. In: Diczjalusz E, Bygdman M (eds) Fertility regulation today and tomorrow, Serono Symposia vol 36. New York Press, pp 95–104

Philliber S G, Philliber W W I 1985 Social and psychological perspectives on volutary sterilization. Studies in Family Planning 16: 1–29

Phillips J M et al 1977 The AAGL survey of sterilization. Journal of Reproductive Medicine 18: 219

Phillips J M et al 1981 The AAGL survey of 1979. Journal of Reproductive Medicine 26: 529

Population Reports 1988 Studies on intrauterine devices. Johns Hopkins University Press, Baltimore

Rinehart W, Piotrow P T 1979 OCs — update on usage safety and side effects. Population Reports Series A, no. 5, A133–A186

RCOG 1982 Late Abortion Survey. Complications of abortion. Alberman E, Dennis J K (eds) RCOG, London

Silvestre L et al 1990 Use of mifepristone. New England Journal of Medicine 322: 645–648

Söderstrom R M 1985 Sterilization failures and their cause. American Journal of Obstetrics and Gynecology 152: 395–403

Steptoe P C 1967 Laparoscopy in gynaecology. E S Livingstone, Edinburgh

Stock R J 1978 Evaluation of sequelae of tubal ligation. Fertility and Sterility 29: 169–175

Swahn M, Bygdeman M 1987 Interruption of early pregnancy with prostaglandins and antiprogestins. In: Diczjlausz E, Bygdeman M (eds) Fertility regulation today and tomorrow, Serono Symposia vol 36. New York Press, pp 109–118

Taylor P J et al 1986 Female sterilization: can the women who seek reversal be identified prospectively? Clinical Reproduction and Fertility 4: 207–215

United Nations 1989 Levels and trends of contraceptive use; as assessed in 1988. United Nations, New York

Van Lith D A F, Wittman R, Keith L G 1984 Early and late abortion methods. Clinics in Obstetrics and Gynaecology 11: 585–602

Vessey M P 1984 The Oxford Family Planning Association Contraceptive Study. Clinics in Obstetrics and Gynaecology 11(3): 743–758

Vessey M P 1989 Oral contraceptives and cancer. In: Filshie M, Guillebaud J (eds) Contraception Science and Practice. Butterworth, London

Vessey M P et al 1983 Tubal sterilization findings in a large survey. British Journal of Obstetrics and Gynaecology 90: 203–209

Whitelaw R G 1979 Ten year survey of 485 sterilizations. Part I Sterilization. British Medical Journal i: 32

WHO 1982a Task Force on Oral Contraception A randomised double blind study of six combined oral contraceptives. Contraception 25: 231–242

WHO 1982b Task Force on Oral Contraceptives A randomised double blind study of two combined and two progestogen only contraceptives. Contraception 25: 243–251

WHO 1982c Task Force on Female Sterilization Minilaparotomy or laparoscopy for sterilization. American Journal of Obstetrics and Gynecology 143: 645–652

WHO 1983a Task Force on Intrauterine Devices IUD insertion following termination of pregnancy. Studies in Family Planning 14: 99–108

WHO 1983b Task Force on Intrauterine Devices IUD insertion following spontaneous abortion. Studies in Family Planning 14: 109–114

WHO 1985 A multinational case control study of ectopic pregnancy. Clinical Reproductive Fertility 3: 131–143

WHO 1987 Mechanism of action, safety and efficacy of IUCDs. Technical Report Series. WHO, Geneva.

22. Hirsutism and virilization

N. M. Duignan

Hirsutism may be defined as 'excessive growth of hair in an abnormal position on the body'. Different investigators have suggested varying criteria for grading the degree of hirsutism, but it remains difficult to quantitate the word 'excessive'; it seems reasonable to use the term hirsutism to describe hair growth that worries the patient. Hirsutism is commonly seen without any evidence of virilism; on the other hand virilism is rarely, if ever, seen without evidence of hirsutism (apart from the neonate). Virilism can be defined as one or more of the following: deepening of the vocal pitch; male-type hairline and scalp thinning; clitoral hypertrophy; breast atrophy; increased musculature. Patients who present with virilization will usually, but not always, also have amenorrhoea; normal menstruation, on the other hand, is frequently present among subjects who present with hirsutism.

PATHOPHYSIOLOGY

Hirsutism may arise as a result of excessive androgen production from the adrenal glands or the ovaries or from an excessive end organ response; virilization, on the other hand, is invariably due to excessive androgen production. It has long been known that androgens are produced in the female by the ovary and the adrenal cortex, and that they are metabolized in the liver. It is now clear that extra-hepatic sites, such as skin, fat and blood, can convert biologically weak precursors secreted by the ovaries or the adrenal glands into more active compounds which cause biochemical changes at cellular level.

Physiology of adrenal androgens

Androgens are secreted from the inner zones of the adrenal cortex, i.e. zona fasciculata and zona reticularis. Although emphasis has hitherto been placed on testosterone as the principal androgenic agent, other steroidal hormones also have a significant effect, either of themselves, or because they are converted into biologically active agents; those which have most been studied in clinical contexts are listed in Table 22.1. Dihydrotestosterone, as the metabolite through which testosterone exerts its biochemical effect at

Table 22.1 Clinically significant androgens

Substance	Biological activity
Dihydrotestosterone	+++
Testosterone	++
Androstanediol	+
Androstenediol	+
Androstenedione	+
Dehydroepiandrosterone	? ±

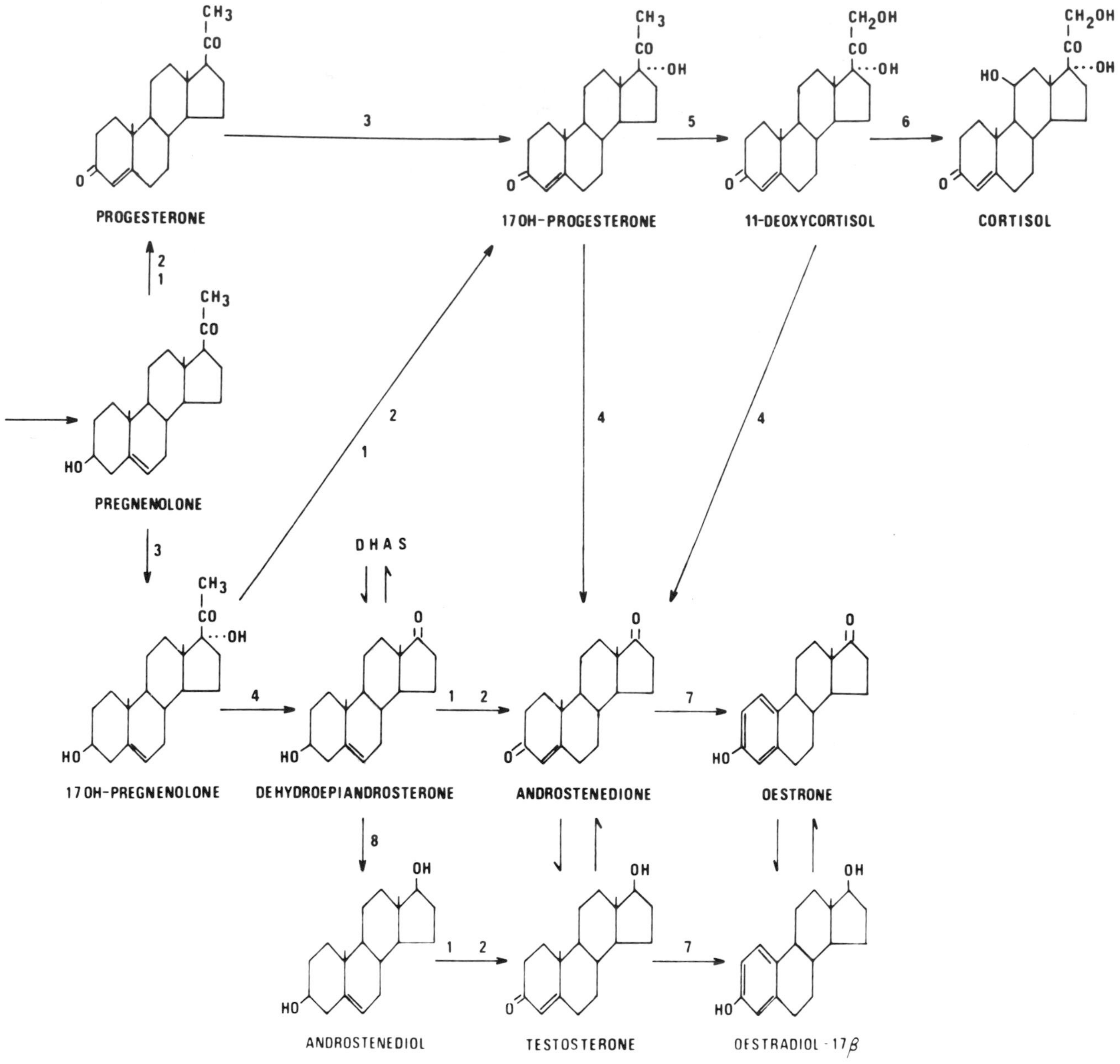

Fig. 22.1 Main pathways of steroid biosynthesis in the adrenal gland. Enzymes: **1** Δ^5-3β-hydroxydehydrogenase; **2** Δ^5-isomerase; **3** 17-hydroxylase; **4** desmolase; **5** 21-hydroxylase; **6** 11β-hydroxylase; **7** 19-hydroxylase and aromatase; **8** 17-hydrogenase.

cellular level, and androstenedione, as a precursor of both androgens and oestrogens, are particularly important.

Approximately 25% of circulating testosterone in women is secreted from the adrenal gland, another 25% from the ovary, while the remaining 50% has an extraglandular origin as the testosterone precursors dehydroepiandrosterone (DHA) and androstenedione, mainly of adrenal origin, are converted to testosterone in blood. While dehydroepiandrosterone sulphate (DHAS) is derived almost entirely from the adrenal glands (Fig. 22.1), androstenedione is also secreted in significant quantities by the ovaries.

The adrenal glands secrete significant quantities of androgen during fetal life, particularly DHAS. Androgen concentrations are very low in the first 5 years of extrauterine life but about the middle of the first decade they begin to rise. This is termed the 'adrenarche' and is clinically manifest by the appearance of pubic and axillary hair. In normal girls androgen levels continue to rise throughout the second decade and are maintained at relatively steady levels until the menopause. Adrenal androgens probably also contribute significantly to the emergence of libido in women and while the secretion of androgens by the adrenal glands decreases after the menopause, this decline is much slower than the secretion of oestrogens by the ovary. In-

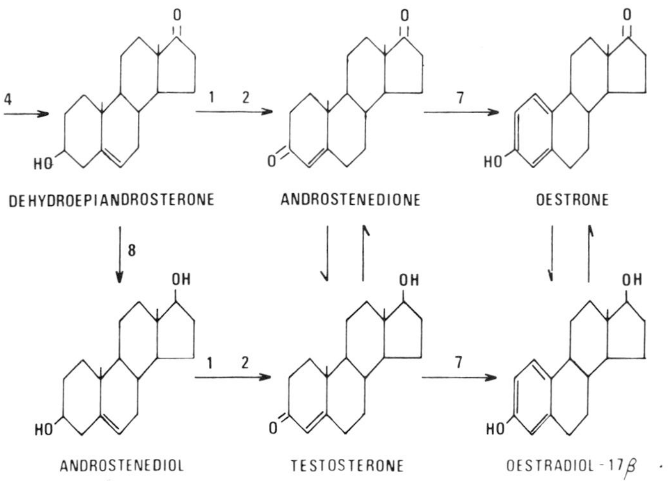

DEHYDROEPIANDROSTERONE ANDROSTENEDIONE OESTRONE

ANDROSTENEDIOL TESTOSTERONE OESTRADIOL-17β

Fig. 22.2 Pathway androgen and oestrogen production in the ovary. Note that DHAS is not secreted by the ovary.

deed, in postmenopausal years the circulating adrenal androgens are a more important source of oestrogens than are the ovaries (McKenna et al 1985).

Ovarian androgen secretion

It has been known for some time that the ovaries were capable of secreting androgens and recent data have been derived from the measurement of androgens in ovarian vein plasma (Kirschner & Jacobs, 1971). Androstenedione is quantitatively the main androgen secreted by the ovary; testosterone and DHA are secreted in smaller amounts. It should be noted that androstenedione, which is a major precursor of testosterone, also has a central place in the synthesis of oestrone and oestradiol (Fig. 22.2).

Peripheral interconversion of androgens

While the adrenal glands and the ovaries are the primary source of androgen secretion in women the peripheral plasma levels and blood production rates result from more than just secretion. Peripheral interconversion of androgens, occurring mainly in the blood, liver and skin, accounts for more than 50% of testosterone production. Of particular interest is the fact that this peripheral interconversion of androgens includes not only the conversion of weak androgens into biologically more active substances, but also the breakdown of inactive androgens into active ones (Fig. 22.3).

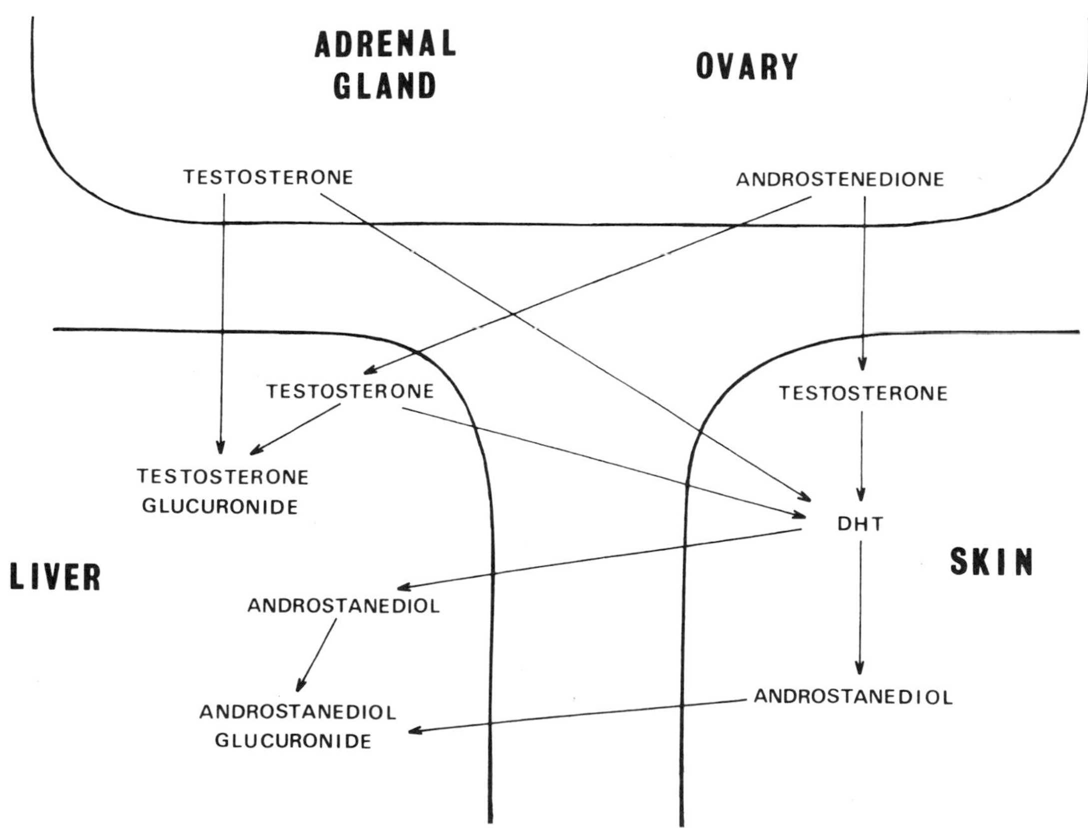

Fig. 22.3 Peripheral conversion, in liver and skin, of testosterone and androstenedione secreted by the adrenal gland and the ovary. Note that the biologically weak androgen androstenedione is converted to dihydrotestosterone (DHT) in skin.

Measurement of androgens

Until relatively recently adrenal androgen secretion has been assessed by the measurement of urinary 17-ketosteroid excretion which comprises mainly DHA, DHAS, androstenedione and breakdown products of testosterone but not testosterone itself. However, the development of sensitive, specific radioimmunoassays now makes measurement of low concentrations of these steroids in blood samples feasible.

Testosterone is a potent androgen which circulates mainly bound to sex hormone-binding globulin (SHBG) but it is only the unbound fraction, approximately 2%, which is biologically active. Oestrogens raise SHBG levels while androgens tend to lower them. Normal testosterone levels may frequently be associated with a suppressed SHBG value, thus giving an elevated free testosterone level. Methods of measuring free testosterone are tedious and cumbersome while SHBG estimation is much easier. Expression of testosterone as a function of SHBG provides an index of free testosterone levels. There is, however, still a place for the measurement of urinary 17-ketosteroids, particularly in pathological situations where abnormal patterns of metabolism may result in the production of an androgen which will not be recognized by the usual battery of radioimmunoassay tests.

CLASSIFICATION

The individual syndromes producing hirsutism or virilization will be outlined and their pathogenesis discussed initially. The investigation and treatment of each syndrome will be subsequently discussed.

The main syndromes giving rise to hirsutism or virilization are as follows:

1. Idiopathic hirsutism.
2. Polycystic ovary syndrome (PCO).
3. Cushing's syndrome.
4. Androgen-secreting adrenal tumours.
5. Masculinizing tumours of the ovary.
6. Adrenal hyperplasia.
7. Acromegaly.
8. Congenital causes.
9. Iatrogenic virilization.
10. Postmenopausal hirsutism.

Idiopathic hirsutism

Idiopathic hirsutism, describes a group of women who present with hirsutism and regular menstruation and who lack any evidence of organic disease. These patients exhibit elevated levels of testosterone and androstenedione while the SHBG level is suppressed and free testosterone levels are elevated. The steroid pattern found in patients with idiopathic hirsutism cannot be accounted for by a simple enzyme deficiency and it appears that the entire androgen biosynthetic pathway has been stimulated, although not in a highly efficient manner, since there is a considerable leakage of precursor into the circulation (McKenna et al 1985).

The source of the excess hormone production in patients with idiopathic hirsitism remains controversial. Northrop et al (1975) suggested that the excess androgen production results equally from the adrenal gland and the ovaries; Oake et al (1974) concluded that the disorder is exclusively explained by adrenal androgen excess while more recently Kirschner et al (1976) suggested that the ovary was primarily responsible. More recently Moore et al (1983) used metyrapone, an inhibitor of 11 β-hydroxylase, to induce hypocortisolism in order to stimulate pituitary secretion of adrenocorticotrophic hormone (ACTH) related peptides. As metyrapone did not perturb adrenal androgen production this assessment provided a method of examining adrenal androgen secretion in response to exogenous stimulation. These workers found that the testosterone response to metyrapone in patients with idiopathic hirsutism was greater than that seen in normal women, indicating an abnormality of adrenal androgens in patients with this syndrome.

In idiopathic hirsutism, oestradiol and oestrone levels are normal. Similarly, the basal levels of luteinizing hormone (LH) and follicle-stimulating hormone (FSH), together with the release of both LH and FSH following the injection of synthetic luteinizing hormone-releasing hormone (LHRH), were no different to normal subjects examined in the follicular phase of the menstrual cycle. These findings are considerably different to those found in patients with PCOS.

PCOS

The true incidence of PCOS is unknown. In a consecutive study of 740 post-mortem examinations of females, including children and postmenopausal women, bilateral polycystic ovaries were found in 26 cases (Sommers & Wadman 1956). The frequency reported among infertile women ranges from 0.6 to 4.3%.

Typically, polycystic ovaries (Fig. 22.4) are enlarged with thickened, curly white, sclerotic capsules and subcapsular follicular cysts of varying size; however, they may occasionally be normal in size. Bisection (Fig. 22.5) reveals numerous cysts in the cortex, and shows the substance of the ovary to be full. Histologically, there is thickening of the tunica albuginea as a result of an increase in the number of collagen fibres, which may penetrate the ovarian stroma. The subcapsular cysts represent poorly developed graafian follicles at varying stages of maturation and regression. Many of these are atretic with the number of cor-

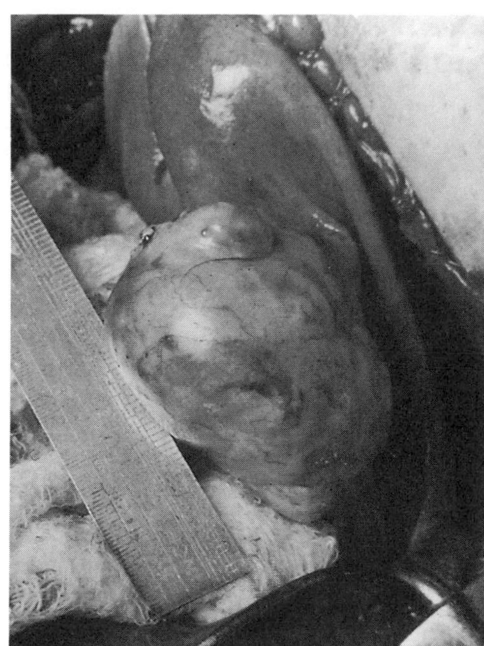

Fig. 22.4 Typical polycystic ovary seen at laparotomy.

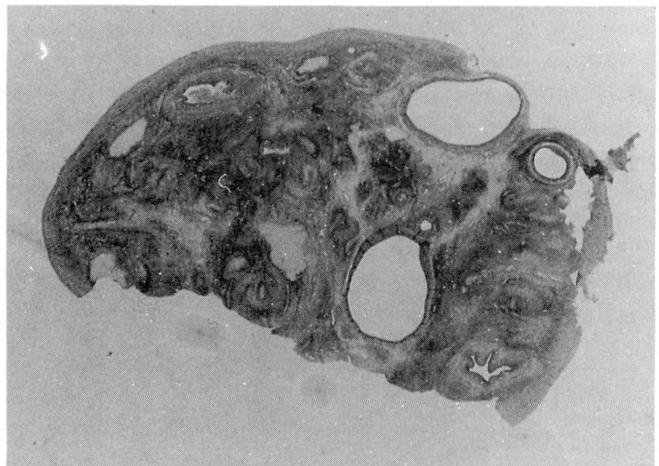

Fig. 22.5 Bisection of polycystic ovary to reveal subcapsular cysts.

pora albicantes and corpora lutea either diminished or totally absent. Marked hypertrophy of the theca interna cells in the walls of the atretic follicles is frequent and islands of luteinized theca cells — sites of androgen production — may be located in different areas of the ovarian stroma. The theca cell hypertrophy, together with the multiple cystic follicles, is characteristic of the microscopic appearance of polycystic ovaries.

The pathogenesis of PCOS remains a matter of controversy. For one thing, histological changes similar to those found in polycystic ovaries have been produced in the gonads of animals treated with androgens; for another, polycystic ovaries have been found in some cases of adrenogenital syndrome, in Cushing's disease, in women with virilizing adrenal or ovarian tumours, in some cases of hyperprolactinaemia and in some insulin-resistance states. The majority of patients with PCOS have been found to exhibit increased androgen secretion and also abnormal gonadotrophin release. On the one hand it has been suggested that these abnormalities were primarily due to abnormal steroidogenesis producing secondary changes in gonadotrophin secretion, while on the other hand it has been suggested that a primary hypothalamic disorder was producing abnormal gonadotrophin release which, in turn, caused both cystic changes in the ovaries and abnormal steroidogenesis.

Oestrone

There is much evidence to support the theory that abnormal circulating oestrogens (increased levels of oestrone and normal levels of oestradiol) bring about the gonadotrophin secretion which is characteristic of PCOS (Table 22.2). Oestrone has been shown to be biologically active in a number of in vivo systems. Obese patients with increased aromatase activity and elevated oestrone levels frequently exhibit an abnormality of gonadotrophin release (Table 22.2). The administration of clomiphene citrate, an anti-oestrogen, frequently leads to follicular development and ovulation, by allowing the release of depressed secretion of FSH from the apparently restraining influence of oestrogens. Since oestradiol levels are normal and oestrone levels are elevated in patients with PCOS, and since the abnormality in gonadotrophin secretion is beneficially altered by the use of the anti-oestrogen, it is likely that the abnormal gonadotrophin secretion is a consequence of hyperoestronaemia.

It has been suggested that patients with idiopathic hirsutism (i.e. women with androgen levels and hirsutism who continue to ovulate regularly) are protected from menstrual disturbances because their oestrone levels remain normal (McKenna et al 1985). In normal women, the ovary

Table 22.2 Frequency of symptoms in 1079 published cases

Symptom	Frequency (%) Mean	Range
Obesity	41	16–49
Hirsutism	69	17–83
Virilization	21	0–28
Amenorrhoea	51	15–77
Infertility	74	35–94
Functional bleeding	29	6–65
Dysmenorrhoea	23	
Biphasic basal temperature	15	12–40
Corpus luteum at operation	22	0–71

From Goldzieher (1973).

produced approximately 80% of circulating oestradiol but only 40% of the circulating oestrone; the remaining 60% of oestrone arises from peripheral conversion of androstenedione, mainly of adrenal origin. Elevated oestrone levels could therefore arise by excessive excretion of oestrone by the ovary, by excessive androstenedione excretion from the adrenal gland, by excessive conversion of normal amounts of androstenedione to oestrone in the presence of increased aromatase activity, or lastly, because of impaired clearance of oestrone. An indirect index of aromatase activity (which converts androstenedione to oestrone) may be provided by expressing oestrone as a function of androstenedione.

Adrenal androgen excess

Several observers have noted that DHAS — a characteristic adrenal androgen — is elevated in PCOS. In patients with PCOS, plasma testosterone, androstenedione and oestrone levels are elevated with a normal oestrone: androstenedione ratio (Table 22.2). This suggests that the elevated oestrone levels occur mainly as a consequence of a normal rate of conversion of the excessive amount of androstenedione available, to yield elevated oestrone levels. Loughlin et al (1985) showed that the incremental testosterone and androstenedione responses following the administration of a single dose of metyrapone at midnight were significantly higher in women with PCOS than in normal women. Similarly Givens et al (1975) reported excessive adrenal androgen responsiveness to exogenous ACTH in PCOS. These observations indicate that an adrenal abnormality does exist in PCOS and McKenna et al (1985) have suggested that the adrenal abnormality was the primary event in the pathogenesis of PCOS.

Obesity

Obesity has long been associated with PCOS. Weight loss has been shown to bring about a reduction in oestrone levels, the return of normal gonadotrophin secretions, and the resumption of regular menstruation. Thus it appears likely that the abnomalities in gonadotrophin secretion and in the ovaries are partly due to the obesity. It would seem that body weight may play the major role in determining whether a patient with mild to moderate adrenal androgen excess demonstrates idiopathic hirsutism or PCOS. Patients with normal adrenal androgen secretion but with marked obesity may also develop PCOS by excessive conversion of normal concentrations of adrenal androgen to elevated oestrone values. As a consequence, LH secretion is stimulated while that of FSH is suppressed; this in turn brings about an excessive stimulation of ovarian androgen production whose conversion to oestrogen is hindered by the failure of proper follicular development. Thus, while hyperandrogenaemia in patients with idiopathic hirsutism may originate entirely in the adrenal glands, in patients with PCOS the eventual hyperandrogenaemia will have two significant sources, the adrenal and the ovary. In contrast, when PCOS develops as a result of obesity the hyperandrogenaemia is solely of ovarian origin.

Abnormal gonadotrophin secretion

Gonadotrophin secretion in the majority of PCOS patients (Yen 1980) is abnormal. Classically the basal levels of LH are elevated while those of FSH are normal or suppressed while the release of LH following injection of LHRH is exaggerated (Duignan et al 1975); furthermore, the ratio of LH:FSH is increased. It is likely that the abnormality in gonadotrophin secretion occurs secondary to the elevated oestrone levels which interfere with the normal feedback mechanism. The fact that the administration of clomiphene citrate, an anti-oestrogen, corrects the gonadotrophin release and allows regular menstruation to occur supports this contention.

Hyperprolactinaemia

About 15% of PCOS subjects have been found also to suffer from hyperprolactinaemia. This coexistence could be merely fortuitous or it may be that the hyperprolactinaemia — either through a direct effect on gonadotrophin-secreting cells or indirectly through a decreased dopamine tone — may also be associated with an increase in the ratio of circulating LH/FSH and the development of PCOS. Alternatively, the association between hyperprolactinaemia and PCOS may be related to the elevated oestrone levels which might increase prolactin secretion.

Conclusion

Classical PCOS may be either primary or secondary. In the primary disorders there is no identifying contributory abnormality such as adrenal hyperplasia, androgen-secreting tumours, or obesity; in secondary PCOS such a predisposing condition coexists. In primary PCOS the abnormal stimulation of the ovary is usually caused by a relative increase in the stimulation by LH and the suppression of FSH. This abnormal gonadotrophin secretion may in turn be caused, either directly or indirectly, by excessive circulating oestrone, prolactin, or both. The excess oestrone may be derived either from excessive availability of androgens (which are converted to oestrone by aromatase in adipose tissue) or from normal levels of androgen in obese patients. The elevated levels of androgen may be derived from either the adrenal glands of the ovaries but it seems likely that the initial elevation in androgen levels is of adrenal origin.

Cushing's syndrome

Cushing's disease (pituitary ACTH excess)

Cushing, who first described this syndrome in 1932, attributed it to pituitary dysfunction but in 1943 Allbright pointed out that overactivity of the adrenal cortex, whether from hyperplasia or tumour, was an invariable feature of this syndrome. In this disorder, hyperstimulation of the adrenal by ACTH gives rise to an excess of both cortisol and androgen.

The disease is more common in women and the androgen excess is probably responsible for some of the typical features such as hirsutism, acne, thinning of scalp hair and, occasionally, clitoral hypertrophy. The essential feature of Cushing's syndrome is the overproduction of cortisol and the diagnosis is dependent on confirming this cortisol excess.

Adrenal tumours

Patients with pure cortisol-secreting adrenal adenomas do not demonstrate evidence of virilization, though they may have increased hair growth of a downy type. The hair distribution is generalized rather than in the typical male pattern, and patients in whom cortisol and androgen excess occur as a consequence of a benign adrenal tumour have features very similar to those described for Cushing's disease. Marked virilization may occur, however, in patients with Cushing's syndrome due to an adrenal carcinoma. These patients exhibit a marked elevation of plasma levels of testosterone and/or androstenedione and/or DHA.

Androgen-secreting adrenal tumours

Androgen-secreting adrenal tumours may occur at any age. In women, they will usually present with the clinical evidence of virilization and menstrual disturbance. Levels of circulating androgens, e.g. testosterone, androstenedione, DHA and DHAS, are increased, and/or urinary ketosteroid excretion rates are elevated. It was formerly believed that normal urinary 17-ketosteroid excretion rates excluded the presence of an adrenal tumour as a cause of virilization but recently a number of virtually pure testosterone-secreting tumours associated with normal urinary 17-ketosteroid excretion have been reported. In almost all patients with virilizing adrenal tumours, plasma testosterone levels are markedly elevated and the main diagnostic problem is distinguishing between an adrenal tumour and an ovarian androgen-secreting tumour.

Masculinizing tumours of the ovary

Masculinizing ovarian tumours are uncommon and account for no more than 1% of all ovarian tumours. Hirsutism may be associated with a Sertoli–Leydig cell tumour (androblastoma, arrhenoblastoma), a pure Sertoli cell tumour, a Leydig (hilus cell) tumour, a gynandroblastoma or, less commonly, with thecal cell tumours or adrenal-rest tumours. The Sertoli–Leydig cell tumour is seen mostly in young women in the second and third decades, and the clinical changes are generally of slow onset. The tumours are almost always unilateral, generally small within the substance of the ovary and frequently near the hilum. The neoplastic mass usually retains the shape of the ovary; a slightly yellow colour may be displayed on the cut surface and small cysts, the result of haemorrhage, may be present.

Three histological types of tumour have been described — the first is a well differentiated tumour, the second an intermediate type and the third a sarcomatoid growth. Patients with the highly differentiated tumours generally show no evidence of virilization while those with the intermediate and sarcomatoid type tumour generally show marked virilization. Plasma testosterone levels are markedly elevated while oestrogen levels tend to be reduced.

Androgenic theca cell tumours presenting with masculinization during pregnancy have been described but are extremely uncommon.

The majority of Leydig cell tumours are known as hilus cell tumours though occasionally a Leydig cell tumour of non-hilar origin may arise. The patients generally present after the menopause with hirsutism as the main manifestation.

Adrenal hyperplasia

Congenital adrenal hyperplasia has been discussed in detail in Chapter 12, but occasionally may not become manifest until after puberty. These patients generally present with hirsutism and oligomenorrhoea or amenorrhoea, though normal ovulatory menstruation may persist for a time in a minority. The commonest form, which is due to a 21-hydroxylase deficiency, is associated with increased plasma DHAS and 17-hydroxyprogesterone. Urinary 17-ketosteroids are always increased.

Acromegaly

Acromegaly is uncommon but will occasionally present with hirsutism. The condition should be suspected if there is associated atypical arthropathy, carpal tunnel syndrome and growth of extremities. Most women will have amenorrhoea and 50% will exhibit hyperprolactinaemia.

Iatrogenic virilization

Hirsutism and/or virilization may develop in some women treated with androgens. While testosterone in the past has been used occasionally in the treatment of disseminated breast carcinoma and endometriosis, it is more frequently used nowadays in the management of frigidity and premenstrual tension. When used for these last two indications, the dosage should not exceed 150–200 mg methyltestosterone by mouth in any 1 month, or 200 mg as an implant. Occasionally, hirsutism may develop even with these dosages. Acne and hirsutism may also develop in women being treated with danazol for endometriosis and therapy may have to be discontinued for this reason. The administration of phenytoin can also cause acne and hirsutism as can drugs that increase prolactin secretion, probably due to the effect of hyperprolactinaemia on the adrenal cortex.

Postmenopausal hirsutism

Postmenopausal women sometimes develop mild hirsutism which generally does not require therapy. This may be due to an increase in free circulating testosterone as SHBG levels fall after the menopause as a result of the reduction in circulating oestrogens.

PRESENTATION

The rare case of hirsutism or virilization prior to puberty is caused by congenital adrenal hyperplasia or a tumour, either of the adrenal gland or the ovary. More commonly, hirsutism will present between the third and fourth decade of adult life.

Idiopathic hirsutism is characterized by the growth of coarse, typically male-type hair in the distribution of normal male secondary sex hair (i.e. in the area of the beard, on the chest wall and abdomen, over the thighs and perineum) while regular ovulatory menstrual cycles are maintained. Acne vulgaris may also be present. Virilization will be absent and the hirsutism develops slowly.

Patients with PCOS may similarly present with hirsutism of slow onset after the menarche. However, in addition, they will also demonstrate all or some of the following features: oligomenorrhoea or amenorrhoea, obesity, infertility and, very rarely, manifestations of virilization. The symptoms noted by Goldzieher (1973) in over 1000 cases are summarized in Table 22.2, and it should be noted that not all patients with PCOS will manifest hirsutism.

Cushing's syndrome, due to pituitary ACTH excess, will typically present with symptoms of hirsutism, acne, thinning of scalp hair and, less frequently, clitoral hypertrophy. The plethoric facies of Cushing's syndrome may in part be contributed to by androgen-induced erythrocytosis. These patients also typically have amenorrhoea and are obese.

Patients with a pure cortisol-secreting adrenal adenoma do not develop virilization, though they may have increased hair growth of a downy type. This hair may be distinguished from androgen-dependent hair by its type (fine and lying along the skin rather than growing away from it) and its distribution which is generalized rather than in the typical male pattern. Patients in whom cortisol and androgen excess occur as a consequence of a benign adrenal tumour have features similar to those already described for Cushing's disease.

When Cushing's syndrome occurs as a result of an adrenal carcinoma, the patient may present with very marked virilization and, in addition, have marked scalp balding, increased muscle mass of a male type, lowering of the pitch of their voice and marked clitoral hypertrophy.

Androgen-secreting tumours of the adrenal gland or ovary can present at any age. The history is usually of short duration and is accompanied by amenorrhoea and signs of virilization (Table 22.3). Occasionally a mass may also be palpable but this is unusual.

Patients with acromegaly and hirsutism will also exhibit signs of associated atypical arthropathy, carpal tunnel syndrome and growth of extremities and will usually have amenorrhoea. When all other syndromes have been excluded, the possibility of iatrogenic hirsutism or virilization as a result of administration of testosterone or other drugs such as danazol must be considered.

INVESTIGATIONS

The first priority in investigation is to take a full history and carry out a proper examination. It is often claimed that hirsutism, in the presence of regular menstruation, is either familial or idiopathic but while this is frequently so it is

Table 22.3 Clinical features and presentation in hirsutism

	Time to presentation	Age at presentation	Virilization	Amenorrhoea/ oligomenorrhoea
Congenital hyperplasia	Months (years)	Childhood (adulthood)	Present	Present
Cushing's syndrome	Months–years	Any	Absent	Present
Androgen-secreting tumours	Months	Any	Present	Present
Idiopathic hirsutism	Years	15–25 years	Absent	Normal
PCOS	Years	15–25 years	Absent	Present

Table 22.4 Hormonal profiles in normal women and patients with idiopathic hirsutism, PCOS and obesity

	Normal women (n = 29)	Idiopathic hirsutism (n = 30)	PCOS (n = 19)	Obesity and amenorrhoea (n = 8)
Testosterone: SHBG ratio	3.1 ± 1.3	5.6 ± 2.9**	9.1 ± 6.8**	5.4 ± 4.2**
Oestradiol: SHBG ratio	5.2 ± 4.7	5.6 ± 3.5	7.5 ± 5.4	8.2 ± 6.9
Androstenedione (nmol/l)	6.0 ± 1.7	7.7 ± 2.6**	9.8 ± 3.3**	5.7 ± 3.0
Oestrone (pmol/l)	178 ± 71	175 ± 87	293 ± 136**	251 ± 123**
Oestrone: androstenedione ratio	34 ± 16	26 ± 15	31 ± 13	50 ± 24**
Basal LH: FSH ratio	1.1 ± 0.5	1.3 ± 0.7	2.7 ± 1.3**	1.7 ± 0.7**
Maximal LH increment after 200 mg LHRH	12.3 ± 11.3	30 ± 55	51 ± 39**	37 ± 32**

Mean ± s.d.
(From McKenna (1988) with permission.
** Significantly different from values in normal women ($p<0.05$; Student's t-test).

not always the case and the problem of hirsutism should be properly investigated even in the presence of normal ovulatory menstruation.

The history alone may suggest adrenal hyperplasia, Cushing's syndrome or even acromegaly and the investigation of an individual patient should take a clear account of the clinical features.

The following investigations may need to be undertaken:

1. Pituitary hormones: FSH, LH and prolactin.
2. Plasma hormones: testosterone and SHBG, androstenedione, 17-hydroxyprogesterone and DHAS, oestrone, oestradiol and progesterone.
3. Urinary steroids.
4. Cortisol and ACTH.
5. Laparoscopy.
6. Ultrasonography and computerized tomography.

The hormonal profiles in normal women and patients with idiopathic hirsutism, PCOS and obesity are summarised in Table 22.4 (McKenna 1988).

Pituitary hormones

Patients with idiopathic hirsutism exhibit normal levels of FSH, LH and prolactin, and the release of FSH and LH after the injection of LHRH is similar to that found in normal women in the follicular phase of the cycle. On the other hand, patients with PCOS have normal or suppressed levels of FSH but elevated levels of LH and release of LH after injection of LHRH is similar to that found amongst normal women in the luteal phase of the cycle, even though the PCOS subjects are tested in the follicular phase. Furthermore, the ratio of LH:FSH of almost 3:1 is significantly greater than that found in normal women. Serum prolactin levels have been found to be elevated in about 15% of PCOS patients while they are normal in those with idiopathic hirsutism.

Plasma hormones

The hormone levels that are elevated in the different syndromes causing hirsutism have already been described. Testosterone levels will be elevated in most circumstances, though not all patients with idiopathic hirsutism or PCOS have elevated levels; the concentrations will be particularly high in patients with congenital adrenal hyperplasia or an androgen-secreting tumour. Androstenedione levels are classically elevated in patients with PCOS and, to a lesser extent, in those with idiopathic hirsutism. 17-Hydroxyprogesterone and DHAS levels will be elevated in patients with congenital adrenal hyperplasia, Cushing's syndrome or androgen-secreting tumours of the adrenal gland. Oestradiol levels are generally normal while oestrone levels are classically elevated in patients with PCOS and also in obese subjects. Progesterone levels can be estimated in patients in whom it is necessary to confirm ovulation.

Urinary steroids

Although the measurement of plasma hormone levels is now routinely used in the assessment of the hirsute patient, measurement of urinary steroids may also provide useful information in certain instances. Urinary 17-ketosteroids will be elevated in patients with adrenal hyperplasia and androgen-secreting adrenal tumours. Traditionally it was believed that normal urinary 17-ketosteroid excretion rates effectively excluded the presence of an adrenal lesion as a cause of virilization. However, a number of virtually pure testosterone-secreting tumours associated with normal urinary 17-ketosteroid excretion have been reported (Givens et al 1974). A formal dexamethasone suppression test is frequently necessary to distinguish between an adrenal tumour and cases of adrenal hyperplasia. After basal studies dexamethasone is administered at a dose of 0.5 mg four times daily for 2 days followed by 2 mg four times daily for a further 4 days. Urinary 17-ketosteroids will promptly be suppressed in patients with adrenal hyperplasia, but where there is an adrenal tumour, while there may be some fall, complete suppression does not occur.

Cortisol and ACTH

Cortisol may be measured by radioimmunoassay in plasma or as urinary-free cortisol in urine. Urinary-free cortisol will be substantially elevated in patients with Cushing's syndrome and, in addition, the normal diurnal variation in plasma cortisol and ACTH will not be present.

Laparoscopy

Laparoscopy can be used to confirm the diagnosis of PCOS; while the procedure is invasive it is more informative than pelvic ultrasonography.

Ultrasonography and computerized tomography

Ultrasonography may be employed as a method of confirming the presence of polycystic ovaries. The anatomical localization of an adrenal tumour is greatly facilitated by the use of ultrasonography, though the more recent use of computerized tomography is much superior.

Other investigative procedures such as arteriography, selective venous sampling of adrenal and ovarian veins, and radioisotope scanning of the adrenals are much more invasive and generally unnecessary.

TREATMENT

Treatment depends on the cause of the hirsutism and it is important to make a proper diagnosis before considering which form of therapy to use. When the hirsutism or virilization occurs as a result of serious pathology, treatment must be directed at curing the primary disease. This treatment may involve hypophysectomy for Cushing's syndrome due to hyperplasia for acromegaly; it may require the surgical removal of adrenal or ovarian tumours, or it may necessitate the use of corticosteroids for virilizing cases of adrenal hyperplasia. When the hirsutism develops as a result of iatrogenic causes then the offending drug should be withdrawn.

However, the great majority of patients presenting with hirsutism will be found to be suffering from either idiopathic hirsutism or PCOS and treatment should be aimed at trying to improve the hirsutism, reducing obesity where necessary, or inducing regular ovulatory cycles in those subjects who wish to become pregnant.

Treatment of hirsutism

Hirsutism may be treated either cosmetically or with hormones; whichever option is chosen it is important that the patient's expectations are reasonable. Many cosmetic measures such as depilatory creams, bleaching, waxing, shaving, plucking and electrolysis can be used to help control hirsutism. Many girls and women tolerate incapacitating hair growth because they fear that if they remove it, it will become worse. It should be stressed that this fear of interfering locally with hair growth lest the condition worsen is ill founded. The psychological impact of a woman having a beard, particularly through the vulnerable teenage years, is devastating. While local measures will bring about an immediate improvement, there will inevitably be a regrowth of hair which has been plucked, removed with creams, waxed or shaved. The rate of return of hair growth, however, varies widely amongst different patients. Electrolysis can destroy hair follicles and this will prevent regrowth of that particular follicle but such treatment will never destroy all hair follicles and if the underlying stimulus to hair growth is not removed then new hair growth is likely to emerge. Nonetheless, cosmetic measures alone will prove adequate for many patients.

Corticosteroids

The use of hormones in addition to cosmetic therapy is worthwhile in many patients, particularly those who present with elevated androgen levels. A hair has a life cycle of approximately 2 years and if hormonal treatment is successful it will slow the rate of established hair growth and prevent new hair growth. However, a significant impact of hormonal therapy may not be seen for at least 6 months.

The administration of dexamethasone 0.5 mg taken at midnight suppresses the early surge of ACTH and reduces the adrenal production of androgen. Approximately 50% of patients will notice a reduction in the number of hairs and in the rate of hair growth within 6 months of commencing treatment. A response to treatment can be predicted by a reduction in the plasma levels of testosterone, the testosterone: SHBG ratio and androstenedione levels. However, dexamethasone should not be used in obese patients as these subjects tend to gain further weight on this therapy. Dexamethasone has the further advantage that it will induce regular menstruation in more than 50% of non-obese patients with PCOS within 3 months of initiation of therapy, (Steinberger et al 1981).

Ovarian inhibition

The administration of oestrogen–progesterone preparations provides a simple and effective method of inhibiting ovarian steroid production; furthermore, oestrogen stimulates the synthesis of SHBG in the liver and also inhibits the enzyme 5α-reductase which converts testosterone to the more biologically active dihydrotestosterone in the skin. However, it should be recognized that oral contraceptive preparations containing norgestrel suppress SHBG levels more severely than those containing norethisterone or one of its precursors; thus a preparation containing 50 μg ethinyloestradiol together with norethisterone is more likely to be beneficial than preparations containing norgestrel. While this therapy will rapidly reduce acne the improvement in hirsutism will only take place after several months of therapy; approximately 30% of patients will derive benefit.

Cyproterone acetate

Cyproterone acetate is an anti-androgenic progestogen and is used in a reversed sequential manner. Cyproterone acetate 50–100 mg is given daily for 10 days from the fifth day of the menstrual cycle; this is accompanied by 50μg oestrogen which is then continued alone for a further 11 days, after which the cycle is interrupted for 7 days. This form of treatment provides regular withdrawal bleeding. Cyproterone acetate has a prolonged half-life and if it is continued throughout the cycle menstruation may not occur for several days after stopping treatment. Furthermore, if cyproterone acetate was used in the absence of oestrogen the possibility of ovulation would exist and if a pregnancy ensued the continued use of anti-androgen would result in feminization of a male fetus.

Cyproterone acetate has been used fairly widely and achieves good results in about 75% of patients who are treated for 12 months.

Spironolactone

Spironolactone has recently been used with some success in the treatment of hirsutism (Molinatti et al 1983). Like cyproterone acetate, this drug may interfere with sexual differentiation of a male fetus and if a patient is exposed to the risk of pregnancy she should be given an oral contraceptive in addition to the spironolactone.

Induction of ovulation

Regular ovulation can be successfully induced in PCOS subjects by administration of clomiphene citrate or, in some cases, by a combination of clomiphene and human chorionic gonadotrophin; by treatment with pituitary gonadotrophins and human chorionic gonadotrophin; by the administration of corticosteroids or by wedge resection of the ovaries. However, while ovarian wedge resection will induce ovulation in 80% of patients, the operation may stimulate the formation of adhesions around the ovaries and tubes and the procedure should rarely be used and only when other forms of treatment are not feasible. Recently multiple ovarian diathermy has been found to be effective in many PCOS patients, at least for a finite time.

Ovulation induction is considered in greater detail in Chapter 6.

KEY POINTS

1. Hirsutism can be described as hair growth that worries the patient. It is commonly seen without any evidence of virilization.
2. Virilization is very rarely seen without hirsutism (apart from in the neonate) and can be defined as one or more of the following: deepening of the vocal pitch, male type hairline thinning, clitoral hypertrophy, breast atrophy, increased musculature.
3. Hirsutism may be a result of excessive androgen production from (a) the adrenal, (b) the ovaries, or (c) from excessive end organ response.
4. Virilization is due to excess androgen production.
5. Idiopathic hirsutism describes a group of women with regular menstruation who lack any evidence of organic disease. They have elevated levels of testosterone and androstenedione with suppressed SHBG.
6. Polycystic ovarian syndrome may present as hirsutism along with any or all of the following: oligomenorrhoea/amenorrhoea, obesity, infertility and occasionally virilization.
7. Classical PCOs are either primary, where there is no contributory androgen producing cause, or secondary, where a cause can be found.
8. Cushing's syndrome is a disorder where hyperstimulation of the adrenal by ACTH gives rise to both an excess of cortisol and androgen.
9. Adrenal tumours, if they are purely cortisol secreting, do not cause virilization unlike benign tumours producing excess androgen and cortisol.
10. Masculinizing tumours of the ovary are uncommon and account for no more than 1% of ovarian tumours.
11. Adrenal hyperplasia usually is diagnosed before puberty but very occasionally may present late.
12. Acromegaly will occasionally present with hirsutism. Most women will have amenorrhoea and 50% will have hyperprolactinaemia.
13. Iatrogenic virilization may develop in women treated with androgens or drugs increasing prolactin secretion. It is also sometimes seen following administration of phenytoin.
14. Postmenopausal hirsutism is probably due to increasing levels of free testosterone as circulating levels of SHBG fall after the menopause.

REFERENCES

Duignan N M, Shaw R W, Glass M R et al 1975 Sex hormone levels and gonadotrophin release in polycystic ovarian disease. Clinical Endocrinology 4: 287–295

Givens J R, Anderson R N, Wiser W L, Coleman S A, Fish S A 1974 A gonadotrophin-responsive adrenocortical adenoma. Journal of Clinical Endocrinology and Metabolism 38: 126–133

Givens J R, Anderson R N, Ragland J B, Wiser W L, Umstot E S 1975 Adrenal function in hirsutism 1. Diurnal change and response of plasma androstenedione, testosterone, 17-hydroxyprogesterone, cortisol, LH and FSH to dexamethasone and 1/2 unit of ACTH. Journal of Clinical Endocrinology and Metabolism 40: 988–1000

Goldzieher J W 1973 Polycystic ovarian disease. Clinical Obstetrics and Gynecology 16: 82–91

Kirschner M A, Jacobs J B 1971 Combined ovarian and adrenal vein catheterization to determine the site(s) of androgen over production in hirsute women. Journal of Clinical Endocrinology and Metabolism 30: 727–734

Kirschner M A, Zucker I R, Jespersen D 1976 Idiopathic hirsutism — an ovarian abnormality. New England Journal of Medicine 294: 637–640

Loughlin T, Cunningham S K, Culliton M et al 1985 Altered androstenedione and oestrone dynamics associated with abnormal hormonal profiles in amenorrhoeic subjects with weight loss or obesity. Fertility and Sterility 43: 720–725

McKenna T J 1988 Pathogenesis and treatment of polycystic ovary syndrome. New England Journal of Medicine 318: 558–562

McKenna T J, Cunningham S K, Laughlin T 1985 The adrenal cortex and virilization. Clinics in Endocrinology and Metabolism 14: 997–1020

Molinatti G M, Messina M, Manieri C, Massucchetti C, Biffignandi P 1983 Current approaches to treatment of virilizing syndrome. In: Molanatti G M, Martini L, James V H T (eds) Androgenization in women. New York, Raven Press, p 179

Moore A, Magee F, Cunningham S K, Culliton M, McKenna T J 1983 Adrenal abnormalities in idiopathic hirsutism. Clinical Endocrinology 18: 391–399

Norththrop G, Archie J T, Patel S K, Wilbanks G D 1975 Adrenal and ovarian vein androgen levels and laparoscopic findings in hirsute women. American Journal of Obstetrics and Gynecology 122: 192–198

Oake R J, Davies S J, McLachlan M S F, Thomas J P 1974 Plasma testosterone in adrenal and ovarian vein blood of hirsute women. Quarterly Journal of Medicine 43: 603–613

Rosenfield R B 1971 Plasma testosterone binding globulin and indices of the concentration of unbound plasma androgens in normal and hirsute women. Journal of Clinical Endocrinology and Metabolism 32: 717–725

Shaw R W, Duignan N M, Butt W R, Logan Edwards R and London D R 1975 Hypothalmic-pituitary relationships in the polycystic ovary syndrome. Serum gonadotrophin levels following injection of oestradiol benzoate. British Journal of Obstetrics and Gynaecology 82: 952–957

Sommers S C, Wadman P J 1956 Pathogenesis of polycystic ovaries. American Journal of Obstetrics and Gynecology 72: 160–168

Steinberger E, Smith K D, Rodriquez-Rigau L J 1981 Hyperandrogenism and female infertility. In: Crosignani P G, Rubin B L (eds) Endocrinology of human infertility: new aspects. London: Academic Press, pp 327–342

Yen S S C 1980 The polycystic ovary syndrome. Clinical Endocrinology 12: 177–208

23. Premenstrual syndrome

P. M. S. O'Brien

INTRODUCTION

Premenstrual syndrome (PMS) is a disorder of unknown aetiology. It has not been proven to be of endocrine origin, nor has it conclusively been demonstrated to depend on the ovarian cycle. However, it seems likely that PMS results as a direct consequence of the hormonal events of the normal ovarian cycle. The main evidence for this is that both bilateral oophorectomy and suppression of the menstrual cycle with analogues of gonadotrophin-releasing hormone (GnRH) eliminate PMS symptoms completely. Secondly, the administration of oestrogen with cyclical progestagen to postmenopausal patients readily induces symptoms in certain women.

To date there is no conclusive evidence that any difference in ovarian hormone status exists in PMS patients compared to asymptomatic women; as yet this has not been proved or refuted. It is clear that nearly all menstruating women exhibit some symptomatic manifestation in the premenstrual phase of the cycle. In the absence of demonstrable endocrine differences, PMS may represent an exaggerated response to the physiological levels of ovarian hormones through the cycle. This may have a demonstrable biochemical basis.

THE SYNDROME

The existence of PMS was first documented by Frank (1931) who suspected that the disorder was related to oestrogen excess. He treated his patients by irradiation of the ovaries with claimed success. Since then numerous aetiological theories have been proposed and a larger number of treatment regimes have been tried. The problem is traditionally thought to affect multiparous women in their mid to late 30s; the symptoms arrive for the first time soon after the birth of their first child. It is considered a disorder of middle-class articulate women, though it is probable that this is the group of women who report their symptoms whilst other groups experience equally severe problems, not recognizing them as such. Research appears to show a higher prevalence of neurosis in PMS patients.

The symptoms of PMS may be multiple and will be considered later in more detail. In addition to these symptoms it has been suggested that exacerbations of certain medical diseases like epilepsy, heart failure and asthma occur more frequently premenstrually. Many behavioural changes are said to occur around this time of the menstrual cycle; for example, suicide attempts, child battering, examination failures, absence from and poor performance at work, alcohol abuse and criminal acts. Indeed, there have been several legal cases where PMS has been cited in defence of severe crime including even murder. Few of the above assumptions have been borne out by adequate scientific assessment.

The prevalence of PMS has been variously reported as ranging from 5 to 95%; this probably reflects the imprecision of diagnostic criteria rather than any biological factor. PMS is unusual in that women usually present themselves with the presumed diagnosis of PMS and it is

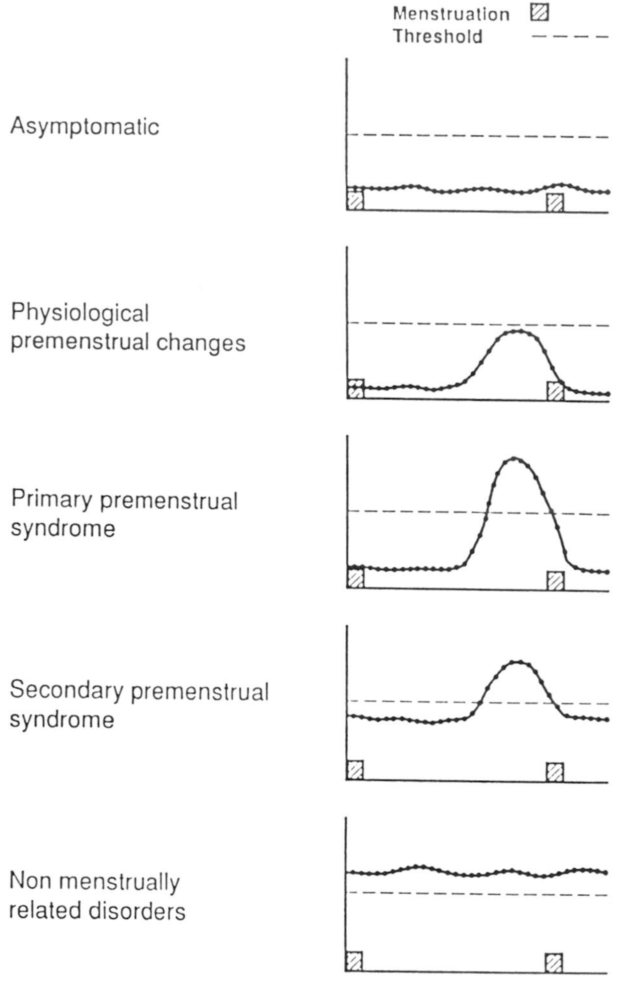

Fig. 23.1 Classification of premenstrual symptomatology.

the clinician's role to determine the validity of this. Many other disorders may be confused (see p. 332) and the diagnosis of PMS itself may be confusing. The following classification may provide some assistance (Fig. 23.1). Women may be asymptomatic, they may have no more than physiological symptoms or may have true primary or secondary PMS. A significant proportion of so-called PMS patients have a psychiatric problem which has been wrongly attributed to the ovarian hormones.

Asymptomatic women

Only 5% of women are completely free from symptoms premenstrually. These are possibly an 'abnormal' group of women.

Physiological premenstrual change

All but 5% of women experience at least one premenstrual symptom. In the majority, these are tolerated and there is no interference with that woman's normal functioning. When symptoms do interfere with such functioning then a woman can be considered to have PMS. It is difficult to quantify this disruption of life — hence the problems in defining the dividing line between physiological and pathological. PMS may be primary or secondary depending on the degree of underlying psychopathology.

Primary PMS

This is a disorder of non-specific somatic, psychological or behavioural symptoms recurring in the premenstrual phase of the menstrual cycle. Symptoms *resolve completely* by the end of menstruation, leaving a symptom-free week. The symptoms are of sufficient severity to produce social, family or occupational disruption. Symptoms must have occurred in at least four of the six previous menstrual cycles.

Secondary PMS

A disorder of non-specific somatic, psychological or behavioural symptoms recurring in the premenstrual phase of the menstrual cycle. Although symptoms remain following menstruation, they should significantly *improve* by the end of menstruation and this improvement should be sustained for at least 1 week.

The symptoms are of sufficient severity to produce social, familial or occupational disruption and should have occurred in at least four of the six previous cycles.

Implied in these definitions is that in secondary PMS there is an underlying psychological disorder whose aetiology is similar to that of common psychiatric disorders such as depression or anxiety. Both primary PMS and the cyclical component of secondary PMS are presumed to be related to the endocrine changes of the ovarian cycle.

Psychological disorder wrongly attributed to PMS

There is a further group of women who will be encountered in the gynaecology clinic; these are women who have continuous or non-cyclical psychological problems wrongly attributed (by patient or doctor) to PMS. It is of course important that such patients do not receive treatment appropriate to PMS and if the severity warrants it they should undergo psychiatric evaluation followed by treatment if necessary.

SYMPTOMS

The character of symptoms in PMS has not been dictated in these definitions principally as they are so numerous and because their timing in the cycle is more important than their specific nature. Over 150 have been recorded in the

Table 23.1 Reported symptoms of PMS

Psychological	Physical
* Aggression	Accident-prone
Agitation	Acne
Anorexia	Asthma
* Anxiety	Bloatedness (actual)
Argumentative	* Bloatedness (feeling of)
Confusion	Blurred vision
* Crying bouts	* Breast swelling
Decreased alertness	* Breast tenderness
Decreased libido	* Clumsiness
* Depression	Constipation
Diminished self-esteem	Diarrhoea
Drowsiness	Diminished activity
Emotional lability	Diminished efficiency
Energetic	Diminished performance
Fatigue	Dizziness
Food craving	Epilepsy
Hopelessness	Finger swelling
Housebound	Flushes
Hunger	Formication
Hypersomnia	* Headache
Impulsive behaviour	Joint pain
Increased libido	Mastodynia
Insomnia	Migraine
* Irritability	Muscle pain
Lack of inspiration	Nausea
Lack of volition	Oedema
Lethargy	Oliguria
Listlessness	Pain — iliac fossa
Loss of attention to appearance	Pain — lower abdomen
* Loss of concentration	Pain — pelvic
Loss of confidence	Polyuria
Loss of judgement	Poor co-ordination
Loss of self-control	* Premenstrual dysmenorrhoea
Malaise	Pruritus
Mood swings	Puffiness
Sadness	Sinusitis
Social isolation	Skin lesions
Suicidal tendency	Sore eyes
* Tension	Sweating
Thirst	Vaginal discharge
Violence	Vertigo
	Vomiting
	Weakness
	* Weight increase (perceived)
	Weight increase (true)

* Commonest symptoms.

research literature (Table 23.1). There are, however common typical psychological symptoms which include irritability, aggression, depression, unexplained crying, tension, anxiety and poor concentration. The key physical symptoms include mastalgia and breast swelling, headache, clumsiness, pelvic pain and, by far the most common, abdominal bloatedness which usually occurs in the absence of weight gain or water retention, though it is often perceived as such.

Measurement and diagnosis

Quantification of PMS is difficult and ideally we would wish to measure:

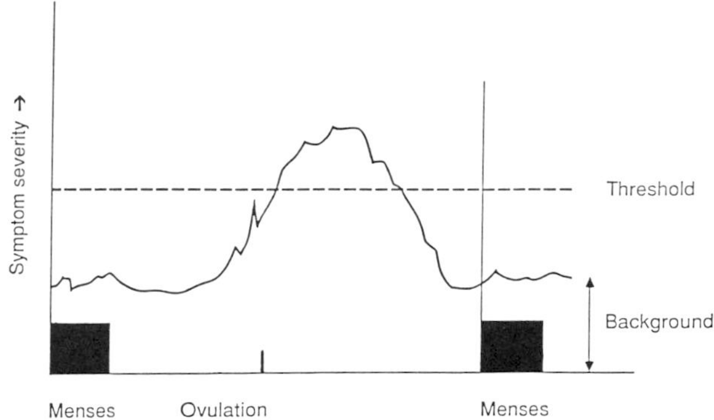

Fig. 23.2 Hypothetical representation of the components of PMS.

1. The cyclical symptoms: their character, timing and severity.
2. The degree of underlying psychological dysfunction.
3. The degree of disruption of that patient's normal functioning and her threshold for complaining (Fig. 23.2).

It is possible to quantify underlying psychopathology using established psychiatric questionnaires. There are many but the simplest of the well established techniques is the General Health Questionnaire (Goldberg & Hillier 1979). The use of this questionnaire appears only to be reliable in PMS patients when completed in the follicular phase of the cycle.

The measurement of the cyclical component of symptoms is best achieved by means either of the Moos' menstrual distress questionnaire (Moos 1985) or specific linear visual analogue scales (Faratian et al 1984).

To measure the threshold for complaining and the degree to which the patient's life is disrupted is less simple; the questionnaire of Steiner and colleagues (1980) goes some way to achieving this.

In clinical practice these three factors are determined from the history and by the self-documentation of symptoms using simple premenstrual calendars (Fig. 23.3a). These however give limited information. They indicate the character of the symptoms and their timing as well as their disappearance following the period. They do not give accurate quantification of symptom severity nor of underlying psychopathology. Even the more complex questionnaires such as the Moos' menstrual distress questionnaire and linear visual analogue scales tell us only of the cyclical component of symptoms and give no indication of underlying psychological problems or the degree to which the symptoms disrupt that patient's normal functioning. The use of premenstrual calendars is the best available compromise, the more sophisticated but cumbersome techniques such as linear visual analogue scales being used only in research. Figure 23.3b demonstrates a typical

Menstrual Chart

Indicate on the chart the days on which symptoms trouble you using the appropriate letter or letters from the key below.

Fill in months (eg. May.)	1	2	3	4	5	6	7	8	9	10	11	12	13	14	15	16	17	18	19	20	21	22	23	24	25	26	27	28	29	30	31
1st Month JULY				T	D T	T	B T	B T	B T	B T	M	M	M	M																T	B T
2nd Month AUGUST	B T	B T	B T	B T D	B T	B	B	B M	M	M	M	M																B T	B T	B T	B
3rd Month SEPTEMBER	D B	T	B T	B T	M	M	M	M																							

Key to symptoms:
D depression. P pain – backache or headache. T tension or irritability. F fatigue. B bloated feeling. M menstruation.

a

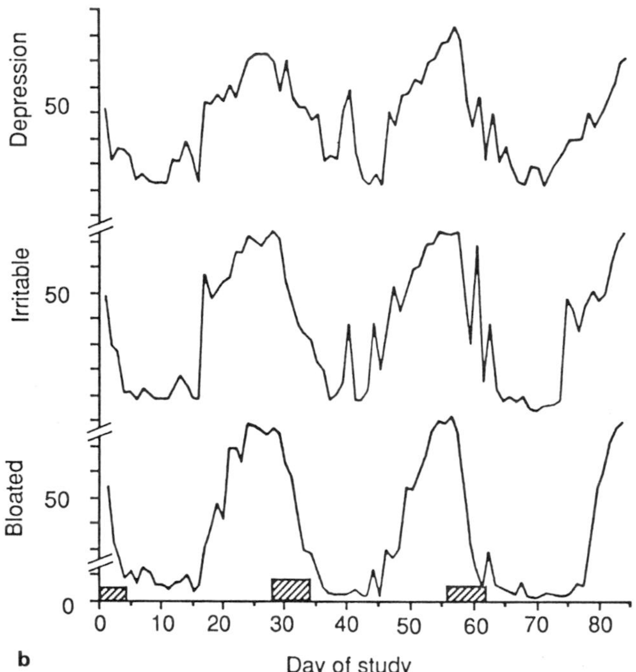

Fig. 23.3 (**a**) Typical premenstrual symptom calendar. (**b**) Visual analogue scores of typical PMS symptoms. Hatched box = menstruation.

record of symptoms obtained from specific visual analogue scales.

Tests

There is presently no objective measure of PMS and unlike other endocrine disorders (if this is one) there is no blood test enabling us to identify PMS patients save to exclude other disorders like the menopause, polycystic ovaries, hyper- and hypothyroidism and anaemia (Table 23.2).

In the difficult case it is of value to use a GnRH depot for 3 months to distinguish to what degree the ovarian cycle contributes to symptoms; those persisting after suppression of the cycle must be the consequence of the underlying psychological disorder and not related to ovarian activity.

Table 23.2 Value of blood tests in PMS

Test	Value in diagnosis
Progesterone, day 21	No value
Oestrogen	No proven value
Sex hormone-binding globulin	Marked differences between symptomatic and asymptomatic patients shown in one study, not confirmed by others
Prolactin	No value
Follicle-stimulating hormone, luteinizing hormone	Excludes perimenopausal women May diagnose polycystic ovaries
Thyroid function tests	Exclusion of hypo- and hyperthyroidism
Electrolytes	No diagnostic value

The following criteria are necessary to diagnose PMS:

1. Symptoms must occur specifically in the premenstrual phase of the cycle.
2. Symptoms must disappear (primary PMS) or improve (secondary PMS) during menstruation.
3. The character of symptoms need not be specific.
4. Symptoms should be of sufficient severity to disrupt the patient's life.
5. Symptoms should have been present in at least four of the previous six cycles.

The above information is obtained from the history and prospectively administered PMS symptom assessment techniques.

AETIOLOGY

The aetiology of PMS is unknown. We have implied that it is related directly to the endocrine events of the ovarian

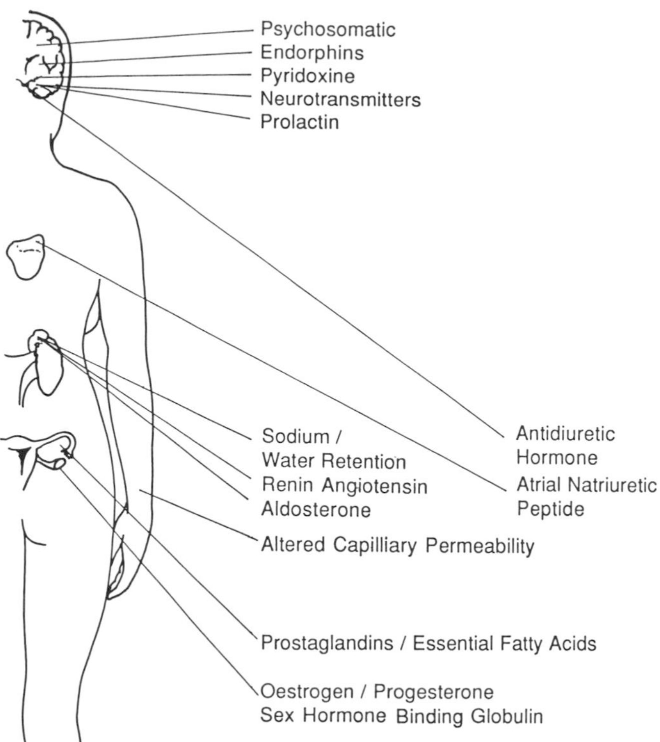

Fig. 23.4 Aetiological theories for PMS.

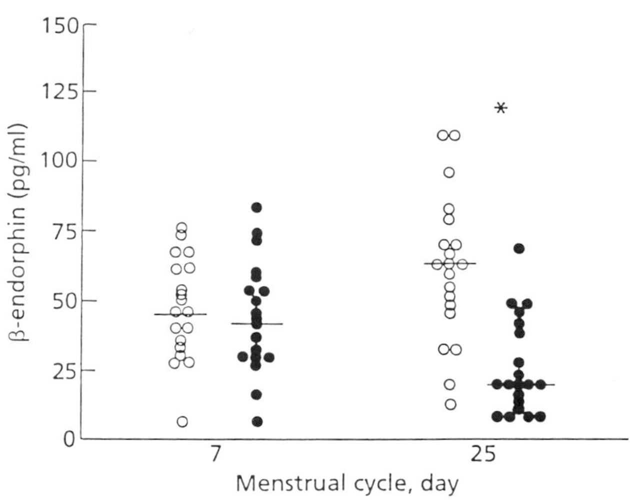

Fig. 23.5 β-endorphin levels in PMS (●) compared with controls (○). The PMS group is significantly different from controls on day 25 ($p < 0.0001$). Bars indicate the median. From Chuong et al (1985) with permission.

cycle. This is probably true but the evidence is mostly inferred. The range of other proposed theories is enormous (O'Brien 1987; Fig. 23.4). The recent and most plausible explanations have included psychoneuroendocrine theories, particularly in relation to the endogenous opioid peptides, prolactin excess, the prostaglandins; theories linked to so-called sodium and water retention including renin, angiotensin, aldosterone, antidiuretic hormone and atrial natriuretic peptide, and finally oestrogen and progesterone imbalance.

Neurotransmitters, endorphins and vitamin B_6

Many neurotransmitters could potentially have a modulatory or mediatory role on neuronal function in PMS. Biogenic amines like serotonin, dopamine and their synthetic pathway cofactors have been considered and more recently a limited amount of evidence for the involvement of the endorphins has become available. Deficiency of vitamin B_6 may be important; vitamin B_6 (pyridoxine) is a cofactor in the final step in the synthesis of serotonin and dopamine from tryptophan. No convincing data have yet demonstrated abnormalities either of brain amine synthesis or deficiency of cofactors like vitamin B_6. Studies of the endorphins have been a little more convincing.

β-endorphin measured in the portal-hypophyseal blood of the rhesus monkey undergoes cyclical variation in the menstrual cycle (Wehrenberg et al 1982). Abnormal levels of endorphins have been demonstrated in various psychological states. It has also been suggested that inhibition of endorphin by naloxone produces PMS-like symptoms. The therapeutic implications of this endorphin withdrawal hypothesis remain uncertain though the proposal must present one of the more plausible explanations for PMS. Chuong and colleagues (1985) have demonstrated diminished luteal phase levels of β-endorphin in women with PMS (Fig. 23.5), and recent data suggest an improvement (but not elimination) in symptoms following the administration of the endorphin inhibitor naltrexone (Chuong 1988).

Prolactin

Because prolactin (in animals) promotes retention of sodium, potassium and water, stimulates the breast and is a so-called stress hormone, many researchers have investigated its role in PMS. Prolactin has not clearly been demonstrated to undergo cyclical change in the normal menstrual cycle, nor do women with PMS demonstrate elevated blood levels of prolactin; moreover, women with hyperprolactinaemia do not report PMS-like symptoms. Therapeutic studies of bromocriptine have failed to demonstrate any significant effect on symptoms, with the notable exception of cyclical mastalgia. Its general role in PMS therapy now seems doubtful (O'Brien & Symonds 1982).

Prostaglandins and essential fatty acids

It has been claimed that specific prostaglandin changes are associated with PMS. Their ubiquitous nature makes them prime candidates to play such an aetiological role but no precise explanation linking prostaglandin activity to PMS has yet been forthcoming. Both inhibition of prostaglandin synthesis and its enhancement using prostaglandin precursors (essential fatty acids) have been claimed to relieve PMS. The underlying theory on which essential fatty acid supplementation is based is complex. However, in the absence of a demonstrable endocrine abnormality in PMS a differential sensitivity to the endocrine changes of the ovarian cycle has been suggested. In in vitro studies, interactions at a cellular and receptor level have been demonstrated between polyunsaturated essential fatty acids and the activity of oestrogen, progesterone, angiotensin II and β-endorphin. Interaction by angiotensin II with essential fatty acids and various prostaglandins has been shown in vivo. Hence defective essential fatty acid/prostaglandin metabolism may give rise to a breakdown in this balance, allowing an exaggerated response to normal circulating levels of these different hormone systems.

Investigation of essential fatty acid levels in PMS has produced interesting but as yet inconclusive information. Abnormalities in essential fatty acid synthesis have been demonstrated in a study by Brush and colleagues (1984) whilst these findings have not been replicated by others (O'Brien & Massil 1990).

Sodium and water retention

There can be few articles on PMS which do not refer to the almost universal acceptance of premenstrual sodium and water retention. It is surprising, then, to find few scientific data which demonstrate such a phenomenon. Whilst women may demonstrate an extremely severe subjective sensation of premenstrual bloatedness, this most frequently occurs in the absence of weight increase, changes in abdominal dimensions or any true water or sodium retention. Preliminary data we have accrued suggest that total body sodium paradoxically tends to *decrease* in women with PMS. The decrease in exchangeable sodium may well give rise to changes in neuronal excitability, accounting for psychological symptoms; similar electrolyte changes have been demonstrated in bipolar psychiatric disorders. It now seems more likely that the symptom of bloatedness exceeds in severity any physical change and that there may be a large 'perceived' component. Alternatively, small and large gut distension may well occur as a result of progesterone-induced relaxation of smooth muscle of the gut. Such a change could well occur in response to progesterone release in the premenstrual phase and indeed one study has demonstrated marked delay in intestinal transit during the luteal phase of the cycle (Wald et al 1981), but this has not been assessed in relation to the symptom of bloatedness.

Endocrine effects on fluid and electrolytes

The lack of premenstrual water and electrolyte shift is paralleled by a similar lack of difference in those hormones which control sodium and water transport. The factors which could promote water retention include excessive production of oestrogen, prolactin, antidiuretic hormone, oxytocin, renin, angiotensin, aldosterone and corticosteroids. Deficiencies of progesterone, atrial natriuretic peptide or renal prostaglandins could also permit water retention by the absence of such a natriuretic effect. No clear differences have been demonstrated in any of these, with the exception of atrial natriuretic peptide. There appear to be abnormally low levels of atrial natriuretic peptide in PMS patients, particularly in the luteal phase (Hussain et al 1990).

Ovarian hormones

It has long been suggested that fluctuation in mood may be related to ovarian hormone imbalance (Dalton 1977). Research into this has produced data which could support theories of oestrogen excess, progesterone deficiency, oestrogen/progesterone imbalance and progesterone excess associated with shortening of the luteal phase. The evidence has been based on a wide range of estimates including vaginal cytology, endometrial histology, plasma and urinary levels of hormones. In most studies the sampling has taken place only once or twice in four phases of the cycle and more rarely on daily samples. The production of ovarian hormones is pulsatile and the amplitude of the progesterone pulses exceeds the differences claimed to have been shown between patients and control subjects.

The least scientific evidence which has been presented has been the supposed improvement of symptoms following replacement therapy of, for example, progesterone. It is unlikely that such purely simple concepts as deficiency or excess of a particular ovarian hormone explain PMS, as oestrogen/progesterone differences are most marked in the first part of the cycle. Thus, factors other than differences in the levels of individual hormones must be important; interactions with other endocrine or biochemical systems may operate or differences in receptor status may be relevant.

A link with ovarian hormone changes, particularly progesterone, seems likely however, since the temporal relationship between progesterone secretion and symptoms is so close. Oestrogen has a direct stimulatory effect on the cerebrum, the breast and the kidney whilst progesterone causes natriuresis and diuresis, and acts on the breast; it could cause abdominal distension through its action on the gut and it is a central nervous sedative. In large doses progesterone causes anaesthesia and in lower doses it probably acts as a minor tranquillizer.

In the absence of conclusive differences in ovarian endocrine status between women who have significant symptoms and those with no more than physiological changes, the following suggestions are made. There is good

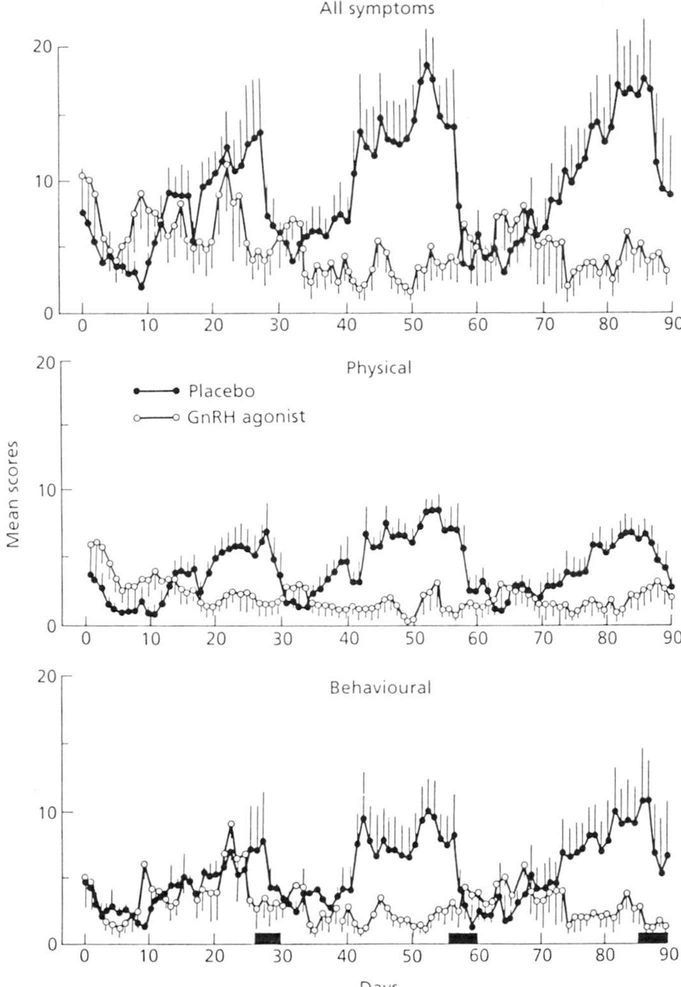

Fig. 23.6 Effect of GnRH analogue on premenstrual symptoms showing virtual complete elimination of symptoms whilst ovarian function is suppressed with continuation of symptoms during placebo. From Muse et al (1984) with permission.

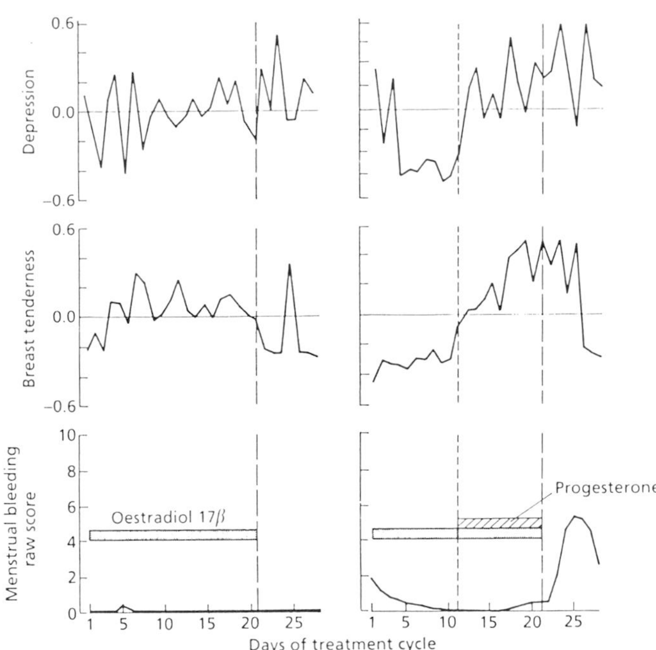

Fig. 23.7 Stimulation of PMS symptoms during treatment of postmenopausal women by oestrogen and progesterone. From Hammarback et al (1985).

evidence to suggest that symptoms are directly linked to ovarian hormone changes. Firstly, ablation of the menstrual cycle by oophorectomy or more conveniently by the administration of analogues of GnRH is associated with a parallel elimination of PMS symptoms (Fig. 23.6; Muse et al 1984). Secondly, in women whose ovarian cycles have ceased (due to menopause or bilateral oophorectomy) and who subsequently receive hormone replacement therapy (HRT), a significant percentage develop PMS symptoms during the progesterone phase of therapy (Hammarback et al 1985) which are so severe that they have to discontinue treatment (Fig. 23.7). It must be noted however that not all women develop such symptoms even when identical dose regimens of HRT are administered; this implies that an additional factor must operate before symptoms are exhibited. This factor is probably identical with that which distinguishes PMS patients from those with physiological changes; there may be a biochemical basis or patients may constitute a psychologically susceptible group. There is currently no explanatory mechanism for this difference though efforts would be most valuably directed towards identifying such a difference, and not the assessment of differing levels of the hormones themselves.

MANAGEMENT

Diagnosis

We have seen that there is no objective means of identifying or quantifying PMS. For practical clinical purposes, dependence is placed on the history, questionnaires, exclusion of certain specific disorders and the use of prospectively administered symptom-rating charts. The simpler charts indicate only the timing and character of the symptoms; the degree to which they disrupt the patient's and her family's life is not objectively quantifiable.

Differential diagnosis

Unlike most medical problems the majority of patients with PMS present to the gynaecologist already self-diagnosed and the doctor's task is to confirm or exclude this diagnosis. Many disorders have been wrongly attributed to PMS (Table 23.3). We have already suggested that physiological premenstrual changes often cause patients to seek advice although symptoms are not particularly severe. Women with psychiatric disorders unrelated to the men-

Table 23.3 Differential diagnosis of PMS

Psychiatric disorders
- May be confused because of the similarity in symptoms and because of the bipolar and periodic nature of some psychiatric disorders, for example manic depressive psychosis
- Many women prefer to 'label' their psychological inadequacies as gynaecological rather than psychiatric
- There are no objective tests but there are many questionnaires. The General Health Questionnaire may help (Goldberg & Hillier 1979)

Intrafamilial and psychosexual problems
- Distinguish between cause and effect

Other causes of breast symptoms
- Cyclical breast pain may be considered part of PMS
- Can be distinguished from non-cyclical breast disease by history
- Non-cyclical disease includes several disorders requiring breast examination and maybe mammography, ultrasonography, aspiration and biopsy
- Breast cancer must, of course, be excluded

Other causes of abdominal bloatedness and water retention
- Only a few women exhibit significant water retention in PMS
- More women have idiopathic oedema which is also cyclical but only occasionally coincides by chance with the menstrual cycle
- Some women call progressive obesity 'PMS bloatedness'
- These can all be distinguished by daily weighing

Endometriosis, pelvic infection and dysmenorrhoea
- Primary dysmenorrhoea occurs with period; it is obtained from the history
- Secondary dysmenorrhoea is related to pelvic pathology
- Laparoscopy will exclude endometriosis or pelvic infection

Medical causes of lethargy and tiredness
- Occasionally anaemia — haemoglobin
- Rarely hypothyroidism or hyperthyroidism

Menopause
- May be confused in patients over 40
- Flushes may uncommonly occur in PMS
- Usually distinguished from history
- Raised follicle-stimulating hormone and luteinizing hormone are usually diagnostic

strual cycle will frequently label their problem as PMS (often they find it more acceptable to label their disorder as gynaecological rather than psychiatric). Similarly, psychosexual problems and intrafamilial discord may be wrongly blamed on PMS and whilst it may well be contributory it is frequently unrelated and PMS is used as a scapegoat.

The essence of diagnosis in all of these disorders is the cyclicity of symptoms. If they are not relieved by the end of menstruation then an alternative explanation must be sought. This is equally true for somatic problems. Non-cyclical breast pain may be due to breast cancer, sclerosing adenosis, trauma, Tietze syndrome or ductectasia or periductal mastitis and may necessitate further investigation such as mammography or biopsy. Cyclical mastalgia is a part of PMS and responds to similar therapeutic measures.

Premenstrual pelvic pain must be distinguished from that due to endometriosis, by laparoscopy if necessary.

Cyclical or idiopathic oedema is a separate problem from PMS though its cyclical nature and frequent association with psychological symptoms may cause confusion. In this disorder, true water retention occurs with huge increases in weight. There is nearly always a history of loop diuretic abuse which is frequently related to secondary hyperaldosteronism. The original reason for the diuretic use may have been for the treatment of premenstrual bloatedness or as an adjunct to diet for weight reduction; both are inappropriate indications for diuretics.

Lethargy due to hypothyroidism or anaemia may rarely be confused with PMS. Anxiety and irritability may result from hyperthyroidism. The presence of other characteristic symptoms will usually distinguish these and the diagnoses can be excluded by the appropriate blood tests.

Two gynaecological problems which are confused with PMS are dysmenorrhoea and the menopause; these are distinctly different problems. The latter is frequently confused in older menstruating women but this can usually be defined by measuring gonadotrophin levels.

Examination

Though the physical examination of the PMS patient will make little contribution to her diagnosis, the importance of opportunistic screening and the exclusion of disorders which may mimic somatic symptoms (i.e. pelvic pain, abdominal bloatedness) cannot be overstressed. Reassurance that there is no breast, cervical or pelvic cancer is of particular value and of course, patients should not receive hormonal therapy without such an examination.

Definitive test for PMS?

When doubt exists this is usually because there are coincident problems and the patient suffers from secondary PMS. It is now possible to identify what proportion of the disorder is due to the ovarian hormone change by administering a depot preparation of a GnRH agonist analogue such as goserelin for 3 months. There may be an exacerbation of symptoms in the first month of evaluation. These should be ignored. By the third month of amenorrhoea, persisting symptoms cannot be due to PMS. Thus, if no symptoms remain at all her diagnosis is primary PMS. If symptoms persist with equal intensity despite this injection her problem has nothing to do with the ovarian cycle and thus she does not have PMS. The relative cyclical and non-cyclical components of secondary PMS can thus be identified.

TREATMENT

The possibility that PMS symptoms may be no more than an exaggerated response to physiological events of the ovarian cycle does not absolve us from the responsibility of determining the best treatment for these patients.

Currently treatment must be offered in the absence of a specific aetiological explanation and must therefore be empirical with little or no scientific foundation on which to base the techniques used.

Treatment depends on the establishment of the correct diagnosis and classification. If we were to treat the woman who wrongly attributes her non-cyclical psychiatric disease to PMS by means of oestradiol implants, failure would be the expected outcome. If we treated a woman with clear-cut primary PMS with minor tranquillizers again we would not succeed. Treatment should thus be aimed at detecting and treating any underlying psychopathology, increasing the patient's threshold for symptoms, and altering her hormonal status even to the extent of removing her own endogenous cycle; the latter approach is usually by endocrine manipulation.

Treatment of any underlying psychological component should be related directly to its nature; thus severe depression, for example, should be treated by antidepressants. Alteration of a patient's threshold to the cyclical events of the menstrual cycle may be achieved less invasively by psychotherapy, counselling or stress management and less conventional methods like hypnosis and possibly even acupuncture. Improvement in the patient's general health and well-being through diet and exercise has also been claimed to achieve these goals. It is probable that measures like these will reduce mild underlying psychological problems, and raise the patient's tolerance to the challenge of her premenstrual changes. The informal psychotherapeutic effect of discussion, counselling and education should not be overlooked.

Placebo effect

When considering claims for drug efficacy it must be remembered that placebo responses in excess of 90% have been reported in some studies (Table 23.4). For instance in the oestrogen implant study of Magos et al (1986) the placebo response during the placebo implant phase was reported as 94% (see Fig. 23.11). Although the placebo effect is seen throughout the 10 months of this study its importance tends to reduce after a few months. Any study of PMS therapy can only be interpreted if adequate placebo controls are included in the study design.

Table 23.4 Examples of the degree of placebo response during placebo phases of representative studies

Treatment	Response(%)	Reference
Oestrogen implants	94	Magos et al (1986)
Lithium	89	Mattsson & Van Schoultz (1974)
Pyridoxine	70	Williams et al (1985)
Progesterone pessaries	60	Sampson (1979)
Progesterone	57	Smith (1975)
Dydrogesterone	53	Haspels (1980)

The range of therapy

The range of proposed therapeutic regimes has been very wide and varied (Table 23.5). This may be blamed partly on the high but short-lived placebo effect in that an apparantly good response is readily observed on most therapy; this leads to enthusiastic and optimistic claims for the regimens employed. Secondly, the lack of long-term benefit leads to the quest for new methods. The range of possibilities includes non-drug, non-hormonal and hormonal methods.

Some of the commonly used agents and methods are discussed.

Table 23.5 Range of treatment approaches for PMS for which success has been claimed

Non-drug	Non-hormonal	Hormonal
Rest	Pyridoxine	Progestogens
Isolation	Essential fatty acids	Progesterone
Psychotherapy	Vitamins	Oral contraception
Education	Diuretics	Testosterone
Yoga	Aldosterone	Danazol
Self-help groups	antagonists	Bromocriptine
Counselling	Clonidine	Hormone implants
Intravaginal electrical	Non-steroidal anti-inflammatories	GnRH analogues
stimulation	Beta-blockers	
Diet	Vitamins	
Music therapy	Music therapy	
Hypnosis	Zinc	
Homeopathy	Tranquillizers	
Acupuncture	Antidepressants	
Stress management	Phenobarbitone	
Nutritional	Lithium	
Manipulation	Immune complexes	
Salt restriction	Antifungals	
Irradiation of ovaries	Naltrexone	
Hysterectomy		
Oophorectomy		

Vitamin B_6

Vitamin B_6 is a cofactor in the final stages of neurotransmitter synthesis, particularly of serotonin and dopapamine, from tryptophan. No abnormalities of these neurotransmitters have yet been identified nor, for that matter, of vitamin B_6 levels or its metabolism. However, several therapeutic trials have been conducted, some controlled. The results of these trials are unfortunately contradictory

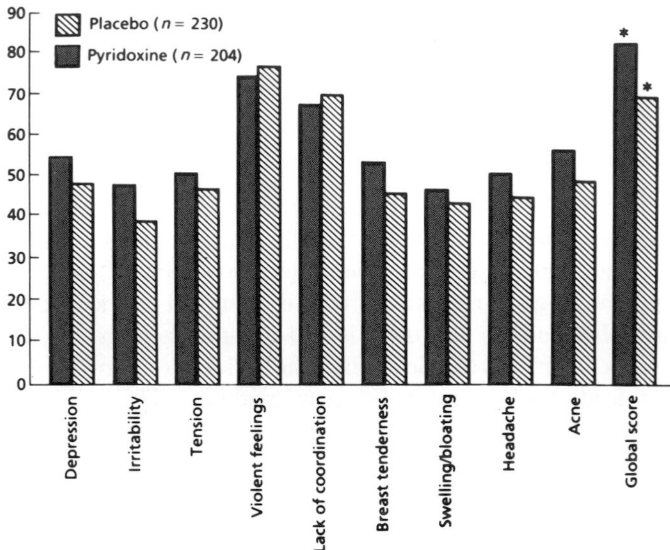

Fig. 23.8 Effect of vitamin B_6 (pyridoxine) and placebo on global symptoms. $^*p < 0.02$. From Williams et al (1985).

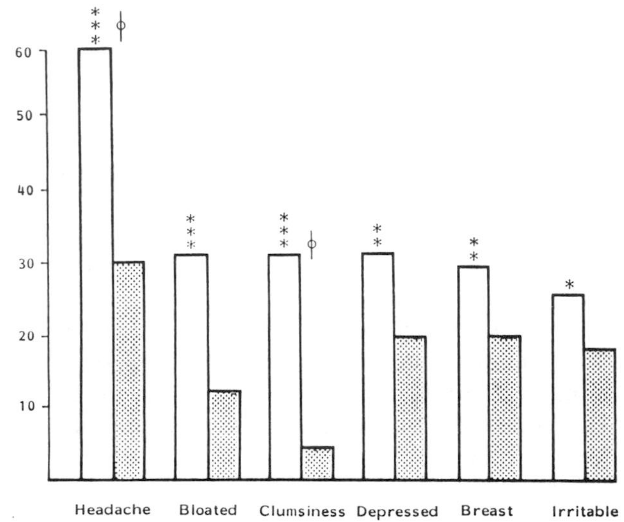

Fig. 23.9 Improvement in PMS symptoms during treatment following supplementation with linoleic and gammalinolenic acid. Although significant improvements are seen when the effect is compared to baseline placebo (*, **, ***) the consistent differences in favour of active therapy (ϕ) are not statistically strong. $^*p < 0.5$; $^{**}p < 0.01$; $^{***}p < 0.001$. significant improvement during treatment over baseline. From Massil et al (1987).

and it is difficult to ascertain how much symptom improvement is due to placebo effect and to what extent there is a true pharmacotherapeutic response. In the trial of Williams et al (1985) — possibly the largest — global symptom assessment showed significant improvement in 82% of patients compared with 70% on placebo (Fig. 23.8). When the effect on individual symptoms was analysed, no clear statistically confirmed improvement could be demonstrated.

There has been some concern about possible side-effects (reversible peripheral neuropathy) at high doses of vitamin B_6. In practice many patients will have self-prescribed vitamin B_6 before consulting their general practitioner or seeing a gynaecologist; if not it is probably safe and worthwhile to try this initially for most patients at a dose of 100 mg daily.

Oil of evening primrose

Oil of evening primrose contains the polyunsaturated essential fatty acids linoleic and gammalinolenic acids. These are the dietary precursors of several prostaglandins, mainly E_2 and E_1. It has been postulated that deficiency of E series prostaglandins and polyunsaturated fatty acids allows an enhanced response to physiological levels of β-endorphin, angiotensin II and the ovarian hormones themselves. Its efficacy in treatment has probably been overstated though there is one recent study demonstrating benefit over placebo for certain symptoms (Fig. 23.9; O'Brien & Massil 1990). It would be reasonable to administer oil of evening primrose at an early stage of therapy; again many patients will have self-prescribed prior to seeking medical treatment. Eight 500 mg capsules are recommended daily; this may be not only difficult to achieve but most patients will find it costly.

Diuretics

The majority of women who experience bloatedness and a feeling of weight increase have no objectively demonstrable premenstrual weight increase, sodium or water retention. Many women who have the separate disorder of cyclical oedema syndrome have developed this as a consequence of inappropriate diuretic therapy for so-called premenstrual water retention. Hence there is a significant risk to diuretic therapy and no rational basis for its use. There is a small group of women who experience true water retention as one of their symptoms and diuretics should be reserved for those with clearly demonstrable oedema or measured weight increase and not those simply with bloatedness. The potential side-effect of cyclical oedema can be minimized by the use of aldosterone antagonists. Spironolactone has been shown to be effective for PMS symptoms, particularly those of swelling (Vellacott & O'Brien 1987).

Hormonal therapy

Oral contraceptive pill

There are no good therapeutic studies of the current lower oestrogen dose preparations nor of the progestogen-only pills. In the majority of studies women who have already been taking higher dose combined pills have been compared with non-pill users. It is thus possible that the inclusion in the control groups of non-reponders and those whose worsening of symptoms caused them to discontinue the pill would bias the results in the pill's favour. With this proviso it would seem that pill users report less PMS than those using barrier contraception. In early studies of the higher dose preparations Cullberg (1972) reported that oestrogen-dominant pills exacerbated symptoms whilst those which were strongly progestogenic were associated with a reduction in PMS. One study of younger women however showed a worsening of symptoms.

The response in an individual woman cannot be predicted. In an overall review of effects on PMS of the combined oral contraceptive pill Smith (1975) concluded that any of the following results could be expected:

1. Complete relief of symptoms.
2. Continuation of symptoms but limited to 1 or 2 days premenstrually.
3 Intolerance of the pill.
4. No change.

It is thus worth trying empirically and assessing the effect of the pill in suitable women. No evaluation of the continuous combined pill has yet been conducted though we will see later the logic of such an approach.

Progestogens

Dydrogesterone and many other progestogens have been advocated on the basis of the unproven progesterone deficiency theory for PMS. There are many uncontrolled studies of these preparations. One double-blind controlled study of dydrogesterone suggested non-significant trends in favour of the active drug. Global retrospective assessment of symptoms appeared to show a superior effect over placebo. A later study by Dennerstein et al, (1986) failed to demonstrate such improvement.

Progesterone

Progesterone pessaries, injections and the oral micronized form have also been advocated as replacement of so-called progesterone deficiency. To date no study of progesterone pessaries has demonstrated benefit superior to that of placebo (Fig. 23.10). At least 10 such studies have now been conducted. The data of Dennerstein et al (1985) suggest that oral micronized progesterone is more effective than identical placebo; however, this conclusion has been criticized on statistical grounds.

Progesterone and progestogen continue to be prescribed because of the large number of anecdotal reports of efficacy; if these hormones are effective it is unlikely that progesterone deficiency is being corrected but more likely that the endogenous endocrine milieu is being disturbed. It is also possible that progesterone is acting as a minor tranqillizer.

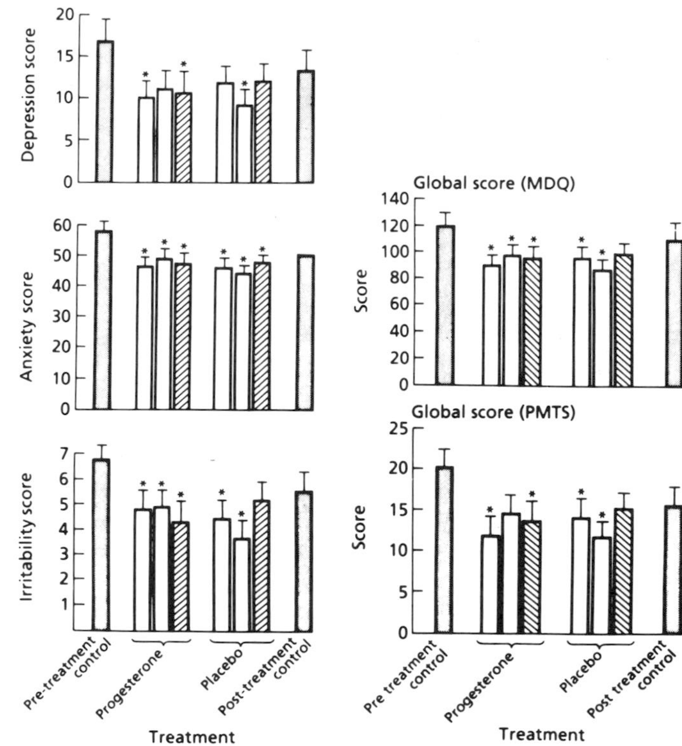

Fig. 23.10 Effect of progesterone suppositories and placebo on irritability, depression, anxiety and global score over 3 months. Although improvement is significant compared with baseline control for both placebo and active therapy, no differences are demonstrable between the two treatments. No abatement of placebo or enhancement of progesterone effect is seen with time. MDQ = Menstrual distress questionnaire; PMTS = premenstrual tension symptoms. From Maddocks et al (1986) with permission.

Bromocriptine

Although prolactin had originally been considered a potential candidate as the pathogenic agent in PMS no studies have demonstrated differences in PMS nor have cyclical changes through the cycle been clearly shown. Several workers have assessed the efficacy of bromocriptine in PMS treatment. The data of the study by Andersen and colleagues (1977) encompass the relevant conclusions to be drawn. Bromocriptine 5 mg daily from day 10 to 26 of the menstrual cycle effectively relieves cyclical breast symptoms but has little effect on the remaining symptoms of PMS.

Suppression of the menstrual cycle

If PMS is the direct or indirect consequence of the ovarian endocrine cycle then elimination of this cycle should confirm this and also offer the ideal means of treatment. In secondary PMS, the cyclical component of what is of course a more complicated phenomenon will be excluded. There are several ways of achieving this. Frank (1931) advocated irradiation of the ovaries and claimed a marked benefit. Oophorectomy (but of course not hysterectomy alone) cures the ovarian component of PMS. Less invasive means of suppressing the endogenous ovarian cycle include the use of continuous combined oral contraception, continuous progestagen, danazol, oestradiol implants and trancutaneous patches, and GnRH analogues. The first two of these have not been formally studied.

Danazol

Mansel & Wisbey (1980) first assessed the effect of danazol on PMS symptoms as part of a study primarily aimed at treating breast pain. No convincing benefit was demonstrated except for the good response for breast symptoms. Subsequent studies have demonstrated benefit for several symptoms at doses of 400, 200 and 100 mg daily (Table 23.6). At 400 mg cycle suppression is usual. In view of the higher incidence of side-effects normally demonstrated with danazol, the lower dose would seem more appropriate but such a dose does not normally suppress the cycle. Serious side-effects of masculinization are largely avoided at both of these doses; the risk of masculinization of a female fetus remains a possibility should pregnancy arise and appropriate mechanical contraception should be advised.

Oestradiol implants and transdermal patches

Suppression of the endogenous ovarian cycle can be achieved by administration of an implant of oestradiol or by use of transdermal patches. Results of studies demonstrating the effect of the oestrogen patches on PMS symptoms have not yet been published, although they do appear to suppress ovulation. One well conducted placebo-controlled study of oestradiol implant therapy has been published by Magos et al (1986; Fig. 23.11). In all, 68 women with clear-cut PMS were assessed in a double-blind parallel group study; 33 received an implant of 100 mg oestradiol plus 5 mg norethisterone for 7 days of the cycle. A total of 35 women received placebos for both implant and norethisterone. Treatment showed high response rates in both groups. The effect of the placebo treatment fell off

Table 23.6 Symptom score after 3 months' treatment with varying doses of danazol compared with placebo

Symptom	Treatment group	Pretrial	After 3 months
Breast pain	Placebo	22.3	12.0
	Danazol		
	100 mg	11.3	0.0 *
	200 mg	18.8	0.0 *
	400 mg	22.5	0.0 *
Irritability	Placebo	21.5	12.0
	Danazol		
	100 mg	18.0	8.0
	200 mg	19.3	0.0 *
	400 mg	17.0	4.0 *
Anxiety	Placebo	14.8	4.0
	Danazol		
	100 mg	1.3	0.0 *
	200 mg	13.3	0.0
	400 mg		
Lethargy	Placebo	23.0	9.0
	Danazol		
	100 mg	14.8	3.0 *
	200 mg	19.3	0.0
	400 mg	14.5	2.0

* $p < 0.05$, Significance of difference between danazol group and placebo. Adapted from Watts et al (1987) with permission.

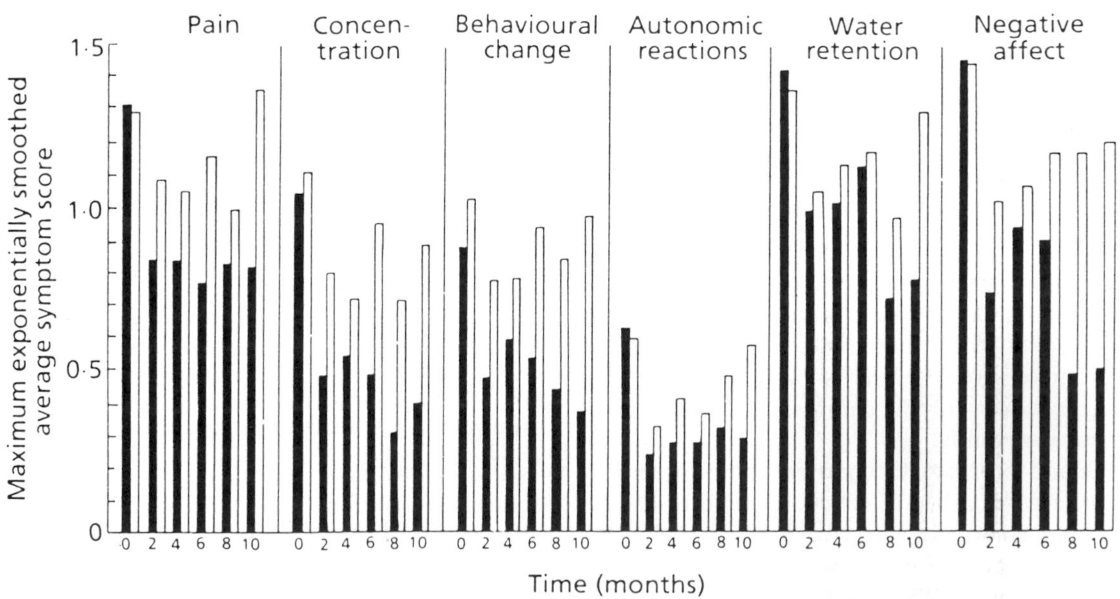

Fig. 23.11 Effect of oestradiol implant and norethisterone (■) on PMS symptoms compared to placebo (□). The marked placebo effect is seen initially but the continued response is only seen during active therapy. From Magos et al (1986) with permission.

after a short interval whilst that of the active implant and norethisterone was maintained throughout the study.

These data are convincing but would have been more scientifically valid if there had been a crossover in the study design and if active implant plus norethisterone had been compared with placebo implant plus active norethisterone; as it stands the norethisterone could have been the active agent, though this seems unlikely.

In practice a significant number of patients withdraw from treatment because of the regeneration of symptoms by the progestagen. Although many patients would be extremely well controlled on oestrogen alone, this is not feasible in the presence of the uterus because of the substantial risk of endometrial hyperplasia and adenocarcinoma. Testosterone implants have also been given when diminished libido is a significant symptom. Most gynaecologists would reserve oestradiol implants for severe cases and in those for whom the menopause is imminent.

GnRH analogues

Agonist analogues of GnRH have been used in several clinical disorders where it is necessary to suppress the gonadal production of steroids. These include prostatic and breast cancer, endometriosis, fibroids and recently their value in PMS has been assessed. In early trials an unclear picture emerged which was probably related to incomplete suppression of ovarian function. Muse et al (1984) demonstrated a clearer result. Daily subcutaneous GnRH 50 μg or placebo was administered for 6 months. This resulted in adequate suppression of the cycle, and elimination of symptoms on active therapy but not placebo (Fig. 23.6). Similar results have been obtained using monthly depot preparations of goserelin.

GnRH analogues have been successfully used in the treatment of endometriosis. When endometriosis is treated with suppression of the menstrual cycle by GnRH analogues the disease and symptoms regress. On discontinuation, menstruation returns, without recurrence of the endometriosis — fortunate though this is, it remains uncertain why. It was hoped that a parallel situation would be seen with PMS and we have recently tested this. Unfortunately, symptoms return with ovarian function in all patients; thus GnRH analogues do not provide a permanent 'cure' for PMS, and this is not surprising. To provide effective therapy the analogue treatment would need to be given indefinitely. Such treatment will be precluded by the genesis of menopausal side-effects, the most worrying of which is osteoporosis. It has been well documented (see Chapter 30) that significant trabecular bone loss occurs after only 6 months of analogue treatment. Whether GnRH analogue plus oestrogen replacement has anything to offer over and above oestrogen replacement alone remains to be determined.

The use of GnRH analogues may have a role in PMS. Elimination of the cycle in this way:

1. allows us to determine to what degree the symptoms are of ovarian endocrine origin;
2. pinpoints which extremely severe patients would benefit from oophorectomy;
3. offers short-term therapy of 6 months in particular circumstances;
4. may be useful for women in whom oestrogens are contraindicated and who are shortly to reach the menopause.

Oophorectomy

There are gynaecologists who will still perform hysterectomy for PMS although hysterectomy alone does not eliminate ovarian function, and thus symptoms persist. There can be few gynaecologists performing oophorectomy without simultaneous hysterectomy. Hysterectomy and bilateral oophorectomy may occasionally be indicated in the most severe cases. It is advisable to evaluate the potential likelihood of success during 3 months' therapy with GnRH analogues. Following hysterectomy, oestrogen without progestagen can be administered without the fear of gestagen-induced PMS.

CONCLUSIONS

If we were to treat PMS only with techniques which have conclusively been shown to be superior to placebo then we would have little to offer PMS patients. Any treatment we

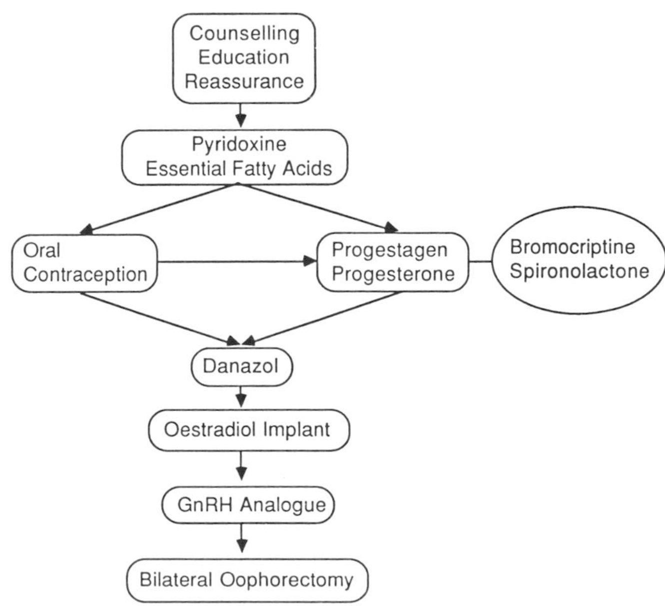

Fig. 23.12 Synopsis of treatment approach to PMS.

do offer will scientifically contradict the majority of statements we have already made and will be essentially empirical (Fig. 23.12). All women with PMS cannot be treated with oestrogen implants, GnRH analogues or oophorectomy. The simpler techniques should be employed initially and referral for gynaecological evaluation should be made after such avenues have been explored. Priority can then be given to patients with true gynaecological problems and those with PMS of such severity to warrant major intervention.

In the absence of a clearly identifiable endocrine abnormality it is possible that PMS should not be considered a gynaecological disorder as it is likely that it represents a psychological or biological predisposition to the normal physiological endocrine events of the ovarian cycle. Although women would prefer to label their problem as gynaecological rather than psychiatric or psychological, gynaecologists, who are often accused of being unsympathetic to women's needs, should not be coerced into dealing with a problem which is not necessarily gynaecological and frequently has a large psychological component.

PMS is a disorder which should be dealt with primarily by the general practitioner, family planning and women's health care units or, for patients with severe secondary PMS, by the psychiatrist. If treatment cannot be achieved by these measures then the gynaecologist may be called upon to manipulate or remove what is possibly normal ovarian function either endocrinologically or surgically.

KEY POINTS

1. Premenstrual syndrome is a disorder of unknown aetiology.
2. The prevalence of premenstrual syndrome has been reported as ranging from 5% to 95% which probably reflects the impression of diagnostic criteria rather than any biological factor.
3. The diagnosis is often confusing and many other disorders may be confirmed.
4. The symptoms are numerous, producing social, familial or occupational disruption, and should have occurred in at least four of the six previous cycles.
5. There are no objective means of identifying or quantifying PMS and for practical purposes dependence is placed on the history, questionnaires and the exclusion of other specific disorders.
6. 5% of women are completely symptom-free premenstrually.
7. All but 5% of women experience at least one premenstrual symptom but many of these are tolerated with no interference to that woman's normal functioning.
8. Primary PMS is a disorder of non-specific somatic psychological or behavioural symptoms recurring in the premenstrual phase and being resolved completely by the end of menstruation.
9. Secondary PMS is a disorder of non-specific somatic psychological or behavioural symptoms recurring in the premenstrual phase of the menstrual cycle, improving but not completely resolving by the end of menstruation.
10. It is implied that in secondary PMS there is an underlying psychological disorder.
11. Treatment is offered in the absence of a specific aetiological explanation and must therefore be empirical and depends upon the establishment of the correct diagnosis.
12. The placebo response is high.
13. If PMS is the direct or indirect consequence of the ovarian endocrine cycle, then elimination of this cycle should confirm the diagnosis and also offer the ideal means of treatment.

REFERENCES

Andersen A N, Larsen J G, Steenstrup O R, Svendstrup B, Nielsen J 1977 Effect of bromocriptine on the premenstrual syndrome. A double-blind clinical trial. British Journal of Obstetrics and Gynaecology 84: 370–374

Brush M G, Watson S J, Horrobin D F, Manku M S 1984 Abnormal essential fatty acid levels in plasma of women with premenstrual syndrome. American Journal of Obstetrics and Gynecology 150: 363–366

Chuong C J, 1988 Clinical trial of naltrexone in premenstrual syndrome. Obstetrics and Gynecology 72: 332–336

Chuong C J, Coulam C B, Kao P C, Bergstal E J 1985 Neuropeptide levels in premenstrual syndrome. Fertility and Sterility 44: 760–765

Cullberg J 1972 Mood changes and menstrual symptoms with different gestagen/oestrogen combinations. Acta Psychiatrica Scandivica 236 (suppl): 1–86

Dalton K 1977 The premenstrual syndrome and progesterone therapy. Heinemann, London

Dennerstein L, Spencer-Gardner C, Gotts G, Brown J B, Smith M A, Burrows G D 1985 Progesterone and the premenstrual syndrome: a double-blind crossover trial. British Medical Journal 290: 1617–1621

Dennerstein L, Morse C, Gotts G et al 1986 The treatment of premenstrual syndrome. A double-blind trial of dydrogesterone. Journal of Affective Disorders 11: 199–205

Faratian B, Gaspar A, O'Brien PMS, Filshie G M, Johnson I R, Prescott P 1984 Premenstrual syndrome: weight, abdominal size and perceived body image. American Journal of Obstetrics and Gynecology 150: 200–204

Frank R T 1931 The hormonal causes of premenstrual tension. Archives of Neurology and Psychiatry 26: 1053–1057.

Goldberg D P, Hillier V 1979 A scaled version of the general health questionnaire. Psychological Medicine 9: 139–145

Hammarback S, Backstrom T, Holst J, von Schoulltz B, Lyrenas S 1985 Cyclical mood changes as in the premenstrual tension syndrome using sequential oestrogen-progestagen postmenopausal replacement therapy. Acta Obstetricia et Gyneocologica Scandinav. 64: 393–397

Haspels A A 1980 A double-blind, placebo-controlled, multicentre study of the efficacy of dydrogesterone (Duphaston). In: van Keep P A, Utian W H (eds) The premenstrual syndrome. MTP Press, Lancaster, pp 81–92

Hussain S Y, O'Brien P M S, De Souza V F, Okonofua F, Dandona P 1990 Reduced atrial natriuretic peptide concentrations in premenstrual syndrome. British Journal of Obstetrics and Gynaecology 97: 397–401

Maddocks S, Hahn P, Moller F, Reid R L 1986 A double-blind placebo-controlled trial of progesterone vaginal suppositories in the treatment of premenstrual syndrome. American Journal of Obstetrics and Gynecology 154: 573–581

Magos A L, Brincat M, Studd J W W 1986 Treatment of premenstrual syndrome by subcutaneous oestradiol implants and cyclical oral norethisterone: placebo controlled study. British Medical Journal 292: 1629–1633

Mansel R E, Wisbey 1980 The effect of gonadotrophin suppression by danazol on symptomatic breast disease. British Journal of Surgery 67: 827

Massil H, Brush M G, O'Brien P M S 1987 A double-blind trial of evening primrose oil in premenstrual syndrome. Proceedings 2nd International Symposium on PMS. Kiawah Island Abstract 47

Mattsson B, Van Schoultz B 1974 A comparison between lithium, placebo and a diuretic in premenstrual tension. Acta Psychiatrica Scandinavica 255 (suppl): 75–84

Moos R 1985 Premenstrual symptoms: a manual and overview of research with the menstrual distress questionnaire. Dept of Psychiatry and Behavioral Sciences, Stanford University School of Medicine, Palo Alto, CA 94304

Muse K, Cetel N, Futterman L, Yen S 1984 The premenstrual syndrome. Effects of 'medical ovariectomy'. New England Journal of Medicine 311: 1345–1349

O'Brien P M S 1987 Premenstrual syndrome. Blackwell Scientific Publications, Oxford

O'Brien P M S, Massil H 1990 Premenstrual syndrome: clinical studies on essential fatty acids. In: Horrobin D F (ed) Omega-6-essential fatty acids: pathology and roles in clinical medicine. Wiley/Liss, New York, pp 523–545

O'Brien P M S, Symonds E M 1982 Prolactin levels in the premenstrual syndrome. British Journal of Obstetrics and Gynaecology 89: 306–308

Sampson G 1979 Premenstrual syndrome. A double-blind controlled trial of progesterone and placebo. British Journal of Psychiatry 135: 209–215

Smith S L 1975 Mood and the menstrual cycle. In: Sachar E J (ed) Topics in psychoendocrinology. Grune & Stratton, New York, pp 19–58

Steiner M, Haskett R F, Carroll B J 1980 Premenstrual tension syndrome: the development of research diagnostic criteria and new rating scales. Acta Psychiatrica Scandinavica 62: 177–190

Vellacott I D, O'Brien P M S 1987 Effects of spironolactone on premenstrual symptoms. Journal of Reproductive Medicine 32: 429–434

Wald A, Van Thiel D H, Hoechsletter I et al 1981 Gastrointestinal transit: the effect of the menstrual cycle. Gastroenterology 80: 1497–1500

Watts J F, Butt W R, Logan Edwards R 1987 A clinical trial using danazol for the treatment of premenstrual tension. British Journal of Obstetrics and Gynaecology 94: 30–34

Wehrenberg W B, Wardlaw S L, Franz A G, Ferin M 1982 β-endorphin in hypophyseal-portal blood: variations throughout the menstrual cycle. Endocrinology 111: 879–881

Williams M J, Harris R I, Dean B C 1985 Controlled trial of pyridoxine in the premenstrual syndrome. Journal of International Medical Research 13: 174–179

24. The menopause

J. W. W. Studd R. Baber

INTRODUCTION

The menopause, occurring on average at the age of 51, is a normal event but it leads to much pathology in excess of that of the normal ageing process. With increased longevity women will now spend a third of their lives in the postmenopausal state of oestrogen deficiency attendant to many long-term symptomatic and metabolic complications. These can largely be prevented by oestrogen replacement therapy which reduces the incidence of osteoporosis, heart attacks, strokes and generally improves the well-being and lifespan of women. It may be the most important development in preventive medicine in the western world for half a century. The tragedy is that less than 10% of women at risk receive this therapy in the UK.

Menopause, derived from the Greek *menos* (month) and *pause* (to stop), refers to the last menstrual period and is generally considered to have occurred after 1 year of amenorrhoea. The climacteric, *klima* (the ladder) is that period of time around the menopause when ovarian function is gradually compromised. Clinically this is the more important event because during this time, periods are often erratic and infrequent, fertility is impaired, menopausal symptoms begin to appear being at their most severe before the periods cease, and the menopause lasts for many years producing the degenerations of prolonged oestrogen deficiency.

The average age of the menopause has not changed for centuries. Aristotle (third century BC), Paulus Aeginata (seventh century AD) and Gilbertus Anglicus (13th century AD) all quote an age of 50 for the menopause. The age of the menopause seems unrelated to socioeconomic factors, race, weight or height although severe malnutrition or cigarette smoking may result in an earlier onset.

The real clinical importance of the menopause today lies in the increasing longevity of 20th century woman. At the time of the Roman Empire the average life expectancy of women was only 23 years whilst from the Middle Ages until the late 19th century only some 30% of women survived to experience the menopause. Today, with the average life expectancy of women approaching 80 years there are 10 million postmenopausal women in the UK and 40 million in the USA. They constitute 20% of the population who will live more than a third of their lives in the endocrinopathy of the postmenopause. The responsibilities and the logistics for treating these patients are considerable.

PATHOPHYSIOLOGY

The ageing of the ovary begins even before birth when a progressive decline in the number of primordial follicles commences. The percentage of growing follicles increases substantially at puberty, is maintained throughout reproductive life and declines in the climacteric period.

Some 10 years before the menopause hypothalamic pituitary activity increases in response to an increased resistance of ovarian follicles and decreased follicular hormone production. This increased activity is manifested by rising plasma levels of follicle-stimulating hormone (FSH) and later, luteinizing hormone (LH). As the menopause draws nearer anovulation and luteal inadequacy become more common resulting in deficient luteal progesterone production and continuing unopposed oestrogen secretion which frequently causes dysfunctional uterine bleeding and endometrial hyperplasia. Finally, ovarian failure occurs, ovarian follicular development ceases, serum oestradiol levels decline and menstruation stops. The ovarian stroma remains active and, with the adrenal cortex, continues to produce some androstenedione and testosterone. The major postmenopausal oestrogen is oestrone, produced by extraglandular conversion of adrenal androgens in peripheral adipose tissue. The rate of production is thus partly dependent on the obesity of the woman.

Consequences of ovarian failure

The major clinical consequences of the climacteric may be attributed to the oestrogen deficiency that follows ovarian failure. There are also frequent psychiatric and environmental components in the symptoms of a 50-year-old woman which should not be obscured or forgotten in any justifiable enthusiasm for oestrogen replacement therapy.

The 'menopausal syndrome' refers to a group of physical and psychological symptoms commonly experienced in the climacteric period (Table 24.1) due to oestrogen deficiency, but as they often predate the menopause, they are also a result of relative oestrogen deficiency as well as to fluctuating levels of ovarian hormones. The symptoms are varied, insidious and can frequently be misdiagnosed as endogenous depression, migraine or general debility. However, vasomotor symptoms and vaginal dryness in association with depression, tiredness, and headaches of recent onset are characteristic enough to enable a confident diagnosis to be made although these may not be the initial presenting symptoms or the most distressing symptoms.

The major long-term sequelae of the menopause include the development of adverse changes in blood lipoprotein concentrations, the generalized atrophy of connective tissues and the progressive reduction in bone mass.

Table 24.1 Frequency of climacteric symptoms in women aged 45–54 years

Complaint	Percentage of women
Irritability	92%
Lethargy	88%
Depression	78%
Flushes and night sweats	75%
Headaches	71%
Forgetfulness	64%
Weight gain	61%
Insomnia	51%
Joint and muscle pain	48%
Palpitations	44%
Crying spells	42%
Constipation	37%
Dysuria	20%
Decreased libido	20%

Short-term symptoms

The characteristic symptoms of oestrogen deficiency include hot flushes, night sweats, headaches, loss of energy and depression. Although they are to some extent self-limiting they can last for more than 10 years. Women frequently speak of a time when they will be 'through the menopause', presumably meaning that these symptoms will have ceased; they fail to recognize that the duration of oestrogen deficiency lasts for as long as life. It equally confusing that these symptoms are often at their worst before the cessation of periods, hence the diagnosis may be delayed or missed completely.

Vasomotor symptoms

The hot flush is well recognized as the most characteristic manifestation of the climacteric. The earliest reference to it comes from the *Ebers Papyrii*, a series of Egyptian texts dated circa 1500 BC. The first medical reference by a physician is probably from Tyler-Smith in 1849 who believed that hot flushes were cases of pathological blushing and supported the view of the toxaemic effect of retained menstrual fluid, thus providing a rationale for the use of leeches as a form of therapy. The hot flushes and night sweats of vasomotor instability occur in some 75% of women. They may be more abrupt and more severe in women whose menopause is induced suddenly, by surgery or radiotherapy. In most women they persist for more than a year, and in 25% of cases they may still be present after 5 years.

Hot flushes may occur at any time of day or night and can be precipitated by a variety of common situations such as sleeping, working, recreation, housework or stress. Prodromal symptoms are common although often difficult for women to describe. Flushes usually begin in the face, neck, head or chest. The initial focal point may be very specific such as the earlobe, forehead or breasts. Subsequent spread is then in any direction and may last from a few seconds to an hour and is extremely variable in frequency and severity. Hot flushes may be associated with episodes of sweating, elevation of skin temperature, irritability, lethargy, insomnia and chronic tiredness. Successful treatment of hot flushes will usually relieve associated symptoms of exhaustion and depression.

The aetiology of the hot flush remains unclear. Oestrogen deficiency seems certain to be involved but a primary role for raised gonadotrophins seems unlikely because hot flushes occur with great severity in women who have undergone hypophysectomy or who have very low plasma FSH levels following treatment with LH-releasing hormone (LHRH) agonists. All the major sex steroids, in-

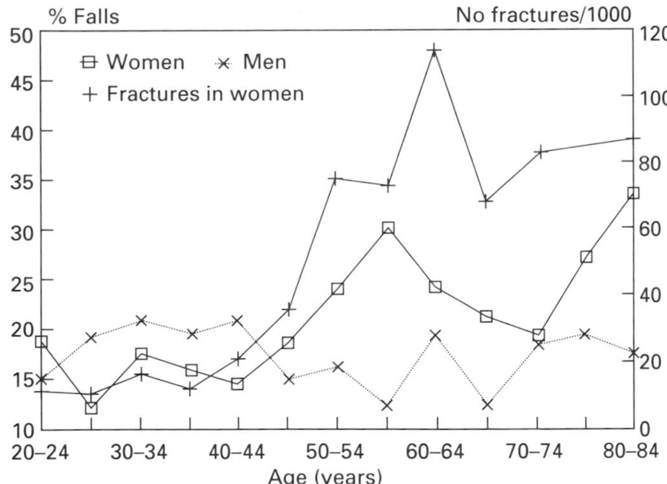

Fig. 24.1 Proportion of women and men reporting falls and the age-specific incidence of distal fracture of the forearm in women. Adapted from Winner et al (1989).

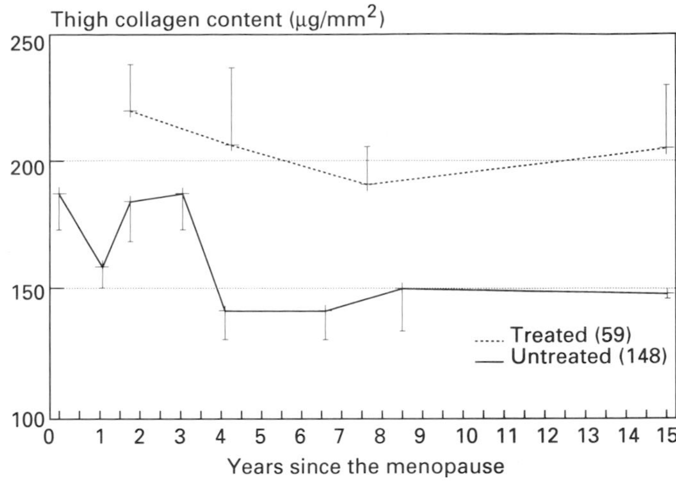

Fig. 24.2 Thigh collagen content after the menopause in 148 untreated women and 59 women treated with oestrogen replacement therapy for over 2 years. Adapted from Brincat et al (1985).

cluding androgens and progesterone, seem to be involved in the aetiology of this peripheral vasomotor instability. Flushes can be severe in orchidectomized men and may be relieved in these men by testosterone replacement therapy.

Hot flushes are not isolated events but are related to the poor vascular control which occurs in hypo-oestrogenic women regardless of whether or not flushes are present. They have particular relevance in older women where the associated insomnia, lethargy and giddiness may lead to falling attacks with the disastrous consequence of femoral neck fracture in osteoporotic women. It seems likely that the giddiness of vasomotor instability is a reason why falls occur more commonly in 60-year-old women than men of the same age (Fig. 24.1). Removal of this locomotor instability by oestrogen therapy should therefore reduce the number of falls and fractures in women with hitherto undiagnosed postmenopausal osteoporosis.

End-organ atrophy

The oestrogen deficiency of the menopause leads to atrophic changes and reduced blood flow in the genital tract and urethra. Prior to oestrogen therapy the blood flow in the postmenopausal woman is 15% of the premenopausal woman but rises fourfold after oestrogen therapy. This relative ischaemia is related to the atrophic changes which occur in the genital tract such as thin skin, sparse hair, introital narrowing and vaginal shortening and dryness. There is reduced elasticity of tissues and diminished vaginal and cervical secretion. Loss of muscle tone leads to pelvic relaxation, uterine descent and anatomical changes around the urethra and bladder neck. The consequences of these changes are increasing dyspareunia and apareunia, genital tract trauma, loss of libido, voiding difficulties, dysuria, urinary frequency, urgency and incontinence. Oestrogen replacement therapy will lead to alleviation of many of these symptoms.

There are other widespread atrophic changes in that women often complain of thin dry skin, brittle nails and loss of hair following the menopause. It is wrong to assume that these observations are merely manifestations of female vanity because these subjective changes actually occur due to generalized loss of collagen. This loss of connective tissue causes the thin transluscent inelastic skin of the older woman (Fig. 24.2) and the frequent muscle and joint pain may also have the same aetiology. The role of collagen loss from the bone matrix in the aetiology of postmenopausal osteoporosis may be of fundamental importance.

PSYCHOLOGICAL CHANGES

Anxiety, irritability and depression commonly arise during the climacteric and are usually the group of symptoms which are worse in the few years before periods cease. Although vasomotor and atrophic changes of the menopause are generally and clearly attributed to hormonal changes there is some dispute about the aetiology of these psychological changes which are often perceived to be environmental rather than hormonal in origin.

Montgomery et al (1987) used a standardized method of psychological assessment to demonstrate the high incidence of psychological disease and the benefits of hormone therapy in women attending a menopause clinic. They revealed that 86% of these self-selected patients had clinical psychiatric illness, which is more than would be seen even at psychiatric outpatients! Many patients improve with oestrogen therapy but it is clear that there is a mixture of endogenous, domestic and also hormonal pathogenesis of depression in these patients and that these women request oestrogens in the hope that some more fundamental environmental cause of depression may be helped.

The highest incidence of depression in middle life arises in the perimenopausal period. It may be that it is not only low levels of oestrogens but fluctuating changes in hormone concentrations such as those seen in the cyclical depression of the premenstrual syndrome that predispose to climacteric depression. This may be mediated by interaction between oestrogens and neurotransmitters. Falling oestrogen levels may reduce dopamine receptor sensitivity or reduce available tryptophan for serotonin synthesis, leading to reduced activity of central nervous system transmitters and consequent depression. Other causes of depression may also occur at the time of the menopause. These include loss of reproductive potential, a perceived loss of femininity, marital disenchantment, the 'empty nest' syndrome and career disappointments.

Depression is twice as common in women as in men and, as this difference begins with puberty and is exacerbated postnatally, premenstrually and perimenopausally, it is believed by many to be the result of a deficiency or change in plasma oestradiol levels. The alternative view is that excessive depression in women is related to the middle-aged woman's role in society and not in any way to her gonadal hormones. The sad result of this dispute is that 40% of middle-aged women are taking tranquillizers or antidepressants rather than replacement oestrogens. This results in more depression, drug dependence, dizziness and falling attacks.

Double-blind trials have shown the beneficial effects of oestrogen therapy on psychiatric disturbances but have been criticized for their poor definition of depression status and the use of non-standardized psychological tests. There is an improvement in depression and anxiety in climacteric women using oestrogens which is greater than placebo but this only seems to occur in those women who are pre-menopausal. There is no clear improvement in the post-menopausal woman. It is possible that oestrogens are most effective in the cyclical depression which occurs in the years when severe premenstrual syndrome blends with the worst years of the climacteric as the menopause approaches.

Both libido and lethargy can be improved by the use of oestrogen replacement, often with the addition of testosterone. Loss of libido in this context is characteristically a loss of interest in normal sexual relations in the presence of an otherwise satisfactory marriage and must be distinguished from dyspareunia which is often atrophic in origin and can easily be treated with oestrogens. Loss of libido has many causes of heart, head and hormones but may arise as a systemic consequence of reduced sex hormone production and also as a local effect of oestrogen deprivation on the genital tract.

LONG-TERM CONSEQUENCES

The long-term consequences of ovarian failure carry a high morbidity and represent a huge burden on any country's health care budget. They include an increased risk of cardiovascular disease and a general decrease in connective tissue leading to osteoporosis and disorders of the bladder. These changes also pose a great challenge as oestrogen-dependent pathology can be prevented and perhaps even reversed by appropriate oestrogen therapy.

Cardiovascular disease

Before the menopause ischaemic heart disease is uncommon in women who do not smoke, do not have hypertension, hyperlipidaemia or diabetes. It is five times more common in men than in premenopausal women but once the menopause has occurred the risk of heart disease in women approaches that in men, suggesting a role for the menopause in this changed risk.

The aetiology of heart disease is of course complex and incompletely understood. However, several studies on the effect of premature menopause on the incidence of heart disease have demonstrated an increased risk which is greater the earlier that cessation of ovarian function occurs. A role for oestrogen deficiency in the aetiology of this disease is strongly suggestive. High plasma levels of low density lipoprotein (LDL) concentrations will increase the risk of heart disease whilst increased high density lipoprotein (HDL) concentrations are cardioprotective.

Prior to the menopause serum LDL levels are lower in women than in men, and serum HDL levels are higher. Following the menopause LDL levels in women rise but do not exceed the levels in age-matched men. Oestrogen in premenopausal women has a protective effect on cardiovascular disease, probably mediated through its effect on the HDL:LDL ratio, but oestrogen may work in other ways such as by a direct effect on blood vessels or by stimulating vasodilation via release of vasoactive peptides and increased blood flow. Oestrogen increases the blood flow in all organs so far investigated including the skin, uterus, vulva and kidneys. It would be surprising if myocardial and cerebral blood flow were not also increased.

Most studies have now demonstrated a reduced risk of heart disease and cerebrovascular disease in post-menopausal women receiving hormone replacement therapy (Ross et al 1984). Oestrogen replacement therapy causes an increase in HDL and a lowering of LDL concentrations and it is possible that these effects are marginally greater with oral therapy following the first-pass liver impact.

Synthetic oestrogens such as ethinyloestradiol or mestranol may be associated with an increase in clotting factors, renin substrate and insulin intolerance and are therefore best avoided, particularly in hypertensive women or those who exhibit other cardiac risk factors. Natural oestrogens such as oestrone or oestradiol do not suffer from this disadvantage nor are they associated with any change in carbohydrate metabolism.

Osteoporosis

The osteoporoses are a heterogeneous group of skeletal disorders characterized by a reduction in bone mass to the extent that there is a significantly increased risk of fracture even in the absence of trauma (Table 24.2). It is important to understand that osteoporosis is not due to loss of calcium as osteoporotic bone is normally calcified. There is merely not enough bone tissue remaining in the skeleton and it is very likely to be primarily a disease caused by a decrease in collagen matrix. The most common cause of this disease is the oestrogen deficiency which occurs in postmenopausal women.

Peak bone mass is reached in the fourth decade of life after which there is an age-related bone loss in both sexes. In women there is an acceleration in the rate of bone loss after the menopause so that by the age of 70 a woman has lost 50% of her bone mass whilst a man only loses 25% by the age of 90.

Table 24.2 Risk factors for the development of osteoporosis

Female
Menopausal
Premature menopause
Primary ovarian failure (i.e. Turner's syndrome)
Thin
Anorexia nervosa
Exercise-induced amenorrhoea
Corticosteroid therapy
Smoking
Sedentary lifestyle
Excessive alcohol and caffeine intake
Nulliparity
Prolonged bedrest
Weightlessness

Fractures are significantly more common in women than men after the age of 40, with approximately 8 fractures among older women for every fracture in men. One in four women at the age of 60 will have had one or more osteoporotic fractures, and one in two women aged 70 will have sustained such a fracture; 25% of women who reach the age of 80 will have sustained a hip fracture. Albright et al (1941) first demonstrated a clear relationship between the menopause, oestrogen deficiency and osteoporosis, postulating that reduced gonadal function led to osteoporosis and demonstrating that treatment with stilboestrol could reverse this pattern. Albright et al also recognized the association between thin skin and postmenopausal osteoporosis and suggested that this may be a disease of protein metabolism. It is unfortunate that this most logical of hypothesis has, until recently, been ignored.

Following the menopause there is increased osteoclastic activity leading to greater resorption of bone. Serum calcium levels remain in the normal range as does the concentration of parathyroid hormone. It has been suggested that calcitonin, a peptide hormone released by the parafollicular cells of the thyroid gland, plays a central role in the aetiology of postmenopausal osteoporosis but most workers have not been able to support this.

Recent studies have largely concentrated on calcium and calcium-related hormones ignoring the organic matrix which is largely collagen and makes up 35% of dry defatted bone mass. It has been suggested that the decline in this organic matrix is the primary pathological event leading to osteoporosis. The coexistence of thin skin with postmenopausal osteoporosis, the osteoporosis of anorexia, steroid-induced osteoporosis and osteogenesis imperfecta provides some evidence that postmenopausal osteoporosis is a generalized connective tissue disorder. Increased bone density and an increased collagen content of the skin both occur with oestrogen therapy but it is not yet determined whether there is a demonstrable increase in the collagenous matrix of bone following the long-term administration of oestrogens. This will await the results of several bone biopsy studies.

Clinical implications

The three most common postmenopausal fractures are those of the distal radius, the vertebral body and the femoral neck. Together they have an incidence of 40% in women over the age of 65. Approximately 0.5% of women over the age of 70 will sustain a Colles' fracture each year, which is 12 times the incidence in age-matched men. Vertebral crush fractures typically involve T8–L4 and may occur spontaneously with normal activity. They cause pain, disability, the deformity known as 'dowager's hump' and loss of up to 15 cm in height. The patient's thoracic organs are thus squeezed into a tiny thoracic cage. The bent spine makes it difficult for the woman to raise her head and she may only stop shrinking when her costal margins rest upon the iliac crests. It is a wretched existence.

A fractured hip is a more dramatic and often terminal complication. Approximately 27% of women who suffer a fractured neck of femur will die within a year of their injury and at least a further 20% will be permanently disabled with loss of independence and dignity. The death

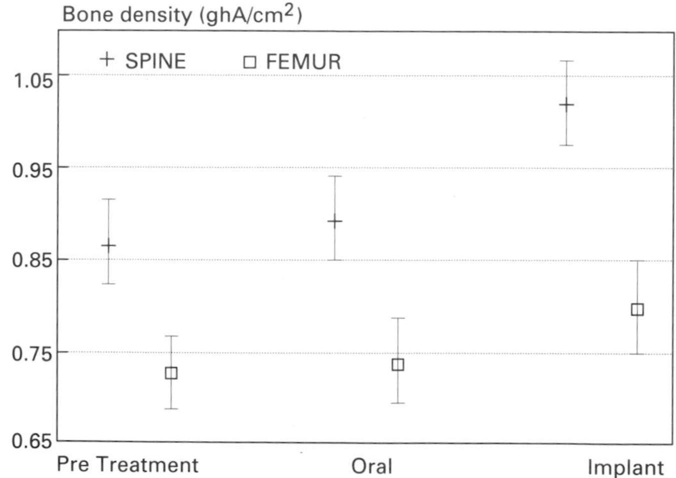

Fig. 24.3 Bone density measurements of the femoral neck and lumbar spine in untreated women, compared with women treated with oral oestrogens or subcutaneous oestradiol implants. Adapted from Savvas et al (1988).

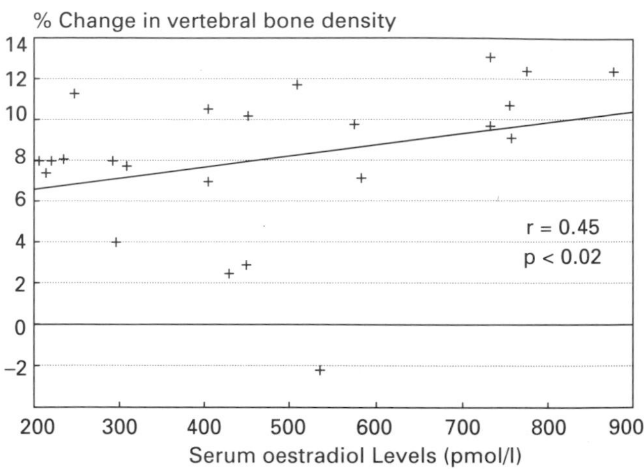

Fig. 24.4 Increase in vertebral bone density compared to serum oestradiol levels in postmenopousal women treated with oestradiol implants. Adapted from Savvas et al (1990).

rate from hip fractures is greater than that of carcinoma of the breast and endometrium combined and the annual cost of non-fatal hip fractures in the UK has been estimated to be about £180 000 000. Postmenopausal osteoporosis is painful, disabling, expensive and preventable.

Many clinical studies have now confirmed Albright's original finding that oestrogen can prevent postmenopausal osteoporosis and epidemiological studies have shown that this will lead to a reduction in fracture incidence. It has been estimated that 5 years of oestrogen therapy will halve a woman's risk of osteoporotic fracture and that as little as 0.625 mg conjugated equine oestrogens is probably sufficient for protection of the skeleton. This dose will not replace bone nor will it suppress the high FSH levels to the premenopausal values (Fig. 24.3). Savvas et al (1988) reported restoration of bone mass with higher serum oestradiol levels achieved by the use of percutaneous oestradiol implants (Fig. 24.4). These data suggest that there is not only a prophylactic role but also a therapeutic role for hormone replacement therapy in the treatment of postmenopausal osteoporosis. Furthermore an increase in bone density occurs if higher oestradiol levels are achieved by percutaneous oestrogen therapy, even in older women with established osteoporosis.

Skin

The skin, one of the largest organs in the body, undergoes changes after the menopause which, although previously attributed to the ageing process, are also due to oestrogen deficiency. Postmenopausal women often complain of thin, dry, flaky skin which bruises easily — symptoms which are rapidly corrected with appropriate oestrogen replacement therapy.

Skin thickness declines after the menopause at the same rate as the decline in bone mass as 30% of skin collagen is lost in the first 10 years following the menopause.

Prospective studies have now shown that skin collagen is lost as a result of ovarian failure, that its loss may be prevented by early use of hormone replacement therapy and that as little as 12 months of oestrogens will restore postmenopausal skin collagen content to its premenopausal level. Both oestrogen and androgen receptors have been identified in the fibroblasts of the skin, the basal cell layer of the epidermis and in osteoblasts, providing evidence for a possible direct action of oestrogen on connective tissues. It is also possible that oestrogens may exert their effects through an intermediary hormone such as growth hormone.

Genitourinary system

The epithelium linings of the vagina and urethra have the highest concentrations of oestrogen receptors in the body and it is no surprise to find atrophic changes in these organs following the menopause. The vaginal skin becomes attenuated and pale as a result of decreased vascularity and may progress to the thin inflamed appearances of atrophic vaginitis. The uterine cervix atrophies and becomes flush with the vaginal vault whilst the uterine body also becomes smaller with a return to the 1:2 corpus:cervix ratio of childhood. The endometrium becomes thin and atrophic although in obese women a proliferative or even hyperplastic endometrium may persist as a result of extraglandular production of oestrogen.

The clinical consequences of genital atrophic changes such as dyspareunia, apareunia and postmenopausal bleeding are well recognized but the effects upon the urinary tract are frequently overlooked. The atrophic bladder and urethra lead to the frequency, dysuria and urgency of the urethral syndrome which may or may not be associated with recurrent infections. The incidence of urinary tract symptoms in women attending menopause clinics is high and many of these women will claim benefit from hormone replacement therapy. It would seem that frequency and urgency cystitis is often helped by oestrogen therapy but stress incontinence is unaffected.

The submucosal vascular plexus and the collagen content of the female urethra contributes to urethral function and is oestrogen-dependent. Postmenopausal women have been shown to have weaker urethral sphincters under stress than perimenopausal women and a correlation has also been demonstrated between urethral pressure measurements and skin collagen content. Increases in urethral pressure have been noted following hormone replacement therapy and may be mediated through an increase in urethral collagen content. Since the oestrogen-dependent increase in skin collagen is maximal in those whose levels are initially lowest it may be that skin collagen measurement or skin thickness could be used as a prognostic index for predicting which patients with urological symptoms might respond to hormone replacement therapy.

Lower urinary tract problems are seemingly increased following the menopause although it is still not clear which symptoms are due to oestrogen deficiency and which are merely age-related. Despite some lack of consensus it remains true that many women will report benefit from hormone replacement therapy and it seems reasonable to employ this therapy as first-line treatment rather than antibiotics, antispasmodics or even repeated urethral dilatations.

Investigation

As public awareness of the consequences of the menopause increases more patients will present to their doctors not merely for relief of short-term symptomatology but also in search of prophylaxis for the long-term consequences. What investigations are required for diagnosis and monitoring of therapy?

The differential diagnosis of climacteric disorders includes premenstrual syndrome, which is more common in the fourth decade of life, depression, migraine and other conditions associated with flushing and sweating such as phaeochromocytoma, carcinoid disease and thyroid disease. These latter all cause additional symptoms and biochemical abnormalities which should make their diagnosis obvious.

The triad of diagnostic features of the menopause are typical symptomatology, amenorrhoea of 12 months' duration and an elevated serum FSH level above 15 iu/l. The diagnosis should usually be apparent by history alone and plasma FSH and oestradiol levels should not often be required for routine clinical diagnosis. Such tests are helpful in problem cases, assessing hysterectomized patients with residual ovaries, those in whom a premature menopause is suspected and to distinguish between climacteric depression that should respond to oestrogen therapy and the depression which needs the opinion of a psychiatrist.

It is important to attempt to establish whether psychological disturbances are due to oestrogen deficiency or result from coincidental social, domestic or economic crises. When diagnosis proves difficult, biochemical tests may be appropriate as high oestrogen levels and low gonadotrophin levels exclude ovarian failure although they do not exclude severe premenstrual syndrome which frequently responds dramatically to oestrogens.

Climacteric depression responds rapidly and well to hormone replacement therapy and therefore if despite this therapy the woman has not responded, it may be assumed that her psychological symptoms are not due to sex hormone imbalance and she would probably be better helped by a psychiatrist.

The monitoring of patients receiving oestrogen therapy usually requires no more than the necessary annual screening of middle-aged women. This would include assessment of blood pressure, breast palpation, mammography, pelvic examination and cervical cytology. The climacteric is usually an easy diagnosis to make and the treatment is straightforward, cheap and safe. It is, therefore, a mistake to insist on intensive screening and monitoring as this imposes expensive obstacles in the way of the patient and the therapy. Is there any justification for pretreatment and annual biochemical and hormonal profiles, endometrial biopsies, or pelvic ultrasound? These have all been recommended but have a commercial ring rather than one of proven medical worth.

Is there a place for bone densitometry or computerized tomography as a routine screening tool? The Royal College of Physicians have made such a recommendation but this is premature. Such investigations are clearly important for research and in patients with suspected or established osteoporosis in order to assess the effectiveness of any treatment. However, women are more than a mere skeleton and even in the presence of a good bone density long-term oestrogen replacement therapy is probably indicated for other aspects of preventive medicine.

Routine pretreatment endometrial biopsy of menopausal patients is inappropriate and such an investigation is only relevant in patients receiving hormone replacement therapy if they experience bleeding other than their regular withdrawal bleed or if they are having an inadequate duration of monthly progestogens. Endometrial cytology has been suggested as a simple means of monitoring the endometrium but was found to be unhelpful in a large study assessing the whole range of histological changes.

Cervical cytological screening programmes established over the past 20 years have been considered effective in reducing both the incidence and mortality of invasive carcinoma of the cervix. Despite the possible low sensitivity of this procedure it remains the most cost-effective technique and all patients attending a menopause clinic for the first time should have a cervical smear performed and then repeated at appropriate intervals.

Carcinoma of the breast affects 1 in 14 women in the UK and 1 in 8 with a family history. The worldwide mortality is 24/100 000 women — a figure unchanged for the past 50 years with approximately 10 000 deaths in the UK each year. Regular mammography after the age of 55 probably reduces mortality from breast cancer by 30%, mainly by increasing the rate of detection of stage 1 disease. In view of the anxiety about breast cancer and oestrogen, whether justified or not, it is important to obtain a baseline mammogram for all menopausal women and for this test to be repeated at regular intervals thereafter.

PREMATURE OVARIAN FAILURE

Premature ovarian failure affects 1% of women under the age of 40 and is thus a relatively common occurrence affecting well over 100 000 women in the UK alone. Its aetiology is often difficult to establish (Table 24.3) but amongst the identifiable causes genetic disorders predominate in those cases which present early and autoimmune disorders are more common in the later-onset presentations.

Table 24.3 The causes of premature ovarian failure

Genetic
Chromosomal
Familial
Metabolic
Immunological
Autoimmune disease
Infection
Environmental
Iatrogenic
Surgical
Chemotherapy
Irradiation
Idiopathic

The diagnosis should always be considered in any woman presenting with a history of primary or secondary amenorrhoea or oligomenorrhoea. Vasomotor disturbances, vaginal dryness, loss of energy and loss of libido also suggest a diagnosis which should be confirmed by an elevated serum level of FSH of above 15 iu/l. An ovarian biopsy is not necessary as the findings will not affect future management and may jeopardize fertility in the young woman who is not menopausal. Women suffering a premature menopause will suffer from an increased risk of cardiovascular disease, cerebrovascular disease and osteoporosis and, because of their age, are more likely to suffer these consequences as they will spend many more years in the postmenopausal state. It is most important that these women are offered oestrogen therapy.

Women with premature menopause may now be able to achieve a pregnancy with ovum donation. Recipients are placed on a hormone replacement regimen of oestrogen and progesterone designed to reproduce the ovarian cycle and prime the endometrium to enable it to receive and implant the embryo. The donor eggs are fertilized by the patient's husband's sperm and the embryo transferred either to the endometrium or into the fallopian tube (Zygote intrafallopian transfer; ZIFT). Excellent results of 27 pregnancies out of 100 ovum donation cycles have been reported (Abdalla et al 1990). This technique offers new hope for a large group of women who were previously unable to conceive and any pregnancy achieved is likely to have a beneficial effect upon the patient's collagen and skeleton.

TREATMENT

Although the majority of women seeking help during the climacteric and postmenopausal years are symptomatic with a clear indication for oestrogen therapy, a number of asymptomatic women will also seek advice to prevent long-term morbidity. Special groups of women to whom oestrogen should be prescribed include those with premature ovarian failure, gonadal dysgenesis or an early iatrogenic menopause as early onset of ovarian function is associated with an early and accelerated increase in the incidence of osteoporosis and ischaemic heart disease.

Treatment of patients without symptoms or risk factors for osteoporosis or arterial disease is currently controversial. Most authorities would favour treatment on the basis that, on current evidence, the benefits far outweigh any disadvantage. Others, particularly physicians, would argue that oestrogens have not yet been used long enough for all potential hazards, particularly malignancies, to become apparent. If hormone replacement therapy prevents hip fractures at 75 but causes breast cancer at 55, there will be no future for it.

Non-hormone treatment

There are many disappointing non-hormonal therapies that have been recommended over the years. Although widely prescribed, hypnotics, sedatives and tranquillizers have not been shown to be capable of relieving symptoms unequivocally due to oestrogen deficiency. Despite this they are frequently prescribed and have been reported in as many as 40% of women attending a menopause clinic. These drugs should best be restricted to women with classical symptoms of an anxiety/depression neurosis and are best withheld from women with suspected climacteric problems until an adequate trial of oestrogen therapy has been implemented.

Clonidine, an alpha-adrenergic agonist has been reported

to be of some benefit in reducing the severity and duration of hot flushes.

A healthy diet and lifestyle are clearly as important after the menopause as before. To be in calcium balance, premenopausal women need 1000 mg of elemental calcium per day; women in the perimenopause require 1200 mg per day and postmenopausal women 1400 mg per day — an amount well above the average daily intake of women in this age group. Dietary correction or calcium supplementation in many women may thus be appropriate and such supplementation has been shown to reduce the daily dosage of oestrogen required to prevent osteoporosis. However, calcium supplementation alone will not prevent or reverse bone loss.

The value of calcitonin in the long-term prevention of osteoporosis remains unproven. An increase in bone mass follows calcitonin therapy but this benefit may be only transient as bone mass declines again after 18 months of treatment.

A sedentary lifestyle can lead to severe bone loss at critical sites. Athletes, cross-country runners and ballet dancers have all been shown to have higher than average bone mass and a slight 0.4% gain in bone mass in postmenopausal women has been described following 1 year of supervised thrice-weekly treadmill walking. Exercise has also been claimed to reduce depression, anxiety and insomnia whilst its benefits on cardiovascular morbidity and mortality are well documented.

Table 24.4 Currently available preparations of natural oestrogens and oestrogen/progestogen combinations suitable for hormone replacement therapy

Route of administration	Drug name	Type of oestrogen
Oral	Hormonin	Oestradiol Oestrone Oestriol
	Questrin Premarin	Oestriol Oestrone Equilin 17 Dihydroequilin
	Progynova	Oestradiol valerate
Vaginal creams	Ovestin Premarin Dienoestrol	Oestriol Oestriol Dienoestrol (synthetic)
Subcutaneous	Oestradiol implants	Oestradiol
Transdermal	Estraderm	Oestradiol
		Type of oestrogen +progestogen
Oral	Menophase	Mestranol + Norethisterone
	Prempak-C	Equilin Oestrone 17 Diydroequilin + Norgestrol
	Cycloprogynova	Oestradiol valerate + Norgestrol
	Trisequens	Oestradiol Oestriol + Norethisterone

Hormonal treatment

Oestrogens

Oestrogen replacement therapy is the logical and appropriate treatment of all climacteric problems caused by ovarian failure. Oestrogen may be administered orally, transvaginally or through the skin as a percutaneous cream or skin patch or as implants (Table 24.4). The pharmacodynamic properties of exogenous oestrogens vary markedly with different routes of administration.

Oral oestrogens

Oral oestrogens are the most widely used and convenient form of treatment. It may not be the best route because the bolus of oestrogen enters directly into the enterohepatic circulation, and the first-pass impact enables the liver to convert one-third of the oestrogen, to oestrone-3-glucoronide and to be excreted in the urine and bile without achieving its desired effects. Thus a ratio of oestrone to oestradiol of 2:1 is achieved with oral therapy whether oestrone or oestradiol is ingested, instead of the physiological ratio of 1:2 that occurs in the premenopausal woman. Oestradiol is the effective oestrogen hence this liver impact explains why oral oestrogens need to be given at higher doses than parenteral oestrogens in order to achieve the same symptomatic relief.

Oral oestrogens cause an increase in sex hormone-binding globulin, cortisol-binding globulin, renin substrate and HDL and a depressant effect on antithrombin III levels. Thus oral oestrogens may be theoretically contraindicated in women with a history of clotting disorders or hypertensive disease. This effect is much more pronounced with synthetic oestrogens which have a greater affinity for oestrogen receptors and a greater resistance to enzymatic conversion. The contemporary view is that ethinyloestradiol and mestranol should not be used for perimenopausal women but it is relevant that a comparison of bioequivalent doses of synthetic and 'natural' oestrogens has not been performed. Ethinyloestradiol has been condemned, rightly or wrongly, because of extrapolation of irrelevant high-dose oral contraceptive data.

Vaginal oestrogen creams

The rate of absorption of oestrogens from the vagina depends partly on the base on which the active ingredient is suspended and partly on the vascularity of the vagina. Vaginal oestrogen creams have long been used to treat atrophic vaginitis by the overcautious on the assumption that they produced a local effect only, but this is not so. Very low doses of vaginal oestrogens do produce significant changes in vaginal cytology without causing a rise in plasma oestrogens but at this dose there is no relief of climacteric symptoms. If a standard daily dose of conjugated oestrogen cream (1.25 mg) is used a plasma level of oestrone and oestradiol higher than that produced by the same dose of oral conjugated oestrogens is found. The plasma level per dose will increase as vascularity improves in response to treatment. These preparations are valuable but should not be used under the misapprehension that they are only effective locally and are, therefore, safe in the few women in whom oestrogens are contraindicated.

Percutaneous oestrogen cream

This mode of delivery is becoming increasingly popular, particularly in continental countries, but unfortunately is not yet available in the UK. The commercial preparations available deliver 3 mg of oestradiol in each daily 5 g applicator of cream. As with other parenteral routes of administration, the liver is bypassed and a physiological oestrone to oestradiol ratio of 1:2 is maintained. Serum oestradiol levels are generally higher than those achieved with oral therapy. Compared with oral oestrogens the serum oestradiol levels rise more slowly, but are maintained for 48 h. Consequently the cream needs to be applied on a daily basis to maintain oestradiol levels. Percutaneous creams have been shown to induce an increase in skin collagen and data are now available which demonstrate that creams are at least as effective in preventing postmenopausal osteoporosis as oral preparations. Although considerable patient motivation is required to use this form of therapy most patients report the cream as easy to use. There are none of the local skin reactions which limit the use of transdermal patches.

Transdermal patches

The ability of the skin to absorb steroids has led to the development of patches using a suitable vehicle which allows penetration through the stratum corneum from which the sex steroid diffuses into the epidermis, papillary dermis and thence to the capillary plexus. The oestradiol transdermal therapeutic system consists of a thin multi-layered unit containing a drug reservoir, a rate-controlled membrane and an adhesive layer.

The patches have surface areas of 5, 10 or 20 cm^2 and administer oestradiol at a controlled rate of 25, 50 or 100 μg/day in vivo. It is claimed that steady-state levels of the drug are obtained if the patches are worn for 72 h and changed twice weekly. The occlusive membrane greatly increases the diffusion of oestradiol through the stratum corneum thus achieving therapeutic efficacy with very low doses of oestradiol. Transdermal oestrogens significantly reduce the incidence of menopausal symptoms, have positive effects on vaginal cytology and do not induce changes in hepatic proteins or in antithrombin III levels and are not associated with changes in urinary calcium:creatinine or hydroxyproline:creatinine ratios. Patches also have a beneficial effect upon bone.

The rapid rise in serum oestradiol levels seen with transdermal patches has also been reported to suppress ovulation; this has been used to treat premenstrual syndrome in the perimenopausal woman (Watson et al 1989). Thus a subsidiary contraceptive role may also be found for this preparation.

Patient acceptability of patches is good as the gastrointestinal side-effects of oral therapy are avoided. There are troublesome skin reactions ranging from hyperaemia to blistering and after a time many women become irritated by the dark rings left behind at the site of the previous patch.

Subcutaneous implants

Subcutaneous implants have been used to treat that climacteric syndrome for 40 years. The technique of insertion is safe and simple and may be performed in outpatient clinics under local anaesthesia. Gonadotrophin levels fall dramatically within 2 weeks and remain suppressed for approximately 6 months if 50 mg oestradiol pellets are used. Oestradiol levels peak at 2–3 months before declining to pretreatment levels after 6 months.

Implants avoid the need for daily patient compliance, give good symptomatic relief, and have few side-effects. Testosterone pellets (100 mg) may be added to oestrogen implants and provide patients with greater relief of the symptoms of lethargy and loss of libido. Implants of oestrogen and testosterone will result in higher bone densities than in a comparable group of postmenopausal women receiving oral therapy and vertebral bone density may be increased in postmenopausal osteoporotic women receiving this therapy by up to 9% in 1 year. It is probable that the higher serum oestradiol levels achieved with implant therapy are responsible for this substantial increase in bone density.

There is some anxiety about the high oestradiol levels which might occur with long-term oestradiol implant therapy. Climacteric symptoms do return after 4–8 months when the plasma hormone profiles are still in the premenopausal range. These symptoms respond to an oestradiol implant and not to a placebo implant. These supraphysiological levels of oestradiol appear in 3.2% of patients and are almost confined to those patients with premenstrual or severe climacteric depression with a history of psychiatric referral and also to patients who have

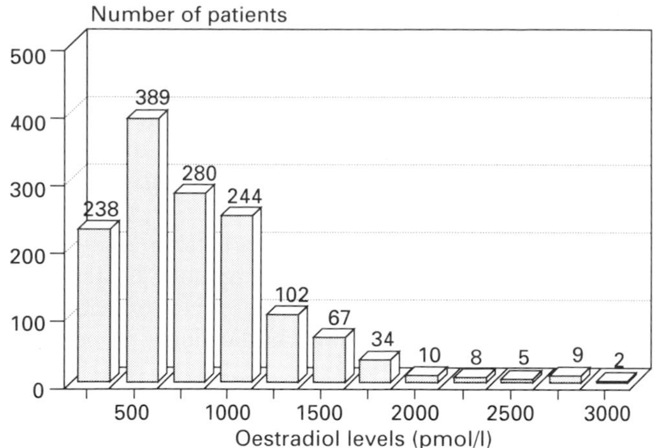

Fig. 24.5 Serum oestradiol levels in 1388 women after treatment with oestradiol implants. Adapted from Garnett et al (1990).

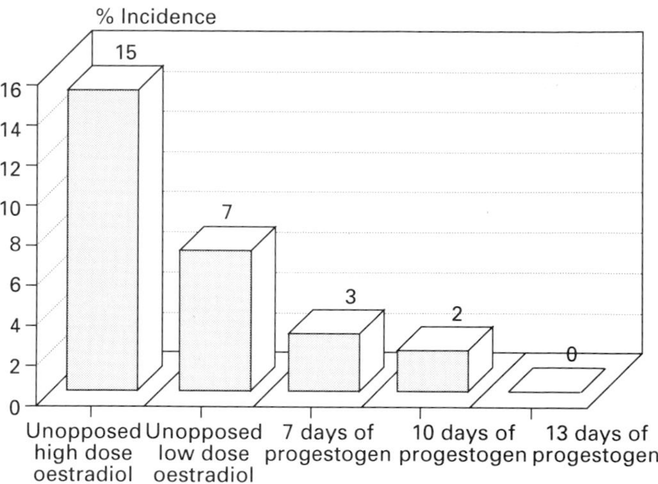

Fig. 24.6 Incidence of cystic hyperplasia in 745 women receiving oestrogen replacement therapy, with different durations of progestogen. Adapted from Sturdee et al (1978).

suffered an early surgical menopause (Fig. 24.5). There is no evidence that these high oestradiol levels are dangerous and indeed may be necessary in patients with severe hormone depression.

Progestogens

Progestogens alone are indicated only in women who cannot receive oestrogen therapy. They are less effective than oestrogen in suppressing hot flushes but have been shown to prevent postmenopausal bone loss. It is claimed that progestogens have a place in the treatment of menopausal patients with a history of breast cancer. The place of progestogen therapy is confused but there probably are enough unwanted side-effects related to progestogen, such as the metabolic effects in lipids and the appearance of premenstrual syndrome symptoms, for it not to be used unless there is a very good reason, such as the prevention of endometrial pathology in women.

Anabolic steroids

Androgens have been used in the prevention and treatment of postmenopausal osteoporosis. Stanozolol has been extensively studied and shown to increase total body calcium in patients with established osteoporosis. Its use in the prevention of postmenopausal bone loss remains to be determined. It is possible that part of the substantial increase in vertebral bone density following the use of oestradiol and testosterone implants may be due to the anabolic effect of the testosterone component.

Combined oestrogen and progestogen therapy

The use of cyclical progestogens to effect a regular medical curettage and prevent endometrial pathology was first described 50 years ago. It was stressed by many, particularly Greenblatt, the father of menopause studies. Unfortunately the advice went unheeded and it needed an American epidemic of endometrial cancer for combination oestrogen/progestogen therapy to be accepted.

Sturdee et al (1978; Fig. 24.6) first showed that although treatment with oestrogens alone resulted in a 15% incidence of endometrial hyperplasia, this was reduced by the addition of cyclical progestogens: a 7-day course resulted in a 4% incidence, a 10-day course in 2% incidence and more than 12 days in 0% incidence (Studd & Thom 1981). A 10- or 12-day course of progestogen is now built into oestrogen/progestogen packs and recent studies have shown that the excess risk of endometrial cancer has been eliminated when this combination is used.

In women who wish to avoid cyclical withdrawal bleeds it is possible to use a regimen of continuous oral oestrogen and progestogen. By adjusting the dose of progestogen appropriately it is possible to obtain 100% amenorrhoea within 6–9 months of therapy although troublesome spotting occurs in about 30% of patients before the amenorrhoea is achieved. No endometrial hyperplasia occurred during a 6-year follow-up.

When administering progestogens the duration of treatment is more important for endometrial protection than the daily dose. The timing of the withdrawal bleed may also be of prognostic significance as patients who bleed before the conclusion of their monthly progestogen course have a proliferative or hyperplastic endometrium whereas those who bled after the progestogen course usually have secretory endometrium.

The obvious conclusion is that cyclical progestogens should be included in a programme of hormone replacement therapy for all women who retain their uterus. However, progestogens are not without side-effects (Table 24.5)

Table 24.5 Common side-effects of hormone replacement therapy related to the use of progestogen

Cyclical bleeding
Premenstrual syndrome Bloating Fluid retention Mastalgia Headaches Depression
Detrimental lipid effects
Dysmenorrhoea

as perhaps 30% of women will produce symptoms of headache, depression, loss of energy and libido, bloatedness and other symptoms similar to the premenstrual syndrome. In high doses they may also adversely affect levels of HDL and LDL, thus negating some of the cardioprotective effects of oestrogen therapy. There is now a search for a safer progestogen but until this is available, cyclical progestogens should always be used in the minimum dose and duration. If the woman has no uterus there is no need for progestogen as there is no good evidence that progestogen protects the breasts.

Complications and contraindications

The main complication is bleeding in patients with a uterus. This may be satisfactory in woman aged 50 but is intolerable 10 years later, particularly if the bleeding becomes more heavy, painful or is associated with premenstrual syndrome symptoms with the progestogen.

There is only one real contraindication which is a recent past history of breast cancer.

Hypertension, varicose veins, previous thrombotic episodes, diabetes, endometriosis and fibroids are classically regarded as contraindications to hormone replacement therapy but there is no evidence that this is so as natural oestrogens did not cause elevation of blood pressure in normotensive or hypertensive women, nor do they alter coagulation, fibrinolysis, platelet behaviour, cause deep vein thrombosis, nor are they insulin-resistant.

The association between exogenous oestrogen use and cardiovascular disease is confused because of inappropriate extrapolation of oral contraceptive data containing relatively large doses of synthetic oestrogens. Numerous studies have now shown a decrease in the incidence of heart attacks and strokes after adjustment for age and systolic blood pressure. Even when risk factors such as family history, hypertension, hyperlipidaemia and previous heart attack is taken into consideration, the overwhelming evidence is that oestrogen therapy reduces incidences of heart attacks. Smoking is the only risk factor unaffected by the benefits of oestrogens.

Progestogens may reduce the beneficial effects of oestrogens by their effect on the HDL:LDL ratio and their use should, therefore, be confined to the minimum safe dose in women with an intact uterus.

Endometriosis and fibroids are responsive to endogenous and exogenous oestrogens and it is possible that hormone replacement therapy may stimulate the activity of these benign gynaecological conditions. In practice, this does not represent a clinical problem as treatment can easily be discontinued. Patients who have undergone a hysterectomy with or without oophorectomy for either of these conditions do not have any contraindications to oestrogen therapy.

Oestrogens were the first substances originating in the body to be implicated as a cause of cancer and almost since oestrogen was first isolated in 1923, a role for it in the genesis of breast and genital tract malignancy has been postulated. Fear of such a link is a major cause for the reluctance of many doctors to prescribe, and patients to seek, hormone replacement therapy.

Unopposed oestrogen therapy is associated with an increased risk of endometrial cancer. This risk is fourfold and should be compared with the fourfold increase being the same as the excess risk found in women who are more than 50 lb (22.5 kg) overweight. The addition of cyclical progestogen therapy for 7–13 days each month will reduce this risk to less than that found in untreated women and combined therapy should thus be offered to all women with an intact uterus.

There is no evidence to implicate hormone replacement therapy in the aetiology of carcinoma of the cervix, nor is there any significant increase in the incidence of epithelial ovarian tumours following oestrogen replacemement therapy. It seems likely that cyclical opposed hormone replacement therapy may confer some protective effect against ovarian cancer in the same way as the oral contraceptive pill.

The available epidemiological evidence relating to breast cancer is confusing but mostly reassuring. The studies are mostly related to the use of oral conjugated oestrogens. Most studies have shown no increased risk or decreased risk of breast cancer but there are recent important studies which show a slight increased relative risk of breast cancer after 5 or 10 years of oestrogen therapy. It is likely that the slight excess can be explained by the increased surveillance, i.e. breast palpation and mammography, that women receiving oestrogen therapy have compared with women who are not under their physician's care for such therapy. This would lead to an increased diagnosis of early-stage tumours. There may also be a confusion of diagnosis in this hormone-dependent tissue in the same way as there was with endometrial hyperplasia and carcinoma 10 years ago. This view is supported by the consistent finding of a significantly decreased mortality from breast cancer in patients receiving oestrogen therapy (Table 24.6). There are high-risk women with a family history of breast malig-

Table 24.6 Mortality in patients using hormone replacement therapy compared with age-specific death rates for England and Wales

Cause of death (ICD 9th revision)	Number of deaths Ratio O/E	95% Confidence limits
Cancer of the breast	0.55	0.28–0.96
Cancer of the endometrium	–	0–1.78
Cancer of the cervix	0.71	0.08–2.56
Cancer of the ovary	1.43	0.62–2.82
Other neoplasms	0.69	0.48–0.96
All neoplasms	0.66	0.50–0.86
Ischaemic heart disease	0.48	0.29–0.74
Cerebrovascular disease	0.65	0.35–1.09
Suicide	2.53	1.26–4.54
All deaths due to injury	1.73	0.95–2.92
Other causes	0.34	0.19–0.57
All causes	0.59	0.49–0.70

Adapted from Hunt et al (1987).

nancy or with benign breast disease. It is not known whether there is any excess risk from these patients. Such women should not be denied treatment but should be offered oestrogen therapy with advice on regular self-examination, physician examination and a mammography.

CONCLUSIONS

The decline in ovarian function which culminates in the menopause gives rise to a hormone deficiency state which causes profound changes in women. Although not all women suffer the distressing short-term sequelae of ovarian failure there is no doubt that all experience oestrogen deficiency which leads to a multi-system disorder ranging from connective tissue loss to psychological disorders.

This hormone deficiency state needs to be recognized for with increasing longevity of the population more and more morbidity and mortality will be seen in those who do not receive hormone replacement therapy. There is poor correlation between the short-term symptoms and long-term consequences of the menopause and at present it is impossible on symptomatology alone to select a group of women who are most in need of long-term oestrogen therapy. With continuing developments, sex hormone replacement is becoming increasingly safe and the benefits even more extensive than once supposed, especially in the prevention of cardiovascular disease and osteoporosis.

Oestrogen replacement therapy may yet prove to be one of the greatest advances in preventive medicine in the western world for half a century.

KEY POINTS

1. Despite increased awareness of its advantages, still only a small proportion of postmenopausal women receive HRT.
2. The major oestrogen postmenopausally is oestrone produced by conversion of adrenal androgens in adipose tissue.
3. There is a high incidence of psychological disorder in women requesting HRT.
4. Genital tract blood flow is reduced by 15% postmenopausally resulting in relative ischaemia and atrophy to the genital tract; this can be corrected by administering oestrogen.
5. Postmenopausally the incidence of ischaemic heart disease increases dramatically, probably related to an increase in low density lipoproteins occurring with falling oestrogen levels.
6. HRT reduces the risk of heart disease and cardiovascular disease.
7. The osteoporosis that occurs postmenopausally results from loss of collagen matrix as the bone is normally calcified.
8. HRT reduces osteoporosis and a 5-year course of treatment is thought to decrease the fracture rate by 50%.
9. Due to the 'first pass effect', the liver excretes 30% of all orally ingested oestrogen.
10. In combined oestrogen or progestogen therapy, the progestogen should be given for at least 10–12 days.

REFERENCES

Abdalla H, Baber R, Kirkland A, Leonard T, Studd J W W 1989 Pregnancies following transfer of frozen thawed zygotes on an ovum donation programme. British Journal of Obstetrics and Gynaecology 96: 1071–1075

Albright F, Smith P, Richardson A 1941 Postmenopausal osteoporosis, its clinical features. Journal of the American Medical Association 116: 2465–2474

Montgomery J, Appleby L, Brincat M et al 1987 Effects of oestrogen and testosterone implants on psychological disorders of the climacteric. Lancet i: 297–299

Ross R, Paganini-Hill A, Mack T 1984 Reduction in fractures and other effects of oestrogen replacement therapy in human populations. Osteoporosis: Proceedings of the Copenhagen International Symposium on Osteoporosis 1: 289–297

Savvas M, Studd J W W, Fogelman I, Dooley M, Montgomery J, Murby B 1988 Skeletal effects of oral oestrogen compared with subcutaneous oestrogen and testosterone in post-menopausal women. British Medical Journal 297: 331–333

Studd J W W, Thom M 1981 Oestrogens and endometrial cancer. In: Studd J W W (ed) Progress in obstetrics and gynaecology, vol 1. Churchill Livingstone, London, pp 182–198

Sturdee D, Wade-Evans T, Patterson M E L, Thom M, Studd J W W 1978 Relations between bleeding pattern, endometrial histology and oestrogen treatment in menopausal women. British Medical Journal 1: 1569–1648

Watson N, Studd J W W, Riddle A, Savvas M 1988 Suppression of ovulation by transdermal oestradiol patches. British Medical Journal 297: 900–901

FURTHER READING

Greenblatt R B (ed) 1986 A modern approach to the peri-menopausal years. W de Gruyter, Berlin

Greenblatt R B, Studd J W W (eds) 1977 The menopause. Clinics in obstetrics and gynaecology. W B Saunders, Oxford

Magos A L, Studd J W W 1990 Hormone implants in gynaecology. In: Studd J (ed) Progress in obstetrics and gynaecology, vol 8. Churchill Livingstone, London, pp 313–334

Studd J W W, Whitehead M I (eds) 1988 The menopause. Blackwell, Oxford

Whitehead M I 1985 The climacteric. In: Studd J (ed) Progress in obstetrics and gynaecology, vol 5. Churchill Livingstone, London, pp 332–361

Zichella L, Whitehead M, Van Keep P (eds) 1987 The climacteric and beyond. Partheon, Lancashire

25. Disorders of male reproduction

F. C. W. Wu

INTRODUCTION

In the last 20 years, rapid progress has been achieved in our understanding of male reproductive physiology with wide-ranging contributions from cell and molecular biologists, urologists and endocrinologists whose efforts have contributed to establishing the discipline of andrology. Some of these advances are beginning to be translated into clinical practice so that the management of male reproductive disorders can be increasingly based on rational scientific principles. Males with reproductive disorders often present to the gynaecologist and family practitioner through the intermediary of their femalc partners. It is therefore important for both the community doctors and hospital specialists to have a high degree of awareness in order to recognize potential problems as well as being cognizant of the newer diagnostic techniques and treatment modalities now becoming increasingly available for male reproductive dysfunctions.

This chapter aims to provide the practising gynaecologist with an overview of clinical andrology with emphasis on male infertility. A description of normal physiology is given as the foundation for explaining pathophysiological mechanisms and as a basis for formulating rational treatment where possible.

PHYSIOLOGY

Spermatogenesis

Spermatogenesis takes place in several hundred tightly coiled seminiferous tubules arranged in lobules (Fig. 25.1) which constitute some 80% of testicular volume in man. Each tubule is like a loop draining at both ends into the rete testis, with which the head of the epididymis is con-

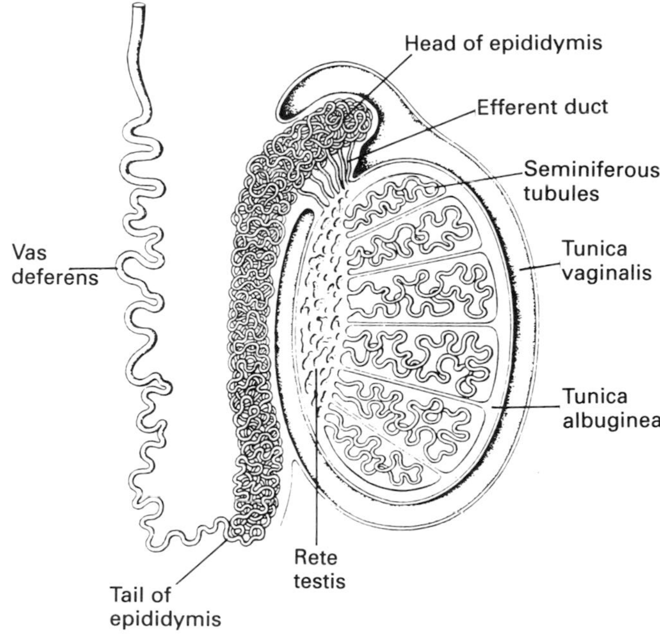

Fig. 25.1 Human testis, epididymis and vas deferens showing efferent ducts leading from the rete testis to the caput epididymis and the cauda epididymis continuing to become the vas deferens (from Dym 1977, with permission).

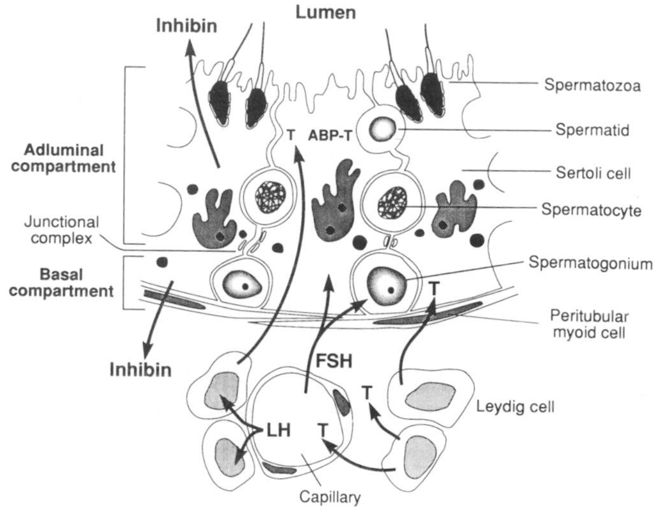

Fig. 25.2 Diagrammatic representation of the anatomical and functional relationships between germ cells, Sertoli cells and Leydig cells. Note the division of the seminiferous epithelium into adluminal and basal compartments by the tight junctions between adjacent Sertoli cells and the bidirectional secretion of Sertoli cell products (e.g. inhibin) into the lumen and interstitial space.
ABP-T = androgen-binding protein T; FSH = follicle-stimulating hormone; LH = luteinizing hormone.

nected by several efferent ducts. Seminiferous tubules are lined by germ cells and Sertoli cells around a central lumen and surrounded by peritubular myoid cells and a basement membrane (Fig. 25.2). Within this seminiferous epithelium resides the most active and dynamic collection of cells in the body but the complicated cellular multiplication and remodelling take place in a virtually avascular environment.

Spermatogenesis is a continuous sequence of highly (spatially and temporally) organized and closely regulated events whereby cohorts of undifferentiated diploid germ cells (spermatogonia) multiply and are then transformed into haploid spermatozoa. The following events, occurring in a precise predetermined sequence and duration, can be observed in the seminiferous epithelium during normal spermatogenesis:

1. Mitotic divisions (at least four) of stem cells to form cohorts of spermatogonia which, at intervals of 16 days, differentiate into primary preleptotene spermatocytes to initiate meiosis.
2. Meiotic reduction divisions of spermatocytes to form round spermatids.
3. Continuous remodelling of Sertoli cells in order to direct the migration of germ cells from basal to luminal positions.
4. Transformation (spermiogenesis) of large spherical spermatids into compact virtually cytoplasm-free spermatozoa with condensed DNA in the head crowned by an apical acrosome cap and tail capable of propelling beating movements.
5. Spermiation or release of spermatozoa from Sertoli cell cytoplasm into tubular lumen.

Cohorts of undifferentiated germ cells, joined to each other by cytoplasmic bridges, progress through these different steps in synchrony so that several generations of developing germ cells are usually observed at any one part of the seminiferous epithelium at any one time. The total duration for a cohort of spermatogonia to develop into spermatozoa is 74 days, during which time at least three further generations of spermatogonia have also successively, at intervals of 16 days, initiated their development.

Sertoli cell function

Sertoli (sustentacular) cells have extensive cytoplasm which spans the full height of the seminiferous epithelium from basement membrane to the lumen (Fig. 25.2). Where adjacent Sertoli cells come into contact with each other near the basement membrane, special occluding junctions are formed which divide the seminiferous epithelium into a basal (outer) compartment which interacts with the systemic circulation and an adluminal (inner) compartment enclosed by a functional permeability barrier, the blood–testis barrier (Fig. 25.2). In the cytoplasmic scaffolding provided by the Sertoli cells, spermatogonia divide by mitosis in the basal compartment while the two reduction divisions of the spermatocytes and spermiogenesis are confined to the unique avascular microenvironment of the adluminal compartment created by the blood–testis barrier. The developing germ cells are therefore completely dependent on Sertoli cells for metabolic support. As germ cells mature, the formation and dissolution of a variety of special junctional connections with adjacent Sertoli cell membrane suggest that functional interactions between them are highly probable. In response to appropriate trophic stimuli [follicle-stimulating hormone (FSH) and testosterone (T)], Sertoli cells secrete a wide range of substances including androgen-binding protein (ABP), inhibin, plasminogen activator, transferrin, lactate, growth factors and a distinctive tubular fluid high in potassium and low in protein which bathes the mature spermatozoa.

Much of Sertoli cell secretion is bidirectional, occurring either from the apex into the lumen or via the base into interstitial fluid and thence into the blood stream. The particular direction of secretion seems to be influenced by hormones and the state of the seminiferous epithelium. Whether any of these secretory products of the Sertoli cell is essential for spermatogenesis or sperm maturation or physiological significance of the direction of secretion is at present unknown. Nevertheless, the fact that both apical and basally secreted products can eventually reach the systemic circulation (e.g. inhibin) provides at least the potential for detecting circulating markers of Sertoli cell function or dysfunction in future.

Unlike the actively dividing germ cells, Sertoli cells do not proliferate in the adult testis. However, the active germ cell division and morphogenesis are matched by the functional diversity and variations of Sertoli cells. Viewed from this perspective, spermatogenesis is a cyclical process which is critically dependent on the periodic changes in Sertoli cell function associated with the constantly changing combination of germ cells in contact with its cytoplasm. Changes in the germ cell complement in contact with any one Sertoli cell occurs at a fixed sequence and interval. Thus the synchronization of these repetitive cyclical changes in Sertoli cell function, associated with the variations in germ cell metabolic requirement as they divide and differentiate, has now become one of the central tenets in our conceptualization of normal spermatogenesis (Sharpe 1986). Although pituitary gonadotrophins provide the primary obligatory trophic support for testicular function as a whole, the classical concept that luteinizing hormone (LH) stimulates Leydig cell steroidogenesis and FSH controls functions in the seminiferous tubules is far too simplistic in the light of our current understanding of spermatogenesis. There is now good evidence that the interstitial and tubular compartments are not functionally distinct but there is a close and complex inter-relationship between them. Thus T from the interstitial Leydig cells stimulates Sertoli cell functions directly or via the peritubular cells. Altered tubular/Sertoli cell function, on the other hand, can induce changes in Leydig cell steroidogenesis, although the identity of the intercompartmental regulator(s) is unknown.

Systemic gonadotrophins are not directly involved in this intricate local intratesticular cross-talking. Furthermore the ability to prepare relatively pure populations of isolated cells from the testis for in vitro studies has demonstrated that individual cell types have receptors for and respond to large variety of hormones and humoral factors. That these factors are produced within the testis and that testicular cells respond to them in concentrations much higher than that found in peripheral plasma provide strong circumstantial evidence to suggest that specific functional interactions between Sertoli–Leydig–peritubular–germ cells exists within the testis. One can envisage interactions in which a particular combination of germ cell types dictates the functional response in adjacent Sertoli cells, which are also under the influence of Leydig cells and peritubular cells. The Sertoli cells in turn govern or initiate the next step in the cytodifferentiation of those germ cells via some paracrine and/or growth factors.

However, at present the nature of these putative paracrine mechanisms are far from clear. To date, T is the only and probably the most important paracrine hormone identified and its presence in sufficient concentrations in the seminiferous tubules is an absolute requirement for spermatogenesis (see below). How much T is required and how it exerts its effects are just some of the fundamental questions that are still unanswered. Despite the large gaps in our existing knowledge, it is becoming increasingly accepted that local co-ordination of the multifarious functions in a variety of different cell types within the testis, orchestrated by the diverse functional capabilities of the Sertoli cells, holds the key to quantitatively normal spermatogenesis.

Hormonal control of spermatogenesis

The hormonal control of spermatogenisis requires the actions of pituitary gonadotrophins LH and FSH. There is general agreement that both LH and FSH are needed for the initiation of spermatogenesis during puberty. However, the specific role and relative contribution of two gonadotrophins in maintaining spermatogenesis are unclear (Sharpe 1987). LH stimulates Leydig cell steroidogenesis, resulting in increased production of T. Normal spermatogenesis is absolutely dependent on T but its mode of action and the amount required remain uncertain. Specific androgen receptors have not been demonstrated in germ cells but are present in Sertoli and peritubular cells. This implies that the actions of androgens on spermatogenesis must be mediated by somatic cells in the seminiferous tubules. The concentration of T in the testis is 50 times higher than that in the peripheral circulation. There is thus a gross over-abundance of T within the normal adult testis and any T-related abnormalities must be due to defects in steroid utilization rather than supply. However, T on its own in hypogonadotrophic conditions can only maintain qualitative normal spermatogenesis when testicular weight and total sperm production remain subnormal (Matsumoto 1989). FSH initiates function in immature Sertoli cells prior to onset of spermatogenesis by stimulating the formation of the blood–test barrier, secretion of tubular fluid and other specific secretory products via FSH receptors which activate intracellular cyclic adenosine monophosphate (AMP). Once spermatogenesis is established in the adult testis, Sertoli cells become less responsive to FSH. However, it can be shown in animals immunized against FSH and in experimentally induced hypogonadotrophic men given gonadotrophin replacement, that both T (LH) and FSH are required for quantitatively normal spermatogenesis. FSH is ineffective on its own without T, but maintains quantitatively normal spermatogenesis in the adult (T-replete) testis by determining the number of spermatogonia available for meiosis. FSH therefore acts either by increasing spermatogonial mitosis or decreasing the number of cells that degenerate at each cell division. T is essential for the subsequent stages from meiosis to spermiogenesis.

Leydig cells

The adult human testis contains some 500 million Leydig

cells clustered in the interstitial spaces adjacent to the seminiferous tubules. The biosynthesis of T in Leydig cells is under the control of LH which binds to specific surface membrane receptors. Steroidogenesis is stimulated through a cyclic AMP/protein kinase C mechanism which mobilizes cholesterol substrate and promotes the conversion of cholesterol to pregnenolone by splitting the C21 side-chain. The subsequent steps in the biosynthetic pathway go through the weakly androgenic intermediates of dehydroepiandrosterone and androstenedione before the principal secretory product of T. T is secreted into spermatic venous system, testicular lymphatics and tubular fluid. Leydig cells also synthesize oestradiol, oxytocin, angiotensin, β-endorphin and prostaglandins but their physiological significance is unknown (for review see Ewing & Zirkin 1983).

T is the most important circulating androgen in the adult male since most dehydrotestosterone is formed locally in androgen-responsive target tissues. T circulates in plasma bound to sex hormone-binding globulin (SHBG) and albumin. The latter binds to all steroids with low affinity (T 3.6×10^4 mol/l) while SHBG is a glycoprotein synthesized in the liver with a molecular weight of 80–94 kDa and a high affinity (8×10^8 mol/l) but low capacity ($3–5 \times 10^{-8}$ mol/l) for T. In man, 60% for circulating T is bound to SHBG, 38% to albumin and 2% is free. Free and albumin-bound T constitute the bioavailable fractions of circulating T but recent evidence suggests that SHBG-bound T may also be extractable in some tissues, namely prostate and testis.

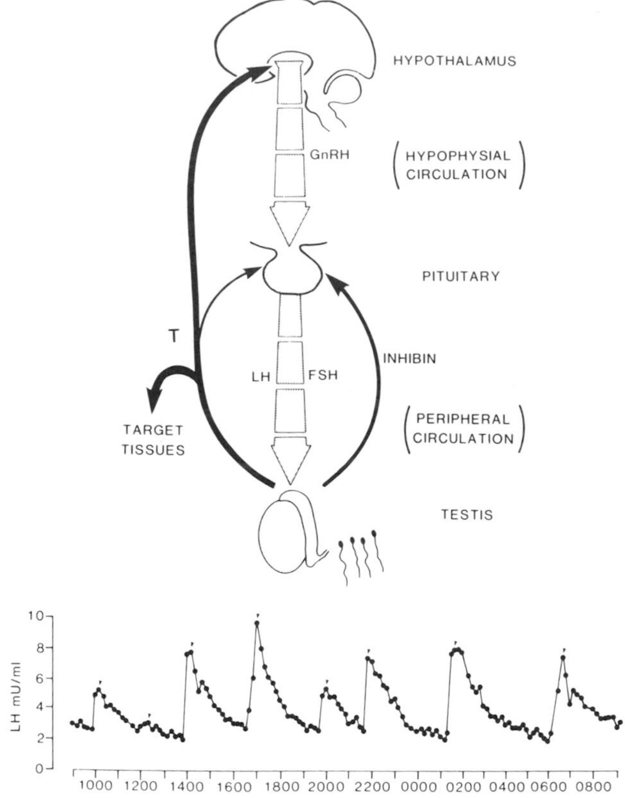

Fig. 25.3 **Top**:Functional relationships in the hypothalamic–pituitary–testicular axis. Gonadotrophin-releasing hormone (GnRH) is secreted into the hypophysial circulation in an episodic manner, represented by a luteinizing hormone (LH) pulse (arrowed below) in the peripheral circulation.
FSH = follicle-stimulating hormone.
Bottom: Peripheral blood LH concentration sampled in an adult male at 10-min intervals for 24 h from 0900 to 0900 h.

Hypothalamic–pituitary–testicular axis

Anterior pituitary gonadotrophin secretion is controlled by hypothalamic gonadotrophin-releasing hormone (GnRH) released into the pituitary portal circulation by axon terminals in the median eminence. The neurosecretory neurones in the medial basal hypothalamus are responsive to a wide variety of sensory inputs as well as to gonadal negative feedback. GnRH stimulates both LH and FSH secretion. In the adult male, GnRH is released episodically into the pituitary portal circulation at a frequency of about every 140 minutes; each volley of GnRH elicits an immediate release of LH producing the typical pulsatile pattern of LH in the systemic circulation (Wu et al 1989; Fig. 25.3). Though also secreted episodically, FSH and T pulses are not apparent in normal men because of the slower secretion of newly synthesized rather than stored hormone, and the longer circulating half-lives. The intermittent mode of GnRH stimulation within a narrow physiological range of frequency is obligatory for sustaining the normal pattern of gonadotrophin secretion. Continuous or high-frequency GnRH stimulation paradoxically desensitizes the pituitary gonadotrophin response because of depletion of receptors and refractoriness of postreceptor response mechanisms.

T exerts the major negative feedback action on gonadotrophin secretion. Its effect is predominantly to restrict the frequency of GnRH pulses from the hypothalamus to within the physiological range. T also acts on the pituitary to reduce the amplitude of LH response to GnRH; this may require the local conversion of T to oestradiol in the pituitary. These inhibitory actions are best seen in agonadal or castrated males where high-frequency and high-amplitude LH pulsatile secretion prevail. Feedback inhibition of pituitary FSH synthesis is also affected by T, particularly at high concentrations, as well as the recently purified glycoprotein Sertoli cell product, inhibin (McLachlan et al 1987). It is believed that tubular damage associated with Sertoli cell dysfunction and a consequently reduced capacity for inhibin secretion is the cause for the FSH rise, with normal LH, commonly found in infertile men.

The spermatozoon

The spermatozoon has a dense oval head capped by an acrosome granule and is propelled by a motile tail (Fig. 25.4). These highly specialized structural features reflect the unique functional activities of the spermatozoon. The acrosome contains enzymes essential for fertilization; the tail contains the energy source and machinery for motility: these combine to deliver the paternal contribution of genetic information in the nucleus to the egg to initiate development of a new individual. The head is made up largely of highly condensed nuclear chromatin, constituting the haploid chromosome complement, and it is covered in its anterior half by a membrane-enclosed sac of enzymes, the acrosome. The area of the sperm head immediately behind the acrosome is important as it is this part which attaches and fuses with the egg. The tail is usually further divided into the mid-piece, principal piece and end-piece. The motor apparatus of the tail is the axoneme which consists of a central pair (doublets) of microtubules of non-contractile tubulin protein enclosed in a sheath linked radially to nine outer pairs of microtubules (Fig. 25.5). Each doublet is also joined by nexin bridges to its neighbour via two adenosine triphosphatase-rich dynein protein arms. This axonemal complex is surrounded by columns of dense fibres which are in turn covered by a helix of mitochondria in the mid-piece, and a fibrous sheath in the principal piece. The dense fibres and the fibrous sheath form the cytoskeleton of the flagellum. Through the hydrolysis of adenosine triphosphate, the dynein arms undergo a series of conformational changes resulting in adjacent doublets sliding over one another. Synchronized movement of groups of microtubules propagating waves of bending motions of the tail is the key to the various modes of co-ordinated sperm motility. Energy for sperm motility is provided by the sheath of mitochondria in the mid-piece of the tail through a second-messenger system involving the calcium-mediated calmodulin-dependent conversion of adenosine triphosphate to cAMP and interaction with adenosine triphosphatase of the dynein.

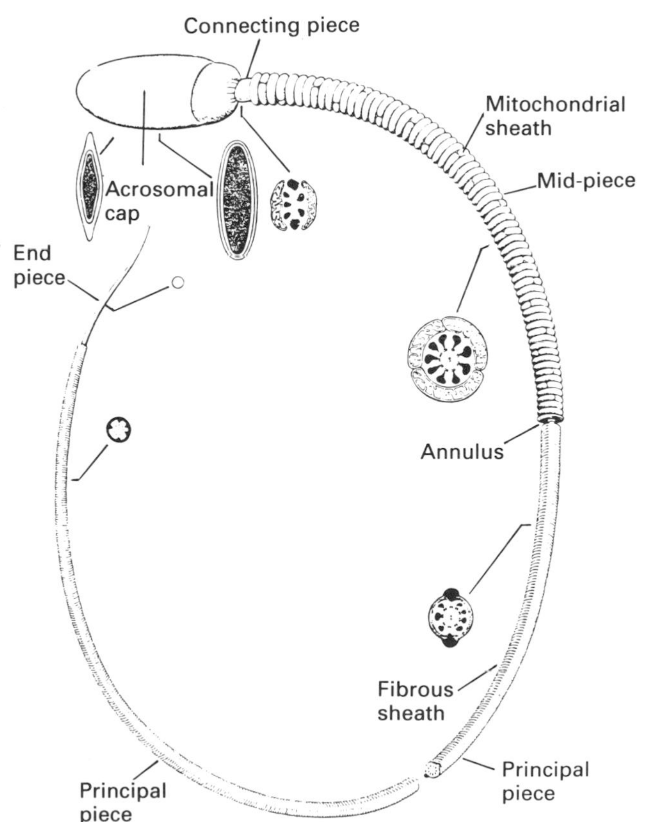

Fig. 25.4 The internal structure of a spermatozoon with the cell membrane removed (from Fawcett 1975).

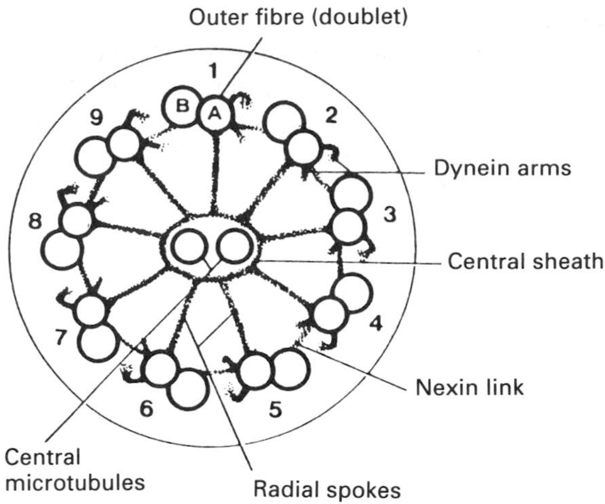

Fig. 25.5 Typical structure of the axoneme of the sperm tail.

Sperm transport and maturation

Spermatozoa are functionally immature and immotile when they are transported out of the testis through the efferent ducts in the caput epididymis. The maturation process continues as the spermatozoa are in transit through the epididymis. The epididymis is a 3–4 m long single coiled tube whose function is under androgen and neural (adrenergic) control. The epididymal epithelium actively reabsorbs testicular fluid but also secretes a hyperosmolar fluid rich in glycerophosphorylocholine, inositol and carnitine. The specific transport of these compounds across the epithelium creates a favourable fluid environment where progressive motility and fertilizing capacity of the spermatozoa are normally acquired. Thus the cytoplasmic droplets decrease in size and move distally along the mid-piece, the acrosome membrane swells, the epididymal glycoproteins are incorporated into the plasma membrane, s–s bonds are formed in the sperm tail cytoskeleton and cyclic AMP content increases. How these changes in the spermatozoa relate to the acquisition of motility and fertility and whether the epididymal epithelium plays an obligatory role is uncertain. Indeed, it has recently been suggested that epididymal transit is not an absolute requirement since pregnancy can be achieved with sperm that have completely bypassed the corpus and cauda epididymis (Silber 1989). It was argued that the time after emergence from the testis may be adequate for sperm maturation, which can be considered merely as a continuation of the intrinsic developmental programme started in the seminiferous epithelium independent of epididymal secretion.

Secretions of the accessory glands form over 90% of the volume of semen and mix with spermatozoa at emission. The seminal vesicles contribute the largest volume of alkaline fluid to the ejaculate and are also the source of seminal fructose, prostaglandins and coagulating proteins. Prostatic secretion contains proteolytic enzymes (which normally liquefy the coagulated proteins in semen within 20–30 min) and are rich in citric acid and zinc. Seminal plasma provides a support medium for transporting male gametes out of the body and for buffering the acidic (<5) pH of the vagina so that a reservoir of functional sperm can be established after ejaculation. Additionally, seminal plasma–sperm interaction at ejaculation may contribute to the continuing process of sperm maturation. The normal storage site of sperm in the male genital tract is the ampulla of the vasa. Unejaculated sperm are mostly leaked out of the vas and voided in urine.

Just as testicular germ cells are subjected to constant attrition, ejaculated spermatozoa have to traverse the cervix, uterus and uterotubal junction before reaching the middle third of the oviduct — the site of fertilization — and at each barrier the sperm population is further reduced so that eventually only 200 or so of the most robust spermatozoa have the opportunity to fertilize the ovum (Harper 1988). It follows that the number of sperm ejaculated does not greatly influence the number entering the fallopian tube, at least not until very low figures are reached.

The cervical canal is the first selective filtering barrier to meet the ejaculated sperm. This barrier is virtually complete except during mid-cycle when oestrogenized cervical mucus glycoprotein fibrils form parallel chains called micelles which permit spermatozoa with active progressive motility to swim through at a rate of 2–3 mm/min. It is believed that crypts of the cervical glands are colonized by migrating spermatozoa, forming sanctuaries from where sperm can be gradually released over a prolonged period. Sperm is transported rapidly through the uterus by uterine myometrium contraction.

The uterotubal junction is the second of the major physical barriers for spermatozoa. The mechanism for selectivity is not clear but may depend on factors other than sperm motility since inert particles can pass through. Once the uterotubular junction has been successfully negotiated, a minority of sperm immediately traverse the oviduct to the ampulla but the majority congregate in the isthmus until ovulation has occurred. At this time, capacitated sperm showing hyperactivated movements of the tail gradually progress towards the fimbriated end, helped on by the muscular contraction of the oviduct wall and the flow of fluid in the oviduct.

Sperm–egg interaction

Capacitation is a series of functional changes occurring either in the female genital tract (uterus and oviducts) or in suitable artificial media in vitro, which render epididymal or ejaculated sperm capable of fertilization. These changes involve the gradual removal or alteration of coating proteins on the plasma membrane which were adsorbed in the epididymis and during contact with seminal plasma. It could therefore be regarded as the reversal or removal of the protective coating acquired during epididymal transit or in the ejaculate. This probably involves destabilizing physicochemical changes in the lipid bi-layer, resulting in increased plasma membrane fluidity of the sperm head and tail. Consequently, receptor sites for egg recognition are exposed and vigorous undulating poorly progressive beating of the sperm tail (hyperactivation) is generated. Capacitation can be bypassed in vitro, using a specific stimulus (e.g. increasing intracellular calcium concentration) to precipitate the acrosome reaction but physiologically acrosome reaction can only take place after the sperm have undergone capacitation in vivo.

At the site of fertilization, capacitated sperm with intact acrosomes penetrate the cumulus to reach the outer zona. Mechanical shearing forces generated by the characteristic flagellar movements of the capacitated sperm are probably the main mechanism responsible for cumulus penetration. Surface hyaluronidase (possibly escaping from the acrosomal membrane) may facilitate cumulus penetration but is not absolutely required.

The zona pellucida is made up of families of sulphated glycoprotein whose structural integrity is maintained by non-covalent forces. Receptors for zona glycoproteins are located on the plasma membrane over the acrosomal cap in acrosome-intact sperm and that over the equatorial segment in the acrosome-reacted sperm. Zona pellucida binding shows a high degree of species specificity and is a classical cell recognition event which may involve an enzyme (galactosyltransferase)-substrate (N-acetyl-glucosamine) type of interaction. Binding of sperm to zona triggers the acrosome reaction, which is an essential step in the fertilization process since only acrosome-reacted sperm can penetrate the zona pellucida and fuse with the oolemma. During the acrosome reaction, the outer acrosome membrane fuses progressively with the inner plasma membrane at a number of sites and vesiculates, forming exit pores (fenestrations) through which the acrosome enzyme matrix is released. Vigorous sperm tail movement assisted by acrosomal enzyme (e.g. hyaluronidase and acrosin) digestion effect penetration through the rigid zona membrane. The sperm head then crosses the perivitelline space and becomes attached to the vitellus, followed by gradual insinuation of the entire sperm tail. The plasma membrane of the postacrosomal region fuses with the egg plasma membrane, upon which the sperm nucleus decondenses and transforms into the male pronucleus. At the same time the egg nucleus completes the second meiotic division, forming the female pronucleus and the second polar body (for review see Yanagimachi 1988).

MALE INFERTILITY

Definition and epidemiology

The currently accepted definition of infertility is the inability to produce a pregnancy after 12 months of unprotected intercourse. However, it should be remembered that only 86% of normal fertile couples achieve a pregnancy in the first year so that some patients being investigated for infertility merely need more time to realize their goal. It should also be appreciated that there is a spontaneous pregnancy rate, albeit decreased, even in those with reduced sperm counts. It follows that most patients are subfertile rather than sterile or infertile and this has important implications in patient management strategies as well as the critical assessment of treatment results. General population surveys in developed countries have indicated that some 8–15% of married couples experience involuntary subfertility (Hull et al 1985). Of these, male factors alone are estimated to be responsible in 30% and contributory in a further 20% of subfertile couples. Thus, male subfertility may affect 5% of men of reproductive age.

Pathophysiology

In the simplest terms, male infertility is a failure to fertilize the normal ovum arising from a deficiency of functionally competent sperm at the site of fertilization. Since less than 0.1% of ejaculated sperm actually reaches the fallopian tube, it might be inferred that defective sperm function rather than inadequate numbers of sperm ejaculated constitutes the most important pathophysiological mechanism in male infertility. Thus specific lesions leading to defective sperm motility or transport and abnormal sperm–egg interaction are probably the key factors responsible for the loss of fertilizing capacity in the gametes. In most instances however, inadequate sperm function is usually but not invariably accompanied by reduced sperm production, suggesting that specific defects in spermatozoa could have arisen from disturbances in regulatory mechanisms which interfere with both germ cell multiplication and maturation in the seminiferous tubules. There is rarely any clinical evidence of systemic gonadotrophin or androgen deficiency in men with male infertility; indeed circulating gonadotrophins are frequently raised. By inference therefore, disturbances in paracrine regulation within the testis could lead to low sperm output (oligozoospermia) from an increased rate of degeneration in the differentiating spermatogonia at successive mitotic divisions, as well as abnormal spermiogenesis giving rise to spermatozoa with poor motility (asthenozoospermia) and/or abnormal morphology (teratozoospermia). The nature of these putative defects in paracrine control remains to be identified but the current hypothesis provides a useful conceptual framework in directing research efforts and planning patient management. Abnormal epididymal function may lead to defective sperm maturation, impairment of sperm transport or even cell death. Interruption of the transport of normal sperm may be due to mechanical barriers between the epididymis and fallopian tube or abnormal coitus and/or ejaculation.

Aetiologies

One of the central problems in male infertility is the difficulty in identifying genuine rather than presumptive aetiological factors. In a World Health Organization (WHO; 1977) survey on the pattern of infertility in 25 countries, 66.6% of males either have no demonstrable cause for their infertility or the aetiology of abnormal semen quality is unidentifiable (Table 25.1). This is confirmed in specialist referral clinics in Edinburgh (for

Table 25.1 Aetiologies of male infertility

Diagnosis	Edinburgh 1979–1982 (%)	WHO 1979–1982 (%)	Melbourne 1979–1980 (%)
Total number	56.3	48.3	6.0
Idiopathic azoo/oligospermia	8.4	16.1 }	7.32
Idiopathic astheno teratozoospermia	19.5	16.8 }	
Varicocele	7.2	17.2	25
Genital tract infection	2.1	4.0	
Sperm autoimmunity	1.8	1.6	5
Congenital (cryptorchidism) chromosomal) disorders	1.2	2.1	1.9
Genital tract obstruction	0.6	1.8	10.8
Systemic/iatrogenic	0.6	1.3	1.0
Coital disorders	1.8	1.0	0.5
Gonadotrophin deficiency	0	0.6	0.6

Edinburgh 1979–1982: from WHO 1979–1982. From Cates et al (1985); Melbourne 1979–1980: from Baker (1989).

couples) and Melbourne (mainly for males), emphasizing the point that only a small minority of infertile men have specific recognizable aetiologies and of these, only a small proportion are treatable.

The aetiological groups can be broadly classified into testicular hypospermatogenesis of known or unknown cause, sperm autoimmunity, genital tract infection, genital tract obstruction, and coital disorders.

Testicular hypospermatogenesis: known aetiology

Chromosome disorders. Normal spermatogenesis is critically dependent on the ordered arrangement of chromosome pairing during cell division. Certain abnormalities of chromosomes may therefore be expected to interfere with spermatogenesis. In over 2000 men attending the Male Subfertility Clinic in Edinburgh over 10 years, the incidence of chromosome abnormalities was 2.2% (Chandley 1979). The frequency of chromosomal abnormalities increased as sperm density declined. Abnormal chromosome karyotypes were found in 15% of azoospermic patients, 90% of whom had Klinefelter's syndrome (47XXY) which accounted for half of the entire chromosomally abnormal group. In oligozoospermic patients, the incidence of chromosome abnormalities was 4%.

Other chromosomal abnormalities encountered more commonly in the infertile male population than newborns included reciprocal X or Y autosomal translocations, XYY and XX males, reciprocal and robertsonian autosomal translocations, supernumerary autosomes and inversion of autosomes.

Chromosomal studies of meiotic germ cells afford an opportunity to study the mechanism by which chromosomal aberrations interfere with spermatogenesis. However, this rarely reveals chromosomal abnormalities involving the germ line exclusively without any detectable changes in somatic karyotype. Though useful as a research tool, meiotic chromosome studies in germ cells require tissues obtained at testicular biopsy and are therefore rarely indicated in routine diagnostic investigations.

Cryptorchidism. The testis which is not in a low scrotal position by the age of 2 years has been found to be histologically abnormal; spontaneous descent rarely occurs after 1 year. It is generally believed that the lower temperature in the scrotum is a prerequisite for normal spermatogenesis. There is no evidence that surgical orchidopexy for an undescended testis improves fertility after 2 years of age. For these reasons, treatment should ideally be undertaken between 1 and 2 years of age. Evidence suggests that fertility may also be impaired in boys with retractile testis who experience spontaneous descent during puberty and a Japanese study showed similar testicular histology between retractile and true cryptorchid testis. It has therefore been suggested that retractile testis is a mild form of cryptorchidism, there being a continuum between abdominal and retractile testes. However, the level of the continuum where treatment is indicated is not clear.

Apart from the association with infertility, cryptorchidism is the only well established risk factor for testicular malignancy. Some 10% of cases have a history of cryptorchidism. The risk of testicular tumour in a patient with a history of undescended testis, whether successfully treated or not, is 4–10-fold higher than in the general population. Other risks of cryptorchidism such as testicular torsion and psychological morbidity also argue for an aggressive approach to treatment in early childhood. For a review on different aspects of cryptorchidism, see the proceedings of a recent symposium (Sharpe et al 1988).

Testicular toxins. The actively dividing male germ cells are one of the most sensitive cell types in the body to toxic effects of radiation, cytotoxic drugs and an increasing number of chemicals. Indeed, male gonadal function is probably the most sensitive index for overexposure to potential toxins (in the workplace, environment, foods, cosmetics and medicines). The classic example is lead which the ancient Romans used to sweeten their food and wine, contributing to the decline in their fertility. The best documented modern example is the pesticide dibromochloropropane (DBCP), which was responsible for azoospermic infertility in half of the male workers in a factory (Whorton et al 1977). The most common example in clinical practice today is sulphasalazine for the treatment of inflammatory bowel diseases. The carrier moiety, sulphapyridine, reversibly impairs sperm motility and sperm function in some patients.

Cytotoxic treatment regimes for Hodgkin's disease, lymphoma, leukaemia and other malignancies damage the differentiating spermatogonia so that most patients become azoospermic after 8 weeks. The degree of stem cell killing governs whether there is recovery of spermatogenesis or not after treatment. This is dependent on the cumulative dose of the drug combinations used. Long-term follow-up has shown that following six or more courses of MOPP (mustine, vincristine, procarbazine and prednisolone), over 85% of patients remained azoospermic and recovery is unlikely after 4 years. Similarly, radiation exposure of over 6 Gy destroys all germ cells with no chance of recovery, while 1–4 Gy produces complete cessation of spermatogenesis with only some stem spermatogonia surviving. There may be recovery after 12–36 months and spermatogenesis may continue to improve for several years but even then it may not be complete. Diagnostic procedures and therapeutic irradiation to other organs such as the thyroid usually expose the testis to <1 Gy.

A number of other drugs are also associated with detrimental effects on spermatogenesis. These include nitrofurantoin, anabolic steroids, sex steroids and anticonvulsants. Recreation drugs such as cigarettes, alcohol and cannabis have all been linked with lower semen quality.

Testicular function is impaired in chronic renal failure; improvement may occur after successful transplantation but not with dialysis. Pyrexial illnesses may non-specifically depress spermatogenesis for some weeks but recovery is complete.

Orchitis. Symptomatic orchitis occurs in 27–30% of males over the age of 10–11 years as a complication of mumps. In 17% of cases, orchitis is bilateral. Seminiferous tubular atrophy is a common sequela of mumps orchitis but recovery of spermatogenesis even after persistent azoospermia for 1 year has been reported (Sandler 1954). The prevalence of infertility after mumps orchitis in unknown but fertility should only be significantly impaired if the orchitis is bilateral.

Gonadotrophin deficiency. Secondary testicular failure due to gonadotrophin deficiency is a rare but important condition to recognize because it is the only category of male infertility consistently treatable by hormone replacement. The diagnosis is prompted by clinical evidence of androgen deficiency and confirmed by low or undetectable levels of gonadotrophin associated with subnormal testosterone. Depending on severity, cause and the time of onset, the clinical features and responsiveness to treatment are variable. The spectrum includes patients with complete congenital deficiency in LH-releasing hormone (LHRH) which results in total failure of testicular and secondary sexual development. Other patients with the so-called fertile eunuch syndrome have less severe or partial LHRH deficiency so that they have larger (4–10 ml) but still underdeveloped testes with more evidence of germ cell activity. In three-quarters of these patients, anosmia or hyposmia and a variety of midline defects can be detected — this is the association known as Kallmann's syndrome. In contrast to these congenital varieties of isolated hypogonadotrophic hypogonadism, postnatally or postpubertally acquired gonadotrophin deficiency may arise from tumours, chronic inflammatory lesions, iron overload or injuries of the hypothalamus and pituitary, so that deficits in other pituitary hormones usually coexist. These patients have developed seminiferous tubules which regressed through lack of trophic support. Their testes volume are significantly larger (10–15 ml) than the former two groups.

Varicocele. The significance of varicocele in male infertility is controversial. Reflux of blood in the internal spermatic vein, usually involving the left side from the renal vein, gives rise to distension of the pampiniform venous plexus and reduction in ipsilateral testicular volume. In infertile patients with unilateral varicocele, varying degrees of non-specific histological abnormalities can be detected in both testes. Increased scrotal temperature, hypoxia, and exposure of the testes to adrenal metabolites have been postulated as possible mechanisms by which spermatic vein reflux can induce seminiferous tubular damage. Since varicoceles can be detected clinically in 15% of young males and semen quality is not different in fertile men presenting for vasectomy with or without varicoceles (de Castro & Mastorocco 1984), it must be emphasized that the condition is not invariably associated with reduced fertility. Therefore the clinician must not automatically assume that the varicocele is directly responsible for infertility without actively excluding other possible aetiologies in a full assessment.

The diagnosis of visible (grade 3) and palpable (grade 2) varicoceles is not difficult when the patient is examined in a standing position. The detection of subclinical (grade 1) varicoceles where spermatic vein reflux can only be detected during the Valsalva manoeuvre requires more experience. This has been aided by the use of Dopplar stethoscope and scrotal thermography.

Testicular hypospermatogenesis: unknown/uncertain aetiology

Azoo/oligozoospermia. Failure of seminiferous tubular function to the extent of producing azoospermia or severe oligozoospermia (<5 million) is usually associated with small (under 15 ml) and soft testes and elevated FSH. Histologically, the tubules may show completely absent or reduced numbers of germ cells, narrow tubular diameter and thickening and hyalinization of peritubular tissue. These changes are non-specific and are not always uniformly distributed throughout the testes. Although the Leydig cells appear normal, there is evidence of malfunction in that near-normal T is maintained only by higher amplitudes of LH pulsatile secretion in these patients (Wu et al 1989). It is however unlikely that T deficiency is the primary cause of defective spermatogenesis.

There is also no evidence to support the contention that abnormalities in pulse frequency of LHRH may be the underlying cause of idiopathic hypospermatogenesis. According to our current view these structural and functional abnormalities are the end-results of the most extreme degrees of disruptions in the paracrine regulation in the testis. These patients usually remain infertile and there is no treatment available. Less severe degrees of oligozoospermia are commonly associated with abnormal morphology and reduced motility.

Asthenozoopermia. Absent or extremely low sperm motility of only 1–2% may result from absence of dynein arms, radial spokes or nexin bridges and dysplasia of fibrous sheath. This is associated with similar defects in respiratory cilia and therefore frequently a history of chronic respiratory infection, bronchiectasis and sinusitis — the immotile cilia syndrome. In addition, some of these patients have situs inversus (Kartagener's syndrome). Based on this classic but extremely rare example, it is now becoming clear that more common but less severe degrees of asthenozoospermia may also be associated with more subtle structural malformations in the axonemal complex, recognizable only with ultrastructural examination and functionally evident as suboptimal sperm movements. Recent quantitative electron microscopic analysis in men with sperm motility disorders has demonstrated a wide variety of structural sperm tail defects of the radial spokes, nexin bridges and disrupted organization of microtubules and fibrous sheath (Hancock & de Kretser, unpublished observations). This suggests that dyskinesis of the flagella (asthenozoopermia) can be caused by malformations of axonemal complex and surrounding structures during spermiogenesis rather than any metabolic or functional defects and is therefore unlikely to respond to drugs aimed at stimulating sperm motility through biochemical mechanisms. Severely degenerate spermatozoa with very low motility have also been found to have arisen during epididymal transit.

Teratozoospermia. Surface morphology directly reflects the maturity and functional integrity of the spermatozoa so that morphological analysis of ejaculated sperm is an important means of assessing spermatogenesis in the testis. Indeed, some workers believe that sperm morphology is the best predictor of spontaneous fertility and in vitro fertilization outcome (Kruger et al 1988). It has been reported that morphology in the individual spermatozoon is positively related to movement characteristics (swimming velocity, sperm head trajectories, flagellar beat frequency) which reflect the vigour of the cell (Morales et al 1988) and its ability to exhibit hyperactivation. Similarly, the ability to undergo the acrosome reaction has also been shown to be significantly higher in sperm with morphologically normal than abnormal sperm heads (Fukuda et al 1989). Ultrastructural studies have also revealed a variety of structural malformations of the acrosome complex, the most extreme example being the round-headed sperm where the acrosome is completely missing, but lesser degrees of acrosomal defects are increasingly being identified. Fertilization blocks in these developmental (morphological) abnormalities, i.e. teratozoospermia, are unlikely to be amenable to treatment by assisted reproductive procedures. These attempts to relate specific functional defects to recognizable structural malformations in individual spermatozoa provide evidence that morphologically abnormal sperm are also functionally impaired. If the information extrapolates to morphologically abnormal sperm in the semen of infertile men, then this could be one reason why teratozoospermia is associated with subfertility. Functional differences between subpopulations of morphologically normal and abnormal sperm may be accentuated after the spermatozoa are separated from seminal plasma. This may be an important reason for the success of in vitro fertilization in treating cases of male infertility with good morphology using sperm subpopulations harvested into artificial media (Kruger et al 1988; Liu et al 1988).

Androgen insensitivity. Low androgen receptor levels in cultured fibroblast from genital or pubic skin has been reported in some oligozoospermic men who have normal male phenotypes (Aiman & Griffen 1982; Morrow et al 1987). Testosterone and LH are usually normal in these patients. This has been regarded as the least severe manifestation of the spectrum of phenotypic abnormalities associated with defects in androgen receptor function. The incidence of this form of androgen resistance in a group of men with azoospermia or severe oligozoospermia has been reported to be 40% (Aiman & Griffen 1982), although this rather high figure has not been confirmed by other workers. Because of the low concentration and instability of the androgen receptor in tissues and its instability during isolation, our understanding of the role of the androgen receptor in regulating spermatogenesis is poor. The recent cloning of the human androgen receptor cDNA has cleared the way for studying possible alterations in androgen receptor expression, structure and function in relation to abnormal spermatogenesis.

Sperm autoimmunity

The significance of immunological infertility due to antibodies against spermatozoa has long been a matter for dispute but is now finally gaining acceptance. Much of this controversy arose because of the inadequacies in differentiating specific antibodies which suppress sperm function from those that are of doubtful clinical relevance. The realization that immunological infertility is a specific disorder caused by sperm membrane-bound immunoglobulin gamma A has resolved some of the discrepancies from earlier data based mainly on sperm agglutination or immobilization tests which correlated with circulating immunoglobulin gamma G or M antibodies and had little direct pathophysiological significance. The newer methods of detecting specific classes of antibody on the sperm surface membrane or seminal plasma have therefore greatly refined the accuracy of this diagnosis and brought it into the realms of potentially treatable infertility.

The incidence of sperm autoimmunity has been reported to be between 2.7 and 23% of men presenting with infertility. This obviously depends on patient selection and method of testing but the true incidence of significant sperm antibody is unlikely to be higher than 5%. Conditions predisposing to sperm autoimmunity include vasectomy, testicular injury or inflammation, genital tract obstruction and family history of autoimmune disease. The incidence of sperm antibody in female partners is not well documented but is believed to be much less common than in males. This however should be regarded as an open issue and more attention should be focused on antibodies in cervical mucus in women with unexplained infertility. It is now the practice of most clinics to screen for sperm antibodies in all male patients except those with testicular failure due to chromosomal abnormalities.

Male patients with significant sperm antibody usually have severely suppressed fertility potential (<0.5%/month pregnancy rate). The major identifiable defect is interference with sperm passage through cervical mucus but there is evidence that fertilization may also be impeded (Dom et al 1981; Clarke et al 1985).

Genital tract infection

Infection in the lower genital tract is an uncommon cause of male infertility in western countries. Gram-negative enterococci, chlamydia and gonococcus are established pathogenic organisms which usually produce unequivocal clinical evidence of infection (adnexitis) such as painful ejaculation, pelvic or sacral pain, urethral discharge, haematospermia, dysuria, irregular tender epididymides and tender boggy prostate. This can be confirmed by semen culture, urethral swabs, and the presence of more than 1 million peroxidase-positive polymorphonuclear neutrophils per millilitre of semen or in expressed prostatic fluid. Inflammation of the accessory glands and excurrent ducts may give rise to disturbed function, formation of sperm antibody and permanent structural damage with obstruction in the outflow tract.

Once the diagnosis of active infection is established, both partners should be treated by appropriate antibiotics (erythromycin, doxycycline or norfloxacin) for 4 weeks.

The entity of asymptomatic prostatitis is poorly defined and there is little evidence to support a genuine role for occult infections in male infertility. There is thus no place for microbiological screening investigations unless there is clinical suspicion of adnexitis. Furthermore, the isolation of non-pathogenic organisms such as staphylococcus, streptococcus, diphtheroids, *Ureoplasma urealyticum* and *Mycoplasma hominis*, which are commensals in the normal urethra, does not warrant the indiscriminate use of antibiotics in the hope of correcting any abnormalities in the semen parameters.

Genital tract obstruction

The combination of azoospermia, normal testicular volume and normal FSH bears the hallmarks of genital tract obstruction. Obstructed sperm transport in the genital tract can be due to congenital or acquired abnormalities. The incidence and relative importance of individual causes of obstruction differ according to geographic locality. In economically advanced countries, postvasectomy and congenital conditions are by far the commonest. In other parts of the world, obstructive azoospermia as a long-term sequelae of genitourinary infections such as gonorrhoea, *chlamydia* and tuberculosis remains one of the most important causes of male infertility.

Three specific congenital abnormalities are recognized. The commonest is agenesis or malformations of the wolffian duct-derived structures: corpus/cauda epididymis, vas deferens and seminal vesicles. Diagnosis is usually quite easy: the scrotal vasa are not palpable or abnormally thin and the ejaculate consists of low volumes (<1 ml) of acidic non-coagulating prostatic fluid devoid of fructose and sperm. Virtually all males with cystic fibrosis are sterile because of this congenital abnormality.

In Young's syndrome, epididymal obstruction is due to progressive inspissation of amorphous secretion in the lumen. In these patients, the high incidence of chronic sinopulmonary infection and bronchiectasis is presumably the consequence of the same abnormality in the respiratory tract.

Obstruction of the ejaculatory duct due to cysts of the verumontanum is a very rare cause of obstructive azoospermia that needs to be differentiated from agenesis of the vasa and seminal vesicles since they have the same abnormal features in the ejaculate but the scrotal vasa are palpable and the condition is treatable.

The existence of partial obstruction, i.e. severe oligozoospermia associated with normal testicular volume and normal FSH, is uncertain. In most instances that have proceeded to scrotal exploration and testicular biopsy, arrest of spermatogenesis rather than extratesticular pathology has been found.

Coital disorders

Inadequate coital technique (including the use of vaginal lubricants with spermicidal properties) and frequency and faulty timing of intercourse may contribute to continuing infertility but are rarely the only aetiological factor in the infertile couple. Erectile and ejaculatory failure may be caused by psychosexual dysfunction, depression, spinal cord injuries, retroperitoneal and bladder neck surgery, diabetes mellitus, multiple sclerosis, vascular insufficiency, adrenergic-blocking antihypertensive agents, psychotropic drugs, alcohol abuse and chronic renal failure. Primary endocrine pathologies such as androgen deficiency, hyperprolactinaemia and hypothyroidism seldom present with infertility without diminished libido and clinical features specific to the hormonal disturbance, e.g. hypogonadism, loss of visual fields and myxoedema. Retrograde ejaculation must be differentiated from aspermia or anejaculation by examination of postejaculatory urine for the presence of spermatozoa.

CLINICAL MANAGEMENT

History

A thorough history is essential for identifying underlying aetiologies and devising individual management strategies. Particular attention should be paid to the following aspects. Previous surgery such as herniorrhaphy in childhood, trauma or torsion suggests possible damage to the vas or testis. Cryptorchidism, especially if bilateral, is associated with severe impairment of fertility and carries an increased risk of testicular malignancy. Although most patients presenting in infertility clinics with a history of cryptorchidism have generally received treatment when younger, orchidopexy is seldom carried out so early as to completely avoid testicular damage. Previous genitourinary infections in the form of orchitis (mumps, syphilis, leprosy, tuberculosis) and epididymitis (gonorrhoea, *Chlamydia*, tuberculosis, schistosomiasis) are serious causes of infertility in a global context. Painful ejaculation, haemotospermia and pain in the perineum are symptoms suggestive of chronic infection in the prostate and seminal vesicles. Delayed onset of puberty may suggest the possibility of gonadotrophin deficiency. A history of recurrent chest infection, sinusitis or bronchiectasis may be obtained in patients with epididymal obstruction (Young's syndrome) or those with absent sperm motility (immotile cilia syndrome) and agenesis of the vasa (cystic fibrosis). Chronic disorders such as renal failure, liver disease, malignancy, diabetes and multiple sclerosis are associated with a variety of testicular and sexual dysfunctions. Because feverish illness can transiently suppress spermatogenesis, the patient should be asked about episodes of pyrexia within the past 6 weeks. Careful enquiry should also be made about occupational or environmental exposure to testicular toxins (herbicides, pesticides, lead, cadmium), radiation, or the use of medications (cytotoxic agents, suphasalazine, nitrofurantoin, anabolic steroids, sex steroids, anticonvulsants, psychotropic and antihypertensive drugs and cimetidine) or recreational drugs (alcohol, tobacco, cannabis). It is important to establish that vaginal intercourse takes place with appropriate frequency and timing without the use of vaginal lubricants which may have spermicidal properties. With experience, it is not difficult to detect the presence of psychosexual dysfunction and varying degrees of more general psychiatric symptoms not uncommonly associated with the stigma and stress of continuing infertility.

Examination

The general physical assessment of height, weight, body habitus and secondary sexual development should be carried out in all patients. If androgen deficiency is suspected (Table 25.2), look for gynaecomastia, cryptorchidism, hypospadias, anosmia and visual field defects. Measurement of testicular volumes by comparison with a series of standard ellipsoids known as the Prader orchidometer (Fig. 25.6) provides a convenient clinical index of seminiferous tubular mass. Normal adult testicular volume is between 15 and 35 ml. Testicular volume is a key finding in differentiating between azoospermia due to seminiferous tubular failure (reduced volumes) and that arising from excurrent duct obstruction (normal volume). Testicular size is also a useful indicator of the degree of testicular development in hypogonadotrophic patients and of testicular atrophy in those with various forms of primary testicular pathologies. If not in the scrotum, the lowest position of the testes should be defined. Irregular contour, induration or abnormal consistency of the testis suggests previous orchitis, surgery or malignancy.

Table 25.2 Clinical features of androgen deficiency

	Before puberty	After puberty
Skeleton	Eunuchoidal proportions	Decreased bone density
Body hair	Lack of pubic, axillary body and facial hair; straight frontal hair line	Decreased facial and pubic hair
Skin	Lack of sebum production; paleness	Atrophic, fine and wrinkled; paleness
Muscles	Underdeveloped	Atrophic
Larynx	Lack of prominence; unbroken high-pitched voice	
Penis	Infantile	
Testes	Underdeveloped — reduced size	Regressed — reduced size
Prostate	Underdeveloped	Regressed
Libido and potency	Not developed	Lost or reduced

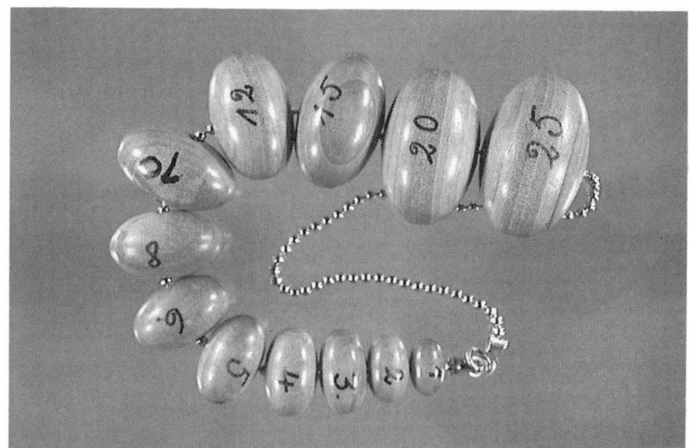

Fig. 25.6 Prader orchidometer for the assessment of testicular volume.

Special attention should also be paid to the palpation of the epididymis and scrotal vas. An enlarged and tense caput epididymis may be palpable in cases of obstructive azoospermia. Irregularity and induration of the epididymis and vas suggest previous infection. In congenital agenesis of wolffian duct-derived structures, the scrotal vasa are either impalpable or extremely thin. The scrotal contents should also be examined with the patient standing so that varicoceles become visible (grade 3) or palpable (grade 2) or are detected as a venous impulse in the spermatic cord during Valsalva manoeuvre (grade 1). Rectal examination may show irregular contour or consistency and tenderness in the prostate in the presence of chronic prostatitis.

Investigations

Semen analysis

Traditionally, the most important starting point for investigating the male contribution to a couple's infertility is the semen analysis (WHO 1987). This remains the case in current practice but it must be emphasized that conventional parameters of semen analysis such as sperm density, percentage of motile sperm, quality of sperm movements and sperm morphology (Table 25.3) are predominantly subjective and at best semi-quantitative evaluations with poor reproducibility. They can therefore provide only a crude index of an individual's potential fertility. Because of the inability of image analysis algorithms to differentiate spermatozoa from leukocytes and cellular debris in the ejaculate, automated computerized methods of semen analysis overestimate sperm concentration and consequently underestimate motility, especially in semen samples from oligozoospermic infertile men. These cannot therefore be recommended as substitutes for the more time-consuming and technically demanding routine semen analysis.

It has already been pointed out that sperm density alone is not critical to fertility until extremely low values (e.g. <5 million/ml) are reached even though samples are, by definition, classified as oligozoospermic if sperm concentrations are less than 20 million/ml. It is therefore not surprising that men of recently proven fertility may have semen parameters falling below the range generally accepted as normal. Conversely, semen parameters in the normal range do not invariably guarantee a favourable prognosis. Thus clinical decisions based on the semen profile should only be taken with due recognition of these limitations.

The poor predictive value of conventional semen analysis highlights one of the major problems in male infertility, which is the lack of a reliable quantitative and objective measure of fertility in men. To remedy this, a number of new tests that evaluate the physiological functions of sperm have been developed.

Table 25.3 Normal values of semen variables

Volume	2.0 ml or more
ph	7.2–7.8
Sperm concentration	20×10^6 spermatozoa/ml or more
Total sperm count	40×10^6 spermatozoa or more
Motility	50% or more with forward progression 25% or more with rapid linear progression within 60 min after collection
Morphology	50% or more with normal morphology
Viability	50% or more live, i.e. excluding dye
White blood cells	Fewer than 1×10^6/ml
Fructose (total)	13 μmol or more per ejaculate
Immunobead test	Fewer than 10% spermatozoa with adherent beads

From WHO (1987).

Sperm function tests

In recent years, new techniques to study individual components of sperm physiology and sperm–egg interaction have been devised in order to provide more objective assessments of sperm function so that fertility potential in a man can be predicted. The rational management of male infertility can therefore be increasingly based on an improved understanding of the precise nature of individual specific defects.

The widespread belief that fertility can best be predicted by sperm motility has prompted attempts to use rather complicated and time-consuming multiple-exposure or time-lapse photography techniques for the measurement of detailed sperm movement characteristics to evaluate male fertility. The application of these methodologies has recently been greatly facilitated by automated systems to characterize the vigour and pattern of swimming movements of large numbers of individual spermatozoa. Several commercial computerized systems such as Cellsoft 2000 (Cryo Resources, New York, USA HTM-2030 (Hamilton Thorn Research, Denvers, MA, USA) and AutoSperm (Amsaten, De Pine, Belgium) are currently available. By digitizing the sperm track analogue signals, which are transmitted to a computer by videomicrography, the stored real-time signals are then subjected to computerized image analysis to provide measurements of sperm movement such as velocity, linearity, lateral head displacement and flagellar beat frequency. However, these measurements are critically dependent on user-selected parameter settings (such as the number of frames, sampling frequency and duration of sampling, the preset thresholds for identifying spermatozoa according to luminosity and size) and algorithms for reconstructing sperm tracks from a series of images. Consequently, this type of sperm movement analysis, though automated, requires some degree of user interaction and therefore cannot be considered to be entirely objective. The true clinical significance and predictive value of individual sperm movement attributes are currently unknown. These techniques therefore remain valuable research tools and cannot be recommended for routine use at present.

The interaction of ejaculated sperm with cervical mucus provides a measure of the functional ability of spermatozoa. It is particularly important in substantiating the clinical significance of antisperm antibody detected by screening tests. The measurement of in vitro sperm penetration into mid-cycle cervical mucus has been standardized in the Kremer capillary tubes (WHO 1987) where a migration distance of <3 cm at 2 h is considered abnormal. The sperm–cervical mucus contact (SCMC) test is a simpler test to detect the presence of sperm antibody, where a positive result will show over 50% of motile spermatozoa displaying a characteristic rapid shaking motion (WHO 1987). When positive, the tests can be performed in conjunction with donor mucus and donor semen to determine the source of the antisperm antibody. These in vitro tests are preferred to the postcoital test which is more difficult to standardize and interpret.

Binding of spermatozoa to the zona pellucida is an early critical event in gamete interaction leading to fertilization. Failure of sperm–zona binding has been observed in some cases of male infertility (Overstreet et al 1980). Assessment of the ability for specific zona binding may therefore be of clinical value but because of the species-specificity of sperm–zona binding, the opportunity to test this function is limited. Recently, human oocytes that failed to fertilize in in vitro fertilization programmes have generated a source of zona pellucida which retains the capacity to bind spermatozoa for a prolonged period when stored in high-salt medium. Such salt-stored zonae have provided the basis for assays of sperm–zona binding (Burkman et al 1988; Liu & Baker 1988). As yet it is too early to know the value of this test in predicting in vitro or in vivo fertility potential.

The acrosome reaction is essential for fertilization so that the rate at which spermatozoa undergo this step may have some bearing on fertility. However, the acrosome status in human spermatozoa has been technically difficult to investigate. In the last few years however, methods using fluoresceinated (pea or peanut) lectin probes directed against the acrosome membrane has been used at the light microscopic level to differentiate between acrosome-intact and acrosome-reacted sperm (Cross et al 1986; Mortimer et al 1987). These can be further refined by incorporating a supravital stain (or hypo-osmotic swelling) to differentiate dead sperm from acrosome-reacted sperm.

It has been reported that the percentage of sperm with normal intact acrosome correlated with fertilization rate in vitro. Whether monitoring the acrosome reaction in vitro has any diagnostic or predictive significance for fertility in vivo remains to be determined. Human spermatozoa only readily undergo the acrosome reaction when in contact with human zona protein and less than 10% of isolated sperm spontaneously acrosome-react during incubation in vitro. Although the poor ability to undergo spontaneous acrosome reaction can be overcome by the use of a biochemical trigger such as ionophores, the lack of a readily available physiological stimulus may limit the potential of these tests.

A biochemically intact plasma membrane is essential for the spermatozoa to undergo capacitation and sperm–egg fusion. A simple test of plasma membrane functional integrity and fluidity may therefore provide useful information not detectable by supravital staining and sperm motility. The hypo-osmotic swelling test is based on the ability of an intact plasma membrane to transport water into the cell when placed in hypotonic media. The distension of the swollen sperm indicated by a characteristic curling of the tail signals the normal functional integrity of the plasma membrane. This ability of spermatozoa to swell has been found to be correlated with the in vitro fertilizing capacity of hamster and human oocytes by some (Jayendran et al 1984; Van der Ven et al 1986) but not others (Chan et al 1985). Further evaluation of this test is clearly required.

Hamster oocytes of which the zona pellucida has been removed by enzyme digestion are able to undergo interspecies fusion with the acrosome-reacted human sperm. This phenomenon has been developed into a bioassay of in vitro fertilization (Yanagimachi et al 1976) which can quantify the ability of human sperm plasma membrane to undergo a sequence of changes including capacitation, acrosome reaction and the generation of a fusogenic equatorial segment capable of interacting with the vitelline membrane of the zona-free hamster oocytes. To circumvent the need for prolonged incubation to capacitate the sperm and the need for a physiological stimulus (zona) for inducing the acrosome reaction, and also to improve the sensitivity of the assay for studying poor quality samples, the divalent cation ionophore A23187 has been used to induce an acute influx of extracellular calcium into the sperm cytoplasm. This rise in intracellular ionic calcium therefore bypasses the need for capacitation and precipitates the acrosome reaction. This modification of the classic hamster oocyte assay can thus identify populations of sperm which are refractory to this specific calcium-mediated stimulus. The rate of sperm–oocyte fusion in the ionophore-stimulated assay has been shown to have good correlations with fertility in unexplained male infertility (Aitken 1985), in donors in a donor insemination programme (Irvine & Aitken 1986) and in in vitro fertilization treatment (Aitken et al 1987). Despite the evidence that this investigation can provide useful information on several key aspects of sperm–egg interaction, the complexity and high costs of the hamster oocyte penetration assay precludes its application as a routine diagnostic test. However, in combination with some measure of sperm movement characteristics, the hamster oocyte penetration assay is currently the best available predictor of in vivo fertility.

Hormone measurements

The measurement of plasma FSH is useful in distinguishing primary from secondary testicular failure and in identifying patients with obstructive azoospermia. In the presence of azoospermia or oligozoospermia, an elevated FSH, particularly with reduced testicular volume, is presumptive evidence of severe and usually irreversible seminiferous tubular damage. Low or undetectable FSH (usually associated with low LH and testosterone with clinical evidence of androgen deficiency) is suggestive of hypogonadotrophism. Conversely, azoospermia with normal FSH and normal testicular volume usually indicates the presence of bilateral genital tract obstruction. Exceptions to these rules occur from time to time. For example, azoospermia or oligozoospermia due to germ cell arrest may be associated with normal FSH while some men with high FSH may have normal spermatogenesis.

Testosterone and LH measurements are indicated in the assessment of the infertile male when there is clinical suspicion of androgen deficiency, sex steroid abuse or steroid-secreting lesions such as congenital adrenal hyperplasia or functioning adrenal/testicular tumours. In men presenting with infertility, testosterone is usually within the normal range although some degree of Leydig cell dysfunction, as evidenced by statistically lower testosterone and higher LH compared to normal, is not uncommon. This may identify those who may be considered for androgen replacement, although this has no bearing on fertility. High LH and testosterone should raise the possibility of abnormalities in androgen receptors while low LH and testosterone suggest hypogonadotrophism.

Hyperprolactinaemia is not a recognized cause of male infertility but prolactin measurement should be undertaken if there is clinical evidence of sexual dysfunction (particularly diminished libido) or pituitary disease leading to secondary testicular failure. Oestradiol measurement is rarely indicated except in the presence of gynaecomastia.

Dynamic tests of pituitary-testicular function such as LHRH, thyrotropin-releasing hormone, human chorionic gonadotrophin stimulation generally do not add to the basal measurements already described. Bearing in mind the episodic nature of LH secretion, the diurnal variation in testosterone and the stress-related secretion of prolactin, it is usually sufficient to repeat their measurements in the morning under resting conditions if necessary.

Chromosome analysis

Buccal smear and/or chromosome karyotyping should be carried out in patients with azoospermia or severe oligozoospermia with testicular atrophy and elevated FSH. Cytogenetic abnormalities, by far the commonest being Klinefelter's syndrome, will be detected in about 10% of this group. If one of the above-mentioned chromosomal abnormalities is identified, a genetic basis for irreversible infertility is assumed so that a clear prognosis and guidelines for alternative management can be offered without delay.

Testicular biopsy

With the use of plasma FSH in recent years to differentiate between primary testicular failure and obstructive lesions, the need for testicular biopsy in the investigation of male infertility has largely been superseded. However, when genital tract obstruction is suspected, testicular biopsy is still useful in confirming normal spermatogenesis and excluding spermatogenic arrest. When the clinical differentiation between spermatogenic failure and obstruction is uncertain (e.g. asymmetrical findings on examination between right and left testes or adnexae), scrotal exploration with testicular biopsy may be helpful. Vasography during scrotal exploration is required to confirm the diagnosis of obstructed ejaculatory ducts. Some would also advocate testicular biopsy with or without scrotal exploration to diagnose partial epididymal obstruction in patients with severe oligozoospermia and normal FSH.

Semen biochemistry

The analysis of biochemical markers of sperm function will probably become the next generation of simple tests of semen quality which could avoid the technical complication and high costs of the currently available bioassays discussed above. At present however, the diagnostic, value and clinical significance of several possible candidates, including the key metabolite for sperm motility, adenosine triphosphate, the acrosomal enzyme acrosin, the lactate dehydrogenase isoenzyme X specifically released by degenerate germ cells and the peroxidative free radicals produced by sperm membrane, all require more detailed study and validation (for review see Aitken 1989). It is envisaged that as more is learned about individual biological defects in sperm function at the biochemical and molecular levels, specific indicators in the semen or blood of individual functional lesions can be simply and economically measured.

The analysis of biochemical markers of accessory gland function has a more established place in current clinical practice. Even so, although a number of specific secretory products of the epididymis, prostate and seminal vesicles can be measured in seminal plasma, only fructose content is generally recognized to be of any value.Undetectable or very low levels of seminal fructose are taken as evidence to corroborate the diagnosis of vasal and seminal vesicle agenesis or blocked ejaculatory ducts in the presence of obstructive azoospermia.

Antisperm antibodies

Currently, the best diagnostic tests are those based on the mixed agglutination reaction where sheep red blood cells or polyacrylamide beads are coated with rabbit antibodies to specific classes of human immunoglobulins which will attach to motile sperm carrying immunoglobulins of the same class on their surface membrane. This permits the detection of immunoglobulin gamma A, G or M on the surface of the sperm head or tail. The direct test uses washed sperm from the patient and the presence of surface-bound antibody, indicated by particulate binding in over 10% of spermatozoa, is considered to be a positive result. It depends on the availability of sufficient numbers of motile sperm in the patient's fresh semen sample and is the standard test in most laboratories currently. The indirect test uses decomplemented patient serum or seminal plasma which is incubated with motile donor sperm. Antisperm antibodies will bind to donor sperm and their presence is detected by attachment of particles to the sperm surface. The indirect test is therefore more convenient for screening large numbers of patients. A positive screening test, however, must be substantiated by investigations to assess the biological significance of sperm antibody. This is usually a test to determine the ability of sperm to penetrate normal mid-cycle cervical mucus (see above).

MANAGEMENT

The management of male infertility remains a difficult and somewhat unsatisfactory experience for patients as well as doctors. The majority of patients present no recognizable or reversible aetiological factors for treatment, while advising those whose semen abnormalities seem more compatible with fertility is fraught with uncertainties due to the poor predictive powers of currently available investigations. Nevertheless, there have been a number of advances in the last few years which are beginning to make a significant impact in our therapeutic capabilities. The approach to management recently proffered by Baker (1989) highlights the scope and limitations of currently available treatments. Accordingly, patients are allocated into three categories: potentially treatable infertility; subfertility due to idiopathic hypospermatogenesis, and untreatable sterility.

Potentially treatable infertility

The number of infertile patients with potentially treatable conditions is unfortunately still small (Table 25.1). Nevertheless, they form a disproportionately important group for whom rational therapies of proven efficacy can be offered.

Testicular toxins

In patients with inflammatory bowel diseases treated by sulphasalazine, changing treatment to 5-aminosalicylic acid removes the toxic agent, sulphapyridine, and leads to a rapid recovery of fertility without deterioration in disease activity. Medications such as nitrofurantoin, anabolic steroids, sex steroids and anticonvulsants and recreation drugs such as cigarettes, alcohol and cannabis should be withdrawn or avoided if possible. Although testicular function should improve in patients with chronic renal failure after successful transplantation, fertility impairment may be perpetuated by the continued use of immunosuppressive agents.

Gonadotrophin deficiency

Patients with gonadotrophin deficiency due to acquired conditions and to a lesser extent, those with partial LHRH deficiency, usually respond to human chorionic gonadotrophin (Profasi 2000 iu i.m. once or twice weekly) alone for 6–12 months (Burger & Baker 1982). During this time the rise in testosterone will virilize the patient and the testes usually increase in size. If there is no sperm in the ejaculate at the end of 12 months, human menopausal gonadotrophin (Pergonal) which contains both FSH and LH should be added, 37.5 iu i.m. thrice weekly initially, increasing to 75 iu thrice weekly if necessary after 6 months. This graded approach may take up to 2 years before one can ascertain if spermatogenesis is established or not. The treatment outcome of gonadotrophin induction of spermatogenesis is variable but in general, 64–76% should show some degree of spermatogenesis and 54–60% could be expected to achieve pregnancies. Previous treatment with testosterone does not appear to compromise the response to subsequent exogenous gonadotrophins (Burger et al 1981).

In patients with more profound degrees of LHRH deficiency, it might be anticipated that the most suitable form of replacement to induce maximal testicular growth and development is to emulate the physiological mode of pulsatile LHRH stimulation of the pituitary and in turn, the testes. This has been made possible by the development of battery-driven portable infusion minipumps which can automatically deliver a desired dose of LHRH at a set time interval. The usual starting regime is the subcutaneous administration of 50 ng/kg/dose of synthetic LHRH (Fertira at 2-h intervals. If testosterone has not reached the normal range by 3 months, the dose should be increased by 50 ng. It is seldom necessary to use more than 200 ng/kg/dose. Possible reasons for treatment failure include non-compliance and unsuspected obstructions in the excurrent ducts; clinically significant antibody formation to LHRH is relatively uncommon and is rarely the cause of treatment failure.

Experience with pulsatile LHRH therapy is still relatively limited because of the small numbers of patients treated. The current impression is that it is achieving a similar degree of success in the induction of fertility as gonadotrophins (Morris et al 1984). However, a report by Liu et al (1988) suggested that pulsatile LHRH therapy for the first 2 years does not accelerate or enhance testicular growth or spermatogenesis compared with human chorionic/menopausal gonadotrophin combination therapy in hypogonadotrophic patients presenting with testes volume <4 ml. This requires confirmation.

Sperm antibody

Treatment of patients with antisperm antibodies by artificial insemination by husband using washed sperm preparations and in vitro fertilization has proven disappointing (Clarke et al 1985). Immunosuppression with high-dose glucocorticoid, including prednisolone 0.75 mg/kg/day for 6 months (Baker 1989) or prednisolone 20 mg b.d. on days 1–10 and 5 mg on days 11 and 12 of the partner's cycle for 6 months (Hendry 1989) has been reported to reduce antibody titres, improve sperm–mucus penetration and achieve significant improvements in pregnancy rates (25–30%) compared to placebo. Cryostorage of semen following significant improvement in quality for later artificial insemination or in vitro fertilization should further amplify the therapeutic benefit. Side-effects are common and are dose-dependent. They may include irritability, sleeplessness, arthralgia, muscle weakness, peptic ulceration, glucose intolerance, cushingoid features and, most disabling of all, bilateral aseptic necrosis of femoral heads (Shulman & Shulman 1982). The high incidence and potentially life-threatening and disabling nature of some of these complications make it imperative that the diagnosis of sperm autoimmunity be fully substantiated by confirmatory biological tests, that other pathologies in both partners be adequately excluded and that the patients be made aware of possible side-effects before embarking on glucocorticoid treatment. Preliminary medical assessment should include blood pressure recording, postprandial blood glucose measurement, chest X-ray and exclusion of active peptic ulceration. A steroid card stating the details of treatment and hospital contact address and telephone number should be carried by the patient at all times during treatment, so that appropriate glucocorticoid replacement can be instituted in case of emergencies.

Genital tract obstruction

Treatment by transurethral endoscopic puncturing of the prostatic cysts offers a good chance of relieving the ejaculatory duct obstruction. However, until recently, the surgical treatment of commoner forms of obstructive azoospermia offered an extremely low rate of success. In the last decade, microsurgical techniques of epididymovasostomy to bypass epididymal obstruction (Silber 1979) have been reported to produce astonishingly good results with patency rates of 78% and pregnancy rates of 56% (Silber 1989). Provided antisperm antibody titres are not high, results of treatment for postinfective cases (especially postgonococcal) are generally more favourable than Young's syndrome where there is a tendency to re-obstruct postoperatively. Pregnancies have also recently been reported in wives of patients with agenesis of the vasa when sperm aspirated from the caput epididymis was used successfully for in vitro fertilization (Silber et al 1988). Unfortunately, these state-of-the-art techniques are extremely expensive and available only in very few centres. Thus for the vast majority of patients with obstructive azoospermia, the outlook remains bleak.

Varicocele

The position of varicocele treatment in the management of the infertile male has continued to generate much controversy. Traditionally, treatment of varicocele is by surgical ligation of the internal spermatic vein above the internal inguinal ring or by microdissection and transection of the venous plexus at the external ring. Between 10 and 20% of patients have persistent or recurrent varicoceles after surgery. Transfemoral embolization of the internal spermatic vein preceded by selective venography to confirm the diagnosis is increasingly used as non-surgical treatment under local anaesthesia. This technique reputedly gives a lower recurrence rate than surgical ligation but is dependent on the availability and expertise of an interventional radiologist.

Results of treatment of varicocele are uncertain. Some studies report a favourable effect of varicocele treatment on semen quality and pregnancy rate (Comhaire 1986) but others found no difference in pregnancy outcome between treated and untreated patients (Rodriguez-Rigau et al 1978; Nilsson et al 1979). These studies have been criticized because of their retrospective and non-randomized design with inadequate numbers of patients to substantiate negative treatment outcomes. Until a proper therapeutic trial is carried out, the significance of varicocele in male infertility must remain an open question.

In the meantime, patients with abnormal semen quality and normal FSH associated with varicocele and no other pathology must be counselled individually: they may or may not have a potentially treatable condition and the outcome of treatment is uncertain. Those with azoospermia and/or elevated FSH have a low probability of improvement and treatment is normally not recommended in this group.

Coital disorders

If semen of good quality can be obtained with masturbation, vibrators or electroejaculation from patients with various coital dysfunctions, and functional spermatozoa recovered from alkalinized bladder urine of appropriate osmolality from the patient with retrograde ejaculation, artificial insemination can be reasonably successful.

Subfertility due to idiopathic hypospermatogenesis

This forms by far the largest group of male patients in infertility clinics (Table 25.1). They have reduced fertility as a result of poor sperm quality reflected by combinations of reduced sperm density, low sperm motility and an increased proportion of abnormal spermatozoa. Despite this, pregnancies can occur in some of these couples without treatment and since semen abnormalities of similar magnitude are not uncommon in men whose partners are current attenders at antenatal clinics, it must be assumed that infertility in these men may be associated with a significant but subtle contribution from their female partners even though they have ostensibly been evaluated as normal by the criteria of current investigations. Clearly, the age of the female partner and the duration of infertility have an important negative influence on the fecundity of these couples in addition to the defects in sperm quality.

Over the years, a wide variety of essentially empirical treatments have been used in attempts to improve fertility in subfertile men. These include testosterone suppression and rebound, gonadotrophins, LHRH, clomiphene, tamoxifen, testolactone, antibiotics, bromocriptine, pentoxiphylline, pancreatic kallikrein, vitamin C, zinc and homologous artificial insemination. However, the vast majority of these regimes have not been subjected to controlled clinical trials and most have fallen into disrepute after a brief period of popularity. The few treatments that were evaluated properly were shown not to be effective in terms of pregnancy rates or improvements in semen parameters. It is imperative that any proposed treatment for male infertility should be subjected to prospective randomized controlled trials because of the significant background treatment-unrelated pregnancy rates (in general about 5% per month) and the tendency of semen variables to show apparent improvements as a result of regression towards the mean. However, the expected treatment-induced increase in pregnancy rates is generally only moderate (20% per month) thus necessitating the inclusion of a very large number of couples in any meaningful clinical trials.

In the last 5 years, in vitro fertilization has been increasingly applied to treat patients with mild to moderate impairments in sperm quality (Yovich et al 1984). This approach was based on the observation that a relatively small number of spermatozoa (100 000–150 000) are required for fertilization in vitro, thus offering the possibility of promoting sperm–egg interaction as a form of assisted conception procedure for patients with oligozoospermic male infertility. It is now generally accepted that fertilization in vitro can be effected by spermatozoa recovered from poor quality semen, albeit at a significantly reduced rate (30–50%) compared to those obtained from normal ejaculates (60–80%). Despite the lower fertilization rate, the overall pregnancy (10–15%) and live birth rates (8–10%) per treatment cycle were not significantly different from that expected with normal semen quality. This also confirms that there is no increase in pregnancy wastage in cases of male infertility.

The fertilization rate declines in proportion with increasing degrees of abnormalities in semen parameters; thus those with single defects in sperm density, motility or morphology have only a moderate reduction in fertilization rate which can be overcome by maximizing the number of follicles recovered for insemination and increasing the number of embryos transferred, while those with multiple defects in semen parameters have significantly poorer results. In attempts to improve the pregnancy rate, gamete intrafallopian transfer has been used to treat oligozoospermic infertility. However the loss of information on the fertilizing capacity of spermatozoa in this procedure is a serious disadvantage. Recently, pronuclear stage pre-embryos have been transferred to the fallopian tubes in the hope that the chance of pregnancy can be maximized while information on fertilization can still be obtained. Micromanipulation techniques have also been applied to place spermatozoa directly into the perivitelline space by injection or zona dissection in order to promote fertilization in vitro (Laws-King et al 1987; Malter & Cohen 1989). Results of these newer methods of treatment are awaited. A further improvement in management is the introduction of appropriate tests of sperm function that can predict the likelihood of fertilization taking place during in vitro fertilization. Hamster oocyte penetration, zona binding assays and detection of acrosome defects are being applied as pretreatment screening investigations: satisfactory results are taken as indications for in vitro fertilization.

It should be made clear that treatment of male infertility by various assisted conception procedures is only moderately successful at present. The predicted live birth rates are certainly not so much higher than spontaneous pregnancy rates in these patients that treatment can be recommended unreservedly. Bearing in mind the considerable financial and emotional investments, it is prudent therefore to counsel in vitro fertilization and related procedures as the last resort for couples with long-standing infertility who have virtually exhausted their spontaneous fertility potential.

Untreatable sterility

Patients with azoospermia or extreme oligozoospermia (<1 million/ml), atrophic testes and elevated FSH have irreversible primary seminiferous tubular failure and are to all intents and purposes sterile. The commonest known aetiologies are Klinefelter's syndrome, cryptorchidism, cytotoxic or irradiation treatment and testicular torsion or trauma. Patients should be informed of their prognosis and counselled regarding the options of continuing childlessness, adoption and donor insemination.

In the cryptorchidic adult presenting with infertility, orchidopexy cannot improve fertility or reduce the risk of malignancy but is directed towards placing the testis in a satisfactory position to facilitate examination and to minimize the risk of trauma and torsion. Ultrasound examination of the testes may help in locating an ectopic or intra-abdominal testis and localized areas of altered echogenicity may indicate malignant change. Testes that could not be placed in a satisfactory scrotal position should be removed and prostheses inserted. No treatment can be offered for those who have had previous treatment but remain infertile. In general, unilateral cryptorchidism is compatible with fertility though at a significantly reduced level.

The differentiation between retractile and true undescended testis in childhood is not easy. It is believed that a retractile testis responds to hormone treatment, presumably due to an androgen-mediated effect in decreasing cremasteric muscle contractility, while a true undescended testis is unresponsive to hormone manipulation and only correctible by surgical orchidopexy. Consequently hormone treatment may be worth a try for all prescrotal testes with a 10–30% chance of full descent, thereby saving an operation. Human chorionic gonadotrophin seems more effective and is much cheaper than LHRH. Hormone manipulation is not suitable for abdominal or high inguinal testes, where surgery should be considered from the outset.

Although the majority of Klinefelter's patients presenting at infertility clinics usually do not complain of symptoms related to androgen deficiency, gynaecomastia may be present in 50% and testosterone is usually in the low normal or slightly below the normal range while bone density may be reduced. Androgen replacement is therefore indicated in some of these patients. A few patients with idiopathic hypospermatogenesis may also come into this category.

KEY POINTS

1. Spermatogenesis is a continuous sequence of highly organized and closely regulated events within the seminiferous tubules. The total duration for development of spermatozoa is 74 days.
2. The presence of testosterone in sufficient quantities in the seminiferous tubules is an absolute requirement for spermatogenesis.
3. Secretions of the accessory glands form over 90% of the volume of semen.
4. Only 200 or so of the most robust spermatozoa reach the site of fertilization.
5. Capacitation is a series of functional changes which render sperm capable of fertilization.
6. Physiologically acrosome reaction can only take place after the sperm have undergone capacitation.
7. Binding of sperm to zona pellucida triggers the acrosome reaction.
8. Only a small minority of infertile men have specific recognizable or treatable aetiologies.
9. Surgical orchidopexy for undescended testis is unlikely to improve fertility after the age of 2 years.
10. Pyrexial illnesses may non-specifically depress spermatogenesis for some weeks but recovery is complete.
11. The significance of varicocele in male infertility is controversial.
12. Azoospermia, normal testicular volume and normal FSH indicates genital tract obstruction.
13. Conventional parameters of semen analysis are subjective, semi-quantitative and poorly reproducible.

REFERENCES

Aiman J, Griffen J E 1982 The frequency of androgen receptor deficiency in infertile men. Journal of Clinical Endocrinology and Metabolism 54: 725–732

Aitken R J 1985 Diagnosis value of the zona-free hamster oocyte penetration test and sperm movement characteristics in oligozoospermia. International Journal of Andrology 8: 348–356

Aitken R J 1989 Assessment of human sperm function. In: Burger H, de Kretser D M (eds) The testis, 2nd edn. Raven Press, New York, pp 441–473

Aitken R J, Thatcher S, Glasier A F, Clarkson J S, Wu F C W, Baird D T 1987 Relative ability of modified versions of the hamster oocyte penetration test, incorporating hyperosmotic medium on the ionophore A23187 to predict IVF outcome. Human Reproduction 2: 227–231

Baker H W G 1989 Clinical evaluation and management of testicular disorders in the adult. In: Burger H, de Kretser D M (eds) The testis, 2nd edition. Raven Press, New York, pp 419–440

Burger H G, Baker H W G 1982 Therapeutic considerations and results of gonadotropin treatment in male hypogonadotropic hypogonadism. Annals of the New York Academy of Sciences 438: 447–453

Burger H G, de Kretser D M, Hudson B, Wilson J D 1981 Effects of preceding androgen therapy on testicular response to human pituitary gonadotropin in hypogonadotropic hypogonadism: a study of three patients. Fertility and Sterility 35: 64–68

Burkman L J, Coddington C C, Fraken D R, Kruger T F, Rosenwaks Z, Hodgen G D 1988 The hemizone assay (HZA): development of a diagnostic test for the binding of human spermatozoa to the human hemizona pellucida to predict fertilization potential. Fertility and Sterility 49: 688–697

Cates W, Farley T M M, Rowe P J 1985 Worldwide patterns of infertility: is Africa different? Lancet ii: 596–598

Chan S Y W, Fox E J, Chan M M C et al 1985 The relationship between the human sperm hypoosmotic swelling test, routine semen analysis and the human sperm zona-free hamster ovum penetration assay. Fertility and Sterility 44: 668–672

Chandley A C 1979 The chromosomal basis of human infertility. British Medical Bulletin 35: 181–186

Clarke G N, Lopata A, McBain J C, Baker H W G, Johnson W I H 1985 Effects of sperm antibodies in males on human in vitro fertilization. American Journal of Immunology and Microbiology 8: 62–66

Comhaire F H 1986 Varicocoele and its role in male infertility. In: Clarke J R (ed) Oxford reviews of reproductive biology, vol 8. Clarenden Press, Oxford, pp 165–213

Cross W L, Morales P, Overstreet J W, Hanson F W 1986 Two simple methods for detecting acrosome-reacted human sperm. Gamete Research 15: 213–226

de Castro M P P, Mastrorocco D A M 1984 Reproductive history and semen analysis in prevasectomy fertile men with and without varicocoeles. Journal of Andrology 5: 17

Dom J, Rudak E, Aitken R J 1981 Antisperm antibodies: their effect on the process of fertilization studied in vitro. Fertility and Sterility 35: 535–541

Dym M 1977 In: Weiss L, Greep R O (eds) Histology, 4th edn. McGraw Hill, New York, p 981

Ewing L L, Zirkin B 1983 Leydig cell structure and function. Recent Progress in Hormone Research 39: 599–635

Fawcett D W 1975 Developmental Biology 44: 394

Fukuda M, Morales P, Overstreet J W 1989 Acrosome function of human spermatozoa with normal and abnormal head morphology. Gamete Research 24: 59–65

Harper M J K 1988 Gamete and zygote transport. In: Knobil E, Neill J (eds) The physiology of reproduction. Raven Press, New York, pp 103–134

Hendry W F 1989 Detection and treatment of antispermatozoal antibodies in men. Reproduction, Fertility and Development 1: 205–222

Hull M G R, Glazener C M A, Kelly N J et al 1985 Population study of causes, treatment and outcome of infertility. British Medical Journal 291: 1693–1697

Irvine D S, Aitken R J 1986 Predictive value of in vitro sperm function tests in the context of an AID service. Human Reproduction 1: 539–545

Jayendran R S, Van der Ven H H, Perez-Pelaez M, Crabo B G, Zavevela L J D 1984 Development of an assay to assess the functional integrity of the human sperm membrane and its relationship to other semen characteristics. Journal of Reproduction and Fertility 70: 219–228

Kruger T F, Acosta A A, Simmons K F, Swanson R J, Matta J F, Oehminger S 1988 Predictive value of abnormal sperm morphology in vitro fertilization. Fertility and Sterility 49: 112–117

Laws-King A, Trouson A, Sathamanthan H, Kola I 1987 Fertilization of human oocytes by micro injection of a single spermatozoa under the zona pellucida. Fertility and Sterility 48: 637–642

Liu D Y, Baker H W G 1988 The proportion of human sperm with poor morphology but normal intact acrosomes detected with pisum sativum agglutinum correlates with fertilization in vitro. Fertility and Sterility 50: 288–293

McLachlan R I, Robertson D M, de Kretser D M, Burger H G 1987 Inhibin — a non-steroidal regulator of pituitary follicle stimulating hormone. Baillière's Clinical Endocrinology and Metabolism 1: 89–112

Malter H E, Cohen J 1989 Partial zona dissection of the human oocyte: a non traumatic method using micromanipulation to assist zona pellucida penetration. Fertility and Sterility 51: 139–148

Matsumoto A M 1989 Hormonal control of spermatogenesis. In: Burger H, de Kretser D (eds) The testis, 2nd edn. Raven Press, New York, pp 181–196

Morales P, Katz D F, Overstreet J W, Samuels S J, Chang R J 1988 The relationship between the motility and morphology of spermatozoa in human semen. International Journal of Andrology 9: 241–247

Morris D V, Adeniyi-Jones R, Wheeler M, Sonksen P, Jacobs H S 1984 The treatment of hypogonadotrophic hypogonadism in men by the pulsatile infusion of luteinizing hormone-releasing hormone. Clinical Endocrinology 21: 189–200

Mortimer D, Curtis E F, Miller R G 1987 Specific labelling by peanut agglutinin of the outer acrosomal membrane of the human spermatozoon. Journal of Reproduction and Fertility 81: 127–135

Nilsson S, Edvinsson A, Nilsson B 1979 Improvement of semen and pregnancy rate after ligation and division of the internal spermatic vein: fact or fiction. British Journal of Urology 51: 591–596

Overstreet J W, Ganagimachi R, Katz D F, Hayashi K, Hanson F W 1980 Penetration of human spermatozoa into the human zona-free hamster egg — a study of fertile donors and infertile patients. Fertility and Sterility 33: 534–542

Rodriguez-Rigau L J, Smith K D, Steinberger E 1978 Relationship of varicocoele to sperm output and fertility of male partners in infertile couples. Journal of Urology 120: 691–694

Sandler B 1954 Recovery from sterility after mumps orchitis. British Medical Journal 2: 795

Sharpe R M 1986 Paracrine control of the testis. Clinics in Endocrinology and Metabolism 15: 185–207

Sharpe R M 1987 Testosterone and spermatogenesis. Journal of Endocrinology 113: 1–2

Sharpe R M, Muller J, Skakkebaek N E 1988 Cryptorchidism. Proceedings of an ESPE Symposium. Hormone Research 30: 129–216

Shulman J F, Shulman S 1982 Methylprednisolone treatment of immunologic infertility in the male. Fertility and Sterility 38: 591–599

Silber S J 1979 Microsurgery of the male genitalia. In: Silber S J (ed) Microsurgery. Williams & Wilkins, Baltimore, pp 259–297

Silber S J 1989 Results of microsurgical vasoepididymostomy: role of epididymis in sperm maturation. Human Reproduction 4: 298–303

Silber S J, Borrero B, Asch O 1988 Pregnancy with sperm aspiration from the proximal head of epididymis: a new treatment for congenital absence of the vas deferens. Fertility and Sterility 50

Van der Ven H H, Jayendran R S, Al-Hasani S, Perez-Pelaez M, Diedrich K, Zaneveld L J D 1986 Correlation between human sperm swelling in hypoosmotic medium (hypoosmotic swelling test) and in vitro fertilization. International Journal of Andrology 7: 190–196

Whorton D, Knauss R M, Marshall S, Milby T H 1977 Infertility in male pesticide workers. Lancet ii: 1259–1261

World Health Organization 1987 WHO Laboratory manual for the examination of human semen and semen-cervical mucus interaction. Cambridge University Press, Cambridge

Wu F C W, Taylor P L, Sellar R E 1989 Luteinizing hormone releasing hormone pulse frequency in normal and infertile men. Journal of Endocrinology 123: 149–158

Yanagimachi R 1988 Mammalian fertilization. In: Knobil E, Neill J (Eds) Physiology of reproduction. Raven Press, New York, pp 135–185

Yovich J L, Stanger J D, Yovich J M 1984 The management of oligospermic infertility by in vitro fertilization. Annals of the New York Academy of Sciences 442: 276–286

Yovich J L, Stanger J D, Key D, Boettcher B 1984 In vitro fertilization of oocytes from women with serum antisperm antibodies. Lancet i: 369–370

SECTION 3

Benign Disease

26. Benign breast disease

J. M. Sackier C. B. Wood

INTRODUCTION

To most women, the idea of breast disease is inseparable from cancer, but in fact the majority of those seen in a breast clinic will have a benign condition. Therefore, the physician has an obligation to reassure a large number of patients that they do not have a malignancy. Many women will attend a clinic purely for reassurance.

Familiarity with the clinical presentation of benign breast conditions is vital to allow rapid diagnosis, treatment and reassurance. However, a high degree of suspicion must always exist as the most innocent seeming lump can turn out to be a cancer.

A wide variety of syndromes come under the umbrella of benign breast disease. The approach to the patient on first presentation will be described initially. After a discussion of the merits of the diagnostic modalities available, the conditions and their treatments will be described.

HISTORY

If the main symptom is of a lump, the doctor should ascertain when it was detected and by whom; whether it has changed in size and if it varies with the menstrual cycle. If pain is a factor, it is important to establish whether the pain was a sequel to finding the lump as this may imply anxiety as the aetiological factor.

A large number of women attend with mastalgia (Preece et al 1976) yet the symptom has historically been attributed a psychological basis. However, in most patients a careful clinical evaluation will reveal a cause. Pain should be characterized by side, site, nature, and degree. Whether or not there are aggravating or relieving factors may be important, e.g. a young girl who develops bilateral pain related to physical exertion may benefit from wearing a firm brassière. The relationship to the menstrual cycle also provides a key to diagnosis.

If a nipple discharge is present the doctor must ascertain whether it is bilateral, the length of history, and which of the seven types is present, that is: milky; multicoloured and sticky; purulent; watery; serous; serosanguineous or bloody.

EXAMINATION

The classical principles of physical examination are nowhere better illustrated than in breast disease where a combination of sensitivity to the patient's concerns and careful assessment are vital. The patient must be comfortable — a semi-recumbent posture is most suitable. The patient should be asked to indicate the site of the lump, pain or discharge. Thorough inspection will reveal scars, lumps, distended veins, visible discharge, and peau d'orange (Fig. 26.1). The brassière should also be examined discreetly for signs of discharge. When the patient raises her arms slowly the nipples should rise symmetrically and any lump or skin tethering may become obvious. The patient should then rest her arms on her lap and the unaffected breast should be palpated first, ensuring that

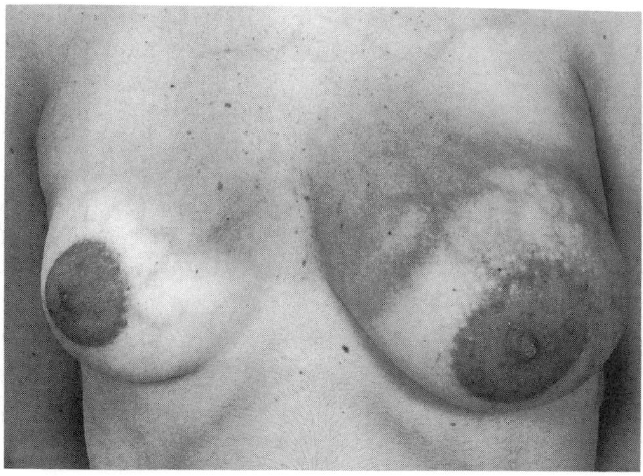

Fig. 26.1 The left breast is clearly larger, more dependent and has visible distended veins. The cause was a giant fibroadenoma.

the four quadrants, axillary tail, axilla and supraclavicular fossae are assessed in turn.

The position of a lump should be noted in relation to the areola using the 'clockface' system for notation. Fixity should be evaluated by moving the lump between finger and thumb with the patient relaxed and while contracting pectoralis major by pressing her hand on to her hip. The consistency of a lump should be defined — it is possible with experience to differentiate a cystic from a solid lesion. An attempt should be made to assess the degree of tenderness of an area reported to be painful and to establish how this section of the breast differs from the surrounding tissue and the other breast.

INVESTIGATIONS

Haematological investigations and a chest X-ray may be indicated as part of the overall evaluation. Cytological examination of a discharge is useful and so manual expression should be delayed until the cytology technician is in the room and ready to fix the slide.

Fine needle aspiration is a fast and effective method for detecting breast cancer but must be interpreted in the light of clinical and radiological findings. The use of local anaesthetic is unnecessary but ethyl chloride spray to the proposed puncture site is appreciated by the patient. An 18 gauge needle and 20 ml syringe should be used, preferably in a gun device. The needle should be introduced over the lesion, the plunger withdrawn and several passes made into the suspicious area. Both a film and a suspension should be made from the material. Tru-cut biopsy has few advantages over fine needle aspiration.

Mammography

This is still the mainstay of breast radiography since first described by Salomon in 1913, but experience is necessary for meaningful interpretation of films.

In recent years there has been concern about the carcinogenic potential of radiation mammography. Data from Hiroshima suggest that it is only in women under 35 years of age that exposure to radiation increases the risk of breast cancer (Tokunaga et al 1984). However, in women less than 35 years old mammography is of limited value as the breast is dense and occult lesions may not be seen. The small number of missed lesions are likely to be medullary or lobular cancers which are slow to metastasize.

There are clear indications that breast screening is of value, with reduction in mortality in every age group (Moskowitz et al 1975). The patient over 35 years with benign breast disease should therefore have a mammogram regardless of whether the presenting complaint merits investigation. She should be warned that the examination

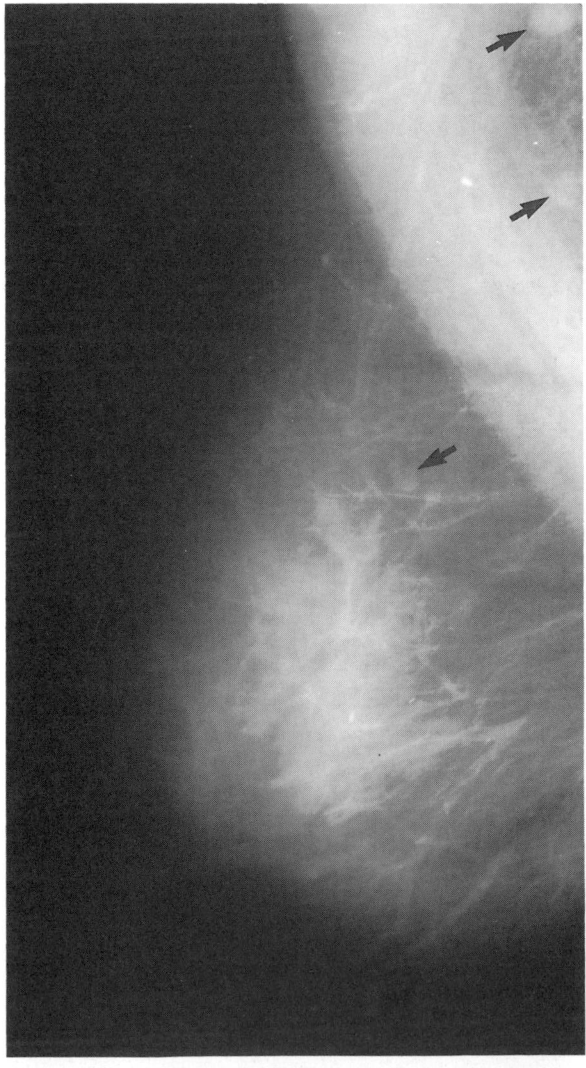

Fig. 26.2 Craniocaudal mammogram showing axillary lymph nodes (arrowed) and an intramammary node with typical central 'nick' (arrowed).

may be uncomfortable as the breasts have to be compressed. The dose of radiation is minimal and is equivalent to visiting Edinburgh Castle for the day. Other indications for mammography, apart from screening, are shown below:

1. Breast lump.
2. Nipple discharge.
3. Pain.
4. Previous breast surgery.
5. Implants or augmentations.
6. Recurrent complaints.
7. Large breasts.
8. Cancerophobia.

Interpretation of the films requires skill, care, and a good magnifying glass. The surgeon should review the X-rays prior to reading the radiologist's report in order to build up his or her own expertise (Fig. 26.2). The craniocaudal views of both breasts should be examined together, allowing direct comparison, and then the mediolateral views assessed. A mammogram reported as normal in the presence of a palpable lump should not deter the surgeon from performing a biopsy.

Microcalcifications may herald an occult neoplasm, but are often benign (Fig. 26.3). If the lesion is impalpable, localization with Frank or Kopans needles or methylene blue (Snyder 1980) enables the surgeon to remove the suspicious area. Through a curved incision in the skin lines of the breast, the surgeon cuts down to the area marked by the dye or needles, removing it with generous margins

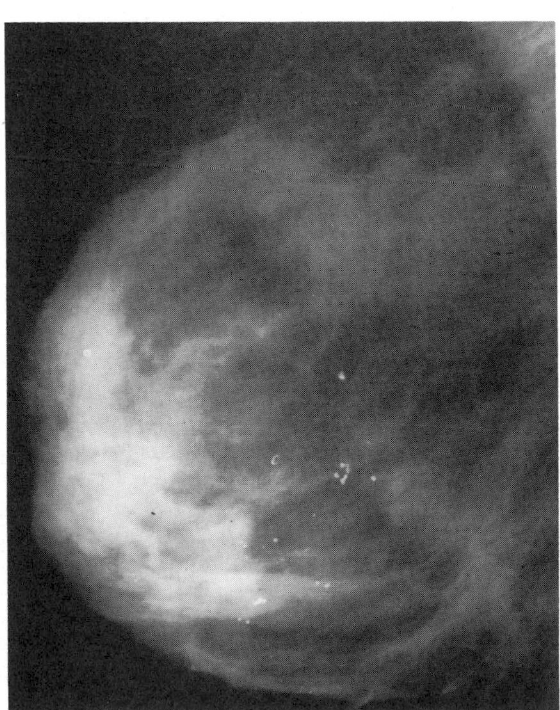

Fig. 26.3 Mammogram showing diffuse, coarse calcification typical of duct ectasia.

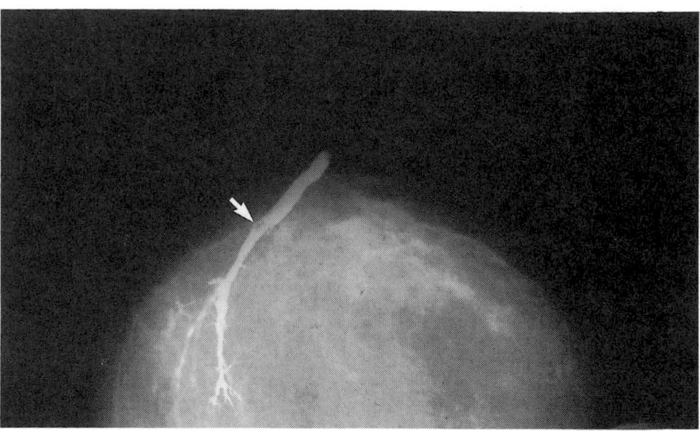

Fig. 26.4 Mediolateral ductogram with one duct outlined by contrast. An intraduct papilloma is visible (arrowed).

(Goldberg et al 1983). The specimen should then be radiographed to ensure that the calcified area has been excised. A useful recent development is the Faxitron unit which may be kept in the operating theatre and which produces an excellent image of the specimen within 5 minutes. In the future, stereotactic localization may greatly enhance the accuracy of the method described above.

Ductography

Introduction of contrast medium into a discharging duct may outline ectasia or intraductal papilloma (Fig. 26.4). It is useful for the patient who continues to have a discharge after surgical exploration.

Thermography

Since its description by Lawson in 1956 this method of detecting lesions by heat emission has decreased in popularity.

Ultrasound

This is useful for differentiating between solid and cystic lesions seen on mammography and to guide fine needle aspirations of lesions (Fig. 26.5). In the young woman, ultrasound may confirm the diagnosis of fibroadenoma and, by measuring a lump, enable the surgeon to monitor successive growth.

FIBROADENOMA

These chronic mammary tumours are called fibroadenomata when the stroma is fibrous, myxomas when myxomatous and when cystic they are known as cystosarcomas. They are common lesions, representing 9–15% of the breast clinic population (Sackier & Wood 1988) and are found in 25% of specimens removed for other reasons.

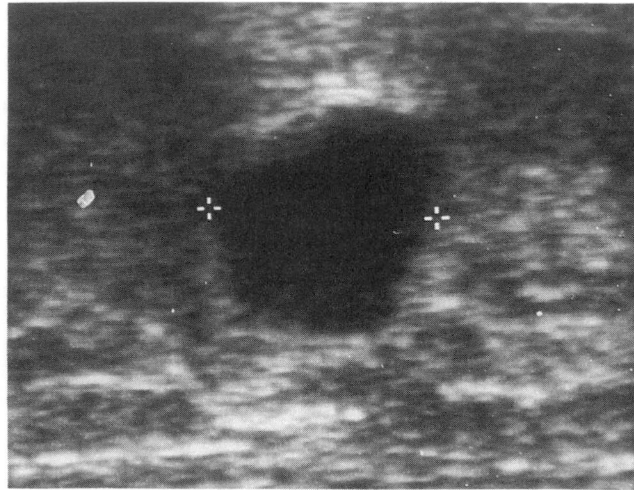

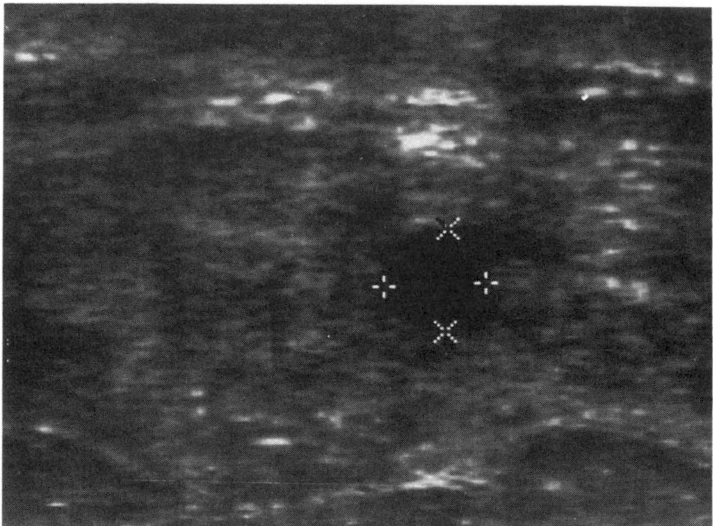

Fig. 26.5 Ultrasound scan showing simple breast cyst.

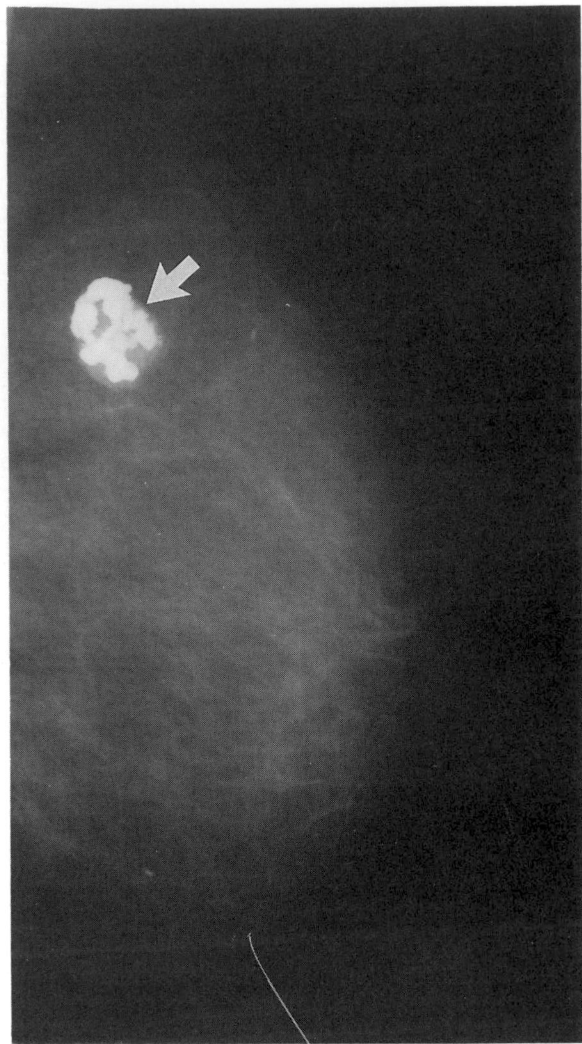

Fig. 26.6 Craniocaudal mammogram with large calcified fibroadenoma visible in upper quadrant (arrowed).

The lesions are firm, smooth, and mobile and bear the descriptive name of 'breast mice'. They are multiple in 15–20% of patients and bilateral in 12%. They are most commonly found in premenopausal women with a mean age of around 25 years.

When presenting in later life the tumours may grow vigorously and achieve considerable size. The condition does not develop after the menopause and women presenting after this have probably had the lesions for years. They may be differentiated from intramammary lymph nodes which are softer. Malignant transformation to carcinoma may occur rarely. Cystosarcoma is a special case and merits separate consideration. Often, cancer in a fibroadenoma has arisen from without and invaded the benign lesion.

If the clinical diagnosis of fibroadenoma is confirmed by cytology and ultrasound or mammography, a young patient may be reviewed 6-monthly as her cancer risk is less than 0.2%. A number of such patients will avoid surgery as the lesion may disappear (Fig. 26.6). These lesions may enlarge during pregnancy and in patients taking the oral contraceptive pill. It may be worthwhile changing such a patient's contraception or reviewing the lesion throughout and after the pregnancy.

A fibroadenoma may be excised for histological confirmation to alleviate a patient's anxiety even if one is certain of the diagnosis or in a young woman who is unwilling to be reviewed regularly. This may often be performed through a circumareolar incision. Only in older patients is it necessary to include a margin of normal breast tissue. Every fibroadenoma should be sent for frozen section to exclude a focus of cystosarcoma phylloides requiring wide resection. Closure with subcuticular polyglycolic acid sutures gives an excellent cosmetic result. Should epitheliosis be a feature of the pathology, close follow-up is recommended.

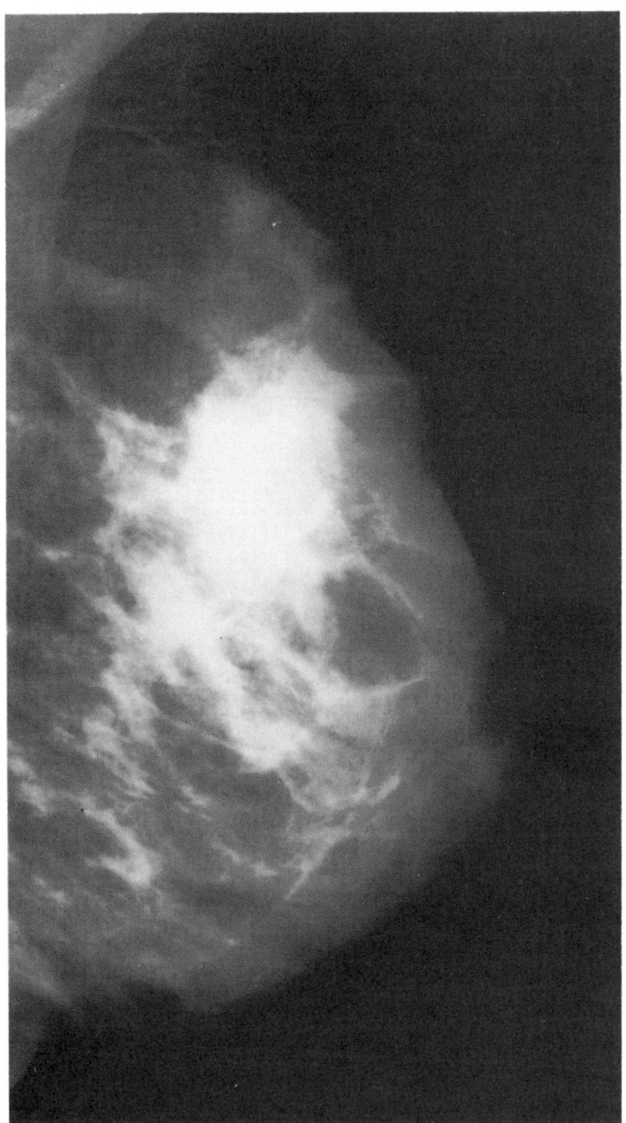

Fig. 26.7 Mammogram demonstrating large calcified cystosarcoma phylloides. This lesion recurred locally twice but remained histologically benign.

Cystosarcoma phylloides

First described in 1838, this fibroadenoma variant is correctly included in any discussion of benign breast diseases. Some remain benign, some arise as malignant tumours, and others become malignant. They occur at an average age of 40 years. For the benign lesions, a wide resection should be performed and the patient reviewed regularly (Fig. 26.7).

BREAST CYSTS

The classical benign cyst may contain as much as 20–30 ml of green/brown fluid. They are often multiple. The cyst contents should be examined cytologically. The patient must be reviewed to ensure that there is no reaccumulation and that the lump has dissipated completely. A watching brief may be employed if all indications are that this is benign. However, any concern should prompt biopsy. Before embarking on excision the surgeon should be aware that this may be a recurrent condition and that a degree of procrastination may avoid multiple operations. Danazol often reduces cyst formation and the pain which accompanies it.

FAT NECROSIS

This may be clinically confused with cancer in the patient with large breasts. There may not be a clear history of breast injury but it is always worth inquiring about road traffic accidents as seatbelt trauma may initiate the lesion. Any concern should prompt excision biopsy.

SKIN LESIONS

The breast is affected by all the skin lesions found elsewhere. Several are listed below:

1. Superficial phlebitis. Occasionally there is a history of trauma. The patient discovers a tender cord, usually in the lateral aspect of the breast (thoracoepigastric vein). A groove may be visible.
2. Mixed tumour of sweat gland origin. Similar to parotid tumours, these are rare, benign neoplasms.
3. Sweat gland adenoma.
4. Sebaceous cyst.
5. Seborrhoeic keratosis.
6. Moles and naevi.

PAIN

The distinction must be drawn between pain referred to the breast from another site (Table 26.1) and true breast pain which is either cyclical or non-cyclical. Nearly 50% of women have some premenstrual breast pain (Mansel 1983). One of the best ways to quantify the problem is to provide the patient with a pain chart to keep for 2 or 3 months (Fig. 26.8).

Table 26.1 Common causes of pain referred to the breast

Tietze's disease: Painful costochondritis syndrome. This usually has no time pattern, is well delineated, unilateral, and affects any age. The pain is often above or below the breast and springing the sternum will recreate the symptoms. Aspirin and reassurance are effective.

Cervical spondylosis: Careful history and examination will reveal the true cause of the pain.

Cardiac pain

Pleurisy

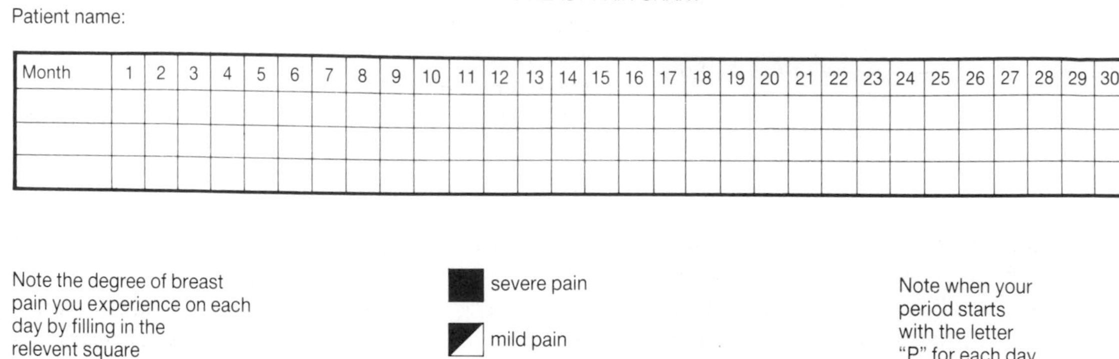

Fig. 26.8 Pain chart to be filled in by the patient for 2 or 3 months prior to review in clinic.

Cyclical pain

This is often bilateral, but slightly more pronounced in the left breast. It usually affects the upper outer quadrants. Generalized lumpiness is common and fibroadenosis falls into this category. The average age of patients is 34 years. The pain is usually described as 'heaviness' or 'tenderness' and tends to occur a week or so prior to the period. This pattern of pain seldom continues after the menopause. A wide range of pathological features are seen if biopsy is performed, including cyst formation, adenosis, dysplasia and epitheliosis.

Non-cyclical pain

These patients are usually older — mean age is 43 years — and pre- and postmenopausal women are similarly affected. Frequently the pain is unilateral, nodularity is absent and the symptom is described as 'drawing' or 'burning'. The most commonly found pathological association is with duct ectasia, although occasionally a cancer will be present.

The management of breast pain

The breast shows variable responses to gonadal steroids. Pregnancy, the menses and administered hormones all alter the growth and regression of mammary tissue. It therefore seems reasonable to assume that manipulation of the female hormones will affect breast dysfunction. Treatment with danazol is efficacious in breast pain (Asch & Greenblatt 1977; Mansel et al 1982). Bromocriptine is not as effective and, although tamoxifen is useful, it has a limited role due to fears of hepatocellular carcinogenicity. A number of other substances have been suggested, including evening primrose oil, but the data are not convincing.

DISCHARGE

The majority of discharges are physiological, a function of increased age (duct ectasia) or due to intraduct papilloma. Hyperprolactinaemia rarely presents as galactorrhoea.

Duct ectasia

This is a disease of the ageing breast with distension of the ducts with debris, subsequent calcification, pain, lumpiness, and discharge of green or brown fluid. A similar discharge may be seen in fibrocystic disease. However, danazol is rarely helpful in duct ectasia. Surgical excision of a single discharging duct may be effective. Hadfield's operation, where the areola is reflected and all the ducts are divided and tied off, will prevent further discharge.

Intraduct papilloma

This is often the source of a bloody discharge in the absence of a palpable mass in the younger patient. Routine ductography is not necessary as careful surgical exploration will reveal the relevant duct.

INFECTION

Although the breast may become infected at any time, it does so most commonly during lactation. This is probably the result of a cracked nipple. Breastfeeding should cease and, if noticed early enough, a course of antibiotics may prove useful. *Staphylococcus aureus* is often the organism responsible so flucloxacillin is a suitable drug. At the first sign of fluctuation, the abscess should be drained through a circumferential incision.

CONGENITAL ABNORMALITIES AND COSMETIC CONSIDERATIONS

A number of developmental anomalies may be seen by the surgeon with a breast practice.

Accessory nipples and breasts

These are found anywhere in the milk line from axilla to groin. Present in 1–2% of the population, they can be the site of all the diseases of normally situated breasts. During lactation, supernumerary breasts may swell and, having no developed duct system, may involute. Excision is warranted when distress is caused.

Asymmetry

The breasts are normally asymmetric but the patient's perception as well as the degree of asymmetry will dictate whether surgical intervention is appropriate. These women are often severely affected psychologically and can benefit enormously from plastic surgery. The absent or deficient areola can be reconstructed by 'borrowing' tissue from the other breast, labia minora grafts or skin tattooing.

Fig. 26.9 Mammogram showing leaking silicone breast prosthesis (arrowed) which caused pain, lumpiness and local inflammation.

Reduction mammoplasty

The young woman with overly large breasts has to buy special clothes, is prone to excoriation of the skin below her breasts and chronic neck and back pain. Surgery should be deferred until she is at least 17 years of age. The results are good in skilled hands and suspension mammoplasty is effective for the woman with sagging breasts.

Augmentation mammoplasty

Modern society projects an image of the desirable woman as possessing large breasts. It is not surprising, therefore, that some patients wish augmentation. Careful screening is required to ensure unnecessary operations are avoided. There are, however, women who do benefit from an increase in breast size by any of the methods currently available, be it silicone implant or inflatable prosthesis. It is as well to bear in mind the complications of this kind of surgery, such as infection, migration of the prosthesis or implantation leakage (Fig. 26.9).

KEY POINTS

1. The majority of women with breast disease have a benign condition.
2. Careful history and examination are particularly important.
3. Fine needle aspiration is a fast and reliable method of excluding breast cancer.
4. Mammography exposes the patient to very low levels of radiation.
5. Mammography is effective in detecting small lesions.
6. Mammography may be uncomfortable as the breasts must be compressed.
7. Fibroadenomata are very common and often multiple.
8. Breast cysts should be aspirated and the fluid sent for cytology.
9. Cyclical breast pain in young women is helped by danazol.
10. Non-cyclical pain is commoner in older women, is most commonly due to duct ectasia but may indicate a cancer.
11. Plastic surgery gives good results in skilled hands, may give considerable benefits but may result in complications.

REFERENCES

Asch R H, Greenblatt R B 1977 The use of an impeded androgen — danazol — in the management of benign breast disorders. American Journal of Obstetrics and Gynecology 127: 130–134

Goldberg R P, Hall F M, Simon M 1983 Preoperative localization of non palpable breast lesions using a wire marker and a perforated mammographic grid. Radiology 146: 833–835

Mansel R E 1983 Classification of mastalgia — the Cardiff system. In: Benign breast disease. Royal Society of Medicine, London, pp 33–41

Mansel R E, Wisby J R, Hughes L E 1982 Controlled trial of the anti gonadotrophin danazol in painful nodular benign breast disease. Lancet i: 928–930

Moskowitz M, Russell P, Fidler J, Sutorius D J, Law E J, Holle J 1975 Breast cancer screening. Preliminary report of 207 biopsies performed in 4128 volunteer screenees. Cancer 36: 2245–2250

Preece P E, Hughes L E, Mansel R E, Baum M, Bolton P M, Gravelle I H 1976 Clinical syndromes of mastalgia. Lancet ii: 670–673

Sackier J M, Wood C B 1988 The treatment of fibroadenoma and phylloides tumours. In: Ioannidou-Mouzaka L, Philippakis M, Angelakis P (eds) Mastology '88. Elsevier, Amsterdam, pp 151–156

Snyder R E 1980 Specimen radiography and preoperative localization of non palpable breast cancer. Cancer 46: 950–956

Tokunaga M, Land C E, Yamamoto T 1984 Breast cancer among atomic bomb survivors. In: Boice J D Jr, Fraumani J F (eds) Radiation carcinogenesis: epidemiology and biological significance. Raven Press, New York, p 45

27. Benign disease of the vulva and vagina

W. P. Soutter

VULVA

INTRODUCTION

This chapter will be confined to discussion of benign conditions and mention of malignant or premalignant disease will be made only in relation to differential diagnosis or management. Premalignant disease is discussed in Chapter 34 and invasive disease in Chapter 39. Similarly, only passing mention is made of sexually transmitted diseases, which are described in Chapter 56. Space does not permit an exhaustive description of all of the many conditions which may affect the vulva. Instead, the emphasis is on common or important conditions (not always the same thing) with the intention of providing the reader with a sound framework upon which to build. More information may be obtained from the excellent books by Dr Marjorie Ridley (1988) and by the late Dr Eduard Friedrich (1983).

Patients with vulval symptoms are met frequently in gynaecological practice. The complaint is often longstanding and distressing and frequently induces a feeling of despair in both patient and doctor. A careful, sympathetic approach and a readiness to consult colleagues in other disciplines are essential. Even when it seems that no specific therapy can be offered, many patients are helped by the knowledge that there is no serious underlying pathology and by a supportive attitude.

ANATOMY AND HISTOLOGY

The vulva includes the mons pubis, the labia majora and minora, the clitoris, the vestibule of the vagina, the bulb of the vestibule and the greater vestibular glands (Bartholin's).

The mons pubis is a pad of fat anterior to the pubic symphysis and covered by hair-bearing skin. The labia majora extend posteriorly from the mons on either side of the pudendal cleft into which the urethra and vagina open. They merge with one another and the perineal skin anterior to the anus. They consist largely of areolar tissue and fat. The skin on their lateral aspects is pigmented and covered with crisp hairs. On the medial side the skin is smooth and has many sebaceous glands. The labia minora are small folds of skin which lie between the labia majora and which divide anteriorly to envelope the clitoris. The medial surfaces contain many sebaceous glands. The clitoris is an erectile structure analogous to the male penis. Partly hidden by the anterior folds of the labia minora, the clitoris consists of a body of two corpora cavernosa lying side-by-side and connected to the pubic and ischial rami, and a glans of sensitive, spongy erectile tissue. The vestibule is that area between the labia minora into which the urethra and vagina open. The bulbs of the vestibule lie on either side of the vaginal opening and are elongated masses of erectile tissue. The greater vestibular glands lie posterior to the bulbs of the vestibule and are connected to the surface by short ducts.

HISTORY

The duration of the complaint, details of the onset and any precipitating factors must be elicited. Information about the treatments used so far is important as many of these women will have already begun to use a variety of local preparations, some of which may be potentially harmful! The use of deodorants, bath gels or biological washing powders may cause an allergic or irritation eczema. Wearing tight clothing, particularly nylon materials, may exacerbate the problem. Depression may be a result of the vulval condition rather than the cause but it will still require treatment. A history of other illnesses or drug treatment may be relevant. The patient should be asked about other skin complaints. Sometimes a further line of enquiry is suggested by the findings on examination.

EXAMINATION

An examination for evidence of systemic disease or of a generalized skin condition is advisable. Pelvic and vaginal examination should be performed unless the patient is too uncomfortable to allow it. Cervical cytology and colposcopic examination of the cervix and vagina may be useful and are mandatory if the vulval condition is thought to be premalignant. The vulva should be examined in a good light, preferably under low magnification. The colposcope is not ideal for this because of the narrow field of view but it is often the best available option.

It is important to take biopsies liberally. These can readily be performed under local anaesthesia (Fig. 27.1) using a disposable 4 mm Stiefel biopsy punch or a Keyes punch. Silver nitrate or Monsel's solution will control the small amount of bleeding which results.

PRURITUS VULVAE

The term 'pruritus vulvae' properly refers to vulval irritation for which no cause can be found. In practice, many gynaecologists use the term to describe this upsetting symptom regardless of whether or not a cause is evident. It should be distinguished from the burning sensation described by some women and discussed later.

Pruritus vulvae is commoner in older women and is most frequently encountered after the age of 40 years. The most common causes are lichen sclerosus and eczema due to an allergy or exposure to an irritant substance. Evidence of

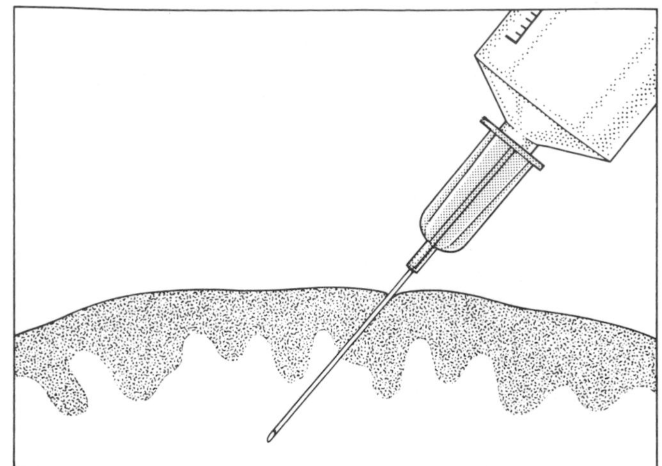

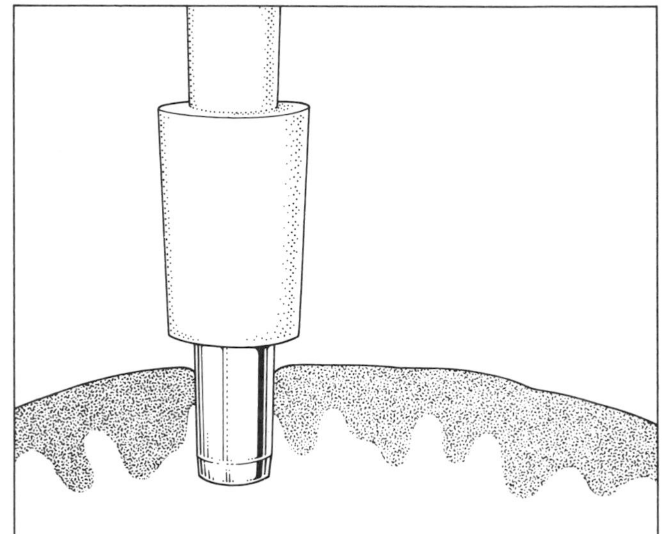

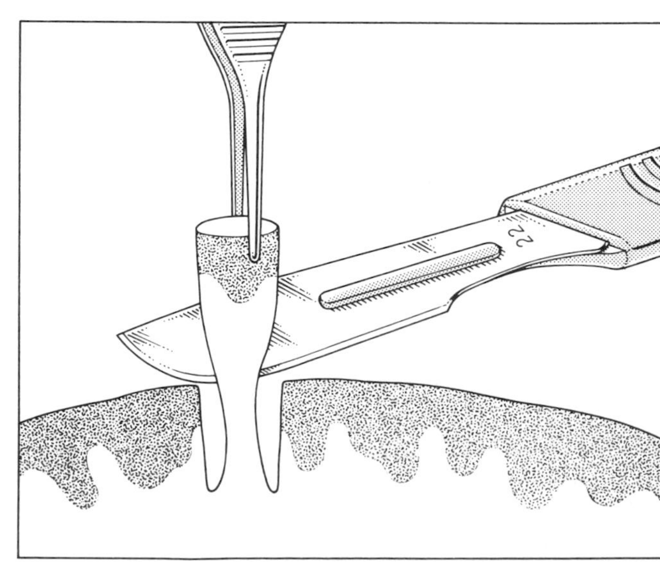

Fig. 27.1 Vulval biopsy under local anaesthesia.

the latter is often obscured by the secondary effects of scratching — a thickening and whitening of the skin. The scratching initiates a vicious cycle, exacerbating the irritation and stimulating more scratching.

A vaginal discharge may give rise to vulval irritation. The discharge may be due to infection but some women seem to experience a profuse physiological discharge. Cautery of the cervix often gives disappointing results in such cases. A bland barrier ointment like zinc and castor oil is sometimes useful in this situation. Threadworm infestation is very common in children and will cause pruritus ani and vulval irritation. Atrophic vaginitis responds to hormone replacement.

Occasionally, a systemic illness may cause pruritus vulvae. Diabetes, uraemia and liver failure are all possible causes to consider.

If no specific cause is found, steps must be taken to remove any possible source of irritation or allergy. Vulval deodorants and perfumed additions to the bath water must be avoided. Simple, unperfumed soap should be used for vulval hygiene and for washing underwear. After washing, the vulva must be dried carefully and gently — if necessary a hair drier set at a low heat can be used. Loose-fitting cotton clothing should be worn to allow the evaporation of sweat. The patient would be well advised not to wear nylon tights.

Potent topical steroids, such as 0.1% diflucortolone valerate or 2.5% hydrocortisone may be used two to three times per day for a few weeks. Thereafter, 1% hydrocortisone will usually suffice to maintain the improvement and to treat relapses. A sedative at night, such as hydroxyzine hydrochloride, can be useful to break the cycle of nocturnal itching and scratching. An antihistamine, terfenadine, taken during the day may help to relieve the itch without causing sedation.

It is important to treat depression appropriately. Even if the patient is not pathologically depressed, she can benefit greatly from sympathetic support and understanding and time must be set aside for this when necessary.

VULVAL PAIN

Vulvodynia is a term applied to a feeling of vulval burning (McKay 1989). Dyspareunia is a frequent complaint and the vagina or perineum may also be involved. When no cause can be found it has been referred to as the 'burning vulva syndrome'. This condition is commonest in younger women. In most cases there is little or nothing to be seen on the vulva. Sometimes, especially with the aid of the colposcope, inflamed minor vestibular glands can be seen. Other minor changes may be visible through the colposcope. Low-grade acetowhite changes (Fig. 27.2) and microvilli on the medial aspect of the labia minora have been attributed, perhaps wrongly, to infection with human papilloma virus but the evidence that these changes contribute to the symptoms is scant. Improvements have sometimes been obtained after laser vaporization of the minor vestibular glands when local inflammation has been evident.

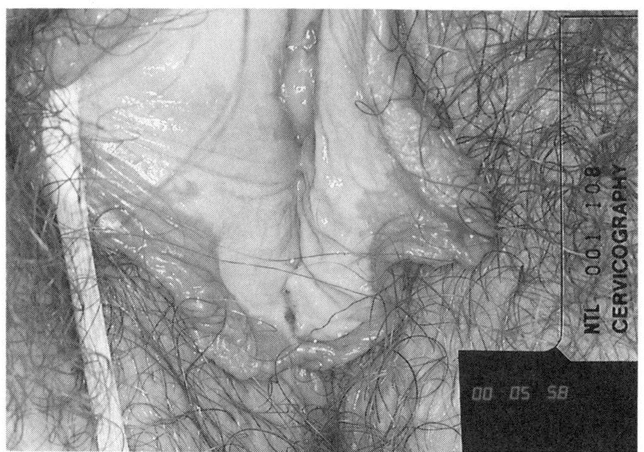

Fig. 27.2 Extensive area of acetowhite change.

Some women complain of vulval or perineal pain. It is not clear if these women should be regarded as a separate group. These are often older patients but both vulvodynia and vulval pain have many different causes so considering them as separate entities is not particularly useful.

Vulvodynia may be caused by vulvovaginal infections, vulval dermatitis or any of the other dermatoses. Neurological causes include spinal cord injury, diabetes and postherpetic neuralgia. Pudendal neuralgia is a syndrome described in men not unlike the vulval pain syndrome of women. No cause is known but it seems likely that some cases of both syndromes may be related to conditions like trigeminal neuralgia and the dystonias.

Some of these women are clinically depressed and can be helped by appropriate therapy. When no abnormality is visible, psychiatric advice should be sought, if only to rule out a psychosis. Once again sympathetic support is essential.

NON-NEOPLASTIC DISORDERS OF THE VULVA

In few areas has there been as much confusion over the terminology used as in that of vulvar 'dystrophies'. The latest recommended scheme is shown in Table 27.1. The non-neoplastic disorders have been separated from the potentially premalignant intraepithelial neoplasia. Only the non-neoplastic disorders will be discussed here.

Lichen sclerosus

This is the commonest condition found in elderly women complaining of vulvar itch but may also be seen in children and less commonly in younger women. The cause is not

Table 27.1 Terminology of disorders of vulval skin and mucosa

Non-neoplastic disorders
Lichen sclerosus
Squamous cell hyperplasia (formerly hyperplastic dystrophy)
Other dermatoses
Vulval intraepithelial neoplasia (VIN)
Squamous VIN
VIN I Mild dysplasia
VIN II Moderate dysplasia
VIN III Severe dysplasia or carcinoma in situ
Non-squamous VIN
Paget's disease

Note 1 Mixed epithelial disorders may occur. In such cases it is recommended that both conditions be reported. For example lichen sclerosus with associated squamous cell hyperplasia (formerly classified as mixed dystrophy) should be reported as lichen sclerosus and squamous cell hyperplasia. Squamous cell hyperplasia with associated vulval intraepithelial neoplasia (formerly hyperplastic dystrophy with atypia) should be diagnosed as vulval intraepithelial neoplasia.

Note 2 Squamous cell hyperplasia is used for those instances in which the hyperplasia is not attributable to another cause. Specific lesions or dermatoses involving the vulva (e.g. psoriasis, lichen planus, lichen simplex chronicus, *Candida* infection, condyloma acuminatum) may include squamous cell hyperplasia, but should be diagnosed specifically and excluded from this category.

From International Society for the Study of Vulvar Disease (1989)

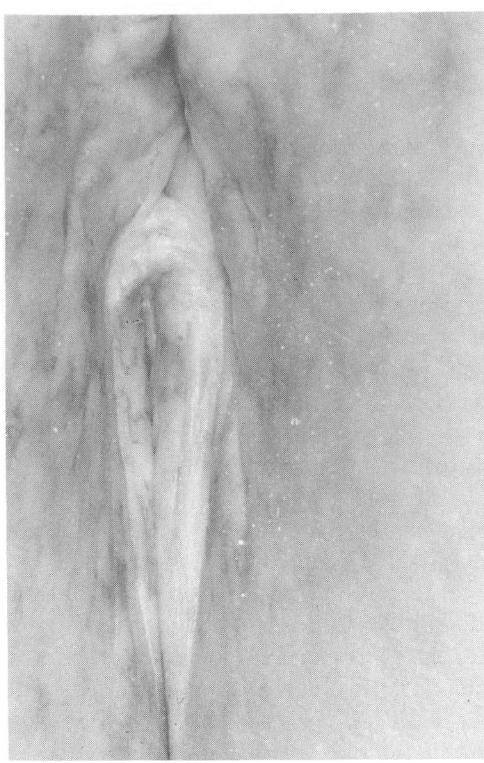

Fig. 27.3 Lichen sclerosus.

known but the condition is associated with autoimmune disorders.

Although it most commonly affects the vulva and perianal skin, lesions do appear elsewhere. The lesion is white and the skin looks thin, with a crinkled surface (Fig. 27.3). The contours of the vulva slowly disappear and labial adhesions form. If the patient has been rubbing the area the skin will become thickened (lichenified). The diagnosis can usually be made clinically but a biopsy should be performed whenever possible. Occasionally, even in a typical case, the histology is not characteristic.

There is much uncertainty about the risk to patients with lichen sclerosus of developing vulval cancer. Vulval intraepithelial neoplasia (VIN) and lichen sclerosus can coexist in the same patient and many patients with invasive carcinoma also have lichen sclerosus in the surrounding skin. About 4% of women with lichen sclerosus develop invasive cancer (Meyrick Thomas et al 1988).

Although there is a 9% prevalence of thyroid disease, pernicious anaemia or diabetes in these patients, screening for these conditions may not be of value as, in most cases, the diagnosis has already been made by the time the patient presents with her vulval complaint (Meyrick Thomas et al 1988).

If the patient is asymptomatic, no treatment is required. Mild itching may be helped by aqueous cream or 1% hydrocortisone ointment applied three times daily. More potent steroids may be required for short periods. If use of an ointment results in maceration, a cream base may be used. Some women benefit from 2% testosterone ointment which should be applied twice or three times per day for 6 weeks. Thereafter the frequency can be reduced to once or twice a week. Excessive dosage will result in clitoral hypertrophy and increased facial hair (Friedrich 1983). There is virtually no place for vulvectomy for this condition as the morbidity is not justified in the face of a high recurrence rate. The same may be said of laser vaporization.

Squamous cell hyperplasia

Squamous cell hyperplasia is a term applied to those women with histological evidence of hyperplasia without any clinical evidence of the cause (Fig. 27.4). Chronic rubbing of otherwise normal skin (lichen simplex), psoriasis, condylomata acuminata and infection with *Candida albicans* are among the diagnoses that must be excluded before this term may be applied. This stipulation is likely to reduce to near zero the number of cases assigned to this category on clinical grounds.

Other dermatoses

These problems are usually seen by dermatologists rather than by gynaecologists but a knowledge of this area will help to identify those patients who should be referred. Space permits only a brief discussion of some of the more common lesions.

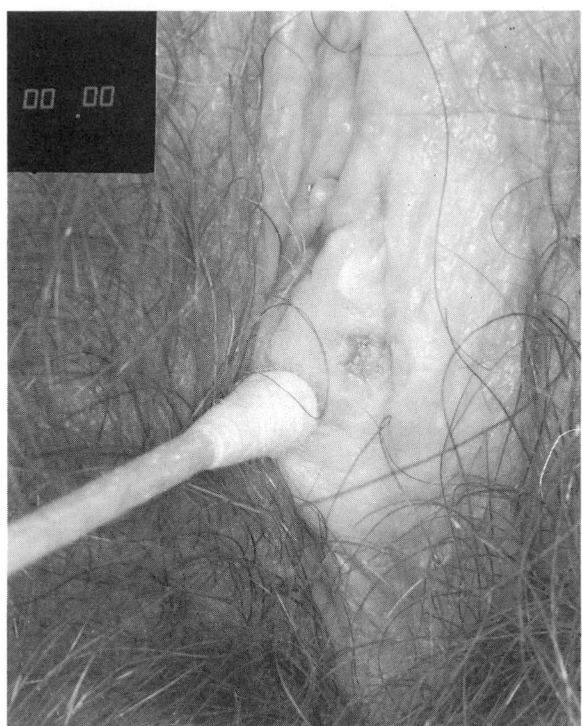

Fig. 27.4 Squamous hyperplasia with a small ulcer caused by scratching.

Allergic or irritant dermatitis

The patient will usually present with vulval itching. The skin is red and swollen and may later become thickened from constant scratching (lichenified). Secondary infection may occur. The list of potential irritants is endless but includes detergents; perfume; synthetic materials; condom lubricants; chlorine in swimming pools; podophyllin; topical antihistamines, anaesthetics or antibiotics. After eliminating exposure to any potential irritant, a 1% hydrocortisone ointment will prove helpful in most cases but sometimes a stronger preparation is needed in the acute phase. Secondary infection may require treatment with local or systemic antibiotics.

Psoriasis

It is unusual for a patient to present with isolated psoriasis of the vulva never having had the abnormality elsewhere. The lesion is red and sharply defined and often has a silvery scaling surface. This last may be absent in moist areas. The mucosal surfaces are rarely involved. Coal tar preparations should not be used on the vulva and treatment is usually begun with a strong steroid ointment (Ridley 1988).

Intertrigo

Any site where the skin remains moist is susceptible to inflammation and secondary infection. The lesions are red, moist and ill defined. Infection with *Candida* is particularly common, especially in obese diabetics. Occasionally psoriasis occurring in a flexure, or seborrhoeic dermatitis may present in a similar fashion but both tend to occur at other sites at the same time. Topical antibiotic therapy may be required in combination with a mild steroid. General measures to keep the area dry and the skin surfaces separated are very helpful.

Lichen planus

This condition may occur on any part of the body and is often found in the mouth. In the skin, it is usually a self-limiting and often asymptomatic condition. The lesions on the vulva are purple-white papules with a shiny surface and regular outline. The histology is diagnostic. If treatment is required, topical steroids are effective.

Erosive lichen planus

This uncommon variant of lichen planus occurs on the mucosal aspects of the labia minora and the vagina. This may cause pain and itching and, if the vagina is involved, may cause bleeding and dyspareunia due to vaginal adhesions. Unfortunately, it is often difficult to establish the diagnosis histologically. Systemic steroids can be helpful but the prognosis is poor as the condition tends to persist. There may be a risk of malignancy.

Vulval ulcers

The causes of benign vulval ulcers are listed below:

1. Aphthous ulcers
2. Herpes genitalis
3. Primary syphilis
4. Crohn's disease
5. Behçet's disease
6. Lipschutz ulcers
7. Lymphogranuloma venereum
8. Chancroid
9. Donovanosis
10. Tuberculosis

Aphthous ulcers

Simple aphthous ulcers, analogous to those seen in the mouth, may be found on the vulva. They are small, painful ulcers with a yellow base, seen mainly on the labia majora. There is no associated constitutional upset and the ulcers are seldom as painful as those found in primary herpes.

Herpetic ulcers

The primary attack of herpes genitalis usually presents as

an extremely painful vulval ulceration together with general malaise, fever and often inguinal lymphadenopathy. Some intact vesicles may still be visible. There is often an associated herpetic pharyngitis. Severe headache should suggest the possibility of viral meningitis. Herpes genitalis is described more fully in Chapter 56.

Syphilitic ulcers

The chancre of primary syphilis is an indurated painless ulcer. There may be several chancres. If secondary infection occurs the ulcer may become tender. The majority occur on the vulva but the cervix may be involved.

Crohn's disease

Crohn's disease may affect the vulva or perineum in 25–30% of cases and this often precedes the appearance of intestinal symptoms by many years. The ulcers look like knife cuts in the skin. Later, when bowel disease is evident, oedema, discharging sinuses and irregular ulcers are more common.

Behçet's disease

Behçet's disease is a chronic condition characterized by oral, genital and ocular ulceration. It may be many years before all of these features are evident. The oral ulcers are often not severe but the vulval lesions can be very erosive. They can last for several months and leave extensive scarring. It can be difficult to distinguish from Crohn's disease and there are no diagnostic histological features. There is no specific treatment. Oestrogen-dominant oral contraceptives are said to have a beneficial effect in some cases and topical and systemic steroids are also used.

Lipschutz ulcers

Lipschutz ulcers affect mainly the labia minora and introitus. They can be acute in onset with an associated fever and lymphadenopathy. Often, no cause can be found but they may be due to Epstein–Barr virus.

'Tropical' infections causing vulval ulceration

Lymphogranuloma venereum, a tropical infection due to certain subtypes of *Chlamydia trachomatis*, causes a painless vulval ulcer which heals after 3–4 weeks. Inguinal lymphadenopathy develops a few weeks later. Chancroid, infection with *Haemophilus ducreyi*, is a very common cause of genital ulceration in tropical parts of the world but outbreaks have occurred in western countries. Donovanosis can cause chronic, spreading ulcers and is most common in South-East Asia and India. Tuberculosis is a rare but important cause of vulval ulceration and inguinal lyphadenopathy.

Disorders of pigmentation

Melanosis vulvae (lentigo) is the commonest pigmented lesion on the vulva, producing asymptomatic, light brown macules which are frequently multiple and can appear anywhere on the vulva. Because they can be difficult to differentiate conclusively from melanoma or VIN, excision biopsy is recommended. Benign naevi may also be difficult to identify with certainty. Biopsy should be the rule for pigmented lesions.

Vitiligo is an area of depigmentation. It does not cause symptoms but may be mistaken for lichenification or lichen sclerosus.

VULVAL NEOPLASIA

VIN are discussed in Chapter 34 and vulval cancer in Chapter 39.

BENIGN TUMOURS

Ectopic tissues

Occasionally, breast tissue may be found on the vulva. It commonly presents during pregnancy as a firm, mobile vulval mass. Endometriosis may also be found on the vulva, often after implantation in a surgical wound such as an episiotomy. This does not always exhibit cyclic changes.

Cystic lesions

Epidermoid and sebaceous cysts can be difficult to differentiate. The distinction is academic as the management of both is excision. Mucinous cysts may arise from the minor vestibular glands (Fig. 27.5) whereas mesonephric cysts are found on the labia majora. Cysts on the anterior part of the vulva may have arisen from peritoneum carried into the vulva by the round ligament (cysts of the canal of Nuck). Cysts may arise around the urethra in Skene's ducts or in suburethral glands.

Bartholin's cyst

These cysts arise from the duct of Bartholin's gland which lies in the subcutaneous tissue below the lower third of the labium majorum. When the duct becomes blocked, a tense retention cyst forms. The patient usually presents only after infection has supervened and a painful abscess has formed. Incision and marsupialization of the abscess and

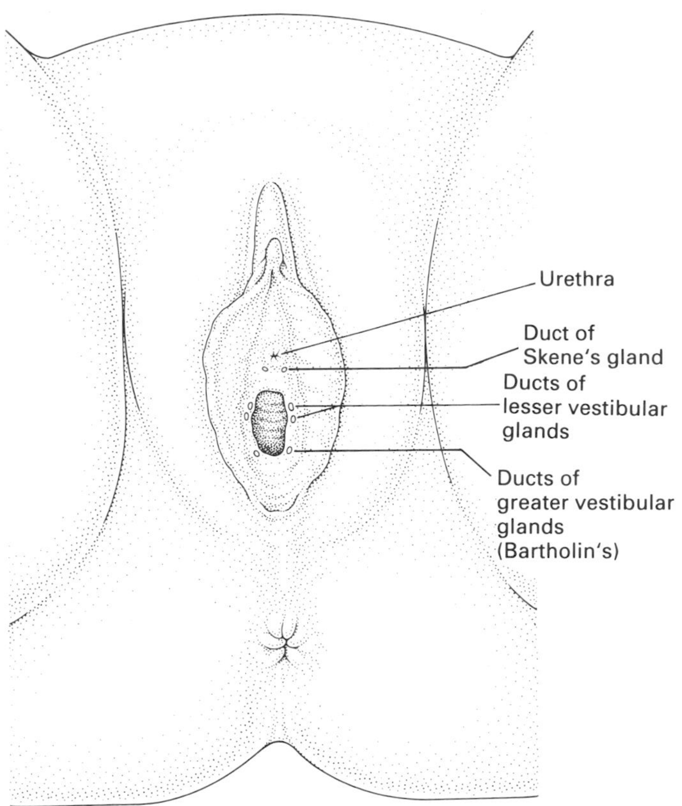

Fig. 27.5 The vulval glands.

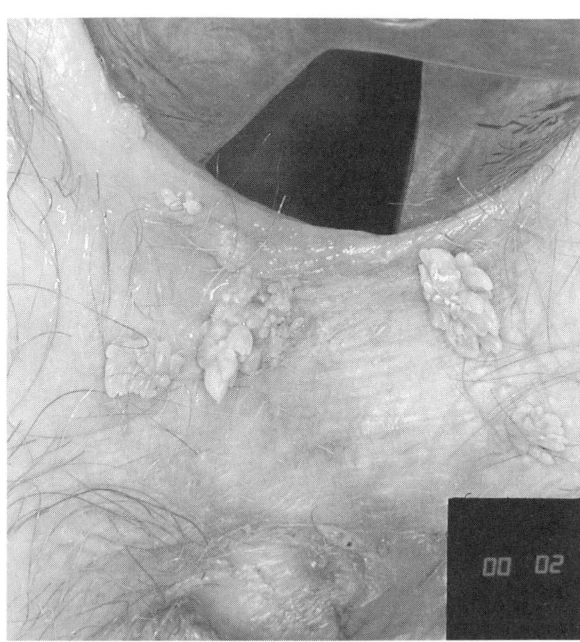

Fig. 27.6 Small genital warts at the fourchette.

antibiotic therapy give excellent results. The pus from the abscess should be sent for culture in media suitable for the detection of gonococcal infection.

Non-epithelial tumours

Lipomas and fibromas are the commonest benign tumours of the vulva which arise from other than the epithelial tissues. The benign angiokeratoma may be difficult to distinguish from a melanoma, especially if the initial red colour has given way to the later brown or black hue and the lesion has begun to bleed due to trauma. Many other benign tumours may be found on the vulva (Fox & Buckley 1988) but the diagnosis is nearly always made on histological rather than clinical grounds.

Epithelial tumours

Squamous papillomata and 'skin tags' are common, benign and similar in appearance. Folliculitis — infection of hair follicles — may be caused by shaving or depilatory creams. Infestation with lice may present in this way. Any precipitating cause should be dealt with. Topical antiseptics or even systemic antibiotics may be required.

Secondary syphilis may present as a maculopapular rash which can affect the vulva. Condyloma lata are sessile papules seen on the vulva and perianal skin. These may ulcerate and are highly infectious. A generalized lymphadenopathy is common at this stage.

Condyloma acuminata are small papules which are sometimes sessile and often polypoid (Fig. 27.6). They are due to infection with human papillomavirus, usually type 6/11. Acetowhite changes and 'microwarts' seen best under low-power magnification have been attributed to human papillomavirus infection but this may not be correct. Microwarts may be no more than a variation of normal. The majority of condylomata acuminata can be treated satisfactorily in the outpatient department by the sparing application of 85% trichloroacetic acid, a very corrosive liquid. Care must be taken not to injure the adjacent normal skin. Podophyllin is less effective and more toxic. If the lesions are large and widespread, removal under general anaesthesia will probably be required using electrodiathermy or carbon dioxide laser. The advantage of the latter is that its greater precision permits removal of the lesion without subsequent scarring and with more rapid healing. Laser treatment of the vulva is discussed more fully in Chapter 34.

The rare keratoacanthoma might well be mistaken for invasive squamous cancer because of its rapid growth over a matter of weeks. Spontaneous involution usually begins after about 6 months. The centre of this well demarcated, regular dome contains a plug of keratin which may suggest the diagnosis but complete excision of the lesion is required for histological confirmation.

TRAUMA TO VULVA OR VAGINA

A torn hymen following a first attempt at intercourse may result in profuse, frightening haemorrhage. Transfusion may be indicated. Suture of the bleeding vessel under general anaesthesia should be accompanied by one or more radial incisions in the hymen to prevent a recurrence.

Trauma is usually the result of falling astride a sharp object like a fence. It may result from sexual abuse, sometimes self-inflicted. It may also occur following normal sexual intercourse, particularly in a postmenopausal woman who has not had intercourse for some time. In these cases the laceration is usually at the vault of the vagina in the posterior fornix.

An indwelling catheter may be necessary and ice packs will give some comfort. Damage to the vagina, rectum, urethra, bladder or ureter may also occur. Pain relief with opiates and replacement of blood loss may be needed urgently. Examination under anaesthesia is often required to determine the extent of the damage. A closed haematoma is best managed conservatively but bleeding lacerations will require suture. Devitalized tissues will need to be excised and tears in bowel or bladder must be repaired in layers. Occasionally a hysterectomy must be performed.

CONGENITAL ABNORMALITIES

Congenital abnormalities of the vulva and vagina are discussed in Chapters 1, 12 and 13.

MISCELLANEOUS CONDITIONS

Occasionally, prolapse of the urethral mucosa will occur, usually in children or elderly women. This can become infarcted. An everted, inflamed portion of the urethral mucosa is called a caruncle. It may be asymptomatic, but it can be painful and cause dysuria and dyspareunia. In elderly women, swelling and erythema of the urethral meatus may just be the result of atrophy which will be improved by oestrogen therapy. Excision or cautery are required for caruncle and urethral prolapse.

VAGINA

INTRODUCTION

Many of the disorders that affect the vagina are discussed in depth elsewhere in this book: congenital abnormalities will be found in Chapters 1, 12 and 13; infections in Chapter 56; psychosexual problems in Chapter 62; atrophic changes in Chapter 24; prolapse in chapter 31; intra-epithelial disease in Chapter 34, and cancer in Chapter 39. The purpose of this short section is to discuss briefly some of these problems as symptom complexes and to refer the reader to those parts of this book where more detailed information may be found.

ANATOMY AND HISTOLOGY

The upper two-thirds of the vagina is derived from the müllerian duct and the lower third from the ectoderm of the cloaca. The vagina is related anteriorly to the bladder above and the urethra below. Posteriorly, the vault of the vagina is covered with the peritoneum of the pouch of Douglas. It thus becomes closely related to loops of small or large bowel. Below this, it is closely related to the anterior wall of the rectum until the perineal body separates it from the anal canal. The ureters run close to the cervix over each side of the vaginal vault to the bladder. Laterally, the vagina is supported by the lower portion of the cardinal ligaments until it reaches the pelvic floor where it is invested by the medial part of the levator ani muscles (pubococcygeus). Lateral to the vagina, most of the tissue is areolar except at the level of the perineal body.

The vagina is lined by stratified squamous epithelium. When the transformation zone of the cervix has extended on to the vagina, clefts or glands partly lined by columnar epithelium will be seen deep to the squamous epithelium.

VAGINAL DISCHARGE

Because there is almost always some escape of vaginal or cervical secretions it can be difficult sometimes to assess the significance of a vaginal discharge and often the patient is just seeking reassurance. The best guide is to ask whether the amount or character of the discharge has altered from the patient's usual pattern.

Physiological discharge

A physiological discharge is usually clear or whitish in colour. Part of this secretion comes from the cervix and, unless the patient is taking an oral contraceptive, the normal cyclical fluctuation may be evident with an increase in flow just before ovulation. Physiological secretion is increased following a pregnancy and women using oral contraception often note an additional loss. Irritation may result from a copious physiological secretion and does not always indicate infection. Similarly, some women find the smell of normal secretion offensive. A marked, recent increase in the volume of discharge, accompanied by irritation suggests the presence of infection. A blood-stained discharge should always arouse suspicion.

Speculum examination will show a healthy-looking vagina with a small amount of mucoid discharge. An area of ectopy (an erosion) may be visible on the cervix but this is a normal finding in premenopausal women and is seldom responsible for symptoms. While a severe case of candidiasis may be associated with the characteristic cottage-cheese discharge, in many cases it is not possible to exclude infection from the clinical appearance. Microscopy and culture are required.

Bacterial vaginosis

Bacterial vaginosis is a common syndrome often overlooked by gynaecologists. It appears to be caused not by one but by several different organisms (see Chapter 56). *Gardnerella vaginalis* is one of these but is often found in asymptomatic women. It would seem either that simultaneous infection with multiple organisms is required or that some hitherto undetected pathogen is the cause.

The characteristic features are a vaginal pH over 5.0 and a fishy odour, made more obvious by adding a drop of 10% potassium peroxide to a drop of the discharge on a slide. Microscopy of the discharge will show 'clue cells': epithelial cells covered by bacteria. Sophisticated gas chromatographic analysis of the discharge adds little to the diagnostic armamentarium save expense. Investigations for other sexually transmitted disease should be instituted (Chapter 56).

Metronidazole is the treatment of choice as a single 2 g dose. This may be repeated in 24 h. In resistant cases, 400 mg b.d. is prescribed for 7 days. The patient must not drink alcohol while taking metronidazole to avoid the risk of an antebuse reaction. Metronidazole often causes nausea and should be taken after food. Further details are given in Chapter 34.

Monilial vaginitis

Candida spp. are frequently found in the vagina of asymptomatic women. Symptoms result when the numbers of organisms increase for reasons which are often not apparent. Diabetic patients, women using oral contraception or taking broad-spectrum antibiotics, pregnant patients and the immunosuppressed are all particularly prone to *Candida* infection.

Such patients will complain of vaginal irritation, dysuria, dyspareunia and a vaginal discharge. The discharge may be recognizable in severe cases when it is thick and white, like cottage cheese. The vulva may be reddened and sore-looking and the vagina and cervix inflamed and covered with adherent lumps of the discharge. Microscopy will show the characteristic hyphae or spores (Fig. 27.7). In cases of doubt, a high vaginal swab should be sent for culture.

A convenient treatment consists of a single 500 mg pessary of clotrimazole with 1% clotrimazole cream for any external lesions. In recurrent cases it may be worth asking the sexual partner to apply clotrimazole to his penis but there is doubt about the value of this approach. Alternatively, the oral agents fluconazole or itraconazole may be

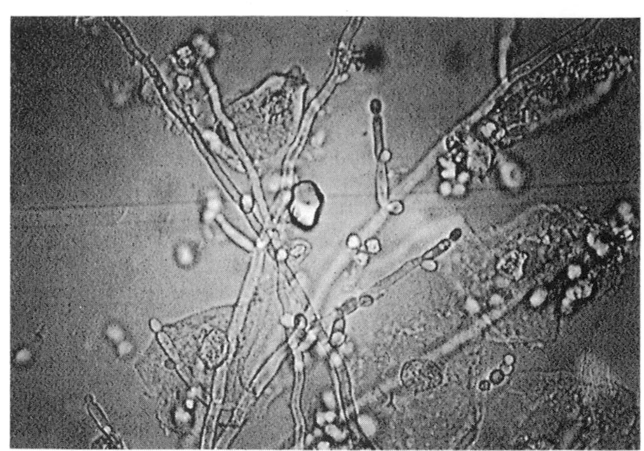

Fig. 27.7 Microscopy of vaginal discharge shows typical hyphae of *Candida*.

prescribed provided the patient is not pregnant and has no evidence of liver or renal impairment.

Trichomonal vaginitis

This condition is caused by a motile protozoon and is sexually transmitted but may be asymptomatic for long periods.

It usually causes a foul-smelling, mucopurulent discharge. The patient may complain of dysuria, dyspareunia and vulvovaginal irritation. The vulva and vagina may be very inflamed. The vagina and cervix are often covered by petechial haemorrhage giving the so-called 'strawberry cervix'.

A wet film will demonstrate the motile organisms, but the diagnosis may be confirmed by culture. As with bacterial vaginosis it may be prudent to screen the patient for other sexually transmitted diseases (Chapter 56).

Treatment is with metronidazole 200 mg t.i.d. for 7 days or as a single dose of 2 g.

Vaginal discharge in children

A vaginal discharge in a young child is often due to infection secondary to atrophic vaginitis. A foreign body is sometimes found or occasionally threadworms are involved. In the older child, evidence of sexual abuse must be sought (Chapter 63). Only very rarely is a vaginal tumour responsible.

The vulva and anus should be inspected for signs of trauma. Atrophic changes should be noted. If possible, swabs should be taken for culture from the vagina and, if indicated, from the rectum and urethra. It is usually possible to perform a gentle rectal examination using the little finger to detect a foreign body in the vagina. In cases of doubt, a general anaesthetic is usually necessary to allow an adequate inspection of the vagina without frightening the child. A paediatric laryngoscope is particularly useful for this.

Any foreign body should be removed and the vagina gently cleansed under general anaesthesia. Appropriate oral antibiotics should be given for any infection. If atrophic vaginitis has contributed, the sparing application of topical oestrogen to the vulva for 2 weeks should suffice.

Miscellaneous causes of vaginal discharge

A number of other problems may present as a vaginal discharge. A foreign body (e.g. a tampon) will cause a purulent, blood-stained discharge whose cause will be all too obvious on speculum examination. A bloody discharge may result from tumours of the vagina, cervix or uterus.

DYSPAREUNIA

Dyspareunia may result from one of many causes, most of which have little to do with the vagina itself. Primary dyspareunia often has a psychological background and may require expert counselling (see Chapter 66). Secondary dyspareunia is more often due to organic disease, especially when the pain is felt only after full insertion has occurred. Pelvic inflammatory disease, endometriosis and pelvic or vaginal tumours are not infrequent causes. Introital, secondary dyspareunia may result from vaginal infection, atrophic changes or follow surgery to the perineum, most commonly an episiotomy. Dyspareunia may result from vulval disease. Radiotherapy to the pelvis or vagina will often cause fibrosis of the pelvic floor and contracture of the vagina. Great care must be taken in the management of these patients to prevent this complication (Chapters 33 and 36).

Examination may reveal spasm of the levator muscles in women with a psychological cause for their symptom but may also be seen in women with a physical cause. Tact and gentleness are essential — it may not be prudent to pursue an attempt at vaginal examination at this stage. Women who complain of dyspareunia due to vulvodynia appear to have no obvious abnormality. Their problem has been discussed earlier in this chapter. A tender perineal scar may be evident in a woman complaining of dyspareunia following childbirth but some of these women also have a psychological overlay which requires help. Occasionally, a tender adhesion may be detected in the vagina. Atrophic changes or vaginal infection may sometimes prove to be the cause.

Retroversion of the uterus is seldom an explanation in itself for dyspareunia. More usually, associated endometriosis or pelvic inflammatory disease is the culprit. An ovarian tumour or a fibroid uterus may present with dyspareunia.

If no cause is evident, laparoscopy is very useful. Quite marked endometriosis or pelvic inflammatory disease may be undetected by bimanual examination. If no pathology is found after a careful inspection of the pelvic organs, the patient may be reassured that no serious disease exists. Specialized investigations may be indicated (Chapter 60) and referral for sexual therapy may be appropriate.

Treatment will depend upon the cause. General advice about coital technique may be helpful, particularly in employing sufficient foreplay to ensure adequate arousal and in adopting coital positions which allow the woman to control insertion and the depth of penetration (see Chapter 66).

ATROPHIC VAGINITIS

Symptoms of vaginal atrophy occur in many women after the menopause. Vaginal dryness, dyspareunia, superimposed infection and bleeding are common problems. These are often associated with symptoms due to atrophy of the lower urinary tract: dysuria, frequency and urgency.

Examination will show pale, thinned vaginal epithelium often with petechial haemorrhage (Fig. 27.8). In extreme cases, the vulva becomes atrophied, the labia shrink and the introitus contracts.

When bleeding has occurred, a cervical smear, examination under anaesthesia and curettage are mandatory to exclude malignancy. Hysteroscopy is a very useful adjunct to these (Chapter 3).

Appropriate hormone replacement therapy will reverse all these symptoms of end organ failure. There is little logic in prescribing an oestrogen cream for local application. It is more expensive, more inconvenient and, dose for dose, has systemic effects that are similar to oral or parenteral therapy.

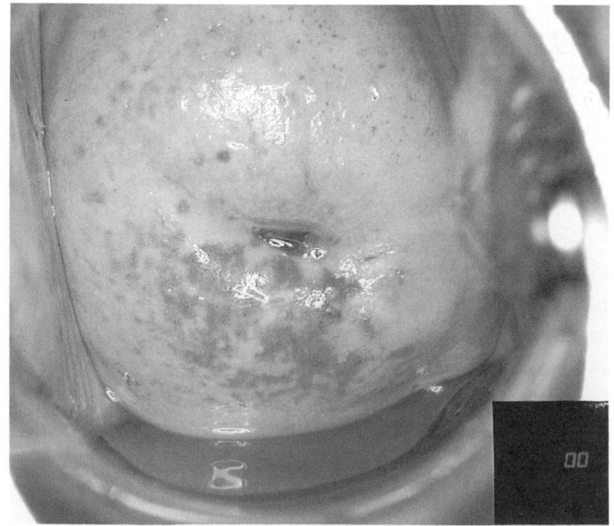

Fig. 27.8 Atrophic changes on the cervix. The epithelium is thin and easily traumatized. On the anterior lip there are small petechial haemorrhages which have coalesced on the posterior lip.

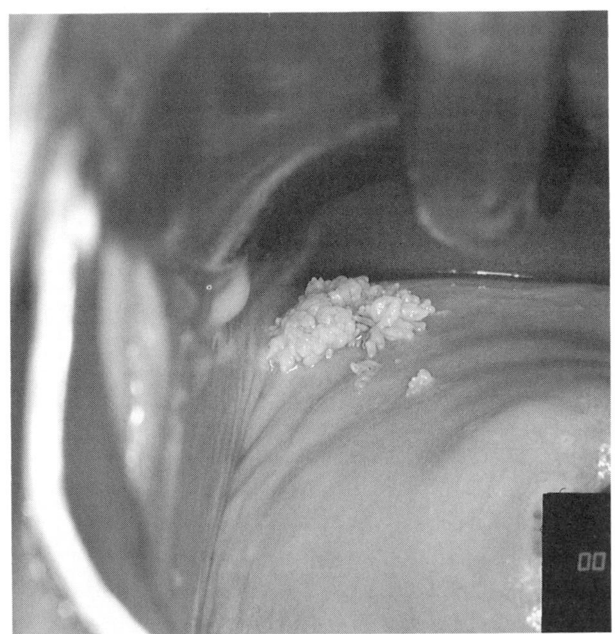

Fig. 27.9 These vaginal condylomata have turned bright white after the application of 5% acetic acid.

Prepubertal children may develop a vaginal discharge, sometimes blood-stained, as a result of secondary infection following atrophic vaginitis (see above).

BENIGN TUMOURS

Tumours in the vagina are uncommon. Condyloma acuminata are by far the commonest seen (Fig. 27.9). The frond-like surface is usually characteristic but it is wise to await the result of a biopsy before instituting treatment.

Endometriotic deposits may be seen in the vagina. They are most common in an episiotomy wound and may lie deep to the epithelium.

Simple mesonephric (Gärtner's) or paramesonephric cysts may be seen, especially high up near the fornices. If asymptomatic, they are best not treated. If treatment is required, marsupialization is effective and safer than excision.

Adenosis — multiple mucus-containing vaginal cysts — is a rare condition which even more rarely gives rise to symptoms. A variety of abnormalities are reported in the daughters of women who took diethylstilboestrol during their pregnancy. Most of these are of no significance (see Chapter 39).

VAGINAL NEOPLASIA

VIN are discussed in Chapter 34 and vaginal cancer in Chapter 39.

KEY POINTS

1. Vulval lesions should be biopsied liberally under local anaesthetic.
2. If no specific cause is found for pruritus vulvae, general advice, sympathetic handling, a steroid ointment and a sedative at night are often helpful.
3. Some patients benefit from antidepressant therapy.
4. There is no place for vulvectomy in the management of lichen sclerosus.
5. Vulval disease may be a manifestation of a systemic disorder.
6. Infection should be excluded in any woman complaining of a vaginal discharge.
7. A vaginal discharge is frequently due to increased physiological secretions.

REFERENCES

Friedrich E G 1983 Vulvar disease, 2nd ed. Saunders, Philadelphia

Fox H, Buckley C H 1988 Non-epithelial and mixed tumours of the vulva. In: Ridley C M (ed) The vulva. Churchill Livingstone, Edinburgh, pp 235–262

International Society for the Study of Vulvar Disease 1989 New nomenclature for vulvar disease. Report of the committee on terminology. American Journal of Obstetrics and Gynecology 73: 769

McKay M 1985 Vulvodynia versus pruritus vulvae. Clinical Obstetrics and Gynaecology 28: 123–133

McKay M 1989 Vulvodynia — a multifactorial clinical problem. Archives of Dermatology 125: 256–262

Meyrick Thomas R H, Ridley C M, McGibbon D H, Black M M 1988 Lichen sclerosus and autoimmunity — a study of 350 women. British Journal of Dermatology 118: 41–46

Ridley C M 1988 The vulva. Churchill Livingstone, Edinburgh

28. Uterine fibroids

C. P. West

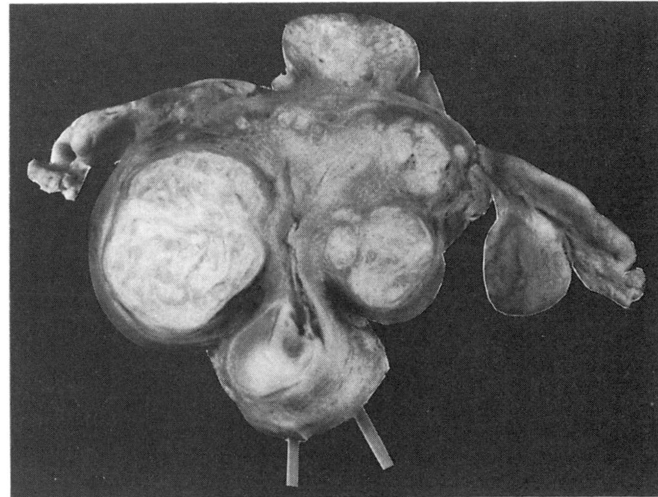

Fig. 28.1 Uterus enlarged by multiple fibroids. The patient presented at 43 years with menorrhagia; she had a 13-year history of primary infertility. Septate vagina and double cervix (marked with rods).

INTRODUCTION

Uterine fibroids are common benign tumours which arise from the uterine myometrium or less commonly from the cervix. They are composed of smooth muscle with a variable amount of connective tissue but are of smooth muscle origin, and thus classified as leiomyomata and also known as myomas. Although inaccurate by histological criteria, the term 'fibroid' is used almost universally to describe these nodular outgrowths which cause enlargement of the uterus and distortion of its normal structure with resulting implications for menstrual and reproductive function.

CLASSIFICATION AND PATHOPHYSIOLOGY

Macroscopically, fibroids are round or oval-shaped tumours, usually firm in consistency, with a characteristic white whorled appearance on cross-section. They may be single but are more commonly multiple and of varying sites and sizes (Fig. 28.1). Tiny 'seedling' fibroids are commonly seen in association with larger tumours and surgical removal of over 120 individual fibroids has been recorded in the literature. Four clinical subgroups are recognized: intramural, subserosal, submucous and cervical.

Intramural fibroids lie within the uterine wall, separated from the adjacent normal myometrium by a thin layer of connective tissue which forms the so-called false capsule. Small nutrient arteries penetrate this capsule although a single larger artery usually provides the major blood supply. Enlargement of a single intramural fibroid gives a globular outline to the uterus (see Fig. 28.10); the increased vascularity gives an appearance similar to that of pregnancy. Large intramural fibroids enlarge and distort the uterine cavity (Fig. 28.1), increasing its surface area although they do not encroach upon the cavity directly.

Subserosal fibroids project outward from the uterine surface, covered with peritoneum. As growth is unrestricted

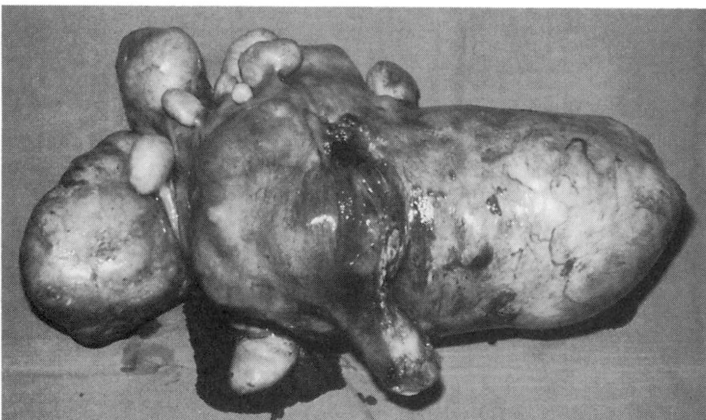

Fig. 28.2 Multiple subserous fibroids, some pedunculated. Specimen width = 350 mm.

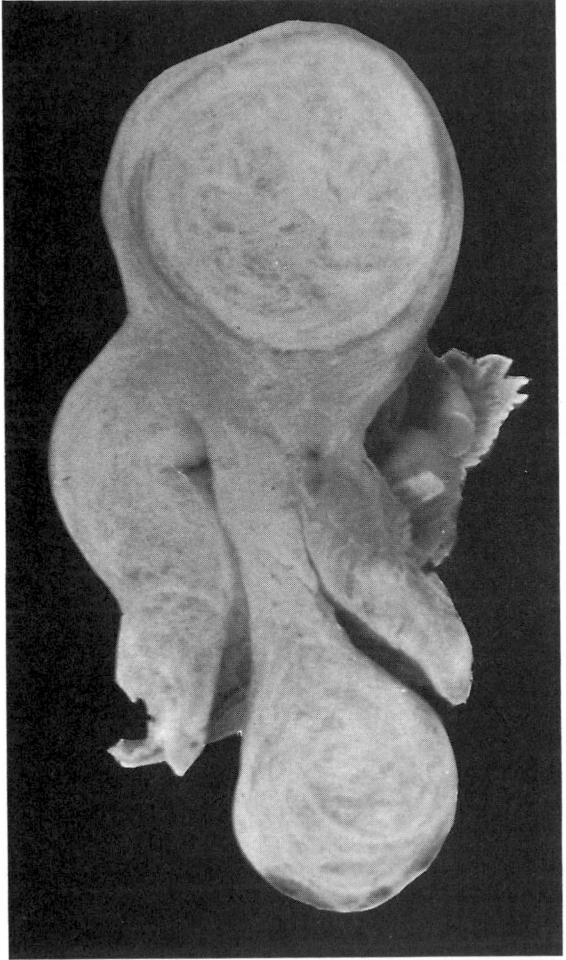

Fig. 28.3 Submucous fibroid protruding through cervix. The patient, aged 44 years, presented with a 3-week history of continuous bleeding; her haemoglobin level was 6.9 g/dl.

by surrounding myometrium they may attain a very large size. Many fibroids in this site become pedunculated (Fig .28.2) and torsion is a potential although rare complication. Sessile subserosal fibroids projecting from the fundal region may become adherent to omentum or bowel, particularly if there has been coincidental inflammatory disease. Fibroids which become attached to the omentum may develop an alternative blood supply, and may rarely become separated from the uterus forming a so-called 'parasitic' fibroid. Subserosal fibroids arising from the lateral uterine wall may lie between the layers of the broad ligament where large tumours may displace the ureters or bulge between the layers of the sigmoid mesocolon, lifting the bowel upwards. Broad ligament fibroids arising from the lateral uterine wall differ from true broad ligament fibroids which have no attachment to the uterus but have their origin in smooth muscle fibres within the broad ligament, for example the round ligament, ovarian ligament or perivascular connective tissue.

Submucous fibroids are less common, comprising around 5% of all leiomyomata. By definition they project into the uterine cavity, are covered by endometrium, and cause irregularity and distortion although uterine enlargement may not be evident. Pedunculated submucous fibroids on a long stalk may prolapse through the cervix (Fig. 28.3) where they may cause intermenstrual bleeding or become ulcerated and infected. Although usually small, submucous fibroids may enlarge to fill the cavity when attempted spontaneous expulsion may result in dilation of the cervix, so that the projecting fibroid resembles a fetal head. Very rarely this has led on to uterine inversion.

Cervical fibroids are relatively uncommon but give rise to greatest surgical difficulty by virtue of their relative inaccessibility and close proximity to the bladder and ureters. Enlargement causes upwards displacement of the uterus and the fibroid may become impacted in the pelvis, causing urinary retention and ureteric obstruction (see Fig. 28.7).

Microscopic appearances

Microscopically, fibroids are composed of smooth muscle cell bundles, also arranged in whorl-like patterns (Fig. 28.4a), admixed with a variable amount of connective tissue although the latter rarely predominates. The relatively poor blood supply to individual fibroids (see below) may result in degenerative changes, particularly within the large tumours. *Hyaline* degeneration (Fig. 28.4b) is the most common, resulting in a smoother and more homogeneous consistency and this may become *cystic* if liquefaction occurs. Much more rarely *fatty* change may develop. This is distinct from the true lipoma of the uterus, which is extremely uncommon. *Calcification* (Fig. 28.5) is a later consequence of degeneration secondary to circulatory impairment and characteristically occurs after the menopause although it may occur earlier in subserosal fibroids with narrow pedicles.

Red degeneration occurs almost exclusively in pregnancy (see Fig. 28.16), causing localized pain and tenderness

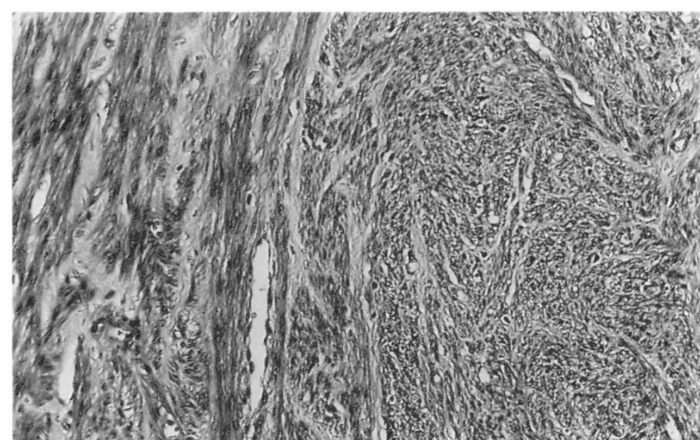

Fig. 28.4a Leiomyoma of uterus. Bundles of elongated smooth muscle cells in both longitudinal (left) and transverse planes (× 160). (Courtesy of Dr K Maclaren.)

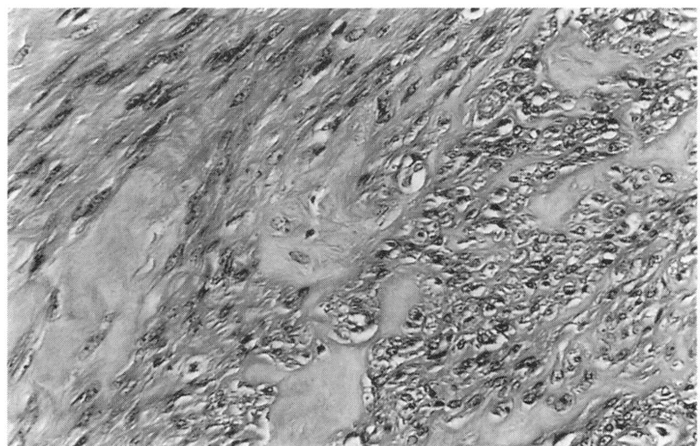

Fig. 28.4b Leiomyoma of uterus showing focal hyalinization. Smooth muscle bundles are separated by dense hyalinized connective tissue (× 320). (Courtesy of Dr K Maclaren.)

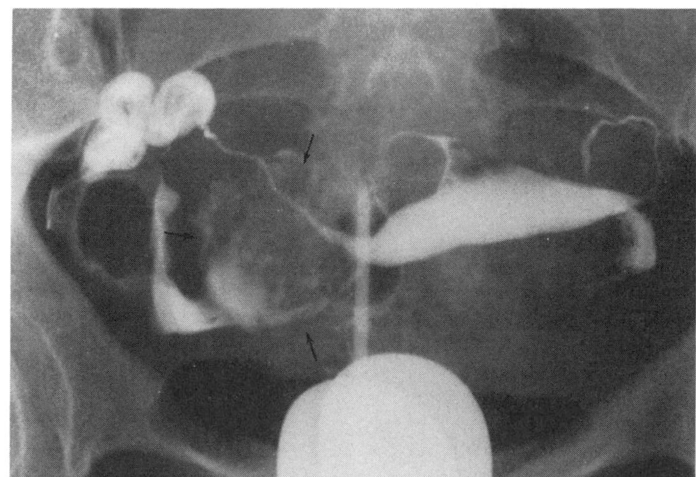

Fig. 28.5a Calcified fibroid seen on hysterosalpingogram. (Courtesy of Dr B Muir.)

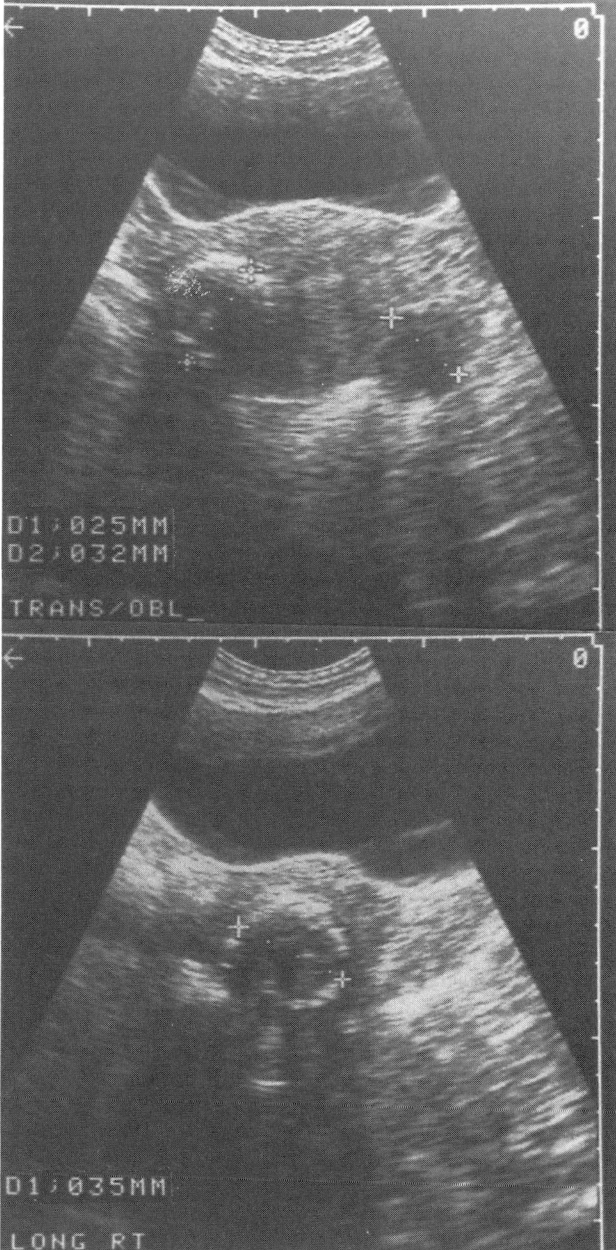

Fig. 28.5b Ultrasound appearance of the uterus shown in Figure 28.5a. **Top** Two fibroids seen in transverse plane with calcified fibroid to left; **bottom** calcified fibroid shown in longitudinal plane.

which may be mistaken for an acute abdomen. Macroscopically, the fibroid appears reddish on cross-section, due to the presence of thrombotic and haemolytic changes within the blood vessels. The exact mechanism involved is not entirely clear. *Sarcomatous* degeneration, discussed on p. 410, is a serious although uncommon complication of fibroid growth.

Fibroids are believed to have an adverse effect on reproductive function by virtue of the resulting enlargement and distortion of the uterus, in particular the endometrial cavity (see Fig. 28.1). Some of the clinical features may be related to the effect of the fibroids on uterine arterial blood supply and venous drainage. Studies of blood flow using isotope clearance (Forssman 1976) and microradiographic studies of vascular patterns within fibroid uteri (Farrer-Brown et al 1971) have demonstrated that fibroids are less vascular than the surrounding myometrium, despite a rich network of surrounding arteries, hence the frequency with which degenerative changes occur. Regardless of their site, fibroids may cause mechanical obstruction to the venous drainage of both the myometrium and the endometrium, resulting in congestion and dilatation of the venous plexuses. Such congestion, if it affects the endometrium, may contribute to heavy blood loss.

AETIOLOGY

The aetiology of uterine fibroids is unknown. They are believed to be unicellular in origin but the initiating factors have not been elucidated. It is presumed that their growth is dependent on ovarian hormones since they do not occur prior to the menarche and normally show a reduction in size after the menopause. This evidence for their oestrogen-dependence has been supported by recent observations that regression occurs in response to the hypo-oestrogenic state induced by agonists of luteinizing hormone-releasing hormone (LHRH) first reported by Filicori and co-workers in 1983 (see West 1988). The potential therapeutic application of such agents is described later (p. 407).

Following on from observations that fibroids are dependent on oestrogen for their continuing growth, it has been suggested that women who develop fibroids have an excess of circulating oestrogen. Support for this theory was found by Witherspoon (1935) who described a relationship between chronic anovulation, endometrial hyperplasia and the development of uterine fibroids. Recent studies have however failed to demonstrate any difference in circulating oestrogen and progesterone concentrations between women with fibroids and healthy controls (Maheux et al 1986). Histological studies have confirmed that hyperplastic changes are commonly present at the margins of fibroids but that these coexist with areas of normal and atrophic endometrium (Farrer-Brown et al 1971). This may reflect local differences in the binding of steroids to fibroid tissue and to normal myometrium, as discussed below. Uterine fibroids do not occur in animal species and thus it has not been possible to provide an animal model for their study. An attempt to induce growth of fibroids in guinea pigs by chronic administration of high doses of unopposed oestrogen resulted in growth of intra-abdominal fibromas which were histologically quite different from leiomyomata and were non-uterine in site (see Miller & Ludovici 1955).

Studies of tissue obtained at hysterectomy have demonstrated that receptors for both oestrogen and progesterone are present in greater concentrations in fibroids than in the adjacent myometrium (Wilson et al 1980), again supporting a role for these hormones in control of fibroid growth. However recent evidence from women rendered hypo-oestrogenic with agonists of LHRH (see West & Lumsden 1989) suggests that oestrogen does not act directly but that its effect on fibroids is mediated by growth factors such as epidermal growth factor (EGF). These factors control cellular proliferation and have been implicated in tumour growth. High-affinity binding sites for EGF are present in the uterus and oestrogen has been shown to influence its binding to fibroids but not to normal myometrium (Lumsden et al 1988). The role of progesterone, if any, in the control of fibroid growth remains unclear.

EPIDEMIOLOGY

It is estimated that around 20% of women of reproductive age have uterine fibroids although presentation occurs most commonly towards the end of their reproductive life. While no hereditary factors have been identified, there are definite racial differences: a ninefold greater incidence has been reported among black women (Witherspoon 1935), where they also present at a younger age. Women with uterine fibroids have had fewer term pregnancies and are generally of lower parity than their contemporaries without this problem but it is not entirely clear whether fibroids are a cause or consequence of low family size. Obesity increases the risk of developing fibroids, while cigarette smoking is associated with a reduced risk (Ross et al 1986). The latter authors found that oral contraceptive users also have a reduced risk compared with users of non-hormonal contraception and this protective effect is related to the duration of usage of the pill and also to its progestogenic content. Similar risk factors are associated with endometrial carcinoma but, unlike the latter, development of fibroids following the menopause has not been described, even in association with the use of hormone replacement therapy. This further supports the evidence that oestrogen alone does not provide the trigger for the initiation of fibroid growth.

PRESENTATION

The clinical presentation of uterine fibroids is dependent in part on the reproductive status of the woman and the site of the fibroids. The symptomatology has been reviewed in detail by Buttram & Reiter (1981). Many fibroids, possibly in excess of 50%, are asymptomatic and discovered at routine pelvic or abdominal examination or during pregnancy.

Menorrhagia

It is uncertain what proportion of women with fibroids

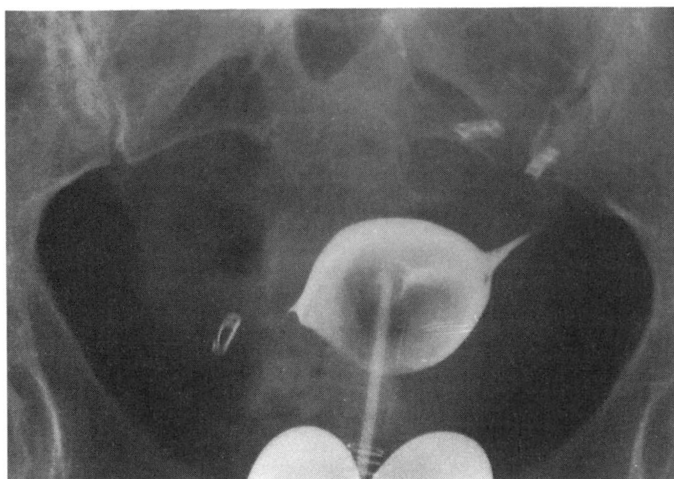

Fig. 28.6 Hysterosalpinogram showing enlargement of uterine cavity and filling defect from intramural fibroid. Extensive endometriosis had complicated laparoscopic sterilization (hence the two clips on the left tube). (Courtesy of Dr B Muir.)

have excessive menstrual loss although estimates vary between 30 and 50%. Investigation of women presenting with menorrhagia has shown the presence of fibroids in only 10% of women with moderately heavy menstrual blood loss (80–100 ml), compared with 40% of those with loss in excess of 200 ml (Rybo et al 1985). Menorrhagia attributable to fibroids may therefore be very heavy, causing significant anaemia. It is important to appreciate that fibroids are not usually a cause of irregular or intermenstrual bleeding and that any disruption of normal cyclicity should not be attributed to the presence of fibroids without first excluding other causes.

The mechanism of the menorrhagia remains a subject of debate. Theories include ulceration and haemorrhage of the endometrium overlying submucous fibroids, enlargement of the total surface area of the endometrium due to mechanical distortion by submucous and intramural fibroids (Fig. 28.6) and stasis and dilatation of the venous plexuses draining the endometrium due to mechanical compression of the venous drainage by fibroids at any site. All these mechanisms may be important and it is now clear that, contrary to some opinions, menorrhagia is not confined only to women with submucous fibroids and that while these may be associated with menorrhagia of greatest severity, they are sometimes asymptomatic. Recent research has implicated disorders of prostaglandin synthesis and metabolism in the aetiology of menstrual disorders (Chapter 14) and this may also be relevant in the presence of fibroids. Fibroids are associated with disordered uterine motility but it is not clear whether this is because of mechanical factors or because of abnormalities of prostaglandin metabolism.

Pelvic pain and pressure symptoms

Fibroids do not usually give rise to pain although, exceptionally, their presentation may be acute on account of torsion or degeneration. Attempted expulsion of a large submucous fibroid through the cervix causes uterine cramp associated with bleeding and may be mistaken for spontaneous abortion, particularly with the clinical finding of a dilated cervix and a protruding mass. Rarely this situation results in uterine inversion. Torsion or painful degeneration presents with an acute abdomen and is commonly confused with complications of ovarian neoplasia. Distinction between these conditions is particularly important in pregnancy complicated by red degeneration of a fibroid in order to avoid subjecting the woman to unnecessary laparotomy.

It is surprising that even in the presence of multiple fibroids menstruation may be painless. They are more often associated with pelvic discomfort and urinary symptoms, attributed to pressure from large fibroids, particularly those arising from the cervix or low down on the anterior uterine wall. Cervical fibroids may present with acute retention of urine (see Fig. 28.7), although this is a fairly uncommon complication.

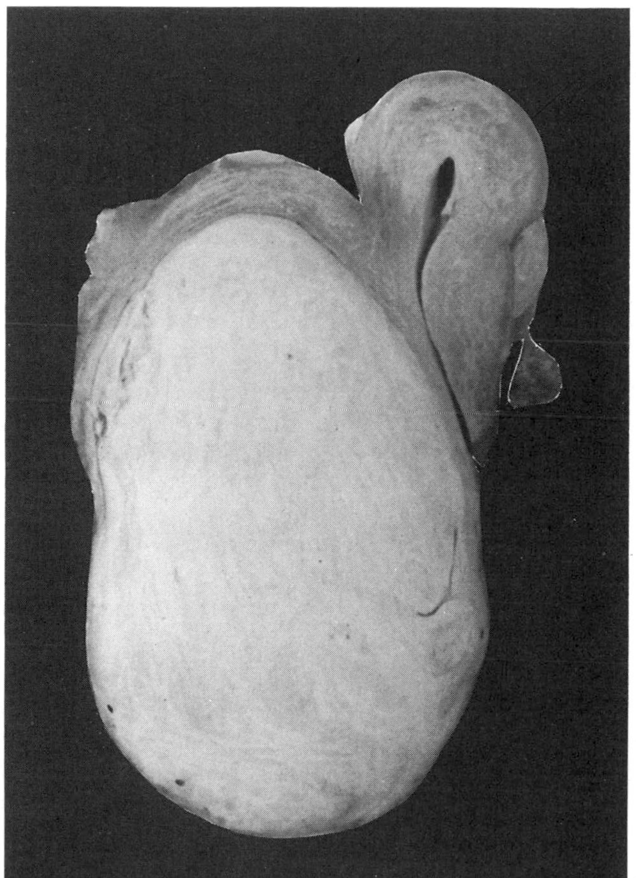

Fig. 28.7 Cervical fibroid growing anteriorly in the supravaginal cervix. Presentation was with frequency of micturition followed by acute urinary retention.

Subfertility

It is estimated that infertility is the major presenting factor or a secondary feature in around 27% of women with fibroids (Buttram & Reiter 1981) and the association of fibroids with low fecundity and childlessness is well recognized. However, when compared with other causes of infertility, they are relatively uncommon, being implicated in approximately 3% of couples. This percentage is higher in negroid races where there is also a high prevalence of pelvic inflammatory disease and the two conditions often coexist. It is probable that a delay in childbearing, whether voluntary or involuntary, may predispose towards the development of fibroids and it is thus mandatory to investigate fully both partners to exclude other factors which may be contributing towards their subfertility. The mechanism whereby fibroids adversely affect conception is unclear but it is likely to be mechanical, by virtue of cornual occlusion or by distortion of the cavity, preventing implantation. In addition, alterations in local blood flow and increases in the binding of steroids to fibroids, compared with myometrium (p. 400), may create unfavourable factors in the local environment which prevent implantation. These mechanisms have yet to be clarified but reports of improved pregnancy rates after myomectomy give support to the belief that in some individuals the presence of fibroids is detrimental to the chance of conception.

INVESTIGATIONS

The range of investigations appropriate to each case of fibroids will vary according to the nature of the individual problem and the proposed plan of management. General assessment must always include a full blood count as many patients with fibroids do not complain of excessive menstruation even when this is present.

Ultrasound should always be used to confirm or clarify the nature of a pelvic mass. Even in relatively unskilled hands it will diagnose pregnancy and differentiate between cystic and solid lesions (Fig. 28.8). With appropriate training and experience, the site and nature of a pelvic mass may be predicted with accuracy in over 80% of cases; difficulty mainly arises in the differentiation of pedunculated fibroids from solid ovarian lesions.

Ultrasound assessment should include examination of the ovaries and kidneys and it is important to look for the presence or absence of free peritoneal fluid as well as to study the nature and consistency of the mass itself. Serial ultrasound examination is of value in monitoring fibroid size during medical or conservative treatment. The volume of individual fibroids (Fig. 28.5b) or of the whole uterus (Fig. 28.8) can be calculated by measuring the diameter in three planes at right angles, using the formula $4/3\pi r3$.

Magnetic resonance imaging is of considerable value in demonstrating the nature of pelvic masses although the technique is very costly and not widely available. Compared with ultrasound, it is a more accurate predictor of the histological features of a tumour. While this is of value in research and in cases of diagnostic difficulty, such a high level of accuracy is not necessary for the routine management of fibroids.

Laparoscopy is of value if the uterus is not larger than a 12-week gestation size and there is associated infertility or pelvic pain. It may reveal the presence of coincidental endometriosis, pelvic adhesions or other tubal pathology.

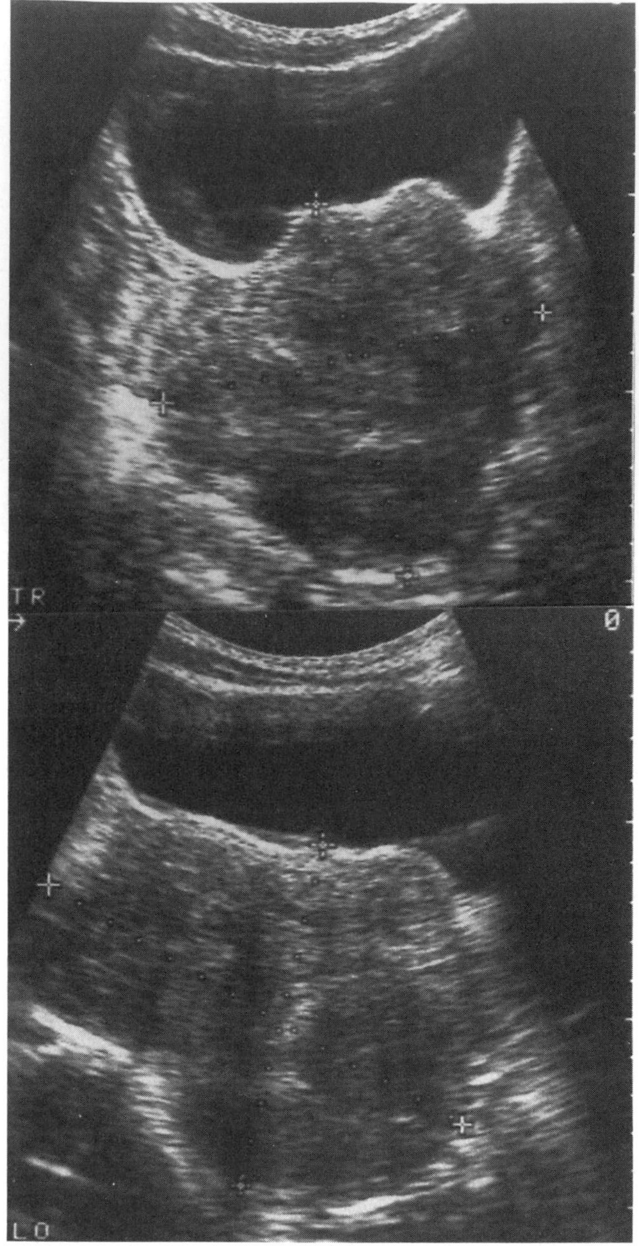

Fig. 28.8 Ultrasound appearance of uterus enlarged by multiple fibroids, showing patchy echogenicity. (Courtesy of Dr B Muir.)

Laparoscopy will also differentiate between a pedunculated fibroid and an ovarian neoplasm in cases where the diagnosis of an adnexal mass is unclear on the basis of clinical and ultrasound findings. It may also be possible, in some circumstances, to remove small fibroids laparoscopically (see p. 406).

Hysterosalpingography or *hysteroscopy* should be carried out routinely in patients with a history of recurrent abortion. Examination of the uterine cavity is also important in an infertile patient with fibroids or in any patient where myomectomy is contemplated in order to identify the presence and site of any submucous fibroids. Not only may these adversely affect implantation but they may be encroaching on to the tubal ostium causing obstruction. Where a filling defect is evident radiologically (e.g Fig. 28.9), direct visualization through the hysteroscope will clarify the diagnosis as well as enabling local hysteroscopic methods of treatment to be performed where appropriate. There is also an increasing place for hysteroscopy in the investigation of menorrhagia and other menstrual abnormalities. In one study quoted by Siegler & Valle (1988), submucous fibroids were visualized hysteroscopically in 13% of patients investigated for abnormal bleeding. Hysteroscopy would not however be appropriate in cases of menorrhagia associated with large fibroids where hysterectomy is the chosen treatment option.

Endometrial sampling by biopsy or curettage is indicated in cases of irregular or intermenstrual bleeding to exclude the present of coexisting endometrial pathology. Where heavy bleeding retains a normal cyclical pattern this is usually unnecessary although curettage may be of diagnostic value in detecting irregularities of the uterine cavity due to submucous fibroids. In this regard, formal curettage has advantages over newer methods of endometrial biopsy as the latter gives less information about the outline of the cavity.

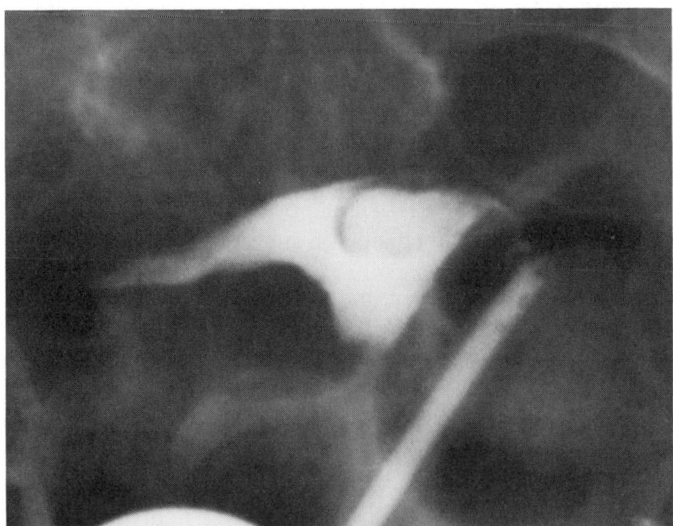

Fig. 28.9 Hysterosalpingogram of a patient presenting with recurrent abortion, showing a filling defect. (Courtesy of Dr B Muir.)

TREATMENT

Recent advances in medical and surgical methods of treatment have increased the potential range of therapeutic options for women with fibroids. It is too early to assess the impact of these developments on our overall gynaecological practice and in particular on the number of hysterectomies performed annually. In deciding about management, the symptoms, reproductive status and attitude of each individual patient should be taken into consideration and the options fully discussed. While surgery remains the treatment of choice for most symptomatic women, alternatives may be appropriate in some situations.

Expectant management

Fibroids are frequently asymptomatic and provided that their nature can be determined with reasonable certainty using the diagnostic methods described above, active treatment is unnecessary. Surgical removal has traditionally been advocated when the uterine size exceeds that of a 12-week pregnancy because of potential confusion with ovarian neoplasia but most pelvic swellings can be confidently diagnosed with the use of ultrasound. Similarly, the risk of sarcomatous change is estimated to be less than 0.1% (see p. 410), making prophylactic removal of a fibroid unjustified. While some gynaecologists and patients will still favour a policy of surgical removal, the mere presence of a fibroid uterus is not known to carry any long-term detrimental effects and spontaneous regression after the menopause may be anticipated. Routine hysterectomy is therefore difficult to justify, particularly in women over the age of 45. Exceptions would include very large fibroids, a rapid increase in size or where there is concern about the nature of the mass.

Hysterectomy

Hysterectomy is the definitive treatment for symptomatic uterine fibroids although the decision to perform hysterectomy should not be undertaken without due consideration of the alternatives; for women who wish to preserve reproductive function, myomectomy or medical treatment must be considered. In most cases total abdominal hysterectomy with ovarian conservation (Fig. 28.10) will be the procedure of choice as uterine enlargement by fibroids makes vaginal hysterectomy inappropriate in most cases. For gynaecologists who favour the vaginal route for routine hysterectomies, consideration may be given to preoperative shrinkage with an LHRH agonist as described below. Similarly, a reduction in volume and vascularity

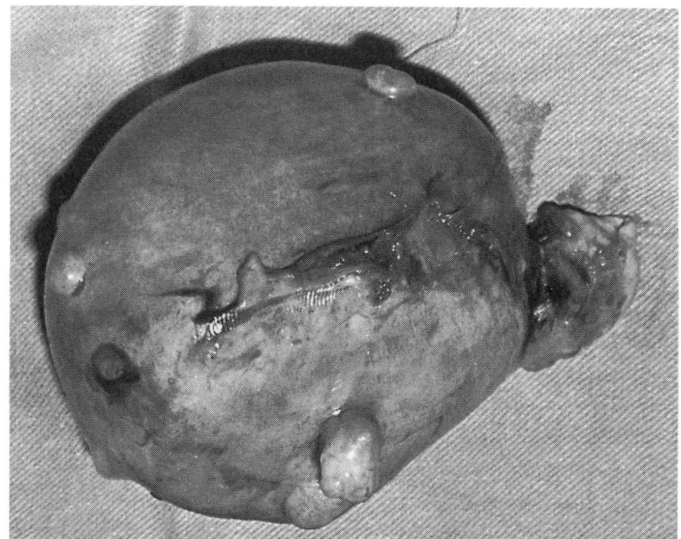

Fig. 28.10 Hysterectomy specimen from uterus enlarged to 16-week gestation size by single intramural fibroid and several small seedling fibroids. Uterine volume = 575 ml.

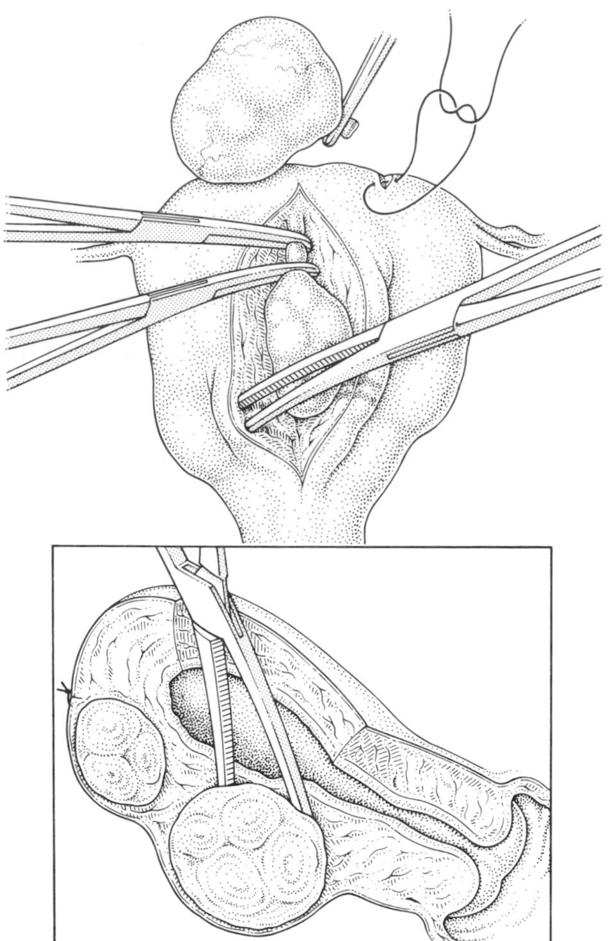

Fig. 28.11 Removal of subserous, intramural, submucous and posteriorly located intramural fibroids through a single anterior incision. (From Buttram & Reiter 1981, with permission.)

may facilitate removal of a very large uterus by the abdominal route.

Abdominal hysterectomy is rendered difficult in the presence of large fibroids arising from the cervix or situated in the broad ligament. It is also more complicated if there are adhesions from previous myomectomies or from associated endometriosis or pelvic inflammatory disease. Difficult access to the pelvis during hysterectomy for large fibroids will be rendered easier by prior enucleation of the fibroids. The ureters may be vulnerable during an operation to remove a broad ligament fibroid and their pathway must always be identified. Regardless of the direction of displacement, they are always extracapsular. In the case of a large cervical fibroid an alternative approach is hemisection of the uterus, followed by enucleation of the fibroid in order to gain access to the uterine arteries and cervix. These techniques are described in detail in Monaghan (1988).

Myomectomy

Removal of individual fibroids was first reported in the middle of the 19th century although current surgical techniques are largely attributable to Victor Bonney who described a personal series of 403 cases. Since then there have been several large published series, reviewed in detail by Buttram & Reiter (1981).

Enucleation of intramural fibroids from their false capsule can be a rapid and simple procedure but may also be associated with considerable technical difficulties, major haemorrhage and a greater postoperative morbidity and mortality than hysterectomy. It is therefore an operation which should be restricted to women who have not completed childbearing. It is most satisfactory where fibroids are solitary or few in number and although removal of as many as 125 individual tumours from one uterus was described by Bonney, such a procedure is tedious and the outcome in terms of reproductive function must be in considerable doubt.

The major problems associated with myomectomy are heavy operative blood loss and postoperative adhesion formation, reducing the chance of successful conception and rendering future surgery more difficult. It is therefore most important that the decision to perform a myomectomy is carefully considered. If operative haemorrhage is very heavy the surgeon may have to resort to hysterectomy and should be reluctant to embark upon surgery if the patient is not willing to consent to the latter alternative. In a woman presenting with infertility, it is sometimes difficult to establish the extent to which the fibroids are interfering with conception and full investigation of both the woman and her partner should be carried out.

As many fibroids which adversely affect conception are

submucous in site, consideration should be given to alternative surgical methods (see below). Subserous fibroids are easily removed with minimal morbidity, particularly if pedunculated (Fig. 28.11) but such fibroids are the least likely to give rise to problems. Some authorities would advise their removal if they are large because of the risk — albeit rare — of acute torsion in pregnancy.

The presence of fibroids in a woman desiring pregnancy at some future date poses particular problems because the risk of new growths occurring after early surgery has to be balanced against any increased technical difficulty that might result from enlargement of the original fibroids should surgery be delayed. The use of interval medical treatment has much to commend it in this situation.

Because of the well recognized morbidity of the procedure of myomectomy, various methods have been advocated to reduce intra- and postoperative complications. Postoperative adhesions are usually a consequence of difficulties with haemostasis and oozing from incision lines and are increased where there are multiple incisions over the uterine body. Adhesions to incisions on the posterior uterine wall are potentially more serious because of involvement of the fallopian tubes and ovaries. To minimize adhesion formation, as many fibroids as possible should be removed through a single incision (Fig. 28.11). Some authorities recommend removal of posterior wall fibroids via the uterine cavity through an incision on the anterior uterine wall. Others avoid opening the uterine cavity unless submucous fibroids are known to be present because of the risk of intrauterine adhesions. Careful obliteration of large cavities left by enucleation of fibroids is very important and opinions vary as to whether redundant myometrium should be removed or preserved. Bonney (Monaghan 1988) described a 'hood' method of closure of the cavity left after enucleation of a very large single posterior tumour (Fig. 28.12), suturing the redundant flap of serosal-covered myometrium over the fundus and low down on to the anterior wall to avoid adhesion formation. Plication of the round ligaments at the end of the procedure to hold the uterus forward in anteversion and the instillation of concentrated solutions of dextran have also been recommended to reduce the risk of postoperative adhesions.

Both mechanical and medical methods have been described to reduce operative blood loss. One such method is the use of the Bonney's myomectomy clamp which is placed across the lower uterus to occlude the uterine arteries (see Fig. 28.12a). It can be used in conjunction with ring forceps to occlude the ovarian blood supply. An alternative is the use of a rubber tourniquet or catheter placed around the uterus through an incision in the broad ligament at the level of the lower segment. Occlusion of the arterial blood supply for prolonged intervals of time may cause ischaemic damage to tissues and release of histamine-like substances into the general circulation has been reported (Monaghan 1988). During a long operation, intermittent release of the clamp or catheter at 10–20-min intervals is recommended. Such occlusive methods are unsuitable for use where there are large cervical or broad ligament fibroids and these are the very tumours which may give rise to greatest difficulty. As an alternative or adjunct to occlusive clamps, local injection of vasopressin is recommended by some authorities although its efficacy has been challenged. Recently, pretreatment with LHRH analogues has been used to reduce the vascularity of the uterus (see

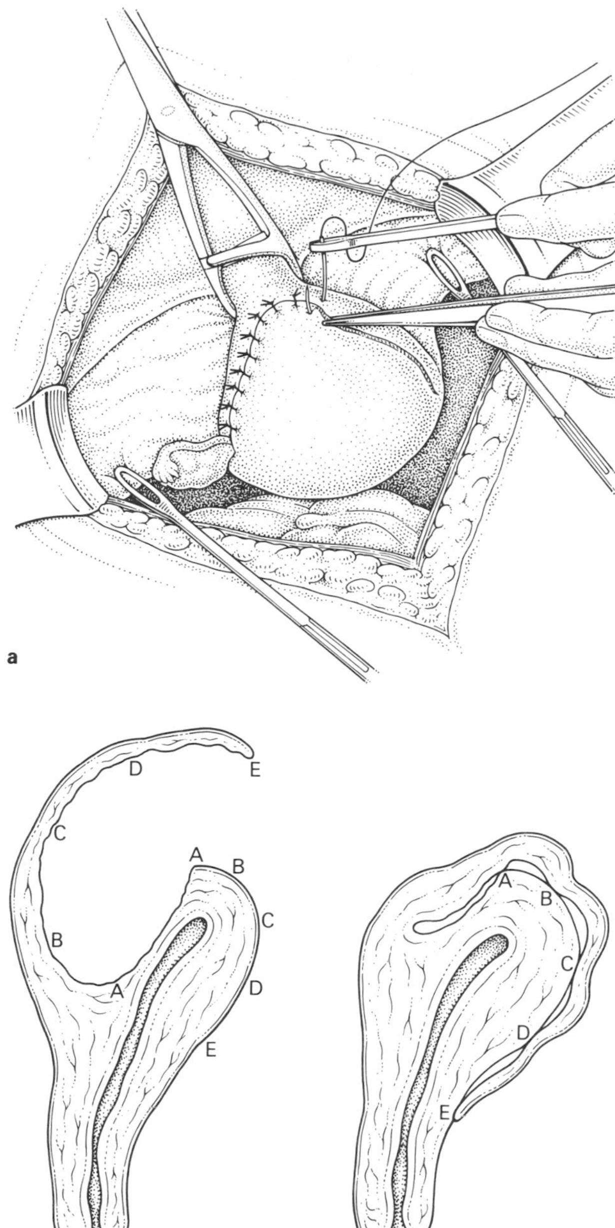

Fig. 28.12a Closure of myomectomy through transverse posterior incision using Bonney's 'hood', showing final anterior suture line and Bonney's clamp in place. **b** Construction of Bonney's hood showing the capsule after enucleation (left) and the hood in place (right). (From Monaghan 1988, with permission.)

below) and this has the advantage of also reducing the size of the fibroids. However their enucleation may be rendered more difficult because the false capsule plane of cleavage between the fibroid and the surrounding myometrium becomes less well defined.

Endoscopic surgical methods

Hysteroscopy

Most submucous fibroids which are protruding through the cervix (see Fig. 28.3) can be removed vaginally with cautery or ligation of the pedicle. If the fibroid is very large, piecemeal removal has been described. However facilities should be available to proceed to hysterectomy if such a procedure is complicated by excessive haemorrhage. Such difficulties might be overcome by preoperative treatment with an LHRH agonist (see below). Diagnostic and therapeutic hysteroscopy (see review by Siegler & Valle 1988) is gaining popularity in the UK and submucous fibroids (such as those illustrated in Figure 28.13) can be resected or, if pedunculated, avulsed under direct hysteroscopic visualization. A urological resectoscope can be used in combination with the hysteroscope and postoperative bleeding is controlled with the balloon of a foley catheter. These procedures may be curative in some cases of menstrual upset or infertility. A newer approach to menstrual dysfunction is endometrial ablation using the neodymium YAG laser, again under hysteroscopic visualization. Currently this technique is very costly and time-consuming and experience of its use in the treatment of fibroids is limited. However it is likely that these hysteroscopic techniques, performed as outpatient procedures with avoidance of major surgery, will become increasingly popular and widespread.

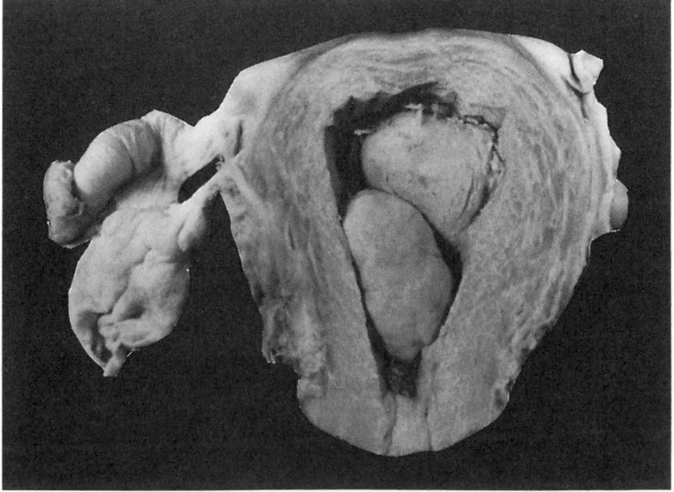

Fig. 28.13 Submucous fibroids (subtotal hysterectomy specimen).

Laparoscopy

Laparoscopy is now a standard investigation for infertility and inevitably many women thus investigated will be found to have small asymptomatic uterine fibroids. Laparoscopic methods of removal of both subserous and small intramural fibroids have been described but as these are unlikely to be interfering with fertility it is not clear whether their removal will carry any long-term advantage for the patient. In theory it may prevent the growth of larger, potentially symptomatic tumours and avoid more major surgical intervention but these advantages have yet to be proven. It is also unlikely that intramural seedlings can be removed by this method.

Medical management

There are two main objectives in the medical treatment of uterine fibroids, namely relief of symptoms and reduction in fibroid size. The ideal end-point of medical treatment would be their complete regression but to date this has not been described. There are few published studies in the literature which have evaluated the role of medical treatments in the management of fibroids and those which have been performed have yielded largely negative results (see review by West & Lumsden 1989). For this reason, medical methods have had a limited role in the management of fibroids.

Progestogens

Progestogens are widely used in the management of dysfunctional uterine bleeding but are generally regarded as ineffective in menorrhagia secondary to fibroids. However they may be specifically indicated in perimenopausal women with fibroids where bleeding is of anovular dysfunction type rather than a direct consequence of the fibroids. There is no evidence that their administration causes any alteration in the size of fibroids despite the antioestrogenic actions of progestogens such as medroxyprogesterone acetate, although degenerative changes have been reported following the administration of high doses.

Androgenic steroids

Androgenic steroids, such as danazol or gestrinone, are useful in reducing or abolishing menstrual blood loss in patients with menorrhagia by virtue of direct effects on the endometrium and negative feedback inhibition of pituitary gonadotrophin release. A small reduction in the volume of uterine fibroids, in the order of 20%, has been reported during therapy with both these androgens, with relief of menstrual symptoms. While such agents may be beneficial for the short-term relief of symptoms, their androgenic properties and side-effects make them unsuitable for long-term use. Their use should be considered in specific clinical situations where short-term symptomatic relief is required.

Prostaglandin synthetase inhibitors

While beneficial in the management of dysfunctional uterine bleeding, prostaglandin synthetase inhibitors have been shown to be ineffective in the treatment of menorrhagia secondary to fibroids. However they may be useful in the relief of pelvic pain in women with fibroids, including painful degeneration.

Oestrogen–progestogen combinations

The role of the oral contraceptive pill in women with fibroids is unclear. Since an early report of enlargement of fibroids during oral contraceptive therapy, its use has been avoided in this situation. The relevance of early studies to modern contraceptive practice must however be questioned as they related to much higher-dose formulations than those which are in current use. In women known to have fibroids, there seems to be no clear contraindication to the use of the pill for contraceptive purposes, provided that uterine volume is monitored and there is no deterioration in its size or in any fibroid-related symptoms. For women without fibroids, there is evidence that long-term use of the oral contraceptive pill has a protective effect against their development (Ross et al 1986). This benefit may be largely attributable to preparations with a relatively high progestogen content. However, this raises the question of whether the pill may be of value in the prevention of further fibroid growth following surgical myomectomy.

The influence of the oestrogen–progestogen combinations used for hormone replacement therapy is also unclear although dose-dependent re-enlargement of fibroids might be expected. It has been suggested that the affinity of weak oestrogens such as oestrone for specific binding sites in fibroids and myometrium is less than for oestradiol and ethinyloestradiol (see Wilson et al 1980) and this may have practical implications in the selection of therapy for the control of menopausal symptoms. Because of the ease of monitoring fibroid size with ultrasound, the use of low-dose oral hormone replacement therapy should not be contraindicated in postmenopausal women with fibroids, particularly if these have been asymptomatic, unless there is any suspicion of coexisting endometrial pathology or sarcomatous change.

LHRH analogues

Agonist analogues of LHRH are the only agents currently available which reliably relieve the symptoms of uterine fibroids and also cause a significant reduction in their size. However this effect persists only for as long as the treatment is administered and cessation of therapy is usually followed by regrowth of the fibroids to their pretreatment size (Fig. 28.14; see review by West 1988). LHRH agonists act by pituitary down-regulation, resulting in suppression of ovarian activity with chronic anovulation, amenorrhoea and lowering of circulating oestrogen concentrations to within or below those normally present in the early follicular phase of the menstrual cycle (Fig. 28.14). The shrinkage of fibroids is therefore a consequence of oestrogen withdrawal and women are likely to experience side-effects of the latter, in particular vasomotor symptoms and vaginal dryness. Because of the potential risk of loss of bone mineral, long-term treatment with LHRH agonists is contraindicated for most women. However they will give effective short-term relief of symptoms, particularly severe menorrhagia, enabling treatment of anaemia prior to surgery. Reduction in the size and vascularity of large fibroids is also of reported benefit prior to hysterectomy or myomectomy.

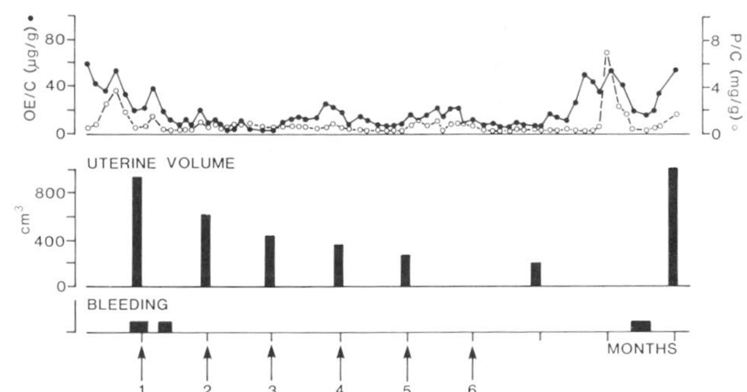

Fig. 28.14 Reversible reduction in uterine volume and amenorrhoea in a patient treated for 6 months with goserelin depot (arrows). Ovarian response was monitored by urinary oestrone glucurone and pregnanediol excretion (expressed as steroid/creatinine ratios: OE/C and P/C.)

After 6 months' treatment with an LHRH agonist, a reduction in fibroid volume by approximately 50% can usually be anticipated; the greatest reduction occurs during the first 3 months with little change thereafter. Bleeding in response to oestrogen withdrawal occurs during the initial treatment cycle but amenorrhoea is usual thereafter (Fig. 28.14). If such treatment is to be used prior to surgery, its optimum duration is around 3–4 months, which should also be sufficient to correct any associated anaemia. Appropriate doses of currently available LHRH agonists include goserelin 3.6 mg by monthly subcutaneous depot injection or intranasal buserelin 900–1200 μg daily, in divided doses. Compliance may be a problem with the nasal spray and as erratic usage may result in stimulation rather than suppression of pituitary-ovarian function, administration by subcutaneous depot is to be preferred.

For women with symptomatic fibroids who are medically unfit for surgery, are known to have extensive pelvic adhesions or who are very obese, long-term therapy with LHRH agonists offers a safer option than surgery. Their use has also been suggested in women who are approaching the age of the natural menopause, where hysterectomy is unlikely to be cost-effective. Opponents of this view argue that this merely hastens the onset of bone loss and may deprive these women of the later benefits of hormone replacement therapy. This decision must rest with the individual woman and her clinician, guided by the severity and chronicity of her symptoms, her age, the size of her uterus and the presence or absence of risk factors for the development of osteoporosis. Some women gain sustained relief of their symptoms following 6 months of treatment with an LHRH agonist, and a single course of therapy with the option of repeat at a later date may give adequate control of symptoms for those who are keen to avoid surgery. In this situation, treatment combinations are currently being investigated with the object of finding an adjunct to LHRH agonists which will protect against bone loss and perhaps augment or prolong regression of the fibroids. Such adjuncts include medroxyprogesterone acetate and low-dose hormone replacement therapy but their efficacy remains to be determined.

Another group of women who would benefit from the use of effective medical therapy are those desirous of pregnancy, particularly those with symptomatic fibroids who wish to delay childbearing and therefore in whom immediate myomectomy may not be desirable. Here short or intermittent courses of an LHRH agonist may successfully control symptoms and delay surgery, preventing further significant enlargement of the fibroids during the period of observation. It is not yet known whether a short course of an LHRH agonist has any beneficial effect in women with fibroids who are immediately desirous of pregnancy. If by virtue of their position small submucous fibroids are a cause of tubal obstruction, relief of this obstruction may lead to pregnancy provided that conception is not delayed.

RESULTS

Assessment of the results of treatment of uterine fibroids must take into consideration the effectiveness of cure of the presenting symptoms, the duration of relief, the need for further treatment, particularly surgery and the morbidity of the treatment method itself. In particular, in those women presenting with infertility or pregnancy loss or where future fertility is desired, the results must be measured in terms of the number and the outcome of any subsequent pregnancies. While hysterectomy gives the best results in terms of symptomatic cure, this will be inappropriate for women wishing to preserve reproductive potential and thus the outcome only of the conservative methods of treatment will be considered here.

Myomectomy

In a comprehensive review of 18 studies, Buttram & Reiter (1981) quoted a 40% conception rate among 1202 women who were desirous of pregnancy. In seven studies of 1941 myomectomies reviewed by the same authors, the spontaneous abortion rate of 19% in 405 pregnancies which followed surgery compared favourably with a rate of 41% in the same women prior to myomectomy. This is still higher than the general population rate. The consensus of opinion favours vaginal delivery rather than elective caesarean section following myomectomy unless the procedure has been very extensive, including opening of the cavity.

Not all women undergoing myomectomy will achieve a pregnancy or even attempt to do so and it is also important to consider the degree and duration of relief of symptoms such as menorrhagia which may have precipitated the decision to perform surgery. Of 285 women in the above-quoted review who complained of heavy menstrual loss, relief was reported in 230 (81%). The recurrence rate of fibroids in these series was 15% for the 2554 women for whom follow-up data were available. Overall 10% of the women required further pelvic surgery — usually hysterectomy — for recurrent or continuing symptoms following myomectomy. These figures justify a conservative approach in selected cases.

Endoscopic methods

There are insufficient published data about the results of endoscopic methods of treatment of uterine fibroids to enable us to reach definite conclusions about their role in current practice. In a review of 371 women treated by hysteroscopic myomectomy for abnormal bleeding, Siegler & Valle (1988) quoted an immediate cure rate of 97% and a recurrence rate of 6%, although duration of follow-up was variable and not specified. Only one patient required a laparotomy for operative complications. This evidence suggests that such methods have a potentially useful role in the management of some women with small fibroids.

LHRH agonists

The impact of LHRH agonists on the overall management of fibroids is also impossible to assess as they are relatively new and their use has until recently been restricted to a few centres. Because of their cost and the risk of premature bone loss, it is clear that they are not a substitute for conventional surgical treatment for the majority of symptomatic women but provide a limited alternative in certain specific situations. Confirmation of their immediate benefit as a preoperative adjunct to surgery is currently under evaluation by controlled clinical trial but longer-term studies are needed to assess their value in preventing postoperative adhesions after myomectomy.

COMPLICATIONS

The complications of uterine fibroids are in part dependent on their site of origin and their size, as discussed on p. 401. For example, torsion is a rare complication of pedunculated subserous fibroids while submucous fibroids may prolapse through the cervix, causing ulceration and infection. Large fibroids arising from the cervix may cause ureteric compression or retention of urine.

Because fibroids are so frequently asymptomatic, especially if small, most of the presenting symptoms described in detail on p. 400 might be regarded as complications rather than an inevitable consequence of their presence, for example menorrhagia, infertility and pregnancy loss. Degenerative changes occur so frequently that they are not usually regarded as a complication, although degeneration occasionally presents with acute pain, particularly in pregnancy. This section will cover the other complications, although they may in most cases be the prime reason for the presentation.

Pregnancy complications

It is usually stated that fibroids increase in size during pregnancy and shrink during the puerperium, although this has not been the finding of recent studies (Aharoni et al 1988) based on serial monitoring by ultrasound (Fig. 28.15). While many pregnancies associated with fibroids proceed uneventfully, there is an increased risk of spontaneous abortion and preterm labour. Pregnancies accompanied by uterine fibroids should therefore be treated as high-risk. These problems may be in part related to abnormalities of uterine contractility and in particular to alterations in blood flow with the fibroids being relatively hypovascular in comparison to the surrounding myometrium. Degenerative changes appear to be very common, in particular the painful red degeneration which is typically associated with pregnancy (Fig. 28.16). Its recognition is important in order to avoid confusion with other acute intra-abdominal conditions and treatment is always conservative, with rest and analgesia. Although rare, torsion of a pedunculated subserous fibroid is more likely to occur in pregnancy and this is the only situation in which removal of a fibroid from the pregnant uterus is ever justified.

Mechanical difficulties due to the site of the fibroids may be encountered during labour and fibroids may be associated with malpresentation of the fetus. If caesarean sec-

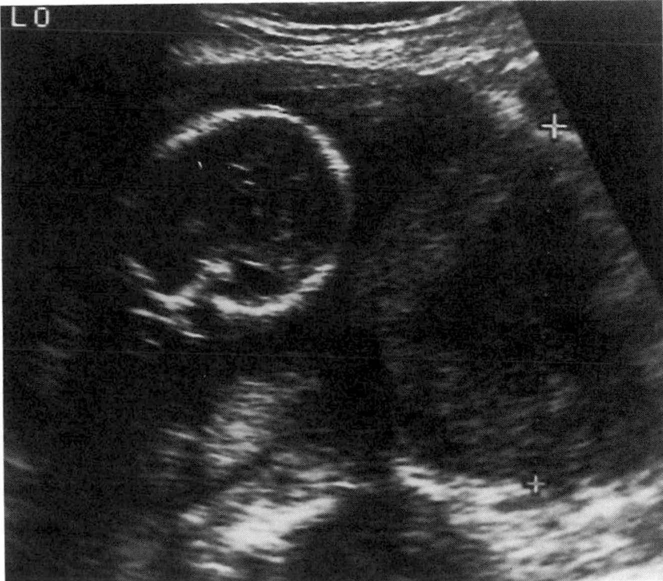

Fig. 28.15 Pregnancy (20 weeks) with lateral fibroid showing degenerative changes. Serial ultrasound measurements showed no change in volume. (Courtesy of Dr B Muir.)

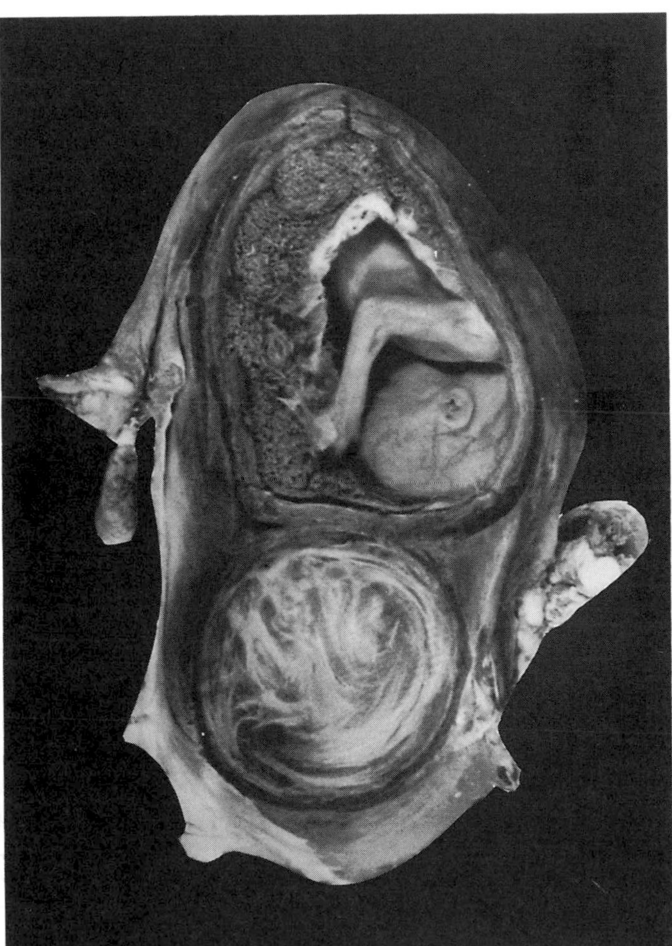

Fig. 28.16 Pregnancy (20 weeks) complicated by painful red degeneration of fibroid (museum specimen.)

tion is required, it is unwise to attempt myomectomy because of the associated vascularity of the procedure. Caesarean hysterectomy may be considered if there are multiple fibroids and the woman has completed her family but the operative morbidity is greatly increased and this procedure would in general be reserved for the emergency situation.

Sarcomatous change

The risk of sarcomatous degeneration is a potentially lethal but uncommon complication of uterine fibroids. Leiomyosarcoma does not inevitably originate in a fibroid uterus and must not be confused with other forms of uterine sarcoma which are totally unrelated to fibroids. Both Corscaden & Singh (1958) and Buttram & Reiter (1981) estimated the risk of sarcomatous change as being in the order of 0.1%, based on the recorded incidence of fibroids in their study populations. Thus, as many cases of fibroids are not diagnosed, even this figure may be an overestimate. Recognition of this complication is nevertheless imperative and among others, Corscaden & Singh emphasize that the majority of cases are symptomatic, with pain, malaise and vaginal bleeding. Rapid enlargement is another suspicious feature and any of these symptoms in a postmenopausal woman should be taken very seriously, particularly as the complication is commoner following the menopause.

Haematological complications

Anaemia secondary to menorrhagia is mentioned above and is more commonly seen in association with fibroids than with menorrhagia due to other causes. In some cases, symptoms of anaemia may be the main presenting feature and the woman may only admit to heavy menstrual blood loss on careful questioning. Paradoxically, fibroids may be associated with polycythaemia and 18 such cases have been described in the literature (see Weiss et al 1975). This is attributed to erythropoietin production by the fibroids and resolves after their surgical removal.

Other unusual complications

Ascites has been described in association with parasitic fibroids which have lost their attachment to the uterus and developed an alternative blood supply from the omentum. This may be related to obstruction of omental blood vessels. Intravenous leiomyomatosis is another rare complication of apparently benign fibroids and metastatic lesions have been described (see Novak & Woodruff 1979). However there is debate about the histological nature of some of these unusual lesions.

KEY POINTS

1. Aetiology is unknown but fibroid growth is thought to be oestrogen dependent.
2. Receptors for both oestrogen and progesterone are present in greater concentrations in fibroids than in the adjacent myometrium but the role of progesterone, if any, is unclear.
3. Incidence in 20% of females of reproductive age. Approximately 50% are asymptomatic, 30–50% present with menorrhagia which can be severe.
4. Factors contributing to menorrhagia may include a mechanical obstruction to venous drainage resulting in congestion and dilatation of venous plexuses; increased total surface area of endometrium; disorders of prostaglandin synthesis and metabolism.
5. The mechanism whereby fibroids affect fertility is unclear (in 30% of women with fibroids, subfertility is a feature).
6. An asymptomatic fibroid uterus is not known to carry any long-term detrimental effects and spontaneous regression after the menopause may be anticipated.
7. Hysteroscopic techniques for removal of submucous fibroids are becoming popular, avoiding major surgery.
8. Medical therapy with GnRH agonists alone is unsuitable for long-term management because of hypo-oestrogenic side effects, and regrowth of fibroids following discontinuation of therapy.
9. Hormone replacement therapy is not contraindicated in postmenopausal women with fibroids.

REFERENCES

Aharoni A, Reiter A, Golan D, Paltiely Y, Sharf M 1988 Patterns of growth of uterine leiomyomas during pregnancy. A prospective longitudinal study. British Journal of Obstetrics and Gynaecology 95: 510–513

Buttram V C, Reiter R C 1981 Uterine leiomyomata: etiology, symptomatology and management. Fertility and Sterility 36: 433–445

Corscaden J A, Singh B P 1958 Leiomyosarcoma of the uterus. American Journal of Obstetrics and Gynecology 75: 149–153

Farrer-Brown G, Beilby J O W, Tarbit M H 1971 Venous changes in the endometrium of myomatous uteri. Obstetrics and Gynecology 38: 743–751

Forssman L 1976 Distribution of blood flow in myomatous uteri as measured by locally injected 133 Xenon. Acta Obstetrica Gynecologica Scandanavica 55: 101–104

Lumsden M A, West C P, Bramley T, Rumgay L, Baird D T 1988 The binding of EGF to the human uterus and leiomyomata in women rendered hypo-oestrogenic by continuous administration of a LHRH agonist. British Journal of Obstetrics and Gynaecology 95: 1299–1304

Maheux R, Lemay-Turcot L, Lemay A 1986 Daily follicle-stimulating hormone, luteinizing hormone, estradiol and progesterone in 10 women harboring uterine leiomyomas. Fertility and Sterility 46: 205–208

Miller N F, Ludovici P P 1955 On the origin and development of uterine fibroids. American Journal of Obstetrics and Gynecology 70: 720–739

Monaghan J M (ed) 1988 Bonney's gynaecological surgery, 9th edn. Baillière Tindall, London

Novak E R, Woodruff J D 1979 Myoma and other benign tumors of the uterus. In: Novak's gynecological and obstetric pathology, 8th edn. W B Saunders, Philadelphia, pp. 260–279

Ross R K, Pike M C, Vessey M P, Bull D, Yeates D, Casagrande J T 1986 Risk factors for uterine fibroids: reduced risk associated with oral contraceptives. British Medical Journal 293: 359–362

Rybo G, Leman J, Tibblin R 1985 Epidemiology of menstrual blood loss. In: Baird D T, Michie E A (eds) Mechanisms of menstrual bleeding. Raven Press, New York, pp. 181–193

Siegler A M, Valle R F 1988 Therapeutic hysteroscopic procedures. Fertility and Sterility 50: 685–701

Weiss D B, Aldor A, Aboulafia Y 1975 Erythrocytosis due to erythropoietin-producing uterine fibromyoma. American Journal of Obstetrics and Gynecology 122: 358–360

West C P 1988 LHRH analogues in the management of uterine fibroids, premenstrual syndrome and breast malignancies. Baillière's Clinical Obstetrics and Gynaecology 2: 689–709

West C P, Lumsden M A 1989 Fibroids and menorrhagia. Baillière's Clinical Obstetrics and Gynaecology 3: in press

Wilson E A, Yang F, Rees E D 1980 Estradiol and progesterone binding in uterine leiomyomata and in normal uterine tissues. Obstetrics and Gynaecology 55: 20–24

Witherspoon J T 1935 The hormonal origin of uterine fibroids: an hypothesis. American Journal of Cancer 24: 402–406

29. Benign tumours of the ovary

W. P. Soutter

Benign tumours of the ovary are common, frequently asymptomatic and often resolve spontaneously. The major concern is to exclude malignancy without causing undue morbidity or impairing future fertility in younger women.

PATHOLOGY (Table 29.1)

Physiological cysts

Physiological cysts are simply large versions of the cysts which form in the ovary during the normal ovarian cycle. They are often found incidentally as a result of pelvic examination or ultrasound scanning. Although they may occur in any premenopausal woman, they are most common in young women. They are an occasional complication of ovulation induction.

Table 29.1 Pathology of benign ovarian tumours

Physiological cysts
Follicular cysts
Luteal cysts
Benign germ cell tumours
Dermoid cyst
Mature teratoma
Benign epithelial tumours
Serous cystadenoma
Mucinous cystadenoma
Endometrioid cystadenoma
Brenner
Benign sex cord stromal tumours
Granulosa cell tumour
Theca cell tumour
Fibroma
Sertoli–Leydig cell tumour

Follicular cyst

Lined by granulosa cells, this is the commonest benign ovarian tumour and is most often found incidentally. A follicular cyst can persist for several menstrual cycles and may achieve a diameter of up to 10 cm. Smaller cysts are more likely to resolve but may require intervention if symptoms develop or if they do not resolve after 8–12 weeks.

Luteal cyst

Less common than follicular cysts, these are more likely to present as a result of intraperitoneal bleeding.

Benign germ cell tumours

Germ cell tumours are among the commonest ovarian tumours seen in women less than 30 years of age. Overall, only 2–3% are malignant but in the under-20s this proportion rises to a third. Malignant tumours are usually solid.

Dermoid cyst (mature cystic teratoma)

The benign dermoid cyst is the only common benign germ cell tumour. It is most common in young women and is bilateral in about 12% of cases. These are usually unilocular cysts less than 15 cm in diameter, lined with epithelium like the epidermis and containing skin appendages and a variety of other tissues including fat, smooth muscle, bone, nervous tissue, respiratory epithelium and apocrine glands among others. They contain sebaceous material and hair.

The cysts are particularly prone to torsion. They may present with rupture or infection. During pregnancy, rupture is more common and may result in a slow leak of fluid into the peritoneal cavity and peritonitis. About 2% contain a malignant component, usually a squamous carcinoma. Most of the cysts occur in women over 40 years old.

Mature solid teratoma

These rare tumours contain mature tissues just like the dermoid cyst, but there are few cystic areas. They must be differentiated from immature teratomas which are malignant (see Chapter 37).

Benign epithelial tumours

The majority of ovarian neoplasia, both benign and malignant, are epithelial in origin. Although benign tumours tend to occur at a slightly younger age than their malignant counterparts, they are most common in women over 40 years.

Serous cystadenoma

This is the most common benign epithelial tumour and is bilateral in about 10%. It is usually a unilocular cyst with papilliferous processes on the inner surface. The epithelium on the inner surface is cuboidal or columnar and may be ciliated. The cyst fluid is thin and serous. They are seldom as large as mucinous tumours.

Mucinous cystadenoma

These constitute 15–25% of all ovarian tumours. They are typically large, unilateral, multilocular cysts with a smooth inner surface. A recent specimen at Hammersmith Hospital weighed over 14 kg! The lining epithelium consists of columnar mucus-secreting cells. The cyst fluid is generally thick and glutinous. It may rarely be complicated by pseudomyxoma peritonei which is more often present before the cyst is removed rather than following intraoperative rupture.

Endometrioid cystadenoma

Most of these tumours are malignant as benign endometrioid cysts are difficult to differentiate from endometriosis.

Brenner

These account for only 1–2% of all ovarian tumours. They probably arise from the surface epithelium. The tumour consists of nests of transitional epithelium in a dense fibrotic stroma. The vast majority are benign, but borderline or malignant specimens have been reported. Almost three-quarters present over the age of 40 and about half are incidental findings, being recognized only by the pathologist. Although some can be large the majority are less than 2 cm in diameter. Some secrete oestrogens.

Benign sex cord stromal tumours

Sex cord stromal tumours represent only 6% of ovarian tumours. They occur at any age from prepubertal children to elderly, postmenopausal women. Many of these tumours secrete hormones and present with the results of inappropriate hormone effects.

Granulosa cell tumours

Most of these are malignant but grow very slowly. Not all produce oestrogens.

Theca cell tumours

Almost all are benign and unilateral. Many produce oestrogens in sufficient quantity to have systemic effects such as precocious puberty, postmenopausal bleeding, endometrial hyperplasia and endometrial cancer. They rarely cause ascites or Meig's syndrome.

Fibroma

These unusual tumours are most frequent around 50 years of age. Most are derived from stromal cells and are similar to thecomas. They are hard, mobile and lobulated with a glistening white surface. Less than 10% are bilateral. While ascites occurs with many of the larger fibromas, Meig's syndrome — ascites and pleural effusion in association with a fibroma of the ovary — is seen in only 1% of cases.

Sertoli–Leydig cell tumours

These are usually of low-grade malignancy. Most are found around 30 years of age. They are rare, being less than 0.2%

of ovarian tumours. They are often difficult to distinguish from other ovarian tumours because of the variety of cells and architecture seen. Many produce androgens and signs of virilization are seen in three-quarters of patients. Some secrete oestrogens. They are usually small and unilateral.

PRESENTATION

Presentation of benign ovarian tumours is as follows:

1. Asymptomatic.
2. Pain.
3. Abdominal swelling.
4. Pressure effects.
5. Menstrual disturbances.
6. Abnormal cervical smear.
7. Hormonal effects.

Asymptomatic

Many benign ovarian tumours are found incidentally in the course of investigating another unrelated problem or during a routine examination while performing a cervical smear or at an antenatal clinic. As pelvic ultrasound is now used more frequently, physiological cysts are detected more often. Where ultrasound was used in trials of screening for ovarian cancer, the majority of tumours detected were benign. Many simple cysts will resolve spontaneously if observed over a period of 2–3 months. Unfortunately it is not possible with ultrasound to differentiate reliably between benign and malignant ovarian disease, especially when the tumour is small (Campbell et al 1989).

Pain

Acute pain from an ovarian tumour may result from torsion, rupture, haemorrhage or infection. Torsion usually gives rise to a sharp, constant pain caused by ischaemia of the cyst. Areas may become infarcted. Haemorrhage may occur into the cyst and cause pain as the capsule is stretched. If the cyst is large, the bleeding may be sufficient to give rise to a haemolytic jaundice so leading the unwary to diagnose malignancy wrongly. Intraperitoneal bleeding mimicking ectopic pregnancy may result from rupture of the tumour. This happens most frequently with a luteal cyst. Chronic lower abdominal pain sometimes results from the pressure of a benign ovarian tumour but is more common if endometriosis or infection is present.

Abdominal swelling

Patients seldom note abdominal swelling until the tumour is very large. A benign mucinous cyst may occasionally fill the entire abdominal cavity. The bloating of which women complain so often is seldom due to an ovarian tumour.

Miscellaneous

Gastrointestinal or urinary symptoms may result from pressure effects. In extreme cases, oedema of the legs, varicose veins and haemorrhoids may result. Sometimes, uterine prolapse is the presenting complaint in a woman with an ovarian cyst.

Occasionally the patient will complain of menstrual disturbances but this may be coincidence rather than due to the tumour. Rarely, sex cord stromal tumours present with oestrogen effects such as precocious puberty, menorrhagia and glandular hyperplasia, breast enlargement and postmenopausal bleeding. Secretion of androgens may cause hirsutism and acne initially, progressing to frank virilism with deepening of the voice or clitoral hypertrophy. Very rarely indeed thyrotoxicosis may occur.

Infrequently, a patient with an abnormal cervical smear will be found to have an ovarian tumour and removal is followed by resolution of the cytologic abnormality. Surprisingly, these are often benign tumours.

DIFFERENTIAL DIAGNOSIS

The differential diagnosis of benign ovarian tumours is as follows:

1. Full bladder.
2. Pregnant uterus.
3. Ectopic pregnancy.
4. Pelvic inflammatory disease.
5. Appendicitis.
6. Fibroids.
7. Ovarian malignancy.
8. Rectal malignancy.
9. Diverticulosis.

A full bladder should be considered in the differential diagnosis of any pelvic mass. In premenopausal women, a gravid uterus must always be considered. Fibroids can be impossible to distinguish from ovarian tumours. Rarely, a fimbrial cyst may grow sufficiently to cause anxiety.

Ectopic pregnancy may present as a pelvic mass and lower abdominal pain, especially if there has been chronic intraperitoneal bleeding. Often a ruptured, bleeding corpus luteum will be mistaken for an ectopic gestation. It is often difficult to differentiate between appendicitis and an ovarian cyst. Co-operation between gynaecologist and surgeon is essential to avoid unnecessary surgery on simple ovarian cysts in young women and the effects this may have upon subsequent fertility. Pelvic inflammatory disease may give rise to a mass of adherent bowel, a hydrosalpinx or pyosalpinx.

If the tumour is ovarian, malignancy must be excluded. In the vast majority of cases this can only be done by a laparotomy. Even then, careful histological examination may be necessary to exclude invasion. Frozen section will only rarely be of value. A pelvic mass may also be caused by a rectal tumour or diverticulitis. Hodgkin's disease may present as a pelvic mass with enlarged pelvic lymph nodes.

INVESTIGATION

The investigations required will depend upon the circumstances of the presentation. The patient presenting with acute symptoms will usually require emergency surgery whereas the asymptomatic patient or the woman with chronic problems may benefit from more detailed preliminary assessment.

Gynaecological history

Details of the presenting symptoms and a full gynaecological history should be obtained with particular reference to the date of the last menstrual period, the regularity of the menstrual cycle, any previous pregnancies, contraception and medication.

General history and examination

Indigestion or dysphagia might indicate a primary gastric cancer metastasizing to the pelvis. Similarly, a history of altered bowel habit or rectal bleeding should be sought as evidence of diverticulitis or rectal carcinoma.

If the patient has presented as an acute emergency, evidence of hypovolaemia should be sought. Hypotension is a relatively late sign of blood loss as the blood pressure will be maintained for some time by peripheral and central venous vasoconstriction. When decompensation of this mechanism occurs, it often does so very rapidly. It is vital to recognize the early signs — cold legs and tachycardia.

The breasts should be palpated and evidence of lymphadenopathy sought in the neck, the axillae and the groins. The chest should be examined for evidence of a pleural effusion. Some patients may have ankle oedema. Very occasionally foot drop may be noted as a result of compression of pelvic nerve roots. This would not occur with a benign tumour but suggests a malignancy with lymphatic involvement.

Abdominal examination

The abdomen should be inspected for signs of distension by fluid or by the tumour itself. Dilated veins may be seen on the lower abdomen. Gentle palpation will reveal areas of tenderness and peritonism may be elicited by asking the patient to cough or alternately suck in and blow out her abdominal wall.

The best way of detecting a mass that arises from the pelvis is to palpate gently with the radial border of the left hand, starting in the upper abdomen and working caudally. This is the reverse of the process taught to every medical student for feeling the liver edge. Use of the right hand alone is the commonest reason for failing to detect pelviabdominal masses.

Shifting dullness is probably the easiest way of demonstrating ascites but it remains a very insensitive technique. It is always worth listening for bowel sounds in any patient with an acute abdomen. Their complete absence in the presence of peritonism is an ominous sign.

Bimanual examination

This is an essential component of the assessment because, even in expert hands, ultrasound examination is not infallible. By palpating the mass between both the vaginal and abdominal hands its mobility, texture and consistency, the presence of nodules in the pouch of Douglas and the degree of tenderness can all be determined (Fig. 29.1). While it is impossible to make a firm diagnosis with bimanual examination, a hard, irregular, fixed mass is likely to be invasive.

Ultrasound

The techniques of ultrasound are discussed in detail in Chapter 5. It can demonstrate the presence of an ovarian

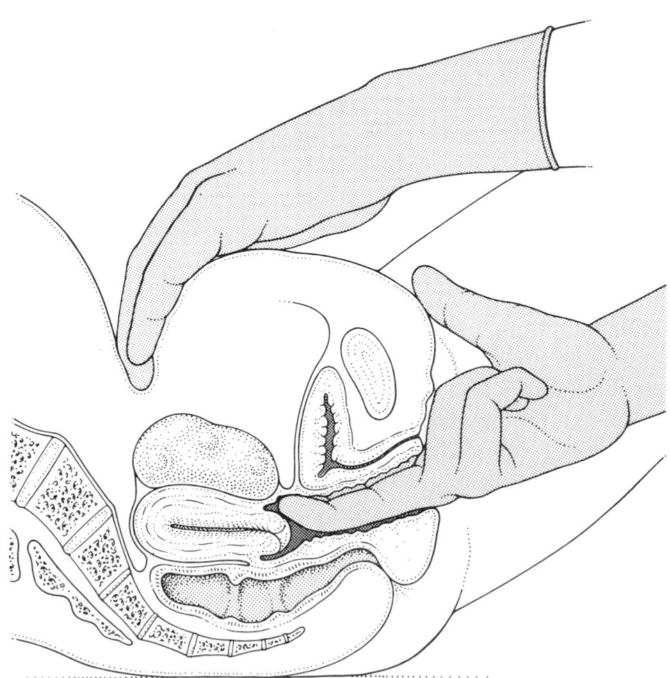

Fig. 29.1 Bimanual examination involves palpating the pelvic organs between both hands.

mass with reasonable sensitivity and fair specificity and although it cannot distinguish reliably between benign and malignant tumours, solid ovarian masses are likely to be malignant. Neither computerized tomography scanning nor magnetic resonance imaging has significant advantages over ultrasound in this situation and both are more expensive.

Radiological investigations

A chest X-ray is essential to seek metastatic disease in the lungs. An intravenous urogram is often performed but is seldom useful. A barium enema is indicated only if the mass is irregular or fixed, or if there are bowel symptoms. A computerized tomography scan is seldom indicated.

Blood test and serum markers

It is always sensible to measure the haemoglobin and an elevated white cell count would suggest infection. Blood may be cross-matched if necessary.

Serum markers have yet to establish a role in the routine management of most ovarian tumours (see Ch. 37). However, a raised serum CA 125 is strongly suggestive of ovarian carcinoma. Women with extensive endometriosis may also have elevated levels but the concentration is usually not as high as is seen with invasive disease. The beta-human chorionic gonadotrophin concentration might be measured to exclude an ectopic pregnancy but trophoblastic tumours and some germ cell tumours secrete this marker.

MANAGEMENT

The management will depend upon the severity of the symptoms; the age of the patient and therefore the risk of malignancy; and her desire for further children.

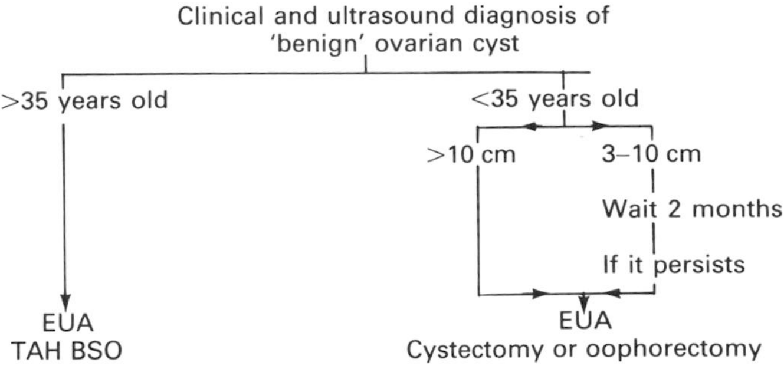

Fig. 29.2 Management of what appears on clinical and ultrasound grounds to be a benign ovarian cyst in an asymptomatic patient. EUA = examination under anaesthesia; TAH BSO = total abdominal hysterectomy and bilateral salpingo oophorectomy in 1981

The asymptomatic patient (Fig. 29.2)

The older woman

Women over 50 years of age are far more likely to have a malignancy (Fig. 29.3) and have little to gain from the conservative management of a definite pelvic mass more than 5 cm in diameter (Rulin & Preston 1987). Even in cases of lesser degrees of ovarian enlargement, malignancy can occur and most are due to benign tumours which should probably be removed.

Premenopausal women

Young women less than 35 years are both more likely to wish to have the option of further children and less likely to have a malignant epithelial tumour. However, ovarian cysts more than 10 cm in diameter are unlikely to be physiological or to resolve spontaneously. A normal follicular cyst may reach 3 cm in diameter and requires no further investigation. A clear unilocular cyst of 4–10 cm identified by ultrasound may be re-examined 8 weeks later for evidence of diminution in size. Resolution of the cyst may be enhanced by use of a combined oral contraceptive. If the cyst

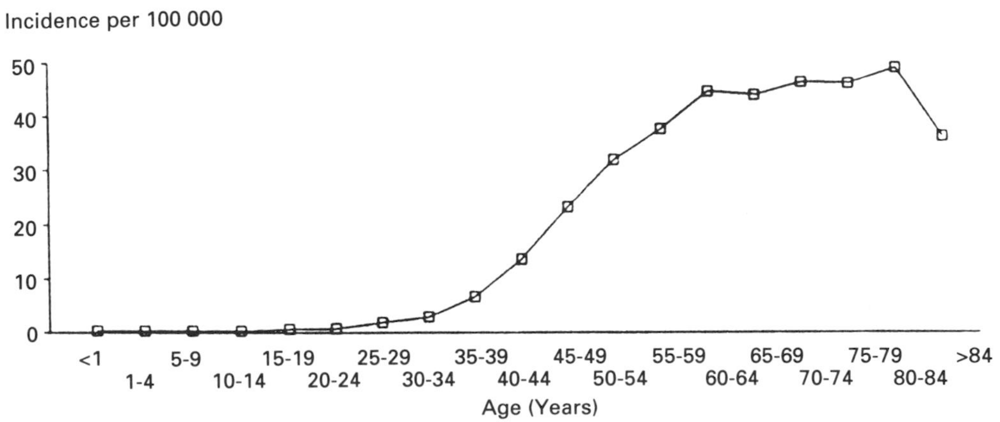

Fig. 29.3 The incidence of ovarian cancer in England and Wales (Office of Population Censuses and Surveys 1985). Note how uncommon ovarian cancer is before the age of 35 years.

does not get smaller, laparoscopy or laparotomy will be indicated.

The role of ultrasound-guided aspiration of unilocular cysts less than 10 cm in diameter remains controversial (De Crespigny et al 1989). A tumour in a young woman that appears to be largely solid on ultrasound is likely to be a germ cell tumour or a malignant teratoma and requires removal.

The indications for observation of an ovarian tumour are given below:

1. Premenopausal woman.
2. Age less than 35 years.
3. Unilateral tumour.
4. Unilocular cyst.
5. Tumour 3–10 cm in diameter.

The patient with symptoms

If the patient presents with severe, acute pain or signs of intraperitoneal bleeding an emergency laparoscopy or laparotomy will be required. More chronic symptoms of pain or pressure may justify pelvic ultrasound if no mass can be felt but ultrasound is unlikely to contribute to the investigation of a woman in whom both ovaries can be clearly felt to be of a normal size.

The pregnant patient

An ovarian cyst in a pregnant woman may undergo torsion or may bleed. Very occasionally, it can prevent the presenting fetal part from engaging. A dermoid cyst may rupture or leak slowly, causing peritonitis. However, an ovarian cyst is usually discovered incidentally at the antenatal clinic.

The pregnant woman with an ovarian cyst is a special case because of the dangers to the fetus of surgery. These have probably been exaggerated in the past and no urgent operation should be postponed solely because of a pregnancy. Thus, if the patient presents with acute pain due to torsion or haemorrhage into an ovarian tumour or if appendicitis is a possibility, the correct course is to undertake a laparotomy regardless of the stage of the pregnancy. However, if an asymptomatic cyst is discovered it is prudent to wait until after 14 weeks' gestation before removing it. This avoids the risk of removing a corpus luteal cyst upon which the pregnancy might still be dependent at an earlier stage.

SURGERY

Examination under anaesthesia

Prior to any laparoscopy or laparotomy for a suspected ovarian tumour, it is prudent to perform a bimanual examination under anaesthesia to confirm the presence of the mass.

Laparoscopy

The indications for laparoscopy are given below:

1. Uncertainty about the nature of the mass.
2. Tumour suitable for laparoscopic surgery.
   a. Age less than 35 years.
   b. Ultrasound shows no solid component.
   c. Simple ovarian cyst.
   d. Endometrioma.
   e. Benign cystic teratoma.

Laparoscopy may be of value if there is uncertainty about the nature of the pelvic mass. Thus it may be possible to avoid a laparotomy when there is no pathology. However, it can be difficult to exclude ovarian disease in the presence of marked pelvic inflammatory disease.

The second indication for laparoscopy is if the patient has a cyst suitable for laparoscopic surgery (Nezhat et al 1989). This applies only to women under 40 years of age (probably under 35 years) in whom the likelihood of malignant disease is very small. The surgery may be performed with scissors and electrocautery but the carbon dioxide laser does offer some advantages. These operations require considerable expertise in laparoscopic manipulation and should not be attempted without appropriate training.

Laparotomy

A clinical diagnosis may not be possible without a laparotomy and even then histological examination is essential for a confident conclusion. Frozen section is seldom of value in this situation as a thorough examination of a tumour is required to exclude invasive disease.

It is essential to explore the whole abdomen thoroughly and to inspect *both* ovaries. If there is any possibility of invasive disease, a longitudinal incision should be used to allow adequate exposure in the upper abdomen. If wider exposure is required after making a transverse incision, the ends of the wound can be extended cranially to fashion a flap from the upper edge of the wound (Fig. 29.4). A sample of ascitic fluid or peritoneal washings should be sent for cytological examination.

In a young women less than 35 years of age an ovarian tumour is very unlikely to be malignant. Even if the mass is a primary ovarian carcinoma it will almost certainly be a germ cell tumour which is responsive to chemotherapy. Thus, ovarian cystectomy or unilateral oophorectomy are sensible and safe treatments for unilateral ovarian masses in this age group (Bianchi et al 1989). It is often said that the contralateral ovary should be bisected and a sample sent for histology in case the tumour is malignant. In practice, most gynaecologists would be unwilling to biopsy an

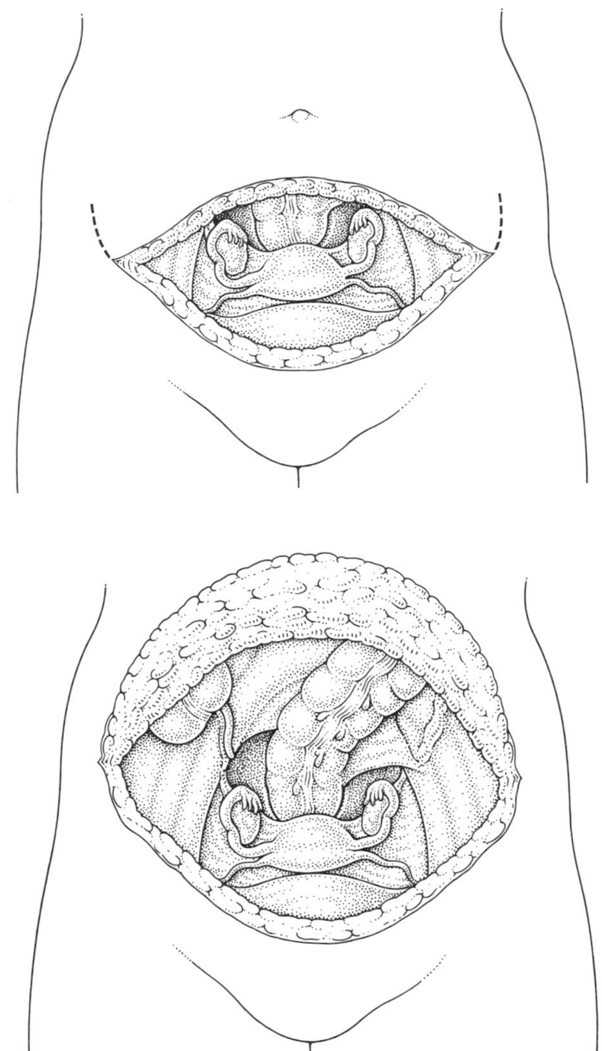

Fig. 29.4 A transverse wound may be enlarged by extending the ends cranially to create a flap from the upper edge.

apparently healthy ovary lest this result in infertility from periovarian adhesions. This would be especially true if the tumour was thin-walled and cystic but even apparently solid tumours may be benign. Bilateral dysgerminomas are not common even allowing for microscopic disease in an apparently normal ovary. Even when the lesion is bilateral, every effort should be made to conserve ovarian tissue. This policy is made possible by the effectiveness of modern chemotherapy for germ cell tumours and is discussed further in Chapter 37.

Because epithelial cancer is so much more likely in a woman over the age of 44 years with a unilateral ovarian mass, she is probably best advised to have a total abdominal hysterectomy, bilateral salpingo-oophorectomy and infracolic omentectomy. However, there is evidence to suggest that unilateral oophorectomy in selected cases of epithelial carcinoma confined to one ovary may give equally good results as the traditional radical approach (Mangioni et al 1989). It would seem reasonable to individualize treatment of women 35–44 years of age where there are greater benefits to the patient from a conservative approach and where the risks may well be less. If conservative surgery is planned, preliminary hysteroscopy and curettage of the uterus are essential to exclude a concomitant endometrial tumour, a thorough laparotomy is especially important and an appropriate plan of action must decided in advance with the patient should more widespread disease be found.

KEY POINTS

1. Asymptomatic, benign ovarian cysts in young women often resolve spontaneously.
2. Ultrasound cannot reliably exclude malignancy.
3. Ovarian cysts are very rarely malignant before the age of 35, especially when less than 10 cm in diameter.
4. Solid ovarian tumours are often malignant — in young women these are usually germ cell or sex cord stromal tumours.
5. Conservative management is appropriate for most young women:
   a. Observation of cystic lesions <10 cm;
   b. Unilateral oophorectomy even of solid lesions.
6. Women over 45 years of age with a unilocular ovarian cyst greater than 5 cm or with any other type of ovarian tumour should usually be advised to have a total abdominal hysterectomy and bilateral salpingo-oophorectomy.
7. A bimanual examination under anaesthesia should be performed prior to any surgery for ovarian tumours to confirm that a mass is still palpable.

REFERENCES

Bianchi U A, Favalli G, Sartori E et al 1989 Limited surgery in non-epithelial ovarian cancer. In: Conte P F, Ragni N, Rosso R, Vermorken J B (eds) Multimodal treatment of ovarian cancer. Raven Press, New York, pp 119–126

Campbell S, Bhan V, Royston P, Whitehead M I, Collins W P 1989 Transabdominal ultrasound screening for early ovarian cancer. British Medical Journal 299: 1363–1367

De Crespigny L C, Robinson H P, Davoren R A, Fortune D 1989 The 'simple' ovarian cyst: aspirate or operate? British Journal of Obstetrics and Gynaecology 96: 1035–1039

Mangioni C, Chiari S, Colombo N et al 1989 Limited surgery in epithelial ovarian cancer. In: Conte P F, Ragni N, Rosso R, Vermorken J B (eds) Multimodal treatment of ovarian cancer. Raven Press, New York, pp 127–132

Nezhat C, Winer W K, Nezhat F 1989 Laparoscopic removal of dermoid cysts. Obstetrics and Gynecology 73: 278–281

Office of Population Censuses and Surveys 1985 Cancer statistics — registration 1981 HMSO, London

Rulin M C, Preston A L 1987 Adnexal masses in postmenopausal women. Obstetrics and Gynecology 70: 578–581

30. Endometriosis

R. W. Shaw

INTRODUCTION

Endometriosis is one of the commonest benign gynaecological conditions. It has been estimated that it is present in between 10 and 25% of women presenting with gynaecological symptoms in the UK and the USA (Tyson 1974). These figures are based on the findings of patients who have undergone laparoscopy for diagnostic indications, e.g. pelvic pain or infertility, or patients undergoing laparotomy. Though it is such a widespread condition much is still poorly understood with regard to its aetiology and pathogenesis and the condition still arouses much interest and controversy.

Definition

Endometriosis may be defined as the finding of tissue outside the uterus that is histologically similar to that of endometrium. Endometrial tissue deep within the myometrium, a condition termed adenomyosis, is a separate pathological entity affecting a different population and with a probable different aetiology.

Prevalence

Continued growth of endometriotic tissue, as with that of the endometrium, is dependent upon oestrogen, thus endometriosis is prevalent in the reproductive years with a peak incidence between 30 and 45 years of age, although it can be found in much younger women. There have been published reports of endometriosis in postmenopausal women where it has been reactivated because of hormone replacement therapy or endogenous sex hormones produced by the ovarian stroma. The apparent increase in this disorder in recent decades stems from more widespread use of laparoscopy in gynaecological practice, particularly in infertile women, in whom the disorder may otherwise be asymptomatic, or for the investigation of pelvic pain.

Endometriosis commonly affects women during their child-bearing years. In the main this is reflected in deleterious sexual, reproductive and social consequences as a result of its associated painful symptoms and infertility. This may extend over several decades of a patient's life, because of its often late diagnosis and its recurrent nature.

PATHOGENESIS AND PATHOPHYSIOLOGY

Endometriosis can be accurately diagnosed by careful visual inspection of the pelvis. Histological confirmation is not mandatory for clinical decision-making but it is helpful if there is uncertainty about the diagnosis, and possibly where there is recurrent disease.

Histology

To make the diagnosis of endometriosis categorically, pathologists require the presence of glands, stroma and evidence of menstrual cyclicity, i.e. tissue, haemorrhage or haemosiderin-laden macrophages. The endometriotic deposits rarely have the identical microscopic appearance or architecture to normal endometrium in situ however. Implants can be composed of isolated scattered glandular and stromal components (Fig. 30.1) rather than exact replication of intrauterine endometrial architecture (Fig. 30.2).

Peritoneal deposits

The morphological characteristics of peritoneal endometriosis are quite varied. The lesion is considered active when there is typical glandular epithelium and active proliferation, or if in the latter part of the menstrual cycle there is some secretory change. Some deposits have areas of oviduct-like epithelium with ciliated cells in association with endometriotic foci. Brown or black coloration of deposits is a function of the amounts of intraluminal debris and haemosiderin. The black pigmented stigmas compose the usual visual criteria for diagnosis of endometriosis and are the late consequence of this cyclical growth and regression of the lesions to the point where tissue bleeding and discoloration by blood pigment have taken place. An ideal environment for implantation and endometrial growth is the ovary because of increased levels of gonadal steroids compared with that of the general circulation. Superficial implants of endometriosis in the ovary resemble implants at other peritoneal sites (Fig. 30.3), however in contrast the texture and structure of large endometrial cysts or endometrial cells which have entered the ovarian stroma are quite different (Fig. 30.4).

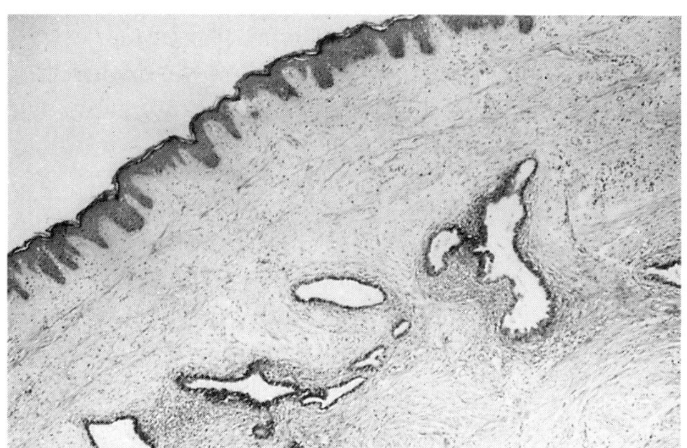

Fig. 30.1 Biopsy of deposit of endometriosis in anterior abdominal wall showing glandular elements beneath the skin (× 40). From Shaw & Marshall (1989) with permission.

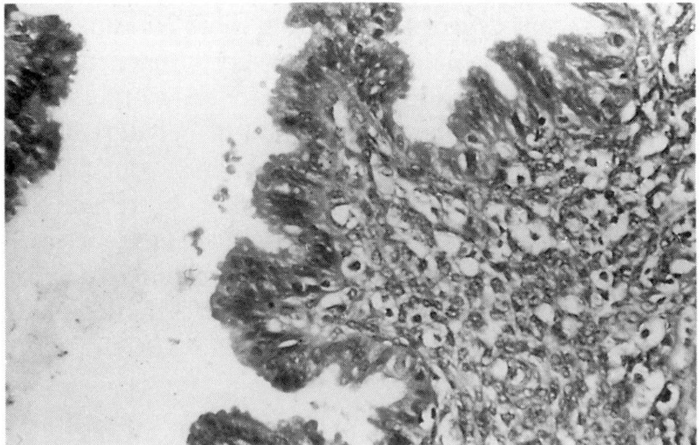

Fig. 30.2 High-power picture of biopsy from endometrial deposit demonstrating glandular structure and macrophages with lipid and haemosiderin accumulation (× 100). From Shaw & Marshall (1989) with permission.

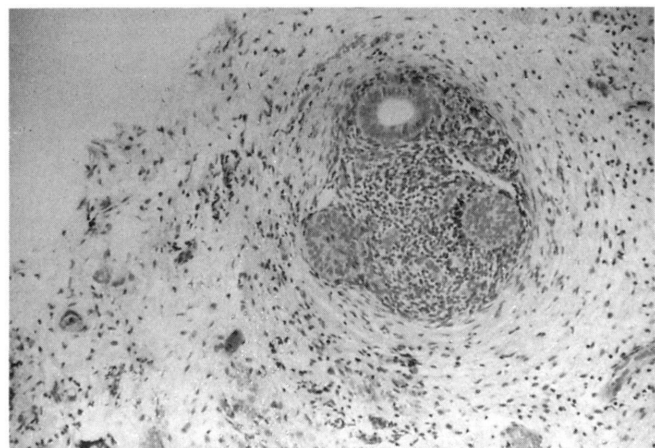

Fig. 30.3 Active endometriosis with glandular and stromal components in a biopsy specimen from a lesion on the uterosacral ligament.

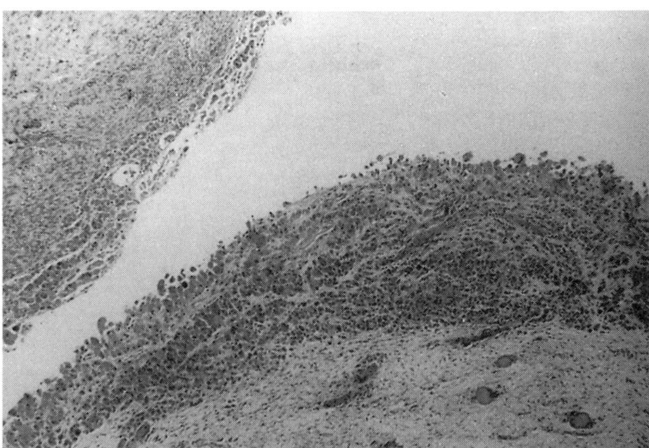

Fig. 30.4 Wall of an endometrial chocolate cyst with extensive fibrosis and haemorrhage but no recognizable endometrial glands or stroma.

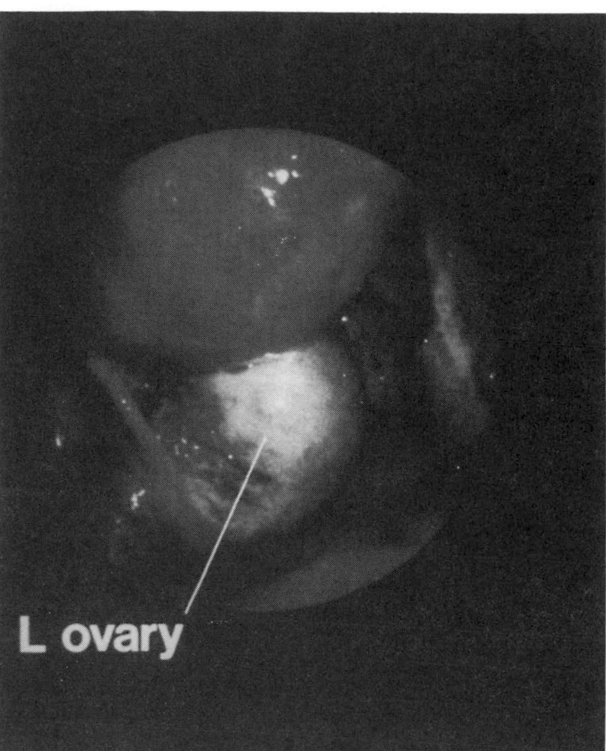

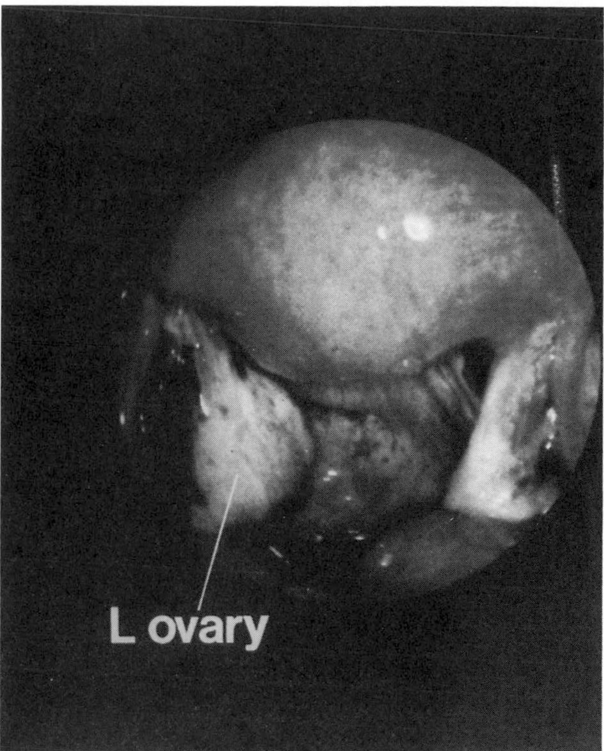

Fig. 30.5 Enlarged left ovary containing a deep-seated endometrioma (**left**) and another ovary with superficial deposits on ovarian capsule (both ovaries) in addition to others on the peritoneal surface in the pouch of Douglas (**right**).

Endometriomas

Endometrial cysts (endometriomas) are often termed 'chocolate cysts' and are filled with a viscous chocolate-coloured liquid, representing debris from cyclical menstruation. Such cysts usually have a well demarcated separation between the cyst wall and the normal adjacent ovarian stroma (Fig. 30.5). The epithelial lining of the endometrioma may resemble the endometrium, but with continual menstrual bleeding without drainage the epithelium becomes flattened and cuboidal without specific distinguishing features, perhaps due to pressure atrophy (Fig. 30.6).

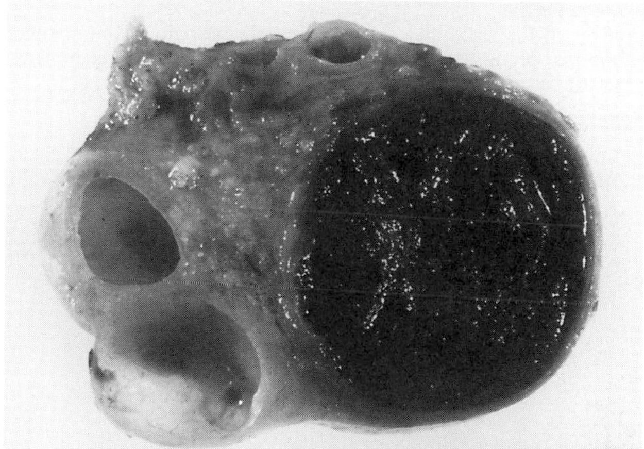

Fig. 30.6 Classical chocolate cyst of ovary (endometrioma) in an ovary containing two other fibrotic walled smaller cysts previously filled with 'chocolate' material prior to section.

Ultrastructure

Endometrial implants do not demonstrate the characteristic ultrastructural changes of the normal endometrium, although the microscopic changes present in endometrium have been observed in ectopic implants. In some individuals there is no evidence of secretory change in deposits; even when these do develop they may not be synchronous with those of the uterine endometrium (Fig. 30.7). The reasons for this probably relate to a deficiency of steroid receptors within the endometriotic tissue and the influence of surrounding scar tissue formation, pressure atrophy and the hormonal independence of the ectopic endometrial glands.

AETIOLOGY

The precise aetiology of endometriosis still remains unknown. Indeed it is often called the 'disease of theories' because of the many postulated mechanisms utilized to explain its pathogenesis (Fig. 30.8). It is likely that no one of these theories would explain all forms of endometriosis.

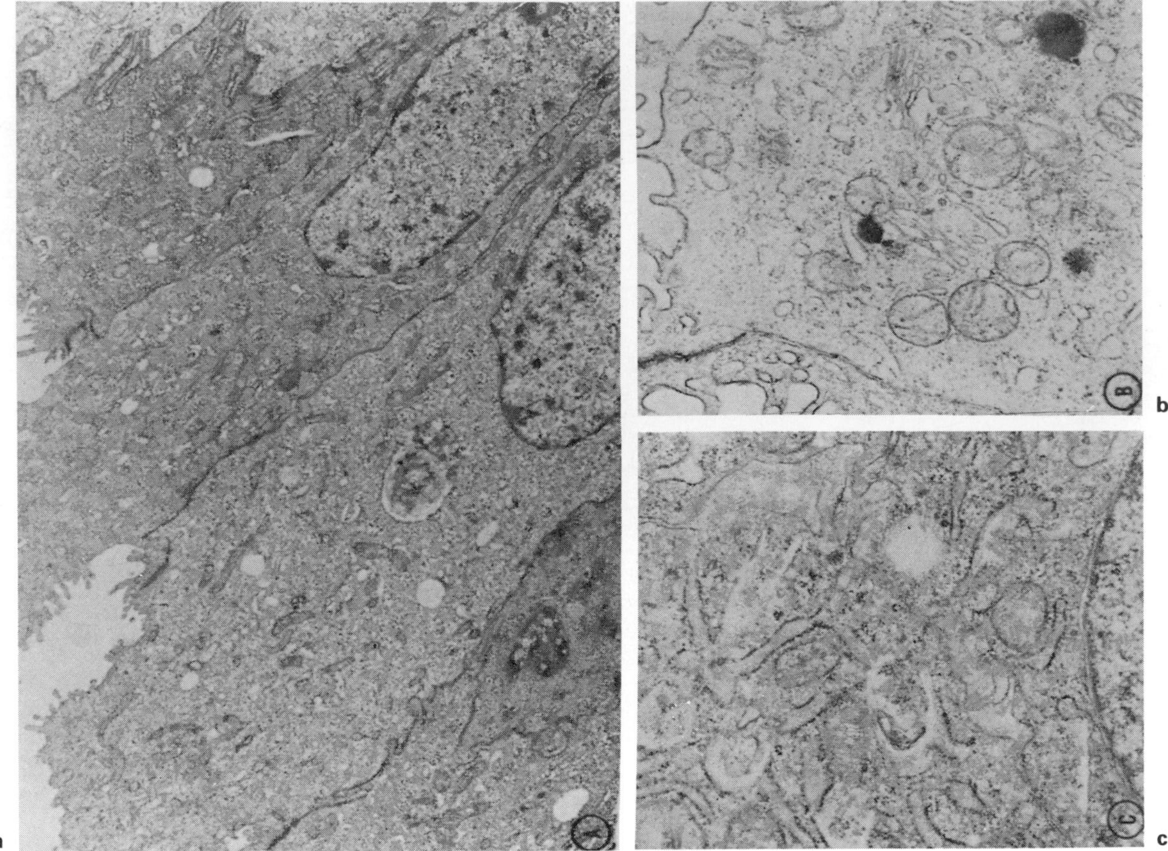

Fig. 30.7 (a) Electron micrograph of an endometrial implant obtained during the early secretory phase of the menstural cycle. (b) Well developed mitochondria, prominent Golgi apparatus and (c) abundant endoplasmic reticulum are apparent in the higher-power views. From Schweppe et al (1984) with permission.

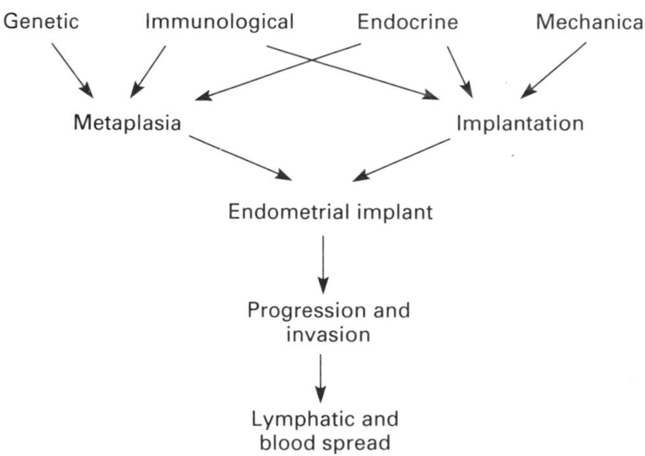

Fig. 30.8 Suggested aetiological factors in the pathogenesis of endometriotic implants.

Retrograde menstruation and implantation

Sampson in a series of publications proposed a theory of retrograde menstruation for the development of endometriosis (Sampson 1927a). This theory suggested that the resultant menstrual regurgitation of menstrual fluid contained some endometrial cells of both stromal and glandular elements, which are deposited on the peritoneal surface of the pelvis during menstruation. In support ot this theory experimental endometriosis has been induced in animals with the replacement of menstrual fluid or endometrial tissue in the peritoneal cavity. In young girls endometriosis has been described associated with abnormalities in the genital tract causing obstruction to the outflow of menstrual fluid (Schifrin et al 1973). However, at laparoscopy, performed during the perimenstrual period, it is not uncommon to find retrograde menstrual fluid within the pelvis in a high percentage of patients (Halme et al 1984). Since this process of retrograde menstruation is quite common then some other mechanism, which may be immunological, may account for the subsequent development of endometriosis in susceptible individuals.

Lymphatic and haematogenous dissemination

Benign vascular and lymphatic embolization to distant sites

outside the peritoneal cavity has been postulated (Sampson 1927b) and indeed endometriotic tissue has been found within lymphatic channels, lymph nodes and pelvic veins, supporting this possible theory. This would explain the finding of endometriosis in such sites as the lung, kidney, joints and skin.

Transformation of coelomic epithelium

This theory, first described by Meyer (1919), postulated the possibility of differentiation by metaplasia of the original coelomic membrane with prolonged oestrogen stimulation towards endometrial-like tissue. It is proposed that these adult cells undergo de-differentiation back to their primitive origin and then transform to endometrial cells. This is an attractive theory which could explain the occurrence of endometriosis in nearly all the ectopic sites in the presence of aberrant müllerian cells. What induces the transformation — whether it be hormonal stimuli, inflammatory irritation or other processes — is uncertain.

Genetic and familial aspects

It has been concluded that there is a statistically higher incidence of endometriosis encountered in first-degree relatives of patients with this disorder, compared to control groups (Simpson et al 1980). In addition there are racial differences in the existence of the disease. This may well suggest some genetic component in its formation.

Autoimmune and immunological factors

Antigens have been identified as being produced by degrading endometrial proteins which have stimulated an immune response characterized by peritoneal irritation and fibrosis. Immunofluorescent assays have demonstrated immunological damage to endometrial cells. In other studies endometrial antibodies have also been discovered in a higher incidence in patients with endometriosis than normal control populations, and there is evidence of decreased cellular immunity to endometrial tissue in the majority of women with endometriosis. This would suggest some immunological aspect which may alter the susceptibility of woman to develop endometriosis (Dmowski et al 1981; Badawy et al 1984).

The conclusion reached from the above theories is that pelvic endometriosis is probably a consequence of transplantation of viable endometrial cells regurgitated at the time of menstruation from the fallopian tubes into the peritoneal cavity. In addition transport of endometrial cells may occur by other routes, and some sites of endometriosis can only be explained by the metaplasia theory.

ENDOCRINOLOGICAL ASPECTS OF ENDOMETRIOSIS

Hormonal responses of endometriotic tissue

Clearly the hormonal dependence of endometriotic tissue comes from the observation that the condition occurs almost exclusively during the reproductive years. Clinical and experimental studies of endometriotic tissue have shown that the response to both endogenous and exogenous oestrogens and progestogens is in a similar manner to that of normally sited endometrium, although the response may be less profound, less predictable and often asynchronous (Schweppe et al 1984). In experimental endometriosis the contained endometrial implants require oestrogen for their further growth and maintenance. The effects of various hormonal agents on both normal and ectopic endometrium are summarized in Table 30.1. Hormonal responsiveness of the tissue is certainly the basis for many of the medical therapies currently in use and discussed later.

Table 30.1 Various hormonal states and their effects upon normal endometrium and ectopic endometrial deposits

Hormonal state	Effects on endometrium	Effects on endometriotic implants
Oestrogenic e.g. exogenous oestrogens	Proliferative activity, hyperplasia	Proliferative activity, hyperplasia
Hypo-oestrogenic e.g. post-menopause, pseudomenopause regimens post-oophorectomy GnRH analogues	Atrophic changes	Atrophy, regression, resorption
Progestational e.g. pregnancy, exogenous progestogens, pseudopregnancy treatment	Secretory activity, decidualization	Secretory activity, necrobiosis and resorption
Androgenic e.g. danazol and its metabolites Gestrinone	Atrophy	Atrophy and regression

GnRH = Gonadotrophin-releasing hormone.

Endocrine disorders in endometriosis

Normal ovarian function occurs in the majority of women suffering from endometriosis, but there are many reports in the literature linking a variety of endocrine abnormalities with endometriosis.

Anovulation

This abnormality often accompanies endometriosis, as does premenstrual spotting (Wentz 1980).

Disordered prolactin secretion

An increased sensitivity to thyrotrophin-releasing hormone (TRH) testing and raised baseline prolactin have been reported in some patients with endometriosis as has galactorrhoea, but these may be coincidental (Muse et al 1982).

Abnormal gonadotrophin secretion

A double mid-cycle peak of luteinizing hormone (LH) in patients with endometriosis has been reported (Cheesman et al 1982) but this finding has not been substantiated by other workers (Bayer & Siebel 1989). There is no proven evidence of hypothalamic pituitary dysfunction in patients with endometriosis.

Luteal phase defect

Luteal phase deficiency has been found in a higher percentage of endometriotic patients with infertility compared to endometriosis patients without infertility (Brosens et al 1978), as has the luteinized unruptured follicle (LUF) syndrome. Brosens et al (1978) reported a high incidence of cycles with luteinized unruptured follicles in women with endometriosis and those with unexplained infertility. The reported correlation between the presence of LUF syndrome and reduced levels of oestradiol and progesterone in peritoneal fluid during the luteal phase fostered the hypothesis that low levels of progesterone in peritoneal fluid favoured the implantation and growth of endometrial cells. Subsequent studies have not confirmed these findings to the same degree but although the relationship of cause and effect is not known, much indirect evidence suggests an association between endometriosis and LUF. Future studies should elucidate the mechanism which associates LUF and endometriosis.

PERITONEAL FLUID ENVIRONMENT IN ENDOMETRIOSIS

It has been suggested that peritoneal fluid volume and its contents may be adversely affected by the presence of endometriotic tissue in the pelvis with possible consequent interference with tubo-ovarian function and/or fertilization and early implantation. The role of peritoneal fluid with regard to steroid content in the luteal phase has already been discussed in relationship to LUF syndrome above.

Peritoneal macrophages

The role of peritoneal macrophages in women with endometriosis has been the source of much interest in recent years. Women with endometriosis associated with infertility have been found to have significantly higher concentrations of macrophages in the peritoneal fluid than either fertile or infertile women without endometriosis (Haney et al 1981). An increased number of peritoneal fluid macrophages has also been reported in women with non-mechanical causes for infertility (Olive et al 1985). These macrophages in patients with endometriosis appear to be highly phagocytic against spermatozoa in vitro, compared with those from fertile women or infertile women without endometriosis (Muscato et al 1982). In addition they are also able to survive better in vitro than those from fertile controls (Halme et al 1986). Peritoneal fluid from patients with endometriosis has also been shown to have a cytotoxic effect on in vivo cleavage of mouse embryos. These findings on the quantitative and qualitative properties of macrophages in peritoneal fluid may explain a mechanism of infertility in patients with endometriosis.

Prostaglandins and prostanoids

The role of prostaglandins and their metabolites in peritoneal fluid in the pathogenesis and symptomatology of endometriosis is controversial. It has been reported that increased levels of prostaglandin $F_{2\alpha}$ ($PGF_{2\alpha}$) are found in the peritoneal fluid of patients with endometriosis (Meldrum et al 1977); also increased peritoneal fluid volume and increased concentrations of the prostaglandin metabolites thromboxin B_2 and 6-keto PGF have been noted. Other investigators have found no increase in either the volume of peritoneal fluid or its concentrations of PGE, $PGF_{2\alpha}$ or metabolites (Rock et al 1982). Conflicting reports may reflect the timing of peritoneal fluid sampling and the quality control of assay systems.

It has been appreciated in recent years that more subtle forms of endometriosis may be present with only minimal evidence of visual changes in the peritoneum. However, if there are changes in the peritoneal fluid prostaglandin content, the mechanism by which these changes influence endometriosis or its association with infertility remains unclear. Increased secretion of $PGF_{2\alpha}$ from endometriotic implants is thought to be the probable main cause of dysmenorrhoea, commonly associated with the disease, and this is supported by the fact that prostaglandin synthetase inhibitors may often be useful in alleviating this symptom.

SYMPTOMATOLOGY

The localization of the endometriotic deposits largely determines the symptoms a patient may experience. In a large series of cases reviewed, Scott & Te Linde (1950) presented the sites where generally endometriosis was commonly detected. The commonest site is the ovary, followed by the pelvic peritoneal surfaces and the posterior aspect of the uterus. The other possible sites involved are seen in only a minority of cases. A more recent study concerned with infertility patients found that the major site involved the ovary in only 54.9% of cases, followed by the posterior leaf of the broad ligament in 35.2% of cases, the anterior and posterior pouch of Douglas in 34% each and the uterosacral ligaments in 28% (Jenkins et al 1986).

Endometriosis is thus outstandingly a pelvic disease with extrapelvic involvement in only a few cases. It is perhaps appropriate to limit discussion mainly to pelvic disease in taking account of clinical presentation and diagnosis.

Pain

The classic symptom of endometriosis is pain, commonly pelvic pain associated with menstruation or in the immediate premenstrual phase. The basis of this pain is uncertain but could reflect stretching of tissues by the menstrual process and an effect from the local production of prostaglandins from endometriotic implants. Pain also relates to tissue damage, and fixity of organs from scar and adhesion formation. What is immediately clear when reviewing patients with endometriosis is the huge variation in the extent of symptomatic distress which does not correlate with the extent of the observed disease. In addition many women who are asymptomatic are found to have endometriosis and in some of these women severe disease is discovered following laparoscopy for infertility or investigation of an incidentally detected ovarian mass. One explanation for this is that in these individuals the disease may have disrupted the pelvic sensation altogether.

Dyspareunia

Another common symptom of endometriosis is deep dyspareunia resulting from the stretching at coitus of the involved pelvic tissues, such as a fixed retroverted uterus, uterosacral ligaments or rectovaginal septum or pressure on involved enlarged ovaries. The presence of endometriotic tissue within these areas however is not always associated with dyspareunia and perhaps less than half the patients who are coitally active admit to this symptom when deposits are found in these areas.

Other symptoms

A wide range of other symptoms has been reported but the common feature is their cyclical nature. Symptoms include bleeding from the genital and urinary system, and cyclical pain and bleeding, particularly in scars. The symptoms of endometriosis related to sites of implants are summarized in Table 30.2.

Table 30.2 Symptoms of endometriosis related to sites of implants

Symptoms	Site
Dysmenorrhoea Lower abdominal pain Pelvic pain Low back pain Menstrual irregularity Rupture/torsion endometrioma Infertility	Reproductive organs
Cyclical rectal bleeding Tenesmus Diarrhoea/cyclic constipation	Gastrointestinal tract
Cyclical haematuria Dysuria (cyclical) Ureteric obstruction	Urinary tract
Cyclical haemoptysis	Lungs
Cyclical pain and bleeding	Surgical scars/umbilicus
Cyclical pain and swelling	Limbs

Table 30.3 Possible mechanisms of causation of infertility with mild endometriosis

Problem area	Mechanism
Ovarian function	Endocrinopathies Anovulation LUF syndrome Altered prolactin release Altered gonadotrophin mid-cycle surge Luteolysis caused by $PGF_{2\alpha}$ Oocyte maturation defects
Coital function	Dyspareunia causing reduced penetration and coital frequency
Tubal function	Alterations in tubal and cilial motility by prostaglandins Impaired fimbrial oocyte pick-up
Sperm function	Phagocytosis by macrophages Inactivation by antibodies
Endometrium	Interference by endometrial antibodies Luteal phase deficiency
Early pregnancy failure	Increased early abortion Prostaglandin-induced or immune reaction

LUF = Luteinized unruptured follicle; PGF_2 = prostaglandin $F_{2\alpha}$.

ENDOMETRIOSIS AND INFERTILITY

If endometriosis is associated with tubal or ovarian damage, or adhesion formation, it is easy to explain its association with future fertility compromise. However, when small deposits of endometriosis are found in asymptomatic infertile patients, controversy exists as to its cause/effect on the relationship. There appears to be an association because endometriosis has been reported in a significant percentage of women undergoing laparoscopy for infertility in various studies, ranging between 15% and 60% (Cohen 1976; Kistner 1977). This compares with an incidence of 2.5–5% in fertile controls. There is little evidence that this relationship is causal and a number of mechanisms have been postulated as to how mild endometriosis can be the causation of infertility. These have already been discussed to some extent in the section on pathogenesis and are summarized in Table 30.3, but it must be stated that there is conflicting evidence that any of the mechanisms described are the cause of the infertility found in patients with mild endometriosis. To investigate this relationship further, it is appropriate to observe whether the treatment of the disease results in improved fertility. This is discussed later in the section treatment.

DIAGNOSIS

Endometriosis should be a differential diagnostic consideration in any patient presenting with infertility, worsening dysmenorrhoea, pelvic pain, dyspareunia or other cycle-associated symptoms related particularly to the bladder or bowel. Currently the only definitive way of confirming the diagnosis is visualization of deposits at laparoscopy. Histological confirmation is not mandatory for clinical decision-making but is essential during research studies.

Pelvic endometriosis

The typical peritoneal endometriotic lesion is described as a powder burn which results from tissue bleeding and retention of blood pigments, producing a brown/black discoloration of the tissue. In the early stages these lesions may appear more pink, red and haemorrhagic and develop into brown/black lesions with increasing time. Eventually, discoloration disappears altogether and a white plaque of old collagen is all that remains of the endometriotic implant. Scarring in the peritoneum surrounding implants is also a typical finding. Apart from encapsulating an isolated implant, the scar tissue may deform the surrounding peritoneum, resulting in development of adhesions between adjacent pelvic structures. These adhesions are commonly found between the mobile pelvic structures, particularly the posterior leaf of the broad ligament and the ovary, and the dependent sigmoid colon and posterior aspect of the vagina and/or cervix.

More recently more subtle laparoscopic appearances have been reported which were confirmed on biopsy as being due to endometriosis (Jansen & Russel 1986; Donnez & Nisolle 1988). The subtle forms are more common and may be more active, and more important than the puckered black lesions which represent the later stages of the disease. The non-pigmented endometriotic peritoneal lesions include:

1. White opacification of the peritoneum. These lesions contain an occasional retroperitoneal glandular structure, scanty stroma surrounded by fibrotic tissue and connective tissue.
2. Red flame-like lesions on the peritoneum, with the appearance of red vesicular excrescences in the broad ligament and uterosacral ligaments, largely due to the presence of active endometriosis surrounded by stroma.
3. Glandular excrescence which closely resemble the mucosa of the endometrium as seen at hysteroscopy — biopsy reveals the presence of numerous glandular elements.
4. Subovarian adhesions condensed in the peritoneum of the ovarian fossa, distinctive from adhesions characteristic of previous salpingitis or peritonitis — this connective tissue often contains sparse endometrial glands.
5. Yellow-brown peritoneal patches called 'café-au-lait spots', found in the cul-de-sac, broad ligament or over the bladder — histologically they are similar to findings of white opacification; the yellow-brown patches indicate the presence of haemosiderin.
6. Circular peritoneal defects of the pelvic peritoneum, uterosacral ligaments or broad ligament. Serial section has demonstrated the presence of endometrial glands in about 50% of these structures.

From the above it is clear that careful laparoscopy by an experienced surgeon is essential if cases are not to be missed. Whenever there is any doubt the need for biopsy confirmation is apparent.

Ovarian endometriosis

The ovary represents a unique site for implantation as levels of gonadal steroids are many-fold higher than those in the general circulation or peritoneal cavity. Superficial implants on the ovary resemble implants in other peritoneal sites. However when endometrial cells enter the ovarian stroma, large endometrial cysts may form, filled with viscous chocolate-coloured liquid — chocolate cysts or endometriomas. The fluid represents the debris from cyclic menstruation. There is usually a well defined separation between the normal adjacent ovarian stroma and the cyst wall. However whilst the epithelial lining of the cyst may initially resemble the endometrium, with increasing time and size pressure atrophy compresses the epithelium to a flat cuboidal pattern.

Non-invasive methods of diagnosis

It is an unsatisfactory situation that in order to diagnose endometriosis with certainty an invasive — albeit minor — surgical procedure in the form of laparoscopy needs to be performed. Whilst this can readily be justified to make the initial diagnosis, if the nature of the disease is of recurrence for the majority of patients throughout their reproductive life, this may involve repeat laparoscopies on many occasions if one is to be certain that the disease process has returned. Attempts have therefore been made to provide a non-invasive test which is highly sensitive and specific for endometriosis. Currently this has eluded investigators.

Serum markers — CA 125

The most widely used serum marker for endometriosis has been the use of the monoclonal antibody OC 125, raised against human ovarian cancer cell-line containing the antigen designated CA 125 (Bast et al 1986). CA 125 is a high molecular-weight glycoprotein found in over 80% of cases of epithelial ovarian carcinoma. Investigation leads to the conclusion that CA 125 is possessed by many tissues present in the pelvis as well as the more distant sites, including the pericardium and the pleura. Moderate elevation of serum CA 125 has been observed in endometriosis, particularly in patients with severe disease (Barbieri et al 1986; Pittaway & Douglas 1989). In these studies serum levels in excess of 35 u/ml were used as a cut-off point, but sensitivity and specificity have proved inadequate for use of CA 125 as a screening test for endometriosis. However, in individuals in whom the disease has been confirmed and treated, an increase in serum levels above 35 u/ml may well be a useful marker of recurrence of the disorder.

Imaging techniques

Ultrasound. Ultrasound examination of the pelvis may be useful in delineating the presence and aetiology of ovarian cystic structures. The characteristic pictures on ultrasound are different when there is a large proportion of blood, e.g. in endometriomas or chocolate cysts, which in a minority of cases may be echo-free; however the walls of the endometriomas are irregular as opposed to the smooth wall of the simple ovarian cyst. The commonest pattern is for the chocolate cyst to contain low-level echoes or lumps of dense high-level echoes representing blood clots. The picture may sometimes be confused if there are several cysts in different phases of evolution.

Computerized tomography (CT) scans and magnetic resonance imaging (MRI). CT provides better definition than ultrasound in many situations but it has not established a role in the assessment of pelvic endometriosis. MRI, which is even more expensive, and currently has been used in only a limited number of patients with ovarian endometriomas, has not proved to be diagnostic since again there has been a significant overlap between endometriomas and cyst adenomas on MRI scanning appearances.

Ultrasound, CT and MRI scanning do not appear to be of any help in the diagnosis of peritoneal endometriosis, which is too small — these techniques are not sensitive enough to detect peritoneal endometriosis.

Immunoscintigraphy. Efforts have been made to use immunoscintigraphic methods to detect deposits of endometriotic tissue on the grounds that these tissue deposits do express CA 125, and if an isotopic labelled OC 125(FAB)2 fragment has been injected then binding to sites of CA 125 expression could be detected (Kennedy et al 1988). Using a gamma camera the sites where binding has occurred can be detected. Results from this method are encouraging but there is still great overlap with binding in other conditions, particularly pelvic inflammatory processes and adhesions.

In summary, whilst there are promising areas of investigations currently being pursued into non-invasive techniques, none at present can stand in place of a laparoscopy.

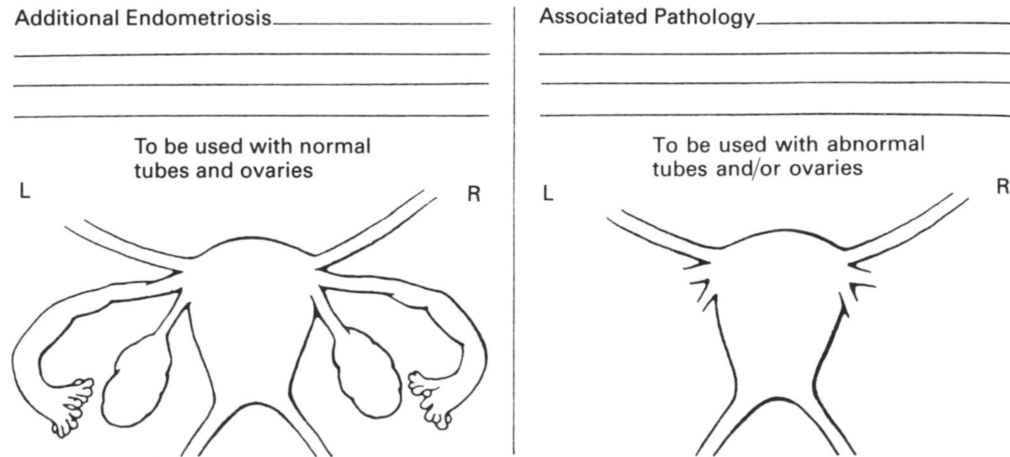

Fig. 30.9 Accurate charting of sites of endometrial deposits is helpful for re-evaluation following treatment or in suspected cases of recurrence. Modified from Revised American Fertility Society Classification of Endometriosis (1985).

CLASSIFICATION SYSTEMS

Over the last three decades various classification systems have been proposed which attempt to standardize criteria from which the severity of endometriosis could be based. Such a system, if available, would help in the critical assessment of performance of various forms of treatment and hopefully provide meaningful prognostic indicators. No classification system so far devised has received uniform acceptance; all have suffered from various pitfalls which make it difficult to compare treatment results. The most recent attempt to provide a standardized classification for uniform use has been the Revised American Fertility Society Classification for Endometriosis (1985) shown in Fig 30.9. This serves to record the sites of deposits accurately and makes some effort to differentiate between superficial and deep-seated disease, as well as the presence or absence of adhesions. Whilst it offers a different weighting to the score given to different types of endometriosis, it must be appreciated that these scores are arbitrary. It is questionable whether a reduction in score of 5 points from 40 to 35 is equivalent to a comparable treatment response with a reduction in 5 points from 10 to 5, for example. Classification of the extent of the disease as mild, moderate and severe is certainly helpful in explaining to the patient the problem and perhaps in determining whether a medical, surgical or combined medical – surgical approach is the most logical treatment step.

The other major pitfall of any scoring system has been the lack of correlation between the score or severity of the disease and its effect on fertility, except when there are adhesions which limit tubal or ovarian mobility.

Provided the above limitations are appreciated, the classification systems do serve some value and are essential in any clinical trial of a new treatment.

TREATMENT

Endometriosis is a particularly difficult disease to treat. Often response to therapy relies on recognition of the disease in its earliest possible stages. With most treatment modalities, recurrence eventually occurs in up to 60% of cases. Thus there is no known permanent cure and eventually clinicians have to proceed to surgical oophorectomy in selected cases; this offers the most effective available treatment to date. In addition in minimal and mild disease (according to American Fertility Society classifications), particularly in asymptomatic cases presenting only with infertility, there exists a controversy as to whether treatment should be given since no control studies have shown a significant increase in fertility rates following such therapy. However, placebo-controlled studies in such cases have shown that endometriosis tends to be a progressive disease (Thomas & Cooke 1986) and hence treatment may at least arrest progression or eradicate disease for significant intervals.

When endometriosis is associated with symptoms, particularly pain, then there can be no doubt that treatment is of benefit, at least in relieving these symptoms. The treatment should be individualized taking into account the patient's age, wish for fertility, severity of symptoms and extent of the disease. An important aspect of therapy is a sympathetic approach with adequate counselling and explanation to the patient which will also ensure her compliance whilst on therapy.

Current treatment is essentially surgical, medical or a combination of both approaches. A combined medical and surgical treatment might utilize medical therapy before, after, or both before and following surgical intervention. This approach may be adopted in patients with moderate to severe disease in whom fertility prospects need to be improved or maintained.

Conservative surgery

Conservative surgical treatment can be carried out either by laparoscopy or by laparotomy; the aim is to conserve as much healthy ovarian tissue as possible as well as restoring the pelvic anatomy to normal. Procedures performed during laparoscopy or laparotomy may involve dissection of endometriotic lesions, diathermy destruction or laser vaporization of deposits, excision and enucleation of endometriomas with ovarian reconstruction, division of adhesions and restoration of pelvic anatomy. For a recent review and results see Sutton (1990).

Radical surgery

Radical surgery is reserved for those patients with severe symptoms, where there is no desired fertility potential, and especially when other forms of treatment have failed. Total abdominal hysterectomy and bilateral salpingo-oophorectomy are performed along with resection of any endometriotic lesions as completely as possible. As the majority of these patients are relatively young, hormonal replacement therapy should be kept to a minimum, as a small percentage of those patients may develop a recurrence of endometriosis when on oestrogen replacement. Combined oestrogen–testosterone implants may minimize the risk of recurrence as well as offering the beneficial effects of the androgens in maintaining libido in young women who are sexually active.

Medical treatment

Ectopic endometrial tissue, as previously described, does respond to endogenous and exogenous ovarian steroid hormones in a fashion sufficiently similar to that of normal

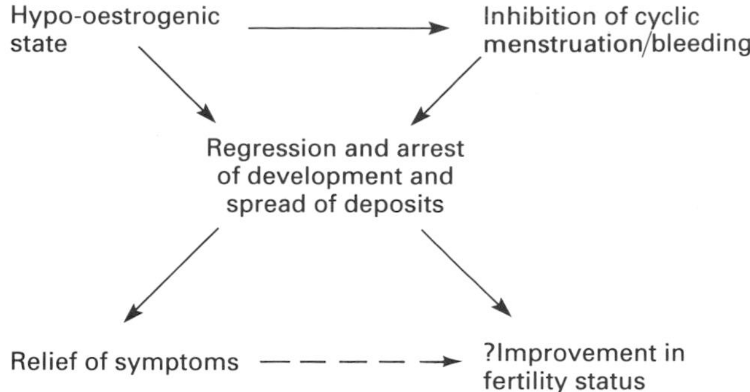

Fig. 30.10 Strategy in the medical treatment of endometriosis.

endometrium. Thus a hormonal approach which suppresses oestrogen–progesterone levels and which prevents cyclical changes and menstruation should be beneficial in its treatment (Fig. 30.10). In the hypo-oestrogenic state following the menopause, atrophy of the normal endometrium and atrophy and regression of endometriotic deposits occur. Administration of progestogens opposes the effect of oestrogen on endometrial tissue by inhibiting the replenishment of cytosolic oestrogen receptors. Progestogens also induce secretory activity in endometrial glands and decidual reaction in the endometrial stroma.

The success of various hormonal therapies depends to a large extent on the localization of the endometriotic lesions. Superficial peritoneal and ovarian serosal implants may respond better to hormone therapy than deep ovarian, deep peritoneal lesions or lesions within organs (e.g. bladder and rectum) which commonly recur after medical therapy and require surgical excision.

The treatment of endometriosis has undergone a remarkable evolution in the last 40 years. In the past testosterone, diethylstilboestrol and high-dose combination oestrogen—progestogen pill preparations were used with some success. However, therapies which induce decidualization (pseudopregnancy regimes) or suppress ovarian function (pseudomenopausal regimes) appear to offer the best chance of inducing clinical remission of endometriosis.

Progestogen treatment

A state of pseudopregnancy can be induced effectively by the use of continuous progestogenic preparations, such as the derivatives of progesterone (dydrogesterone or medroxyprogesterone acetate) or derivatives of 19-nor-testosterone (norethisterone, norethisterone acetate, norgestrel, ethynodrel and lynoestrenol).

The use of progestogens induces a hyperprogestogenic–hypo-oestrogenic state. Treatments are available orally or injected as depot formulation and are administered for 6–9 months. The results achieved appear to be comparable to those achieved with combined oral oestrogen–progestogen preparations in the past. The side-effects most commonly seen with progestogen usage include breakthrough bleeding, weight gain, abdominal bloating, oedema and acne.

Following treatment with injectable medroxyprogesterone acetate depot, the return of ovulation may remain suppressed for several months. Thus it should not be given to patients wishing to conceive.

The adverse effects of progestogens on low and high density lipoproteins have still to be fully evaluated in relation to the type and duration of progestogen usage in the treatment of endometriosis.

Combined oestrogen–progestogen preparations

Kistner (1959) introduced the regimen of continuous combined oral contraceptives in order to reproduce the hormonal milieu of pregnancy. One of the higher-dose 50 μg ethinyloestradiol combined oral contraceptives may be administered continuously for 6–9 months. If breakthrough bleeding occurs, changing to another preparation with higher prostestogenic content or increasing the dose of the original preparation to 2 tablets daily may be advocated.

Side-effects such as weight gain, headaches, breast enlargement and/or tenderness, nausea and depression may occur. The risk of thromboembolism is increased and contraindications for the use of this form of therapy are the same as those for combined oral contraception.

Danazol

Danazol is an isoxazol derivative of 17-alpha ethinyl testosterone. Because of its base structure it has both androgenic and anabolic properties. Danazol is currently one of the most widely used medical treatments for endometriosis. Its mechanism of action is complex and includes suppression of the hypothalamic–pituitary axis with interference of pulsatile gonadotrophin secretion and inhibition of mid-cycle gonadotrophin surge but no change in basal gonadotrophin levels. It achieves a direct inhibition of ovarian steroidogenesis by inhibiting several enzymatic processes and competitive blockage of androgen, oestrogen and progesterone receptors in the endometrium. An increase in free testosterone occurs because of a reduction in sex hormone-binding globulin and this explains many of danazol's androgenic side-effects. The increase in free testosterone may also contribute towards its direct action on inducing endometrial atrophy. The degree of endocrine changes described above is dose-related.

In the treatment of endometriosis danazol is administered in a dose range of between 400 and 800 mg daily titrated by the induction of amenorrhoea and tolerance. In the case of mild to moderate endometriosis there is a highly effective symptomatic improvement in over 85% of cases (Dmowski & Cohen 1978).

Objective resolution of endometriotic lesions has been observed at post-treatment laparoscopic evaluation in between 70 and 95% of patients, depending upon the stage of the disease (Barbieri et al 1982). However, recurrence rates of up to 40% have been reported in the 36 months after completion of a course of danazol — annual recurrences in the first, second and third years were 23, 5 and 9% respectively (Dmowski & Cohen 1978).

Danazol therapy should be commenced in the early follicular phase of the menstrual cycle. It is recommended that the patient should use additional barrier methods of contraception in order to avoid the drug being administered during early pregnancy where continued use could lead to androgenization of the developing female fetus. The drug dosage should be related to the patient's clinical staging, response and severity of side-effects, starting with a dose of 400 mg/day in mild disease and 600–800 mg/day in moderate to severe cases for a recommended treatment course of at least 6 months.

Danazol is associated with side-effects related to its androgenic and anabolic properties. These include weight gain, acne, oily skin, fluid retention, muscle cramps and mood changes. Less commonly, hirsutism, depression, hot flushes, skin rash and deepening of voice are noted. The incidence and severity of these side-effects are dose-related. It is recommended that patients discontinue treatment if they develop any hirsutism, a skin rash or experience deepening of the voice.

Metabolic side-effects include elevation of low density lipoproteins and reduction of high density lipoproteins and cholesterol concentrations (Fahraeus et al 1984). These effects are quickly reversed after ceasing treatment. In addition, changes in liver enzymes are noted — danazol is contraindicated in patients with liver disease.

Gestrinone

Gestrinone is a synthetic trienic 19-norsteroid (13-ethyl-17-alpha-ethinyl-17-hydroxy-gona-4, 9, 11-triene-3-one). It has been shown in recent clinical trials to be another effective clinical treatment for endometriosis (Thomas & Cooke 1987). The drug exhibits mild androgenic, marked, antiprogestogenic and anti-oestrogenic as well as moderate antigonadotrophic properties. The combined effect is to induce progressive endometrial atrophy. Gestrinone has a high binding affinity for progesterone receptors; it also binds to androgen receptors but not to oestrogen receptors (Azadian-Boulanger et al 1984). The combined endocrine effect of gestrinone therapy is similar to that of danazol in that the mid-cycle gonadotrophin surge is abolished — although basal gonadotrophin secretions are not significantly reduced — together with inhibition of ovarian steroidogenesis, and reduction of sex hormone-binding globulin levels. Gestrinone has a prolonged half-life and may be administered orally at a dosage of 2.5–5.0 mg twice-weekly for a period of 6–9 months in patients with endometriosis. This dosage schedule effectively induces endometrial atrophy with 85–90% of patients becoming amenorrhoeic within 2 months.

Whilst gestrinone has only recently been introduced for the treatment of endometriosis, current controlled open studies appear to show that it compares favourably with danazol in terms of both symptomatic relief and resolution of endometrial deposits (Azadian-Boulanger et al 1984; Mettler & Semm 1984).

The side-effects, occurring in up to 50% of patients, include weight gain, breakthrough bleeding, reduced breast size, muscle cramps and — uncommonly — hirsutism and voice hoarseness.

Gonadotrophin-releasing hormone (GnRH) agonist

Surgical castration is known to be an effective therapy for severe endometriosis. Thus the possibility of inducing a reversible medical castration with the continued administration of GnRH agonists is currently being investigated as an alternative therapy in endometriosis. Modification of the native GnRH molecule with substitution, particularly in positions 6 and 10, with alternative amino acids produces agonistic analogues with a reduced susceptibility to degradation and hence a prolonged therapeutic half-life (Fig. 30.11). Continued administration of these analogues induces pituitary gonadotrophin desensitization and down-regulation and an eventual state of hypogonadotrophic–hypogonadism. Reduced gonadotrophic stimulation of the ovaries leads to cessation of follicular growth and reduction in ovarian steroidogenesis, with circulating oestradiol 17β levels falling to those observed in the low range of the early follicular phase or post-menopausal range (50–150 pmol/l).

A large number of data have now appeared in the literature from both controlled trials and randomized comparative trials of GnRH analogues and danazol (for review, see Shaw 1988). These trials have all confirmed the value of GnRH analogues for the treatment of endometriosis. Rapid and effective symptomatic relief is achieved with these agents as well as a marked degree of resolution of the endometrial deposits in the majority of patients. However for both symptomatic relief and the resolution of endometrial deposits there is essentially no significant difference in comparative trials between the GnRH analogues and danazol. However, patient acceptability and the profile of side-effects may be slightly in favour of the GnRH analogues (Matta & Shaw 1987; Henzl et al 1988; (Table 30.4).

Further comparative studies are needed to define these issues more fully. Side-effects of GnRH include those which are predictable from induction of a significant degree of hypo-oestrogenism. These include hot flushes in vir-

	1	2	3	4	5	(6)	7	8	9	(10)	
	Pyro – GLU	– HIS	– TRP	– SER	– TYR	– GLY	– LEU	– ARG	– PRO	GLY – NH_2	LHRH

	Position 6	Positions 9/10	
Nonapeptides	D – SER (Bu^t)	PRO – NET	Buserelin
	D – LEU	PRO – NET	Leuprolide
Decapeptides	D – TRP		Tryptorelin
	$(D – NAL)_2$		Nafarelin
	D – SER (Bu^t)	AZA – GLY	Goserelin

Fig. 30.11 Amino acid sequence of native luteinizing-hormone releasing hormone (LHRH) and some of the agonistic gonadotrophin-releasing hormone (GnRH) analogues used in the treatment of endometriosis.

Table 30.4 Principal side-effects experienced in patients randomized to receive buserelin or danazol for 6 months

	Buserelin	Danazol
Dose	400 μg t.d.s. intranasally	600–800 mg orally daily
Number of patients	39	18
Symptoms		
Hot flushes	74%*	22%
Breakthrough bleeding	23%	55%*
Headaches	20%	39%
Vaginal dryness	23%*	5.5%
Superficial dyspareunia	5.2%*	Nil
Weight gain (>3 kg)	Nil	66%*
Acne/oily skin	Nil	39%*

From Matta & Show (1987).
* $P \leq 0.05$ between treatments.

tually all patients and headaches, and less commonly atrophic vaginitis, vaginal dryness and reduced libido.

Dosage varies depending on the analogue used and its formulation but includes nafarelin 200 μg twice daily intranasally, buserelin 300–400 μg three times daily intranasally and goserelin 3.6 mg depot monthly.

Metabolic side-effects include (as in the menopause) increased excretion of urinary calcium; over a 6-month period there is a 3–5% loss in vertebral trabecular bone density of the lumbar spine as assessed by CT (Matta et al 1987). In most patients the bone density changes are completely reversible following a 6-month course of therapy with GnRH analogues. However the implications of such changes in calcium homeostasis with prolonged and repetitive treatment with GnRH analogues must be further investigated. Nevertheless, GnRH analogues appear to be well tolerated and an effective means of treating endometriosis and offer an alternative to other current medical treatments.

Combination of medical and surgical therapy

There is perhaps more speculation as to the value of pre- or postoperative medical therapy than hard data. Individual gynaecologists have a 'belief' in one or the other even though their own data do not suggest advantages of one method over the other.

It is the frequency of recurrent endometriosis after medical or surgical therapy and the documentation of microscopic disease together with differences in vascularity between various lesions that have encouraged the use of combination therapy.

Preoperative therapy might help reduce somewhat the size of an endometrioma prior to surgical removal since medical therapy alone will never succeed. Preoperative treatment will also reduce vascularity and may subsequently aid dissection of implants and adhesive processes. The role of postoperative medication is to eliminate any residual macro- or microscopic disease.

The duration of such therapies is uncertain since no true randomized comparative trials exist, but most gynaecologists prescribe a 3-month treatment course preoperatively and between 3 and 6 months postoperatively depending upon the amount of macroscopic disease left following attempted surgical removal.

RECURRENT ENDOMETRIOSIS

The natural course of the disease remains a mystery. It has been suggested that in only one-third of cases is the disease progressive, whilst in the remainder the endometriosis remains in a steady state or eventually even resolves spontaneously.

In many instances after medical suppression of the disease or after surgical destruction of all visible deposits, residual viable (microscopic) implants can regenerate once ovarian function is re-established. In other cases new disease develops at new sites, perhaps indicating the potential for an entire 'field change' within the pelvic peritoneum. The degree of differentiation of a lesion may also correlate with persistence of disease following medical therapy. Two-thirds of those lesions which were most highly differentiated disappeared following 6 months of medical therapy, whilst three-quarters of poorly differentiated lesions persisted (Schweppe 1984). However as far as therapeutic options are concerned there is no essential difference between primary and recurrent endometriosis. The choice of treatment in a patient with recurrent disease is not determined by the manifestations of the disease as such whether it is (primary or recurrent), but by the extent of distortion of the pelvic anatomy and severity of symptomatology. In many instances repeat medical therapy or repeat conservative surgery is appropriate, but with severe symptoms and repeat recurrence a radical surgical approach may become necessary in due course.

KEY POINTS

1. Endometriosis is most commonly found inside of the pelvis but rarely it has been described in sites such as the urinary tract, lungs and umbilicus.
2. Endometriosis is one of the commonest gynaecological conditions and is present in between 10 and 25% of women presenting with gynaecological symptoms in the UK and the USA.
3. The growth of endometriotic tissue depends on oestrogen, thus endometriosis occurs almost exclusively in the reproductive years, with a peak incidence between 30 and 45 years of age.
4. The theories of aetiology of endometriosis include Sampson's theory of retrograde menstruation and implantation and Meyer's theory of transformation of coelomic epithelium. Immunological factors are also thought to be important.
5. The peritoneal fluid in women with endometriosis contains higher concentrations of more active macrophages and higher concentrations of prostaglandins than in normal women. These factors may be important in explaining the link between infertility and endometriosis.
6. Endometriosis that is associated with tubal and ovarian damage and the formation of adhesions can compromise fertility. The link between mild endometriosis and infertility is more controversial.
7. The only way to diagnose endometriosis is by direct visualization at laparoscopy or laparotomy; histological confirmation is also important.
8. The typical peritoneal endometriotic lesion is described as a powder burn, but recently, non-pigmented lesions have been described.
9. The medical treatment of endometriosis involves suppressing oestrogen-progesterone levels to prevent cyclical changes and menstruation and include progestogens, gestrinone, danazol and gonadotrophin-releasing hormone analogues.
10. The surgical treatment of endometriosis is either minimally invasive, such as laparoscopic diathermy or laser vaporization; or radical, when total abdominal hysterectomy and bilateral salpingoophorectomy are performed.
11. The natural course of the disease is not clearly defined, but perhaps in a third of cases the disease is progressive whilst in the remainder the disease remains in a steady stage or may even resolve spontaneously.

REFERENCES

Azadian-Boulanger G, Secchi J, Tournemine C, Sakiz E, Vige P, Henrion R 1984 Hormonal activity profiles of drugs for endometriosis therapy. In: Raynaud J P, Ojasoo T, Martini L (eds) Medical management of endometriosis. Raven Press, New York, pp 125–148

Badawy S Z A, Cuenca V, Stitzel A, Jacobs R D B, Tomar R H 1984 Autoimmune phenomena in infertile patients with endometriosis. Obstetrics and Gynaecology 63: 271

Barbieri R L, Evans S, Kistner R W 1982 Danazol in the treatment of endometriosis: analysis of 100 cases with a 4-year follow-up. Fertility and Sterility 37: 737–749

Barbieri R L, Niloff J M, Bast R C, Shaetzl E, Kistner R W, Knapp R C 1986 Elevated serum concentrations of CA-125 in patients with advanced endometriosis. Fertility and Sterility 45: 630–634

Bast R C, Feeney M, Lazarus H, Nadler L M, Colvin R B Knapp R C 1986 Reactivity of a monoclonal antibody with human ovarian carcinoma. Journal of Clinical Investigation 68: 1331

Bayer S R, Siebel M M 1986 Endometriosis: clinical symptoms and infertility. In: Rolland R, Chandha D R, Willemsen W P (eds) Gonadotrophin down-regulation in gynecological practice. Alan R Liss, New York, pp 103–133

Brosens I A, Koninckx P R, Correleyn P A 1978 A study of plasma progesterone, oestradiol-17β, prolactin and LH levels and of the luteal phase appearance of the ovaries in patients with endometriosis and infertility. British Journal of Obstetrics and Gynaecology 85: 246–250

Cheesman K L, Ben-Nun I, Chatterton R T, Cohen M R 1982 Relationship of luteinizing hormone, pregnanediol-3-glucuronide, and estradiol-16-glucuronide in urine of infertile women with endometriosis. Fertility and Sterility 38: 542–544

Cohen M R 1976 Endoscopy. In: Greenblatt R B (ed) Recent advances in endometriosis. Excerpta Medica, Amsterdam, pp 18–31

Dmowski W P, Cohen M R 1978 Antigonadotrophin (danazol) in the treatment of endometriosis: evaluation of post-treatment fertility and 3-year follow-up data. American Journal of Obstetrics and Gynecology 130: 41–48

Dmowski W P, Steele R W, Baker G F 1981 Deficient cellular immunity in endometriosis. American Journal of Obstetrics and Gynecology 141: 377–383

Donnez J, Nisolle M 1981 Appearance of peritoneal endometriosis. In: IIIrd Laser Surgery Symposium, Brussels

Fahraeus L, Larsson-Cohn U, Ljungberg S, Wallentin L 1984, Profound alterations of the lipoprotein metabolism during danazol treatment in pre-menopausal women. Fertility and Sterility 42: 52–57

Halme J, Becher S, Wing R 1984 Accentuated cyclic activation of peritoneal macrophages in patients with endometriosis. American Journal of Obstetrics and Gynecology 148: 85–90

Halme J, Becker S, Haskill S 1986 Altered life span and function of peritoncal macrophages: a new hypothesis for pathogenesis of endometriosis. Society of Gynecologic Investigation, Toronto, Abstract 48

Haney A F, Muscato J J, Weinberg J B 1981 Peritoneal fluid cell populations in infertility patients. Fertility and Sterility 35: 696–698

Henzl M R, Corson S L, Moghissi K, Buttram V C, Bergquist C, Jacobson C 1988 Administration of nasal nafarelin as compared with oral danazol for endometriosis. New England Journal of Medicine 318: 485–489

Jansen R P S, Russel P 1986 Nonpigmented endometriosis: clinical laparoscopic and pathologic definition. American Journal of Obstetrics and Gynecology 155: 1154--1159

Jenkins S, Olive D L, Haney A F 1986 Endometriosis: pathogenic implications of the anatomic distribution. Obstetrics and Gynaecology 67: 335–338

Kennedy S H, Soper N D W, Mojiminiyi O A, Shepstone B J, Barlow D H 1988 Immunoscintigraphy of ovarian endometriosis. A preliminary study. British Journal of Obstetrics and Gynaecology 95: 693–697

Kistner R W 1959 The treatment of endometriosis by inducing pseudopregnancy with ovarian hormones: a report of 58 cases. Fertility and Sterility 10: 539–545

Kistner R W 1977 Endometriosis. In: Sciarra J (ed) Gynecology and Obstetrics, vol 1. Harper & Row, Hagerstown

Matta W H, Shaw R W 1987 A comparative study between buserelin and danazol in the treatment of endometriosis. British Journal of Clinical Practice 41 (Suppl 48): 69–73

Matta W M, Shaw R W, Hesp R, Katz D 1987 Hypogonadism induced by luteinizing hormone releasing hormone agonist analogues: effects on bone density in premenopausal women. British Medical Journal 294: 1523–1524

Meldrum D R, Shamonki I M, Clark K E 1977 Prostaglandin content of ascitic fluid in endometriosis: a preliminary report. 25th Annual meeting of the Pacific Coast Fertility Society, Palm Springs, California

Mettler L, Semm K 1984 Three-step therapy of genital endometriosis in cases of human infertility with lynestrenol, danazol or gestrinone administration. In: Raynaud J P, Ojasoo T, Martini L (eds) Medical management of endometriosis. Raven Press, New York, pp 233–247

Meyer R 1919 Uber den Staude der Frage der Adenomyosites Adenomyoma in Allgemeinen und Adenomyometitis Sarcomastosa. Zentralblatt fur Gynäkologie 36: 745–759

Muscato J J, Haney A F, Weinberg J B 1982 Sperm phagocytosis by human peritoneal macrophages: a possible cause of infertility in endometriosis. American Journal of Obstetrics and Gynecology 144: 503–510

Muse K, Wilson E A, Jawad M J 1982 Prolactin hyperstimulation in response to thyrotropin releasing hormone in patients with endometriosis. Fertility and Sterility 38: 419–422

Olive D L, Weinberg J B and Haney A F 1985 Peritoneal macrophages and infertility: the association between cell number and pelvic pathology. Fertility and Sterility 44: 772–777

Pittaway D E, and Douglas J W 1989, Serum CA-125 in women with endometriosis and chronic pelvic pain. Fertility and Sterility 51: 68–70

Revised American Fertility Society Classification of Endometriosis 1985 Fertility and Sterility 43: 351–352

Rock J A, Dubin N M, Ghodgaonkar R B, Bergquist C A, Erozan Y S, Kimball A W Jr 1982 Cul-de-sac fluid in women with endometriosis: fluid volume and prostanoid concentration during the proliferative phase of the cycle — days 8–12. Fertility and Sterility 37: 747–752

Sampson J A 1927a Peritoneal endometriosis due to menstrual dissemination of endometrial tissue into peritoneal cavity. American Journal of Obstetrics and Gynecology 14: 422

Sampson J A 1927b Metastatic or embolic endometriosis due to menstrual dissemination of endometrial tissue into the venous circulation. American Journal of Pathology 3: 93–109

Schifrin B S, Erez S, Moore J G 1973 Teenage endometriosis. American Journal of Obstetrics and Gynecology 116: 973–980

Schweppe K W 1984 Morphologie und Klinik der Endometriose. F K Schattauer Verlag, Stuttgart, pp 198–207

Schweppe K W, Wynn R M, Beller F K 1984 Ultrastructural comparison of endometriotic implants and entopic endometrium. American Journal of Obstetrics and Gynecology 148: 1024–1039

Scott R B, Te Linde R W 1950 External endometriosis: the scourge of the private patient. Annal of Surgery 131: 706

Shaw R W 1988 LHRH analogues in the treatment of endometriosis — comparative results with other treatments. Clinical Obstetrics and Gynaecology 2: 659–675

Shaw R W, Marshall J C (eds) 1989 LHRH and its analogues. Wright, London

Simpson J L, Elias S, Malinak L R, Buttram V C Jr 1980 Heritable aspects of endometriosis I: genetic studies. American Journal of Obstetrics and Gynecology 137: 327–331

Sutton C 1990 Advances in the surgical management of endometriosis. In: Shaw R W (ed) Endometriosis. Parthenon Publishing, Camforth, pp 209–226

Thomas E J, Cooke I D 1987 Impact of gestrinone on the course of asymptomatic endometriosis. British Medical Journal 294: 272–274

Tyson J E A 1974 Surgical considerations in gynaecologic endocrine disorders. Surgical Clinics of North America 54: 425–442

Wentz A C 1980 Premenstrual spotting: its association with endometriosis but not luteal phase inadequacy. Fertility and Sterility 33: 605–607

31 Vaginal prolapse

S. L. Stanton

CLASSIFICATION

A prolapse is a protrusion of an organ or structure beyond its normal anatomical confines. This is classified according to its anatomical location and it is convenient to start from the anterior and move to the posterior vaginal wall.

The following classification is used: descent of the urethra (urethrocele), bladder (cystocele), uterus and cervix, vault, small bowel (enterocele) and rectum (rectocele) into the vagina and sometimes beyond (Fig. 31.1). An enterocele may contain omentum as well as small bowel. Some amount of vaginal wall laxity is normal and prolapse is a matter of degree rather than being absolute. It is graded according to whether it is slight (when there is some movement on coughing) or marked (where prolapse appears at or beyond the introitus). Uterine descent is graded differently: first-degree indicates some descent within the vagina, second-degree indicates that the cervix appears at the introitus and third-degree or procidentia indicates that the uterus is entirely outside the introitus, usually bringing with it some cystocele, enterocele and rectocele. When a hysterectomy has been performed, descent of the vaginal vault is called vault prolapse.

Prolapse is common and may be associated with urinary symptoms. It is benign, but third-degree uterine prolapse

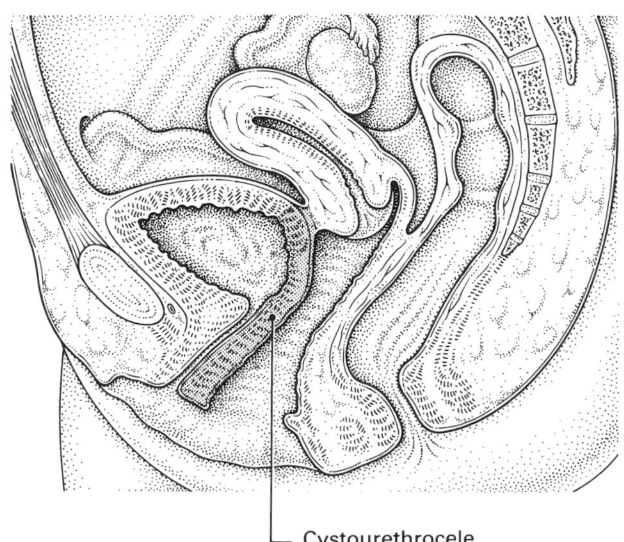

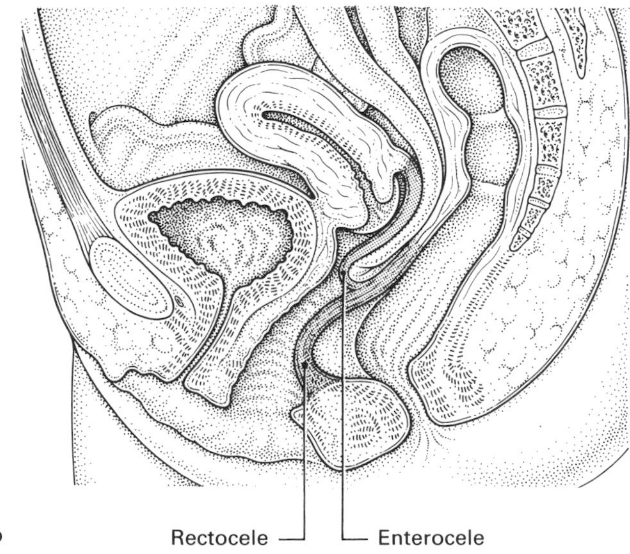

Fig. 31.1 **a** Cystourethrocele. **b** Rectocele and enterocele.

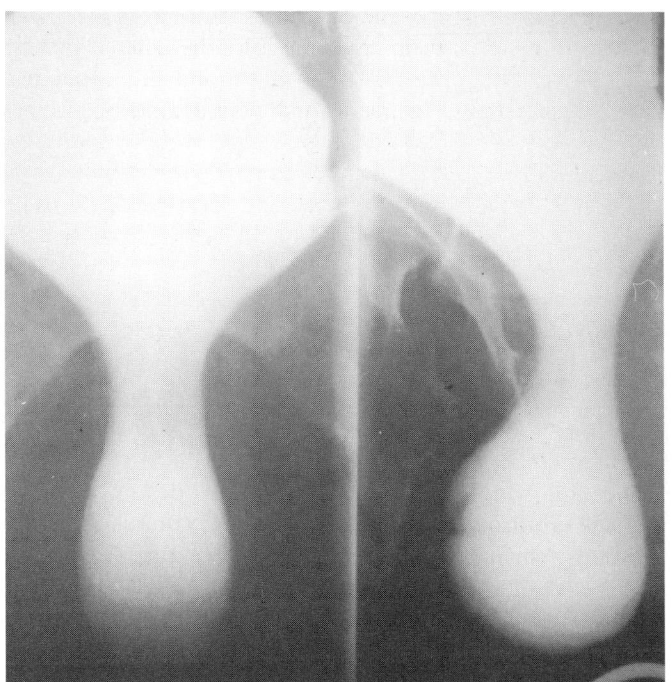

Fig. 31.2 X-ray showing marked cystocele with ureterovesical junctions outside the vagina.

with a cystocele may cause ureteric obstruction and therefore is potentially fatal (Fig. 31.2). The ureters are also at risk of being traumatized during vaginal hysterectomy.

INCIDENCE

Cystourethrocele is the most common prolapse, followed by uterine descent and then rectocele. A urethrocele occurring on its own is rare. The enterocele is more common following abdominal or vaginal hysterectomy or colposuspension.

Approximately 20% of patients waiting for gynaecological surgery are due to have repair of prolapse (Stallworthy 1971). The incidence rises in the elderly, constituting 59% of one series of patients who underwent major gynaecological surgery (Lewis 1968). With improved general health, better care in labour and shorter duration of first and second stages and a tendency towards smaller families, it is likely that prolapse may become less common.

PELVIC ANATOMY

The pelvic viscera are supported by the pelvic floor, which is composed of muscle, fascia and ligamentous supports.

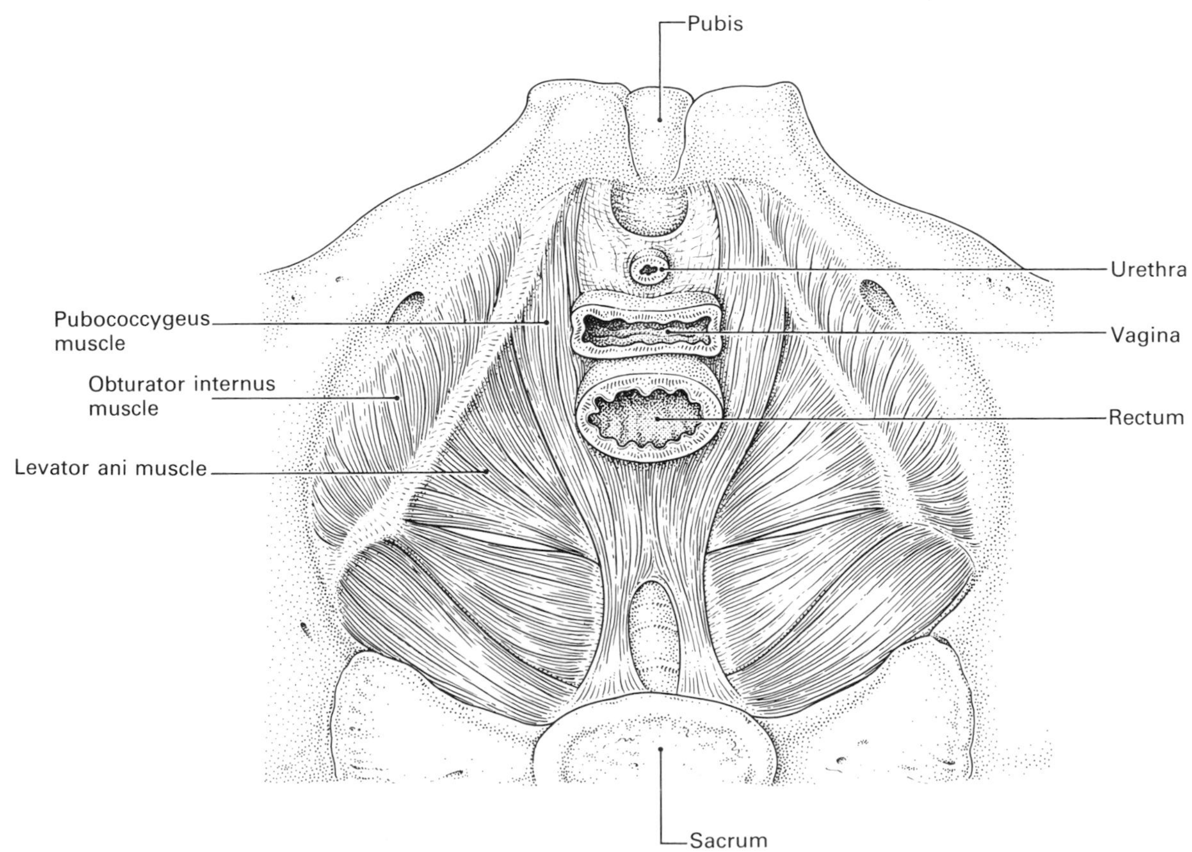

Fig. 31.3 Pelvic floor muscles from above.

Pelvic floor

The pelvic floor includes the levator ani, internal obturator and piriform muscles, and superficial and deep perineal muscles (Fig. 31.3). The levator ani (which is in two parts — pubococcygeal and iliococcygeal) is covered by pelvic fascia and arises from the pelvic surface of the pubic bone (lateral to the symphysis pubis) and posteriorly from the ischial spine. In between, it takes origin from the internal obturator fascia (tendinous arch). The pubococcygeal muscle fans out and forms two parts which are inserted differently. The anterior fibres decussate around the vagina and pass to the perineal body and anal canal. Although anteriorly the fibres of the pubococcygeal muscle are in close relation to the urethra, they are not structurally attached to it (Gosling 1981). Posterior fibres join the raphe formed by the iliococcygeal muscle. The deeper fibres of each side unite behind the anorectal junction to form the puborectal muscle, which slings the anorectal junction from the pubic bone. The fibres of the iliococcygeal muscle proceed downwards medially and backwards to be inserted into the last two pieces of the coccyx and into a median fibrous raphe that extends from the tip of the coccyx to the anus. The muscle is supplied by the anterior primary rami of S3 and S4.

The coccygeal muscle is a flat, triangular muscle arising from the ischial spine and in the same place as the iliococcygeal muscle. It is inserted into the lateral margin of the lower two pieces of the sacrum and the upper two pieces of the coccyx. Its nerve supply is the anterior primary rami S3 and S4.

Both of these muscles act as support for the pelvic viscera and as sphincters for the rectum and vagina. Contraction of the pubococcygeal muscle will also arrest the urinary stream.

These muscles are aided by the muscles of the urogenital diaphragm — the superficial and deep perineal muscles that originate from the ischial rami and are inserted into the perineal body (Fig. 31.4) They are supplied by the perineal branch of the pudendal nerve (S2 to S4) and brace the perineum against the downward pressure from the pelvic floor. The muscles are covered superiorly by fascia continuous with that over the levator ani and internal obturator muscles and inferiorly by fascia called the perineal membrane.

Pelvic ligaments

The pelvic ligaments are condensations of pelvic fascia that sling the cervix, uterus and upper part of the vagina from the walls of the pelvis. They include the following:

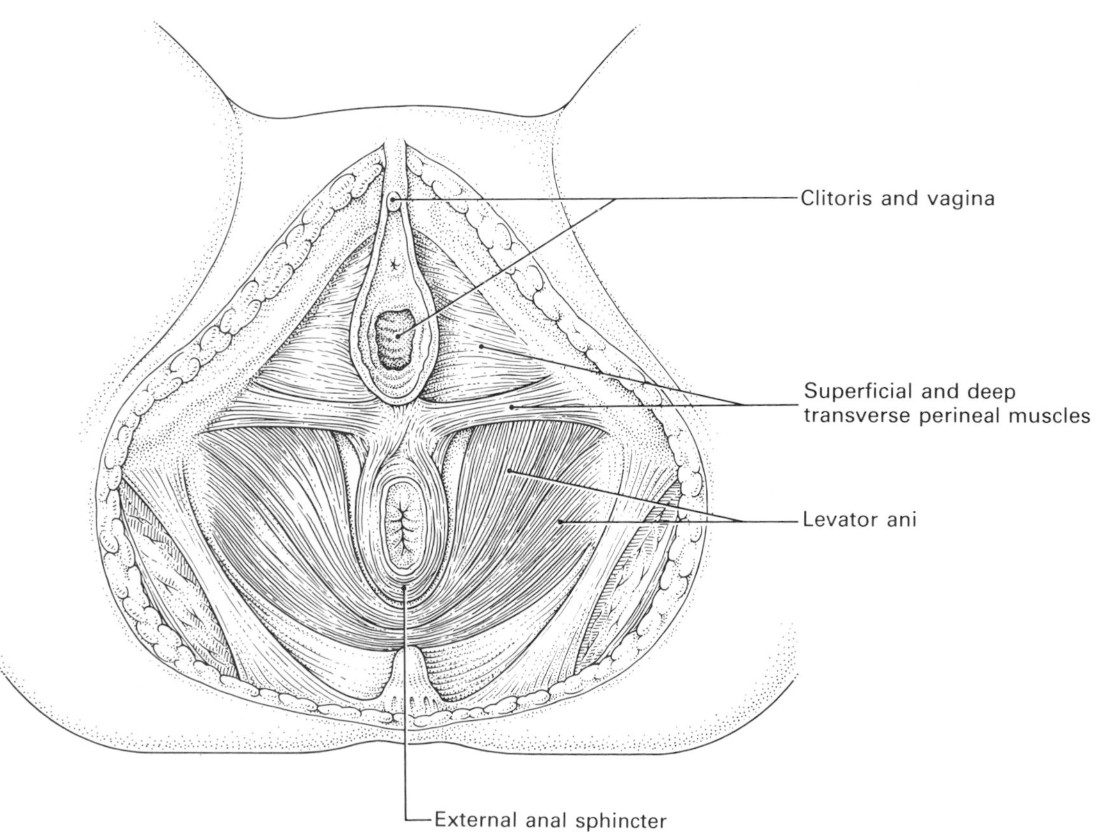

Fig. 31.4 Superficial and deep perineal muscles.

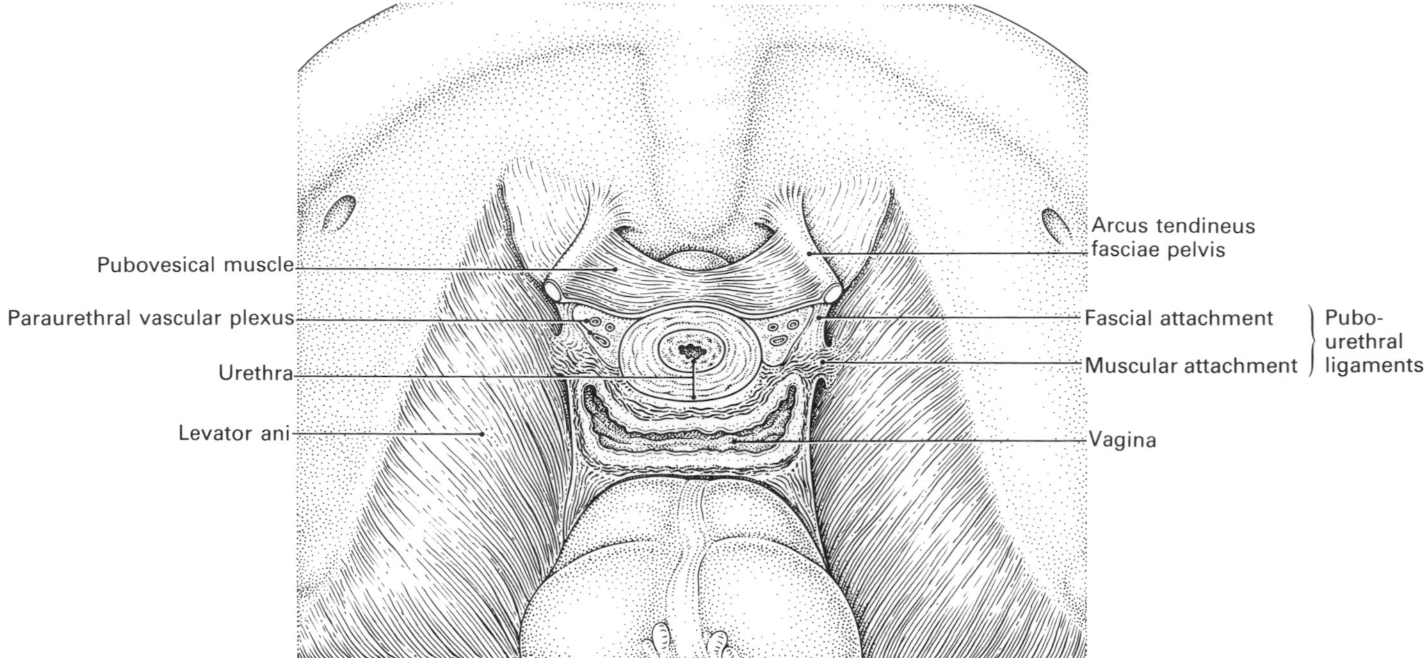

Fig. 31.5 Posterior pubourethral ligaments.

1. The pubocervical ligament (pubocervical fascia) extends from the anterior aspect of the cervix to the back of the body of the pubis.
2. The lateral cervical ligament (transverse cervical, Mackenrodt or cardinal ligaments) extends from the lateral aspect of the cervix and upper vagina to the pelvic side walls. It is the lower part of the broad ligament and nerves and vessels pass through from the pelvic side walls to the uterus. The ureter passes underneath it to the ureterovesical junction. The upper edge of the broad ligament contains the ovarian vessels.
3. The uterosacral ligament extends from the back of the uterus to the front of the sacrum.
4. The posterior pubourethral ligament extends from the posterior inferior aspect of the symphysis to the anterior aspect of the middle third of the urethra and on to the bladder (Fig. 31.5). It maintains elevation of the bladder neck and prevents excess posterior displacement of the urethra (Gosling 1981). It may facilitate micturition and is important in maintaining continence.
5. The round ligament, which is not ligamentous but is formed of smooth muscle, passes from the uterine cornu through the inguinal canal to the labia majus. It is believed to keep the uterus anteflexed but probably plays little part in actually supporting the uterus.

Structures involved in prolapse

A cystocele occurs because the bladder descends through the pubocervical fascia and attenuates the overlying vaginal skin. A large cystocele will carry both the ureterovesical junctions and the lower end of the ureters with it, so that these protrude outside the vagina. This can result in ureteric obstruction and ureteric damage occurs when these structures are not recognized at surgery.

A urethrocele occurs because of loss of support by the pubocervical fascia and posterior tubourethral ligaments. The latter are probably the most important structures supporting the urethrovesical junction and maintaining continence.

Descent of the uterus and cervix occurs when the lateral cervical ligaments become weakened. Sometimes, particularly in prolapse associated with nulliparity, the cervix elongates and the uterus descends without any cystocele but with an enterocele; condensations of pelvic fascia are inadequately developed and lack their normal resilience.

Vault prolapse occurs following abdominal or vaginal hysterectomy, due to failure to support the vault adequately using the lateral cervical ligaments or to inadequate strength of these ligaments, or to failure to correct an enterocele at time of hysterectomy. It usually contains small bowel or omentum and may accompany uterine descent or follow a colposuspension. It used to be a common sequel to vaginal hysterectomy until its prevention was noted and a prophylactic high fascial repair performed (Hawksworth & Roux 1958). Failure despite this may be caused by the presence of deep uterovesical and uterorectal peritoneal pouches.

A rectocele represents weakness in the posterior vaginal wall, allowing protrusion of the rectum into the vaginal canal. The rectum descends through the rectovaginal septum and carries attenuated vaginal wall in front of it. There is separation of the posterior fibres of the pubococcygeal muscle.

AETIOLOGY

Congenital weakness of pelvic fascia ligaments can account for a small percentage of prolapse, especially when spina bifida or bladder exstrophy is present. Congenital shortness of the vagina or deep uterovesical or uterorectal peritoneal pouches are also responsible (Jeffcoate 1967). However the most common factors are antecedent childbirth and the menopause. Prolapse can occur during pregnancy. Keettel (1941) reported an incidence of between 1 in 10 000 and 1 in 15 000 pregnancies. Factors included prolonged and difficult labour, bearing down before full dilatation, multiparity, laceration of the lower genital tract in the second stage, forceful delivery of the placenta during the third stage and inadequate repair of pelvic floor injuries.

Electrophysiological studies of the pelvic floor by Snooks et al (1984), Swash (1984), Allen et al (1990) and Sayer et al (1990) have shown that there are denervation changes in the pelvic floor (and anal sphincter) following vaginal delivery and that these may account for temporary and sometimes permanent urinary or faecal incontinence.

Where prolapse and stress incontinence coexist it is likely that collagen is weaker and there is less denervation than in those without prolapse.

The role of positions other than squatting for delivery is believed by some clinicians to be instrumental in causing prolapse. Indeed in countries where squatting is the normal position for delivery and where women return early to heavy physical work, little prolapse is found.

Some women, especially black women, form keloid as a response to injury and this may explain why prolapse is comparatively rare in the black race.

After childbirth, menopause (with oestrogen deficiency) is probably the most significant factor in prolapse incidence. Lacking oestrogen, the tissues of the female genital tract become atrophic and weakened. This may be aggravated by anything which raises the intra-abdominal pressure, e.g. chronic cough, constipation or heavy lifting.

PRESENTATION

Symptoms

Symptoms of prolapse depend not necessarily on the size but on the site and type of prolapse. Discomfort experienced with prolapse is usually caused by abnormal tension on nerves in the tissues that are being stretched.

Cystocele and cystourethrocele

Prolapse of the bladder and urethra may lead to dragging discomfort, the sensation of a lump in the vagina and urinary symptoms, the commonest of which is stress incontinence. This will be present if there is undue mobility and descent of the urethrovesical junction or if repeated operations have produced scarring around the urethra and bladder neck leading to inadequate urethral closure. About 50% of patients with urethral sphincter incompetence and stress incontinence have a cystourethrocele; therefore prolapse is not the sole cause of this condition. Retention of urine can occur if a large cystocele is present and the bladder neck is anchored normally. This leads to overflow incontinence and failure to diagnose retention. It can be corrected temporarily by manually replacing the prolapse. If sufficient urine is being voided but a chronic residual urine remains, the patient may complain of frequency and inadequate emptying and a urinary tract infection may supervene.

Urgency and frequency are found in association with cystocele and its correction may relieve these symptoms, although not invariably. It is therefore unwise to perform a repair operation just for these symptoms, especially without the exclusion of other causes of urgency and frequency (e.g. detrusor instability) beforehand. It is important to realize that a patient with incontinence may develop frequency and urgency as a self-induced habit to keep the bladder empty. The patient voids at frequent intervals, believing that incontinence is better controlled if the bladder is kept as empty as possible. From time to time while endeavouring unsuccessfully to find a toilet, she may experience urgency. If this pattern is repeated, urgency becomes an established symptom. Certainly these symptoms are often linked and cure of one may lead to cure of both (Stanton et al 1976).

Uterine descent

Uterine descent may cause low backache which is relieved by lying flat or temporarily using a ring pessary to support the prolapse. A patient with procidentia may complain of protrusion of the cervix and a blood-stained, sometimes purulent vaginal discharge.

Enterocele or vault prolapse

An enterocele or vault prolapse may produce only vague symptoms of vaginal discomfort. Since an enterocele is often associated with other prolapse, it can be difficult to ascribe separate symptoms to it. Rarely, dehiscence of the vault may occur and the patient complains of acute pain; small bowel may be seen at the vulva (Fig. 31.6). This can strangulate and is an acute abdominal emergency.

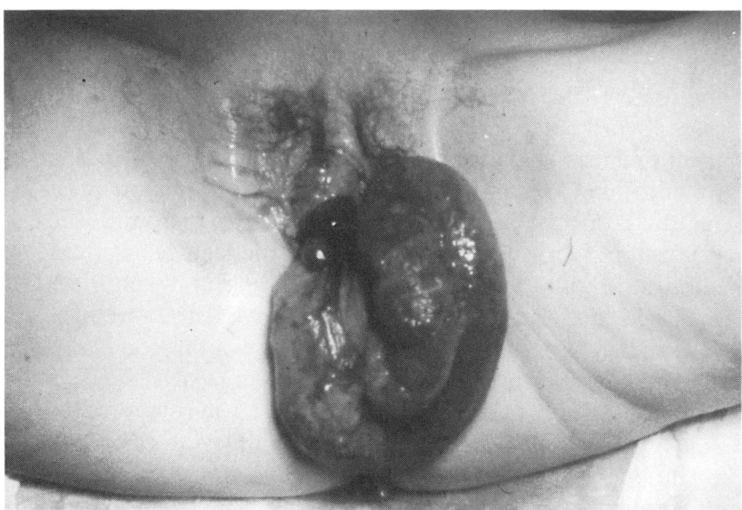

Fig. 31.6 Dehiscence of the vault and presentation of small bowel at the vulva.

Rectocele

This gives rise to symptoms of backache, a lump in the vagina and incomplete bowel emptying; the patient may have discovered that digital reduction of the rectocele allows completion of bowel action.

Signs

Certain predisposing conditions to prolapse such as chronic cough and constipation may be present. A patient complaining of prolapse should be examined in the lithotomy or left lateral position using a Sims' speculum. Stress incontinence is most likely to be demonstrated if the bladder is full. The patient is asked to cough or bear down and any anterior wall prolapse or uterine descent will be demonstrated by retracting the posterior vaginal wall. Sometimes the patient may have to stand up to show prolapse or stress incontinence. Enterocele and rectocele can be demonstrated by using the speculum to retract the anterior vaginal wall. If the rectocele protrudes and obscures an enterocele, it can be reduced by the examining finger and an enterocele will be either seen at the tip of the examining finger or felt as an impulse on coughing. Further differentiation can be made by asking the patient to cough while the rectum and vagina are simultaneously examined. If the cervix protrudes outside the vagina, it may be ulcerated and hypertrophied, with thickening of the epithelium and keratinization. Carcinoma of the cervix is not a sequel to long-standing procidentia but may be a coincidental finding. A full pelvic examination should always be performed to exclude a pelvic mass that might cause prolapse.

Differential diagnosis

A variety of conditions can mimic prolapse of the anterior of the vaginal wall, such as congenital anterior vaginal wall cyst (e.g. remnant of the mesonephric duct system or Gartner's duct), a urethral diverticulum, metastases from a uterine tumour (e.g. choriocarcinoma or adenocarcinoma) and an inclusion dermoid cyst following trauma or surgery. Procidentia can be confused with a large cervical or endometrial polyp or chronic uterine inversion.

INVESTIGATION

A mid-stream specimen of urine should be sent for culture and sensitivity before any treatment is undertaken. When urinary symptoms are present, cystometry and uroflowmetry are advisable. If frequency is a nuisance, a urinary diary should be completed, early-morning urine sent for acid-fast bacilli culture and cystoscopy under general anaesthesia to assess bladder capacity may be required. If there is a procidentia, a renal ultrasound scan and blood urea are necessary.

TREATMENT

It is important to ensure that the woman's symptoms are caused by prolapse and not by other pelvic or spinal conditions. The patient should be told that provided there is no urinary tract obstruction or infection, prolapse carries no risk to life. It is preferable to have completed childbearing because a successful pelvic floor repair can be disrupted by a further vaginal delivery. Coital activity must be taken into account and narrowing of the vagina carefully avoided. Obese patients should be referred to a dietician for dietary control and chronic cough and constipation should be corrected as far as possible. Ulceration of the cervix (after first excluding any neoplastic lesion) may be managed by reducing the uterine prolapse and applying oestrogen cream, if not contraindicated. The ulcer will usually heal within 7 days.

Prevention

Shortening the first and particularly second stage of delivery with an increase in operative intervention and a decline in parity are likely to decrease the incidence of prolapse. The role of episiotomy is uncertain and controversial. Postnatal exercises have little proven scientific evidence to support their benefit but are traditionally advised. Hormone replacement therapy given at the time of menopause may help prevent development of postmenopausal prolapse but is unlikely to alter established prolapse.

Medical

Before safe anaesthesia and surgery, prolapse was managed by a variety of ingenious pessaries of differing shapes and sizes. Today the role of the pessary is more restricted and is indicated below.

1. During and after pregnancy (awaiting involution of tissues).
2. As a therapeutic test to confirm that surgery might help.
3. When the patient has not completed her child-bearing, or is medically unfit or refuses surgery and prefers conservative management.
4. For relief of symptoms while the patient is awaiting surgery.

Older pessaries were made of vulcanized rubber and had to be changed every 3 months. Today the modern pessary is made of inert plastic and can be left in place for up to a year provided there are not adverse symptoms or signs. The most common pessary is ring-shaped and is available in a variety of sizes. Shelf pessaries are also helpful. The two main complications are vaginal ulceration (if the pessary is too large or there is loss of vaginal sensation) and incarceration leading to vaginal discharge and bleeding (when the pessary has been forgotten and not changed for several years).

When prolapse occurs during pregnancy, reposition of the prolapse and insertion of a ring pessary with additional vaginal packing if necessary and bedrest may be sufficient.

Physiotherapy and electrical stimulation of pelvic floor muscles have a minor role in the management of established prolapse.

Surgical

The surgical repair of prolapse is one of the oldest gynaecological procedures, dating back to the 19th century. The majority of operations are performed through the vagina and the abdominal route is reserved for recurrence. The aims of surgery are to correct the prolapse, to maintain continence and to preserve coital function.

Cystourethrocele

Traditionally an anterior colporrhaphy or anterior repair corrects cystocele or cystourethrocele and stress incontinence. Nowadays it is less frequently used for stress incontinence, because it has a lowered success rate compared to urethrovesical suspension procedures. The essential features are a vertical anterior vaginal wall incision and dissection to display the proximal two-thirds of the urethra, the urethrovesical junction and part of the bladder base. The urethrovesical junction is repositioned higher in

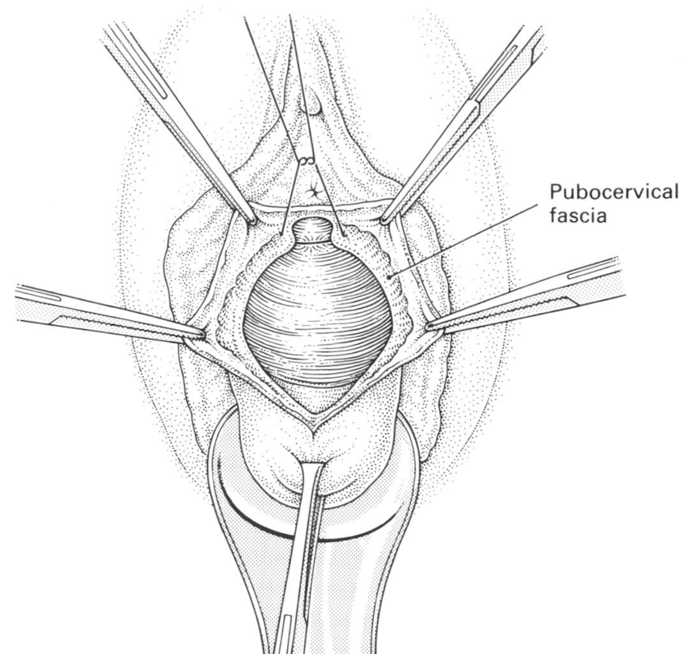

Fig. 31.7 Fascial repair in an anterior colporrhaphy.

the pelvis using one or two Kelly sutures (Fig. 31.7). The cystocele is then reduced by insertion of several interrupted sutures in the overlying pubocervical fascia which is found attached to the underside of the vaginal skin. Surplus vaginal skin is excised and the wound closed with an interrupted or continuous suture.

There are many variations on this procedure. Pacey (1949) emphasized the importance of locating the edge of the pubococcygeal muscle and coapting this in the midline. Ingelman-Sundberg (1946) advocated cutting the pubococcygeal muscle behind the mid-point and uniting the anterior portion in the midline to form a further support for the bladder neck, whilst laterally fixing the posterior portion of the muscle.

Approximately 50% of patients will encounter urinary retention following an anterior repair, so many gynaecologists now use a suprapubic catheter. This allows the patient to void spontaneously and is more comfortable and less prone to urinary infection than a urethral catheter. The catheter is clamped on the second postoperative day and removed when the patient is voiding amounts greater than 200 ml with a residual urine volume of less than 150 ml.

One of the most important complications that can occur following an anterior colporrhaphy is the development of incontinence in a patient who was hitherto dry. It is said to be due to correction of the cystocele and removal of the valve mechanism present at the bladder neck. I think this is unlikely and that incontinence is more likely to be caused by interference with the sphincter mechanism during dissection leading to inadequate support and elevation of that region.

If the cystocele coexists with a first- or second-degree uterine prolapse and a rectocele, a Manchester repair can be performed. This is an older procedure and less commonly used today. It consists of amputation of the cervix, and an anterior and posterior repair. Its disadvantages are:

1. The uterus is left behind, and this can prolapse further or may contain unsuspected disease, or be the future site for a carcinoma. Bonnar et al (1970) found unsuspected lesions in 26% of uteri removed at hysterectomy for prolapse.
2. It does not effectively allow enteroceles to be corrected.

The Burch colposuspension can correct very effectively a cystocele, where this is complicated by the presence of stress incontinence due to urethral sphincter incompetence (Burch 1961; Fig. 31.8). The lateral fornices are approximated and sutured to the ipsilateral iliopectineal ligaments, producing elevation of the bladder neck and reduction of a cystourethrocele (Stanton et al 1976; Stanton & Cardozo 1979). Enterocele formation is a complication of this procedure.

Uterine prolapse

The vaginal hysterectomy is the preference today for correction of uterine prolapse unless the patient wishes to conserve the uterus in which case a Manchester operation can be performed.

The vaginal hysterectomy can be combined with an anterior or posterior colporrhaphy and correction of an enterocele by coaptation of the uterosacral ligaments is usually accomplished. Indeed most surgeons carry out prophylactic coaptation of these ligaments at the time of hysterectomy to avoid a future enterocele and vault prolapse.

A vaginal hysterectomy is indicated:

1. For uterine prolapse where the uterus is smaller than 14 weeks in size (a larger uterus can be removed by morcellation).
2. For recurrent uterine prolapse following a Manchester repair.
3. When the patient is obese. Pitkin (1976) has shown that abdominal wound complications are seven times more common in women weighing more than 90 kg who have undergone abdominal hysterectomy. With a vaginal hysterectomy, there is no difference in morbidity or length of stay when comparing obese women and those of normal weight (Pitkin 1977).
4. Where a painful abdominal wound is undesirable and early ambulation is advantageous (e.g. in pulmonary disease or the elderly).
5. Where non-malignant uterine pathology (e.g. dysfunctional uterine bleeding) exists and where it is technically feasible to remove the uterus.

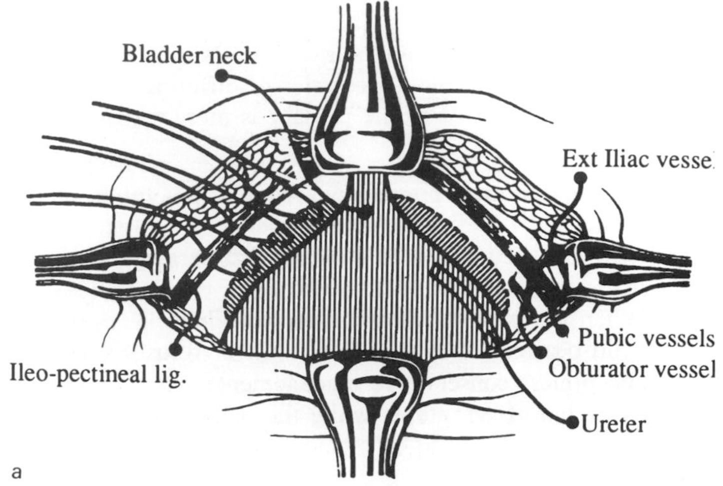

a

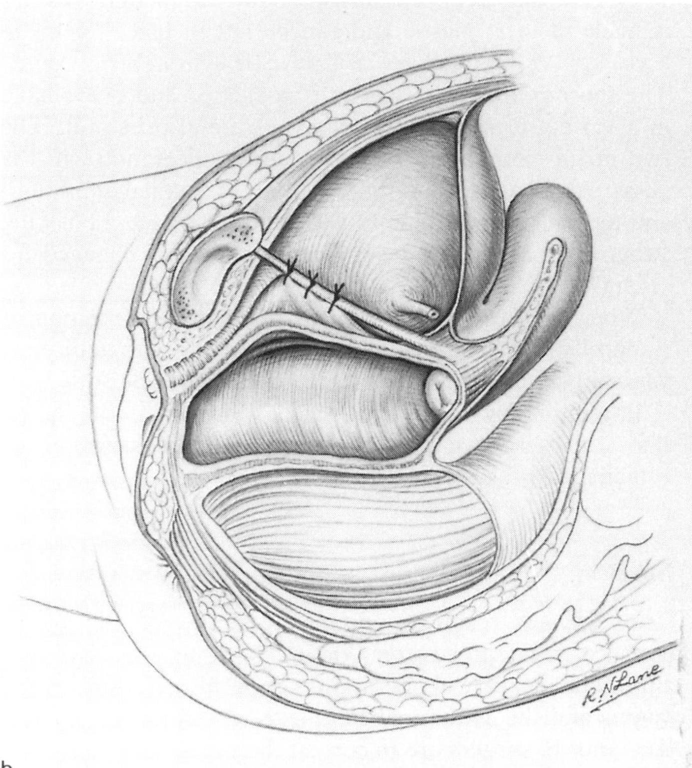

b

Fig. 31.8 Burch colposuspension. **a** Plan view; **b** sagittal view at the end of the procedure.

The assessment for vaginal hysterectomy is important. The subpubic arch should be sufficiently wide to accommodate two fingers which will allow the operator access to the uterus. There should be sufficient vaginal capacity to allow surgery to be carried out and clinical experience, with the help of an episiotomy, will determine this. Unless morcellation is intended, the uterus should not be larger than 14 weeks in size. It is wise to avoid vaginal hysterectomy, where there is likelihood of bowel adhering to the fundus of the uterus, following previous pelvic surgery or where ventrosuspension has been performed.

The principles of vaginal hysterectomy include careful upward displacement of the bladders and ureters, ligation of each main pedicle and repair of any enterocele. The ovaries are inspected and if there is ovarian pathology or the woman is over 50 years of age, vaginal oophorectomy can be easily accomplished at the same time (Sheth 1991). The pedicles are then approximated to each other in pairs to reform the roof of the vault. The uterosacral ligaments are united and the vaginal skin closed, first securing the posterior fornix skin to the new vault. If a vaginal hysterectomy alone is performed, bladder drainage is unnecessary.

When the woman wishes to retain her uterus, a uterosacropexy (similar to colposacropexy) is performed. The junction of the cervix and uterus is attached to the anterior longitudinal ligament over the first sacral vertebra by inorganic tissue such as Terylene, which should then be peritonealized.

Enterocele or vault repair

Most enteroceles can be repaired at the time of abdominal surgery, by coaptation of the uterosacral ligaments. The more extensive procedure described by Moschowitz has the danger of inclusion of a ureter when inserting the pursestring sutures into the pouch of Douglas peritoneum, and as there is little inherent strength in this peritoneum, it seems an unnecessary procedure.

The initial decision to use the vaginal suprapubic route of access depends on the patient's general state and whether or not she wishes to continue intercourse. The vaginal route is simpler, provides a relatively pain-free postoperative recovery but may preclude intercourse if an over-enthusiastic repair is performed. In an older patient, it is frequently impossible to find adequate or convincing uterosacral ligaments to bring together. The sacrospinous fixation operation (Nichols 1982) does not compromise vaginal size, but the surgery is carried out under limited visibility and damage to pudendal vessels is a recognized hazard. If intercourse is not intended, it is easier to obliterate the vagina, placing successive pursestring sutures to include the uterosacral ligaments and then the levator ani and finally the superficial perineal muscles.

Where there is recurrent prolapse and intercourse is intended, most clinicians prefer the abdominal route. With the colposacropexy (Birnbaum 1973; Fig. 31.9) the vault is attached by a non-absorbable mesh (Terylene or Teflon) to the anterior longitudinal ligament of the first sacral vertebra. Care has to be taken here because of the venous plexus in front of this ligament. The mesh is peritonealized, to avoid bowel becoming trapped underneath it.

If the enterocele or vault prolapse is recurrent, Zacharin's (1985) vaginal repair of enterocele can be carried out (Fig. 31.10). This is an extensive synchronous abdominal and vaginal procedure. The levator muscles are exposed from above and enterocele is dissected out from below. The abdominal surgeon identifies both ureters. The levator hiatus is closed and the vagina reformed and sutured to the levator plate, to re-establish vaginal function and permit intercourse.

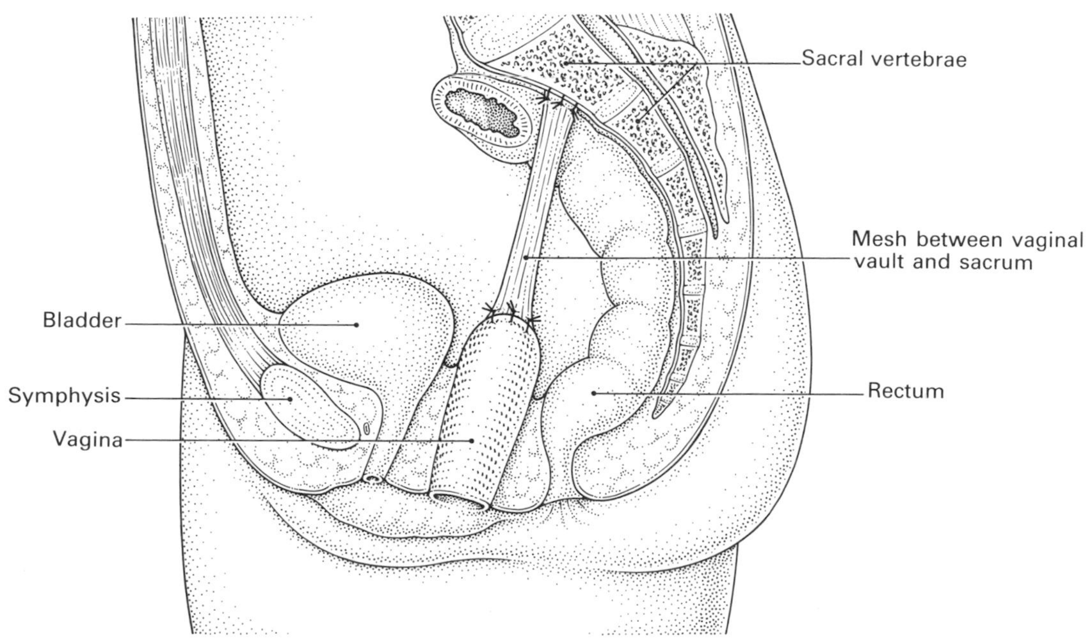

Fig. 31.9 Colposacropexy.

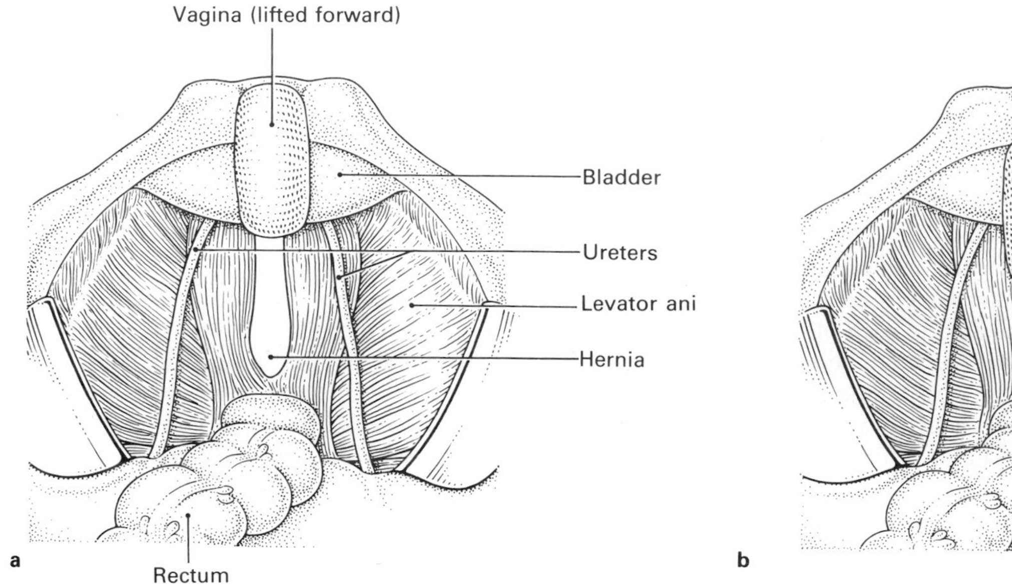

Fig. 31.10 Zacharin (1985) enterocele repair.

These procedures were critically reviewed by Wall & Stanton (1988).

Rectocele

Some clinicians maintain that the pelvic floor repair or correction of incontinence by anterior colporrhaphy is incomplete without the addition of a posterior colporrhapy. Jeffcoate (1959) showed in a group of women who had an anterior and posterior repair that 30% had apareunia or severe dyspareunia. In a later paper, Francis & Jeffcoate (1961) incriminated the posterior colporrhaphy as the main cause for this and showed that omission of the posterior colporrhaphy did not compromise the result of prolapse repair. It is reasonable therefore to restrict this operation only to patients with symptomatic and demonstrable rectocele, or those who have a small rectocele and are due to have a colposuspension, which often aggravates posterior wall prolapse.

The technique of posterior colporrhaphy involves dissection of the levator ani muscles and rectum via a vertical posterior vaginal wall incision. The levator muscles and then the superficial perineal muscles are sutured together; any excess vagina skin is cautiously excised and the wound closed with a continuous locking stitch to avoid vaginal wall shortening.

Bladder drainage may be required especially in elderly patients because they often take longer to resume spontaneous micturition following pelvic surgery.

To minimize the risk of postoperative infection by anaerobic organisms, 1 g metronidazole is given rectally 2 h prior to surgery. Prophylactic subcutaneous heparin against deep vein thrombosis should be employed if the patient is over 35 years of age, obese, a heavy smoker or has a past history of deep vein thrombosis.

CONCLUSION

Prolapse (and its surgical correction) is a common gynaecological entity. The number of neighbouring structures that can be involved render it a complicated condition to assess and treat adequately. The clinician must be aware of the important association of urological symptoms and should carefully investigate them and decide whether abdominal or vaginal surgery is more appropriate.

KEY POINTS

1. Prolapse is benign except when third-degree uterine prolapse may be associated with ureteric obstruction.
2. Prolapse is due to denervation associated with childbirth, collagen weakness and oestrogen deficiency at the menopause.
3. Only about 50% of patients with a cystourethrocele have stress incontinence.
4. A large enterocele may require prompt surgery as vault dehiscence with extrusion of bowel can occur.
5. Surgery is the most usual form of treatment for prolapse and should be deferred until childbearing and vaginal delivery have been completed.
6. The anterior repair is a reliable cure for a cystourethrocele but is unreliable for the correction of stress incontinence.

REFERENCES

Allen R, Hosker G, Smith A Pelvic floor damage and childbirth: a neurophysiological study. British Journal of Obstetrics and Gynaecology 97: 770–779

Birnbaum S J 1973 Rational therapy for the prolapsed vagina. American Journal of Obstetrics and Gynecology 115: 41–419

Bonnar J, Kraszewski A, Davis W 1970 Incidental pathology at vaginal hysterectomy for genital prolapse. British Journal of Obstetrics and Gynaecology 77: 1137–1139

Burch J C 1961 Urethro-vaginal fixation to Cooper's ligament for correction of stress incontinence. American Journal of Obstetrics and Gynecology 100: 768–774

Francis W, Jeffcoate T N A 1961 Dyspareunia following vaginal operations. British Journal of Obstetrics and Gynaecology 68: 1–10

Gosling J 1981 Why are women continent? Proceedings of symposium 'The incontinent woman'. Royal College of Obstetricians and Gynaecologists, London

Hawksworth W, Roux J 1958 Vaginal hysterectomy. British Journal of Obstetrics and Gynaecology 65: 214–228

Ingelman-Sundberg A 1946 Operative technique in stress incontinence of urine in the female. Nordisk Medicine 32: 2297–2299

Jeffcoate T N A 1959 Posterior colpoperineorrhaphy. American Journal of Obstetrics and Gynecology 773: 490–502

Jeffcoate T N A 1967 Principles of gynaecology, 3rd edn. Butterworths, London

Keettel W C 1941 Prolapse of the uterus during pregnancy. American Journal of Obstetrics and Gynecology 42: 121–126

Lewis A C 1968 Major gynaecological surgery in the elderly. Journal of the International Federation of Gynaecology and Obstetrics 6: 244–258

Nichols D 1982 Sacrospinous fixation for massive eversion of the vagina. American Journal of Obstetrics and Gynecology 142: 901–904

Pacey K 1949 Pathology and repair of genital prolapse. Journal of Obstetrics and Gynaecology of the British Empire 56: 1–15

Pitkin R M 1976 Abdominal hysterectomy in obese women. Surgery, Gynecology and Obstetrics 142: 532–536

Pitkin R M 1977 Vaginal hysterectomy in obese women. Obstetrics and Gynecology 49: 567–569

Sayer T, Dixon J, Hosker G, Warrell D 1990 A study of paraurethral connective tissue in women with stress uncontinence of urine. Neurourology and Urodynamics 9: 319–320

Sheth S 1991 Place of oophorectomy at vaginal hysterectomy. British Journal of Obstetrics and Gynaecology 98: 662–666

Snooks S, Swash M, Henry M, Setchell M 1984 Injury to innervation of the pelvic floor musculature in childbirth. Lancet ii: 546–550

Stallworthy J A 1971 Prolapse. British Medical Journal 1: 499–500, 539–540

Stanton S L, Cardozo L D 1979 Results of colposuspension operation for incontinence and prolapse. British Journal of Obstetrics and Gynaecology 86: 693–697

Stanton S L, Williams J E, Ritchie D 1976 Colposuspension operation or urinary incontinence. British Journal of Obstetrics and Gynaecology 83: 890–895

Swash M 1984 Ano-rectal incontinence: electrophysiological tests. British Journal of Surgery (suppl): S14–S22

Wall L, Stanton S L 1988 Alternatives for repair of post hysterectomy vault prolapse and enterocele. Contemporary Obstetrics and Gynecology Sept. 32–48

Zacharin R 1985 Pelvic floor anatomy and the surgery of pulsion enterocele. Springer Verlag, Vienna

SECTION 4

Oncology

32. The epidemiology of gynaecological cancers

N. E. Day

The principal aim of studying the epidemiology of a cancer is to understand how prevention might be effected, both through the identification of the factors responsible for the differences in risk across populations and population subgroups and by rigorous evaluation of mass screening modalities.

GENERAL OVERVIEW

This chapter will consider the epidemiology of cancer of the ovary, the cervix uteri and the corpus uteri. On a global basis, cancer of the cervix is the second most common cancer in women after breast cancer, accounting for about 15% of all cancers in women; it was estimated that in 1980 some 500 000 cases occurred worldwide (Parkin et al 1988). In many developing countries, notably in Africa and Latin America, cervical cancer is the most common cancer among women. Cancer of the ovary and endometrium are seldom more than the fifth or sixth most common cancers either in developed or developing countries.

Table 32.1 gives an overview of the frequency of these different cancers throughout the world, expressed in terms of the probability (as a percentage) of developing the cancer before age 75, given that death has not intervened earlier. A 15–20-fold variation is seen for both cervical and endometrial cancer; ovarian cancer, in contrast, shows only a two- to threefold variation in risk. As will be described

Table 32.1 Probability of developing cancer at different locations before age 75 in selected populations across the world

	Cervix uteri (%)	Corpus uteri (%)	Ovary (%)
Brazil — Recife	7.7	0.8	0.6
Colombia — Cali	5.3	0.7	0.9
Puerto Rico	1.6	1.0	0.7
Canada			
British Columbia	0.9	1.9	1.2
Manitoba	1.5	2.5	1.5
USA			
Detroit — Black	1.9	1.2	1.0
— White	0.9	2.7	1.4
Iowa	0.9	2.4	1.4
San Francisco — Chinese	1.3	1.6	0.9
China — Shanghai	1.1	0.4	0.5
Hong Kong	2.6	0.8	0.6
India			
Bombay	2.2	0.2	0.8
Madras	4.7	0.2	0.5
Israel — all Jews	0.4	1.2	1.4
Japan — Osaka	1.8	0.3	0.5
Singapore			
Chinese	1.9	0.6	0.9
Malay	1.2	0.5	1.0
Indian	3.1	0.4	0.4
Denmark	1.9	1.9	1.7
Finland	0.7	1.5	1.1
France - Lière	1.4	1.2	0.9
GDR	2.5	1.7	1.4
Norway			
Urban	1.9	1.5	1.7
Rural	1.3	1.4	1.7
Spain — Zaragoza	0.6	0.9	0.6
UK			
South Thames	0.9	1.1	1.3
Mersey	1.7	0.9	1.3
Scotland	1.2	0.8	1.3
New Zealand			
Maori	2.9	1.7	1.0
Non-Maori	1.2	1.2	1.2

From Muir et al (1987).

later, the variation in risk for cervical cancer is explicable in terms of differing levels of risk behaviour and mass screening across populations, indicating how both primary and secondary prevention are feasible. For endometrial cancer, worldwide variation in risk demonstrates a major role for environmental and lifestyle factors, and hence the potential for primary prevention; unfortunately specific factors have not yet been delineated precisely enough for intervention measures to be identified. For cancer of the ovary, the global pattern of risk is too amorphous to suggest where preventive efforts might be effective.

Mortality rates for cancer of the cervix and endometrium are not helpful for comparisons of risk on an international basis, since mortality statistics often fail to distinguish between these two subsites of the uterus, and deaths are often attributed to cancer of the uterus not otherwise specified. Failure to recognize this limitation of mortality statistics can lead to some gross errors in their interpretation.

CERVICAL CANCER

Age aspects and time trends

The major factors which affect the epidemiology of cervical cancer in a population are the level of sexual activity and the degree of effective mass screening. In populations without mass screening and with incidence rates relatively constant over time, the change in incidence with age follows a typical pattern, rising rapidly in the age-span 25–40 years, before which it is rare; the incidence then reaches a plateau and may even begin to decline in the sixth and seventh decades of life and later. Figure 32.1 gives data from Norway, displaying this typical pattern.

Departures from this pattern would normally indicate changing patterns of screening or of sexual lifestyle. Illustrating this phenomenon are data from the Birmingham Cancer Registry from 1960 to 1982 (Fig. 32.2). A rapid increase in the 25–34 age group, a marked decline in the 40–54 age group and stability in the rates over age 55 reflect the upsurge in sexual activity among younger women in the 1960s and the introduction of systematic screening activity in the middle-age range. Before screening became widespread in the UK, considerable variation in the rates of cervical cancer among birth cohorts could be closely related to the infection rates of sexually transmitted diseases among these cohorts (Beral 1974).

In Scandinavia, the major change in both incidence and mortality rates since the late 1950s can be closely linked to the different approaches in the five different countries to the introduction of mass screening (Hakama 1982; Laara et al 1987; Fig. 32.3). Finland and Iceland introduced nationwide mass screening in the mid 1960s, Denmark and Sweden introduced screening in a few counties in the mid to late 1960s with coverage extending later, and in Norway organized screening was confined to one county.

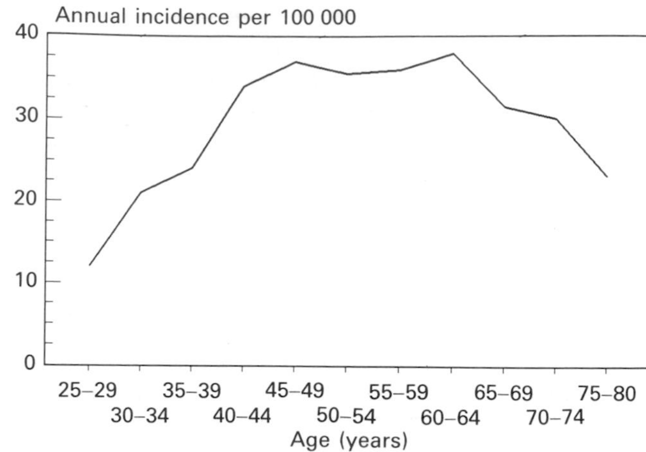

Fig. 32.1 The incidence of cervical cancer in an unscreened population in which the rate is not changing with time (Muir et al 1987).

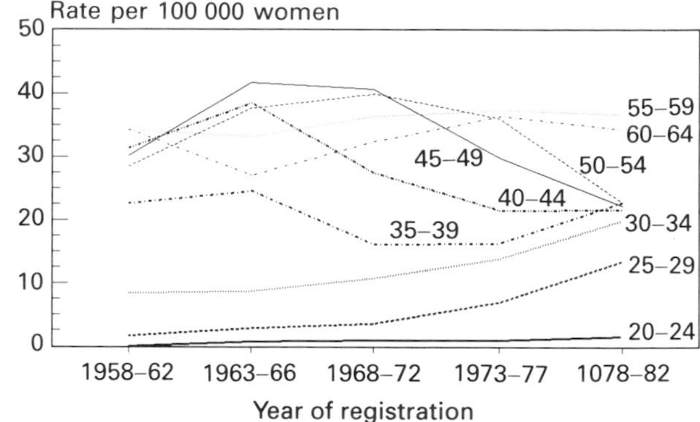

Fig. 32.2 Changing incidence rates in different age groups as a result of screening activity and changes in the underlying prevalence. These data are from the Birmingham Cancer Registry.

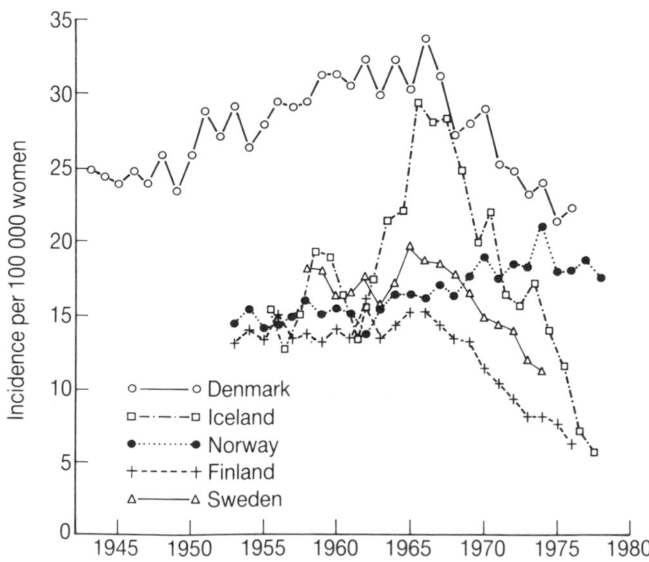

Fig. 32.3 The effect of different screening policies on changing rates of cervical cancer in the Nordic countries. Modified from Hakama (1982).

It is of interest to note that in countries where cervical cancer is common, it is commoner in 25–34-year-old women than any other cancer in any other country in the world (Muir et al 1987). This demonstrates the extraordinary sensitivity of the tissues of the cervix to the oncogenicity related to early sexual activity. The plateauing of the rates after age 40 is analogous to the evolution of lung cancer risk among ex-smokers and suggests that in the third and fourth decade of life either cervical tissue loses its sensitivity or exposure is largely reduced.

In the UK the incidence of several sexually transmitted diseases appears to have declined since the start of the AIDS epidemic (Johnson & Gill 1989). This decline might be expected to reverse the increasing trend of cervical cancer seen in young women.

Aetiological factors

It has been recognized for many years that the major risk factors of cervical cancer relate to sexual activity, as exemplified by the high rates seen among prostitutes and the virtual absence of the disease among nuns. Other exposures which have been proposed as risk factors for cervical cancer include cigarette smoking, oral contraception, immunosuppression and dietary factors.

Sexual activity

The two main behavioural aspects of sexual activity which modify risk for the disease are age at first intercourse and the number of sexual partners (Table 32.2). The effect of age at first intercourse has suggested to some authors that young cervical tissue is more sensitive to oncogenic change; an alternative and simple explanation would derive from multistage models of carcinogenesis. Many epithelial cancers exhibit a risk which increases with some high power (about 4) of either duration of exposure or time since first exposure. This behaviour would imply a difference in risk of two- to threefold between women starting sexual activity at 16 as opposed to those starting at age 21, in line with the results shown in Table 32.2.

Both of these factors point to the role of a sexually transmitted agent; further support is given to this hypothesis by the apparent high risk for monogamous women whose male partner has had many sexual partners. A later section discusses the agent most likely to be the specific aetiological factor.

Table 32.2 Relative risk for cervical cancer associated with factors reflecting sexual lifestyle after adjustment for other sexual factors, smoking, number of births and Pap smears

Number of sexual partners	Relative risk	Age at first intercourse	Relative risk
1	1.0	>21	1.0
2	1.5	20–21	1.9
3–4	2.2	18–19	2.2
5+	2.8	<18	2.5

Modified from Brinton et al (1987).

Transmissible agents

The viruses on which attention is now focused are the human papillomaviruses (HPV), particularly HPV16 and 18. Previously, herpes simplex virus type 2 (HSV2) had been extensively investigated but neither the epidemiological nor the experimental data relating HSV2 to cervical cancer have proved convincing (Munos & Bosch 1989).

Evidence for the role of HPV16 and 18 is still accumulating and must be considered not definitive yet. A major problem has been the different sensitivities and specifications of the laboratory techniques used to identify the presence of the virus. A recent monograph (Munos et al 1989) reviews the position and the results available at the end of 1988. The introduction of polymerase chain reaction techniques, with their greatly enhanced sensitivity, is in the process of changing the picture completely. It is certainly plausible to speculate that in the near future definitive evidence will emerge that HPV, particularly types 16 and 18, is the dominant cause of cervical cancer. The perspective for primary prevention would then be radically changed.

Smoking

A large number of studies have found a higher incidence of cervical cancer among smokers than among nonsmokers. The IARC concluded that although there was considerable consistency among the studies, a causal role for tobacco smoking in the development of cervical cancer could not be inferred (IARC 1986a). The problem is that of confounding, basic to epidemiological data founded on observational studies. Smoking is known to be related to sexual activity and many sexually transmitted diseases are two to three times more frequent in smokers than nonsmokers. In order to examine the relationship of smoking to cervical cancer, one has first to remove the effect of the specific sexually related aetiological factor (i.e. the transmissible agent) which at present is impossible to do since the identity of the agent is unknown (see later section). If one adjusts for some surrogate variable such as number of sexual partners, one will have a very inefficient control of confounding (Tzonou et al 1986). It will not be until the specific transmissible agent has been unequivocally identified and correct adjustment has been made for it that the role of smoking can be unambiguously addressed.

Oral contraception

Studies relating oral contraception to cervical cancer risk suffer from the same problem of interpretation, with oral contraception use related both to level of sexual activity and to the risk of infection by a sexually transmissible agent. The increased risk for cervical cancer seen among women who take oral contraceptives cannot at present be taken to indicate a causal role for oral contraceptive use.

Immunosuppression

An increased risk of cervical cancer has been seen among women given immunosuppressive therapy following renal transplant (Hoover 1977). A similar increase is seen in women following treatment for Hodgkin's disease (Kaldor et al 1987), where both the original malignancy and the therapy (both radiotherapy and chemotherapy) could have been immunosuppressive.

Dietary factors

There is some evidence that diets low in beta-carotene or vitamin C can lead to higher cervical cancer risk. The data come from retrospective questionnaire studies and so suffer from the recognized deficiencies of this method of data collection. Moreover, cigarette smoking and a diet low in fruit and fresh vegetables are often positively associated, so that there is scope for considerable confounding (Munos & Bosch 1989).

Screening for cervical cancer

The use of cervical cytology to identify precancerous lesions in healthy, asymptomatic women, as opposed to its use for diagnostic purposes, was introduced in the USA and parts of Scandinavia in the 1950s. Clinical enthusiasm for the discovery of early lesions outran the quality of evidence demonstrating that mass screening could reduce morbidity and mortality from the invasive disease, with the result that its application was often not within a proper epidemiological context (e.g. the target population was undefined; uptake rates were incorrectly estimated by being based on slides read rather than on women screened). Consequently, population benefits were often not achieved.

In some populations, notably much of Scandinavia and parts of Scotland (Day 1984), the organization of cervical cytology services had a public health rather than a clinical orientation and the effect on rates of the disease was impressive. Falls of 60% or more in both death and incidence rates from the disease were seen in, for example, Finland, Iceland and the Grampian region of Scotland (Hakama 1982; MacGregor et al 1986; Laara et al 1987). The basic question now with cervical cancer screening is how, using current knowledge of the natural history of the disease, population-based screening can be optimally effected within the health care delivery system of the respective population.

The natural history can be represented in simplistic terms:

Normal epithelium → Atypia detectable by cervical cytology → Ivasive cancer

The classification of atypia has changed frequently and depends on whether it is based on histological or cytological grounds. Carcinoma-in-situ, dysplasia and cervical intraepithelial neoplasia (CIN) are descriptions of tissue, not of individual cells, and so should refer only to a histological specimen. Much discussion has centred on the nature of the CIN lesions, to what extent they progress, how rapidly, and whether CIN I, or even CIN II is a genuine precursor state or simply an indicator of a high-risk individual. It appears undeniable that too many CIN lesions are found for them all to progress to malignancy, and that the rate of regression is higher for CIN I than for CIN II. It is also apparent that the great majority of squamous invasive cancers (which constitute 90% or more of invasive cancers in unscreened populations, although the introduction of the term 'adenosquamous' is a complicating factor) pass through a stage in which atypia could be detected cytologically.

The question of how long they remain in this preinvasive, detectable stage was investigated in an international study co-ordinated by the IARC (1986b). A number of centralized screening centres in Europe and Canada identified women who had developed cervical cancer after at least one normal cytological smear. Incidence rates (or relative incidence rates) were calculated for invasive cancer in terms of the years that had elapsed since the last negative smear, and the number of previous negative smears. These rates were expressed as a proportion of the rate observed in the absence of screening and so expressed the reduction in risk produced by screening. These are in fact the proportions of lesions that progress from normality to invasion in that number of years, or less. The results are given in Table 32.3. They clearly indicate that screening every 3 years is virtually as effective as screening every year (Table

Table 32.3 The reduction in risk of cervical cancer among women who have had at least two normal cytological smears

Time since last negative smear (in months)	Relative risk
<12	0.07
12–23	0.08
24–35	0.13
36–47	0.19
48–59	0.31
60–71	0.31
72–119	0.63
120+	1.0

Table 32.4 Percentage reduction in cumulative risk of invasive cervical cancer in the age range 35–64, with different screening frequencies

Screening frequency (in years)	% Reduction in cumulative risk	No of tests in 35–64 age range
1	93.3	30
2	93.3	15
3	91.4	10
5	83.9	6
10	64.2	3

32.4). The only justification for annual screening is to compensate for inadequacies in the screening process which are better rectified by direct action. The joint UICC–IARC monograph on cervical screening concluded that:

> The main unknown question concerning cervical screening at present relates to the treatment of early atypical lesions, many of which will regress. Markers which identified the lesions which would progress would be of great utility, both in avoiding unnecessary treatment and in preventing undue delay in treatment. Use of HPV markers for this purpose appears a promising line of research.

Conclusions

Cervical tissue is highly sensitive to the carcinogenic action of sexual contact, a sensitivity which shows itself in the unusually high rates seen in young women — higher than the rates for any other malignancy in that age group — and in the large differences among populations. Enough is known at present for primary prevention to be possible; the probable identification of subtypes of HPV as the principal aetiological agent suggests that, before long, primary prevention will be feasible as well as possible. Secondary prevention by cytological screening has been demonstrated to be effective on a population basis, the extent of effect seen in different populations reflecting the appropriateness of the organization.

OVARIAN CANCER

The overall variation throughout the world in rates for ovarian cancer is less than for any other of the more common malignancies (Table 32.1). The highest rates are seen in Scandinavia and the lowest in Asian populations, but the range is little more than threefold. Differences are minor between, for example, blacks and whites in the USA or urban and rural populations in Europe.

A range of different cancers are classified as of ovarian origin. In women under 30 years of age, germ cell tumours, teratomas and dysgerminomas are seen, but over the age of 30 the great majority of ovarian malignancies are adenocarcinomas. Most of the following discussion refers to the last group. These have been extensively subclassified (serous, mucinous and endometrioid being the major types) but there is little evidence that different histological subtypes behave differently epidemiologically. They will be treated as a single entity.

Age aspects and time trends

The age distribution of ovarian cancer shows a steady rise in incidence to the mid-50s, after which the incidence remains roughly constant (Fig. 32.4). Time trends in incidence in western countries in the last 30 years have not shown any marked variation. Analysis of the Danish Cancer Registry material collected from 1943 to 1982 indicates little change in incidence by years of birth for women born in this century, but a rapid increase in the risk from the 1860–1869 decade of birth cohort to the 1900–1909 birth cohort (Ewertz & Kjaer 1988). Mortality from ovarian cancer in Denmark shows a somewhat different picture with a decrease in risk seen over successive decades of birth from 1910 to 1950. This decrease appears related to survival, with an improving stage at diagnosis being seen for younger women.

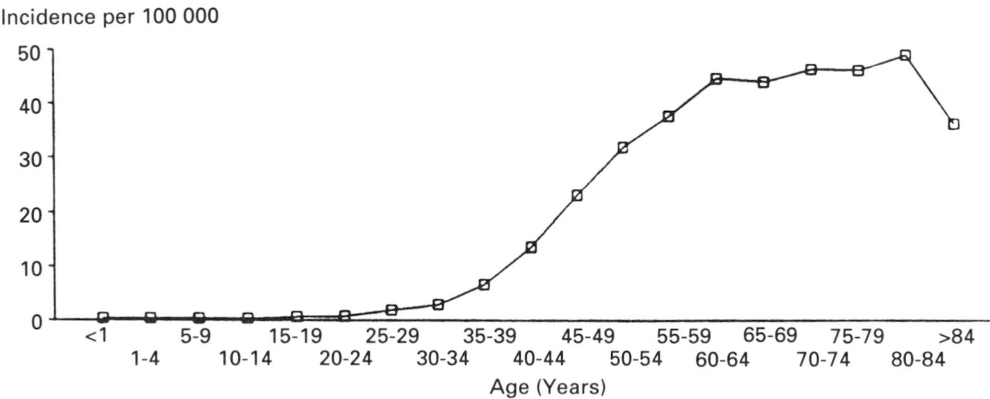

Fig. 32.4 The age-specific incidence of ovarian cancer in England and Wales (Office of Population Censuses and Surveys 1985).

Aetiological factors

The main factors affecting risk for ovarian cancer so far identified have been reproductive, that is parity and use of oral contraceptives. For associated factors, including age at menarche, menopause and first or last birth, the evidence is less clear.

Parity

One of the largest studies to report on parity was a prospective study of 60 565 women in Norway (Kvale et al 1988) among whom 445 cases of ovarian cancer arose in the period 1961 to 1980, of which only 12 were germ cell tumours. The relative risks for parity 0 to parity 5+ are given in Table 32.5, together with the relative effects of age at first birth, age at last birth, age at menarche and age at menopause. Each of these last four factors can be seen to have a negligible effect, a finding in agreement with most previous studies. The effect of parity is clear, however, with a smoothly decreasing risk with increasing parity.

This effect of parity is seen at the population level. Beral et al (1978) examined changes in mortality over time for both England and Wales and the USA on a birth cohort basis. Considerable variation was seen among birth cohorts, virtually all of which could be explained by the average completed family size for each birth cohort (Fig. 32.5). This elegant finding suggests that the relationship with parity is primarily with the number of children a woman chooses to have, rather than an intrinsic child-bearing capacity, and also that other environmental factors that have been changing over time have little role in ovarian cancer. It should be noted that this study refers to cohorts of women who would have used oral contraceptives rarely.

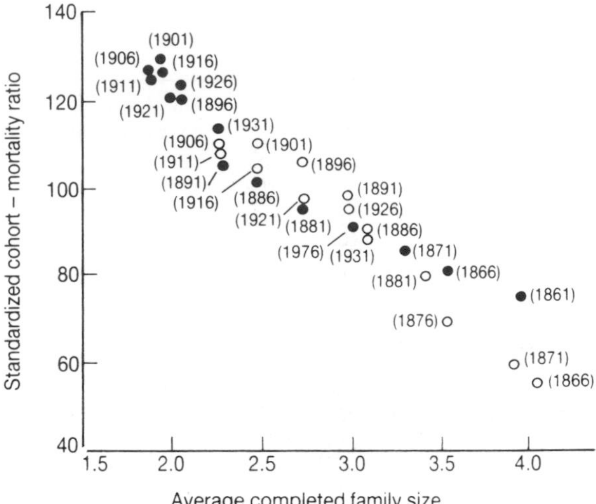

Fig. 32.5 Age-standardized mortality ratios from ovarian carcinoma are plotted against the average completed family size for different generations of women in England and Wales (●) and the USA (○). Each point represents a separate birth cohort with the mid-year of birth shown in brackets. Modified from Beral et al (1978).

Table 32.6 Risk of ovarian cancer with respect to oral contraception use showing the results of a case control study in San Francisco

Oral contraceptive use	Relative risk
Never used	1.0
Ever used	0.74
Duration of use	
1–12 months	0.97
13–36 months	0.81
>36 months	0.40

From Wu et al (1988).

Oral contraception

The second factor associated with reproduction is use of the contraceptive pill. Typical results, from a study in the USA (Wu et al 1988), are given in Table 32.6. Table 32.7 gives the results by number of full-term pregnancies. The effects of parity and of oral contraceptive use are independent of each other, combining in approximately multiplicative fashion. Furthermore, the relative reduction in risk for a given number of years of oral contraceptive use does

Table 32.5 Reproductive risk factors for ovarian cancer showing observed to expected (Obs:Exp) ratios from a prospective study of 425 women in Norway

Parity	Obs:Exp	Age at first birth	Obs:Exp	Age at last birth	Obs:Exp	Age at menarche	Obs:Exp	Age at menopause	Obs:Exp
0	1.50	<20	0.79	<25	1.04	<13	0.95	<46	1.04
1	1.32	20–24	0.98	25–29	0.94	13	0.91	46–47	1.00
2	0.89	25–29	0.93	30–34	1.06	14	1.13	48–49	0.97
3	0.76	30–34	1.30	35–39	0.99	15	0.93	50–51	0.93
4	0.73	>34	0.80	>39	0.97	16	0.93	52–53	1.07
						>16	1.04	>53	1.08

Modified from Kuale et al (1988).

Table 32.7 Relative risk of ovarian cancer by both oral contraceptive use and parity

Months of oral contraceptive use	Number of pregnancies 0	1–2	>3
<12 months or never used	1.00	0.63	0.55
13–36	0.82	0.35	0.68
>36	0.13	0.34	0.23

From Wu et al (1988).

Table 32.8 Risks for ovarian cancer by duration of ovulation results of a case control study in San Francisco

Years of ovulation	Relative risk
<25	1.00
25–29	1.58
30–34	2.48
>34	3.26

From Wu et al (1988).

not diminish after oral contraceptive use ends, but appears to continue indefinitely (although follow-up studies over several decades have not yet been performed).

Years of ovulation

The findings on parity and oral contraceptive use support the hypothesis of Fathalla (1971) that duration of active ovulation is of major importance in determining ovarian cancer risk. The results of the American study were expressed in these terms, as shown in Table 32.8 (Wu et al 1988).

It is of interest to note that one might predict on the basis of multistage models of carcinogenesis that a difference between 25 and 35 years of 'exposure' would generate a difference in risk of $(25/35)^4$ i.e. about fourfold, close to that seen in Table 32.8. The main epidemiological findings in terms of age, parity and oral contraceptive use are explicable if the ovarian epithelium is at risk during the cellular proliferation associated with ovulation but not when the ovary is quiescent.

The lack of effect of age at menarche and age at menopause probably results from the large number of anovulatory cycles around both ages, so that data on onset and cessation of ovulation are very imprecise.

Other environmental factors

Other factors which have been investigated and for which no good evidence exists for an effect on risk (in either direction) include non-contraceptive oestrogens, alcohol and tobacco. Coffee has occasionally been implicated but the data appear weak.

In Singapore, the China-born Chinese have rates similar to those seen in China, whereas the rates in the Singapore-born are nearly twofold higher. Similar changes are seen among Chinese and Japanese migrants to the USA (Lee et al 1988). However, in the overall epidemiological picture, there are no large differences in risk between populations to suggest that major environmental risk factors remain to be identified.

Genetic factors

Genetic factors clearly play an important role in the development of ovarian cancer. In a national study in the UK, based on the 1939 household registration, the risk was substantially elevated among women with a first-degree relative with the disease. The increase in risk was largest if the relative developed the disease under age 50, when the relative risk lay between six- and 10-fold (Ponder et al 1989). If two or more close relatives are affected, the lifetime risk rises to about 40% (as compared with the figures in Table 32.1), much of which occurs before the age of 50. This value of 40% is close to the chance of 50% of inheriting a putative gene. It is thought that perhaps 1% of all cases in the UK may belong to this very high-risk group. The specific gene or genes have not yet been identified.

Screening for ovarian cancer

Attention has been given in the past decade to the development of both immunological and imaging techniques for the early detection of malignancy. Initial small-scale studies have demonstrated that at least some asymptomatic tumours can be detected using either ultrasound screening or a number of tumour markers (primarily CA125; Jacobs & Oram 1989; Scott et al 1989). Until large-scale randomized trials have been conducted, however, there is no justification for including ovarian screening in a national health programme.

Conclusions

Epidemiological studies have not identified major environmental causes, nor do they suggest that factors which could form the focus for intervention studies are likely to be identified in the near future. The only prospect for primary prevention appears to be in the manipulation of ovulation by judicious use of oral contraceptives. Such an approach clearly requires to balance both increased and decreased risk for a range of diseases. There is no immediate prospect of population-based mass screening.

ENDOMETRIAL CANCER

As seen in Table 32.1, the incidence of endometrial cancer varies widely, the lowest rates being seen in Asian populations and the highest among white North American women. It is noteworthy, however, that on migration to the USA, the rates in Asian populations rise very markedly to approach those seen in the local white population. This rise is steeper than for almost any other cancer site. Endometrial cancer is rare until age 35, when it rises to reach a plateau at 55 years (Fig. 32.6).

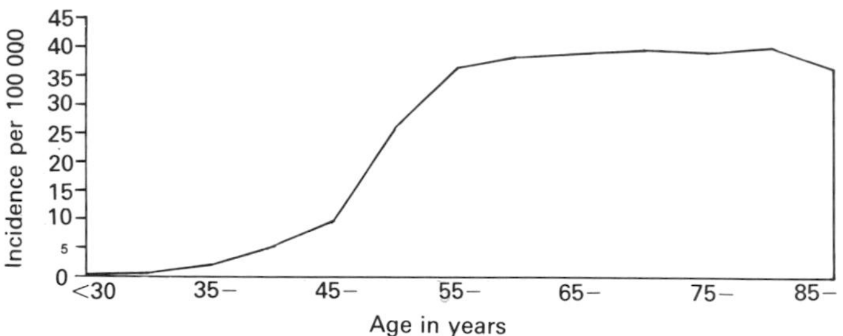

Fig. 32.6 The incidence of endometrial carcinoma in different age groups in England and Wales in 1981 (Office of Population Censuses and Surveys 1985).

Aetiological factors

The main risk factors identified for endometrial cancer relate to hormonal status and reproductive history. Early age at menarche and low parity increase risk as for breast cancer but of greater importance are late menopause, the use of oestrogen replacement therapy and obesity. Table 32.9 present the levels of risk that have been observed for these last factors.

Table 32.9 Risk factors for endometrial cancer

	Daily dose (mg)	Relative risk
Oestrogen replacement therapy (unopposed)		
Mack et al (1976)	<0.625	5.0
	>0.625	9.48
Weiss et al (1979)	<1.25	6.5
	>1.25	7.6
	Weight (kg)	**Relative risk**
Obesity		
Premenopausal women		
Henderson et al (1983)	<59.0	1.0
	59.0–67.9	1.5
	68.0–77.0	2.0
	77.1–86.1	9.6
	86.2	17.7
Postmenopausal women		
La Vecchia et al (1984)	<52.9	1.0
	52.9–66.0	1.6
	66.1–79.2	3.3
	>79.3	7.6

Table 32.10 Protective factors for endometrial cancer

		Relative risk
Cigarette smoking (ever/never)		
Levy et al (1987)	Premenopausal	0.5
	Postmenopausal	0.4
	Years of use	**Relative risk**
Combined oral contraceptive use		
Henderson et al (1983)	0	1.0
	<2	0.75
	2–3	0.79
	4–5	0.28
	>5	0.14

In contrast to the increase in risk associated with the above factors, a decrease in risk for endometrial cancer has been seen both for cigarette smokers and for users of the combined oral contraceptive (rather than sequential-type oral contraceptives). Table 32.10 indicates the degree to which risk has been reduced.

These results have been combined by Key & Pike (1988) into a single hypothesis, that risk for endometrial cancer is directly related to the cumulative degree of endometrial mitotic activity, and that mitotic activity of the endometrium increases directly with levels of unopposed oestrogen up to a certain upper limit, beyond which further increases in oestrogen levels produce no further mitotic response. Progestogens greatly reduce the rate of mitotic activity. The quantitative consequences of this hypothesis are displayed in Figure 32.7, which can also be considered to be a summary of the observed risk differentials associated with the different factors.

Endometrial cancer is also associated with conditions which are themselves associated with obesity, including diabetes and hypothyroidism, but the associations are through obesity.

These findings suggest a major potential for primary prevention, mainly through weight loss but also through the use of combined oral contraceptives. A major unknown in the epidemiology of endometrial cancer is the extent to which hormone replacement therapy (in which a progestogen is included with the oestrogen) would increase risk. Given the considerable benefits in terms of osteoporosis and cardiovascular diseases resulting from hormone replacement therapy, the issue is of considerable importance.

Screening for endometrial cancer

There are no immediate prospects for mass screening and secondary prevention. Although a number of instruments have been developed for endometrial sampling without anaesthesia for diagnostic purposes (Iverson & Segadal 1985), none has been evaluated in an asymptomatic population.

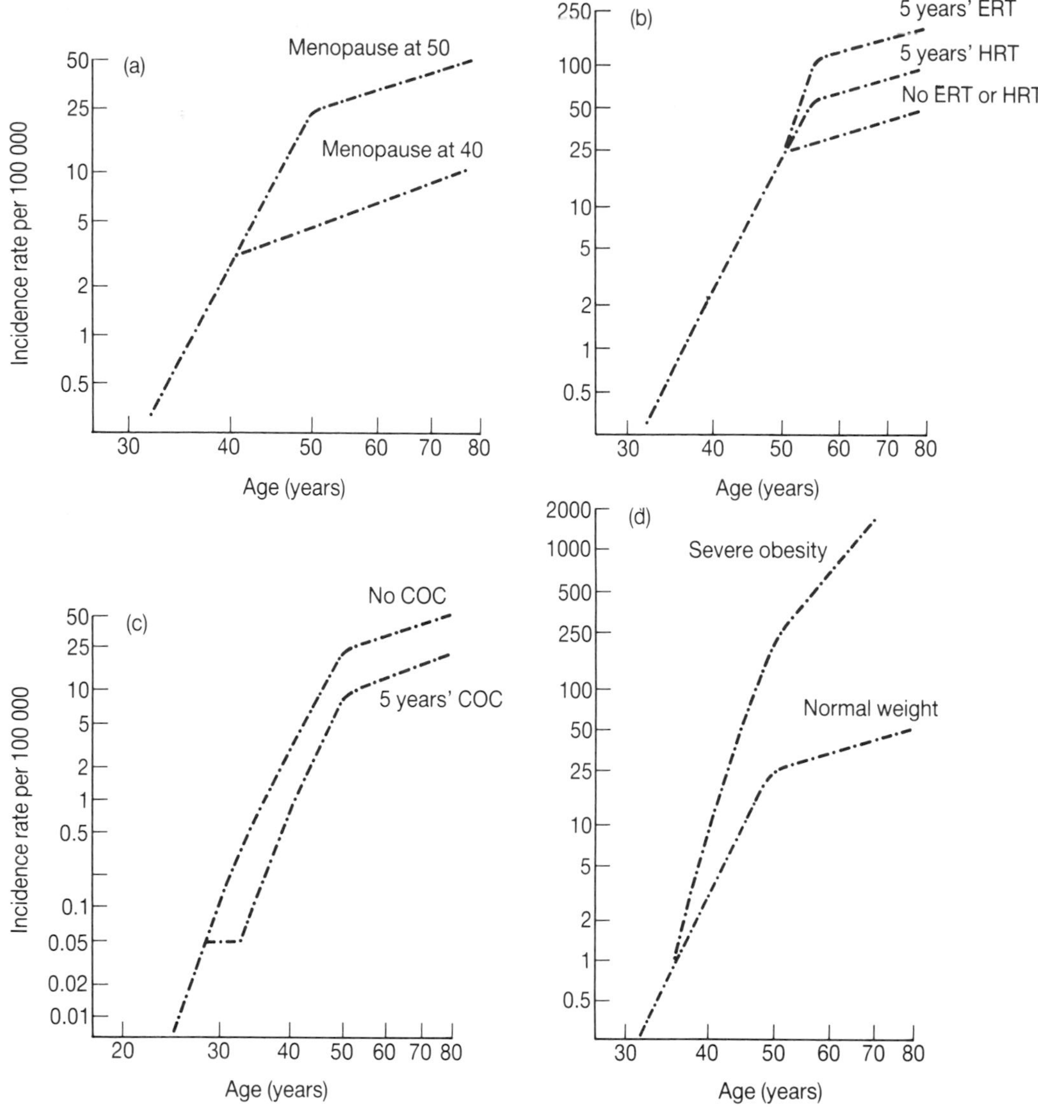

Fig. 32.7 Predicted effects of different hormone events on the risk of endometrial cancer: (**a**) menopause at age 50 years or at age 40 years; (**b**) 5 years of oestrogen replacement therapy (ERT) or combined hormone replacement therapy (HRT) starting at age 50 or no oestrogen hormone therapy; (**c**) 5 years of combined oral contraception (COC) from age 28 years or no COC; (**d**) extreme obesity (anovular from 35 years of age) or normal weight. Modified from Key & Pike (1988).

KEY POINTS

1. On a global basis, cancer of the cervix is the second most common cancer in women after breast cancer.
2. Cancer of the ovary and endometrium are seldom more than the fifth or sixth most common cancers either in developed or developing countries.
3. Large variations in the incidence of both cervical and endometrial cancer are seen worldwide but ovarian cancer shows only a two- to threefold variation in risk.
4. The major factors which affect the epidemiology of cervical cancer in a population are the level of sexual activity and the degree of effective mass screening.
5. In Scandinavia, the major change in both incidence and mortality rates since the late 1950s can be closely linked to the different approaches in the five different countries to the introduction of mass screening.
6. The two main behavioural aspects of sexual activity which modify risk for the disease are age at first intercourse and the number of sexual partners.
7. Although a large number of studies have found a higher incidence of cervical cancer among smokers a causal role for tobacco smoking in the development of cervical cancer cannot be inferred.
8. Screening every 3 years is virtually as effective as screening every year. The only justification for

annual cytology is to compensate for inadequacies in the screening process which are better rectified by direct action.
9. The decreased risk of ovarian cancer associated with increasing parity is related primarily to the number of children a woman chooses to have, rather than to her intrinsic fertility. Other environmental factors that have been changing over time have little role in ovarian cancer.
10. Oral contraceptive use reduces the risk of ovarian cancer and the relative reduction in risk does not diminish after oral contraceptive use ends.
11. Duration of active ovulation is of major importance in determining ovarian cancer risk.
12. Possibly 1% of all cases in the UK may belong to a very high-risk group with a strong family history.
13. Until large-scale randomized trials have been conducted there is no justification for including ovarian screening in a national health programme.
14. On migration to the USA, the rates of endometrial carcinoma in Asian populations rise very markedly to approach those seen in the local white population.
15. The risk for endometrial cancer is directly related to the cumulative degree of endometrial mitotic activity which increases directly with levels of unopposed oestrogen up to a certain upper limit.

REFERENCES

Beral V 1974 Cancer of the cervix: a sexually transmitted infection. Lancet i: 1037–1040

Beral V, Fraser P, Chilvers C 1978 Does pregnancy protect against ovarian cancer? Lancet i: 1083–1087

Brinton L A, Hamman R F, Higgins G R et al 1987 Sexual and reproductive risk factors for invasive squamous cervical cancer. Journal of the National Cancer Institute 79: 23–31

Day N E 1984 The effect of cervical cancer screening in Scandinavia. Obstetrics and Gynecology 63: 714–718

Ewertz M, Kjaer S K 1988 Ovarian cancer incidence and mortality in Denmark 1943–82. International Journal of Cancer 42: 690–697

Fathalla M F 1971 Incessant ovulation — a factor in ovarian neoplasia. Lancet ii: 163

Hakama M 1982 Trends in the incidence of cervical cancer in the Nordic countries. In: Magnus K (ed) Trends in cancer incidence. Hemisphere, New York

Henderson B E, Casagrande J T, Pike M C, Mack T, Rosario T, Duke A 1983 The epidemiology of endometrial cancer in younger women. British Journal of Cancer 47: 749–756

Hoover R 1977 Effects of drugs: immunosuppression. In: Hiatt H H, Watson I D, Winsten J A (eds) Origins of human cancer. Cold Spring Harbor Laboratory, New York

IARC 1986a Tobacco smoking. IARC monograph on the evaluation of the carcinogenic risk of chemicals to man, vol 38. IARC, Lyon

IARC 1986b Screening for cervical cancer — the duration of low risk following negative cervical cytology. British Medical Journal 293: 659–664

Iverson O E, Segadal E 1985 The value of endometrial cytology. A comparative study of the Gravlee jet-washer, Isaacs cell sampler and Endoscann versus curettage in 600 patients. Obstetrical and Gynecological Survey 40: 14–20

Jacobs I J, Oram D A 1989 Potential screening tests for ovarian cancer. In: Sharp F, Mason W P, Leake R E (eds) Ovarian cancer: biological and therapeutic challenges. Chapman and Hall Medical, London

Johnson A M, Gill O N 1989 Evidence for recent changes in sexual behaviour in homosexual men in England and Wales. Philosophical Transactions of the Royal Society of London B 325: 153–161

Kaldor J, Day N E et al 1987 Second malignancies following testicular cancer, ovarian cancer and Hodgkin's disease: an international collaborative study among cancer registries. International Journal of Cancer 39: 571–585

Key T J A, Pike M C 1988 The base effect relationship between unopposed oestrogens and endometrial mitotic rate: its central role in explaining and predicting endometrial cancer risk. British Journal of Cancer 57: 205–213

Kvale G, Hensel I, Nilsen S, Beral V 1988 Reproductive factors and risk of ovarian cancer: a prospective study. International Journal of Cancer 42: 246–252

Laara E, Day N E, Hakama M 1987 Trends in mortality from cervical cancer in the Nordic countries in relation to organised mass screening. Lancet i: 1247–1249

La Vecchia C, Franceschi S, Decarli A, Gallus G, Tagnoni G 1984 Risk factors for endometrial cancer at different ages. Journal of the National Cancer Institute 73: 667–675

Lee H P, Day N E, Shanmugaratnam K 1988 Cancer incidence in Singapore: time trends 1968–82. IARC Scientific Publication no 91. IARC, Lyon

Levy F, La Vechia C, Decarli A 1987 Cigarette smoking and the risk of endometrial cancer. European Journal of Cancer and Clinical Oncology 23: 1025–1029

MacGregor J E, Moss S, Parkin D M, Day N E 1986 Cervical screening in North East Scotland. British Medical Journal 290: 1543–1546

Mack T M, Pike M C, Henderson B E et al 1976 Estrogens and endometrial cancer in a retirement community. New England Journal of Medicine 294: 1262–1268

Muir C, Waterhouse J, Mack T M, Powell J, Whelan S (eds) 1987 Cancer incidence in five continents, vol 5. IARC, Lyon

Munos N, Bosch F X 1989 Epidemiology of cervical cancer. In: Munos N, Bosch F X, Jensen O M (eds) Human papilloma virus and cervical cancer. IARC Scientific Publication no 94. IARC, Lyon

Munos N, Bosch F X, Kaldor J M 1989 Does human papilloma virus cause cervical cancer? The state of the epidemiological evidence. British Journal of Cancer 47: 1–5

Office of Population Censuses and Surveys 1985 1981 Cancer statistics — registrations. HMSO, London

Parkin D M, Laara E, Muir C S 1988 Estimate of the worldwide frequency of 16 major cancers in 1980. International Journal of Cancer 41: 184–187

Ponder B A J, Easton D F, Peto J 1989 Risk of ovarian cancer associated with family history. In: Sharp F, Mason W P, Leake R E (eds) Ovarian cancer: biological and therapeutic challenges. Chapman and Hall Medical, London

Scott I V, Milford Ward A, Selby C, Whitehead S, Wilcox M 1989 Development of population-based studies in ovarian cancer screening. In: Sharp F, Mason W P, Leake R E (eds) Ovarian cancer: biological and therapeutic challenges. Chapman and Hall Medical, London

Tzonou A, Kaldor J M, Smith P G, Day N E, Trichopoulos D 1986 Misclassification in case control studies with two dichotomous risk factors. Revue d'Epidémiologie de Santé Publique 34:10–17

Weiss N S, Szekely D R, English D R, Schweld A I 1979 Endometrial cancer in relation to patterns of menopausal oestrogen use. Journal of the American Medical Association 242: 261–265

Wu M L, Whittemore A S, Paffenberger R S et al 1988 Personal and environmental factors related to epithelial ovarian cancer I. Reproductive and menstrual events and oral contraceptive use. American Journal of Epidemiology 128: 1216–1228

33. The principles of radiotherapy and chemotherapy

H. E. Lambert

RADIOTHERAPY

Radiotherapy is the therapeutic use of ionizing radiation. It is mainly used for treating malignant tumours including gynaecological cancers, in particular carcinoma of the cervix.

RADIATION PHYSICS

When living matter absorbs radiation energy, ionization of biological molecules occurs. Ionization is the result of radiation energy ejecting one or more electrons from an atom. Ionizing radiation as used for treatment is either electromagnetic or particulate.

Electromagnetic radiation

X-rays and gamma rays are identical types of electromagnetic radiation. X-rays for treatment purposes are produced by a machine called a linear accelerator which accelerates electrons to high kinetic energy then stops them abruptly on a target usually made of tungsten or gold. Part of the kinetic energy of the electrons is converted to X-rays. Gamma rays are emitted naturally by radioactive isotopes such as ^{60}cobalt as they decay to reach a stable form.

Gamma rays and X-rays are characterized by a short wavelength and high frequency. They consist of a stream of photons (packets of energy) which are absorbed in tissue and at high acceleration have sufficient power to break chemical bonds. This leads to biological change and can result in the death of a cell — hence their use in the treatment of cancer.

Particulate radiation

This consists of atomic subparticles, i.e. electrons (negative charges), protons (positive charges), neutrons (no charge) and negative π mesons. At present, only electrons are used commonly in radiotherapy, having been accelerated to high energy in a linear accelerator from which the tungsten target has been removed so that X-rays are not produced.

The gray

Radiation energy absorbed in tissue is measured in grays (Gy). One gray is the equivalent of 1 J/kg. Previously radiation energy was measured in rads, 1 Gy being equivalent to 100 rad. Particulate radiation causes ionization directly and X-rays and gamma rays indirectly by giving up their energy to eject fast-moving electrons from atoms.

RADIOBIOLOGY

The study of ionizing radiation on living matter is called radiobiology. The principal critical target in a cell is DNA. When this is damaged, cell metabolism and reproduction are affected. Ionizing radiation will act on both normal and cancer cells and the problem for radiotherapy is to eliminate cancer cells without permanently damaging vital tissues. Recovery of normal tissue is usually better than that of malignant tissue as long as the overall dose is not too large and it is given over a period of time. It is therefore the practice to fractionate the dose of radiation over several days or weeks.

SCHEDULING AND DOSE OF RADIOTHERAPY

Dose fractionation

Fractionated external beam therapy is usually given once-daily 4–5 times a week. To improve cure rates, particularly in rapidly growing tumours, treatment can be accelerated by giving larger doses per fraction over a shorter time. This will increase the cell kill per fraction but will also interfere with normal cellular repair. Acceleration is also carried out using normal-sized fractions twice daily separated by at least 6 h. Hyperfractionation, in which three or more small fractions are given each day, is also being examined. The theoretical reason for increasing the number of daily fractions is to allow sufficient time for normal tissue to regenerate but insufficient for tumour cells.

Dose prescription

The radiation dose prescribed includes the total dose to be given, the total number of fractions, the total time and the dose per fraction. For example: 50 Gy in 25 fractions given 5 times weekly in 5 weeks at 2 Gy per fraction.

For radical curative treatment, the greater the tumour volume, the higher the radiation dose necessary to eliminate the cancer. For example, 50 Gy in 5 weeks is sufficient for microscopic foci in 90% of patients but 65–70 Gy in $6\frac{1}{2}$–7 weeks is needed to destroy a 2 cm mass. When there is no likelihood of cure but the patient is symptomatic, palliative radiotherapy has a valuable role to relieve pain. Doses are smaller and treatment time is reduced. If radiation fails, repeat treatment is of no value and will cause severe injury to normal tissues.

RADIOTHERAPY TECHNIQUES

Several techniques are used in the management of gynaecological cancer:

1. *Teletherapy* is external irradiation where the tumour is at a long distance — usually 100 cm — from the source of ionizing radiation.
2. *Brachytherapy* is either intracavitary or interstitial (inserted directly into tissues) therapy where there is a 'short' distance between source and tumour (e.g. in the vagina and cervical canal).
3. *Instillation of radioactive fluids* into the pleural and peritoneal cavity, or more rarely by intra-arterial infusion to the tumour site.

Teletherapy — external irradiation

Teletherapy is used to treat large volumes such as those required for carcinoma of the cervix where the volume includes the tumour itself, the parametria and the regional lymph nodes. The size of the treatment volume and the overall dose will be influenced by the age and general condition of the patient. For example, arteriosclerosis or bowel disease such as diverticulitis both reduce bowel tolerance. Small bowel tolerates only relatively low doses of radiation but its mobility enables it to move in and out of the treatment area thus reducing the dose it receives. Damage to small bowel can result from surgical adhesions causing small bowel fixation. Care must also be taken with the rectum and pelvic colon which will inevitably be partly in the treatment volume.

Treatment planning

The aim of planning is to deliver a homogeneous dose to the tumour volume while giving a low dose to surrounding normal tissues. The volume is measured in three dimensions — superior–inferior, anterior–posterior and right to left laterally. The dose of radiation which will be tolerated by normal tissues within the tumour volume must be known. Particular attention must be given to critical organs, such as the kidney or spinal cord, which tolerate only low doses of radiation. Accurate tumour localization is essential and is assessed by both clinical and surgical findings, with additional information from X-rays, ultrasound and computerized tomography (CT) scanning and magnetic resonance imaging when appropriate.

Planning procedure

The patient is placed on a mobile couch beneath a simulator — a diagnostic X-ray machine connected to a television screen which emulates a treatment machine (Fig. 33.1). The simulator defines the limits of the treatment volume, using a beam of light in place of the X-rays of the treatment machine. It will also take X-ray films for a permanent record.

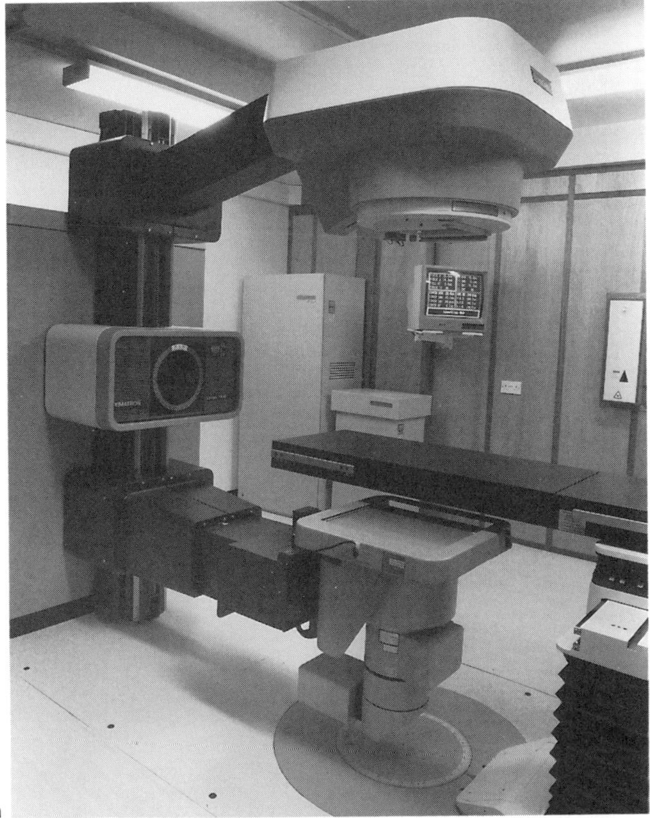

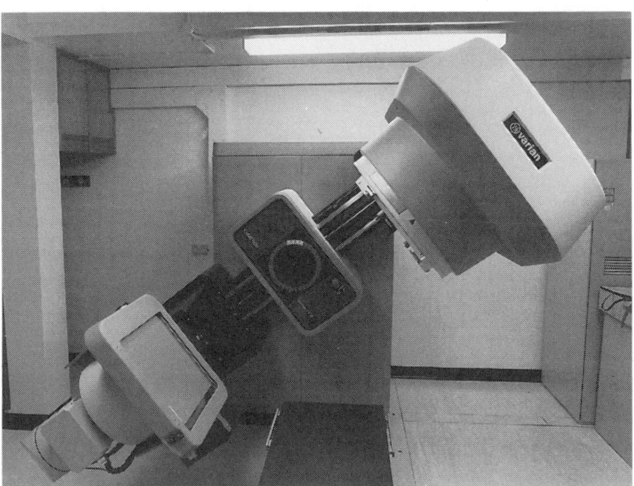

Fig. 33.1 (**a**) A Ximatron simulator with couch (manufactured by Varian TEM). (**b**) The gantry rotated.

The patient is positioned carefully with the help of a laser beam to ensure accurate replication at each treatment session. Cross-wires mounted in the light beam from the simulator define the size of the area to be treated (Fig. 33.2). This is marked on the patient with a semi-permanent dye, usually gentian violet, which will not wash off easily during the treatment period. The body contour at the volume centre is measured using pliable wire or more accurately with CT. On to this contour the tumour volume will be drawn either on paper or by using a CT planning computer.

For the tumour to receive an adequate dose without overdosing the skin or other tissues, several fields arranged at different entry points to the body are used (Fig. 33.3). A planning computer (Fig. 33.4) calculates field sizes, the dose from each field, and the angles of the treatment machine to give a homogeneous distribution to the tumour. The computerized plan of the final radiation dose delivered to the pelvis for carcinoma of the cervix by a three-field arrangement is shown in Figure 33.5.

Lead or brass compensators may be placed in the path of the radiation beam to absorb unnecessary radiation. The most frequently used compensators are wedge-shaped (Fig. 33.6). The wedges are made with angles from 15 to 60° to vary the amount of radiation absorbed. Sometimes compensators need to be designed specially for individual patients.

Choice of machine

The intensity of a beam of radiation decreases with depth in tissue but high-energy machines spare skin by delivering more radiation below the skin surface at the same time reaching deeply situated tumours. Such machines include those with a ^{60}Co source releasing gamma rays of 1.3 meV energy, or linear accelerators which deliver X-rays of 4–8 meV.

Implementation of the plan

Treatment is carried out in a specially protected room, preventing radiation of personnel outside. The patient lies on the treatment couch in the same position as established with the simulator (Fig. 33.7). The machine angle, size of field, and the use of wedges are carefully prepared for each treatment field. Radiographers, who set up and treat patients, use a control console outside the treatment room to start and stop the radiation, to set the dose and the time. Treatment time for each field is short, usually less than 1 min. As the patient has to be alone during this time she is supervised using a television camera or a very thick lead glass window. A microphone enables patients to talk to staff and if they are distressed the treatment is stopped immediately so the radiographers can re-enter the room. There are many safety precautions to prevent acciden-

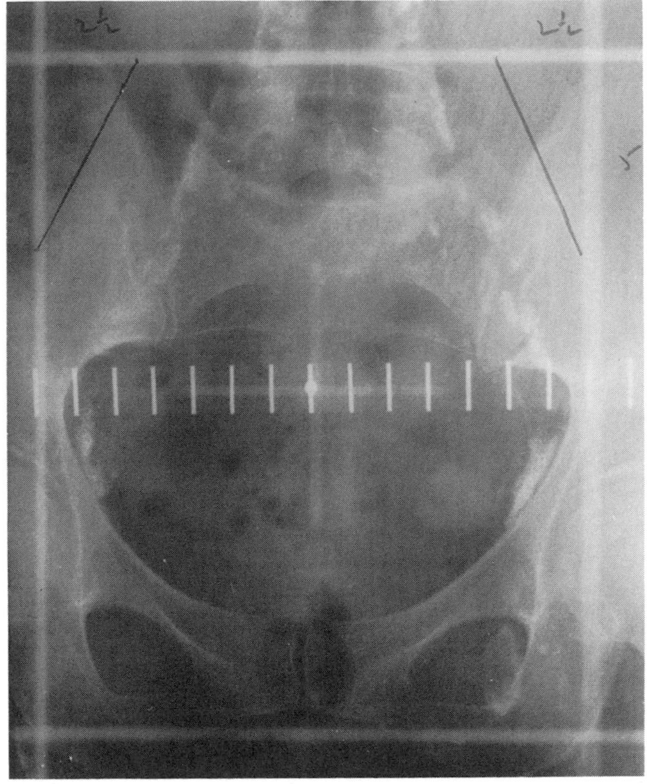

a

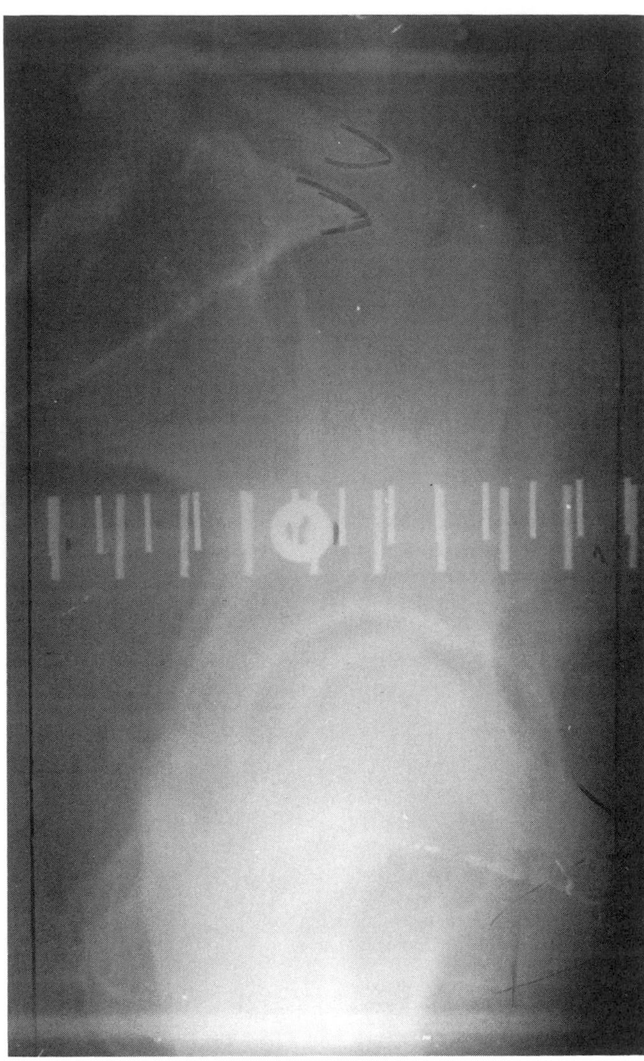

b

Fig. 33.2 (**a**) Anteroposterior X-ray of the treatment area, the pelvis, showing the superior, inferior and lateral margins. The triangular areas are protected from the beam. The patient has had a lymphangiogram. (**b**) Lateral X-ray of the treatment area.

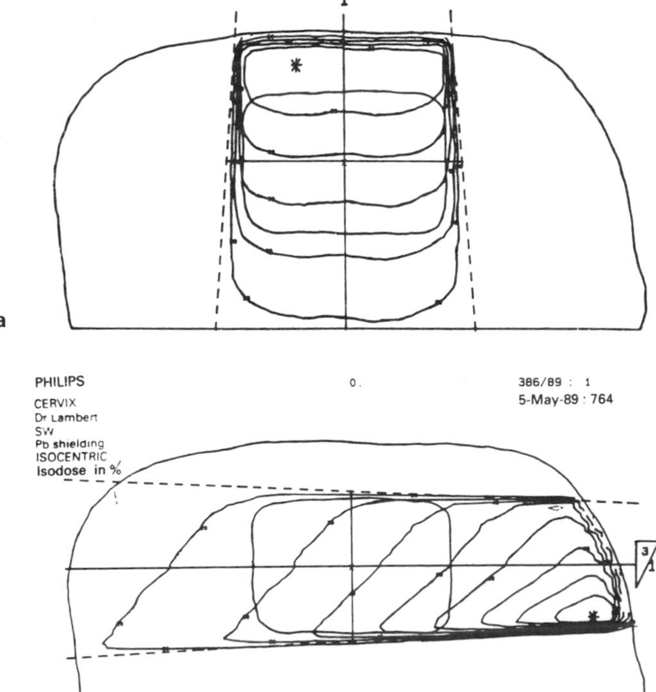

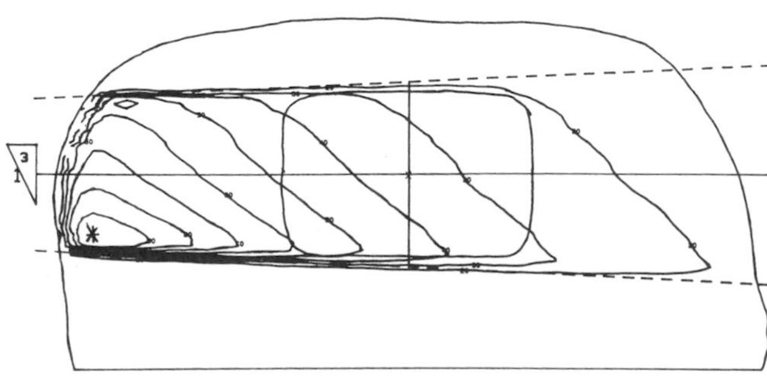

Fig. 33.3 Computer simulations of the isodose pattern of (**a**) the anterior field; (**b**) the left lateral field; (**c**) the right lateral field.

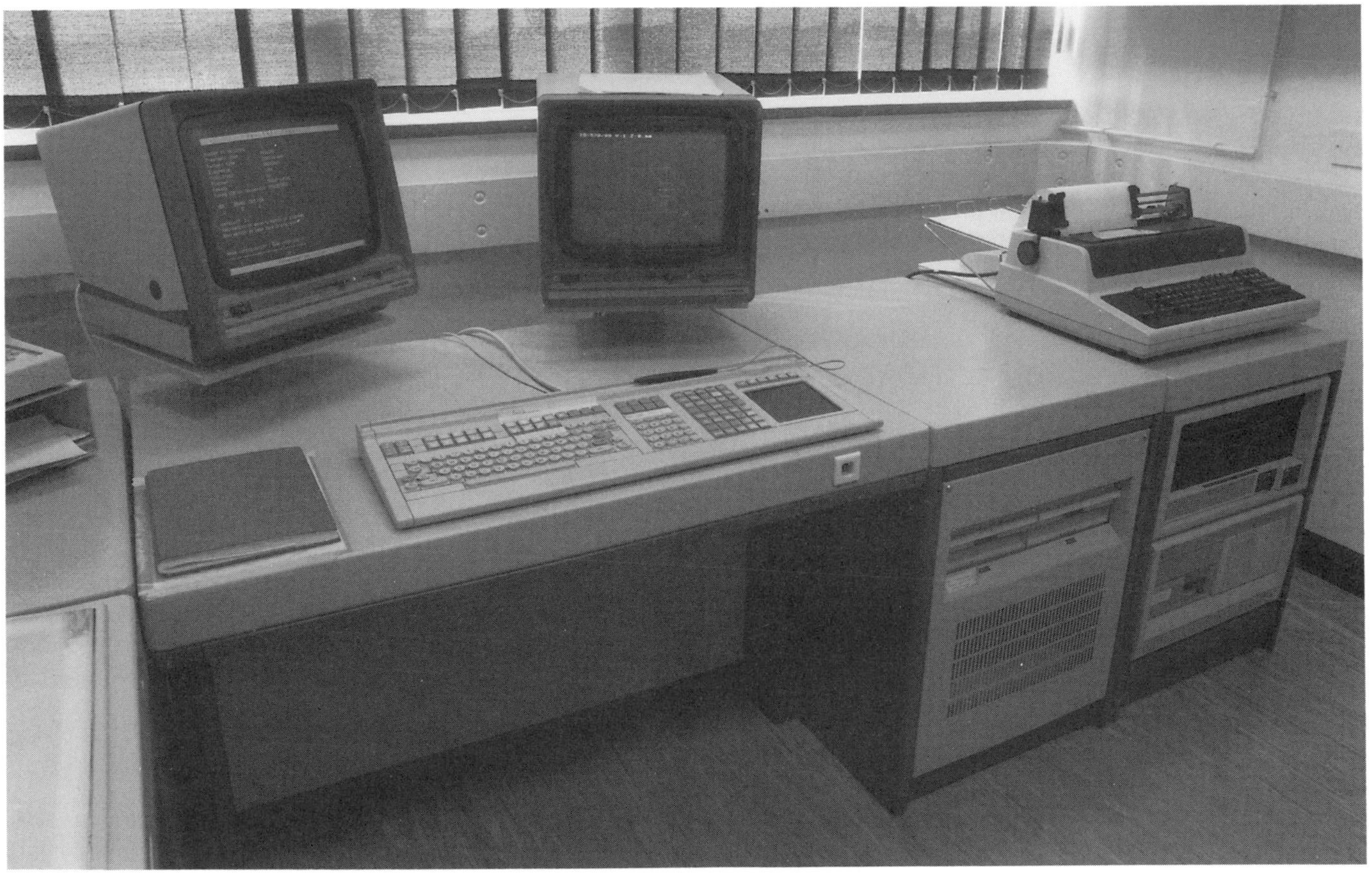

Fig. 33.4 The planning computer. A plan of the volume being prepared is shown on one screen and instructions are shown on the second. A permanent record is produced as in Figures 32.3 and 32.5.

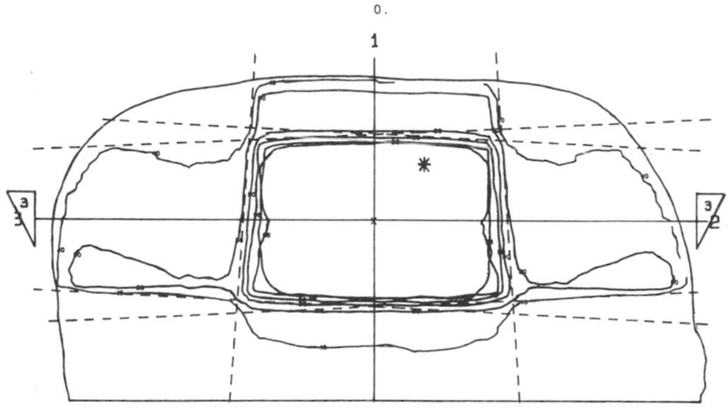

Fig. 33.5 The final tumour volume is shown, derived from the summation of the isodoses from all three fields.

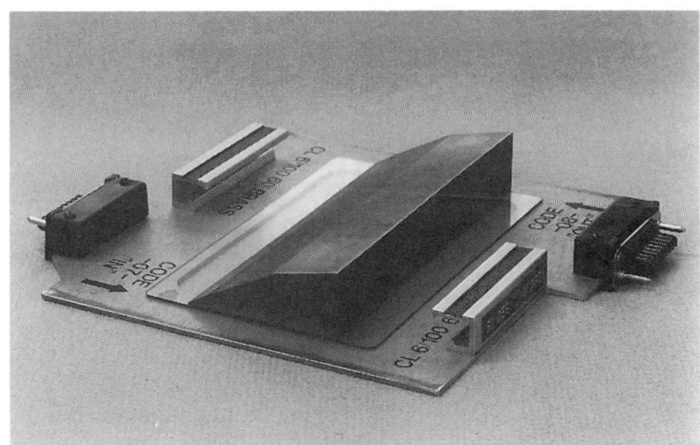

Fig. 33.6 A 60° wedge compensator.

tal overdosage and treatment machines are checked frequently.

Intracavitary brachytherapy

Brachytherapy enables a very high dose of radiation to be given close to a radioactive source with a very rapid fall-off further away. This method is suitable for treating small tumour volumes. Until recently, the energy source used was radium-226 but because of its long half-life — approximately 1600 years — and because it produces radon, a radioactive gas, it has been replaced by other radioactive isotopes such as caesium-137 (^{137}Cs) which has a half-life of 33 years and produces no toxic gases.

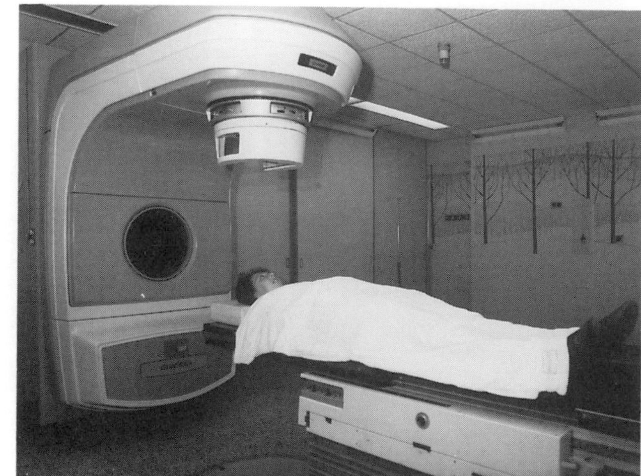

Fig. 33.7 Patient lying on the couch of a 6 Mev Varian Linear Accelerator.

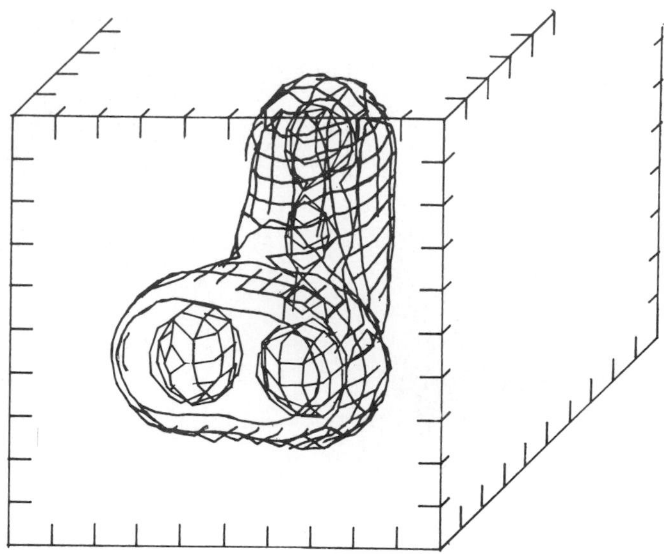

Fig. 33.8 The volume from the summation of three brachytherapy sources — an intrauterine tube and two vaginal ovoids. This shows the limits of the treatment volume and the rapid fall-off of the dose.

Brachytherapy methods

The commonest method of giving intracavitary radiation for gynaecological tumours is with the Manchester system in which a single uterine tube containing ^{137}Cs is passed through the cervix into the uterine cavity so that the inferior margin is flush with the external cervical os and smaller tubes, containing ^{137}Cs in plastic vaginal ovoids, are inserted into the lateral vaginal fornices. The tumour volume treated by these three radioactive sources is shown in Figure 33.8. This is a low dose rate treatment lasting for several days.

Most radiotherapy centres have replaced the direct insertion of radioactive sources into a patient with an after-loading system. This system allows time to be taken over the positioning of source trains without hazard to the operator. Only after the accuracy of their placement has been verified with X-ray films are the radioactive sources inserted.

In manual after-loading systems (Fig. 33.9), the active sources are inserted after the patient has returned to the ward so eliminating radiation risk to theatre staff. Remote after-loading systems are preferred as they allow complete staff protection. The patient is treated in a protected room for approximately 20 h in the case of the Selectron, which uses ^{137}Cs, or for a few minutes with high dose rate systems like the High Dose Selectron which uses ^{60}Co, or the

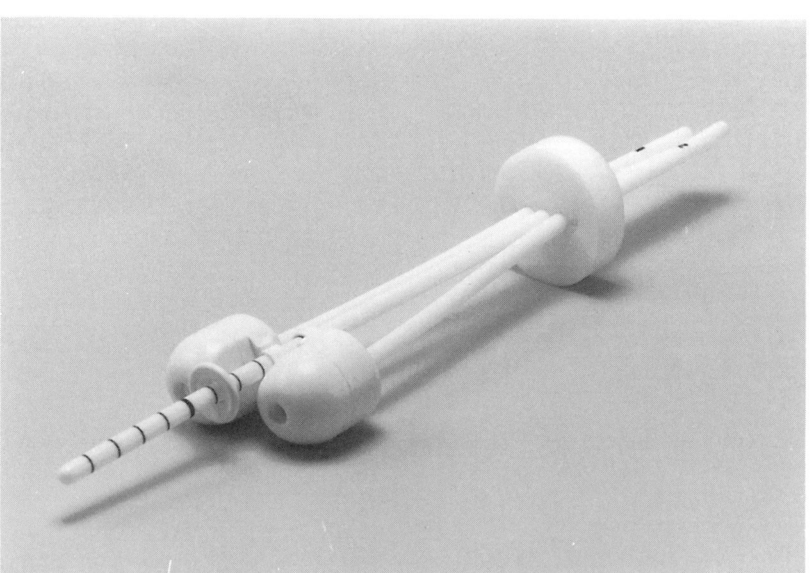

Fig. 33.9 The Amersham manual after-loading system for treating carcinoma of the cervix. There are three trains — a central one for the uterine tube and two lateral trains for the vaginal ovoids.

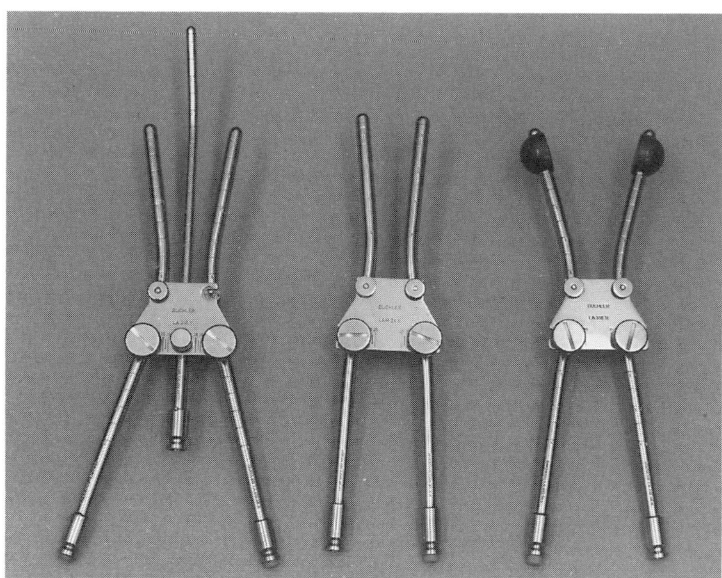

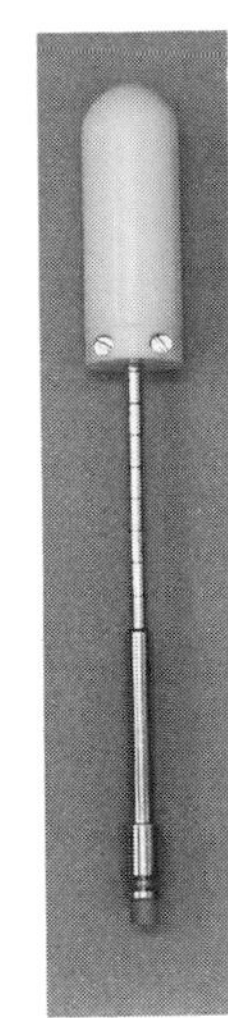

Fig. 33.10 (**a**) Source trains for remote high dose rate after-loading (Buchler). From left to right: a central uterine and two vaginal source trains; vaginal source trains without and with ovoids. (**b**) A vaginal obturator.

Buchler machine using iridium-192 (Figs 33.10 and 33.11). With high dose rates severe damage to normal tissues could result but this is avoided by both reducing and fractionating the total dose. All the techniques described are equally effective.

Intracavitary brachytherapy

The procedure is carried out under general anaesthetic. A pelvic examination, including cystoscopy and proctoscopy, is performed. For cervical cancer, the cervix is dilated and the uterine length measured with a sound to ascertain the length of the uterine tube required. The width of vaginal vault is assessed to decide on the size of applicator or applicators to be inserted. The bladder is catheterized. The uterine tube is inserted first and then the vaginal applicators. A gauze pack keeps the sources in place and away from the rectum to reduce the rectal dose which can be checked with a dosimeter. A computer using information from X-rays is a better way of measuring the doses given to both the treatment volume and to normal tissues (Fig. 33.8).

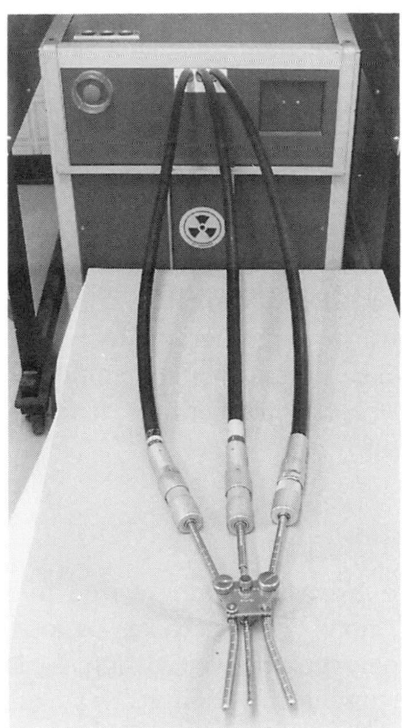

Fig. 33.11 Attachment of source trains to a safe containing the radioactive sources.

For carcinoma of the cervix, the dose to be given to the patient can be calculated at reference point A which in theory estimates the normal tissue dose where the ureter crosses the uterine artery. It is 2 cm lateral to the cervical canal and 2 cm superior to the lateral fornix. In practice this point is measured from the X-rays as 2 cm lateral to the centre of the uterine radioactive source and 2 cm superior to its inferior margin. A newer method of describing the given dose recommended by the ICRU (International Commission on Radiation Units and Measurements) measures the size of the tumour volume receiving full radiation dose. If the sole method of treatment is by intracavitary radiation, a dose of 80 Gy is given in two fractions but after external irradiation only one fraction of 20–30 Gy is required.

Interstitial brachytherapy

In some areas, treatment of small tumours with sparing of normal tissues can best be carried out by the insertion di-

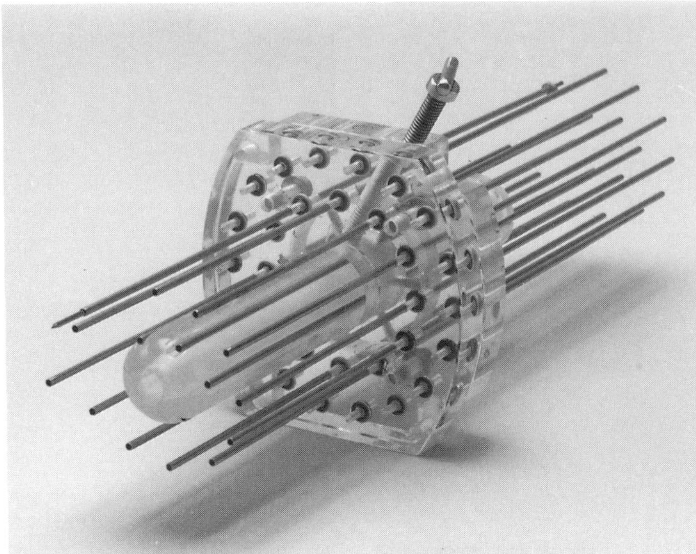

Fig. 33.12 A template (the 'Hammersmith hedgehog') for the interstitial treatment of carcinoma of the vagina.

rectly into the tumour of radioactive sources as needles, wires or seeds. An example is the insertion of radioactive needles for early cases of vaginal carcinoma. One such technique is to use a template (Fig. 33.12) which allows the insertion of guide tubes which can be after-loaded with active sources once X-rays have confirmed the correct position of the guides. Templates increase the accuracy of implants by ensuring that the sources are distributed in a regular fashion giving a uniform dose to the treatment volume without 'hot' or 'cold' spots. The isotopes commonly used for this procedure are ^{192}Ir, ^{137}Cs, and ^{125}I. For a radical course of treatment, doses such as 60 Gy are given in 6 days.

Instillation of radioisotopes in solution

Radiotherapy for small-volume disease in the peritoneal, pleural or pericardial space can be given as a solution of radioisotopes. Early ovarian cancers have been treated using radioactive isotopes of either gold or phosphorus linked to carrier colloids. This gives a high dose of radiation but only to a depth of 4–6 mm, limiting therapy to small deposits on the pleural or peritoneal surfaces. Radioactive labelled monoclonal antibodies have been used in the same way in the hope that the antibody will target the radiotherapy to the tumour site.

RADIATION DAMAGE

The dose of radiation is limited by the tolerance of normal tissue. Large single fractions of radiation cause more damage than multiple small fractions for the same total dose.

Normal tissue reactions occur both early and late. Early reactions take place during or immediately after a course of radiotherapy but recovery is usually rapid. Late reactions occur from 1 year onwards, are permanent and usually slowly progressive. Skin, bowel and bone marrow proliferate rapidly and so are particularly susceptible to acute reactions during treatment. Tissues which divide slowly, such as kidney, show late reactions because the damage to DNA only becomes apparent when cells divide.

Skin

Except when the vulval or anal region is included, radiation damage to skin is largely avoided when treating pelvic tumours as megavoltage machines deliver their maximum dose below the skin surface and the use of multiple treatment fields reduces the dose to any particular area of skin. Epidermal cells turnover in 2–3 weeks so any damage becomes apparent after that time. Erythema may be followed by dry desquamation or, with more severe damage, by moist desquamation. The basal cells are usually spared allowing the skin to regrow.

Gastrointestinal mucosa

Cells in the intestinal mucosa are replaced every 3–6 days leading to diarrhoea when bowel is included in the treatment volume such as the pelvis or abdomen. Late but rare complications to both small and large bowel include bleeding, stenosis and malabsorption. These may require special diets and nutritional support with vitamin supplements or, exceptionally, surgical intervention such as excision of damaged bowel with or without a stoma. The poor blood supply after radiation damage makes surgery difficult and the security of bowel anastamoses uncertain.

Bone marrow

The bone marrow is very sensitive to radiation and frequent blood counts are essential when large volumes of marrow are included in the treatment fields as for example in whole abdominal radiotherapy for ovarian carcinoma. The white blood count and platelet count are affected early while anaemia occurs later because of the longer life span of red blood cells.

Other organs

Late damage to liver and kidneys due to damage of the vascular supply may cause cirrhosis or loss of renal function. Ureteric damage and vesicovaginal fistulae are rare. Bladder changes including telangiectasiae are common and occasionally cause haemorrhagic cystitis. The ovaries are particularly sensitive to radiation and even small doses can cause ovarian failure.

CONCLUSION

Ionizing radiation is a sophisticated technique used for the treatment of cancer. It requires both highly technical machinery and expertise from specially trained personnel — engineers, physicists, doctors and radiographers. Side-effects are usually slight but complications can occur even after ideal treatment.

CHEMOTHERAPY

Cytotoxic chemotherapy developed from the realization that the effects on bone marrow cells of mustard gas used in World War I could be extended to the treatment of cancer. In the 1940s methotrexate and other anti-metabolite drugs were discovered and since that time many drugs have been found that are of potential use in cancer therapy. Of these, approximately 40 drugs are now in general use.

CLASSIFICATION

The most common classification of cytotoxic chemotherapy is one based on their biochemistry. Drugs are divided into alkylating agents, anti-metabolites, vinca alkaloids, antibiotics and miscellaneous (not belonging to any of the other groups).

DRUG EVALUATION

Before cytotoxic drugs can be used to treat cancer in humans they must first be tested for both their efficiency and toxicity in animals. A promising drug is then studied in patients with advanced cancer to obtain pharmacological information (phase 1). Sensitive tumours are identified in phase 2 before a large number of patients with responsive tumours are treated to define further the drug's role (phase 3).

PHARMACOLOGY

When considering the pharmacology of a drug the following aspects must be investigated: absorption, distribution, metabolism and excretion. Drugs can only be taken orally if well absorbed from the alimentary tract. Parenteral administration — intravenous, intramuscular or intra-arterial — is the optimal route for most cytotoxic drugs. Of these, intravenous is by far the commonest route used. Occasionally, in superficial tumours, cytotoxic drugs are given topically (5-fluorouracil) or by injection directly into the tumour (bleomycin).

The metabolism of drugs within the body is often unknown but several, including 5-fluorouracil, are metabolized in the liver. Most drugs are excreted in urine but a few are excreted in the alimentary tract via the bile duct. Only a very few drugs cross the blood–brain barrier, e.g. the nitrosoureas and etoposide. This barrier can be overcome by intrathecal administration, and methotrexate is given this way in the treatment of lymphatic leukaemia (Table 33.1).

CYTOTOXIC DRUGS USED COMMONLY IN GYNAECOLOGY

Alkylating agents (including the platinum compounds)

These drugs cross-link DNA strands by forming covalent bonds between highly reactive alkylating groups and nitrogen groups on the DNA helix. This either prevents division of the helix at mitosis or results in an imperfect division and cell death.

The most frequently used alkylating agents are cyclophosphamide, chlorambucil and melphalan. Newer agents include treosulfan and ifosfamide. Many alkylating agents may be taken orally. Cyclophosphamide is inactive until it is converted into its active metabolite in the liver (Table 33.1).

The toxic effects of alkylating agents are listed in Table 33.2. In particular, they can cause vomiting if given in large doses but this is seldom intractable. Most cause significant myelotoxicity which can be cumulative. Alopecia is most marked with cyclophosphamide and ifosfamide. Both these last drugs are excreted in the urine in the form of active metabolites which can cause a severe chemical cystitis when given in high doses unless mesna (sodium 2-mercaptoethanesulphonate) is administered at the same time to protect the bladder mucosa. In addition, ifosfamide may cause a fatal encephalopathy and must be given only after reference to a treatment nomogram.

Platinum agents

Cisplatin and carboplatin, drugs containing the metal platinum, act in a fashion similar to alkylating agents. Both are given intravenously but, because of its severe nephrotoxicity, cisplatin requires a forced diuresis.

Cisplatin causes severe nausea and vomiting which require potent anti-emetic therapy. Peripheral neuropathy can be disabling and is usually dose-related. Cisplatin has little myelotoxicity except for anaemia which frequently has to be corrected with blood transfusion.

Carboplatin has very little nephrotoxicity or neurotoxicity and also causes less vomiting. It may be given to outpatients as it only requires a half-hour infusion unless vomiting, which is often delayed, is severe. Carboplatin is myelotoxic, a particular problem being thrombocytopenia. Impaired renal function increases myelotoxicity.

Anti-metabolites

These compounds closely resemble essential metabolites for

Table 33.1 Cytotoxic drugs: dosage, routes of administration and excretion

Cytotoxic drug	Route of Administration	Dosage* (as single agent)	Excretion
Alkylating agents			
Chlorambucil	Oral	10 mg/day or 10–14 days per month	Urine
Cyclophosphamide	Oral, i.v.	Oral 100–200 mg/day	Bile
		i.v. 500–1000 mg weekly	Urine
		High dose 20–40 mg/kg	
Ifosfamide	i.v.	8–10 g/m^2 over 5 days 2–4 weekly	Urine
Melphalan	Oral	0.2 mg/kg/day × 5 4-weekly	Urine
Treosulfan	i.v., oral	5 g/m^2 i.v. 3-weekly	Urine
Platinum compounds			
Cisplatin	i.v.	50–120 mg/m^2 weekly to 4-weekly	Urine
Carboplatin	i.v.	400 mg/m^2 4-weekly	Urine
Anti-metabolites			
Methotrexate	Oral, i.m., i.v.	e.g. 100–1000 mg/m^2 with folinic acid rescue	Urine Bile
		or 2.5–5 mg/day orally	
5-Fluorouracil	Oral, i.v.	Loading dose 12 mg/kg/day ×3	Urine
		Maintenance 3–15 mg/kg/week	
Vinca alkaloids			
Vincristine	i.v.	1–2 mg weekly	Bile
Vinblastine	i.v.	0.1–0.2 mg/kg weekly	Bile
Vindesine	i.v.	3–4 mg/m^2 weekly	Bile
Antibiotics			
Anthracyclines			
Doxorubicin (Adriamycin)	i.v.	60–75 mg/m^2 3-weekly (Total dose <450 mg/m^2)	Bile
Epirubicin	i.v.	75–90 mg/m^2 3-weekly	Bile
Mitozantrone	i.v.	14 mg/m^2 3-weekly	Bile
Other antibiotics			
Actinomycin D	i.v.	0.5 mg/day × 5 4-weekly	Bile
Mitomycin	i.v.	4–10 mg 6-weekly	Urine
Bleomycin	i.m., i.v. i.p.	10–60 mg weekly	Urine
	Malignant effusions	60 mg i.p.	
		Maximum total dose 300 mg	
Miscellaneous			
Dacarbazine (DTIC)	i.v.	250 mg/m^2/day × 5 3-weekly	Urine
Etoposide (VP16)	Oral, i.v.	60–120 mg/m^2/day × 5 4-weekly	Urine
Lomustine (CCNU)	Oral	120 mg/m^2 6–8-weekly	Urine

* The doses shown are for general information only. The appropriate dose will vary in different circumstances and specific protocols should be consulted for detailed guidance.

the synthesis of nucleic acids and proteins. They are incorporated into natural metabolic pathways and enzyme systems and disrupt the cellular mechanism. Each anti-metabolite acts at different sites in the pathway of nucleic acid synthesis.

Methotrexate

Methotrexate is a folic acid antagonist. It inhibits the enzyme dihydrofolate reductase which reduces dihydrofolate to tetrahydrofolate, the precursor of co-enzymes essential for the formation of purines and pyrimidines, the nitrogen bases of DNA. These effects are bypassed by giving folinic acid. Folinic acid rescue is given from about 12 h after the methotrexate dose to all patients receiving 100 mg or more.

The commonest complication with methotrexate is oral ulceration. Because it is excreted in urine, the dose must be reduced in women with renal impairment or with large fluid collections such as ascites which delay excretion (Tables 33.1 and 33.2).

5-Fluorouracil

5-Fluorouracil is a pyrimidine analogue which blocks thy-

Table 33.2 The major toxic effects of some commonly used cytotoxic drugs

Agents	Nausea and vomiting	Myelosuppression	Renal toxicity	Neuropathy	Others
Alkylating agents					
Chlorambucil	—	Moderate	—	—	Stomatitis, pulmonary fibrosis, hepatitis — all rare
Cyclophosphamide	Moderate	Moderate	Haemorrhagic cystitis	—	Alopecia; cardiomyopathy — rare; pulmonary fibrosis — very rare
Ifosfamide	Severe	Mild	Haemorrhagic cystitis	—	Alopecia; central nervous system; confusion, tonic–clonic spasm and (rarely) coma
Melphalan	Mild–moderate	Moderate	—	—	Pulmonary fibrosis — rare
TreosulphanI	Oral: moderate i.v: nil	Moderate	—	—	Pulmonary fibrosis — very rare
Platinum compounds					
Cisplatin	Very severe	Mild	Severe	Moderate	Ototoxicity; hypomagnesaemia
Carboplatin	Moderate	Moderate–severe	Mild	Rare	Ototoxicity — mild
Anti-metabolites					
Methotrexate	Mild	Mild–moderate	Severe with high doses	—	Stomatitis; hepatitis with high doses
5-Fluorouracil	Mild	Moderate	—	—	Mucositis; dermatitis; alopecia — high doses only
Vinca alkaloids					
Vincristine	—	—	Bladder atony (rare)	Severe	Constipation; paralytic ileus; convulsions — rare; alopecia
Vinblastine	Mild	Moderate	—	Mild	Alopecia
Vindestine	Mild	Mild	—	Moderate	Alopecia; stomatitis; severe constipation; convulsions rarely
Antibiotics					
Anthracyclines					
Doxorubicin	Severe	Moderate	—	—	Alopecia — severe; cardiomyopathy — severe (if total dose > 450 mg/m^2)
Epirubicin	Moderate	Moderate	—	—	Alopecia; mucositis; cardiomyopathy — moderate
Mitozantrone	Mild	Moderate	Mild	—	Cardiomyopathy —mild
Other antibiotics					
Actinomycin D	Moderate	Moderate–severe	—	—	Alopcia; mucositis; diarrhoea; fever; myalgia
Bleomycin	—	—	—	—	Fever; skin changes; pulmonary fibrosis and interstitial pneumonia
Mitomycin	—	Severe (delayed)	—	—	Stomatitis
Miscellaneous					
Dacarbazine (DTIC)	Severe	Severe	—	—	Photosensitivity; rare — fever, alopecia, hepatitis
Etoposide (VP16)	Moderate	Severe		—	Alopecia
Lomustine (CCNU)	Moderate	Severe (delayed)	Rare	—	—

midine synthesis and inhibits the incorporation of uracil into DNA. Myelosuppression and mucositis are the most common toxic effects but, unless very high doses are given, are not usually severe (Table 33.2).

Vinca alkaloids

Vincristine, vinblastine and vindesine are derived from the periwinkle plant, *Vinca rosea*. They act during the metaphase of mitosis, probably through toxicity to the microtubules of the mitotic spindle.

Peripheral and autonomic neuropathy are particular problems with vinca alkaloids, particularly vincristine. In addition, they are very irritant and are best injected into a fast-flowing drip. Vincristine is one of the very few chemotherapeutic drugs that is not myelotoxic.

Etoposide

Etoposide is a semi-synthetic derivative of podophyllotoxin that acts on cells in G2 in the cell cycle. Toxicity is shown in Table 33.2.

Antibiotics

Many antibiotics inhibit tumour cell division. Actinomycin D and doxorubicin (Adriamycin) form irreversible complexes with DNA. Bleomycin breaks up DNA chains thus interfering with DNA replication.

Doxorubicin (Adriamycin)

Doxorubicin is a widely used anthracycline but causes marked alopecia and is myelosuppressive. It should always be given as a fast-running infusion as it is very irritant and will cause a necrotic ulcer if injected subcutaneously. Cardiomyopathy results from high cumulative doses unless the total dose is limited to 450 mg/m^2. As it is excreted in bile, an elevated bilirubin is an indication to reduce the dose. Newer anthracycline drugs epirubicin and mitozantrone appear to be as effective as doxorubicin but are much less cardiotoxic (Tables 33.1 and 33.2).

Bleomycin

Bleomycin is commonly included in multi-drug regimens. It is not myelotoxic but sometimes causes a febrile reaction. Increased pigmentation of flexures is common. The most important toxic effect is a pulmonary fibrosis which is dose-related and not often seen at a cumulative dose less than 300 mg/m^2.

Hormones

Progestins such as medroxyprogesterone acetate are used in endometrial cancer. There is little evidence that high doses are more effective than 200 mg b.d. Although widely regarded as free of side-effects and toxicity, many patients do complain of fluid retention and there is some concern that prolonged use may increase the risk of cardiovascular disease. Tamoxifen, an anti-oestrogen widely used in breast cancer, may have a role in endometrial cancer (see Ch. 37). Glucocorticoids are often useful as anti-emetics and in terminal care.

ROUTE OF ADMINISTRATION

Most cytotoxic drugs are given orally or intravenously. The intramuscular and intra-arterial routes are sometimes used and drugs are also instilled into the peritoneal or pleural cavities.

Oral chemotherapy

Only a few drugs, mainly alkylating agents, are well absorbed by the oral route. Administration may be continuous on a daily basis but is usually intermittent; for example chlorambucil 10 mg daily for 14 days every 28 days, to allow recovery of normal cells.

Systemic chemotherapy

With intravenous and intramuscular administration, drugs are normally given at intervals of 1–4 weeks. This pulsed treatment allows the bone marrow to recover and, although some cancer cells will also recover, there is a net loss of cancer cells in every cycle.

Intrapleural and intraperitoneal chemotherapy

Chemotherapy can been given into both the pleural and peritoneal cavities. Bleomycin has been used in this way for recurrent ascites or pleural effusions but it acts mainly by stimulating an inflammatory reaction and forming adhesions. Tetracycline is equally effective. Cytotoxic drugs given systemically are far more effective at dealing with ascites and do not cause 'pocketing' from adhesions.

Recently, use of the intraperitoneal route has been explored as a method for giving high concentrations of drugs in large volumes of peritoneal dialysate. The peritoneal cavity acts as a reservoir, releasing the drugs slowly into the systemic circulation. This results in very high and prolonged local concentrations of drug. However, absorption of cytotoxic drugs directly into tumour nodules is limited as the drug penetration will be only 3–6 cells deep. Some agents are unsuitable because they cause a severe, local chemical peritonitis. Cisplatin can be given by this route but if the dose is too high, systemic complications ensue. This technique is still experimental.

SINGLE-AGENT AND COMBINATION CHEMOTHERAPY

Drugs can be used alone or in combination. Combination chemotherapy in conditions such as Hodgkin's disease or germ cell ovarian tumours can be curative and are much more effective than single-agent regimens. However, combination regimens have yet to show clear-cut advantages in epithelial cancers.

The theoretical advantages of combination chemotherapy are:

1. Drugs acting at different cell sites can be combined to give a synergistic effect.
2. The ability of tumour cells to develop resistance to cytotoxic therapy is reduced.
3. Drugs with different toxicities can be combined to avoid the cumulative toxic effects of each individual drug.

SEQUENTIAL THERAPY

An alternative mechanism for preventing development of drug resistance is to give different drugs in turn. This also allows for a shorter treatment time as severely myelotoxic drugs can be alternated with those which are not. This approach has been effective in treating germ cell tumours and trophoblastic disease (Ch. 40) but not in epithelial tumours.

DURATION OF THERAPY

The optimal duration of chemotherapy is unknown. A palpable tumour will contain 10^9–10^{12} cells but even a clinically undetectable mass will still have 10^8 cells so further chemotherapy is still needed. However, prolonged chemotherapy will cause toxicity. The bone marrow can become hypoplastic and the risk of developing leukaemia or other second cancers is increased. In practice, chemotherapy is usually given for 6–12 months.

Rarely where tumours release a specific tumour marker, such as beta-human chorionic gonadotrophin in trophoblastic disease, marker measurements allow the treatment period to be more accurately defined for each patient. Sufficiently sensitive and specific tumour markers are not yet developed for the common gynaecological tumours.

CALCULATION OF DOSE

To give equivalent dosage to patients, the dose of cytotoxic drugs is based on an estimate of the patient's surface area (m^2) calculated from height and weight. When myelotoxicity is encountered, the dose is modified to prevent severe leukopenia or thrombocytopenia in subsequent courses. With renal or hepatic impairment, doses are reduced for drugs excreted by the kidneys or metabolized by the liver.

TOXIC EFFECTS

The tissues affected by cytotoxic drugs include:

1. Bone marrow.
2. Injection site.
3. Skin, hair and mucosa.
4. Gastrointestinal tract.
5. Reproductive system.
6. Heart.
7. Lungs.
8. Liver.
9. Renal system.
10. Nervous system.

A knowledge of these toxic effects is essential for the safe management of cytotoxic chemotherapy. The most common toxicities for each of the commonly used drugs are shown in Table 33.2. Patients in a poor general condition will not tolerate intensive chemotherapy and, unless there are very exceptional circumstances, chemotherapy is not given in the presence of infection.

Myelosuppression

Myelosuppression occurs with almost all drugs from their action on bone marrow stem cells — the exceptions being vincristine and bleomycin. The blood count must therefore be checked regularly and before each course of treatment. Granulocytes have a life span of 4–5 days, so leukopenia can appear soon after treatment has been given and, if severe (less than 0.5×10^9/l), can result in infections not only from infective organisms such as *Staphylococcus aureus* but also from opportunistic organisms which normally cause no problems in healthy individuals. Fungal infections also occur. Infections need to be treated aggressively as they can be life-threatening. Additional treatment is sometimes required including bowel sterilization and granulocyte transfusions. Granulocyte colony-stimulating factors which have recently been investigated increase the tolerance of bone marrow to chemotherapy, reducing the incidence of secondary infections. Reductions in platelet count also occur soon after treatment. Platelet transfusion relieves spontaneous bleeding from severe thrombocytopenia (less than 25×10^9/l). Anaemia usually occurs only after several courses of chemotherapy because of the long half-life of red blood cells. Blood transfusion may be required.

Prolonged chemotherapy, particularly with alkylating agents such as chlorambucil, has been associated with an increased incidence of myelogenous leukaemia. This is dose-related.

Alimentary tract toxicity

Nausea and vomiting are a common occurrence with chemotherapy, marked with doxorubicin but most particularly severe with cisplatin. This is principally due to a central nervous system effect. Anti-emetic therapy includes steroids, high-dose metoclopramide and other drugs such as the phenothiazines. The most effective agents are the newly released 5-hydroxytryptamine antagonists.

Mouth ulcers are particularly common with the antimetabolites methotrexate and 5-fluorouracil. This ulceration can also affect small bowel mucosa and in extreme cases result in infection leading to septicaemia.

Injection site

Some drugs given intravenously can give rise to phlebitis or thrombosis (e.g. vincristine and doxorubicin). This can be avoided by giving bolus injections into a free-running infusion. If such drugs leak out of the vein, they can result in marked morbidity including large painful ulcers and loss of function.

Skin and hair

Alopecia is a common problem with cyclophosphamide and the antibiotic cytotoxic drugs, in particular doxorubicin. The hair will regrow after chemotherapy is stopped but a wig will be required in the intervening period.

Hyperpigmentation of the skin can occur with treosulfan or bleomycin.

Reproductive system

Chemotherapy causes infertility, but young women successfully treated for germ cell tumours have had normal pregnancies. Depending on the drugs given, fertility may return after some years but recovery is rare after procarbazine (used in Hodgkin's disease) and cyclophosphamide. Menstruation may cease permanently in women approaching the menopause, but there is usually only temporary cessation in young women.

Cytotoxic drugs during pregnancy, particularly in the first trimester, can result in abortion or congenital abnormalities. In theory, genetic damage to the fetus or to ova could cause abnormalities in later generations.

Heart

Doxorubicin can cause cardiomyopathy. This results initially in electrocardiogram changes or tachycardia but can lead to heart failure. The risk is dose-related. By keeping the total dose below 450 mg/m^2 and not using it in cases of impaired cardiac function, cardiotoxicity is rarely seen. The newer anthracycline drugs epirubicin and mitozantrone are less cardiotoxic. Cyclophosphamide is cardiotoxic when given in high doses after radiotherapy to the thorax.

Lungs

Bleomycin can cause pulmonary fibrosis and severe respiratory distress. Therefore, chest X-rays and respiratory function tests are essential before treatment. Anaesthesia after bleomycin also carries an increased risk and anaesthetists need to be aware that the drug has been given in the past.

Liver

Toxic effects to the liver are not common. Methotrexate can cause hepatocellular damage resulting in abnormal liver function tests and very rarely jaundice, so caution must be exercised in patients with impaired hepatic function. Care must also be taken with drugs activated in the liver like cyclophosphamide or excreted in the bile (e.g. doxorubicin).

Renal system

Nephrotoxicity is a serious complication of cisplatin and resulted in fatalities until forced diuresis was found to reduce renal damage. The toxicity is dose-related. To avoid serious renal damage the serum creatinine should be measured before every course. If it increases by more than 25% over the pretreatment value a creatinine or ethylenediaminetetraacetic acid clearance should be performed. If the clearance is less than 60 ml/min, the dose should be reduced by 50%. If the clearance is less than 40 ml/min, cisplatin should be discontinued. Carboplatin, an analogue of cisplatin, has virtually no renal toxicity.

The effect of metabolites from cyclophosphamide and ifosfamide on bladder mucosa has been mentioned previously.

Nervous system

Neurotoxicity is a common toxic effect with vincristine but is less common with other vinca alkaloids. It causes peripheral neuropathy which gives tingling initially but loss of sensation and difficulty with walking can occur later. Vincristine can also affect the autonomic nervous system causing severe constipation. This has been mistaken for a surgical emergency. Cisplatin also causes a dose-dependent peripheral neuropathy and high-tone deafness.

ROLE OF CHEMOTHERAPY

Chemotherapy can be given with either curative or palliative intent. It is the definitive mode of treatment in trophoblastic and germ cell tumours of the ovary and has a major role in the palliation of recurrent and advanced gynaecological malignancies, particularly of the ovary and cervix.

Adjuvant chemotherapy, given in addition to surgery or radiotherapy, is used in carcinoma of the ovary where disease is known or suspected to be present after surgery with the intent of prolonging disease-free survival. Neoadjuvant chemotherapy is given prior to definitive surgical or radiation therapy to reduce tumour bulk. It is currently being investigated in advanced cervical cancer.

CONCLUSION

The role of chemotherapy in gynaecological cancer is limited. Only the rare trophoblastic and germ cell tumours are cured by drugs. Its use in solid tumours is peripheral to surgery and radiotherapy and will remain so unless new drugs with greater activity and tolerable toxicity become available. The present drugs in use show considerable toxicity and can be life-threatening. They should only be given under specialist supervision.

Probably the most important contribution from chemotherapy is improved quality and duration of survival. This is particularly noticeable in patients with advanced ovarian carcinoma, even though the 5-year survival figures have hardly been improved.

KEY POINTS

1. Most radiotherapy is given in the form of electromagnetic radiation as either X-rays from a linear accelerator or as gamma rays from a radioactive isotope such as ^{60}cobalt, ^{137}caesium or ^{192}iridium.
2. Tumour tissue recovers more slowly from radiation damage than does normal tissue so radiotherapy is usually given in many fractions over weeks to exploit this difference.
3. Teletherapy is used to treat large volumes and several fields are used with different entry points to the body to reduce the dose to skin and other normal tissues.
4. Intracavitary brachytherapy is used to treat small volumes as there is a very rapid reduction in the dose of radiotherapy with increasing distance from the source.
5. Brachytherapy may be given at a low dose rate, lasting for several days, or at intermediate or high dose rates lasting for hours or minutes.
6. The main radiation complications following treatment of gynaecological cancers are to the gastrointestinal tract, the bladder and the bone marrow.
7. There are several different alkylating agents, each with a different toxicity spectrum but with similar anti-tumour activity.
8. Cisplatin has little myelotoxicity but causes severe nausea and vomiting, and can cause nephrotoxicity and peripheral neuropathy. Carboplatin has almost no nephrotoxicity or neurotoxicity but is myelotoxic and particularly prone to cause thrombocytopenia.
9. Although combination chemotherapy is much more effective than single-agent regimens in conditions such as Hodgkin's disease or germ cell ovarian tumours, a clear-cut advantage is not yet apparent in epithelial ovarian cancers.
10. Every cytotoxic agent has a characteristic pattern of toxicity which must be taken into account in its use, particularly in combinations.
11. Cytotoxic drugs should only be prescribed by those with specialized knowledge of their use as toxicity can be fatal.
12. Chemotherapy can be curative in trophoblastic disease and ovarian germ cell tumours but may only extend survival in other gynaecological malignancies such as ovarian carcinoma where cure rates are disappointing.

FURTHER READING

Rankin E M, Kaye S B 1990 Principles of chemotherapy. In: Sikora K, Halnan K E (eds) Treatment of cancer, 2nd edn. Chapman & Hall, London, pp 127–146

Stewart S, Kam K C 1990 Radiotherapy techniques, planning and equipment. In: Sikora K, Halnan K E (eds) Treatment of cancer, 2nd edn. Chapman & Hall, London, pp 827–852

34. Premalignant disease of the lower genital tract

W. P. Soutter

THE CERVIX

TERMINOLOGY OF CERVICAL PREMALIGNANCY

The terminology used to classify squamous cell lesions on the cervix has changed over the years in an attempt to reflect changing views of their nature (Table 34.1). Scheme 1 represents the original terms in use until Richart (1967) suggested scheme 2, incorporating the term 'cervical intraepithelial neoplasm' (CIN), to indicate the concept of cervical premalignancy as a continuum of change. Later, milder lesions thought to be due to human papillomavirus (HPV) infection were identified. The Bethesda terminology attempts simplification by grouping CIN I with HPV as a lesion with low potential for malignant change. The Bethesda terminology does not yet have wide support in the UK.

Adenocarcinoma-in-situ is recognized more frequently than before. It has become relatively more important where screening has reduced the numbers of squamous cancers without affecting the incidence of adenocarcinoma.

Table 34.1 Different terminologies for squamous cell cervical lesions

Scheme 1	Scheme 2	Bethesda scheme
	HPV changes	Low-grade lesions
Mild dysplasia	CIN I	Low-grade lesions
Moderate dysplasia	CIN II	High-grade lesions
Severe dysplasia	CIN III	High-grade lesions
Carcinoma-in-situ	CIN III	High-grade lesions

HPV = Human papillomavirus; CIN = cervical intraepithelial neoplasia.

PATHOLOGY OF CERVICAL PREMALIGNANCY

Cervical intraepithelial neoplasia

The diagnosis of CIN is based upon the architectural and cytological appearances of the cervical epithelium.

Architectural features include differentiation, stratification and maturation, terms which are closely related but not synonymous. The proportion of the thickness of the

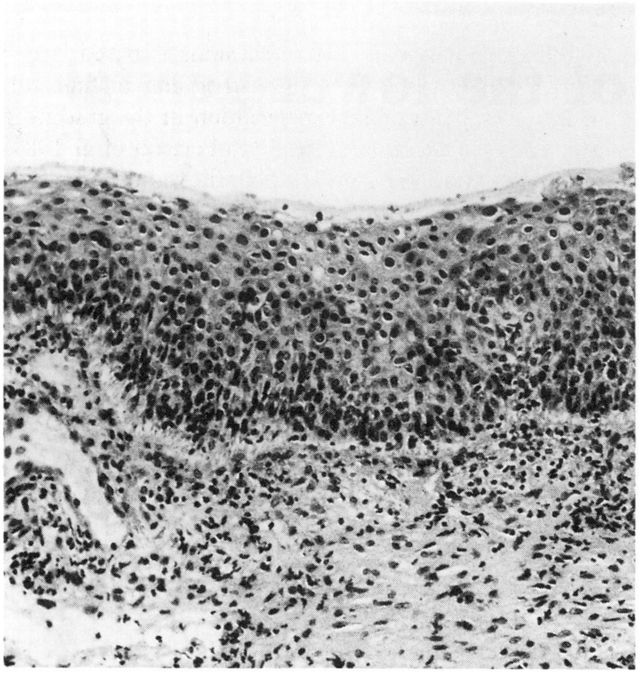

Fig. 34.1 CIN I — haematoxylin and eosin × 170 (by kind permission of Dr M. C. Anderson).

epithelium showing differentiation is a useful feature to be taken into account when deciding the severity of a CIN. It is not the most important criterion despite the fact that it is one of the easiest to assess. In CIN I (Fig. 34.1) at least the upper half of the epithelium usually shows good differentiation and stratification whereas in CIN III differentiation may be very slight or even absent (Fig. 34.2).

Nuclear abnormalities are the most important combination of features to be taken into account when assessing CIN. The nuclei are examined using similar criteria to those employed by the cytologist in assessing a cervical smear: nuclear cytoplasmic ratio, hyperchromasia, nuclear pleomorphism and variation in size of nuclei. Both the overall number of mitotic figures and their height in the epithelium are assessed. The more superficially the mitotic figures are found, the more severe the CIN is likely to be. Abnormal configurations (three-group metaphases and multipolar mitotic figures) are more likely to be found in severe forms of CIN.

CIN may affect the gland crypts as well as the surface epithelium (Fig. 34.3). Anderson & Hartley (1980) showed

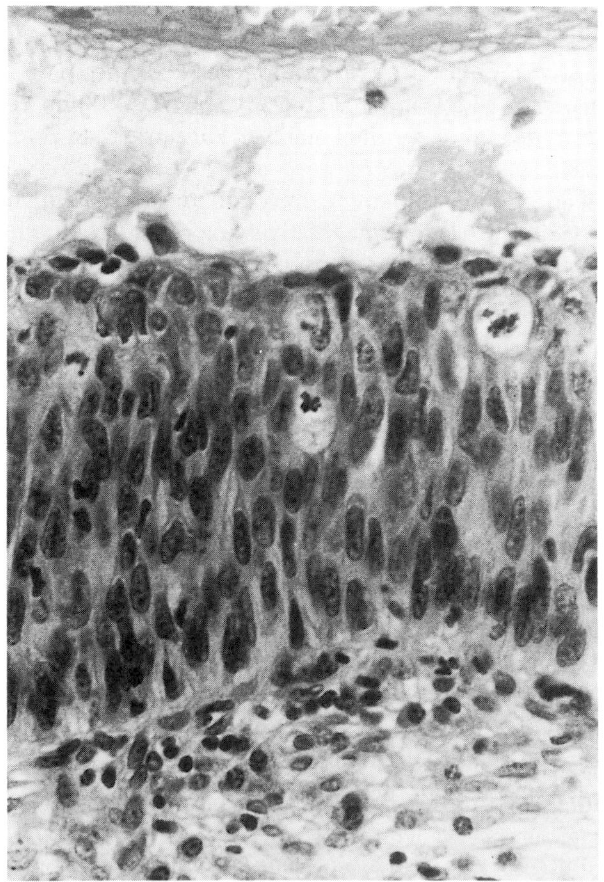

Fig. 34.2 CIN III — haematoxylin and eosin × 170 (by kind permission of Dr M. C. Anderson).

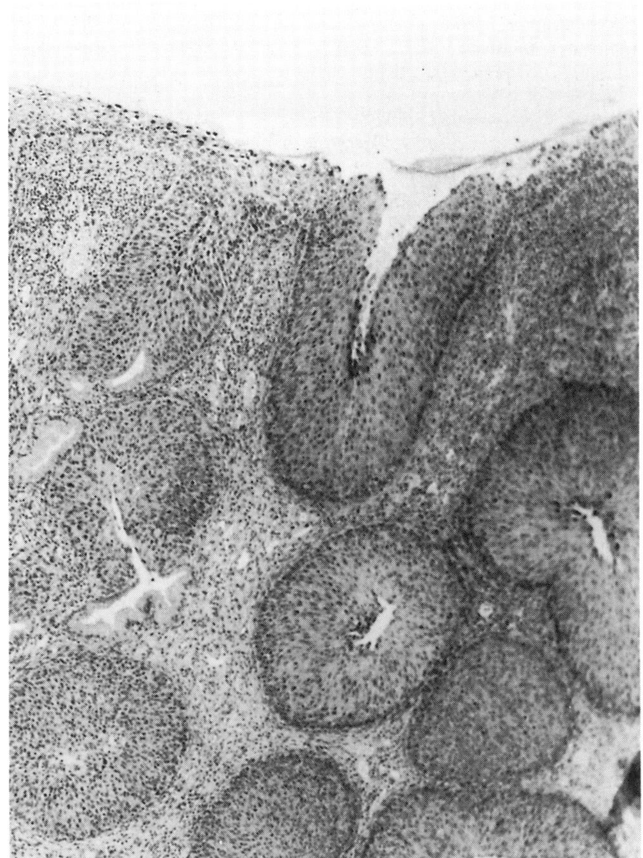

Fig. 34.3 CIN in gland crypts. The morphology of the abnormal epithelium in the involved crypts is similar to that on the surface. Normal columnar epithelium is recognizable in some crypts. Haematoxylin and eosin × 90 (by kind permission of Dr M.C. Anderson).

that the mean depth of crypt involvement in women with CIN III was 1.25 mm and that the mean plus 3 standard deviations (taking in 99.7% of the population) was 3.8 mm. These figures suggested that treatment to a depth of 5 mm into the stroma would be sufficient to eradicate most CIN; however, practical experience has shown that treatment to 10 mm gives much better results without increasing morbidity (Soutter et al 1986a).

Adenocarcinoma-in-situ (AIS)

This underdiagnosed lesion is characterized by columnar cells with large hyperchromatic nuclei and prominent nucleoli (Fig. 34.4). The nuclei may be stratified and show abnormal mitotic figures. There is often gland budding and a 'back-to-back' arrangement. In some cases, the whole of a gland may be involved but often the lesion occurs as a sharply demarcated area in the deep portions of the glands. It may be multifocal. Early invasion is said to have occurred when these lesions are seen lying more deeply in the stroma than the normal glands.

The vast majority of women with AIS are detected by abnormal cytology although in only half of these is an abnormality of the glandular cells recognized. In the remainder, the smear contains a squamous abnormality (Andersen & Arffmann 1989). In two-thirds of cases there is associated CIN or invasive squamous cancer and it is usually only the squamous lesion which is recognized. There are no specific colposcopic features which identify AIS. It is often not detected until a cone biopsy or hysterectomy is performed.

In the great majority of cases, the lesion lies in the transformation zone, close to the squamocolumnar junction (SCJ). Isolated AIS high in the endocervical canal some distance from the SCJ is rare. It follows that a cone biopsy with a good margin of excision in the endocervical canal will be adequate treatment for most cases of AIS.

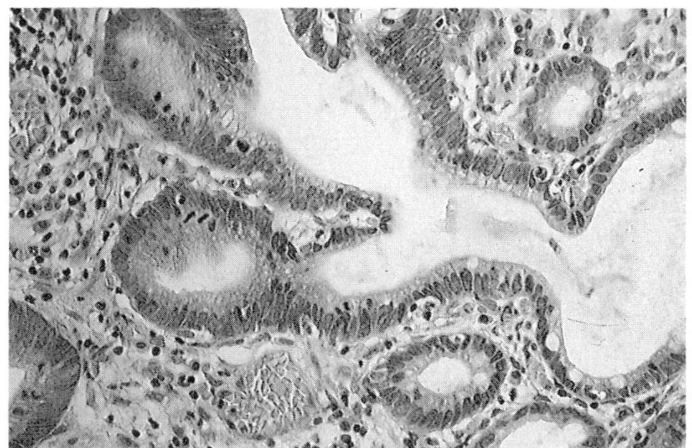

Fig. 34.4 A focal area of AIS showing gland budding, large hyperchromatic nuclei and nuclear stratification (by kind permission of Dr J. Pryse Davies).

Diagnostic precision

The histological diagnosis of these lesions is based largely upon subjective criteria. It is not surprising to find substantial inter- and intraobserver variation in the grading of CIN and the identification of AIS (Robertson et al 1989). Although the variation is greatest at the mild end of the spectrum there is still a considerable amount of disagreement over severe lesions.

The scope for disagreement is inevitably increased when comparing two samples from the same lesion. In a study performed at Hammersmith Hospital, London, there were substantial differences between the colposcopically directed punch biopsy diagnosis and that based on a laser cone biopsy (Skehan et al 1990). This relative imprecision of histological grading of CIN makes it virtually impossible invariably to distinguish by punch biopsy a woman with CIN I from one with CIN III. This should be borne in mind when considering any discussion of the natural history of different grades of CIN and different treatment policies.

MALIGNANT POTENTIAL OF CIN

Progression from CIN III to invasion

The malignant potential of CIN III is amply demonstrated by McIndoe et al (1984) in a crucial paper. A group of 131 patients who had been treated for CIN III and who continued to produce abnormal cytology for more than 2 years after the initial treatment were followed for 4–24 years. After 20 years' follow-up, 36% of these women had developed invasive disease.

Progression from CIN I to CIN III or invasion

Studies of progression from CIN I to CIN III are blighted by the difficulty in accurately determining the grade of the initial lesion. Those reports that relied upon cytology only to determine the initial diagnosis and to document progression or regression are invalidated by the poor correlation between the grade of cytologic abnormality and that of the histology (Soutter et al 1986b). Basing the diagnosis of CIN I upon a colposcopic assessment without punch biopsy, progression to CIN III was observed in 26% of women within 2 years (Campion et al 1986).

Which lesions to treat?

Given the clear malignant potential of untreated CIN III, the difficulty in identifying CIN I accurately and the high progression rate in women whose CIN I was not treated, it seems to be prudent to treat all women with CIN regardless of the grade of abnormality. There is no justification for treating subclinical HPV lesions.

SCREENING FOR CERVICAL PREMALIGNANCY

The objective of cervical screening is to reduce the incidence and the mortality from cervical cancer. When the screening programme detects early invasive disease it can be said to have been only partly successful since the treatment of these early lesions carries a substantial morbidity, is not universally successful and is expensive. The objectives of cervical screening can only be achieved by detecting cervical premalignancy.

Cervical cytology

Cervical cytology is the only well established screening method. When a properly organized programme is implemented, substantial reductions in both incidence and mortality from cervical cancer are achieved (Anderson et al 1988). The vital elements of a successful programme are obtaining wide cover of the population at risk and taking effective action when a cytological abnormality is discovered.

To achieve wide cover, the confidence of the target population must be won. They must know about the programme, what it aims to achieve and how, and they must be convinced that the programme will be successful. If the quality of a cytology service is high, 3-yearly smears are virtually as effective as annual smears (IARC Working Group 1986). Currently in the UK, the proportion of a screened population with positive smears (moderate–severe dyskaryosis) is highest in women aged 25–35 years (Fig. 34.5). A rational programme would therefore recommend 3-yearly smears for all at-risk women between 20 and 60 years of age.

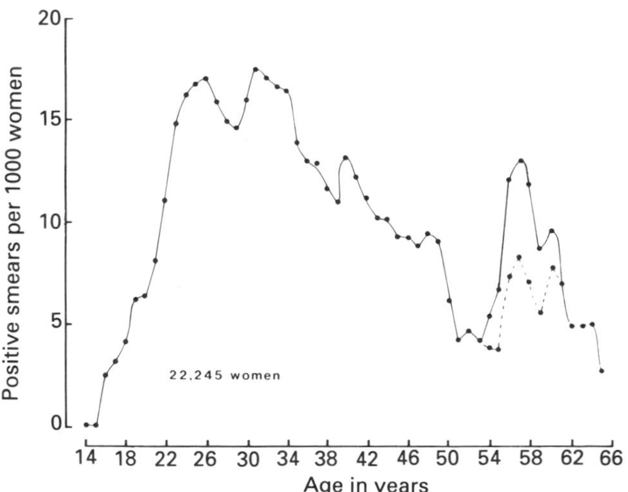

Fig. 34.5 Positive smears per 1000 women examined compared with age, plotted as a 3-year moving average — Queen Elizabeth Hospital, Gateshead, 1983. The second peak among the older women is due to smears being taken from women with symptoms and signs of malignancy. The dashed line corrects for this. From Soutter et al (1984) with permission.

In spite of the success achieved by cervical cytology, it is not without its shortcomings. A satisfactory sample must include cells from the relevant part of the cervix. The cytologist must scan the whole slide carefully to detect one of what may be a small number of abnormal cells. The assessment and definition of cytologic abnormality are subjective with considerable interobserver variation. The process is laborious and tiring with considerable scope for operator error, especially when the workload is high.

The imprecision of cervical cytology is evident from the many studies which report CIN II–III or invasive disease in about 50% of women with smears showing only mild dyskaryosis (Soutter et al 1986b). The high risk associated with a mildly dyskaryotic smear is further illustrated by a prevalence of invasive cancer of 561/100 000 women in a group of 1781 patients with mild dyskaryosis followed up cytologically for 2–12 years (Robertson et al 1988). This should be compared with the annual incidence of cervical cancer in the UK of 15.8/100 000 women.

There have been few satisfactory investigations of the accuracy of cervical cytology. Although false-negative rates from 2.4 to 26% have been estimated by a variety of different types of study, there have been few in which a large asymptomatic population has been screened by cytology and the results of cytology corroborated by an alternative test like colposcopy. In an ongoing study of this sort which has enrolled over 400 women, the sensitivity of cytology has been low (0.52) but the specificity high (0.94). There is clearly scope for a more accurate and less labour-intensive screening method.

Cervicography

Cervicography is a method of detecting cervical pathology which uses the same principles as colposcopy. The cervix is visualized, 5% acetic acid is applied and, after allowing 1 min for the effect of the acetic acid to become apparent,

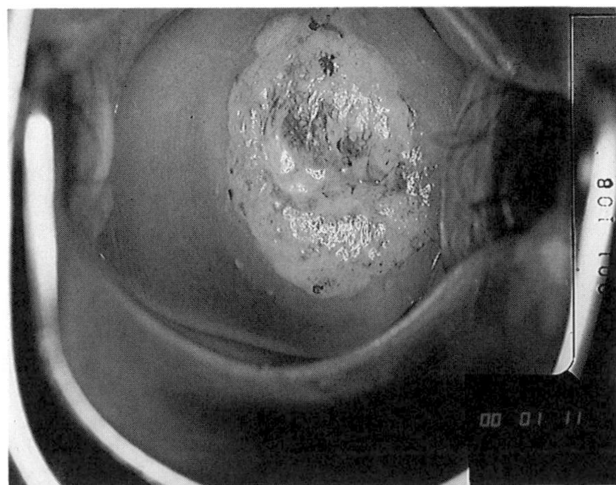

Fig. 34.6 Cervigram showing CIN III. A strongly staining acetowhite lesion with well demarcated, regular edges is seen.

two photographs are taken of the cervix using a specially designed camera (Fig. 34.6). The film is developed as 35 mm slides and these are projected and interpreted by an experienced reviewer. Slides from between 30 and 50 patients can be reported in an hour. The sensitivity of this method is high (89%) but initial reports suggested low specificity. With increased experience and minor modifications to the reporting technique, the specificity is now more satisfactory (92%; Campion et al 1990). This promising technique is likely to be taken up first in countries which have no established cervical cytology service or where it can be added to an established cytology screening programme either as an additional primary screening method or as a secondary screen of women with equivocal cytology.

Other new methods

A number of innovative methods of identifying abnormal cells by computer image analysis or by the use of novel techniques for detecting changes in the molecular biology of the cell membrane are under investigation. None has so far been tested in a large study of asymptomatic women. One promising method, based upon DNA hydrolysis, appears to offer good sensitivity and specificity (Sincock et al 1987). An interesting feature of this technique is that it detects an abnormality in apparently normal cells in women with CIN or cancer. More work is needed to confirm these interesting data.

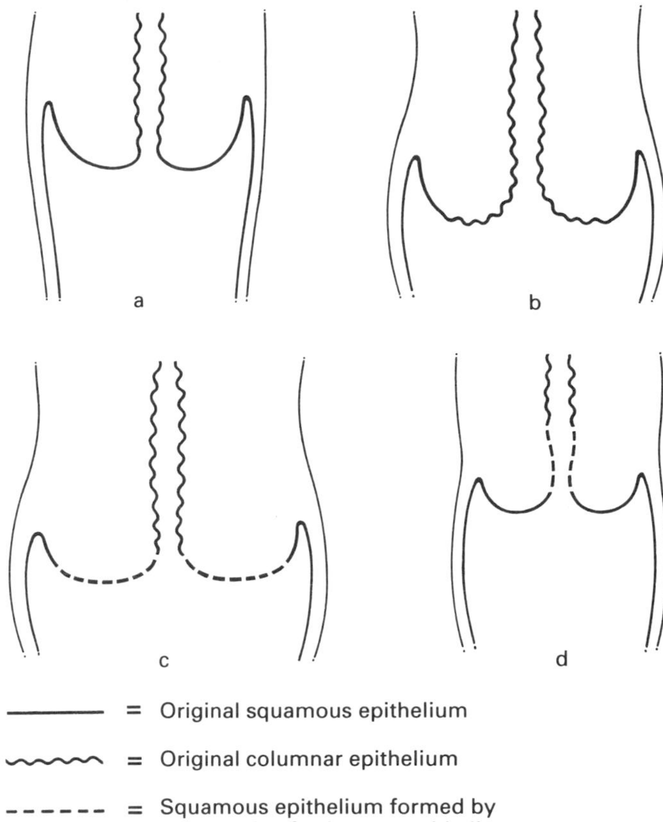

Fig. 34.7 The different stages in the development and involution of the cervix. (**a**) Before puberty the ectocervix is covered with squamous epithelium and columnar epithelium is usually confined to the endocervical canal. (**b**) The cervix enlarges and everts when oestrogen levels rise. This exposes columnar epithelium on the ectocervix. (**c**) The columnar epithelium on the ectocervix is replaced with squamous epithelium by a process of metaplasia. (**d**) Following the climacteric when oestrogen levels fall, the cervix shrinks drawing the squamocolumnar junction up the canal.

COLPOSCOPY OF THE CERVIX

The basis of colposcopy

Eversion of the cervix

At puberty, during pregnancy or when the combined oral contraceptive pill is taken, the cervix enlarges. As it does so, there is a tendency to eversion and to the exposure of columnar epithelium on the ectocervix (Fig. 34.7). The thin columnar epithelium appears red and the result is what is so often erroneously referred to as a 'cervical erosion'.

Squamous metaplasia

The columnar epithelium on the ectocervix is gradually replaced by a process of squamous metaplasia spreading from the SCJ towards the cervical canal. The normal end-result of this transformation is the replacement of the ectopic columnar epithelium with mature squamous epithelium (Fig. 34.7c). If squamous epithelium now covers the entrance to a cervical crypt and the columnar cells continue to secrete mucus in the crypt, a nabothian follicle results. This is the only clinical evidence of the prior existence of columnar epithelium in that area. When the cervix shrinks in the months and years following pregnancy and after the menopause, it gradually inverts, drawing the new SCJ up the endocervical canal (Fig. 34.7d).

The transformation zone

The region of the cervix in which this process of metaplasia occurs is called the transformation zone. In some women the transformation zone may extend on to the vaginal walls. A common source of confusion in colposcopy is the loose use of the term 'transformation zone' when referring to that part of the true transformation zone where metaplastic or dysplastic epithelium can be seen colposcopically.

The genesis of squamous cervical neoplasia

Squamous neoplasia results from a disruption of the normal

metaplastic process. Thus, CIN develops as a confluent lesion confined to an area of the cervix contiguous with the SCJ. It is this characteristic localization which enables the colposcope to be used in the assessment of CIN.

The role of colposcopy

Prior to the advent of colposcopy, cytologists recommended referral to a gynaecologist only after two successive severely dyskaryotic smears were obtained. The reason for this delaying policy was because a knife cone biopsy would be required to determine whether or not there was a premalignant lesion on the cervix and this operation had potentially serious consequences for the future obstetric prospects of the young women in whom these abnormalities were most often found.

That conservative policy is no longer justifiable. With colposcopy, the women who require treatment can be identified and those who do not can be reassured. In addition, the treatment can be carefully tailored to remove only the minimum of cervical tissue. Most women with CIN can be treated in the outpatient clinic with methods that do not prejudice their future fecundity. With the recognition that mild cytological abnormalities are associated with a high prevalence of significant histological abnormalities, it is apparent that the indications for referral need to be revised (Table 34.2). Nowadays, no woman with abnormal cytology should be treated without prior colposcopy.

Although the majority of women sent for colposcopy have abnormal smears, a suspicious-looking cervix is sufficient reason for referral even if the smear is negative. Such women sometimes have invasive cancer.

The colposcopic method

A detailed description of the author's personal method may be found elsewhere (Soutter 1989). Space permits only an outline description here.

Bimanual examination and the smear

A bimanual examination is essential to aid detection of frank invasive disease of the cervix, a uterine or an ovarian mass. A bivalve speculum is then introduced and a smear is taken. Deferring the smear until after the colposcopic inspection may reduce the risk of removing the epithelium one wishes to study (see below) but unfortunately it provides a less satisfactory sample for the cytologist (Griffiths et al 1989). Only if the os is narrowed or the SCJ out of sight up the canal is an endocervical brush used.

Preacetic acid examination

If the view of the cervix is obscured by a discharge this should be removed gently with saline. The preliminary inspection should include both the cervix and upper vagina. At this stage of the examination there are three objectives: to identify leukoplakia; to exclude obvious evidence of invasive disease; and to identify viral condylomata.

Leukoplakia must be identified prior to the application of acetic acid after which it may be impossible to differentiate from acetowhite epithelium. Because the hyperkeratinization of leukoplakia may conceal invasive disease, biopsy is mandatory.

Invasion is often obvious from the bizarre appearances of the surface of the cervix, which may appear grossly irregular, either raised or ulcerated (Fig. 34.8). This disorganization of the surface is usually recognizable even when atypical vessels cannot be identified or the area subsequently fails to turn white after the application of acetic acid. The atypical vessels seen on invasive lesions run a bizarre course and are often corkscrew- or comma-shaped

Table 34.2 Management of abnormal cervical cytology

Papanicolaou class		Histology	Action
I	Normal	0.1% CIN II–III	Repeat in 3 years (unless clinical suspicion)
II	Inflammatory	6% CIN II–III	Repeat in 6 months (colposcopy after 3 abnormal)
	Borderline nuclear changes	20–37% CIN II–III	Repeat in 6 months (colposcopy after 2 abnormal)
III	Mild dyskaryosis	50% CIN II–III	Colposcopy
	Moderate dyskaryosis	50–75% CIN II–III	Colposcopy
IV	Severe dyskaryosis 'Positive' 'Malignant cells'	80–90% CIN II–III 5% Invasion	Colposcopy
V	Invasion suspected	50% Invasion	Urgent colposcopy
Abnormal glandular cells		? Adenocarcinoma of the cervix or endometrium	Urgent colposcopy

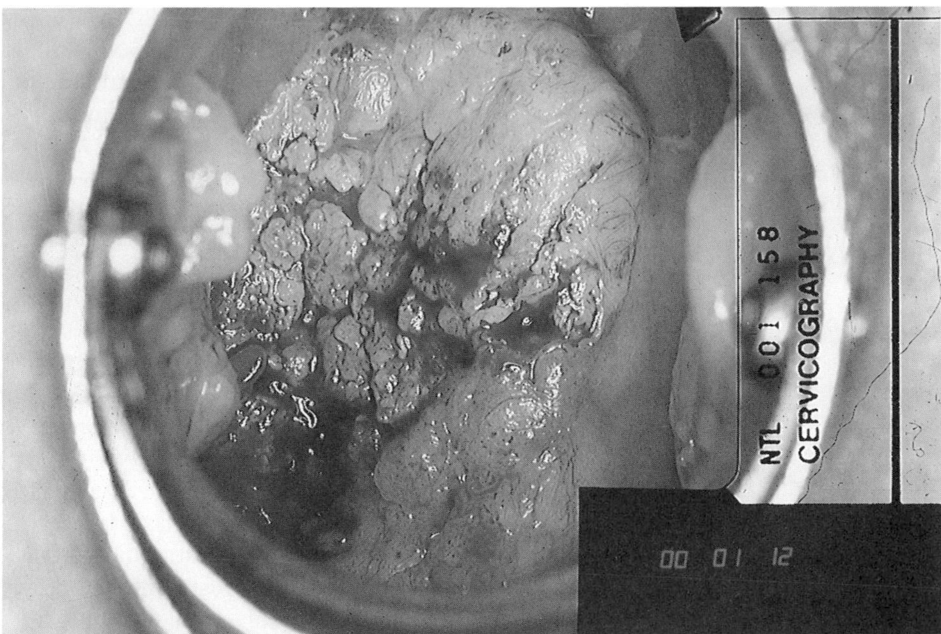

Fig. 34.8 A cervigram of a stage Ib cervical cancer showing the irregular surface.

(Fig. 34.9). They are large in diameter, abruptly appearing on and disappearing from the surface. They do not branch dichotomously like normal vessels.

Condylomata are usually obvious from their regular frond-like surface (Fig. 34.10) but biopsies should be taken, especially when they are located within the active part of the transformation zone where it is more difficult to be sure of their benign nature.

Acetic acid examination

A low-power inspection. Having completed the first inspection of the cervix, 5% acetic acid should be applied liberally and gently. This turns abnormal epithelium white, producing the so-called 'acetowhite' changes of CIN. It is important to allow sufficient time to elapse for faintly staining areas to show up. While waiting for any colour changes to occur, the cervix and vaginal fornices are inspected under low power in order to have the widest field of view possible so that areas of faint acetowhite may be observed against the contrasting background of normal epithelium. After about 30 s it is usually possible to proceed. If a lesion has become visible, its outer limits should be determined first.

Identifying the SCJ. Next, the position of the SCJ must be ascertained to define the upper limits of the abnormality. Failure to identify the SCJ correctly is one of the main pitfalls in colposcopy. It is important to note that the SCJ is marked by the lower limit of normal columnar epithelium, not the upper limit of squamous, as these do not always lie at the same level. The higher the SCJ ap-

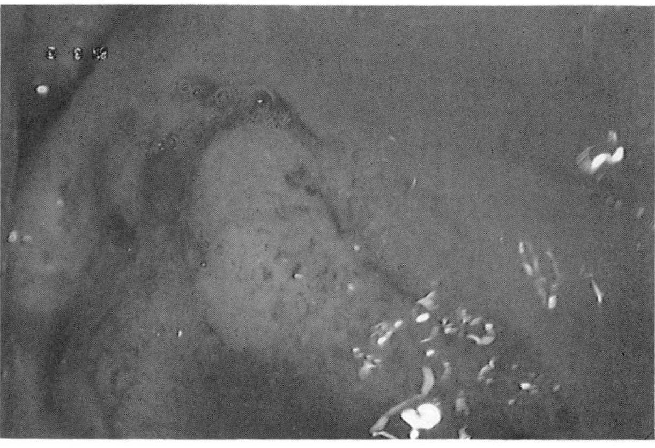

Fig. 34.9 This high-power view of a cervical tumour shows some short atypical vessels in the lower centre of the picture and longer stretches of atypical vessels both above this area and in the bottom left-hand corner. Note also the irregular surface.

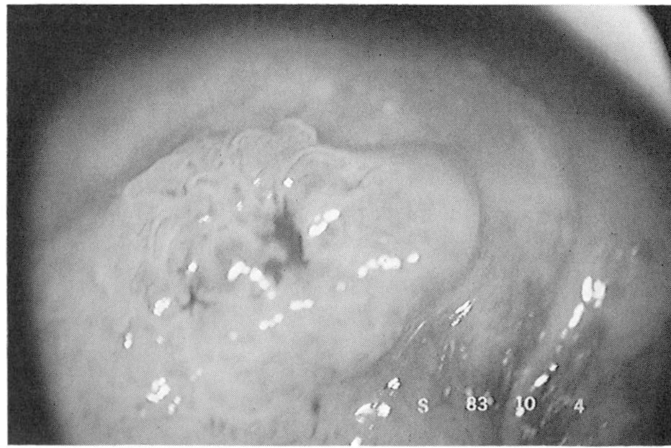

Fig. 34.10 A high-power view of a large cervical condyloma prior to the application of acetic acid. Note the regular form and the microvilli with looped capillaries on the top of the condyloma.

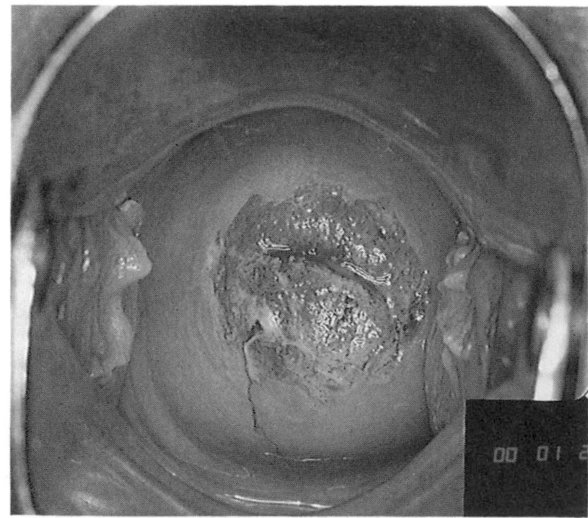

Fig. 34.11 A cervigram of a normal cervix with a large ectropion. The central portion of the cervix around the os is covered with normal columnar epithelium.

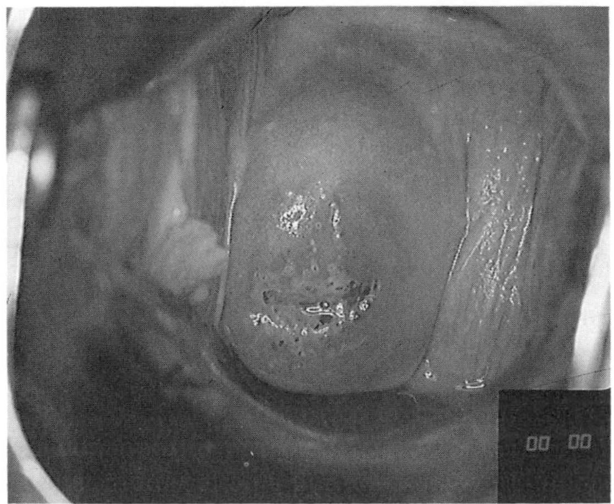

Fig. 34.12 This cervigram shows an area of faintly acetowhite epithelium around the cervical os; however, it is seen most clearly on the anterior lip in this photograph.

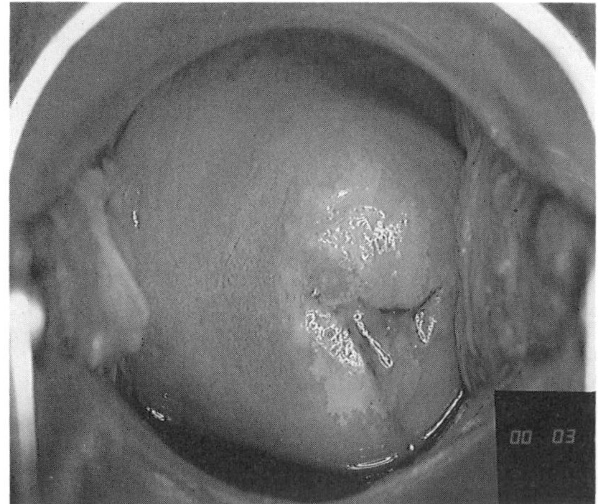

Fig. 34.13 A large, faintly acetowhite lesion with an irregular edge is visible on both lips of the cervix. Two satellite lesions are visible on the posterior lip at 6 o'clock below the main lesion.

pears to lie in the canal the more difficult it becomes to assess the lesion accurately and, except when the cervix is very patulous, 5 mm represents the limit above which colposcopic evaluation becomes unsafe.

Determining the nature of the lesion. It is necessary only to decide whether or not a lesion with malignant potential is indeed present and whether invasion may have already occurred. It is preferable to adopt a very conservative approach to the latter objective and to regard cases of severe CIN III as being potentially invasive. When determining the significance of a lesion, the colposcopist assesses the colour, the margins and the vascular markings.

Non-malignant epithelium that becomes acetowhite. Not all areas of acetowhite change are abnormal. Columnar epithelium will blanch briefly after exposure to acetic acid. It may be identified by its villous or furrowed surface (Fig. 34.11). Squamous metaplasia has a glassy white appearance but can be hard to distinguish from CIN I (Fig. 34.12). After any form of treatment, the cervix may develop areas of acetowhite, sub epithelial fibrosis. This can be recognized by the radial arrangement of lines of fine punctation.

Wart virus lesions. Considering the difficulties the histopathologist has in differentiating CIN from wart virus lesions it is no surprise that flat viral lesions are difficult to identify with certainty colposcopically. In general, they have faint, very irregular margins and isolated satellite lesions (Fig. 34.13). In early condylomata, looped capillaries in small villi may be seen (Fig. 34.10). The delicate fronds of fully formed condylomata are usually easy to identify but all raised lesions on the active transformation zone must be biopsied lest they be invasive cancer.

Features of CIN. CIN are usually distinct acetowhite lesions with clear margins (Fig. 34.6). They often show a mosaic vascular pattern with patches of acetowhite separated by vessels like red weeds between white flagstones. Where the vessels run perpendicular to the surface, punctation is seen as the vessels are viewed end-on. This appears as red spots on a white background. In general, the more quickly and strongly the acetowhite changes develop, the clearer and more regular the margins of the lesion, and the more pronounced the mosaic or punctation, the more severe is the lesion likely to be. However, not all features will be equally marked and many CIN III lesions show only a strong matt-white colour.

Features of invasion. Frank, early invasion is often obvious before acetic acid is applied (see above) but microinvasion may not become apparent until after the application of the acid. Although atypical vessels may be seen, the only indication of invasion is often a very marked mosaic pattern or coarse punctation — large-diameter, widely separated red spots (Fig. 34.14).

Because even expert colposcopists will fail to identify correctly every case of early invasion (Bekassy et al 1983), excisional treatment which removes the whole lesion for

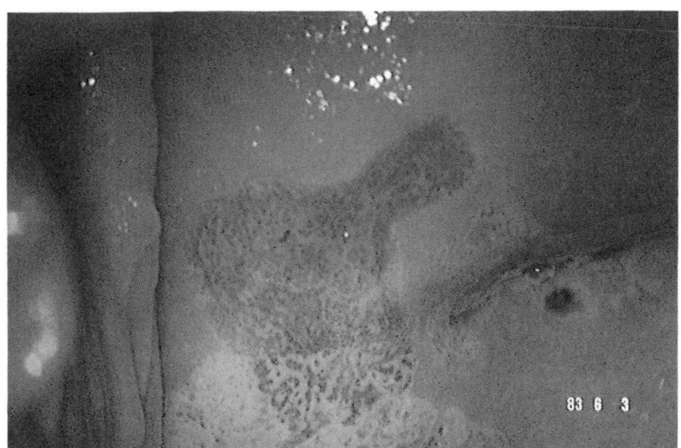

Fig. 34.14 This microinvasive lesion is a good example of coarse punctuation.

histological assessment merits wider use to avoid the risk of undertreating invasive disease.

Pitfalls in colposcopy

The first pitfall — the false SCJ caused by an abrasion

The SCJ should be identified by observing the *lower limit of normal columnar epithelium*, not the upper limit of squamous. The reason for this is the ease with which CIN and metaplastic epithelium can be detached from the underlying stroma, particularly at the SCJ where the unwary may mistakenly regard the upper limit of acetowhite change as synonymous with the SCJ. Careful inspection of the red epithelium at this junction will reveal a flat surface covered by spidery and often whorled blood vessels characteristic of exposed stroma. This can be distinguished from columnar epithelium which has a soft, velvety-looking surface and blanches briefly when exposed to acetic acid.

The second pitfall — the SCJ in the canal

When the SCJ lies within the endocervical canal, if the upper part of the lesion is inspected from too acute an angle the assessment of both the length of the endocervical canal involved with CIN and the severity of the lesion becomes unreliable.

The third pitfall — the previously treated cervix

When a cervix has been treated previously for any reason, the topography of the transformation zone will have been altered. Areas of metaplasia, CIN or invasive disease in the canal or in cervical glands may have escaped destruction and may persist as isolated iatrogenic skip lesions surrounded by columnar epithelium, or covered by new squamous epithelium (Fig. 34.15). Such patients should always be treated by an excisional method.

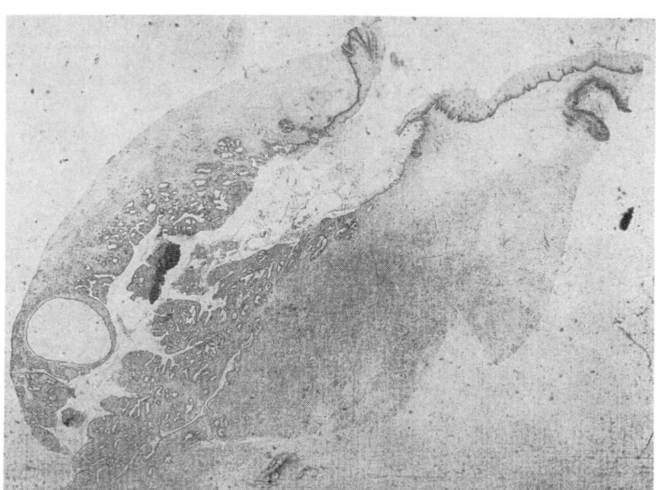

Fig. 34.15 An iatrogenic skip lesion can be seen in this cone biopsy performed in spite of normal, satisfactory colposcopy because of severe dyskaryosis in a woman who had previously been treated with cervical electrodiathermy. The ectocervical end of this cone biopsy to the bottom and left is covered with normal squamous epithelium. The SCJ is near the external os and the lower canal is lined by columnar epithelium but halfway up the canal, near the nabothian cyst on the right, is an isolated area of CIN III. In deeper sections this was shown to be an invasive tumour.

The fourth pitfall — glandular lesions

It cannot be assumed that the rules of colposcopy apply to women with adenocarcinoma or AIS. AIS cannot be identified colposcopically so a cone biopsy is an essential investigation in the management of a patient with abnormal glandular cells in her smear. Many of these patients also have CIN which requires treatment in its own right. A cone biopsy which completely excises AIS is probably adequate therapy.

TREATMENT OF CIN

Detailed descriptions of the techniques discussed may be found elsewhere (Monaghan 1987). CIN was originally treated by radical hysterectomy but it soon became evident that this was unnecessary and simple hysterectomy became the method of choice. In time, it was realized that cone biopsy was just as effective and now hysterectomy is reserved for those with difficult-to-treat recurrent disease or who have additional indications for hysterectomy. The introduction of colposcopy and a better appreciation of the limited location of CIN led to the introduction of more conservative methods of treatment.

Table 34.3 Methods of ablative treatment of CIN: in chronological order, with the longest established methods first

Method	Anaesthesia	Restrictions
Radical electrodiathermy	GA	Vaginal extension of CIN?
Cryotherapy	None	CIN III; large lesions
Laser vaporization	LA	None
'Cold' coagulation	None	Vaginal extension of CIN

GA = general anaesthesia; LA = local anaesthesia

Ablative methods

A large number of ablative methods are available (Table 34.3). The chief advantage of these (with the exception of radical electrodiathermy) is that general anaesthesia is not required. Cryotherapy is the one method most often associated with unsatisfactory results but this has usually been due to inappropriate case selection. A disadvantage common to all these techniques is that they depend heavily upon the exclusion of invasion by colposcopy and directed biopsy. In addition, they are not applicable to all patients — some will always require an excisional treatment. The indications for excisional treatment of CIN are listed below:

1. Any suspicion of invasive disease.
2. Any suspicion of a glandular abnormality.
3. SCJ not clearly visible.
4. History of any previous cervical surgery.
5. Elective method of treating any case of CIN?

Excisional methods

Knife cone biopsy was supplanted as the standard treatment by ablative techniques partly because of the complications and partly because of the need for general anaesthesia. Complications are listed below.

1. Intraoperative haemorrhage.
2. Secondary haemorrhage.
3. Pelvic infection.
4. Cervical stenosis.
5. Cervical incompetence.

The complications of laser cone biopsy are fewer than those of knife cone biopsy; the technique is far more precise (Larsson et al 1983) and the distortion of the cervix that results is much less, suggesting that there will be fewer problems in any subsequent pregnancies. In addition, laser cone biopsy can very often be performed under local anaesthesia (Partington et al 1987).

The ability to perform laser cone biopsy under local anaesthesia, the observation that the complications were no greater than in laser vaporization (Partington et al 1989) and anxieties about invasive cancer being missed led to a widening of the indications for excisional therapy and to the suggestion that laser excision should replace vaporization for most patients. The advent of large loop electrodiathermy excision of the transformation zone (LLETZ) made excisional treatment quicker and reduced the cost of the equipment required (Prendiville et al 1989). This technique employs a blended diathermy current and a loop of very thin stainless-steel wire (Fig. 34.16 and 34.17).

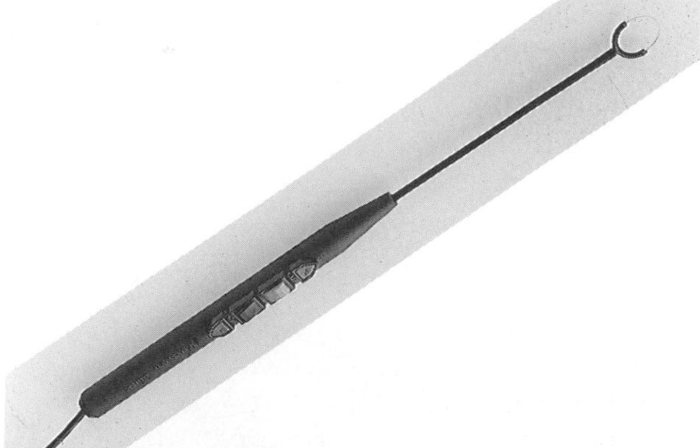

Fig. 34.16 One of the varieties of large wire loops used for LLETZ. (Figure supplied by Valleylab UK.)

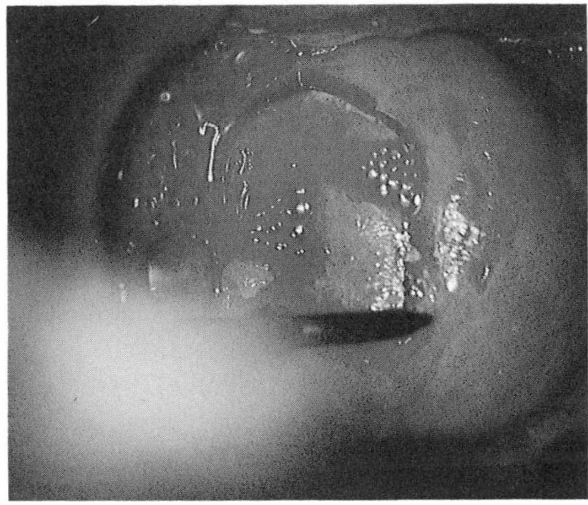

Fig. 34.17 A cone biopsy being taken with LLETZ. (Figure supplied by Valleylab UK.)

Choice of technique

None of the different methods of treating CIN is more effective than any of the others when used appropriately by a well trained and experienced operator. Each has particular advantages of cost or ease of use or speed or precision. The particular method chosen will depend upon local circumstances. It seems sensible to the author to choose a method which will allow abnormalities to be excised under local anaesthesia. In spite of its greater capital cost, the laser does have the advantage that it may be used both to excise and to vaporize lesions when it is appropriate to do so. An example of the latter are large lesions which extend on to the sides of the cervix or beyond the cervix into the fornices.

Results of treatment

Treated adequately, no more than 5% of patients treated for CIN will have recurrent disease within 2 years (Soutter et al 1986a). Thereafter, the number of recurrences is small. However, long-term follow-up is necessary as these women remain at a higher risk of CIN or invasive cervical cancer than the general population (Burghardt & Holzer 1980). In that study, the prevalence of invasive cancer in women treated by cone biopsy after colposcopic assessment was 574/100 000 during a follow-up of 4–20 years. All of the cancers were detected within 11 years. In addition, the same rate of residual vaginal intraepithelial neoplasia of the vaginal vault was observed in the 11 years after hysterectomy following incomplete excision by cone biopsy. A further 2.21% were found to have recurrent CIN but the authors did not specify how long after the initial treatment these were discovered. In the light of the results of this and other similar studies, annual cytological follow-up of patients treated for CIN by any method would seem to be prudent for at least 10 years.

THE VAGINA

TERMINOLOGY AND PATHOLOGY OF VAIN

The terminology and pathology of vaginal intraepithelial neoplasia (VAIN) is analogous to that of CIN (VAIN I–III). The main difference is that vaginal epithelium does not normally have crypts so the epithelial abnormality remains superficial until invasion occurs. The common exception to this is found following surgery — usually hysterectomy — when abnormal epithelium can be buried below the suture line or in suture tracks.

NATURAL HISTORY OF VAIN

VAIN is seldom seen as an isolated vaginal lesion. It is more usual for it to be a vaginal extension of CIN. In most cases it is diagnosed colposcopically prior to any treatment during the investigation of an abnormal smear. However, it may not be recognized until after a hysterectomy has been performed. When this happens, abnormal epithelium is likely to be buried behind the sutures used to close the vault. Consequently a portion of the lesion will remain invisible and unevaluable (Fig. 34.18). In the series reported by Ireland & Monaghan (1988), 28% of those treated surgically proved to have unexpected invasive disease. Untreated or inadequately treated VAIN may progress to frank invasive cancer (Woodman et al 1984). Very rarely, VAIN may be seen many years after radiotherapy for cervical carcinoma when it is probably a new lesion. Care must be taken in these women to ensure that postradiotherapy changes are not being misinterpreted as VAIN.

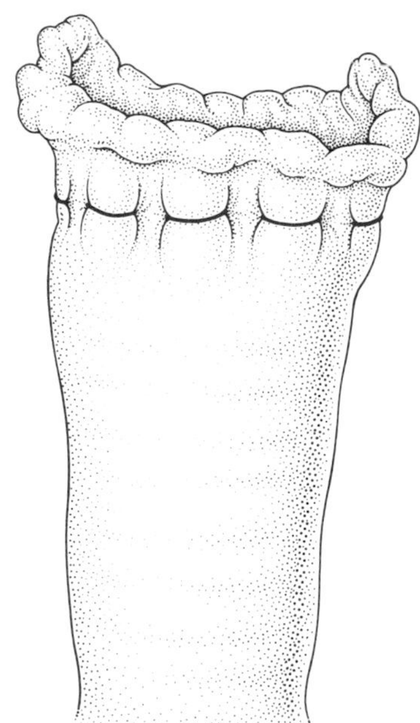

Fig. 34.18 Sutures in the vaginal vault isolate a cuff of the vagina above the suture line.

COLPOSCOPY OF THE VAGINA

Colposcopy of the vagina is more difficult than the cervix, partly because of the greater area of epithelium to be examined, partly because the surface of the vaginal epithelium is very irregular and partly because it is very difficult to view the vaginal walls at right angles. If the patient has had a hysterectomy it is very difficult to see into the angles of the vagina and impossible to visualize epithelium that lies above the suture line or vaginal adhesions. The colposcopic features of VAIN are very similar to those of CIN except that mosaic is seen less often (Fig. 34.19).

TREATMENT OF VAIN

Carbon dioxide laser

Provided invasive disease has been excluded, laser vaporization is a satisfactory way of treating VAIN in women who have not undergone previous surgery. However, the report of invasive disease developing in 2 out of 14 posthysterectomy patients treated with the laser illustrated the dangers of overlooking disease buried above the suture line (Woodman et al 1984). Thus, although the

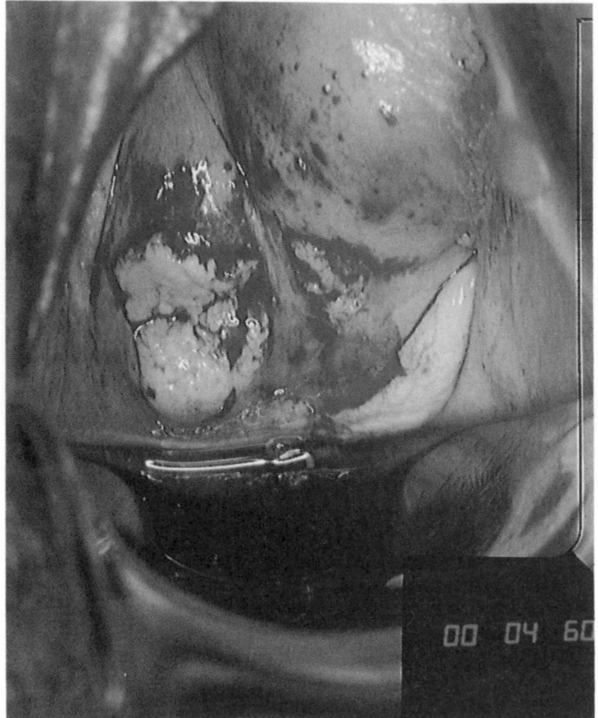

Fig. 34.19 VAIN after a hysterectomy. A patch of dense acetowhite epithelium is easily visible in the centre of the figure in the left vaginal angle. A second area of VAIN can be seen just above the speculum, spreading out of the right angle.

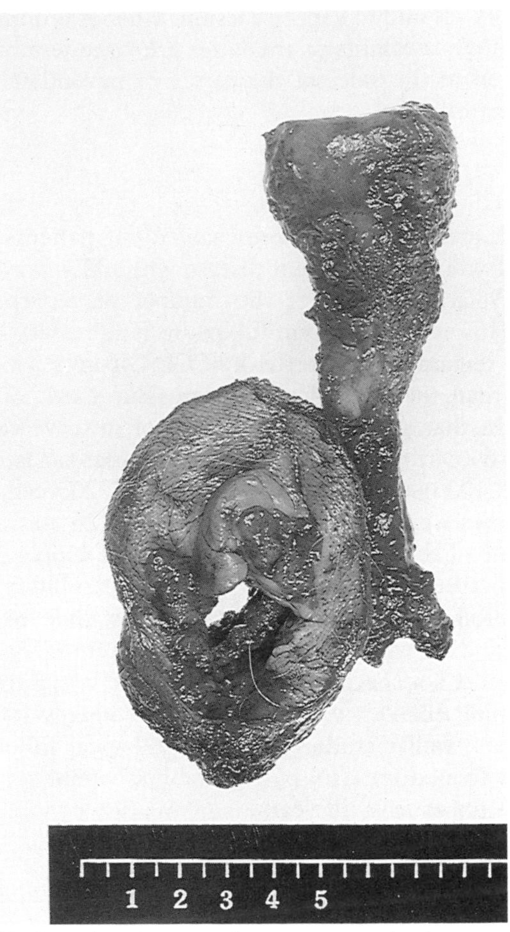

Fig. 34.20 A total vaginectomy, hysterectomy and vulvectomy performed by the vaginal route in an elderly woman with severe irritation from extensive VAIN and VIN 20 years after radiotherapy for cervical cancer (units in cm).

laser may be useful in reducing the size of a lesion or in treating women who have not had a hysterectomy, it should not be used as the sole method of treatment in VAIN of the vaginal vault following hysterectomy. The same applies to the use of topical 5-fluorouracil.

Partial or total vaginectomy

Surgical excision of VAIN gives far more satisfactory results (Ireland & Monaghan 1988) and is the only effective option available to patients previously treated with radiotherapy. The patients in Ireland & Monaghan's series were treated by an abdominal operation or by a combined abdominal and vaginal approach. This necessitates extensive pelvic dissection which can be avoided by a vaginal approach (Fig. 34.20). While the latter procedure is often very straightforward, it can prove to be extremely taxing in patients with a narrow introitus and no laxity of the vaginal vault.

Where the lesion involves a large area of the vagina there may be a place for laser vaporization to reduce the size of the lesion. The entire lesion is vaporized under general anaesthesia and, some months later when the effect of the laser treatment can be assessed, the vault of the vagina is excised. When this approach is unsuccessful and in older patients, total vaginectomy or radiotherapy is required.

Radiotherapy

There can be no doubt that intracavitary radiotherapy is a highly effective treatment for VAIN (Hernandez-Linares et al 1980; Woodman et al 1988). The two major concerns about this form of therapy are the possibility of radiation-induced cancer and the effects it may have upon coital function. Radiation-induced second cancer in the vaginal vault may occur but it is probably an extraordinarily rare event (Choo & Anderson 1982; Boice et al 1985). Brachytherapy to the vault of the vagina is unlikely to cause major coital problems if the patient and her spouse are encouraged to resume normal sexual relations as soon as possible (Woodman et al 1988). Where the area of disease is more extensive, no method of therapy is likely to be free of the risk of inducing sexual dysfunction.

Conclusions

The management of VAIN after hysterectomy in a young woman is likely to be surgical. If the lesion is extensive, prior laser therapy may be helpful in reducing the extent of disease. In older patients, especially when access is difficult, surgery offers few additional benefits but carries a potential for greater morbidity. Radiotherapy is therefore likely to be the treatment of choice. Whatever the circumstances it would be sensible for such patients to be evaluated and treated by those with experience of this unusual but troublesome condition.

THE VULVA

Vulval intraepithelial neoplasia (VIN) is seen more commonly than was the case 10–20 years ago. It is not certain whether this represents a real increase or is simply the result of a greater awareness of the problem.

PATHOLOGY OF PREMALIGNANT DISEASE OF THE VULVA

Both squamous VIN and adenocarcinoma-in-situ (Paget's disease) occur on the vulva. The latter is very rare. The histological features and terminology of VIN are analogous to those of CIN and VAIN. In the same way, the histological appearance of Paget's disease is similar to the lesion seen in the breast. In a third of cases of Paget's disease, there is an adenocarcinoma in underlying apocrine glands and these carry an especially poor prognosis (Creasman et al 1975).

NATURAL HISTORY OF VIN

Forty per cent of women with VIN are younger than 41 years (Buscema et al 1980). Although histologically very similar to CIN and often occurring in association with it, VIN is said not to have the same malignant potential (Buscema et al 1980; Kaufman & Gordon 1986b). However, this opinion is based largely on studies of women who have been treated by excision biopsy or vulvectomy. This may not be true of untreated or inadequately treated patients; 5 such women progressed to invasive cancer in 2–8 years (Jones & McLean 1986).

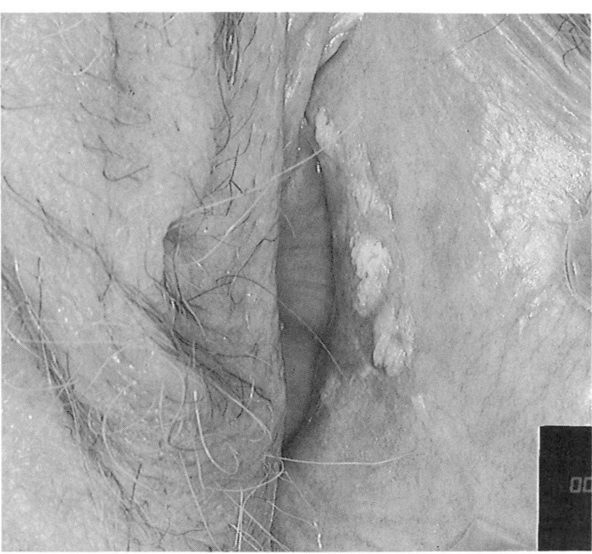

Fig. 34.21 Small patches of VIN III appearing as leukoplakia.

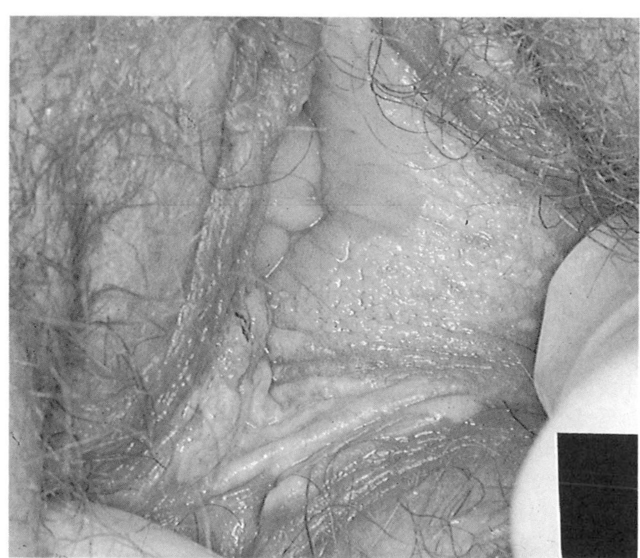

Fig. 34.22 An area of VIN III on the labium minorum seen as a slightly raised, whitish lesion with a granular surface.

DIAGNOSIS AND ASSESSMENT OF VIN

Intraepithelial disease of the vulva often presents as pruritus vulvae but 20–45% are asymptomatic and are frequently found after treatment of preinvasive or invasive disease at other sites in the lower genital tract, particularly the cervix (Jones & McLean 1986; Kaufman & Gordon 1986a).

These lesions are often raised above the surrounding skin and have a rough surface. The colour is variable — white, due to hyperkeratinization; red, due to thinness of the epithelium, or dark brown, due to increased melanin deposition in the epithelial cells (Fig. 34.21 and 34.22).

However, the full extent of the abnormality is often not apparent until 5% acetic acid is applied (Fig. 34.23). After 2 min, VIN turns white and mosaic or punctation may be visible. While these changes may be seen with the naked eye in a good light, it is much easier to use a hand lens or a colposcope. Toluidine blue is also used as a nuclear stain but areas of ulceration give false-positive results and hyperkeratinization gives false negatives.

Adequate biopsies must be taken from abnormal areas to rule out invasive disease. This can usually be done under local anaesthesia in the outpatient clinic using a disposable 4 mm Stiefel biopsy punch or a Keyes punch.

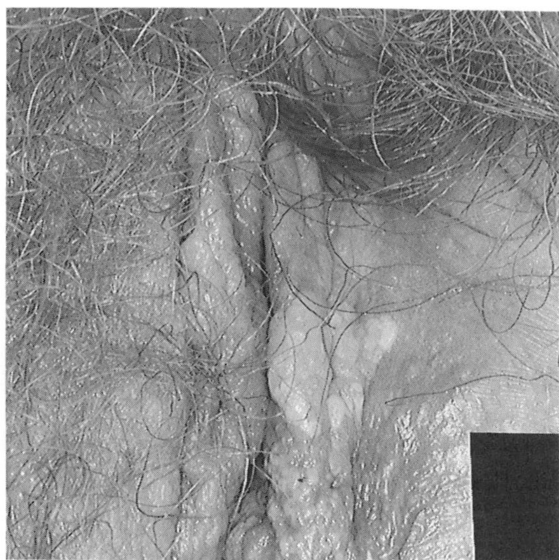

Fig. 34.23 A small patch of VIN III after the application of acetic acid.

TREATMENT OF VIN

The treatment of VIN is difficult. Uncertainty about the malignant potential, the multifocal nature of the disorder and the discomfort and mutilation resulting from therapy suggest that recommendations should be cautious and conservative in order to avoid making the treatment worse than the disease. The youth of many of these patients is a further important consideration. None the less, the documented progression of untreated cases to invasive cancer underlines the potential importance of these lesions (Jones & McLean 1986). If the patient has presented with symptoms, therapy is required. Asymptomatic patients, particularly under the age of 50 years, are probably best observed closely with biopsies repeated if there are any suspicious changes.

Surgery

If the lesion is small, an excision biopsy may be both diagnostic and therapeutic. If the disease is multifocal or covers a wide area, a skin graft may improve the cosmetic result of a skinning vulvectomy (Caglar et al 1986). However, the donor site is often very painful and a satisfactory result can be obtained in many patients without grafting.

Carbon dioxide laser

An alternative approach is to vaporize the abnormal epithelium with the carbon dioxide laser. Careful control of the depth of destruction is essential for good cosmetic results (Reid 1985). The first surgical plane is recognized by moving the laser beam rapidly in parallel lines until bubbles of silver opalescence can be seen beneath the surface char. This is accompanied by a crackling sound. The basement membrane may then be exposed by wiping off the char with a moist swab. Further light application of the laser will expose yellowish tissue that looks like a chamois cloth. This is the papillary dermis and marks the second plane. Vaporization to the first or second surgical planes is sufficient for viral disease or for vulval dystrophy without atypia causing otherwise intractable pruritus vulvae. Healing is usually complete within 14 days and the cosmetic result is excellent.

The third plane is the superficial reticular dermis and is identified by the presence of whitish fibres like soggy thread. This is the deepest level from which normal healing can take place by epithelialization from skin appendages in the base of the crater. The fourth plane, the deep reticular dermis, contains most of the hair follicles and apocrine glands. These look like grains of sand when exposed by the laser but are usually largely destroyed by the time they become visible. Skin grafting is necessary if the dermis is destroyed to this level.

Given the very irregular surface of the vulva, it is very difficult to achieve a uniform depth of destruction. Moreover, the depth of treatment required for VIN is still unclear (Dorsey 1986). In some cases hair follicles may be involved for several millimetres below the surface (Mene & Buckley 1985) but it may not always be necessary to destroy the whole depth of involved appendages (Dorsey 1986). In any case, treatment of the whole vulva to such a depth would result in a third-degree burn which would need skin grafting. A practical policy is to treat the abnormal areas to the second or third surgical planes. This usually heals well after 4 weeks. If VIN in a follicle grows on to the surface after this treatment and gives rise to symptoms, the localized area of recurrence can be treated more deeply.

Results

Assessment of the results of treatment should include a consideration of the length of follow-up. Surgical excision is associated with recurrence rates of 13–43% (Jones & McLean 1986; Shafi et al 1989). Short-term results from patients treated by laser were very promising (Leuchter et al 1984) but longer follow-up showed a recurrence rate similar to surgery (Shafi et al 1989). Close observation and rebiopsy are essential to detect invasive disease among those who relapse. Early invasion was detected in 3 (14%) of 21 patients with persisting signs of disease (Shafi et al 1989). Repeated treatments are commonly required.

VIN — CONCLUSIONS

VIN is becoming more common, especially in young women. The treatment must be carefully tailored to the individual to avoid mutilating therapy whenever possible.

In view of the uncertainty about the malignant potential of these lesions, there is a place for careful observation — especially of young women without severe symptoms. However, it must not be forgotten that some of these patients will develop vulvar cancer if untreated so the importance of close follow-up must be emphasized to the patient and her general practitioner.

PAGET'S DISEASE

This is an uncommon condition, similar to that found in the breast. Pruritus is the presenting complaint. The lesion is indistinguishable clinically from squamous intraepithelial neoplasia and the diagnosis must be made by biopsy.

Associated malignancies

In approximately one-third of patients there is an adenocarcinoma in the apocrine glands (Boehm & Morris 1971; Creasman et al 1975). This has a poor prognosis if the groin lymph nodes are involved with no women surviving 5 years (Boehm & Morris 1971). Excluding underlying adnexal carcinomas, concomitant genital malignancies are found in 15–25% of women with Paget's disease of the vulva (Degefu et al 1986). These are most commonly vulval or cervical, but transitional cell carcinoma of the bladder (or kidney), and ovarian, endometrial, vaginal and urethral carcinomas have all been reported (Degefu et al 1986).

Treatment

The treatment of Paget's disease is very wide local excision usually involving total vulvectomy because of the propensity of this condition to involve apparently normal skin (Creasman et al 1975). The specimen must be examined histologically with great care to exclude an apocrine adenocarcinoma.

KEY POINTS

1. Both squamous (CIN) and glandular (AIS) premalignant lesions are seen on the cervix.
2. The diagnostic precision of small biopsies is not good. Invasive disease is not always detected and CIN II–III may be substantially undercalled.
3. After 20 years, about one-third of women with CIN III will develop invasive disease if untreated.
4. Progression of CIN I to CIN III or worse may occur in 26% of women within 2 years.
5. A well organized cervical cytology screening programme which reaches a large proportion of the population at risk and which includes effective action when abnormal smears are detected will reduce the incidence and mortality of cervical cancer.
6. The four pitfalls in colposcopy are:
    1. The false SCJ caused by an abrasion.
    2. The SCJ in the canal.
    3. The previously treated cervix.
    4. Glandular lesions.
7. The majority of women with CIN can be treated in the outpatient department.
8. Excisional methods provide the whole lesion for histology without increasing the discomfort or complications for the patient.
9. Most cases of VAIN are seen after hysterectomy.
10. VAIN hidden above the vaginal suture line cannot be evaluated and early invasive cancer is common.
11. Surgical excision (preferably by the vaginal route) or intracavitary radiotherapy are the most effective treatments.
12. The malignant potential of VIN is uncertain.
13. Treatment of VIN is mutilating and should be limited for the most part to symptomatic patients.

REFERENCES

Andersen E S, Arffmann E 1989 Adenocarcinoma in situ of the uterine cervix: a clinico-pathologic study of 36 cases. Gynecologic Oncology 35: 1–7

Anderson G H, Boyes D A, Benedet J L et al. 1988 Organisation and results of the cervical cytology screening programme in British Columbia, 1955–85. British Medical Journal 296: 975–978

Anderson M C, Hartley R B 1980 Cervical crypt involvement by intraepithelial neoplasia. Obstetrics and Gynecology 55: 546–550

Bekassy Z, Alm P, Grundsell H, Larsson G, Åstedt B 1983 Laser miniconisation in mild and moderate dysplasia of the uterine cervix. Gynecologic Oncology 15: 357–362

Boehm F, Morris J M 1971 Paget's disease and apocrine gland carcinoma of the vulva. Obstetrics and Gynecology 38: 185–192

Boice J D, Day N E, Andersen A et al. 1985 Second cancers following treatment for cervical cancer. An international collaboration among cancer registries. Journal of the National Cancer Institute 74: 955–975

Burghardt E, Holzer E 1980 Treatment of carcinoma-in-situ: evaluation of 1609 cases. Obstetrics and Gynecology 55: 539–545

Buscema J, Stern J, Woodruff J D 1980 The significance of histologic alterations adjacent to invasive vulvar carcinoma. American Journal of Obstetrics and Gynecology 137: 902–909

Caglar H, Delgado G, Hreshchyshyn M M 1986 Partial and total skinning vulvectomy in treatment of carcinoma in situ of the vulva. Obstetrics and Gynecology 68: 504–507

Campion M J, McCance D J, Cuzick J, Singer A 1986 The progressive potential of mild cervical atypia: a prospective cytological, colposcopic and virological study. Lancet ii: 237–240

Campion M J, di Paola F M, Vellios F 1990 The value of cervicography in population screening. Journal of Experimental and Clinical Cancer Research 9 (suppl): FC/107

Choo Y C, Anderson D G 1982 Neoplasms of the vagina following cervical carcinoma. Gynecologic Oncology 14: 125–132

Creasman W T, Gallacher H S, Rutledge F 1975 Paget's disease of the vulva. Gynecological Oncology 3: 133–148

Degefu S, O'Quinn A G, Dhurandhar H N 1986 Paget's disease of the vulva and urogenital malignancies: a case report and review of the literature. Gynecological Oncology 25: 347–354

Dorsey J H 1986 Skin appendage involvement and vulval

intraepithelial neoplasia. In: Sharp F, Jordan J A (eds) Gynaecological laser surgery. Perinatology Press, New York, pp. 193–195
Griffiths M, Turner M J, Partington C K, Soutter W P 1989 Should smears in a colposcopy clinic be taken after the application of acetic acid? Acta Cytologica 33: 324–326
Hernandez-Linares W, Puthawala A, Nolan J F, Jernstrom P H, Morrow C P 1980 Carcinoma in situ of the vagina: past and present management. Obstetrics and Gynecology 56: 356–360
IARC Working Group on Evaluation of Cervical Cancer Screening Programmes 1986 Screening for cervical squamous cancer: duration of low risk after negative results of cervical cytology and its implication for screening policies. British Medical Journal 293: 659–664
Ireland D, Monaghan J M 1988 The management of the patient with abnormal vaginal cytology following hysterectomy. British Journal of Obstetrics and Gynaecology 95: 973–975
Jones R W, McLean M R 1986 Carcinoma in situ of the vulva: a review of 31 treated and five untreated cases. Obstetrics and Gynecology 68: 499–503
Kaufman R, Gordon A 1986a Squamous cell carcinoma in situ of the vulva. Part I. British Journal of Sexual Medicine 13: 24–27
Kaufman R, Gordon A 1986b Squamous cell carcinoma in situ of the vulva. Part II. British Journal of Sexual Medicine 13: 55–58
Larsson G, Gullberg B, Grundsell H 1983 A comparison of complications of laser and cold knife conisation. Obstetrics and Gynecology 62: 213–217
Leuchter R S, Townsend D E, Hacker N F, Pretorius R G, Lagasse L D, Wade M E 1984 Treatment of vulvar carcinoma in situ with the CO_2 laser. Gynecologic Oncology 19: 314–322
McIndoe W A, McLean M R, Jones R W, Mullins P R 1984 The invasive potential of carcinoma in situ of the cervix. Obstetrics and Gynecology 64: 451–458
Mene A, Buckley C H 1985 Involvement of the vulval skin appendages by intraepithelial neoplasia. British Journal of Obstetrics and Gynaecology 92: 634–638
Monaghan J 1987 (ed) Operative surgery — gynaecology and obstetrics. London, Butterworth Scientific
Partington C K, Soutter W P, Turner M J, Hill A S, Krausz T 1987 Laser excisional biopsy under local anaesthesia — an outpatient technique? Journal of Obstetrics and Gynaecology 8: 48–52
Partington C K, Turner M J, Soutter W P, Griffiths M, Krausz T 1989 Laser vaporisation versus laser excision conisation in the treatment of cervical intraepithelial neoplasia. Obstetrics and Gynecology 73: 775–779
Prendiville W, Cullimore J, Norman S 1989 Large loop excision of the transformation zone (LLETZ). A new method of management for women with cervical intraepithelial neoplasia. British Journal of Obstetrics and Gynaecology 96: 1054–1060
Reid R 1985 Superficial laser vulvectomy II. The anatomic and biophysical principles permitting accurate control over the depth of dermal destruction with the carbon dioxide laser. American Journal of Obstetrics and Gynecology 152: 261–271
Richart R M 1967 Natural history of cervical intraepithelial neoplasia. Clinics in Obstetrics and Gynecology 10: 748–784
Robertson A J, Anderson J M, Swanson Beck J et al. 1989 Observer variability in histopathological reporting of cervical biopsy specimens. Journal of Clinical Pathology 42: 231–238
Robertson J H, Woodend B E, Crozier E H, Hutchinson J 1988 Risk of cervical cancer associated with mild dyskaryosis. British Medical Journal 297: 18–21
Shafi M I, Luesley D M, Byrne P et al. 1989 Vulval intraepithelial neoplasia — management and outcome. British Journal of Obstetrics and Gynaecology 96: 1339–1344
Sincock A M, Evans-Jones J, Partington C K, Steel S J 1987 Quantitative assessment of cervical neoplasia by hydrolysed DNA assay. Lancet ii: 942–943
Skehan M, Soutter W P, Lim K, Krause T, Pryse-Davies J 1990 Reliability of colposcopy and directed punch biopsy. British Journal of Obstetrics and Gynaecology 97: 811–816
Soutter W P 1989 A practical approach to colposcopy. In: Studd J (ed) Progress in obstetrics and gynaecology, vol 7. Churchill Livingstone, London, pp. 355–367
Soutter W P, Brough A K. Monaghan J M 1984 Cervical screening for younger women. Lancet ii: 745
Soutter W P, Wisdom S, Brough A K, Monaghan J M 1986a Should patients with mild atypia in a cervical smear be referred for colposcopy? British Journal of Obstetrics and Gynaecology 93: 70–74
Soutter W P, Abernethy F M, Brown V A, Hill A S 1986b Success, complications and subsequent pregnancy outcome relative to the depth of laser treatment of cervical intraepithelial neoplasia. Colposcopy and Gynecologic Laser Surgery 2: 35–42
Woodman C B J, Jordan J A, Wade-Evans T 1984 The management of vaginal intra-epithelial neoplasia after hysterectomy. British Journal of Obstetrics and Gynaecology 91: 707–711
Woodman C B J, Mould J J, Jordan J A 1988 Radiotherapy in the management of vaginal intraepithelial neoplasia after hysterectomy. British Journal of Obstetrics and Gynaecology 95: 976–979

35. Malignant disease of the breast

M. D. Brooks S. C. A. Fraser S. R. Ebbs M. Baum

EPIDEMIOLOGY

Cancer of the breast is the most common malignancy affecting women in North America and most of Europe. Here it comprises the leading cause of death for females under 55 years of age. Incidence rates of breast cancer are approximately six to seven times higher in the western world than in most of Asia and Africa. Westernized countries have shown a small increase in recent years but socioeconomic changes in Japan have been accompanied by a rapid rise in incidence. The recent rise is generally less marked in the high-risk populations of the world than in the low-risk countries, implying that environmental causes predominate. Whilst diet may be the first factor to spring to mind, other cultural or behavioural patterns related to contraception or child-bearing could be implicated. In high-risk areas the small rise in the registration of breast cancers has not been accompanied by changes in mortality from the disease, suggesting that this might be a result of earlier detection of less aggressive tumours. In the USA and the UK it is estimated that currently about 1 in 13 women will develop breast cancer.

AETIOLOGY AND RISK FACTORS

Demographic factors

Women have a 100 times greater incidence of breast cancer than men. The incidence increases sharply until around the time of the menopause. In the postmenopausal years the rate continues to increase but more slowly in regions of the world which have a high incidence. In low-risk areas, the incidence plateaus or even declines after the menopause. The age-related death rates for England and Wales are shown in Figure 35.1. Racial characteristics appear of lesser importance than environmental factors; immigrants gradually assume the incidence rates of their adopted land. For example, Japanese migrants to the USA suffer the high risk associated with their new home whilst Japanese women living in Hawaii have an incidence rate midway between that of Japan and the USA. Within any particular country an increase in socioeconomic status is accompanied by an increase in incidence. This is thought to account for much of the rise in incidence seen in the USA as black women attain a higher socioeconomic status.

Family history

The risk of developing breast cancer for a woman who has a first-degree relative with the disease is increased two or

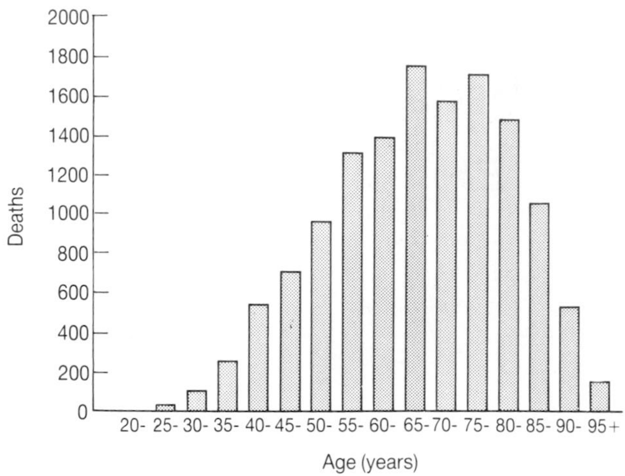

Fig. 35.1 The age-related death rate from breast cancer in England and Wales in 1988. From Office of Population Censuses and Surveys.

three times. This appears to be determined partially by the number of relatives affected. In some families the hereditary risk of breast cancer may reach 50%, being inherited as an autosomal dominant trait. Often such cancers occur before the menopause and bilaterally. The alterations seen in the risks of migrants suggests that whilst genetic factors predispose to breast cancer, its initiation requires exposure to an environmental factor.

Past medical history

Once a woman has developed a breast cancer the chances of a further breast cancer developing are increased about fourfold. Whether the benign diseases of the breast, grouped under the banner of aberrations of normal development and involution (ANDI) by Hughes et al (1987), constitute a risk for the subsequent development of breast cancer remains a controversial issue. In a study involving over 10 000 women, Dupont & Page (1985) found no increased risk for these benign conditions in the absence of either a positive family history or the presence of cellular atypia in the benign biopsy material. Other studies have indicated an increased risk of breast cancer for women with a history of previous ovarian, endometrial, colorectal or salivary tumours, malignant melanomas, soft tissue sarcomas or primary biliary cirrhosis.

Menstrual and reproductive history

Both early age at menarche and late menopause are independent risk factors for the development of breast cancer, suggesting that both result in an increased exposure to carcinogens. Bearing children reduces the risk of breast cancer with a maximal protective effect being achieved by bearing a full-term pregnancy at a young age, implying that the breasts might in some way be matured by such an event. A woman who has had a child before age 25 has approximately half the risk of developing breast cancer of a nullipara or one whose first pregnancy occurred over the age of 30. The effect of abortion or miscarriage is unclear, with evidence currently suggesting that such events might carry a small but increased risk.

Menopause beyond the age of 55 years doubles the risk. Protection against breast cancer appears to be conferred by an artificial premature menopause below the age of 45 years. The exact role of endogenous hormones is unclear with no consistent differences demonstrated between breast cancer cases and controls in circulating or excreted hormone levels. The influence of steroid binding proteins such as sex hormone-binding globulin has been neglected and calculation of biologically available levels of hormones might be more appropriate.

Dietary risk factors

Fat consumption plays an important role in the stimulation of breast cancer in some experimental animal models. For example, changes in diet by Japanese migrants suggests that increased fat intake in early life might be a possible aetiological factor, although correlations have also been demonstrated in various populations directly between the incidence of breast cancer and the intake of sugar and meat, and inversely with cereals, seafoods and selenium.

Recent studies have suggested that a modest regular intake of alcohol may be associated with an increased risk of breast cancer. The putative mechanism is alcohol stimulation of liver enzymes which results in alterations in its ability to metabolize oestrogens.

Exogenous hormones

The contraceptive pill

The results of studies are conflicting and up until now it has been impossible to determine whether oral contraceptive use predisposes to breast cancer. Problems in the interpretation of the results include the simultaneous administration of oestrogens and progestagens which may have opposing actions in this context. If the hormones are acting as initiators of the cancer there will be a possible latent period of 15 years before the true hazards are revealed. It seems more likely that the pill may be functioning as a promoter resulting in an acceleration in the clinical presentation of cases: more breast cancers might then be found in younger women and fewer in older women.

In spite of all these caveats new data are beginning to

emerge that long-term use of oral contraceptives may have a significant effect on breast cancer incidence. However, these data relate mainly to older high-dose formulations and the risk seems to be less with modern low-dose pills. More information is required to settle this matter.

Hormone replacement therapy

Individual studies on this aspect have also yielded conflicting evidence and again there are the problems of a variety of preparations containing varying proportions and absolute doses of oestrogens and progestagens with the literature confounded by publication bias. A recently performed overview of all available studies (Armstrong 1988) shows no increase in breast cancer risk for 'ever use' of oestrogen by postmenopausal women. Only when the relative risk for the highest dose category in every study or for women with a positive family history is overviewed was there evidence that the risk of breast cancer might be increased. There is no evidence for any association between breast cancer and breastfeeding, thyroid disease, rauwolfia derivatives (dopamine antagonists which could lead to elevation of prolactin, e.g. reserpine), or diazepam.

Other factors

Exposure to ionizing radiation carries an increased dose-related risk. Sensitivity varies with age, being maximal in childhood. Although the normal latent period of breast cancer appears to be 15 years, those exposed at a very young age do not realize the increased risk until they reach the age at which breast cancer normally develops. Routine mammography carries a negligible risk of subsequent breast cancer.

For postmenopausal women a high body mass index confers a higher risk of breast cancer and it has been suggested that obesity might act through peripheral production of oestrogen by adipose aromatase.

The extremely dense dysplastic mammographic pattern may identify a subgroup at risk. The influence of psychological stress upon the development of breast cancer remains speculative.

PREVENTION OF BREAST CANCER

The identification of risk factors for the development of breast cancer has suggested ways to reduce the incidence of the disease. Logical actions would be to encourage childbirth at a young age, reduce the intake of dietary fat and discourage obesity. Cuzick et al (1986) have suggested that the amount of biologically available oestrogen is the key factor in the aetiology of breast cancer. They postulate that tamoxifen, which appears to function at least partially by blocking the effects of oestrogen on the breast cancer cell, might be a useful method of preventing breast cancer although they counsel caution against the possible long-term side-effects of the drug. A pilot study has been proposed on a high-risk group.

Prophylactic mastectomy is currently the standard treatment in many centres for in situ carcinoma because of the risk of subsequent invasive carcinoma. It appears from both cadaver studies and the follow-up of women with palpable carcinoma in situ that, after subcutaneous mastectomy, there is a great likelihood of breast tissue remaining which could become malignant. This suggests that total mastectomy would be necessary if amputation is thought to be justified.

PATHOLOGY

Two common forms of invasive breast cancer occur: ductal carcinoma and lobular carcinoma. In addition, several 'special' forms of breast cancer have been described and there has recently been an increased appreciation of in situ carcinoma.

Invasive lobular carcinoma

About 5% of breast cancers are of this type. The microscopic appearance is characterized by a fibrous matrix through which run loose strands of small tumour cells in a linear arrangement known as Indian filing. The tumour cells also tend to grow circumferentially around ducts and lobules (targetoid growth).

Clinically the disease usually presents as an ill defined tumour in the upper outer quadrant of the breast. Synchronous or metachronous bilateral carcinomas are not uncommon. Rarely are calcifications seen on mammography. Although overall the prognosis appears similar to invasive ductal carcinoma, when lobular cancer metastasizes, several unusual patterns of spread occur. Central nervous system metastases usually take the form of a meningeal infiltration. In the abdomen, diffuse retroperitoneal or serosal spread occurs and the microscopic appearance of signet ring cells deposited in abdominal organs may cause diagnostic difficulty, especially in view of the tumour's predilection to spread to ovaries and uterus.

Invasive ductal carcinoma

This category encompasses all the tumours that do not otherwise fall into a special category. About 70–80% of breast cancers are of this type. Attempts have been made to define prognostic subgroups from the microscopic characteristics of the tumour. Grading assesses the degree to which carcinoma departs both in its architecture and cytology from the normal breast epithelium. The tendency to form tubules, pleomorphism of cells, frequency of hyperchromatic nuclei and mitoses are awarded points and three grades of malignancy are determined from the sum. High-grade malignancies carry the worst prognosis. Many other histological predictive indicators such as ploidy, vessel or nerve invasion have also been described.

Special forms

Tubular carcinoma

This term describes a variant of ductal carcinoma where over 75% of the neoplastic elements resemble normal breast ductules. In pure form it is a rare tumour (approximately 2%) although a higher proportion occurs amongst the small mammographic-detected malignancies. As might be anticipated, such a well differentiated tumour carries a favourable prognosis.

Medullary carcinoma

These are uncommon, solid, circumscribed tumours with a marked lymphocytic infiltrate and again have a relatively favourable prognosis. Often patients with medullary carcinoma are young.

Mucinous (colloid or gelatinous) carcinoma

This is characterized by accumulated, abundant, extracellular mucus secretion around clumps of tumour cells lying in slender strands or papillary clusters. This tumour is thought to have a favourable prognosis. It comprises between 1 and 2% of breast cancers.

Papillary carcinoma

This is a rare, usually well circumscribed carcinoma whose invasive pattern is predominantly in the form of papillary structures often with foci of intraduct papillary growth. It is generally found in the elderly and classically presents with a nipple discharge.

In situ carcinoma

When this term was originally applied to the breast by Foote & Stewart in 1941 it was felt that these lesions inevitably progressed to invasive cancer. Increasingly detected by mammography, more has been learnt about their biology, but knowledge still remains somewhat rudimentary. Two basic types have been described, — lobular carcinoma in situ (LCIS) and ductal carcinoma in situ (DCIS).

LCIS. This involves breast lobules. Microscopically this type has a distinct appearance as cells originating from the acini and terminal ducts proliferate to fill the acinar lumen and enlarge the affected lobules. Found primarily in premenopausal women, its status as either a marker of risk or as a premalignant lesion remains the subject of controversy. Such women have an increased risk of invasive cancer over the general population by perhaps a factor of 10; however cancers that subsequently develop are usually ductal rather than lobular and just as likely to be in the contralateral breast. There remains a division of opinion as to whether patients should be managed just by close observation or by bilateral mastectomy.

DCIS. This is related to small terminal ducts. This description encompasses a wide variety of disease from a microscopic cluster of a few cells to that of an appreciable size which is easily palpable clinically. Although generally viewed as an intermediate stage between benign and malignant, the risk of developing invasive carcinoma after biopsy alone is approximately 20–30% — about the same as LCIS. However the clinical presentation of the subsequent cancer contrasts with that occurring after LCIS by usually being found at the diagnostic biopsy site. Because of the limited malignant potential, complete excision may be sufficient for the microscopic variant. The palpable form of the disease (over 1 cm diameter) is best regarded as an invasive tumour and treated with appropriate surgery. If wide excision is selected, it appears that radiotherapy is needed to reduce an unacceptable incidence of local recurrence.

BREAST SCREENING

The prognosis of breast cancer is related to the stage of the disease at the time of diagnosis and treatment. A number of studies have shown that mortality may be reduced in certain subgroups of a population screened for early breast cancers.

The most important screening modalities are clinical examination and mammography. Mammography is the most sensitive of all methods presently available, capable of detecting both in situ and invasive disease. Clinical examination lacks both the sensitivity and specificity of mammography but may be reserved for subsequent investigation of those women recalled after suspicious radiography.

Breast self-examination, although an apparently simple and cheap form of screening, requires a population both well motivated and well informed, together with an efficient system of self-referral. The evidence that self-examination has a place in this field is lacking. On the other hand the evidence for mammography-based screening is more clearly defined.

The first large randomized, controlled study of breast screening was the Health Insurance Plan (HIP) of Greater New York which began in 1963 and which randomized 62 000 women aged 40 to 64. The study group were offered four consecutive annual physical examinations and two-view mammography, whilst the other was not. There was a 40% reduction in mortality from breast cancer in screened women over 50 years of age (Shapiro 1977). As may be expected, smaller tumours with a lower incidence of lymph node involvement were detected amongst the screened population. No reduction in mortality was shown for women in the 40–50 year age group. Even amongst the screened group, more aggressive cancers continued to develop between the annual visits.

A similar reduction in mortality in women over 50 was found in a randomized controlled trial conducted within two Swedish counties in which 134 867 women were enrolled (Tabar et al 1985). This study used single-view mammography every 24 months for women aged 40–49 and every 33 months for women aged 50–74. There was a 40% reduction in mortality for the older group. Additional support for these findings has come from other investigations in USA, Holland, Italy and the UK.

This evidence has encouraged the establishment of a UK national screening programme along guidelines set down by the Forrest (1987) report which advocated screening for all women aged 50-64 employing single-view oblique mammography at 3–yearly intervals. The logistics of a national programme are immense and the cost benefits as yet unproven. The inevitable over-sensitivity of mammography leading to a possibly unacceptable number of false positive results has emphasized the need for strict quality control. The psychological morbidity of such screening is unknown. Whether national screening will alter breast cancer mortality remains to be seen.

PRESENTATION

Breast lump

By far the commonest presentation of mammary cancer is a lump in the breast. The mass is usually painless and is discovered either by chance, for example when washing, or during self-examination. Occasionally pain or discomfort has developed and a lump is found subsequently. Not infrequently the lump is discovered by others, such as the husband or a member of medical staff during routine clinical examination.

The lump is most commonly found in the upper outer quadrant of the breast including the axillary tail. Tumours are seen with decreasing frequency in the central and upper inner areas followed by the inferior quadrants. Simultaneous bilateral carcinomas are uncommon (0.1–2% of cases).

Lymph node enlargement

Lymphadenopathy may be palpable in the axilla and uncommonly may be the only sign of occult carcinoma. Lymph node metastases are less frequently felt above and below the ipsilateral clavicle.

Nipple discharge

Nipple discharge is not a frequent sign or symptom of malignancy. Tumours associated with discharge probably constitute less than 2% of the total and a mass will usually be present. Multiduct or bilateral discharge is more often associated with physiological disorders (e.g. duct ectasia). Single duct discharge indicates a local cause such as intraduct papilloma or carcinoma. The discharge appears serous or bloody in either case.

Skin changes

The stroma around an infiltrating carcinoma exhibits a marked fibrosis causing shortening of Cooper's ligaments adjacent to the tumour and dimpling of the overlying skin. The contour of the breast is thus gradually altered. Similarly a tumour deep to the areola pulls on the nipple inverting it (Fig. 35.2). Infiltration and blockage of the dermal lymphatics by tumour produces oedema in the overlying skin (peau d'orange).

Paget's disease

Progression of intraepithelial carcinoma from a primary tumour within the breast through proximal ducts to the surface of the nipple produces a progressive centrifugal destruction of the nipple and surrounding skin. This is known as Paget's disease and appears as a slowly growing red, raw or dry, scaly patch replacing the nipple and areola. Although an underlying carcinoma is palpable in only 40% of patients, characteristic changes are seen on mammography.

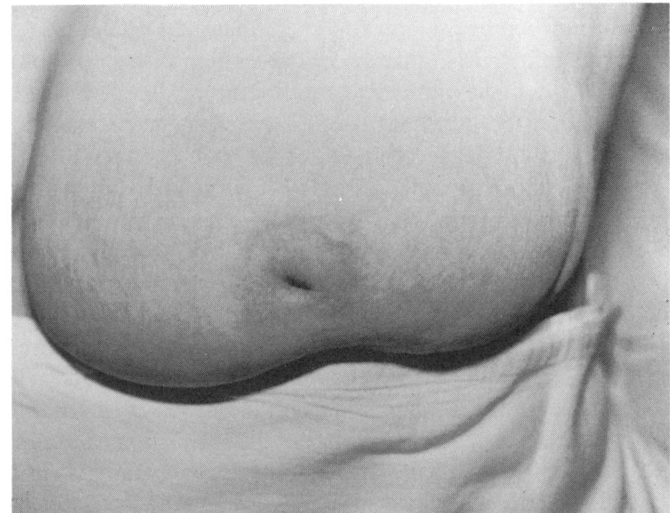

Fig. 35.2 A carcinoma of the left breast causing skin and nipple retraction.

Inflammatory carcinoma

This uncommon but dramatic variant of mammary carcinoma constitutes between 1.5 and 4% of all cases. Clinical signs and symptoms resemble acute infection with erythema, swelling, pain and tenderness. Clinical progression is swift with early nodal and systemic dissemination.

Breast cancer in pregnancy

Presentation may be delayed during pregnancy and lactation as physiological breast enlargement can mask parenchymal abnormalities. Conversely, palpable masses may be misinterpreted as normal breast adaptation for lactation. Breast tumours therefore tend to be more advanced when found during pregnancy; however the prognosis is similar to the non-pregnant population when matched for age and stage.

Advanced disease

Breast cancer presenting at an advanced stage may reach an enormous size with ulceration and fixation to the chest wall without obvious dissemination. In contrast, multiple metastases in the liver, lungs, brain and skeleton may arise without palpable evidence of a breast primary.

Subclinical disease

Screening programmes are now revealing an increasing number of subclinical, mammographic cancers that constitute a new and possibly more curable presentation of the disease.

DIFFERENTIAL DIAGNOSIS

The differential diagnosis of breast cancer includes a number of benign, neoplastic and inflammatory conditions that can mimic malignancy. Most benign breast tumours are well defined clinically, radiographically and ultrasonographically but confusion may arise, particularly in middle and older age groups.

Although occasionally associated with underlying intraduct carcinoma, nipple discharge is more commonly seen with inflammatory lesions (e.g. duct ectasia), intraduct papillomata, endocrine disease (e.g. hyperprolactinaemia) or drug therapy (e.g. psychotrophics). Plasma cell mastitis and breast abscess produce changes similar to inflammatory carcinoma, whilst the periductal fibrosis associated with duct ectasia mimics malignancy by inversion of the nipple.

Dermatitis or eczema of the areola may suggest Paget's disease but in the former the nipple is usually spared. Lastly, traumatic fat necrosis can produce marked fibrosis which may simulate carcinoma on both clinical and mammographic examination.

INVESTIGATION

Radiography

Soft tissue radiography of the breast has been in clinical use for over 30 years and remains the method of choice for demonstrating the primary lesion. Two systems are employed, — xeromammography and film/screen.

Xeromammography utilizes a radioelectric process wherein a precharged selenium-coated plate is exposed to X-rays. Bipolar charged particulate dust is then sprayed on to the plate adhering to areas of residual charge. A print is then taken from the coated surface of the plate. This process produces images of fine detail with edge enhancement giving sharp delineation of the breast architecture. Because of improvements in film/screen mammographic quality together with lower radiation dosage and increased convenience, xeromammography is now of lesser importance.

Film/screen mammography employs the conventional radiochemical reaction of X-ray photon on photographic plate. The breast is held between compression plates for standard views but fine magnified detail is possible with localized pressure. The indications for mammography are given below:

1. *Assessment of known malignancy*
   a. Multifocal disease in the same breast?
   b. Synchronous disease in the contralateral breast?
   c. Follow-up after treatment of the primary lesion.
2. *Clinical uncertainty*
   a. Assessment of clinically suspicious lesion.
   b. Malignancy arising within benign breast disease.
3. *Investigation of nipple abnormality*
   a. Nipple discharge.
   b. Paget's disease.
4. *Investigation of occult primary*
5. *Screening*
   a. General population.
   b. High-risk population (positive family history).
6. *Localization of impalpable lesions*
   Impalpable but mammographically suspicious areas may be localized prior to surgical excision either by dye injection or more commonly by placing a percutaneous hooked needle alongside the lesion.

Radiographic signs of malignancy

Malignant microcalcifications are generally of variable size and density. Branching forms are common, indicating their intraductal position. A malignant cluster of fine calcification may be seen within an opacity lying amid an area of parenchymal distortion (Fig. 35.3). Benign calcifications are usually larger, less clustered and may be hollow.

Comparison of similar views will reveal areas of parenchymal asymmetry between breasts. The edge of a malignant opacity is ill defined with straightening and dis-

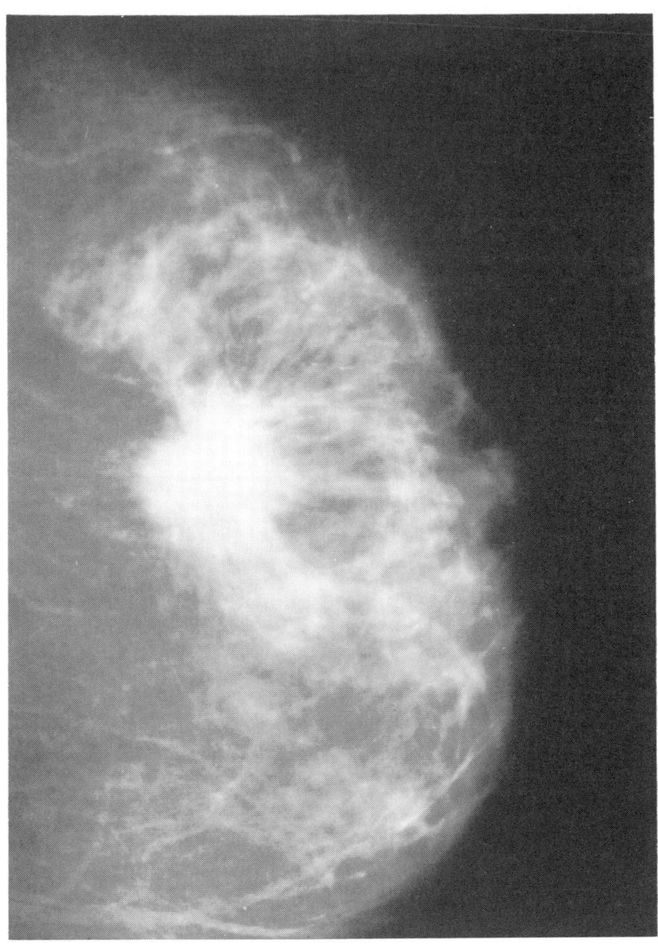

Fig. 35.3 Mammogram showing a large spiculated mass lying centrally. This was a carcinoma.

tortion of the surrounding fibrous septa. Benign lesions appear well defined, often with a clear halo of compressed fat around them. Well circumscribed malignant tumours of the colloid or medullary type simulate benign lesions radiographically. Oedema in the skin over a tumour produces skin thickening. Skin and nipple distortion are clearly demonstrated.

Ultrasound

A variety of ultrasound techniques are available and as definition improves so does its clinical application. Ultrasound has advantages over radiography in certain areas:

1. In younger dense breasts when radiography would constitute a cumulative radiation hazard.
2. For the definition of benign cystic and solid lesions.
3. For patient comfort.

Sensitivity and specificity are not as high as in mammography and ultrasound is therefore best reserved as a complementary examination.

Thermography

Breast thermography records infrared radiation from the surface of both breasts. Increased vascularity within a tumour produces a 'hot spot'. Unfortunately, this technique lacks specificity and is not used in standard practice.

Assessment of metastatic disease

Conventional and specialized imaging techniques are needed, including chest and skeletal X-rays and computerizied tomography, particularly for pulmonary, mediastinal and cerebral metastases. Scintigraphy is used to display skeletal metastases. Hepatic secondaries are well demonstrated by either ultrasound or scintigraphy although computerized tomography can also be extended into the abdomen.

STAGING

Breast cancer is now staged by the TNM system according to UICC criteria (Table 35.1). A comparison with the previously used Manchester classification is shown in Table 35.2. The relative survival figures are shown in Figure 35.4.

TREATMENT

As understanding of breast cancer has altered, so too has the primary treatment. The trend toward conservation rather than radical surgery is a recognition of the concept of biological predeterminism; the desire not to mutilate has to be balanced against the aim of obtaining local control

Table 35.1 The UICC TNM staging system for breast cancer

T Tumour size	
T0	Impalpable
T1a/b	2 cm
T2a/b	2–5 cm
T3a/b	>5 cm
T4a	Direct chest extension
T4b	Skin infiltration or oedema or peau d'orange or satellite nodules in the same breast
T4c	T4a + T4b
(a = No deep fixation; b = with deep fixation)	
N Nodal status	
N0	No palpable nodes
N1a	Palpable homolateral axillary nodes Clinically non-malignant
N1b	Palpable homolateral axillary nodes Clinically malignant
N2	Palpable fixed malignant nodes
N3	Clinically malignant homolateral clavicular nodes or oedema of arm
M Metastases	
M0	No clinically apparent distant metastases
M1	Distant metastases apparent

Table 35.2 Manchester and UICC staging systems

Manchester stage	UICC stage		
I	T1a	N0	M0
	T2a	N0	M0
II	T0	N1	M0
	T1a	N1	M0
	T2a	N1	M0
III	T3	N0,1,2	M0
	T0,1,2,	N2	M0
	T1b,T2b	N0,1,2	M0
	T4	N0,1,2	M0
IV	Any T	N3	or M1

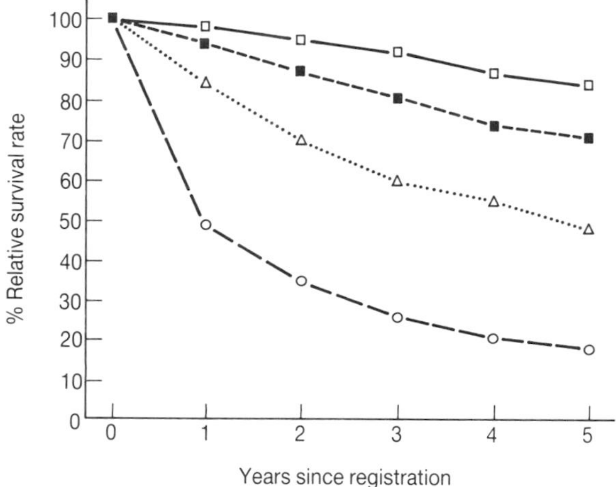

Fig. 35.4 The relative percentage survival by stage is shown for women registered with the Thames Cancer Register 1975–1980. □ = stage I; ■ = stage II; △ = stage III; ○ = stage IV.

from primary treatment. Accurate staging is also important so that appropriate systemic treatment can be chosen. It is now recognized that a multidisciplinary approach at the outset will simplify management and pool both knowledge and prejudices alike. The objectives of primary therapy are to control local disease, achieve accurate staging and obtain prognostic information.

Early disease

The presence of distant metastases at the time of diagnosis is notoriously difficult to predict, so that the surest diagnosis of early, curable disease is retrospective. Axillary nodal involvement implies that distant spread is likely but does not rule out prolonged survival. Knowledge of node status is only obtained reliably at surgery, therefore any operation should include at least sampling of axillary nodes for histology. Local recurrence is still best prevented by removal of the primary tumour and the axillary nodes (Fig. 35.5).

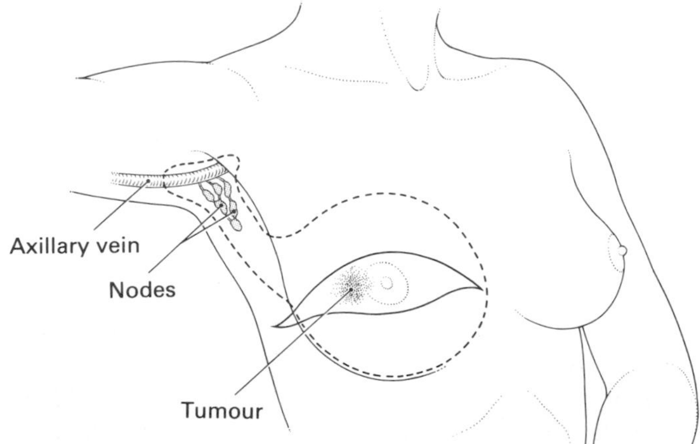

Fig. 35.5 Simple mastectomy with removal of axillary nodes up to the axillary vein. The dashed line shows the extent of the excision through the horizontal ellipse.

Primary therapy

Until the late 1970s, the standard treatments of a potentially curable primary tumour were radical mastectomy; Patey mastectomy, or total mastectomy plus radiotherapy. Since then, a number of randomised controlled trials have shown that wide local excision (WLE; Fig. 35.6) with radiotherapy is associated with no worse a survival or local recurrence rate than mastectomy alone in selected cases. In the 1990s, WLE is the preferred surgical therapy, with the following exceptions:

1. Where adequate local excision is either impossible or would result in poor cosmesis.
2. In diffuse multifocal disease.
3. In disease involving the nipple.

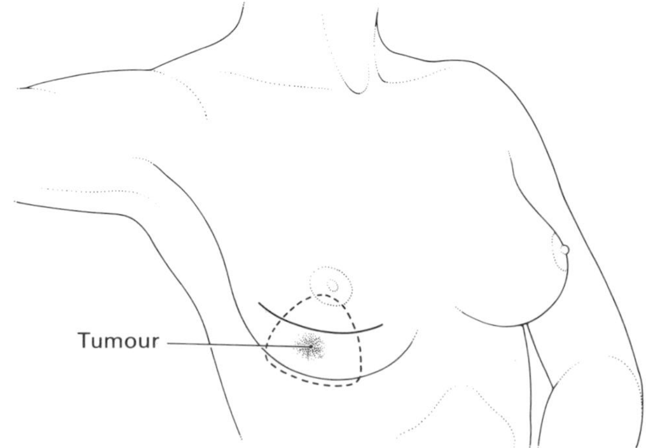

Fig. 35.6 Wide local excision through an incision in Langer's lines.

Generally, where there is the possibility of reasonable cosmesis, breast preservation is desirable.

Those at greatest risk of local recurrence have tumours of greater than 3 cm diameter with tumour close to resection margins and with poor differentiation on histology. Radiotherapy of the residual breast is required after WLE irrespective of the margins of excision, because the incidence of microscopic residual disease has been as high as 30% in some series.

To control local disease in the axilla, two policies are possible: sampling and irradiation, or surgical dissection alone. Axillary dissection exposes the medial cutaneous nerve to risk of damage and it should never be combined with radiotherapy because of consequent lymphoedema of the arm.

It is assumed that any woman would prefer the less mutilating surgery of WLE rather than mastectomy. However, psychological studies have produced less clear-cut results. The close follow-up of the conserved breast may result in severe anxiety for some women and the risk of a local recurrence is an important consideration. The clinician must discuss the options with the patient at all stages and accommodate her wishes provided that she has been fully informed of the consequences.

Reconstruction is often possible if mastectomy is unavoidable, and can be done either at the time of initial surgery or as a secondary procedure. Time tends to reduce demand for the latter. Insertion of a silicone prosthesis in the subpectoral plane to create a mound can be augmented by more complex plastic surgical procedures such as the raising of a latissimus dorsi flap followed by reconstruction of the nipple. Local recurrence is neither made more likely nor concealed by reconstruction.

In the elderly patient, some early empirical studies suggested a role for tamoxifen treatment alone for the primary disease. The few randomized trials so far reported have equivocal results which have been confounded by the trial designs, and the Cancer Research Campaign (1988) trial of tamoxifen versus tamoxifen plus surgery has not yet reached a firm conclusion. However, for frail old women with a limited life expectancy, tamoxifen 40 mg/day is a reasonable alternative to surgery.

Adjuvant therapy

Since Beatson's observations in 1896, variations on the theme of castration have improved the outlook for premenopausal women undergoing surgery. This effect seems confined to those with involved axillary nodes. A similar improvement in outlook is achieved by combination chemotherapy following surgery but there is some evidence to suggest that this is due at least in part to a chemical castration. The development of tamoxifen in the 1970s allowed a less drastic alternative. Subsequent randomized controlled trials by the Nolvadex Adjuvant Treatment Organisation (1988), the Cancer Research Campaign (1988) and the Scottish Cancer Trials Office (1987) have all confirmed that adjuvant tamoxifen prolongs survival and delays recurrence for pre- and postmenopausal women. With the luteinizing hormone-releasing hormone agonist Zoladex a reversible, safe 'oophorectomy' has become available.

For postmenopausal women, the options are clearer. Tamoxifen 10 mg b.d. for 2 years or more delays recurrence and prolongs survival in node-positive and node-negative women whether or not the tumour contains oestrogen receptors. The drug is non-toxic and rather than simply blocking oestrogen receptors, it may have a more complicated mechanism involving local polypeptide growth factors. Adjuvant chemotherapy has no significant benefit for postmenopausal women.

The standard treatment of any woman with curable breast cancer is adequate local control of the primary, sampling or removal of the axillary nodes, radiotherapy in selected cases, then adjuvant treatment. Postmenopausal women should have tamoxifen. Premenopausal women with involved nodes should be offered chemotherapy or preferably randomized into one of the current trials comparing chemotherapy, tamoxifen and Zoladex.

Preclinical cancers

It is not yet known if excision biopsy of impalpable lesions detected by mammographic screening should be augmented by another modality of treatment. A number of centres favour excision biopsy and radiotherapy although a proportion of DCIS treated conservatively do recur locally. A national UK trial for screen-detected DCIS has been agreed and will involve local excision of focal lesions with randomization to either postoperative radiation or tamoxifen. When multifocal, DCIS is always treated successfully by mastectomy.

Breast cancer in pregnancy

Breast cancer arising in pregnancy usually presents at a more advanced stage, for reasons discussed earlier in this chapter. As the optimum treatment for a premenopausal woman may involve surgery, radiotherapy and chemotherapy, fetal damage can result. Generally, an early pregnancy should be terminated and a later one induced as soon as the fetus is viable, prior to the commencement of treatment. Obviously there may be important social considerations in individual cases.

Advanced disease

Advanced breast cancer is not curable. The majority of

locally advanced tumours demonstrate distant metastases within a few years, so the objective of treatment of these and patients with known distant metastases is to limit tumour progression, relieve pain and preserve a good quality of life for as long as possible. This is best achieved using systemic therapy backed up by specific local measures where necessary. Hormonal therapy is usually tried before cytotoxic therapy but radiotherapy and other measures may be required for locally symptomatic lesions.

In premenopausal women, ablative hormonal therapy or cytotoxic therapy are the choices. Zoladex has removed the need for oophorectomy. Postmenopausal women are more likely to respond to tamoxifen or other additive endocrine therapy. Tamoxifen was originally introduced as a treatment for advanced disease and achieves an overall response rate of 35%. When relapse occurs, progestagens have few side effects and, one stage on from these, aromatase inhibitors such as aminoglutethimide are well tolerated if the initial nausea, vomiting and rash settle.

Although it is true that knowledge of the oestrogen receptor and progesterone receptor status of the tumour may allow a more rational choice of first-line treatment for advanced disease, in practice this is seldom determined because a reliable assay is available in only a few centres and sufficient material can be obtained only at superficial sites. Slow-growing local, regional or bony disease is always worth a trial of endocrine therapy whereas rapidly progressive inflammatory carcinoma, visceral metastases and life-threatening complications demand urgent chemotherapy; the disease is invariably oestrogen receptor-negative in such cases.

In both pre- and postmenopausal women, unless the patient is moribund, the question of cytotoxic chemotherapy will eventually arise. Regimens abound, and on average, any regime will only prolong the patient's life by a further 3 months. However, the quality of life improves considerably during a response. The problem is finding a regimen which is both effective and universally tolerated. Outpatient chemotherapy has its own problems and is best left in the hands of a medical or radiation oncologist.

The treatment of problems commonly encountered in advanced disease is summarised in Table 35.3 For long bone fractures and vertebral collapse, the appropriate orthopaedic treatment should not be altered just because the patient has breast cancer. Orthopaedic treatment will need augmentation with radiotherapy to limit local progression and treat pain. In most cases, it is both humane and cost-effective to attempt treatment of locally troublesome lesions to allow the patient to continue an independent existence for as long as possible.

Secondaries can arise anywhere and must be assessed promptly by the surgeon to see if treatment will help; this means that a patient with advanced disease must be monitored closely.

Table 35.3 Treatment of the complications of advanced breast cancer

Complication	Treatment
Vertebral collapse	Radiotherapy plus decompression
Long bone fracture	Internal fixation plus radiotherapy
Hypercalcaemia	Rehydration, calcium-lowing agents
Pleural effusions	Drainage plus pleural cytotoxics plus pleurodesis
Liver pain, cachexia	Oral corticosteroids
Cerebral secondaries	Dexamethasone Radiotherapy
Rampant local disease	Chemotherapy Radiotherapy

Pain control is perhaps the most important aspect of management. Terminal care teams are invaluable and should be involved at an early stage.

Advanced disease causes considerable distress not only to the unfortunate patient, but also to her attendants and relatives. The general practitioner and hospital staff must be in close contact to ensure that the management is appropriate, effective and humane.

KEY POINTS

1. Breast cancer is the most common cancer affecting women in the developed world. It is the commonest cause of death for women under 55 years of age.
2. The largest numbers of cases are seen in women between 65 and 80 years of age.
3. Environmental factors play an important part in determining the incidence.
4. A family history of breast cancer in a first-degree relative increases the risk of developing breast cancer.
5. Early age at menarche and a late menopause are independent risk factors.
6. Childbirth before the age of 25 reduces the risk of breast cancer.
7. Benign breast disease probably does not predispose to breast cancer.
8. The modern low-dose contraceptive pill probably does not increase the risk of breast cancer but more data are required.
9. The evidence for the effect of hormone replacement therapy on breast cancer is conflicting but tends to suggest no increased risk.
10. Mammographic breast screening appears to reduce the mortality in women over 50 years of age but does result in a large number of false positive tests.
11. Most patients present with a lump in the breast, but skin changes or inversion of the nipple may be the first sign.

12. Breast cancer presents at a more advanced stage in pregnancy but otherwise the prognosis is unchanged.
13. *In selected cases*, wide local excision plus radiotherapy to the breast give the same survival and local recurrence rates as mastectomy.
14. Adjuvant tamoxifen for 2 years or more gives a clear survival advantage to postmenopausal women.
15. Premenopausal women with nodal disease should have chemotherapy, tamoxifen or Zoladex.

REFERENCES

Anon 1989 Cancer risks of oral contraception. Lancet i: 21–22

Armstrong B K 1988 Oestrogen therapy after the menopause: boon or bane? Medical Journal of Australia 148: 213–214

Baum M 1988 Breast cancer: the facts. Oxford University Press, Oxford

Cancer Research Campaign adjuvant breast trial working party 1988 Cyclophosphamide and tamoxifen as adjuvant therapies in the management of early breast cancer. British Journal of Cancer 57: 604–607

Cuzick J, Wang D Y, Bulbrook R D 1986 The prevention of breast cancer. Lancet i: 83–86

Dupont W D, Page D L 1985 Risk factors for breast cancer in women with proliferative breast disease. New England Journal of Medicine 312: 146–151

Early Breast Cancer Trialists' Collaborative Group 1988 Effects of adjuvant tamoxifen and cytotoxic therapy on mortality in early breast cancer: an overview of 61 randomized trials among 28 896 women. New England Journal of Medicine 319: 1681–1691

Forrest A M P 1987 Report to health ministers of England, Wales, Scotland and Northern Ireland from working group on breast cancer screening. HMSO, London

Hughes L E, Mansel R E, Webster D J T 1987 Aberrations of normal development and involution (ANDI): a new perspective on pathogenesis and nomenclature of benign breast disorders. Lancet ii: 1316–1319

Nolvadex Adjuvant Treatment Organisation (NATO) 1988 Controlled trial of tamoxifen as single adjuvant agent in the management of early breast cancer. British Journal of Cancer 57: 608–611

Schnitt S J, Silen W, Sadowsky N L, Connolly J L, Harris J R 1988 Ductal carcinoma in situ (intraductal carcinoma) of the breast. New England Journal of Medicine 318: 898–903

Scottish Cancer Trials Office 1987 Adjuvant tamoxifen in the management of operable breast cancer: the Scottish trial. Lancet ii: 171–175

Shapiro S 1977 Evidence on screening for breast cancer from a randomised trial. Cancer 39: 2772–2782

Simpson H W, Candlish W, Pauson A W, McArdle C S, Griffiths K, Small R G 1988 Genesis of breast cancer is in the premenopause. Lancet ii: 74–76

Tabar L, Gad A, Holmberg L H et al 1985 Reduction in mortality from breast cancer after mass screening with mammography. Lancet i: 829–832

Wolfe J N 1976 Risk for breast cancer development determined by mammographic parenchymal pattern. Cancer 37: 2486–2492

36. Malignant disease of the cervix

M. C. Anderson C. A. E. Coulter W. P. Mason W. P. Soutter J. Tidy

EPIDEMIOLOGY

Invasive carcinoma of the cervix constitutes 4% of female malignancies. In England and Wales in 1983, 5400 cases of carcinoma-in-situ of the cervix (cervical intraepithelial neoplasia (CIN III) and 3879 of carcinoma of the cervix were registered (Office of Population Censuses and Surveys Copes 1987). Although there were fewer cases of invasive carcinoma of the cervix than in 1978, registrations of CIN III had increased by almost 40%.

The incidence of CIN III in England and Wales is 21 per 100 000 women compared with 13 per 100 000 for invasive carcinoma. Throughout the world, the incidence of invasive disease varies widely: the cumulative risk of developing carcinoma of the cervix is 5.5% in Columbia by the age of 74, compared with 1.5% in England and Wales and 0.5% in Spain and Israel. Worldwide, cervical cancer is the second commonest cancer in women and is very nearly as common as breast cancer.

Age at presentation

In England and Wales, the incidence of invasive cervical cancer has risen in the 25–34-year-old group from approximately 6 per 100 000 in 1968 to about 16 per 100 000 in 1981 (OPCS 1985). The age-related distribution now shows a distinct shoulder due to this rising rate in younger cohorts (Fig. 36.1) and in 1981, 31% of cases were in women under 45 years old.

It has been said that younger women have more aggressive disease but there is no evidence of that in women treated before 1981 (Meanwell et al 1988). There remains an anxiety that a poorer prognosis is apparent only in pa-

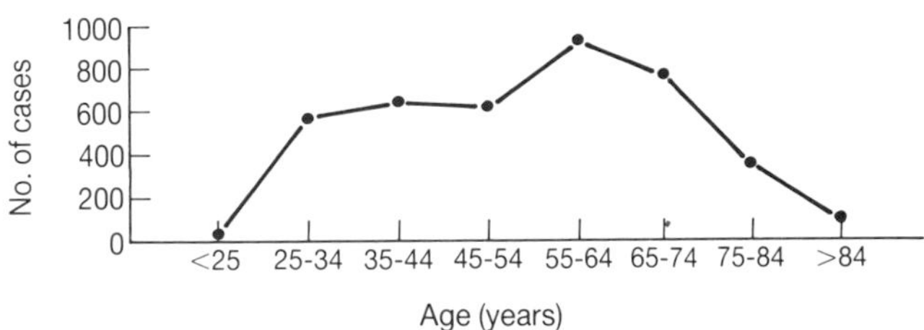

Fig. 36.1 A graph of the age-related distribution of cervical cancer in England and Wales in 1981 has a distinct shoulder because of a sharp increase in the younger cohorts of women. About 31% of cases are in women less than 45 years of age (OPCS 1985).

tients treated more recently (Dattoli et al 1989). The worse prognosis applied equally to women treated with surgery or with radiotherapy.

ANATOMY

The stratified squamous epithelium of the vagina and ectocervix meets the columnar epithelium of the uterine cavity at the squamocolumnar junction. In premenopausal women, this squamocolumnar junction is usually situated just inside the external cervical os and can be readily visualized using a colposcope. The position of the squamocolumnar junction tends to lie inside the canal after the menopause. It is the site of origin of the vast majority of preinvasive and invasive cervical neoplasia.

Lymphatic drainage

The regional lymph drainage of the female genital organs follows a relatively well defined pattern. Cervical tumours spread via the parametrial lymphatics to the internal (hypogastric) and external iliac nodes which surround the corresponding iliac vessels on the pelvic side wall. The lymph vessels ascend towards the network of nodes around the common iliac vessels on each side and amalgamate in a plexus surrounding the aorta and vena cava. The inferior margin of the aortic nodes is at the lower border of the fourth lumbar vertebra. The common iliac vessels commence to the right of the midline at the upper border of the same vertebra and pass to the front of the sacroiliac joint on each side before bifurcating into external and internal branches.

AETIOLOGY

An association between sexual behaviour and the subsequent development of cervical carcinoma was suggested by physicians working in the 18th and 19th centuries. Since these early reports there has been considerable interest in the risk factors associated with cervical neoplasia and the possibility that a sexually transmissible agent may be involved in the process.

Sexual history

Two factors related to sexual behaviour — age at first intercourse and number of sexual partners — have been examined extensively. Rotkin (1973) reported a 50% excess of cases of cervical neoplasia in women who started sexual intercourse before their 20th birthday, supporting the proposal that the adolescent cervix may be more vulnerable to potential oncogenic agents. Several other studies, however, have found a history of multiple sexual partners to be more significant than early age of first intercourse. Harris et al (1980) recorded a 14.2-fold increased risk of developing severe dysplasia with a past history of six or more partners and this finding has been confirmed by others. There appears to be little correlation between the number of sexual acts and cervical neoplasia amongst women with two or less lifetime partners (Harris et al 1980).

Smoking

A strong epidemiological link between smoking and cervical neoplasia has been demonstrated in studies which have controlled adequately for sexual behaviour (but see Ch. 32). A 12.7-fold greater risk of developing carcinoma-in-situ has been found after 12 years of smoking. The products of smoking, cotinine and nicotine, are found in higher concentrations in cervical mucus than in serum from women with CIN. However, little is known about the direct effects of these agents on human epithelia. There are few data on the role of nitrosamines, the chemical carcinogens linked with the development of other smoking-related cancers, in the cervix.

Smoking reduces the number of Langerhans cells present in the cervical epithelium in a dose-dependent manner. These cells, originally derived from macrophages, play a role in local immune surveillance within epithelia. Because their role is not fully understood, it is difficult to speculate upon the ways in which the reduction of Langerhans cells may contribute to cervical neoplasia.

Contraception

No definite association between oral contraception and cervical neoplasia has been clearly demonstrated. Studies which have shown an increased risk in oral contraceptive pill users have often failed to control adequately for the sexual history of the women involved (Beral et al 1988). A lower incidence of cervical neoplasia has been demonstrated in women using a diaphragm, suggesting that a transmissible agent may be involved.

Male factor

In view of the association between sexual behaviour and cervical neoplasia it would be expected that factors relating to the male partner may influence the outcome. Kessler (1984) described a 2.7-fold increased risk of developing cervical neoplasia for a woman whose husband had previously been married to a woman with cervical carcinoma. Recent evidence seems firmly to refute the proposal of an association between penile and cervical cancer. The sexual history of the male partner may also influence the risk of a woman developing cervical neoplasia; a history of 15 or more partners is associated with a 7.8-fold increased risk of the current female partner developing cervical neoplasia

(Buckley et al 1981). Several potent immunosuppressive agents are present in human seminal plasma. These may influence the development of cervical neoplasia by reducing the local immune response to viral infections or to cells transformed by other agents.

Infective agents

Agents that are known to infect the lower female genital tract have been studied in an attempt to find a link with cervical neoplasia. Of the non-viral agents, *Trichomonas vaginalis* and *Chlamydia trachomatis* have been studied recently. A twofold increased incidence of antibodies against *Chlamydia trachomatis* was found in women with CIN when compared with controls. However, most research interest has concentrated upon viral agents. Both Epstein–Barr virus and cytomegalovirus are thought to infect the cervix but neither has been linked to the development of cervical neoplasia. Early work on herpes simplex virus type 2 (HSV-2) did demonstrate a possible link with cervical neoplasia. In the laboratory, HSV-2 has been shown to be a very weak oncogenic virus; however, analysis of many cervical tumours has failed to show any evidence of HSV-2 DNA. Despite early case-controlled studies linking previous infection with HSV-2 to cervical neoplasia, large population studies have shown that the presence of HSV-2 antibodies is related to sexual activity rather than cervical neoplasia.

Human papillomaviruses

Recent research has concentrated on the possible link between certain types of human papillomavirus (HPV) and cervical neoplasia. These are small DNA viruses which have no outer, lipid-containing viral membrane. They cannot be grown in cell culture and so the development of adequate type-specific antibodies has been difficult. The distinction between different HPV types is based therefore upon differences in DNA sequence (Howley & Schlegel 1988).

Over 50 different HPV types have now been described, of which at least nine infect the lower female genital tract. The sexual transmission of these viruses from male to female and female to male has been shown to occur. The HPV types which infect the lower reproductive tract can be divided into two groups. One group, which includes types 6, 11, 31, 35, 42 and 50, is found in condylomata acuminata, low-grade CIN and only rarely in invasive tumours. The second group includes types 16, 18 and 33, and is associated with low-grade CIN that progresses, advanced CIN and invasive tumours.

HPV types 16 and 18 have the ability to transform cells in culture which can then cause tumours in immunocompromised animals. The transforming ability seems to depend upon two proteins produced by HPV 16 and 18 — the E6 and E7 proteins. The E7 protein has structural and functional homologies with two well known viral transforming proteins, SV40 large T and E1A of adenovirus. All three proteins bind the product of the retinoblastoma gene, a putative anti-oncogene. This may be the mechanism by which these proteins bring about cellular transformation. Integration of HPV-DNA into the host genome may be an important early event in the neoplastic process. The majority of cervical carcinomas examined have integrated-HPV sequences whereas integration is uncommon in normal tissue and CIN. When integration occurs the circular HPV-DNA is usually opened in the region which encodes for the E1 and E2 proteins. This will prevent any transcription of genes downstream from the break (e.g. E2) but will allow transcription of the upstream E6 and E7 proteins. The loss of E2 transcription may lead to the autonomous expression of E6 and E7 since it is E2 that controls early gene expression. This uncontrolled expression of the transforming proteins may be important in cellular transformation brought about by HPVs 16 and 18.

The prevalence of HPV infection in the normal population has, until recently, been difficult to quantify. Early studies had used techniques which were only capable of detecting relatively large numbers of HPV molecules. The development of a method by which DNA may be selectively amplified in vitro, the polymerase chain reaction, may allow a more accurate estimation of the prevalence of HPV infection to be made. Using this method HPV 16 was found in 70% of women with normal cervical cytology. If a high prevalence is proved to exist, it would seem that some other factor must be involved if there is a link between HPV infection and cervical neoplasia.

Conclusions

There is a wealth of epidemiological evidence to suggest that the risk of developing cervical neoplasia is associated with sexual behaviour and that a sexually transmissible agent may be involved in the process. Many such agents have been studied but none has a proven role. Until more information is available, the causal role of particular HPV types in cervical neoplasia must be treated cautiously.

PATHOLOGY

Malignant tumours of the cervix may be of squamous or glandular type; squamous cell carcinomas account for about 90% of invasive carcinomas and most of the remainder are adenocarcinomas. Preinvasive lesions are discussed in Chapter 34.

Squamous cell carcinoma

Early stromal invasion

The earliest recognizable stages of invasion arising from CIN are minute prongs of malignant cells pushing through the basement membrane into the cervical stroma. As these become slightly larger, better differentiated cells may be recognized in the invasive islands and a lymphocytic infiltrate and loosening of the stroma may be seen. This earliest invasion (early stromal invasion; ESI) is often a multifocal phenomenon, occurring from either the surface epithelium or involved crypts. These lesions are adequately treated by cone biopsy.

Microinvasive carcinoma

Eventually, the invasive foci amalgamate and become measurable, at which stage the lesion is referred to as microinvasive carcinoma (Fig. 36.2). This term ought to be used to describe squamous cell tumours which have become invasive but have not yet become capable of metastasis. A diagnosis of microinvasive carcinoma on section would then mean that treatment need not be radical. However, because of uncertainties and lack of precision in defining the histological criteria of microinvasive carcinoma this cannot yet be accepted as true. Although the International Federation of Gynaecologists and Obstetricians (FIGO) defines stage Ia2 (microinvasive carcinoma) as a lesion which when measured in two dimensions has a maximum depth of invasion of not more than 5 mm and a maximum width of not more than 7 mm, tumours at the larger extreme of this range do have some metastatic potential.

For practical purposes, it is advised that conservative treatment should only be contemplated in examples where invasion is not greater than 3 mm from the nearest basement membrane and lymphatic channel involvement is not seen. Lesions larger than this, particularly when lymphatic channel involvement is seen, are probably best treated by radical hysterectomy.

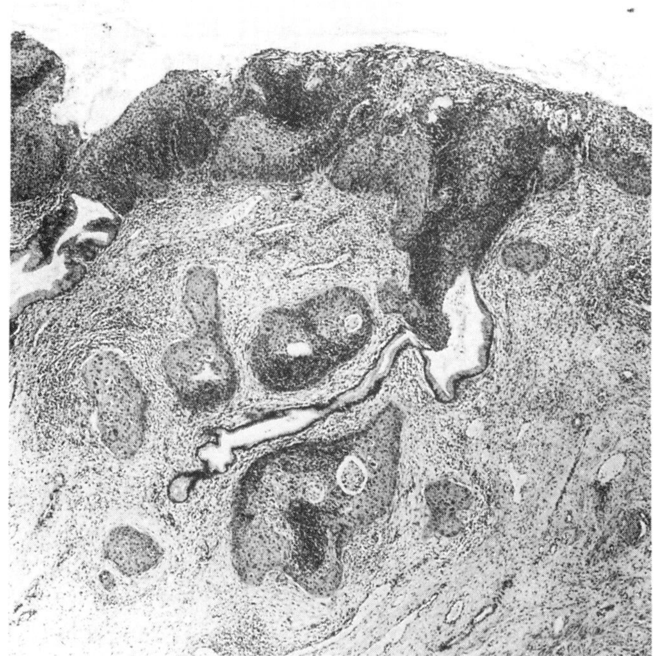

Fig. 36.2 Microinvasive carcinoma showing multiple foci of invasion arising from a gland crypt. The invasive islands are irregular in outline and partly show better differentiation than the overlying CIN. Haematoxylin and eosin ×42.

Invasive squamous cell carcinoma

By the time they become clinically apparent, most squamous cell carcinomas involve the external os and are visible on speculum examination. Some, however, remain entirely within the canal and are classified clinically as endocervical carcinomas. A squamous cell carcinoma may be either predominantly exophytic, growing out from the surface often as a papillary or polypoid excrescence, or mainly endophytic, infiltrating the surrounding structures. Ulceration and excavation are frequently seen.

The simplest and most widely used classification of squamous cell carcinoma subdivides the tumours into three groups: large-cell keratinizing; large-cell non-keratinizing and small-cell non-keratinizing. These categories have been adopted by the World Health Organization. This classification depends on the histological cell type of the tumour whereas, from a clinical point of view, the grade (degree of differentiation) may be more important. Some so-called small-cell non-keratinizing carcinomas contain argyrophil cells and are akin to the small-cell anaplastic (oat cell) carcinoma of the bronchus with a correspondingly poor prognosis.

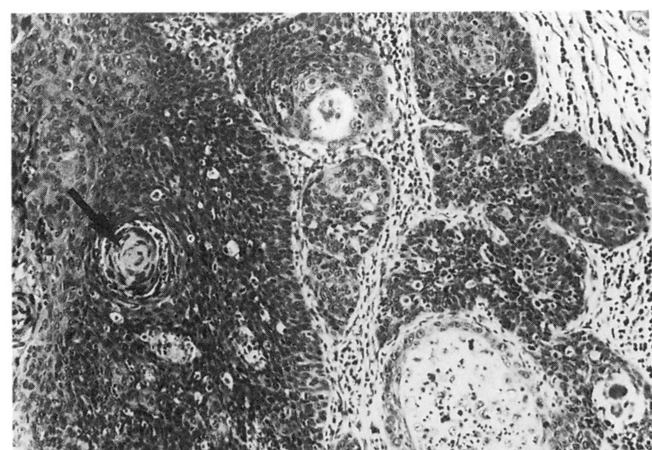

Fig. 36.3 Invasive squamous cell carcinoma. The invasive islands are composed of poorly differentiated cells but an attempt at formation of a keratin pearl is marked by an arrow. Haematoxylin and eosin ×160.

Invasive squamous cell carcinoma of the cervix infiltrates the tissue as irregular islands and cords of cells (Fig. 36.3). The intervening stroma often shows a dense chronic inflammatory reaction, representing an immune response by the host against the tumour.

Verrucous carcinoma is a rare variant of keratinizing squamous carcinoma. Progressive local invasion occurs but it rarely metastasizes to the lymphatic system. The relatively low mitotic rate in these tumours renders them rather resistant to radiotherapy. Surgery is therefore the treatment of choice.

Adenocarcinoma

Malignant tumours of glandular origin comprise 10–15% of cervical tumours. This figure is increasing, representing both an absolute increase in the number of cases of adenocarcinoma and an increase in proportion of glandular tumours (Gallup & Abell 1977; Shingleton et al 1981).

Adenocarcinoma-in-situ was reported over 30 years ago and is being seen with increasing frequency. Microscopically, adenocarcinoma in-situ generally retains the architectural pattern of the normal endocervical crypts, replacing the normal epithelium by an atypical epithelium showing loss of polarity, increased nuclear size, nuclear pleomorphism and anisokaryosis, mitotic activity, reduction in cytoplasmic mucin and, frequently, stratification (Fig. 36.4). The glandular abnormalities of the cervix appear to form a continuous spectrum of disease in exactly the same way as the squamous abnormalities. The less severe forms are referred to as glandular atypias, often divided into mild and severe.

A number of different histological patterns are found in invasive adenocarcinoma of the cervix. The endocervical type accounts for up to 90%. It is composed of crowded glands of variable size and shape with budding and branching of the epithelium (Fig. 36.5), somewhat resembling that of normal endocervical epithelium. The terms 'adenoma malignum' and 'minimal deviation adenocarcinoma' have been used to describe a carcinoma in which the glandular pattern is particularly well differentiated and there is virtually no atypia of the epithelial cells. Tumours of endometrioid, clear cell, mucinous and papillary patterns are also seen.

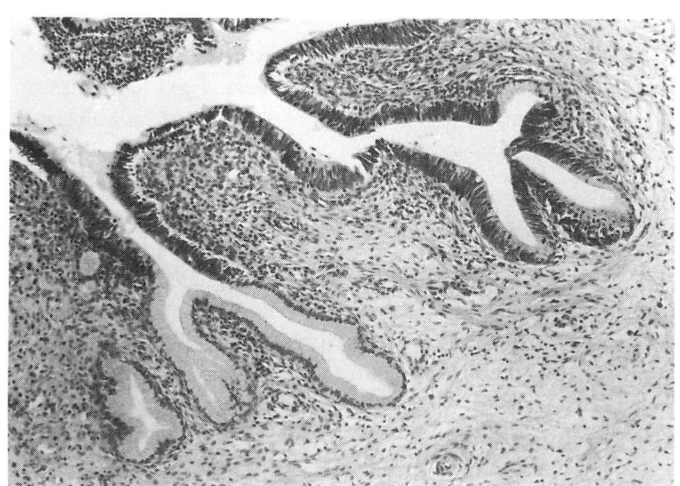

Fig. 36.4 Adenocarcinoma-in-situ. The abnormal epithelium follows the architectural outline of the normal crypts but the epithelium shows marked nuclear crowding, with loss of polarity and reduced mucin production. Haematoxylin and eosin ×160.

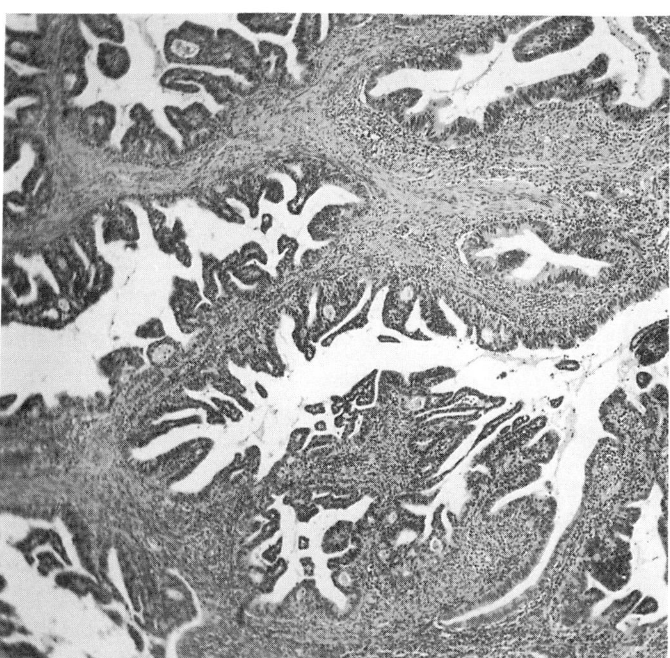

Fig. 36.5 Invasive adenocarcinoma of the cervix. Although the architectural pattern bears a superficial resemblance to normal cervical crypts, the pattern is excessively complex and papillary, with associated cellular abnormalities. Haematoxylin and eosin ×100.

NATURAL HISTORY

Carcinoma of the cervix spreads predominantly by either direct invasion or lymphatic permeation. The tumour may invade into the vaginal mucosa or into the myometrium of the lower uterine segment. It seems that while spread into the parametrial tissues may occur as a continuous wave of infiltrating tumour, initially at least, it is more common for there to be scattered foci of tumour in the parametrium which only gradually become palpable as they coalesce. Only 5% of small primary lesions which involve less than 20% of the cervix have histological evidence of parametrial disease, usually in parametrial nodes. In contrast, 48% of tumours invading more than 80% of the cervix are associated with parametrial extension which is confluent in 23% (Burghardt et al 1988). If lymphatic spaces within the tumour are invaded, spread to the pelvic nodes may occur more often. The incidence of node involvement increases

Table 36.1 Increased incidence of nodal metastases with stage

Stage	% Positive nodes	
	Pelvic	Para-aortic
Ib	16	7
II	30	16
III	44	35
IV	55	40

with the stage, grade and volume of the tumour (Table 36.1).

Survival following surgical treatment is closely related to the proportion of cervix involved. For example, 70% of patients with positive nodes survive for 5 years if the tumour invades less than 20% of the cervix but only 54% survive if it involves more than 60% (Pickel et al 1988).

Forty per cent of patients with carcinoma of the cervix die with uncontrolled pelvic disease leading to ureteric obstruction. Direct involvement of bone within the pelvis is common. Blood stream metastases also occur and tend to be observed in poorly differentiated tumours and the higher stages of disease. The most common sites are the lungs, bones and liver.

CLINICAL STAGING

The FIGO classification is the most widely used (Table 36.2; FIGO 1988). It is recommended that bimanual examination under anaesthesia should be performed by more than one examiner. The intravenous urogram findings may be included, as may cystoscopy, but neither special imaging techniques nor subsequent operative findings alter the staging.

Surgical staging has been advocated, particularly to assess involvement of the para-aortic nodes. However, this delays the commencement of radiotherapy. The transperitoneal approach to the nodes combined with radiotherapy increased the incidence of bowel damage and is not recommended. The postoperative risk is less with a retroperitoneal approach but it is unlikely that the information gained will lead to changes in management which will improve the prognosis. If para-aortic nodes are enlarged on imaging, fine-needle aspiration cytology may be performed under computerized tomography (CT) or ultrasound control without the necessity for surgery.

Table 36.2 The FIGO staging classification for cervical cancer

Stage	Description
0	Preinvasive carcinoma (carcinoma-in-situ, CIN)
I	Carcinoma confined to the cervix (corpus extension should be disregarded)
Ia	Preclinical carcinoma of cervix diagnosed only by microscopy
Ia1	Minimal microscopically evident stromal invasion
Ia2	Microinvasive carcinoma — lesions detected microscopically that can be measured; depth of invasion from the base of the epithelium from which it originates should not be greater than 5 mm. The horizontal spread must not exceed 7 mm. Larger lesions should be staged as Ib
Ib	Lesions of greater dimensions than stage Ia2 whether seen clinically or not. Preformed space involvement should not alter the staging but should be specifically recorded so as to determine whether it should affect treatment decisions in the future
II	Carcinoma extending beyond the cervix and involving the vagina (but not the lower third) and/or infiltrating the parametrium (but not reaching the pelvic side wall)
IIa	Carcinoma has involved the vagina
IIb	Carcinoma has infiltrated the parametrium
III	Carcinoma involving the lower third of the vagina and/or extending to the pelvic side wall (there is no free space between the tumour and the pelvic side wall)
IIIa	Carcinoma involving the lower third of the vagina
IIIb	Carcinoma extending to the pelvic wall and/or hydronephrosis or non-functioning kidney due to ureterostenosis caused by tumour
IVa	Carcinoma involving the mucosa of the bladder or rectum and/or extending beyond the true pelvis
IVb	Spread to distant organs

DIAGNOSIS AND INVESTIGATION

Presenting symptoms

The most common presenting features are postcoital or intermenstrual bleeding. A foul-smelling vaginal discharge may be the initial symptom. Anaemia may result from heavy vaginal bleeding. Pelvic and leg pain is uncommon in early tumours but often occurs during later stages of the disease due to spread to the pelvic side wall or invasion of the lumbosacral plexus.

Tumours which spread into the bladder may cause haematuria or frequency of micturition. Spread of tumour into the rectum may cause tenesmus or rectal bleeding. Fistula formation may occur into either organ.

Clinical examination and initial investigations

The physical examination should include careful examination of the supraclavicular and inguinal nodes, and palpation of the abdomen for enlarged liver or kidneys. A preliminary speculum examination of the cervix should be performed prior to gentle digital examination. A smear may be taken from the cervix for cytology and a punch biopsy performed if there is an obvious lesion present. However, it should not be forgotten that the smear may be negative in the presence of invasive disease and a superficial biopsy may not confirm the diagnosis.

Bimanual examination may reveal a hard, friable, irregular, enlarged cervix which becomes fixed as the tumour spreads into the parametria. Rectovaginal examination is the best way of assessing parametrial and posterior spread. Mandatory investigations are a full blood count, urea and electrolytes, liver function tests, intravenous urogram and chest X-ray.

Examination under anaesthesia

Ideally, examination under anaesthesia should be performed by the gynaecologist and radiotherapist jointly. Rectovaginal examination is repeated in order to stage the tumour clinically. If there is any suspicion of rectal spread, proctoscopy and sigmoidoscopy are performed. Cystoscopy is not essential in patients who have early-stage disease but must be performed if the disease appears locally advanced. If histological confirmation of diagnosis is lacking, a knife biopsy should be obtained rather than a punch. The length of the uterine cavity is measured and curettings are taken from the endocervix and from the endometrial cavity.

Additional investigations

Other investigations may be performed but do not alter the FIGO staging of disease. Lymphangiography is not a routine test for staging. When assessed by surgical lymphadenectomy, lymphangiography correctly identified only 61% of women with positive nodes and 78% of those without nodal metastases (Lagasse et al 1979). Nodal disease was detected following lymphadenectomy in 21% of the women with negative lymphangiograms. Lymphangiography helps the planning of radiation fields and may be used to monitor the completeness of lymphadenectomy but does not appear to be sufficiently accurate to be considered a routine diagnostic test.

CT scanning and abdominopelvic ultrasound may be used to estimate the size and extent of the primary tumour and to detect nodal disease. Neither is sufficiently accurate to merit routine use. Transrectal ultrasound probes may give greater accuracy in the future. Currently the most promising imaging method is magnetic resonance imaging. Although it appears to give reliable information about the primary tumour, it is unable to identify small metastatic deposits in lymph nodes.

TREATMENT OF MICROINVASIVE DISEASE

No further treatment is required in young women if a colposcopically directed cone biopsy completely excises the lesion; if the depth of invasion is less than 3 mm, and if there is no marked lymph space involvement (Creasman et al 1985). However, in women who have completed their family, a total hysterectomy is often performed. If marked lymphatic space involvement is present or if invasion extends beyond 3 mm there is a possibility of metastatic spread and more radical treatment should be considered.

TREATMENT OF INVASIVE CERVICAL CANCER

The definitive treatment for carcinoma of the cervix may involve either surgery or radiotherapy or a combination of both. Each patient should be staged and discussed jointly although certain principles of management will develop in every unit. In many centres, surgery is performed on the younger patient with lower-volume stage Ib disease. This allows conservation of the ovaries, the preservation of a more normal vagina and avoidance of the long-term bowel and bladder sequelae sometimes seen after radiotherapy. Radiotherapy is then used for the older and less fit patients regardless of the size of the tumour; for women with bulky stage Ib and IIa tumours, or for more advanced disease.

Surgery

It is of great importance that the surgical procedure is carried out in a unit in which the Wertheim hysterectomy is regularly performed as this operation may be associated with mortality and considerable morbidity in less experienced hands.

Preoperative care

It is not usually necessary to prepare the bowel rigorously, but a mild aperient and a small enema if necessary do ensure that the pelvis is not filled with distended loops of bowel and help to make the patient's first few postoperative days more comfortable. Cross-matching 4 units of blood is a sensible precaution as occasionally blood may be needed rapidly. A single dose of a broad-spectrum antibiotic given prophylactically with the premedication does reduce the risk of infective complications.

The value of subcutaneous heparin is less certain. It may not be as effective in reducing thromboembolic complications in women with gynaecological cancers and these patients have a greater risk of haemorrhage. A compromise adopted by some is to defer the start of the prophylactic heparin until the first postoperative day. Anti-thrombotic stockings are useful provided they are worn correctly.

Some patients may benefit especially from preoperative physiotherapy. This applies particularly to smokers. The anaesthetist should be consulted and warned about any potential difficulties. Epidural analgesia is a very valuable adjunct to the general anaesthetic, reducing blood loss and causing some constriction of the bowel which thus occupies less space in the operative field. It may also be used to give postoperative analgesia.

The surgical procedure

Either a midline or a high transverse incision may be used. The procedure commences with the lymphadenectomy — the para-aortic nodes are resected first and the dissection continues caudally until all of the iliac nodal groups have been resected (Figs 36.6 and 36.7). During the lymphadenectomy both ureters are reflected medially attached to the parietal peritoneum. Any fixed and enlarged nodes are subjected to frozen section. If they are positive, the procedure is abandoned and the patient treated by irradiation. Resection of enlarged, mobile nodes should not preclude continuing with the procedure.

Following the lymphadenectomy, the bladder is reflected inferiorly, the ureteric tunnels are defined and the uterine vessels divided (Fig. 36.8). The ureters are mobilized and reflected laterally by division of the small vessels running forwards to the bladder. The rectovaginal space is opened up and the rectum displaced posteriorly to define the uterosacral ligaments on each side of the rectum. These are divided as far posteriorly as possible. The cardinal ligaments, parametrial and paravaginal tissues are clamped and divided close to the pelvic side wall taking care not to damage the internal iliac vein. In this way the uterus, cervix and upper third of the vagina are resected together with the related parametrial and uterosacral tissues. The more radical the resection of the parametria, the more common are postoperative voiding problems. This is why less radical procedures are sometimes adopted in patients with small lesions. Suction drains are inserted into the pelvis.

Exenterative surgery — removing the bladder or rectum

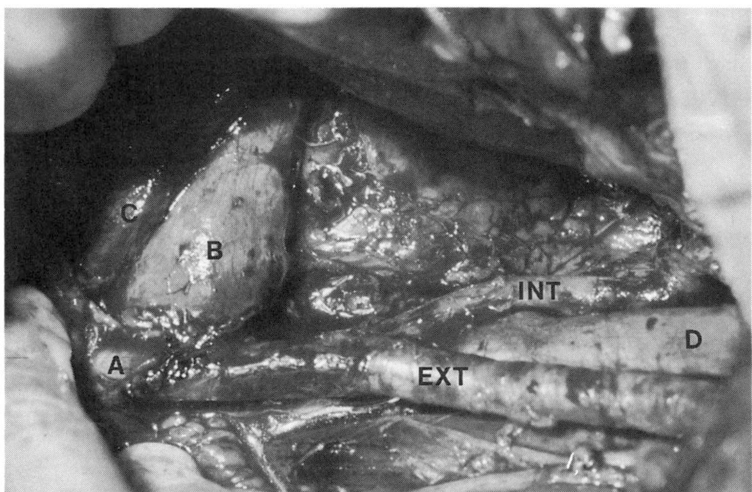

Fig. 36.6 The pelvis is viewed obliquely from the right. The right common iliac artery (A) is seen crossing over the left common iliac vein (B) as it runs behind the left common iliac artery (C). The right external iliac vein (D) can be seen first medial to the artery below the inguinal ligament. It then runs behind the common iliac artery and (not shown) joins the vena cava lateral to the artery. EXT = right external iliac artery; INT = right internal iliac artery.

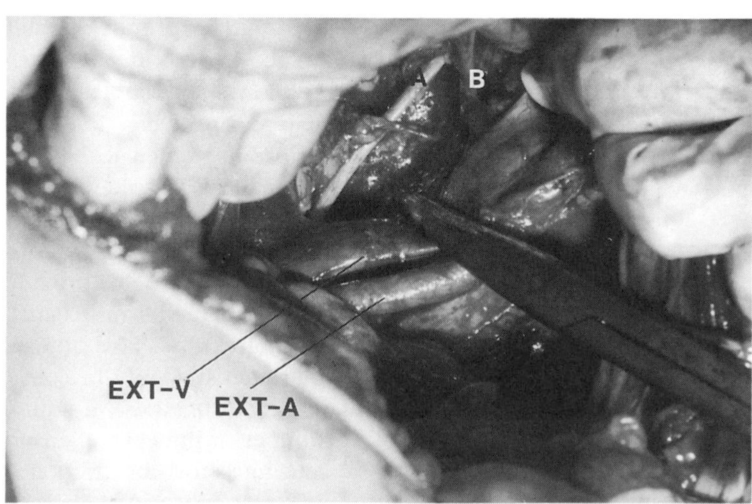

Fig. 36.7 The obturator nerve (A) and an abnormal obturator vein (B) are visible. EXT-A = right external iliac artery; EXT-V = right external iliac vein.

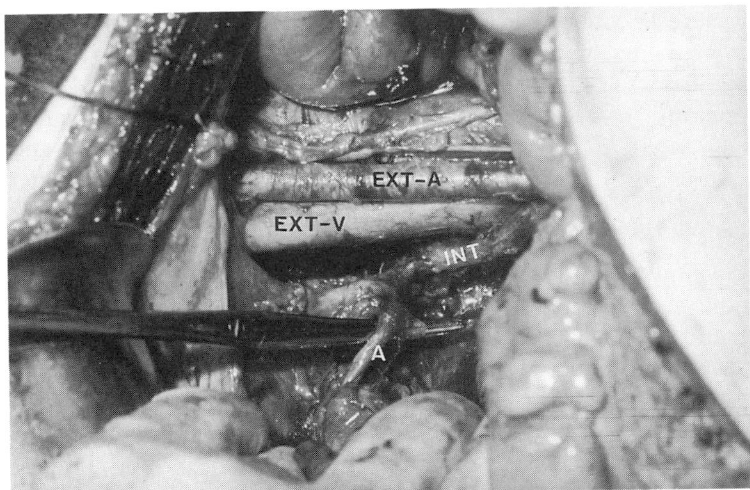

Fig. 36.8 Pelvis viewed from the left. The right uterine artery (A) is displayed by the forceps close to its origin from the internal iliac artery (INT). EXT-A = right external iliac artery; EXT-V = right external iliac vein.

or both with the uterus — is usually reserved for women with a small central recurrence usually following radiotherapy. The quicker the recurrence becomes evident after the initial therapy, the worse the prognosis and the less the likelihood of benefit from exenteration. Selective exenteration, conserving either bladder or rectum, is sometimes possible. With proper patient selection the results of exenterative surgery can be very worthwhile.

Postoperative care

The pulse and blood pressure must be monitored with great care. The urinary output should exceed 30 ml/h and the intravenous fluids should be carefully adjusted to achieve this. Frusemide is rarely required. Any diminution in the urine output should be regarded as a possible sign of hypovolaemia due to occult blood loss and the vital signs and peripheral circulation should be examined closely.

The drains should be kept in place until the loss is minimal. The urinary catheter is best left in situ for 10 days. The residual urine volume should be checked by catheterizing the patient after she has 'emptied' her bladder herself. If the residual volume exceeds 100 ml, the bladder should be catheterized intermittently and the patient taught to do this herself so that, if the problem does not resolve rapidly, she may be discharged to continue self-catheterization at home.

The patient should be encouraged to mobilize as soon as possible by both nursing staff and physiotherapist. As her general condition improves, opportunities should be created to allow her to discuss her feelings and her fears for the future. The effect of her illness and the operation upon her life at home and at work, and upon her self-image and sexuality are topics she may well wish to talk about. Experienced, caring nursing staff have a particularly important role in this aspect of her recovery.

Complications of surgery

The immediate complications of surgery include haemorrhage and damage to the urinary or intestinal tract. Lacerations of the main pelvic veins or the vena cava will require careful repair with fine prolene or vicryl sutures. Vascular clamps may be invaluable. Ligation of one or both internal iliac arteries may be required but the results of this procedure are often disappointing. Pressure with a hot pack for 2 min controls the bleeding in most cases and allows preparation to be made for a further attempt to deal with the problem. Often, the field is cleared and the loss reduced by this manoeuvre sufficiently to expose the lacerated vessel. Prompt replacement of blood loss is essential and fresh frozen plasma should be given if more than 4 units of blood are required. If postoperative bleeding occurs, the site should be identified with arteriography as bleeding from pelvic vessels can be arrested by selective arterial embolization. Damage to ureter, bladder or bowel seldom gives rise to problems provided it is recognized and repaired at the time.

The most feared postoperative complication is pulmonary embolism. There may be no evidence of a deep venous thrombosis in the legs, the clot having arisen in the pelvic veins. If there is any doubt about the diagnosis a VQ scan should be performed as an emergency but heparin therapy should be started whenever there is strong clinical suspicion. In the absence of a pulmonary embolism, it is probably wise to obtain confirmatory evidence before starting therapy for a suspected deep venous thrombosis.

Ureteric and bladder fistulae follow 2–5% of Wertheim hysterectomies. A trial of conservative management is sometimes worthwhile but the patients usually prefer to opt for early surgical repair. Far more common than ureteric fistulae is the atonic bladder with loss of bladder sensation. This almost invariably rectifies itself in time but some women do need to undertake intermittent self-catheterization for several months.

Combinations of surgery and radiotherapy

If multiple lymph modes are found to be involved histologically or if the resection margins were narrow, postoperative radiotherapy should be considered. There is little evidence that radiotherapy increases survival in this situation but it may reduce the incidence of pelvic failure. Morrow reported that 84% of the recurrences in non-irradiated cases were found in the pelvis compared with 50% in irradiated cases (Morrow et al 1980).

In spite of radical surgery, radiotherapy can be given safely but the dose is usually limited to 4500 cGy in 24 fractions over 5 weeks. The 5-year survival for node-negative patients is 80–90% whereas for node-positive patients it drops to 50%.

Preoperative intracavitary therapy is sometimes given but there is no evidence that this improves survival. Doses of 3500 cGy to point A are given in one or two low dose rate insertions and surgery is performed 3–4 weeks later.

Radiotherapy

Radiotherapy for carcinoma of the cervix is given by intracavitary and external beam irradiation. The rapid fall-off in dose from intracavitary therapy gives effective treatment to the cervix and surrounding tissues whilst the small bowel, rectum and bladder receive a relatively low dose.

External beam treatment is used to control spread within the pelvis, particularly to lymph nodes, and contributes to primary tumour control. As the disease becomes more advanced, the balance between intracavitary and external beam treatment alters. Although it is possible to manage early-stage disease by intracavitary treatment alone, more advanced disease requires the combination of both techniques.

Intracavitary therapy

More details of intracavitary therapy are given in Chapter 33. Hollow radiopaque intrauterine and intravaginal tubes which act as carriers of the radioactive material are placed in the uterine cavity and the vaginal fornices under general anaesthesia (Fig. 36.9). These after-loading systems allow the applicators to be positioned accurately before the radioactive sources are inserted and avoid exposing theatre staff to unnecessary radiation. The sources may then be inserted either manually or remotely using a semi- or fully automated device so that staff exposure is minimal or zero. High- or low-energy sources may be used (see Ch. 33).

The dose is expressed at representative points in the pelvis. Point A is defined as the point 2 cm lateral to the central uterine canal and 2 cm above the external cervical os. This point is considered to lie in the paracervical region close to the uterine artery and the ureter. Point B is 5 cm lateral to the central uterine canal and 2 cm above the cervical os. The dose to point B is usually about one-third of the dose given to point A due to the rapid fall-off in dosage with intracavitary insertions.

In the Manchester system, 6600–7600 cGy were prescribed to point A in two treatments each lasting 70 h 4–7 days apart. The currently used Amersham system is a modification of this technique. Various improvements have been implemented which allow for better staff protection and better geometrical arrangements of the radioactive sources.

If intracavitary irradiation is to be the only modality of treatment, a dose of 8000 cGy is given to point A in three insertions with an interval of 1 week between each insertion. Following external beam therapy, a dose of 2000–2500 cGy is given to point A in a single insertion.

Patients with small-volume stage I tumours are treated by intracavitary treatment alone but more advanced disease requires a combination of an intracavitary dose and external beam therapy. The rationale for the different techniques is that the risk of lymph node involvement increases with the size of the tumour and the proportion of cervix involved.

External beam therapy

External beam therapy is normally given first because it shrinks the tumour mass thus allowing a more satisfactory dose distribution from the intracavitary sources. A homogeneous dose of radiation is given to the pelvis through either three or four fields. The treatment volume extends from the junction between L4 and L5 to cover the common iliac nodes, to the lower border of the obturator foramen radiologically or the lower margin of the pubic symphysis by palpation. If the disease extends down the vagina the lower border must be taken to the introitus which must be defined with a marker placed at a vaginal examination with the patient in the treatment position. The lateral margins of the field should lie 1 cm outside the bony margins of the pelvis.

The radiotherapy apparatus used is most commonly a linear accelerator working at an energy of 4 million electronvolts (MeV) or greater. A cobalt unit may be used but gives a less satisfactory dose at depth and less well defined field margins. The dose to the rectum must not exceed 6000 cGy. The dose given to the pelvis varies depending upon the stage of the disease. Stage IIb–IVa cases receive 5000 cGy to the whole pelvis in 5 weeks in 25 fractions. If bulky disease is present in one parametrium a further 500 cGy may be given in 3–5 fractions to this

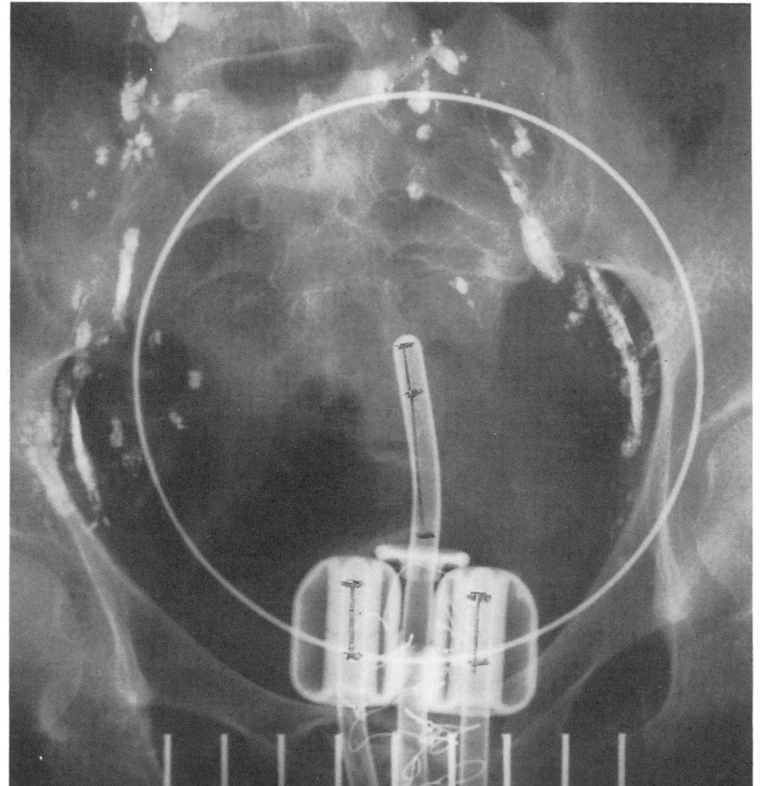

a

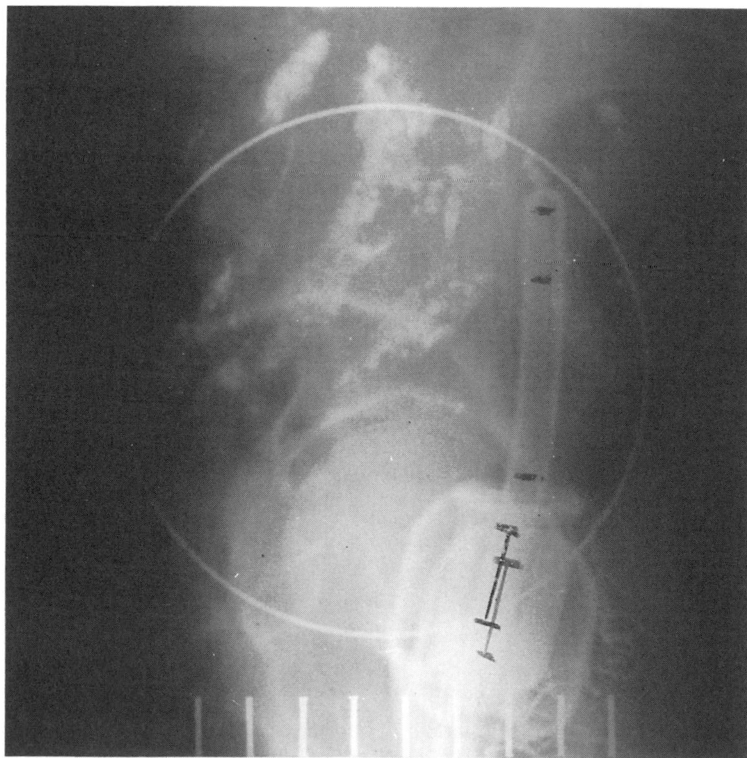

b

Fig. 36.9 These X-rays show an Amersham tube and ovoids in position. Contrast material can be seen in the lymph nodes from a previous lymphangiography.

area. Following this a caesium insertion is performed and a further 2000 cGy given to point A. If an insertion is not possible the central dose may be taken to 5500–6000 cGy using external beam therapy alone.

About 35% of stage III patients have involved para-aortic nodes. However, it is difficult to assess the nodes accurately and to treat involved nodes effectively. Piver & Barlow (1977) treated biopsy-positive para-aortic nodes to more than 5500 cGy; 20% of patients died of the complications of treatment, usually small bowel stenosis. If para-aortic node treatment is contemplated, lymphography or CT scanning should be performed with directed fine-needle aspiration of suspicious nodes.

In patients with disease outside the pelvis (stage IVb), the treatment should be directed to relieving symptoms. If pelvic symptoms such as bleeding or offensive discharge are predominant, palliative treatment may be given to a small volume using opposed fields and giving a 3000 cGy midline dose in six treatments over 3 weeks. If pain is due to para-aortic node spread into the underlying vertebrae, palliative radiotherapy can be given but a high dose (5000 cGy midline dose in 5 weeks) is needed for control. If there is bone pain due to blood-borne metastases, a 1-week course of palliative radiotherapy may be given to a dose of 2500–3000 cGy in five treatments.

Results of radiotherapy

Tumour bulk and clinical stage are major predictors of the response to treatment (Table 36.3). Substantial tumour regression during external beam therapy predicts a high chance of local tumour control and survival. If at the time of intracavitary treatment substantial tumour is still present, surgery or chemotherapy should be considered.

Table 36.3 Results of treatment by radiotherapy

Stage	5-year survival	
	Kottmeir	Fletcher
I	65–90%	91% (includes Ia)
IIa	45–65%	83.5%
IIb	45–65%	66.5%
IIIa	20–35%	45%
IIIb	20–35%	35%
IV	0–15%	14%

Radiotherapy complications

During radiotherapy most patients will suffer from diarrhoea. A low-residue diet is suggested and anti-diarrhoeals such as Lomotil, codeine phosphate or loperamide are prescribed. The radiation reaction usually settles down within 2–3 weeks of completion of all therapy but a minority of patients will continue to need anti-diarrhoeal drugs.

If diarrhoea is associated with colicky pain or nausea, the possibility of small bowel damage must be considered and the treatment suspended. Treatment may be restarted at a lower daily dose but if the problem persists radiotherapy may have to be abandoned.

Urinary symptoms are less common. If they are a problem, infection must be excluded. Occasionally anticholinergic agents may be helpful.

Late complications are related to dose and pre-existing problems. Some 5–10% of patients develop long-term problems which are usually related to the small or large bowel but may involve the urinary tract. These include subacute obstruction, diarrhoea due to radiation colitis and haematuria due to radiation cystitis. The symptoms are often quite mild. Patients at high risk of developing radiation complications are those with poor nutritional status and recent weight loss, previous pelvic or abdominal surgery, severe vascular disease or pelvic inflammatory disease.

Complications may develop at any time after treatment but symptoms of bowel damage occur on average after about 10 months and bladder symptoms after 22 months. Bowel and bladder symptoms should always be investigated and it must not be assumed that they are due to recurrent malignant disease.

Management of complications must be individualized and early detection is of the greatest importance. Small bowel obstruction following radiotherapy should be managed conservatively only in its initial stages. If prolonged or repeated episodes occur, surgical intervention is imperative. Rectosigmoid constriction can normally be diagnosed from the clinical history and readily confirmed by barium studies. It can be managed without the need for a permanent colostomy in the majority of patients.

Vesicovaginal fistulae will occasionally occur in patients who have been treated entirely appropriately. Repair of such fistulae involves the provision of an alternative blood supply to the area either by omental or myocutaneous grafting.

Chemotherapy

Radiotherapy and surgery are the only modalities which can cure cervical cancer but chemotherapy can cause tumour regression. Single agents that have significant response rates include cisplatin, bleomycin and methotrexate. Combination regimens have been developed using these drugs and, as with ovarian cancer, cisplatin combinations appear to have the highest response rates.

These regimens have been used on patients with locally advanced or metastatic disease and are now being investigated as adjuvant therapy in patients with locally advanced disease who normally have a high failure rate after conventional therapy. Blake et al (1986) achieved a projected 66% 5-year survival rate for patients with stage III disease. Preliminary results in similar trials suggest a possible role for chemotherapy in carcinoma of the cervix in the future but this should still be regarded as experimental therapy not to be used outside a trial protocol.

SPECIAL TREATMENT PROBLEMS

Carcinoma of the cervical stump

Subtotal hysterectomy is now rarely performed but this problem may occur in older patients. External beam radiotherapy to the usual dose should be given if bowel tolerance allows. To obtain a satisfactory dose, a medium caesium tube should be inserted together with ovoids. If this is not possible the external beam dose must be increased. The results are comparable with those in patients with an intact uterus.

Carcinoma after simple hysterectomy

Invasive carcinoma may be found after a hysterectomy for presumed preinvasive disease or when cervical pathology was not suspected. Pelvic irradiation should be given to a dose of 4500 cGy in 5 weeks and vault irradiation given thereafter. If patients are treated appropriately the survival rate is similar to that for patients treated with an intact uterus, provided the lesion was originally stage I.

Carcinoma of the cervix during pregnancy

Management will depend on the stage at diagnosis, the gestational age and the wishes and beliefs of the patient and her partner (Table 36.4). When fetal survival is desired, delivery should be delayed until the fetus is mature rather than just potentially viable.

Table 36.4 The management of cervical cancer during pregnancy.

Trimester	Stage I	Stage II and onwards
First	Wertheim's hysterectomy	Vaginal termination & radiation
Second	Termination of pregnancy by hysterotomy & Wertheim's hysterectomy	Prostaglandin termination & radiation
Third	Caesarean at 34/52 & Wertheim's hysterectomy	Caesarean at 34/52; Start radiotherapy after 10 days

Haemorrhage

If a patient presents with massive bleeding, bed rest and vaginal packing may arrest the haemorrhage. If this is not successful, treatment should begin with an intracavitary application giving 2000 cGy to point A. The haemoglobin in such a patient, and in any other, should always be restored to above 12 g/dl as patients with a haemoglobin of less than that have a poorer survival.

Recurrence after radiotherapy

The patient should be assessed jointly with a gynaecologic oncologist to ensure that the possibility of surgical salvage is not overlooked. The prognosis for those few women with a central pelvic recurrence alone is relatively good with exenterative procedures and such women should be carefully assessed and considered for such procedures in recognized gynaecological oncology units.

FOLLOW-UP

The continuing follow-up of these patients is of great importance to evaluate results, provide reassurance and to give symptomatic relief to patients whose treatment has failed. It is recommended that there should be 3-monthly follow-up for 3 years, 6-monthly follow-up for 2 years and annual visits thereafter.

Counselling should be provided to support the patient throughout her treatment and should be continued to cope with all aspects of readjustment, including the prevention of sexual problems that tend to develop in these women and their partners. Premenopausal patients will have suffered functional ovarian ablation and may be treated with hormone replacement therapy if they are troubled by menopausal symptoms. Younger patients with a good prognosis should be encouraged to take hormone replacement therapy to reduce the risk of osteoporosis and cardiovascular disease.

Radiotherapy will cause the vagina to contract and it is important to remind patients who were sexually active to try and resume activity, often with the help of lubricants, within a couple of months of the completion of treatment. Dilators can be used to maintain vaginal patency. Patients need to be reassured that coitus will not cause the tumour to become active and that the cancer cannot be communicated to their partner.

KEY POINTS

1. In England and Wales the incidence of cervical cancer is rising in the younger age groups. In 1981 31% of cases were in women aged less than 45 years.
2. The cause remains unknown, but is related in some way to sexual intercourse. No infective agent has been implicated with certainty.
3. Conservative treatment of microinvasive lesions should only be contemplated where invasion is not greater than 3 mm from the nearest basement

membrane and lymphatic channel involvement is not seen.

4. Squamous cell carcinoma is the most common type and has a similar prognosis to adenocarcinoma. Undifferentiated tumours have a poor prognosis.
5. Metastatic spread is mainly lymphatic and involvement of the parametria is initially focal rather than confluent.
6. The size of the primary tumour and the proportion of the cervix it occupies are the most important indications of prognosis after the status of the lymph nodes.
7. Overall, half of the women with cervical cancer die within 5 years.
8. Examination under anaesthesia is an essential step in determining the extent of disease and in deciding on the optimum method of therapy.
9. Magnetic resonance imaging gives the best estimate of the size of the tumour but is not reliable in identifying nodal disease.
10. Surgery is most often performed on the younger patient with lower-volume stage Ib disease.
11. Radiotherapy is used for the older and less fit patients regardless of the size of the tumour; for women with bulky stage Ib and IIa tumours, or for more advanced disease.

REFERENCES

Beral V, Hannaford P, Kay C 1988 Oral contraceptive use and malignancies of the genital tract: results from the Royal College of General Practitioners' oral contraception study. Lancet ii: 1331–1335

Blake P R, Branson A N, Lambert H E 1986 Combined radiotherapy and chemotherapy for advanced carcinoma of the cervix. Clinical Radiology 37: 465–469

Buckley J D, Harris R W C, Doll R, Vessey M P, Williams P T 1981 Case-control study of the husbands of women with dysplasia or carcinoma or the cervix uteri. Lancet ii: 1010–1014

Burghardt E, Haas J, Girardi F 1988 The significance of the parametrium in the operative treatment of cervical cancer. In: Burghardt E, Monaghan J M (eds) Operative treatment of cervical cancer. Clinical Obstetrics and Gynaecology, vol 2. Baillière Tindall, London, pp 879–888

Creasman W T, Fetter B F, Clarke-Pearson D L, Kaufmann L, Parker R T 1985 Management of stage Ia carcinoma of the cervix. American Journal of Obstetrics and Gynecology 153: 164–172

Dattoli M J, Gretz H F, Beller U et al 1989 Analysis of multiple prognostic factors in patients with stage Ib cervical cancer: age as a major determinant. International Journal of Radiation Oncology Biology and Physics 17: 41–47

FIGO 1988 Annual report on the results of treatment in gynaecological cancer, vol 20. Stockholm, International Federation of Gynaecology and Obstetrics

Gallup D G, Abell M R 1977 Invasive adenocarcinoma of the uterine cervix. Obstetrics and Gynecology 49: 596–603

Harris R W C, Briton L A, Cowdell R H et al 1980 Characteristics of women with dysplasia or carcinoma in situ of the cervix. British Journal of Cancer 42: 359–369

Howley P M, Schlegel R 1988 The human papillomaviruses. American Journal of Medicine 85: 155–158

Kessler II 1984 Natural history and epidemiology of cervical cancer with special reference to the role of herpes genitalis. In: McBrien D C H, Slater T F (eds) Cancer of the uterine cervix. Academic Press, London, pp 31–37

Lagasse L D, Ballon S C, Berman M L, Watring W G 1979 Pretreatment lymphangiography and operative evaluation in carcinoma of the cervix. American Journal of Obstetrics and Gynecology 134: 219–224

Meanwell C A, Kelly K A, Wilson S et al 1988 Young age as a prognostic factor in cervical cancer: analysis of population based data from 10 022 cases. British Medical Journal 296: 386–391

Morrow C P, Shingleton H M, Austin M J et al 1980 Is pelvic radiation beneficial in the postoperative management of stage Ib squamous cell carcinoma of the cervix with pelvic node metastases treated by radical hysterectomy and pelvic lymphadenectomy. Gynecologic Oncology 10: 105–110

Office of Population Censuses and Surveys 1985 Cancer statistics: registrations in England and Wales 1981. MB1 no 13. HMSO, London

Office of Population Censuses and Surveys 1987 Cancer statistics: registrations in England and Wales 1983. MB1 no 15. HMSO, London

Pickel H, Haas J, Lahousen M 1988 Prognostic factors in cervical cancer on the basis of morphometric evaluation. In: Burghardt E, Monaghan J M (eds) Operative treatment of cervical cancer. Clinical Obstetrics and Gynaecology, vol 2. Baillière Tindall, London, pp 805–816

Piver M S, Barlow J Jr 1977 High dose irradiation to biopsy confirmed aortic node metastases from carcinoma of the uterine cervix. Gynecologic Oncology 3: 168–175

Rotkin I D 1973 A comparison review of key epidemiological studies in cervical cancer related to current searches for transmissible agents. Cancer Research 33: 1353–1367

Shingleton H M, Gore H, Bradley D H, Soong S-J 1981 Adenocarcinoma of the cervix. I. Clinical evaluation and pathologic features. American Journal of Obstetrics and Gynecology 139: 799–814

37. Carcinoma of the ovary and fallopian tube

M. C. Anderson H. E. Lambert W. P. Soutter

EPIDEMIOLOGY

Carcinoma of the ovary is commoner in developed areas, such as Europe and the USA, than in the Third World. In England and Wales, deaths from carcinoma of the ovary have nearly doubled since 1941 with over 3700 women dying from this tumour in 1983 (Ponder et al 1990). Deaths from ovarian cancer now outnumber those from carcinoma of the cervix and body combined.

Most ovarian tumours are of epithelial origin. They are uncommon before 35 years of age but the incidence increases rapidly with age thereafter to a peak in the 50–70-year-old age group. Just under half occur in women aged 45–65 years (Fig. 37.1). Only 3% of ovarian cancers are seen in women younger than 35 years and the vast majority of these are non-epithelial cancers such as germ cell tumours.

AETIOLOGY

The aetiology of ovarian carcinoma is unknown. Epithelial tumours are associated with nulliparity; an early menarche; a late age at menopause, and a long number of years of ovulation. The low frequency of ovarian carcinoma in highly parous women is thought to be due to the sup-

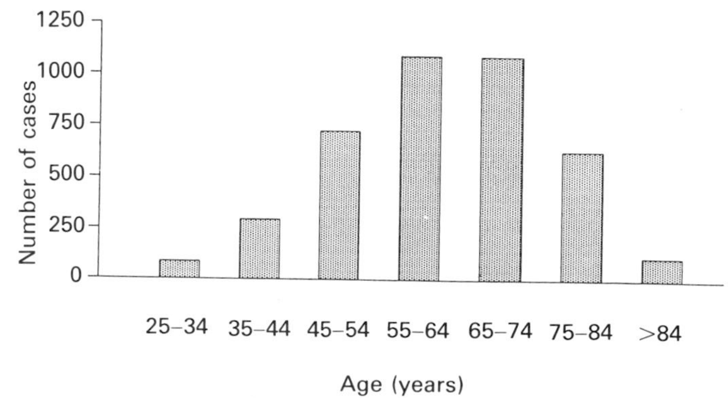

Fig. 37.1 The age distribution of ovarian cancer in England and Wales in 1981 (Office of Population Censuses and Surveys 1988).

pression of ovulation. There is now evidence that oral contraceptives may play a powerful protective role (Villard-Mackintosh et al 1989).

In about 1% of cases there is a family history of ovarian, endometrial or breast cancer. A woman who has two or more close relatives affected by ovarian cancer has about a 40% chance of developing the disease. Half of this risk occurs before the age of 50.

CLASSIFICATION OF OVARIAN TUMOURS

Ovarian tumours can be solid or cystic. They may be benign or malignant and in addition there are those which, while having some of the features of malignancy, lack any evidence of stromal invasion. These are called borderline tumours.

The most commonly used classification of ovarian tumours was defined by the World Health Organization (Serov et al 1973). This is a morphological classification that attempts to relate the cell types and patterns of the tumour to tissues normally present in the ovary. The primary tumours are thus divided into those that are of epithelial type (implying an origin from surface epithelium), those that are of sex cord gonadal type (also known as sex cord stromal type or sex cord mesenchymal type and originating from sex cord mesenchymal elements), and those that are of germ cell type (originating from germ cells). A simplified version of the World Health Organization classification is given in Table 37.1.

Table 37.1 Histological classification of ovarian tumours

Epithelial tumours	85%
Serous tumours	40%
Mucinous tumours	10%
Endometrioid tumours	20%
Clear cell (mesonephroid) tumours	5%
Brenner tumours	
Mixed epithelial tumours	
Undifferentiated carcinoma	
Unclassified epithelial tumours	
Sex cord gonadal tumours	6%
Granulosa-theca cell tumours	
Sertoli–Leydig cell tumours	
Gynandroblastoma	
Germ cell tumours	2%
Dysgerminoma	
Yolk sac tumour	
Teratomas	
Immature	
Mature	
Miscellaneous tumours	
e.g. lymphoma	<1%
Secondary (metastatic) tumours	6%
e.g. breast, gastrointestinal, endometrial	

Figures are estimates of the proportion of malignant ovarian tumours made up by the group in question

PATHOLOGY OF EPITHELIAL TUMOURS

Well differentiated epithelial carcinomas tend to be more often associated with early-stage disease, but the degree of differentiation does correlate with survival, except in the most advanced stages. Diploid tumours tend to be associated with earlier-stage disease and a better prognosis. Histological cell type is not of itself prognostically significant. Comparing patients stage for stage and grade for grade, there is no difference in survival in different epithelial types. However, mucinous and endometrioid lesions are likely to be associated with earlier stage and lower grade than serous cystadenocarcinomas.

Serous carcinoma

Gross features

The majority of serous carcinomas show a mixture of solid and cystic elements, although a significant minority are predominantly cystic. Serous carcinomas have a propensity to bilaterality, ranging from 50 to 90%.

Microscopical features

The better differentiated tumours have an obviously papillary pattern with unequivocal stromal invasion; psammoma bodies (calcospherules) are often present (Fig. 37.2). None of these features is diagnostic of serous tumours alone.

Endometrioid and clear cell carcinomas and, to a lesser extent, mucinous carcinomas may all form papillary structures. The term 'papillary carcinoma of the ovary', therefore, should not be used as a diagnosis.

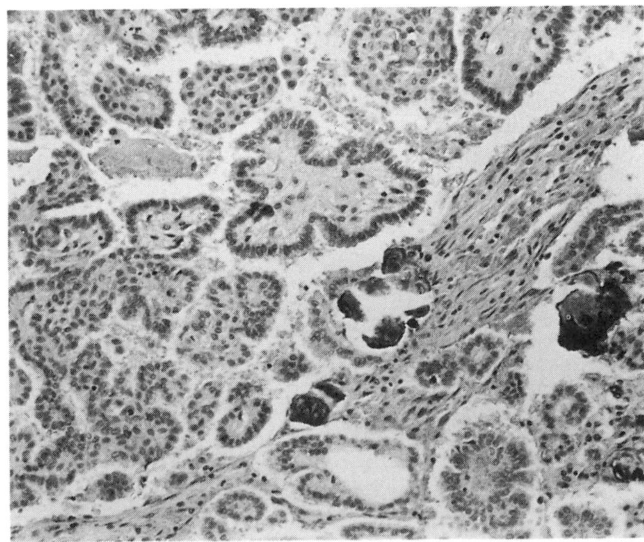

Fig. 37.2 Serous papillary cystadenocarcinoma: a well differentiated (grade 1) serous carcinoma. The papillary pattern is obvious and a group of psammoma bodies is present at the lower right. Haematoxylin and eosin × 180.

At the other end of the spectrum is the anaplastic tumour composed of sheets of undifferentiated neoplastic cells in masses within a fibrous stroma. Occasional glandular structures may be present to enable a diagnosis of adenocarcinoma to be made. All gradations between these two are seen, sometimes in the same tumour.

Mucinous carcinoma

Gross features

Malignant mucinous tumours comprise about 10% of malignant tumours of the ovary. They are typically multilocular, thin-walled cysts with a smooth external surface, containing mucinous fluid. The locules vary in size and often the tumour may be composed of one major cavity with many smaller daughter cysts apparently within its wall. Mucinous tumours are amongst the largest tumours of the ovary and may reach enormous dimensions: a cyst diameter of 25 cm is quite commonplace.

A mucinous cystadenocarcinoma may look the same as a benign tumour. Some malignant tumours may exhibit obvious solid areas, perhaps with necrosis and haemorrhage. The more advanced carcinomas will show the stigmata of ovarian malignancy, with adhesions to adjacent viscera and malignant ascites.

Microscopical features

Mucinous adenocarcinomas present a variety of histological appearances (Fig. 37.3). The better differentiated examples are composed of cells that retain a resemblance to the tall, picket-fence cells of the benign tumour, although stromal invasion is present. As differentiation is lost, the cells become less easily recognizable as of mucinous type and their mucin content diminishes.

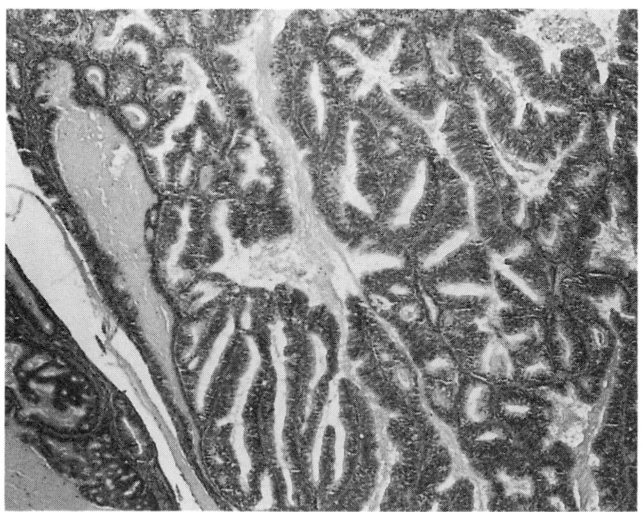

Fig. 37.3 Mucinous adenocarcinoma of the ovary. Haematoxylin and eosin × 180.

Endometrioid carcinoma

These are ovarian tumours that resemble the malignant neoplasia of epithelial, stromal and mixed origin that are found in the endometrium (Czernobilsky et al 1970).

Gross features

There is little to characterize an ovarian tumour as being of endometrioid type by naked-eye examination. Most are cystic, often unilocular, and contain turbid brown fluid. The internal surface of the cyst is usually rough with rounded, polypoid projections and solid areas, the appearances of which are usually distinct from those of the papillary excrescences seen in serous tumours.

Microscopical features

Endometrioid carcinomas resemble the endometrioid carcinomas of the endometrium (Fig. 37.4). The pattern is predominantly tubular and may resemble proliferative endometrium. The epithelium is tall and columnar, with a high nuclear:cytoplasmic ratio. Endometrioid carcinomas of the ovary are more likely to be papillary than are primary endometrial carcinomas. Some 5–10% of cases are seen in continuity with recognizable endometriosis. Ovarian adenoacanthomas, with benign-appearing squamous elements, account for almost 50% in some series of endometrioid tumours.

Associated endometrial carcinoma

It is important to note that 15% of endometrioid carcinomas of the ovary are associated with endometrial carcinoma in the body of the uterus. Although this is sometimes due to a primary in one site and a secondary at the other, in most cases these are two separate primary tumours.

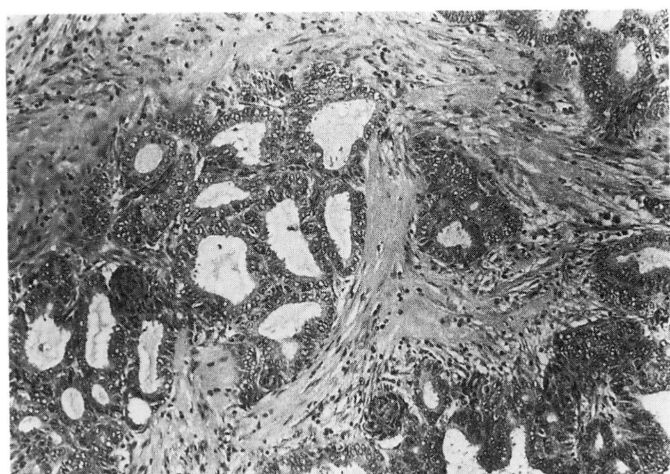

Fig. 37.4 Endometrioid carcinoma of the ovary. Haematoxylin and eosin × 180.

Clear cell carcinoma (mesonephroid)

These are the least common of the malignant epithelial tumours of the ovary, accounting for 5–10% of ovarian carcinomas (Anderson & Langley 1970).

Gross features

There is nothing characteristic about the gross appearances of the clear cell tumour to distinguish it from the other cystadenocarcinomas of the ovary. Most are thick-walled, unilocular cysts containing turbid brown or blood-stained fluid, with solid, polypoid projections arising from the internal surface. About 10% are bilateral.

Microscopical features

Clear cell carcinomas of the ovary are characterized by the variety of their architectural patterns, which may be found alone or in combination in any individual tumour (Fig. 37.5). The appearance from which the tumours derive their name is the clear cell pattern but, in addition, some areas show a tubulocystic pattern with the characteristic 'hob-nail' appearance of the lining epithelium. The third major pattern is papillary.

Association with endometriosis and endometrioid tumours

Because there is a very strong association between clear cell tumours of the ovary and ovarian endometriosis, and because clear cell and endometrioid tumours frequently coexist, it has been suggested that the clear cell tumour may be a variant of endometrioid tumour.

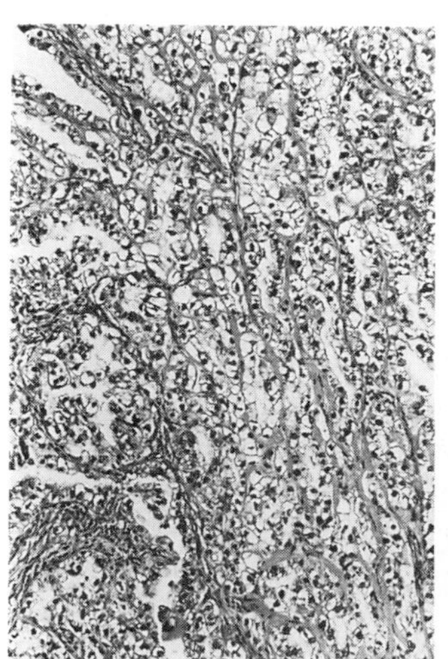

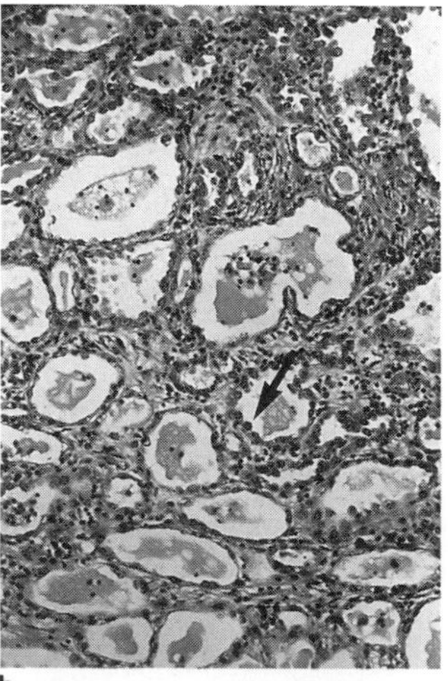

Fig. 37.5 Clear cell carcinoma of the ovary. (**a**) A moderately differentiated glandular pattern composed entirely of clear cells. Haematoxylin and eosin × 170. (**b**) A tubulocystic area showing prominent 'hob-nail' cells (arrow). Haematoxylin and eosin × 230.

Borderline epithelial tumours

Some 10% of all epithelial tumours of the ovary are of borderline malignancy (Ovarian Tumour Panel of the Royal College of Obstetricians and Gynaecologists 1983). These show varying degrees of nuclear atypia and an increase in mitotic activity, multilayering of neoplastic cells and formation of cellular buds, but no invasion of the stroma. Most borderline tumours remain confined to the ovaries and this may account for their much better prognosis. Peritoneal lesions are present in some cases and although a few are true metastases, many remain stationary and even regress after removal of the primary. The histological diagnosis of borderline malignancy can be difficult, particularly in mucinous tumours (Fig. 37.6). Most borderline tumours are serous or mucinous in type. Other borderline tumours are rare.

NATURAL HISTORY

Approximately two-thirds of patients present with disease spread beyond the pelvis. This is probably due to the insidious nature of the disease but may sometimes be due to a rapidly growing tumour. The advanced stage at presentation is responsible for the poor prognosis: the overall 5-year survival is approximately 25%.

Metastatic spread

The pelvic peritoneum and other pelvic organs become involved by direct spread. The peritoneal fluid, flowing to lymphatic channels on the undersurface of the diaphragm, carries malignant cells to the omentum, to the peritoneal surfaces of the small and large bowel and liver and to the parietal peritoneal surface throughout the abdominal cavity and on the surface of the diaphragm. Metastases on the

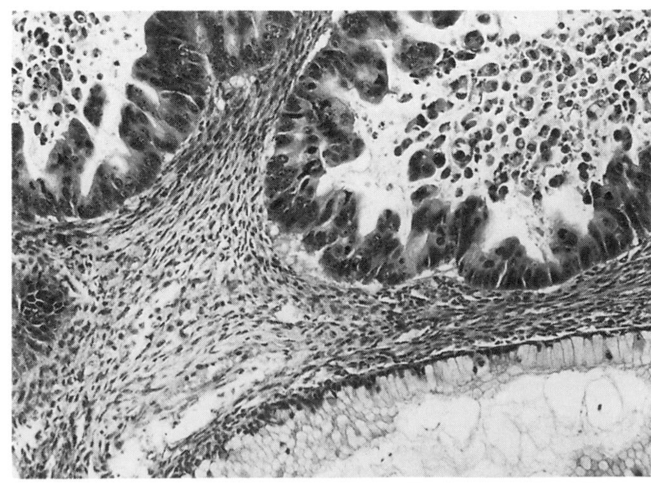

Fig. 37.6 A borderline mucinous tumour with multilayering of the epithelium but no evidence of stromal invasion.

undersurface of the diaphragm may be found in up to 44% of what otherwise seems to be stage I–II disease. Intraperitoneal metastases are superficial and seldom involve the substance of the organ beneath.

The tumour may spread along the lymphatics that run with the ovarian vessels to the para-aortic region at the level of the renal vessels or via the broad ligament to pelvic nodes (Table 37.2). Spread may also occur to nodes in the neck or groin. Haematogenous spread usually occurs late, mainly to the liver and the lung. Metastases to bone and brain are sometimes seen.

Table 37.2 Pelvic and para-aortic lymph node metastases

	Nodes involved	
	Pelvic Nodes	Para-aorticnodes
Stage I–II	19%	15%
Stage III–IV	66%	66%

CLINICAL STAGING

The staging of ovarian cancer as redefined by FIGO in 1989 is shown in Table 37.3 (FIGO 1988). The major change was the introduction of three substages of stage III. As before, the parenchyma of the liver must be involved to classify the patient as stage IV. A pleural effusion does not put the patient in stage IV unless malignant cells are found in the pleural fluid.

Table 37.3 FIGO stage for primary ovarian carcinoma

Stage I	Growth limited to ovaries
Ia	Growth limited to the one ovary; no ascites; no tumour on external surface; capsule intact
Ib	Growth limited to both ovaries; no ascites; no tumour on external surfaces; capsule intact
Ic	Tumour either stage Ia or Ib but tumour on surface of one or both ovaries; or with capsule ruptured; or with ascites present containing malignant cells; or with positive peritoneal washings
Stage II	Growth involving one or both ovaries with pelvic extension
IIa	Extension and/or metastases to the uterus or tubes
IIb	Extension to other pelvic tissues
IIc	Tumour either stage IIa or IIb but tumour on surface of one or both ovaries; or with capsule ruptured; or with ascites present containing malignant cells; or with positive peritoneal washings
Stage III	Growth involving one or both ovaries with peritoneal implants outside the pelvis or positive retroperitoneal or inguinal nodes. Superficial liver metastasis equals stage III Tumour is limited to the true pelvis but with histologically proven malignant extension to small bowel or omentum
IIIa	Tumour grossly limited to the true pelvis with negative nodes but with histologically confirmed microscopic seeding of abdominal peritoneal surfaces
IIIb	Tumour with histologically confirmed implants on abdominal peritoneal surfaces, none exceeding 2 cm in diameter; nodes are negative
IIIc	Abdominal implants greater than 2 cm in diameter or positive retroperitoneal or inguinal nodes
Stage IV	Growth involving one or both ovaries with distant metastases. If pleural effusion is present there must be positive cytology to allot a case to stage IV Parenchymal liver metastasis equals stage IV

DIAGNOSIS

Abdominal pain and discomfort are the commonest presenting complaints and distension or feeling a lump the next most frequent. Patients may complain of indigestion, urinary frequency, weight loss or, rarely, abnormal menses or postmenopausal bleeding. A hard abdominal mass arising from the pelvis is highly suggestive, especially in the presence of ascites. A fixed, hard, irregular pelvic mass is usually felt best by combined vaginal and rectal examination (Fig. 37.7). The neck and groin should also be examined for enlarged nodes.

Haematological investigations include a full blood count, urea, electrolytes and liver function tests. A chest X-ray is essential. If the patient has bowel symptoms, a barium enema will help to differentiate between an ovarian and a colonic tumour and to assess bowel involvement from the ovarian tumour itself. An intravenous pyelogram is sometimes useful.

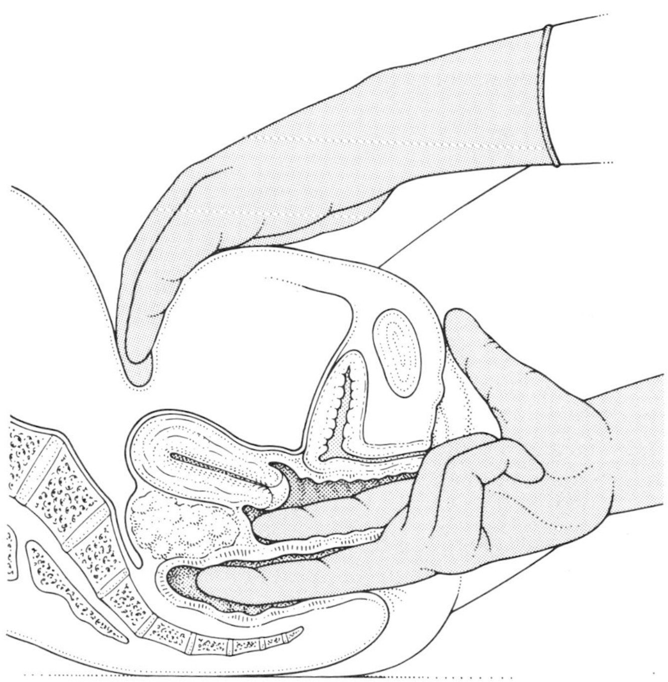

Fig. 37.7 A combined vaginal and rectal examination allows more accurate assessment of the pouch of Douglas.

Imaging techniques

These are discussed in greater detail in Chapter 5. Ultrasonography may help to confirm the presence of a pelvic mass and detect ascites before it is clinically apparent. In addition, it is a relatively reliable technique for examining the hepatic parenchyma and may detect enlarged lymph nodes. However, ultrasound is not reliable in discriminating between benign and malignant tumours and its main role is in identifying solid tumours in young women.

Computerized axial tomography is of limited value and is more expensive than ultrasonography. Magnetic resonance imaging is particularly useful for examining the pelvis but is not widely available. Radioimmunoscintigraphy has some value in detecting spread of ovarian tumour within the abdomen but is not used routinely. None of these techniques will detect small peritoneal metastases.

Lymphangiography is accurate only to a degree as it cannot detect micrometastases and false-positive results are frequent. The most accurate method for assessing lymph node involvement is biopsy at the time of surgery.

Cytology

In patients with pleural effusion or ascites, the fluid may be examined for the presence of malignant cells. It is seldom justifiable to perform a paracentesis for cytology. That can be deferred until the laparotomy. Fine-needle aspiration of clinically suspicious lymph nodes in the groin or neck can be very valuable.

Markers for epithelial tumours

So far, none of the markers available is suitable for the early detection of epithelial carcinoma. The most useful is CA 125, derived from a human ovarian cancer line. However, it may be increased in women with endometriosis. Rapidly falling levels of CA 125 in response to chemotherapy indicate a better prognosis than when they remain elevated or fall only slowly. A rise in CA 125 may precede clinical evidence of recurrent disease by several months in some cases. However the values can be normal in the presence of small tumour deposits.

Carcinoembryonic antigen is abnormal most often in mucinous cystadenocarcinoma but the tumour-associated antigens OCCA and OCA are raised in both serous and mucinous cystadenocarcinoma. Sensitivity may be increased by using a panel of tumour markers. Many new tumour markers are being investigated and may prove useful.

Screening

Much effort has been devoted to developing methods of detecting early ovarian cancer in asymptomatic women. A major difficulty is an ignorance of the natural history of early disease: it is not known how long an ovarian cancer will remain in an early, curable stage.

Ultrasound studies have detected numbers of benign ovarian tumours but relatively few malignant lesions. One encouraging finding has been that a majority of the malignancies detected were in an early stage. However, over 2% of the screened women in one study were referred for a laparotomy or laparoscopy but did not have ovarian cancer. Just under half of these did have benign ovarian tumours but the remainder had physiological ovarian cysts or non-ovarian masses (Campbell et al 1989). With longer experience and more refined techniques, such as colour Doppler imaging, the false-positive rate may be reduced.

An alternative approach has been to use serum CA 125 estimations as an initial screening tool, reserving pelvic examination and ultrasound for those with abnormal marker levels. It is premature to draw any conclusions about these studies and screening should only be offered in the context of a clinical trial at the present time. A possible exception is the woman with two close relations who have ovarian, breast or endometrial cancer.

SURGERY

The exploration

Surgery is the mainstay of both the diagnosis and the treatment of ovarian cancer. A vertical incision is required for an adequate exploration of the upper abdomen. Before any manipulation of the tumour, a sample of ascitic fluid or of peritoneal washings with normal saline must be taken for cytology.

The whole abdomen must be inspected carefully with special attention being given to the omentum, the sub-diaphragmatic areas, anterior abdominal wall, the paracolic gutters, the surface of the large and small bowel and the pelvic organs. If accessible, the pelvic and para-aortic nodes are palpated.

The therapeutic objective

The therapeutic objective of surgery for ovarian cancer is the removal of all tumour or, if this is not possible, the reduction of residual masses to less than 1.5 cm diameter. Griffiths and his co-workers (1979) showed that women with residual masses <1.5 cm following surgery did as well as those whose metastases were small from the outset. They subsequently demonstrated a further improvement in survival when all macroscopic disease was removed. These results have been confirmed by others but the benefit of cytoreduction is less in women with extensive preoperative disease (>10 cm) or ascites (Hacker et al 1983; Webb 1989) or who require bowel resection (Webb 1989). Thus, although the patient will derive substantial symptomatic relief from extensive cytoreduction (Blyth & Wahl 1982), this may not always translate into improved survival.

Early disease

The resection of all visible tumour usually requires a total hysterectomy and bilateral salpingo-oophorectomy but in a woman younger than 35 years whose family is not complete and who has a unilateral tumour and no ascites, unilateral salpingo-oophorectomy is justifiable after careful exploration to exclude metastatic disease (Mangioni et al 1989). Biopsy of the healthy-looking contralateral ovary is not justifiable in these circumstances (see Ch. 29).

If the tumour is found to be poorly differentiated or if the washings are positive, a second operation to clear the pelvis may be advisable. If an ovarian endometrioid carcinoma is diagnosed histologically, hysteroscopy and endometrial curettage at a later date will exclude a coexistent tumour in the endometrial cavity.

Resection of disease in the upper abdomen

Even if no disease is apparent in the upper abdomen, infracolic omentectomy is advisable because microscopic spread can be present when the omentum looks normal. Even when the omentum is extensively infiltrated it is usually possible to free it from adherent loops of small bowel and to separate it from the transverse colon and stomach. If a limited area of the small bowel or its mesentery is involved it can be resected. However, multiple or extensive resections of small bowel are limited by the need to preserve a functional length of intestine and such patients will still have a poor prognosis.

Resection of disease in the pelvis

If the pelvic tumour is large or densely adherent to the pelvic side wall and the colon, it is usually easier to enter the retroperitoneal space at the pelvic brim in order to ligate the ovarian vessels, dissect the ureter from the pelvic peritoneum and mobilize the tumour. The mass can often be freed from the bladder and rectum by peeling the tumour-bearing visceral peritoneum off the underlying organ, but sometimes resection of part of the bladder or removal of the sigmoid colon and rectum is necessary. In the latter instance, primary re-anastomosis is often possible. The uterine vessels may then be ligated at the pelvic side wall and a hysterectomy performed.

Lymphadenectomy

Observing a high incidence of pelvic and para-aortic node metastases in their patients, Burghardt and his colleagues (1989) attempted a complete clearance initially of only the pelvic nodes and more recently of pelvic and para-aortic nodes to the level of the renal vessels. It remains to be seen whether radical lymphadenectomy will make a major impact upon the survival of women with this dreadful disease.

Feasibility and morbidity of cytoreductive surgery

The proportion of patients optimally cytoreduced depends upon the attitudes and experience of the surgical team. If it is felt that patients will not benefit from prolonged and difficult operations, no more than a biopsy will be done, leaving most patients with massive residual disease. Not surprisingly, an enthusiastic and determined surgical team with experienced anaesthetic and nursing colleagues will successfully cytoreduce patients with advanced disease more often than those with less experience or enthusiasm. Between 66 and 98% of women with advanced disease are said to be amenable to optimal surgery. A reasonable target to aim for is 75%.

The postoperative morbidity is surprisingly low for a poor-risk group and seems to relate more to the experience of the team looking after the patient than to the amount of surgery performed.

Intervention debulking surgery

An alternative approach to initial aggressive surgery is a planned second laparotomy after 2–4 courses of cytoreductive chemotherapy in those women who respond. The chemotherapy is then resumed as soon as possible after the second operation. The evidence to date on this approach is not encouraging.

Second-look surgery

The objectives of second-look surgery are firstly to determine the response to previous therapy in order to document accurately its efficacy and to plan subsequent management, and secondly to excise any residual disease. While there is no doubt that second-look surgery gives the most accurate indication of the disease status — laparotomy being more accurate in this respect than laparoscopy — neither the surgical resection of residual tumour nor the opportunity to change the treatment has any effect on the patient's survival. Until an effective consolidation therapy becomes available, second-look procedures have no place outside clinical trials.

RADIOTHERAPY — EPITHELIAL TUMOURS

Indications for radiotherapy

No treatment is required for stage I disease localized to the ovaries which does not penetrate the capsule and is well differentiated. In all other cases of stage I or stage II disease chemotherapy or radiotherapy is given following surgery. Radiotherapy should encompass the whole peritoneal cavity to be effective.

In stage III disease, Dembo and his colleagues in Toronto have found that irradiation to the whole abdomen and pelvis is effective where there is minimal disease after surgery — no macroscopic disease in the upper abdomen and less than 2–3 cm residual disease in the pelvis (Dembo 1987).

Radiotherapy is ineffective in more advanced disease. In stage IV carcinoma of the ovary it can be useful as a palliative procedure, for example in the treatment of painful bone metastases.

Radiotherapy technique

Anterior and posterior stationary fields encompass the peritoneal cavity from the diaphragm to the pelvic floor (Fig. 37.8). The liver is not shielded unless the dose to this organ exceeds 30 Gy as this could lead to hepatic failure. The kidneys are particularly sensitive to radiation and, to keep their dose to a maximum of 20 Gy, they are protected by inserting lead blocks in the treatment beam (see Ch. 33). The total dose is usually not more than 30 Gy to the abdomen in 25 daily fractions. A top-up dose may be given to the pelvis to bring the dose in this area to 40 Gy.

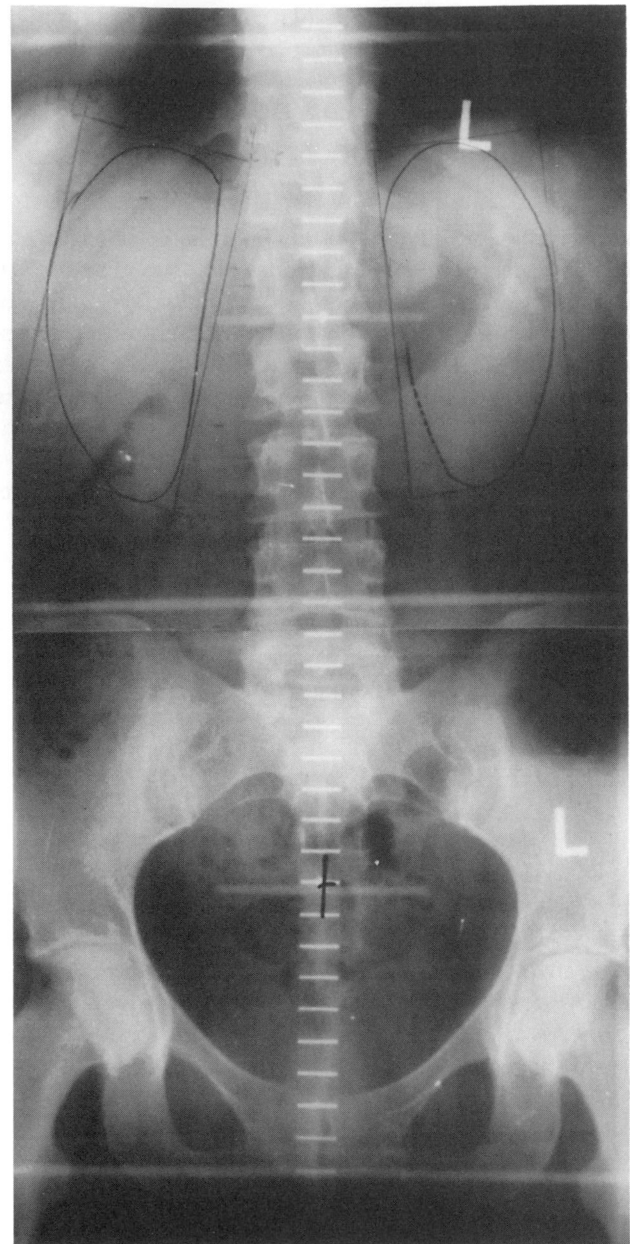

Fig. 37.8 The field for whole abdominal radiotherapy.

Complications of radiation therapy

As a large amount of bone marrow is included within the treatment fields, leukopenia and thrombocytopenia are common.

Some nausea, vomiting and diarrhoea will occur during treatment but anti-emetic therapy such as metoclopramide, a low-fibre diet and anti-diarrhoeal therapy, for example codeine phosphate 30 mg 1–3 times a day, all help.

Late complications are mainly gastrointestinal. Severe bowel stenosis or haemorrhage requiring surgical intervention occur in around 5% of cases. As complications are more likely following multiple abdominal operations, radiotherapy should be avoided in such patients.

Radioactive isotopes

Radiotherapy for early carcinoma of the ovary can be given intraperitoneally using radioactive isotopes of either gold or phosphorus linked to carrier colloids. The radioactive substances are absorbed directly on to the peritoneal surface and are taken up by macrophages. A high dose of radiation is given but only to a depth of 4–6 mm, limiting therapy to small peritoneal deposits, and it is not useful for large deposits within the abdomen. Although cure rates of 90% in stage I disease have been reported, in the absence of randomized studies there is no real evidence of any benefit.

Monoclonal antibodies (e.g. HMFG1, HMFG2, AUA1 and H17E2) react with antigens produced by ovarian carcinomas. Using ^{131}iodine or ^{90}yttrium, radioactive labelled monoclonal antibodies given intraperitoneally can image ovarian tumours and are being assessed for intraperitoneal therapy. Each patient needs to be assessed with a panel of antibodies to find which bind to the patient's tumour. In theory, small residual tumours within the peritoneal cavity will receive a high dose of radiation with a low dose to normal organs.

Radiotherapy — conclusions

Postoperative abdominopelvic radiotherapy may be of

value in the management of some patients with early carcinoma of the ovary. Intraperitoneal, colloid-bound, radioactive isotopes have no established place in the management of ovarian cancer.

CHEMOTHERAPY — EPITHELIAL TUMOURS

Chemotherapy plays a major role in the treatment of epithelial ovarian carcinoma. Surgery alone is justified only in stage I disease when the capsule is intact. Most other cases receive either chemotherapy or total abdominal radiotherapy (Table 37.4). Although radiotherapy may be given in those stage IIb and stage III cases with no macroscopic disease or with a pelvic residuum of less than 2–3 cm, chemotherapy is the more usual treatment. Radiotherapy has no place in the management of bulky residual disease.

Table 37.4 The postsurgical treatment of epithelial ovarian cancer

Stage of cancer	Treatment
Stage Ia intact capsule grade 1–2	No further treatment
Stage Ib–IIIa with minimal residuum	Chemotherapy or ? whole abdominal radiotherapy
More than minimal residuum	Chemotherapy

Single agents

The alkylating agents have been the most commonly used drugs in carcinoma of the ovary for several decades. These include melphalan, chlorambucil, cyclophosphamide, thiotepa and, more recently, treosulfan and ifosfamide. The response rate varies with the circumstances in which the drug is used but is in the range of 35 to 65%. The toxicity of these agents is discussed in Chapter 33. Other active drugs include the anti-metabolites 5-fluorouracil and methotrexate, and the anti-tumour antibiotic doxorubicin (Adriamycin).

Cisplatin (cis-dichlorodiammineplatinum) is a heavy-metal compound which produces better response and survival rates in patients with stage III and IV epithelial ovarian carcinoma than cyclophosphamide (median survival 19 compared with 12 months; Lambert & Berry 1985). However, it can cause severe vomiting and renal damage unless given with adequate hydration and can also cause hearing loss and peripheral neuropathy. An analogue of cisplatin called carboplatin (JM8, Paraplatin) is equally effective in ovarian cancer. The new agent has the advantage that there is less nausea and vomiting and no significant renal toxicity. Neurotoxicity is rare and hearing loss is usually subclinical. The lack of renal toxicity avoids the need for intravenous hydration, so it can be given on an outpatient basis. However, leukopenia and thrombocytopenia are the dose-limiting side-effects, especially in the presence of renal impairment when dose reductions are necessary. Platinum analogues are the best single agents available at present for treating cancer of the ovary.

Combination chemotherapy

In spite of the theoretical advantage of combination chemotherapy (Ch. 33), very few trials show a statistically significant improvement in survival. This may be due in part to the small numbers of patients studied and in part to the inclusion of women with bulky disease in whom the prognosis is poor and therefore in whom differences between therapies may not emerge.

Cisplatin combinations produce better response and survival rates than non-cisplatin multi-agent regimens (Neijt et al 1984; Peto & Easton 1990) but because relatively few patients have been entered into comparative studies, it is still not clear whether platinum-containing combinations are better than single-agent cisplatin. Neijt and his colleagues (1987) were unable to show any survival advantage for cyclophosphamide (CHAP5) over cisplatin (CP). The Gruppo Interegionale Cooperativo Oncologico Ginecologia (1987) compared CAP (cyclophosphamide, Adriamycin, cisplatin) with CP and with P (cisplatin alone) in over 500 patients with stage III–IV disease. The survival rates were not significantly better for the patients treated with the combinations. However, meta-analysis does show an improvement in 2-year survival for cisplatin combinations over single-agent cisplatin (odds ratio 0.65, 95% confidence limits 0.45–0.94; Peto & Easton 1990).

Intracavitary chemotherapy

Chemotherapeutic agents may also be administered into either the pleural or peritoneal cavities. The intraperitoneal use of drugs like melphalan, 5-fluorouracil and cisplatin in large volumes of fluid is of interest because of the differential between the intraperitoneal and intravenous concentrations that can be obtained with drugs which are cleared slowly from the peritoneal cavity but quickly from the systemic circulation. Cisplatin is the best drug currently available because it is both effective and lacks intraperitoneal toxicity (Ozols 1989). This treatment remains experimental and is only suitable for very small peritoneal deposits because of the poor penetration obtained (1–3 mm).

OTHER TREATMENTS

Hormonal therapy

Cytoplasmic oestrogen and progesterone receptors have been detected in malignant ovarian tumours, but the use of progestogens has met with little success except in a very few isolated cases. Tamoxifen and luteinizing hormone-releasing hormone analogues have also been used in a few patients with advanced ovarian cancer and some stabilization has been observed. Hormone therapy has little role in the management of ovarian cancer.

Immunotherapy

The role of immunotherapy in ovarian carcinoma has aroused interest but has no proven benefit at the present time. Combinations of BCG (bacille Calmette-Guérin), *C. parvum* or, more recently, alpha-interferon with chemotherapy have shown some encouraging results.

Corynebacterium parvum has also been used intraperitoneally but can cause profound peritoneal irritation, fibrosis and bowel obstruction. Intraperitoneal recombinant alpha-interferon has more recently been used with mixed results.

RESULTS — EPITHELIAL TUMOURS

Borderline epithelial tumours

The 5-year prognosis is good but the death rate continues to rise slowly thereafter. The 5-year survival rate for serous tumours is 90–95% and for mucinous tumours is 81–91%. By 15 years the rates are only 72–86 and 60–85% respectively. The poorer survival for borderline mucinous tumours may be simply an indication of the greater difficulty in distinguishing this group from well differentiated mucinous adenocarcinomas. Survival is related to stage; at 5 years for stage I it is nearly 100% but for stage III only 65—87%. The 10-year survival for stage I is 73–95%.

Invasive epithelial cancer

The 5-year survival rate for epithelial ovarian cancer ranges from 60 to 70% in stage I disease to 10% in stage III–IV but, since the majority of patients present with advanced disease, the overall 5-year survival in the UK is only 23% (Office of Population Censuses and Surveys 1988).

One problem in comparing present-day results with old data is that, with improved surgical staging, there is some reclassification of patients from stage I to stage III, improving the results in both stages, without affecting overall survival — the 'Will Rogers phenomenon'. Most studies do show some prolongation of median survival in patients who are left with only minimal residual disease following surgery.

Platinum-based drugs are the most effective single agents currently available but, although cisplatin combination regimens provide higher initial response rates than cisplatin alone, this benefit has not been sufficiently long-lasting to affect 5-year survival rates.

NON-EPITHELIAL TUMOURS

Non-epithelial tumours constitute approximately 10% of all ovarian cancers. Because of their rarity and their sensitivity to intensive chemotherapy, it is especially appropriate to refer these patients for specialist care.

Sex cord stromal tumours

Granulosa and theca cell tumours

The most common sex cord stromal tumours are the granulosa and theca cell tumours. Even so, they account for only about 1.5% of all ovarian tumours and 5–10% of solid ovarian tumours. They often produce steroid hormones, in particular oestrogens, which can cause postmenopausal bleeding in older women and sexual precocity in prepubertal girls. The hormones may cause cystic glandular hyperplasia, or occasionally carcinoma of the endometrium. Most secrete inhibin which shows promise as a marker in the follow-up of these tumours.

Theca cell tumours are usually benign. The majority of those that are invasive contain a malignant granulosa cell element. Granulosa cell tumours occur at all ages, but are found predominantly in postmenopausal women. Most present as stage I. Bilateral tumours are present in only 5% of cases.

Pathology. Granulosa cell tumours are normally solid although, when they become large, cystic spaces may develop and some tumours are predominantly cystic. Like

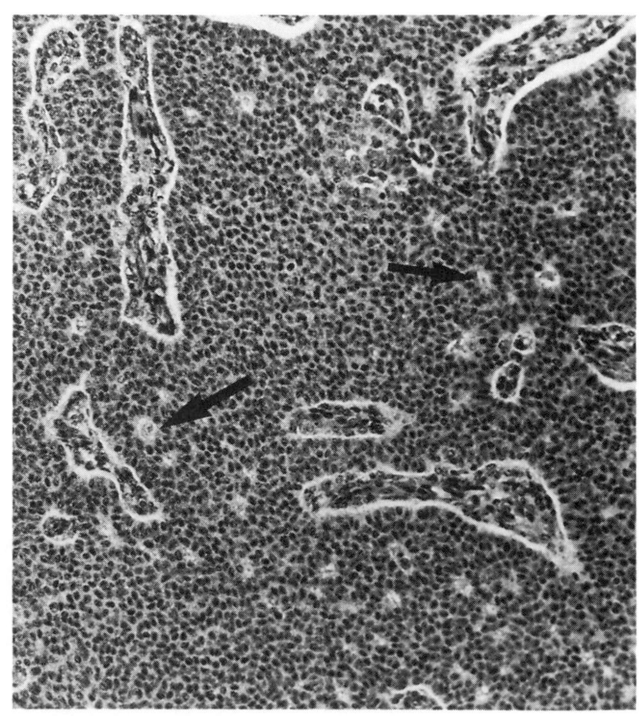

Fig. 37.9 A granulosa cell tumour showing a microfollicular pattern. Arrows show Call–Exner bodies. Haematoxylin and eosin × 170.

most tumours of the sex cord–stromal tumour group, the cut surface is often yellow, reflecting the presence of neutral lipid which is related to sex steroid hormone production. Areas of haemorrhage are also common.

A variety of histological appearances are seen in granulosa cell tumours: follicular, insular, trabecular, moiré-silk and diffuse (sarcomatoid). These may occur separately but are more usually found in combination. The most characteristic pattern is the microfollicular, in which the tumour cells are arranged in large groups in which are numerous Call–Exner bodies, small rounded cavities that often contain dense eosinophilic material of basement membrane type or nuclear debris (Fig. 37.9).

Treatment. The surgical treatment is the same as for epithelial tumours. Unilateral oophorectomy is indicated only in young women with stage I disease. Additional therapy is required in women with advanced or recurrent disease. Total abdominal irradiation has been the treatment of choice but chemotherapy as for epithelial tumours is being used more frequently. The 5-year survival is around 80% overall but late recurrence is common, making the assessment of adjunctive therapy difficult.

Sertoli–Leydig cell tumours

Half of these rare neoplasia produce male hormones which can cause virilization. Rarely oestrogens are secreted. The prognosis for the majority who have localized disease is good and surgery as for granulosa cell tumours is the treatment of choice. Chemotherapy may be used for metastatic or recurrent disease.

Germ cell tumours

Dysgerminomas

Dysgerminomas are uncommon ovarian tumours accounting for about 1% of all primary malignant ovarian tumours in a Caucasian population. Originating in the germ cells, 90% occur in young women less than 30 years old. They behave in a similar way to seminoma in men, spreading mainly by lymphatics to para-aortic, mediastinal and supraclavicular glands. All cases need to be investigated by chest X-ray, computerized tomography scanning or lymphangiogram. Serum alpha-fetoprotein and beta-human chorionic gonadotrophin should be assayed to exclude the presence of elements of choriocarcinoma, endodermal sinus tumour or teratoma.

Pathology (Gordon et al 1981). Dysgerminomas are solid tumours which have a smooth or nodular, bossellated external surface. They are soft or rubbery in consistency, depending upon the proportion of fibrous tissue contained in them. They may reach a considerable size; the mean diameter is 15 cm. Approximately 10% are bilateral; they are alone among malignant germ cell tumours in having a significant incidence of bilaterality.

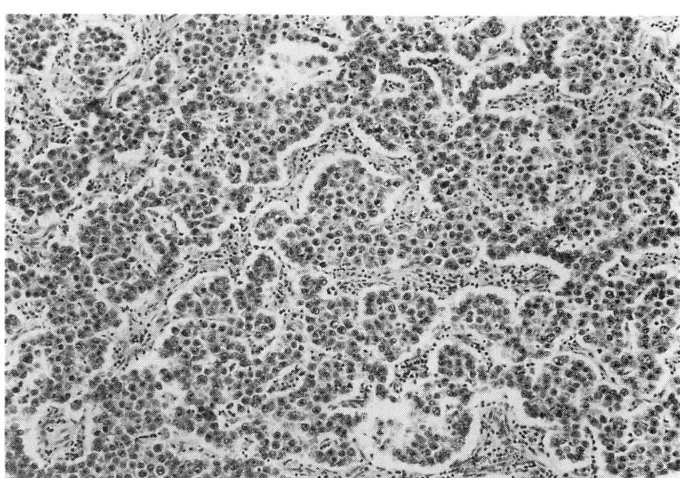

Fig. 37.10 A dysgerminoma with the typical large, pale round cells separated by fibrous septa in which a lymphocytic infiltrate is prominent. Haematoxylin and eosin × 200.

Dysgerminoma is composed of groups of large, round tumour cells separated by fibrous tissue septa infiltrated by lymphocytes (Fig. 37.10). The tumour cells possess abundant, pale, slightly eosinophilic cytoplasm which contains glycogen, lipid and alkaline phosphatase — the last being situated predominantly in the periphery of the cell. A minimal lymphocytic response, a high mitotic count, capsular penetration, intraovarian lymphatic or vascular invasion are all associated with a decreased survival.

Immature teratoma, yolk sac tumour or choriocarcinoma are found in 6.7–13.8% of dysgerminomas. Very thorough sampling of all dysgerminomas must be undertaken by the histopathologist to exclude the presence of these more malignant germ cell elements as this indicates a worse prognosis.

Treatment. A germ cell tumour should be suspected prior to surgery if a young woman has what appears to be a predominantly solid tumour on ultrasound examination. Such patients should be referred to a gynaecological oncologist.

Pure dysgerminomas have a good prognosis as 75% are stage I tumours. In young women with stage Ia disease, unilateral oophorectomy is performed. If the malignant nature of the tumour is recognized before or during the laparotomy, some authorities recommend biopsy of the other ovary. If both ovaries are affected, conservation of some ovarian tissue may be attempted in young women. In older patients, hysterectomy and bilateral salpingo-oophorectomy are recommended.

Although radiotherapy has been used for metastatic or recurrent disease, chemotherapy is the treatment of choice as fertility is likely to be preserved. Chemotherapy is used for stage Ib–IV and for recurrent disease. Mixed dysgerminomas are treated in the same way as malignant teratomas. The regimens used are discussed below.

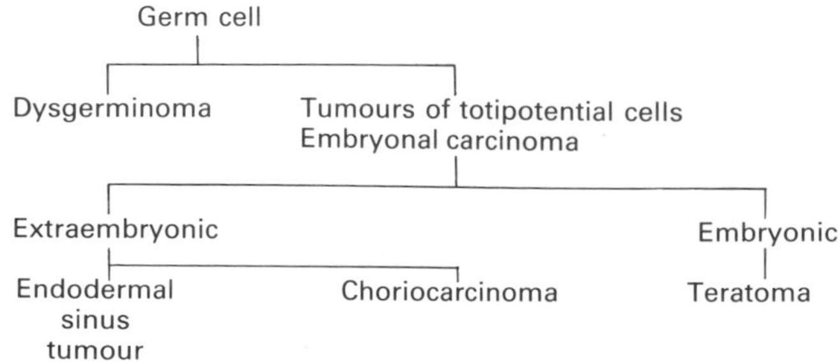

Fig. 37.11 The derivation of germ cell tumours.

Other germ cell tumours

Germ cell tumours other then dysgerminoma also occur in young women under 30 years old. Their very poor prognosis has been greatly improved by combination chemotherapy. Their derivation from germ cells is shown in Figure 37.11. Mature teratomas are benign, the most common being the cystic teratoma or dermoid cyst.

Pathology of yolk sac (endodermal sinus) tumours (Kurman & Norris 1976). Yolk sac tumour is the second most common malignant germ cell tumour of the ovary, comprising 10–15% over all and reaching a higher proportion in children. It may present as an acute abdomen due to rupture of the tumour following necrosis and haemorrhage.

The tumour is usually well encapsulated and solid. Areas of necrosis and haemorrhage are often seen, as are small cystic spaces. Its consistency varies from soft to firm and rubbery and its cut surface is slippery and mucoid.

The yolk sac tumour is characterized by the presence of a variety of patterns. The background of the tumour is a loose vacuolated network of microcysts lined by flat cells of mesothelial appearance. The most characteristic feature is the endodermal sinus (Schiller–Duval body). A constant finding is para-aminosalicylic acid-positive hyaline globules containing alpha-fetoprotein and other metabolic products of the normal yolk sac.

Pathology of immature teratomas. These tumours are solid and often malignant. It should be noted that solid teratomas are not all of immature type. Immature teratomas are composed of a wide variety of tissues and comprise about 1% of all ovarian teratomas.

The tumours are unilateral in almost all cases and appear as solid masses that have smooth and bossellated surfaces. The cut surface shows mainly solid tissue, although small cystic spaces are visible. The tumour is very heterogeneous; areas of bone and cartilage may be apparent and hair may be seen. The most conspicuous feature is usually the soft, pale pink to cream-coloured immature neural tissue. Both the gross appearance and the histology may resemble a benign teratoma due to the presence of these mature elements. The amount of embryonal tissue, its degree of atypia and mitotic activity correlate with the prognosis.

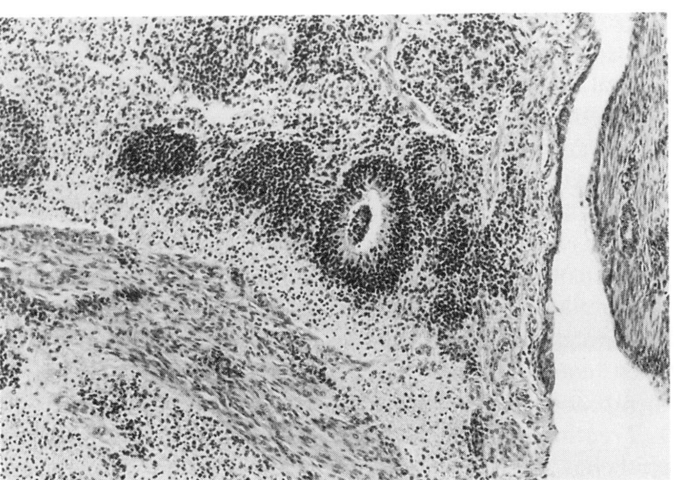

Fig. 37.12 An immature teratoma with prominent neuroectodermal tissue and a well formed rosette. Haematoxylin and eosin × 170.

Rosettes of tightly packed neuroectodermal cells with dark nuclei are usually the most conspicuous feature (Fig. 37.12).

A careful search must be made for elements of yolk sac tumour and choriocarcinoma; the presence of these may have a bearing on prognosis and treatment, particularly if the teratoma is of low grade. Blood levels of beta-human chorionic gonadotrophin and alpha-fetoprotein should be estimated to exclude their presence even when the tumour appears to be a straightforward immature teratoma.

Chemotherapy for non-epithelial tumours

The main treatment for these tumours is combination chemotherapy, following conservative surgery to establish the diagnosis, remove the primary lesion and to stage the disease. VAC (vincristine, actinomycin D and cyclophosphamide) is recommended for dysgerminoma and moderately differentiated teratomas (stage II and early stage III). The more toxic PVB (cisplatin, vinblastine and bleomycin) or PEB (etoposide instead of vinblastine) are suggested for all cases of poorly differentiated teratoma, endodermal sinus tumour and choriocarcinoma. Recurrent disease following chemotherapy seldom responds to further treatment. Prior radiotherapy seems to reduce the efficacy of chemotherapy.

The projected 5-year survival is in the region of 77% (Newlands & Bagshaw 1987) and normal pregnancies following chemotherapy are common in these patients if conservative surgery was possible (Bianchi et al 1989).

OVARIAN CARCINOMA — CONCLUSIONS

Epithelial ovarian carcinoma is still a difficult tumour to treat, partly because of its late presentation and partly because no truly effective therapy has yet been developed.

Surgery remains the most important part of the management. Prolonged survival is only possible when the surgeon can excise the tumour virtually completely. Chemotherapy has had a major impact on the rare germ cell tumours. Although it is less effective in the common epithelial malignancies it does extend substantially the life expectancy of many patients.

The value of other approaches, such as radiotherapy, is controversial. Immunotherapy has not yet established a role in the treatment of this disease. In order to improve the survival rate for ovarian cancer, research effort needs to be directed towards early diagnosis and to more effective drug therapy.

CANCER OF THE FALLOPIAN TUBE

Primary carcinoma

Primary carcinoma of the fallopian tube is extremely rare, comprising only 0.3% of gynaecological malignancies. Although it may occur at any age, it is most common after the menopause. It is usually unilateral. It spreads like ovarian carcinoma and metastasizes frequently to pelvic and para-aortic nodes.

Pathology

Because of the histological similarity between serous ovarian carcinoma and primary tubal carcinoma, strict criteria must be applied before the diagnosis of tubal carcinoma can be made. Carcinoma of the fallopian tube usually distends the lumen with tumour. The tumour may protrude through the fimbrial end and the tube may be retort-shaped, resembling a hydrosalpinx. It is typically very similar to the serous adenocarcinoma of the ovary histologically (Fig. 37.13). The predominant pattern is papillary, with a gradation through alveolar to solid as the degree of differentiation decreases.

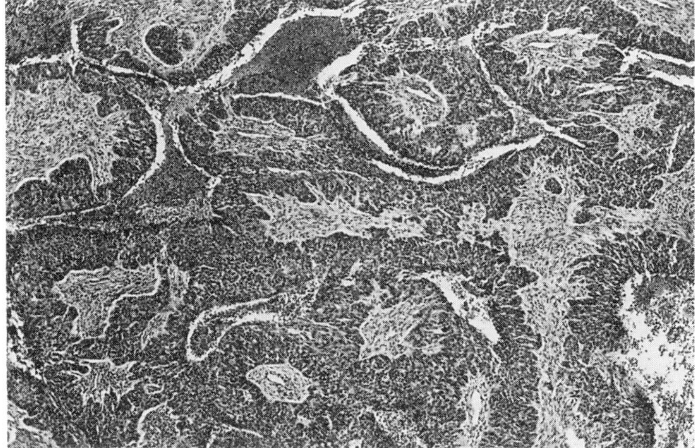

Fig. 37.13 A rather poorly differentiated serous adenocarcinoma of the fallopian tube in which the papillary pattern is still recognizable. Haematoxylin and eosin × 100.

Clinical presentation and management

Cancer of the fallopian tube will often present with postmenopausal bleeding and should be considered particularly if the patient complains of vaginal bleeding, a watery discharge and abdominal pain. Unexplained postmenopausal bleeding or abnormal cervical cytology without any obvious cause demands a careful bimanual examination and pelvic ultrasound. Laparoscopy may be required in doubtful cases.

The clinical staging is the same as for ovarian cancer and the management is very similar with surgery to remove gross tumour and postoperative chemotherapy for patients with metastatic disease. The prognosis appears to be similar to ovarian cancer.

Metastatic carcinoma

Secondary spread to the fallopian tube from malignancies in the ovary, gastrointestinal tract and breast are not uncommon. The treatment is determined by the management of the primary tumour.

KEY POINTS

1. About half of the women with ovarian cancer are aged 45–65 years and the number of deaths from this tumour equal those from cervix and endometrium combined.
2. The use of oral contraceptives protects against the development of ovarian cancer.
3. A small proportion of women with ovarian cancer do have a family history of this disease and their close relatives also have a high risk of developing ovarian carcinoma.
4. Population screening for ovarian cancer is not yet justified with the techniques evaluated so far.
5. Surgical resection of all visible epithelial ovarian cancer is an important part of the patient's management.
6. Chemotherapy of epithelial ovarian tumours with platinum agents, either alone or in combination, will prolong the patient's life but are unlikely to result in an improved long-term survival.
7. Chemotherapy for germ cell tumours is effective, even in advanced or recurrent cases. A young woman with a solid ovarian tumour should be referred to a gynaecological oncologist. If the diagnosis is made postoperatively, she should always be referred to a specialist team.
8. Primary carcinoma of the fallopian tube is treated like ovarian carcinoma.

REFERENCES

Anderson M C, Langley F A 1970 Mesonephroid tumours of the ovary. Journal of Clinical Pathology 23: 210–218

Bianchi U A, Favalli G, Sartori E et al 1989 Limited surgery in non-epithelial ovarian cancer. In: Conte P F, Ragni N, Rosso R, Vermorken J B (eds) Multimodal treatment of ovarian cancer. Raven Press, New York, pp 119–126

Blyth J G, Wahl T P 1982 Debulking surgery. Does it increase the quality of survival? Gynecologic Oncology 14: 396–408

Burghardt E, Lahousen M, Stettner H 1989 The significance of pelvic and para-aortic lymphadenectomy in the operative treatment of ovarian cancer. In: Burghardt E, Monaghan J M (eds) Operative treatment of ovarian cancer. Baillière Tindall, London, pp 157–165

Campbell S, Bhan V, Royston P, Whitehead M I, Collins W P 1989 Transabdominal ultrasound screening for early ovarian cancer. British Medical Journal 299: 1363–1367

Czernobilsky B, Silverman B B, Mikuta J J 1970 Endometrioid carcinoma of the ovary. A clinicopathologic study of 75 cases. Cancer 26: 1141–1152

Dembo A J 1987 Epithelial ovarian cancer: radiotherapy for minimal disease. In: Sharp F, Soutter W P (eds) Ovarian cancer — the way ahead. Royal College of Obstetricians and Gynaecologists, London, pp 409–425

FIGO 1988 Annual report on the results of treatment in gynaecological cancer, vol 20. FIGO, Sweden

Gordon A, Lipton D, Woodruff J D 1981 Dysgerminoma; a review of 158 cases from the Emil Novak ovarian tumor registry. Obstetrics and Gynecology 58: 497–504

Griffiths C T, Parker L M, Fuller A F J 1979 Role of cytoreductive surgical treatment in the management of advanced ovarian cancer. Cancer Treatment Reports 63: 235–240

Gruppo Interegionale Cooperativo Oncologico Ginecologia (1987) Randomised comparison of cisplatin with cyclophosphamide/cisplatin and with cyclophosphamide/doxorubicin/cisplatin in advanced ovarian cancer. Lancet ii: 353–359

Hacker N F, Berek J S, Lagasse L D, Nieberg R K, Elashoff R M 1983 Primary cytoreductive surgery for epithelial ovarian cancer. Obstetrics and Gynecology 61: 413–420

Kurman R J, Norris H J 1976 Endodermal sinus tumour of the ovary: a clinical and pathologic analysis of 71 cases. Cancer 38: 2404–2419

Lambert H E, Berry R J 1985 High dose Cis-platinum compared with high dose cyclophosphamide in the management of advanced epithelial ovarian cancer stage III and IV: a report from the North Thames Co-operative Group. British Medical Journal 290: 889–893

Mangioni C, Chiari S, Colombo N et al 1989 Limited surgery in epithelial ovarian cancer. In: Conte P F, Ragni N, Rosso R, Vermorken J B (eds) Multimodal treatment of ovarian cancer. Raven Press, New York, pp 127–132

Neijt J P, Ten Bokkel Huinink W W, Van der Burg M E L et al 1984 Randomized trial comparing two combination chemotherapy regimens (Hexa-CAF vs CHAP 5) in advanced ovarian carcinoma. Lancet ii: 594–600

Neijt J P, Ten Bokkel Huinink W W, Van der Burg M E L et al 1987 Randomized trial comparing two combination chemotherapy regimens (CHAP-5 v CP) in advanced ovarian carcinoma. Journal of Clinical Oncology 5: 1157–1168

Newlands E S, Bagshaw K D 1987 Advances in the treatment of germ cell tumours of the ovary. In: Bonnar J (ed) Recent advances in obstetrics and gynaecology. Churchill Livingstone, Edinburgh, pp 143–156

Office of Population Censuses and Surveys 1988 Monitor MB1 88/1 Cancer survival 1981 registrations. HMSO, London

Ovarian Tumour Panel of the Royal College of Obstetricians and Gynaecologists 1983 Ovarian epithelial tumours of borderline malignancy: pathological features and current status. British Journal of Obstetrics and Gynaecology 90: 743–750

Ozols R F 1989 Intraperitoneal chemotherapy: current status and future studies. In: Conte P F, Ragni N, Rosso R, Vermorken J B (eds) Multimodal treatment of ovarian cancer. Raven Press, New York, pp 283–291

Peto J, Easton D 1990 Randomized cancer trials — past failures, current progress and future prospects? Cancer Surveys 8: 511–533

Ponder B A J, Easton D F, Peto J 1990 Risk of ovarian cancer associated with a family history. In: Sharp F, Mason W P, Leake R E (eds) Ovarian cancer: biological and therapeutic challenges. Chapman Hall, London, pp 3–6

Serov S F, Scully R E, Sobin L H 1973 International classification of tumours no 9. Histological typing of ovarian tumours. World Health Organization, Geneva

Villard-Mackintosh L, Vessey M P, Jones L 1989 The effects of oral contraceptives and parity on ovarian cancer trends in women under 55 years of age. British Journal of Obstetrics and Gynaecology 96: 783–788

Webb M J 1989 Cytoreduction in ovarian cancer: achievability and results. In: Burghardt E, Monaghan J M (eds) Operative treatment of ovarian cancer. Baillière Tindall, London, pp 83–94

38. Malignant disease of the uterus

M. A. Quinn   M. C. Anderson   C. A. E. Coulter

INTRODUCTION

Carcinoma of the endometrium has traditionally been the poor relation of gynaecological malignancies with the majority of cases being treated outside major oncology centres. Such an approach has stemmed from a belief that this cancer carries a uniformly good prognosis, despite the fact that 5-year survival figures approximate those of cancer of the cervix which more often presents at a late stage than endometrial cancer. More than 1200 women in England and Wales died from this cancer in 1983 and it is a sad fact that the best therapy for this disease has yet to be defined and that treatment protocols still rely heavily on historical data rather than being based on prospective randomized trials. Confusion and controversy relate to a number of basic areas in the management of patients with corpus cancer, including the place of radiation therapy, of radical surgery and of adjuvant treatment with hormones. This chapter aims to give an overview of existing information relating to the natural history of the disease and thereby to provide a rational approach to the care of women with this cancer.

EPIDEMIOLOGY

The median age of patients with endometrial cancer is 61 years, with 75–80% of women being postmenopausal and 3–5% being less than 40 years old.

Geographical and racial variation in incidence

The incidence of corpus cancer varies markedly, not only from country to country, but between different racial groups in one geographical area. The highest incidence is in white North Americans who have a rate approximately seven times higher than the Chinese. Women of Spanish descent in Los Angeles have a relative risk of developing endometrial cancer of 0.69 compared to white women, whilst Spanish women in Latin America have a relative risk of 0.2.

Risk factors in postmenopausal and premenopausal women

Factors known to increase the likelihood of developing the disease are listed below.

1. Obesity.
2. Impaired carbohydrate tolerance.
3. Nulliparity.
4. Late menopause.
5. Unopposed oestrogen therapy.
6. Functioning ovarian tumours.
7. Previous pelvic irradiation.
8. Sequential oral contraceptives with dimethisterone.
9. Family history of carcinoma of breast, ovary or colon.

Most of these relate to postmenopausal women. Women under 40 years of age who develop endometrial cancer have a high incidence of anovulation, especially due to polycystic ovarian syndrome, and are often obese — 45% of women in one series weighed more than 80 kg (Quinn et al 1985a). Premenopausal women over 40 years of age do not seem to share the same risk factors as younger women; in particular, this group has a low incidence of nulliparity and in approximately 25% of cases, a corpus luteum will be identified on histological examination of the excised ovaries.

Body weight

Most of the known risk factors for the development of this cancer share a common basis — excessive unopposed oestrogen stimulation of the endometrium. The major circulating oestrogen in postmenopausal women is oestrone, derived from aromatization of peripheral androgens, mainly Δ4-androstenedione. This conversion takes place in a wide variety of body sites, particularly in fat and muscle. A doubling in body weight results in a doubling of peripheral conversion, and although oestrone is bound less avidly by endometrial oestrogen receptors than oestradiol, continuous exposure allows nuclear uptake and resultant protein synthesis and cell growth to occur. This influence of body weight on circulating oestrogens is further amplified by the association between reduced levels of sex hormone-binding globulin and obesity, which leads to an increase in free oestrogen being available to target organs.

Carbohydrate metabolism

The mechanism by which disturbed carbohydrate metabolism influences the risk of development of endometrial cancer is unclear. One study has shown that postmenopausal women with diabetes mellitus have increased oestrogen and reduced gonadotrophin levels independent of body weight (Quinn et al 1981). Whether women with endometrial carcinoma have an altered oestrogen metabolism independent of the effect of weight remains controversial.

Oestrogen production by ovarian tumours

The ovarian tumours classically associated with oestrogen production are the granulosa-theca cell tumours with approximately 10% of cases (reported range 2.5–23%) being associated with endometrial cancer and 50% (reported range 22–72%) with endometrial hyperplasia. Ovarian epithelial cancers, however, may also be responsible for steroid production, probably by a process of stromal luteinization due to locally produced human chorionic gonadotrophin. In one series, 7 of 9 mucinous carcinomas, 5 of 6 endometrioid carcinomas and all 8 Krukenberg tumours were associated with an increase in oestrogen secretion (Rome et al 1981).

Exogenous oestrogens and antioestrogens

The association between exogenous oestrogens and endometrial cancer is discussed in Chapter 24. The administration of unopposed oestrogens leads to a risk of developing endometrial cancer from seven to 10 times that of the general population, whilst the addition of a progestagen to oestrogen therapy for 12–14 days each month reduces the risk to less than that of the general population.

One area of recent concern has been the possible association of adjuvant tamoxifen therapy in breast cancer patients with an increased risk of endometrial cancer. This situation requires clarification, especially in the light of the known association between breast and endometrial cancer.

Radiotherapy

Pelvic irradiation is an unusual predisposing factor for the development of endometrial cancer; most cases in the literature have occurred in patients treated for carcinoma of the cervix. It is important to remember that young women treated for cancer of the cervix by radiotherapy need hormonal replacement and that this should always be with oestrogen and a progestagen rather than oestrogen alone.

SCREENING

The methods available to screen asymptomatic woman for endometrial neoplasia are listed below.

1. Endometrial biopsy.
2. Aspiration curettage.
3. Endometrial lavage.
4. Endometrial brush sponge.
5. Endometrial aspiration.
6. Papanicolaou smear of cervix.

7. Vaginal pool smear.
8. Progestogen challenge test.

Given the number of available devices and tests, it can be surmised that no one method is perfect and that no data currently available support the value of these tests in reducing the morbidity and mortality of the disease.

Endometrial sampling

Endometrial sampling techniques involve the use of various ingenious devices to obtain a sample of endometrial tissue for histological or cytological examination. The former is easier for the pathologist to interpret. Most studies have been performed in patients about to undergo diagnostic curettage and the value of these instruments as a tool for screening the asymptomatic population is not yet clear. Koss et al (1982) compared the use of the Mi-Mark Helix and Isaac's aspirator in screening just over 2000 asymptomatic women, 80% of whom were postmenopausal. Adequate samples for assessment were obtained in 80% of women screened, with a fall-off in successful sampling with advancing age. Eight cancers were detected by endometrial sampling. One cancer was missed and another was detected by vaginal cytology in a patient in whom the endometrial sampling procedure could not be performed. The sensitivity of the technique was 80%.

Vaginal or cervical cytology

The use of Papanicolaou smears to detect endometrial cancer has been evaluated mostly in symptomatic patients and the pick-up rate of cervical scrapes and posterior fornix samples in such patients is about 50% (Voupala 1977). The experienced cytopathologist may identify a number of features which warrant a recommendation for further investigations. Such features include the presence of numerous histiocytes in a postmenopausal smear, the presence of proliferative cells in the luteal phase of the menstrual cycle or in a postmenopausal women, and the presence of atypical or malignant glandular cells.

Should fractional curettage and hysteroscopy fail to indicate the origin of atypical glandular cells then diagnostic laparoscopy (with pelvic washings) or even laparotomy may be required to discount a tubal or ovarian origin.

Progestogen challenge test

The progestogen challenge test is based on the hypothesis that endometrial cancer is oestrogen-dependent and that a withdrawal bleed following postmenopausal progestogen administration is indicative of the presence of oestrogen-stimulated endometrium (Gambrell et al 1980). The role of this test in a population setting is yet to be defined.

PATHOLOGY

Malignancy may develop in either the glands or stroma of the endometrium. Endometrial adenocarcinoma, derived from the endometrial glandular cells, is overwhelmingly the most common malignant tumour arising in the body of the uterus; the stroma is the origin of the much rarer endometrial stromal sarcomas. The even more uncommon malignant mixed müllerian tumour is composed of both glandular and stromal elements. The sarcomas are discussed separately.

Endometrial carcinoma is usually seen as a raised, rough, perhaps papillary area, occupying at least half the endometrium. Endometrial carcinomas often arise in the fundal region of the uterus; the internal os is rarely involved early in the disease. Myometrial invasion may be obvious to the naked eye. There seems to be no correlation between the degree of exophytic growth of the tumour within the uterine cavity and the presence of myometrial invasion.

Endometrial carcinoma is not a single tumour; it is a group of distinct subtypes (Poulsen et al 1975):

1. Adenocarcinoma not otherwise specified (endometrioid).
2. Adenocarcinoma with benign squamous change (adenoacanthoma).
3. Adenosquamous (mixed) carcinoma.
4. Papillary serous adenocarcinoma.
5. Clear cell carcinoma.
6. Squamous cell carcinoma.

Endometrioid adenocarcinoma

The commonest endometrial carcinoma is referred to as endometrioid adenocarcinoma (Fig. 38.1), the glandular pattern of which generally resembles that of normal proliferative phase endometrium, although sometimes showing extreme

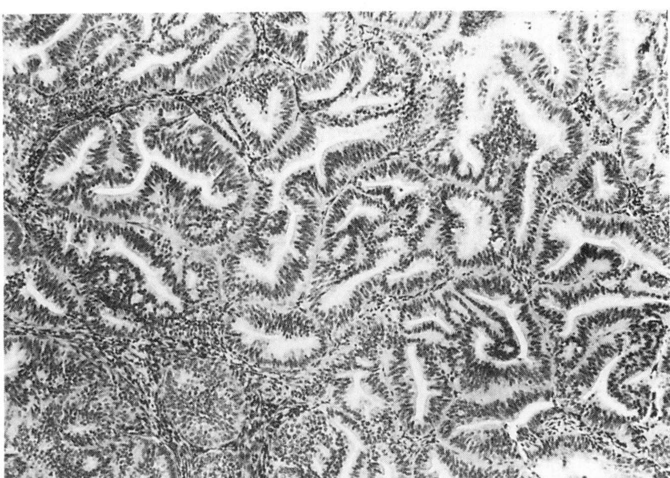

Fig. 38.1 A well differentiated (grade 1) endometrial carcinoma of endometrioid pattern. Haematoxylin and eosin ×170.

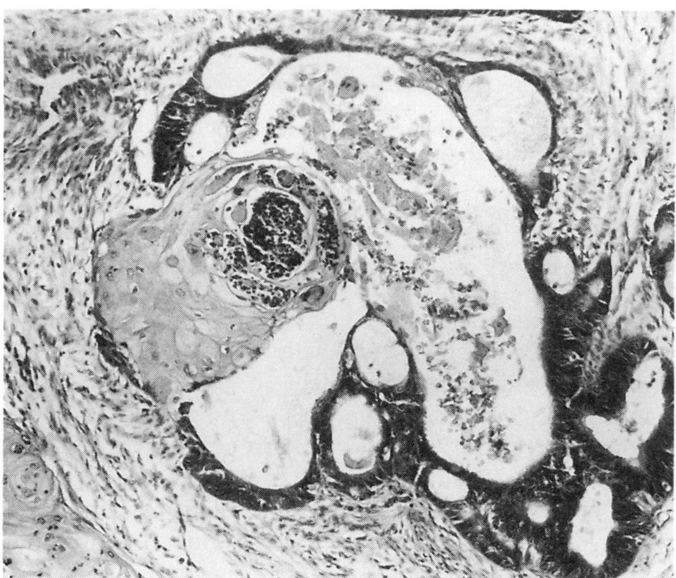

Fig. 38.2 Adenocarcinoma with benign squamous metaplasia (adenoacanthoma). Haematoxylin and eosin ×195.

complexity of the glands and cribriform pattern. Multi-layering of the epithelial cells is nearly always seen.

Endometrial adenocarcinoma with squamous metaplasia (adenoacanthoma)

Up to 25% of endometrioid-pattern endometrial adenocarcinomas contain areas of squamous metaplasia. Those tumours in which the squamous component is morphologically benign are commonly termed 'adenoacanthoma' (Christopherson et al 1983). The squamous change is seen as islands of typical squamous epithelium, very often situated within the gland lumina or as surface or diffuse squamous metaplasia (Fig. 38.2).

Adenosquamous carcinoma

An adenosquamous carcinoma is a carcinoma of the endometrium composed of malignant glands with a morphologically malignant squamous element. Histologically, the glandular element always predominates, making up at least 70% of the tumour.

Papillary serous and clear cell carcinomas

Less common variants of endometrial adenocarcinoma are the papillary serous and clear cell carcinoma. These are both associated with a poor prognosis.

PRESENTATION AND DIAGNOSIS

Presenting symptoms

The vast majority of women diagnosed as having endometrial cancer present with abnormal bleeding. The remainder have a discharge or pain, or are referred because of an abnormal screening test. Postmenopausal bleeding is the most common presenting symptom as 75–80% of women with the disease are in this age group. Diagnostic curettage in the patient with postmenopausal discharge due to a pyometra will reveal a carcinoma in about 50% of cases, and it is usually in these women that the rare pure squamous carcinoma is found. The presence of pain is usually an indicator of metastatic disease.

The most common mistake made which delays the diagnosis is to assume that vaginal spotting is due to atrophic vaginitis. Any woman who bleeds after the menopause has a 10–20% risk of having a genital cancer. A cervical smear and diagnostic curettage should be performed in all cases, no matter what the clinical diagnosis may be. The same is required for a woman on hormone replacement therapy with irregular bleeding.

The woman with premenopausal endometrial carcinoma usually presents with irregular bleeding but over one-third of premenopausal patients present with heavy but regular periods (Quinn et al 1985a).

Diagnosis and assessment

All patients with abnormal bleeding and a normal cervical smear should undergo fractional curettage or hysteroscopy or both to evaluate the status of the endocervix. Fractional curettage involves curetting the endocervix thoroughly up to the internal os. The length of the uterine cavity is assessed using a sound, the cervix is dilated and the cavity curetted. Samples of tissues from these two sites need to be assessed separately by the pathologist. The presence of stromal invasion of the cervix or carcinomatous tissue contiguous with endocervical glands are the only real criteria by which to diagnose cervical involvement by a primary endometrial tumour.

The role of hysteroscopy in evaluating endocervical spread of endometrial cancer is not yet well defined. Proponents of this technique argue that the visual demonstration of spread to the endocervix is accurate whilst its detractors argue that subepithelial spread will be missed and that there is a danger of cancer cells being flushed through the fallopian tubes into the peritoneal cavity. Until firm data are available, fractional curettage should be the diagnostic aid of choice.

Assessment of the endocervix is not merely academic. Patients with endometrial tumour involving the cervix have a higher risk of metastases to other pelvic organs and to lymph nodes, and a survival rate about 25% less than those with tumour confined to the corpus. Even involvement of the lower uterine segment carries a higher risk than disease confined to the fundus, with 14% of such patients having pelvic nodes involved — more than triple the rate for fundal disease (Creasman et al 1987).

PROGNOSTIC FACTORS

A multitude of prognostic factors has been identified in this disease. Most are closely inter-related, so that multivariate analysis has been required to determine the importance of any one factor. Known prognostic factors in patients with endometrial adenocarcinoma are listed below.

1. Age.
2. Body morphology.
3. Stage of disease.
4. Histological subtype.
5. Degree of differentiation.
6. Myometrial invasion.
7. Peritoneal cytology.
8. Lymph node involvement.
9. Steroid receptor status.
10. Ploidy status.
11. Capillary-like space involvement.

Age and body morphology

Older women with endometrial carcinoma are more likely to die of the disease than their younger counterparts. Although this may be due to the fact that the older patient is more likely to have a poorly differentiated and deeply invasive tumour, this does not seem wholly to account for the difference in survival.

Patients who are obese with high cholesterol levels and diabetes, who have signs of hyperoestrogenism such as oestrogenic vaginal smears and who have a late menopause and a history of anovulatory infertility are more likely to have well differentiated, superficially invasive tumours and a better prognosis (Bokhman 1983). The good prognosis of patients who have been taking oestrogens is almost certainly related to this same situation.

Stage of disease

The current FIGO (International Federation of Gynaecology and Obstetrics) staging criteria are shown in Table 38.1; the stage distribution and 5-year survival of over 14 000 patients reported by FIGO (1988) are shown in Table 38.2. It should be noted that the overall survival (65.1%) has changed little in the last 20 years and, stage for stage, survival is similar to that of carcinoma of the cervix.

Table 38.1 FIGO staging of carcinoma of the corpus uteri (until 1989)

Stage	Description
I	The carcinoma is confined to the corpus
Ia	The length of the uterine cavity is 8 cm or less
Ib	The length of the uterine cavity is more than 8 cm
II	The carcinoma has involved the corpus and the cervix but has not extended outside the uterus
III	The carcinoma has extended outside the uterus but not outside the true pelvis
IV	The carcinoma has extended outside the true pelvis or has obviously involved the mucosa of the bladder or rectum. A bullous oedema as such does not permit a case to be allotted to stage IV
IVa	Growth has spread to adjacent organs such as urinary bladder, rectum, sigmoid or small bowel
IVb	Growth has spread to distant organs

Table 38.2 FIGO stage distribution and 5-year survival

Stage	Percentage	% 5-year survival
I	74.0	72.3
II	13.5	56.4
III	6.2	31.5
IV	2.8	10.5
Unstaged	3.5	47.8

Modified from FIGO (1988) with permission.

Histological subtype

Most authors now agree that areas of squamous metaplasia do not imply a worse prognosis. On the other hand, the presence of *malignant* squamous components (adenosquamous carcinoma) may be associated with a poorer outcome. Some institutions report an increasing proportion of these tumours overall, whilst others report an association of increasing age, increasing stage and poorer glandular differentiation, all of which may contribute to a reduced survival. Whether adenosquamous histology is an independent variable associated with a poor outcome is not yet clear.

There is little debate about the poor prognosis of patients with clear cell cancers who, even with stage I disease, have an overall survival of less than 50%. This tumour is more common in black women which may partially account for their poorer survival compared to whites. Serous papillary carcinoma of the endometrium, histologically similar to serous papillary cancer of the ovary, has a very poor prognosis and a pattern of spread more akin to ovarian than endometrial malignancy.

Degree of differentiation

The 5-year survival rate of patients with grade 3 tumours is 20% less than that of patients with better differentiated cancers. Higher-grade tumours are more likely to be associated with myometrial invasion. Approximately 25% of grade 1 tumours are confined to the endometrium compared with only 10% of grade 3 lesions.

Myometrial invasion

The depth of myometrial invasion is an excellent guide to the likelihood of spread to lymph nodes and beyond. In early disease it is probably the single most important prognostic factor, with recurrence developing in almost 50% of patients with deeply invasive cancers.

Peritoneal cytology

Positive peritoneal washings are present in approximately 12–15% of all cases of endometrial cancer, with half of these having no histological evidence of extrauterine spread. The interpretation of peritoneal cytology can be very difficult but the unequivocal presence of malignant cells in peritoneal washings is a very ominous sign.

Lymph node involvement

The surgicopathological study carried out by members of the Gynaecologic Oncology Group (Creasman et al 1987) has given a valuable insight into the patterns of spread of endometrial cancer as well as the importance of various prognostic factors.

Seventy of the 621 patients (11%) with disease clinically confined to the corpus had metastases to either pelvic or para-aortic nodes, or both (Table 38.3). Twice as many patients with an enlarged uterus (>8 cm) had positive pelvic nodes (Table 38.4). Histological subtype seemed to be associated with para-aortic but not pelvic node involvement, with serous papillary and clear cell cancers having the highest risk of spread to para-aortic nodes.

Both grade of tumour and depth of myometrial invasion were associated with nodal involvement. Well differentiated tumours with superficial invasion of the myometrium were associated with a 3% prevalence of positive pelvic nodes and 1% positive para-aortic nodes, while 34% of poorly differentiated and deeply invasive tumours had positive pelvic nodes and 23% had positive para-aortic nodes. Depth of myometrial penetration is a more important guide to the likelihood of nodal metastases than tumour grade.

Other factors significantly associated with lymph node involvement include tumour size, capillary-like space (CLS) involvement, adnexal involvement, positive peritoneal cytology and isthmic or cervical involvement by tumour. It is important to note that macroscopic involvement of nodes was seen in only 10% of cases subsequently proven to have nodal spread.

Table 38.3 Incidence of nodal involvement when disease is clinically confined to corpus

Positive nodes	Percentage
Pelvic nodes only positive	6
Para-aortic nodes only positive	2
Pelvic and para-aortic nodes positive	3

Table 38.4 Risk factors for nodal involvement in endometrial cancer

Uterine size >8 cm
Poorly differentiated adenocarcinoma
Adenosquamous, clear cell and serous papillary cancers
Myometrial invasion
Positive peritoneal cytology
Isthmic or cervical involvement
Tumour size
Spread outside the uterus
Capillary-like space involvement

Steroid receptor status

Receptors for oestrogen (ER) and progesterone (PR) were first identified in endometrial tissue in 1975. Approximately 79% of cases will have 'cytoplasmic' ER and in 70% of cases 'cytoplasmic' PR are present (Table 38.5). Tumours which are of high grade or deeply invasive are more likely to be receptor-negative or to have only low levels of receptors. Patients with advanced disease or with clear cell or serous papillary tumours are also more likely to have receptor-negative tumours. A number of studies have now convincingly shown that receptor status is an important independent indicator of prognosis.

Ploidy status

Studies of the ploidy status of a variety of gynaecological malignancies indicate that aneuploid tumours carry a significantly worse prognosis them diploid tumours. Iversen (1986) studied 75 samples of endometrial cancer by flow cytometry and compared outcome with other variables such as receptor status, tumour grade, surgical stage and degree of myometrial invasion. Ploidy was found to be the best predictor of survival, followed by surgical stage.

Table 38.5 Soluble ('cytoplasmic') steroid receptors in endometrial carcinoma

	ER +ve	PR +ve
Overall	79%	70%
G1	92%	84%
G2	76%	68%
G3	56%	44%
Adenosquamous	72%	68%
Clear cell	58%	50%
Serous papillary	53%	27%

ER = oestrogen receptors; PR = progesterone receptors.

Capillary like space involvement

Hanson and his co-authors (1985) found CLS involvement in 16 of 111 stage I endometrial tumours. Although associated with poorly differentiated and deeply invasive cancers, CLS involvement was an independent prognostic factor. CLS involvement increases the rate of pelvic lymph node spread by a factor of four and para-aortic node spread by a factor by two (Creasman et al 1987).

MANAGEMENT

The number of women who are medically unfit and unable to undergo surgery is shrinking. This, together with the inaccuracy of clinical staging (Table 38.6) and the importance of prognostic factors which can be identified surgically, has led to the introduction by FIGO of a surgicopathological staging scheme (Table 38.7).

Table 38.6 Comparison of clinical and surgical staging in endometrial carcinoma

Clinical staging	Number	Surgical staging		Change of stage
		Lower	Higher	
Ia	34	4	18	47.8%
b	12	0	2	16.6%
II	8	4	1	62.5%
III	5	1	2	60.0%
IVa	1	0	0	0
b	2	0	0	0

Adapted from Cowles et al (1985) with permission.

Table 38.7 FIGO surgical staging of endometrial carcinoma (from 1989)

Stage		Description
Stage	Ia G123	Tumour limited to endometrium
	Ib G123	Invasion < ½ myometrium
	Ic G123	Invasion > ½ myometrium
Stage	IIa G123	Endocervical glandular involvement only
	IIb G123	Cervical stromal invasion
Stage	IIIa G123	Tumour invades serosa and/or adnexae and/or positive peritoneal cytology
	IIIb G123	Vaginal metastases
	IIIc G123	Metastases to pelvic and/or para-aortic lymph nodes
Stage	IVa	Tumour invades bladder and/or bowel mucosa
	IVb	Distant metastases including intra-abdominal and/or inguinal lymph node

G123 refers to the grade of the tumour. For example, a grade 2 tumour invading to the serosal surface of the uterus with no metastatic disease would be stage IIIa G2.
From FIGO (in press).

Stage I

The treatment of choice in patients with endometrial cancer is total abdominal hysterectomy and bilateral salpingo-oophorectomy, especially since clinical staging is so inaccurate (Cowles et al 1985). Given the inaccuracy of clinical staging together with the facts that up to 30% of endometrioid tumours will have their grading changed once hysterectomy samples are available and that about 25% of cases will have the histological subtype reassigned, preoperative irradiation should be withheld, especially since there are no published data to show improved survival compared to postoperative irradiation. Some patients may avoid irradiation which they did not really require.

Preoperative evaluation

Prior to surgery a thorough history and full medical examination should be undertaken. Special attention should be paid to the lymph node-bearing areas in the neck and groin, to the breasts and axillae, and to the detection of any ascites, masses or organomegaly within the abdomen. During vaginal examination, the distal anterior vagina should be carefully inspected and palpated since sub-urethral metastases are not uncommon.

Preoperative tests required in these patients, who are often obese and medically unfit, will include a full blood examination, tests of liver and renal function, electrolytes, CA 125 level, chest X-ray, intravenous pyelogram, and urinalysis for sugar and protein. The incidence of CA 125 levels above the normal range increases with increasing spread of disease so that virtually all patients with clinical stage IV disease will have raised levels.

Preoperative anaesthetic consultation is imperative for these patients, not only from a medical point of view, but also to provide the woman with valuable information on the type of anaesthetic she will receive, what this will involve, what 'accessories' she will have when she goes to the recovery room (intravenous lines, central lines, oxygen mask, epidural line etc.) and how long she will stay in the recovery room.

Likewise, it is the surgeon's responsibility to ensure that the patient is fully informed about the procedure: the type of incision, use of washings, criteria for lymphadenectomy and possible complications should all be discussed, as well as the potential need for adjuvant treatment following surgery. Patients with endometrial cancer should be admitted at least 48 h prior to operation. Blood should be cross-matched (packed-cells) and a low residue diet commenced, laxatives given, and a liquid diet prescribed for the day before surgery. The bowel should be clean and empty by the time she reaches the operating room as 1% of these patients will have a colonic cancer diagnosed at the laparotomy and an empty bowel considerably reduced postoperative abdominal discomfort. Subcutaneous heparin should be commenced the night before planned surgery and continued until the patient is mobile. Alternatively an intravenous bolus can be given with the anaesthetic induction. Because of possible dehydration occurring as a result of laxative and enema use, it is wise to insert an intravenous line on the evening prior to surgery to ensure optimal fluid balance during the operation.

Operative approach

A midline sub-umbilical incision, which can be extended above the umbilicus if required, is the incision of choice; a transverse incision will not allow adequate exposure of the upper abdomen and should be avoided. In the obese patient it is best not to straighten out the abdominal wall by pulling up the panniculus of fat over the pubic symphysis; retraction of this excess fat is often tiring, exposure can be suboptimal, and the incidence of wound infection in the skin fold is very high. Immediately the abdominal cavity is entered, 100 ml of sterile saline or Hank's solution should be instilled into the pelvis to bathe the uterus, bladder and pouch of Douglas, and then aspirated. The specimen should be mixed with 1000 units of heparin to prevent a clot forming which could trap malignant cells.

Once the peritoneal washings have been taken, a thorough laparotomy should be performed, with particular attention being paid to the liver, omentum, uterine adnexae and retroperitoneal node-bearing areas. A simple total hysterectomy and bilateral salpingo-oophorectomy should then be completed. Removal of a vaginal cuff, once thought to be mandatory, does not reduce the recurrence rate or improve survival, nor does radical hysterectomy. Likewise, manoeuvres to occlude the cervix and fallopian tubes to prevent intraoperative spill of tumour are unnecesary.

The uterus can now be opened off the operating table and the depth of myometrial invasion assessed. The specimen should then be placed on ice and sent immediately to the pathology laboratory for histology and receptor analysis. Alternatively, a piece of the carcinoma can be snap-frozen in liquid nitrogen and stored for receptor analysis at a later date. At this point a decision as to lymph node removal is made. This should be considered in patients with poorly differentiated disease; adenosquamous, clear cell or serous papillary tumours; lesions which invade more than one-third of the myometrium and those which are seen to involve the cervix or adnexae.

Patients with these high-risk tumours who are medically fit should then have the pelvic and para-aortic nodes removed. The side walls of the pelvis should be explored for any obviously enlarged nodes and these should be removed and sent for frozen section; if positive for tumour, further pelvic nodal excision is unnecessary but the para-aortic nodes should be sampled. For the 90% of patients without grossly enlarged nodes, block dissection of external and internal iliac nodes together with obturator nodes should be performed followed by removal of the anterior fat pad overlying the aorta from the bifurcation to the level of the duodenum. The peritoneum over these areas should be resutured and vacuum drains left along the pelvic vessels to be removed once drainage is less than 100 ml/24 h.

The abdominal incision must be closed by some form of mass closure technique, which will reduce the incidence of burst abdomen and postoperative hernia. The Smead–Jones technique is recommended.

Radiotherapy

Radiotherapy is usually given after surgery. It is more effective combined with surgery than when given alone (Bickenback 1967). However, if the patient is not fit for surgery, two caesium insertions delivering 6000 cGy to point A may be used for well differentiated tumours. If the curettings were poorly differentiated, 4500 cGy may be

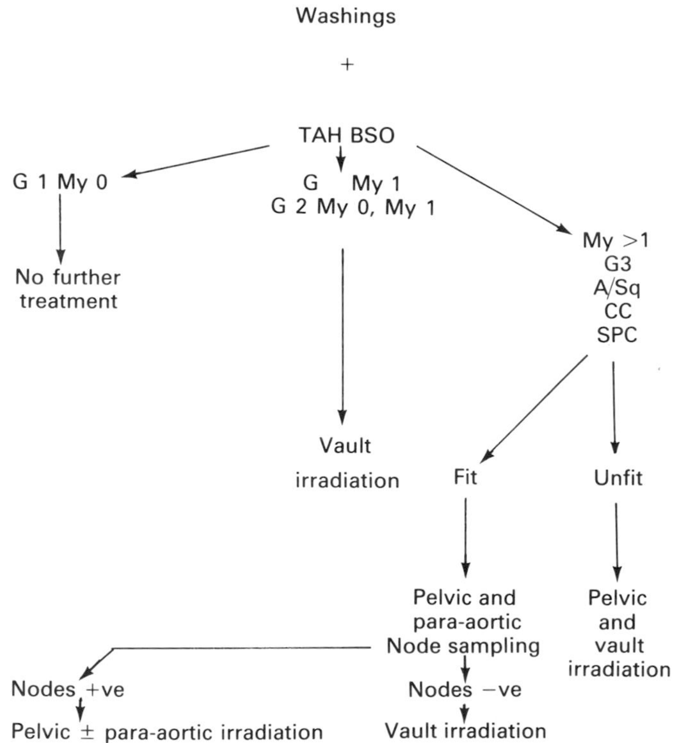

Fig. 38.3 Protocol for the management of stage I endometrial carcinoma.
TAH BSO = total abdominal hysterectomy and bilateral salpingo-oophorectomy.
G1 = well differentiated endometrioid adenocarcinoma;
G2 = moderately well differentiated endometrioid carcinoma;
G3 = poorly differentiated endometrioid carcinoma.
My 0 = No myometrial invasion; My 1 = less than one-third myometrial invasion.
A/Sq = Adenosquamous carcinoma; CC = clear cell carcinoma;
SPC = serous papillary carcinoma.

given in 5 weeks to the whole pelvis. This is followed by a single insertion delivering 2000–2500 cGy to point A.

Postoperative vault irradiation reduces the incidence of vault recurrence (Graham 1971) and is omitted only in superficial well differentiated tumours (Fig. 38.3). A 2000–2500 cGy dose is given to the surface of the vagina. External beam therapy is reserved for women with poor prognostic factors such as poorly differentiated tumours or deep myometrial invasion (Bean et al 1978). The technique is similar to that used for cervical cancer, delivering no more than 4000 cGy in 25 fractions over 5 weeks.

Stage II

The management of patients with endometrial cancer involving the cervix depends on whether spread is microscopic or macroscopic. Should the cervix be obviously involved with tumour, either a radical hysterectomy and bilateral pelvic lymphadenectomy with para-aortic node sampling should be performed in the surgically fit patient or radiation should be used. If radiation is chosen, 5000 cGy is given to the whole pelvis in $5\frac{1}{2}$ weeks, followed by a single insertion giving 2000 cGy to point A. In this latter instance, the addition of extrafascial hysterectomy 6 weeks after pelvic irradiation and intracavity brachytherapy may improve survival.

In those patients in whom spread to the cervix is occult, with the diagnosis being made on hysteroscopy or endocervical curettage, management should be identical to those patients with high-risk stage I disease.

Stage III

The rare patient with parametrial extension of disease or vaginal involvement should have a computerized tomography scan of the pelvis and upper abdomen performed. Should the disease be confined to the pelvis then radiation therapy is the treatment of choice, given in a manner similar to stage II. On the other hand, when there is clinical spread to the adnexae a laparotomy should still be undertaken to define accurately the extent of the disease and to remove as much tumour as possible. Following removal of the pelvic disease, omentectomy and lymphadenectomy should be performed together with multiple peritoneal biopsies, in a similar fashion to the surgical approach in patients with ovarian malignancies. Any remaining disease should be biopsied and tissue sent for receptor analysis. Patients with metastases to the tubes or ovaries found incidentally at surgery have a 5-year survival of approximately 80%, about five times higher than when other pelvic structures or the vagina is involved.

Stage IV

The lungs are the most common site of metastases in patients presenting with extrapelvic disease, followed by peripheral lymph nodes and bladder. Over 20% of patients will have disease at multiple sites. Management needs to be individualized, with the primary aim being control of symptoms and local control of tumour growth. Radiation therapy, cytotoxic drugs and hormonal therapy may all be required.

The use of whole abdominal irradiation with a pelvic boost for patients with intra-abdominal spread which has been optimally debulked has been reported to be very successful, with a 5-year survival of over 70% (Greer and Hamberger 1983).

Adjuvant progestogen therapy

Because of the known response of advanced and recurrent endometrial cancers to progestational agents, the use of such therapy in the absence of residual disease has seemed an attractive proposition, especially as adjuvant hormonal treatment seems to reduce the recurrence risk in patients with postmenopausal breast cancer. A number of trials have been undertaken in patients with stage I and stage II disease using a variety of progestogens, a variety of routes of administration and a variety of time periods during which the hormone has been prescribed. No properly randomized trial has shown a survival benefit, but all published studies suffer from the inclusion of patients with low-risk tumours, thereby decreasing the — likelihood of detecting a therapeutic benefit in the treated group (Kneale 1986). The current Clinical Oncology Society of Australia–New Zealand–UK trial of adjuvant medroxyprogesterone acetate has aimed to overcome this problem by including only high-risk patients and an answer (requiring 1300–1500 patients) is expected by the mid 1990s.

Recurrent disease

Approximately 70% of all recurrences following primary treatment present within the first 2–3 years. Early recurrences carry a grave prognosis presumably because of the inherent aggressiveness of the tumour. The common sites of treatment failure are lungs, bone, inguinal and supraclavicular nodes, vagina, liver and peritoneal cavity.

Local pelvic recurrence tends to occur in the non-irradiated patient and, if isolated, is curable by radiation in 25–50% of cases. Radiotherapy is also of great value for palliation of symptoms, particular relief of pain and discomfort due to bony and nodal metastases.

The patient with a late central pelvic recurrence following surgery and irradiation should be managed in a similar fashion to the patient with recurrent cervix cancer. Assessment of spread by computerized tomography scanning, intravenous pyelography and cystoscopy should allow a number of patients to be considered for exenterative surgery. However, the older age of these patients and the greater prevalence of medical disorders mean that few are suitable for exenteration.

Progestational therapy has been used in patients with recurrent endometrial carcinoma for many years. The response rate is probably around 15 or 20%. A 52% response rate may be expected in patients with grade 1 adenocarcinoma as opposed to a 15% response rate in patients with grade 3 cancers (Kohorn 1976). Tumours which recur more than 3 years after primary treatment are more responsive to progestogens, whilst recurrences which are widespread, are intra-abdominal or have been previously irradiated show lower response rates. The factors associated with tumour response to progestogens are listed below:

1. Tumour differentiation.
2. Disease-free interval.
3. Site of recurrence.
4. Number of metastases.
5. Prior irradiation.
6. Steroid receptor status.

Approximately 80% of PR positive and 70% of ER positive tumours respond to progestogen treatment, whilst only 11% of PR negative and 5% of ER negative tumours respond. Unfortunately, recurrent tumour is often inaccessible for biopsy and only data on the primary tumour are available. None the less, this gives an excellent guide to response (Quinn et al 1985b). An alternative approach to prediction of response has been taken by Stratton et al (1989) who used the subrenal capsule assay to predict response. All 10 tumours found to be resistant to medroxyprogesterone acetate in this model were from patients who subsequently failed to respond to the hormone. To date, there is no scientific information as to whether the dose or the progestogen used is important.

Tamoxifen is an anti-oestrogen which also has the ability to increase intracellular PR content and is an attractive drug for use in patients with advanced disease; response rates to tamoxifen alone vary from 0 to 60% (Quinn & Campbell 1989). These probably depend on previous treatment, with higher response rates seen in patients previously responding to progestogens. The use of combination therapy has been studied by Rendina et al (1984) who added tamoxifen to medroxyprogesterone acetate in patients who relapsed or initially failed to respond to the progestogen. Patients who relapsed after an initial response to medroxyprogesterone acetate had a 62% response to the combination whilst 48% of patients who initially had no response to medroxyprogesterone acetate, responded to the combination. Whether tamoxifen and progestagens should be given simultaneously or sequentially awaits further clarification. Aminoglutethimide, an aromatase inhibitor which causes adrenal blockade, has also been used successfully in advanced endometrial cancer (Quinn 1989).

The use of cytotoxic therapy in patients with advanced endometrial cancer is a less attractive option than hormonal therapy since many of these women are elderly and medically unfit. Nonetheless, cytotoxic agents do have a role following failure of hormonal therapy. Single agents known to have activity include Adriamycin (response rate 19–38%), cisplatin (response rate 4–42%), cyclophosphamide (response rate 21%) and hexamethylmelamine (response rate 30%). Combination therapy has so far not proven superior to single-agent therapy (Thigpen et al 1987). It has been suggested that steroid receptor-negative tumours are more sensitive to cytotoxic therapy but this awaits confirmation.

UTERINE SARCOMA

Sarcomas of the uterus are often highly malignant but rare tumours with an incidence of approximately 2/100 000 women over the age of 20 years. They account for 3–5% of all uterine cancers. These tumours are more common in black women and in women who have undergone previous pelvic irradiation. The literature relating to these tumours is beset by differences in histological classification. This situation is further complicated by difficulties in determining the malignant status of some of the smooth muscle tumours. No staging system for these tumours has been proposed by FIGO but a potential clinical staging scheme which would allow a comparison of results from different centres and a rational approach to therapy is given below.

Stage I Sarcomas confined to the uterus.
Stage II Sarcomas involving the corpus and cervix.
Stage III Sarcomas which have spread beyond the uterus, but not outside the pelvis.
Stage IV Sarcomas which have spread outside the pelvis or into the bladder and/or rectum.

Endometrial stromal sarcomas

Low-grade endometrial stromal sarcoma

The low-grade endometrial stromal sarcoma has previously been known as endolymphatic stromal myosis, endolymphatic stromatosis or stromal endometriosis. This neoplasm arises from endometrial stroma, from adenomyosis and occasionally from pelvic endometriosis (Hendrickson & Kempson 1987).

The tumour may be polypoid and protrude into the uterine cavity, but an infiltrating growth pattern is more characteristic, resulting in an area of thickening of the uterine wall. Microscopically (Fig. 38.4), the cells of the tumour resemble those of normal endometrial stroma; nuclear atypia is usually slight. The most striking feature of the low-grade endometrial stromal sarcoma, and the origin of the alternative name of endolymphatic stromal myosis, is the nature of the infiltrating margin of the tumour. Broad rounded bands and sharp finger-like

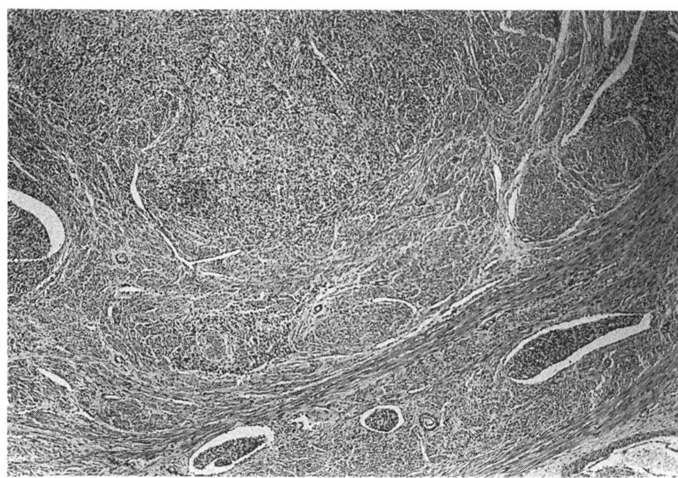

Fig. 38.4 A low-grade endometrial stromal sarcoma with prominent lymphatic channel involvement. Haematoxylin and eosin ×64.

processes of stromal cells infiltrate extensively into the myometrium, between the muscle fibres and particularly into the lymphatic spaces. Mitotic figures are generally less than 10 per 10 high-power fields.

This lesion is almost always not diagnosed until the time of hysterectomy, with abnormal vaginal bleeding being the most common symptom. In approximately 1 in 3 cases extra-uterine spread is detected at operation into the broad or cardinal ligaments, the adnexae or to other intra-abdominal organs. The aim of surgery should be to remove all visible disease. The ovaries should be removed, especially in the premenopausal patient. This neoplasm is an intermediate-type malignancy with late recurrence being common. The recurrence rate in early-stage disease has been reported to be as high as 50% in some series (Piver et al 1984) and adjuvant progestational therapy or pelvic irradiation is indicated.

High-grade endometrial stromal sarcoma

The uterus harbouring a high-grade stromal sarcoma is usually enlarged and the tumour appears as a polypoid mass extending into the uterine cavity from the endometrium. The mass is characteristically round with a smooth surface, a feature that often distinguishes this tumour from the rather unusual polypoid variant of endometrial carcinoma, which has a rough or papillary surface. Necrosis of the tumour is often a prominent naked-eye feature.

Microscopically, the resemblance to endometrial stromal cells is less obvious than is seen in the low-grade endometrial stromal sarcoma (Fig. 38.5). The cells are oval or spindle-shaped and may show considerable pleomorphism. Mitotic figures are numerous, always exceeding 10 per 10 high-power fields and often amounting to as many as 40 or 50 per 10 high-power fields. The tumour is richly vascular but blood vessel and lymphatic channel involvement is much less frequently seen than in the low-grade variant. Areas of necrosis are frequently present.

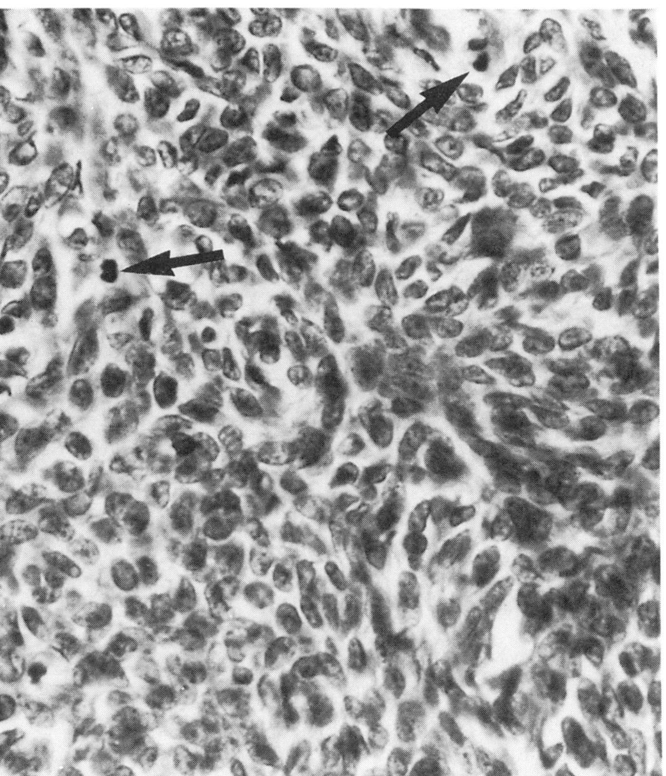

Fig. 38.5 A high-grade endometrial stromal sarcoma. Nuclear crowding and pleomorphism are apparent and, although mitotic figures (arrowed) are not conspicuous, this tumour contains more than 10 mitotic figures per 10 high-power fields. Haematoxylin and eosin ×650.

High-grade endometrial stromal sarcoma is an aggressive tumour which occurs most commonly following the menopause and usually presents as abnormal vaginal bleeding or discharge. The treatment of choice is total abdominal hysterectomy and bilateral salpingo-oophorectomy. The overall survival of patients with this rare sarcoma is less than 50%. Adjuvant pelvic irradiation is used in the hope of improving local control. Adriamycin or progestagens (Katn et al 1987) may be used in recurrent disease.

Malignant mixed müllerian tumour

The malignant mixed müllerian tumour is composed of malignant glands in malignant stroma (Fortune & Östör 1987). In the past, different terms have been used to describe it; those that contain homologous mesenchymal elements have been called 'carcinosarcoma' and those with heterologous elements have been known as 'mixed mesodermal tumours'.

Grossly, the neoplasm characteristically distends the uterine cavity and occasionally protrudes through the ex-

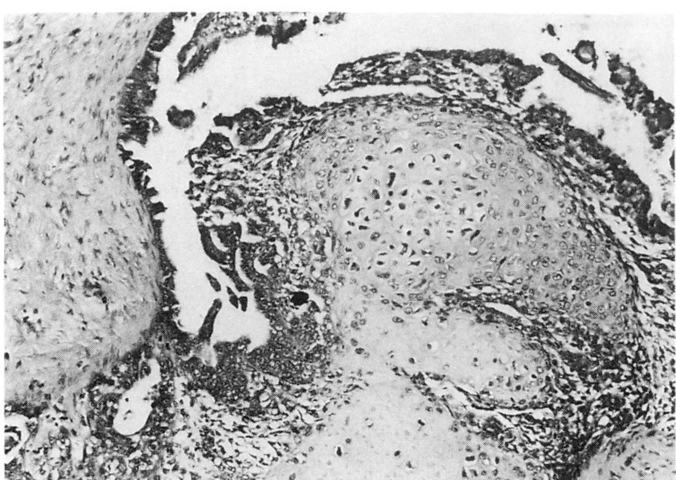

Fig. 38.6 Malignant mixed müllerian tumour. Malignant papillary epithelium and malignant cartilage are both present in this illustration. Haematoxylin and eosin ×195.

ternal cervical os. Areas of haemorrhage and necrosis are often prominent and myometrial invasion may be very obvious as many of these tumours do not seem to be recognized until they have reached a fairly advanced stage. Multicentric tumour masses may be found.

The microscopic features of the malignant mixed müllerian tumour are striking and characteristic (Fig. 38.6). Both the epithelial and mesenchymal elements are malignant. Most frequently the carcinomatous element is of an endometrioid pattern, although often poorly differentiated. On occasion, squamous cell carcinoma is the sole epithelial component. The stromal element may be homologous or heterologous. The homologous malignant mixed müllerian tumour contains a mesenchymal element that is composed of cell types that are normally found in the uterus, such as leiomyosarcoma, endometrial stromal sarcoma, fibrosarcoma and the often encountered undifferentiated sarcoma. The heterologous elements are rhabdomyosarcoma, osteosarcoma and chondrosarcoma.

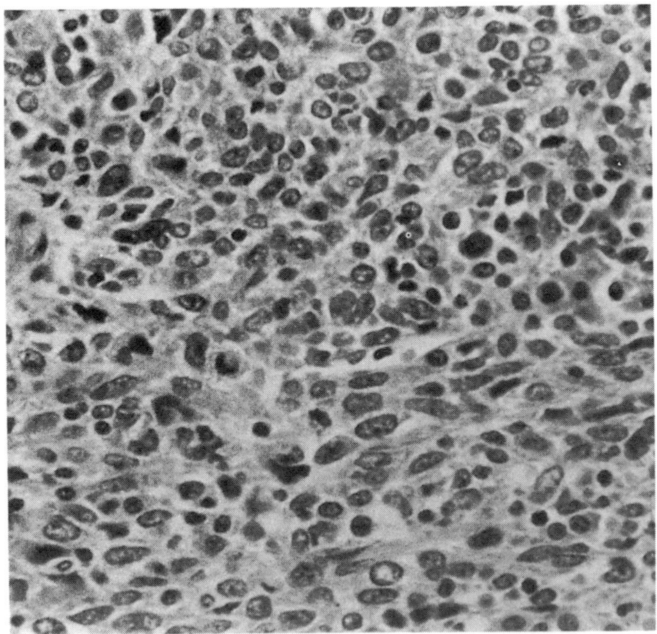

Fig. 38.7 Leiomyosarcoma. Although a few cells are spindled, most are poorly differentiated and show marked nuclear pleomorphism. Haematoxylin and eosin ×720.

The average age of patients with these aggressive cancers is 60 years and presentation is usually with abnormal bleeding, pain or a mass. These tumours have a similar pattern of spread and prognosis to poorly differentiated adenocarcinomas with spread to the cervix and regional nodes being common (Gallup et al 1989). They should be managed in a similar fashion to endometrial cancer, with pelvic and para-aortic node sampling being utilized in the medically fit patient. Postoperative pelvic irradiation improves local pelvic control. Cisplatin, Adriamycin and cyclophosphamide is the combination of choice for patients with recurrent or advanced disease.

MYOMETRIAL TUMOURS

Leiomyosarcoma

This tumour is the malignant counterpart of the leiomyoma and is the most common pure sarcoma of the uterus (Hendrickson & Kempson 1987). Its incidence is commonly quoted as 0.67/100 000 women and its stated frequency as a percentage of smooth muscle tumours of the uterus ranges from 0.13 to 6%; this 50-fold variation implies that different diagnostic criteria are being employed. Although the true figure is unknown because the presence of benign leiomyomas goes unrecognized in many women, it might be reasonable to suggest that perhaps 2 or 3 women per 1000 with smooth muscle tumours of the uterus have a leiomyosarcoma.

The gross appearance of a leiomyosarcoma may not differ significantly from that of a leiomyoma. Leiomyosarcomas have been described as having a cut surface that appears paler, perhaps more yellow, than a leiomyoma, with areas of haemorrhage and necrosis. Adhesions and evidence of gross invasion into the surrounding myometrium may be present, but this is seldom of diagnostic value. Leiomyosarcomas are frequently found in uteri that contain leiomyomas, but they can also occur singly, and are more likely to be solitary than a leiomyoma. The peak age incidence of leiomyosarcoma is about 10 years later than leiomyoma.

Microscopically, well differentiated leiomyosarcomas are composed of elongated cells with regular nuclei that are little different from those of leiomyoma (Fig. 38.7). At the other end of the spectrum, a poorly differentiated leiomyosarcoma is composed of rounded and pleomorphic cells that have virtually no resemblance to normal smooth muscle cells. Areas of necrosis and haemorrhage, sometimes obvious to the naked eye, are also seen microscopically.

The 5–10% of leiomyosarcomata which arise from a fibroid have a better prognosis than those which originate in normal myometrium. This is especially true if the surrounding muscle is not involved. Some 20% of patients are nulliparous. A history of pelvic irradiation is uncommon (5%) and the majority of patients present with menometrorrhagia or postmenopausal bleeding. Other presenting symptoms include vaginal discharge, pelvic pain or pressure and weight loss. Rarely, a sarcoma is detected when fibroids enlarge rapidly. In over 80% of cases the diagnosis is not made until hysterectomy is performed, with the remainder being detected on curettage.

In those patients in whom a pre-operative diagnosis is made, the treatment of choice is total abdominal hysterectomy and bilateral salpingo-oophorectomy. Washings from the pelvis should be taken. Given the propensity for leiomyosarcomata to spread within the abdomen and to lymph nodes, a full staging procedure similar to that for patients with ovarian cancer and including pelvic and para-aortic lymphadenectomy is performed on fit patients.

The role of adjuvant treatment, either radiotherapy or chemotherapy, has not been accurately defined in patients with early-stage disease. Recurrences are more common with tumours with more than 10 mitoses per 10 high-power fields and in patients with positive washings or lymph node involvement. Adjuvant pelvic irradiation improves local pelvic control but does not influence survival. Although cytotoxic agents such as vincristine, actinomycin and cyclophosphamide in combination, as well as Adriamycin and DTIC either alone or in combination, have proven activity in advanced or recurrent cases, their use in an adjuvant setting has not been shown to improve survival in any randomized trials. Cisplatin is also active in these tumours.

Other myometrial tumours

Atypical smooth muscle tumours include leiomyoblastoma, clear cell leiomyoma and epithelioid leiomyoma. The majority of patients are premenopausal and present with irregular bleeding, pain and abdominal distension. The diagnosis is usually made following hysterectomy. Recurrences occur in approximately 10% of cases and are more likely when the mitotic count is more than one per 10 high-power fields.

Intravenous leiomyomatosis refers to the rare situation in which there are fibrous growths into uterine veins and beyond. Again, most women are premenopausal and these growths may be oestrogen-dependent. Occasionally the major veins are involved and a direct surgical approach offers the best chance of cure. Benign metastasizing leiomyoma is similar but venous infiltration is absent and nodules are usually found in the pulmonary circulation. Progression is more common in the younger patient and respiratory failure may ensue. Again, oestrogen dependence has been suggested. Leiomyomatosis peritonealis disseminata occurs in premenopausal women, often with a history of oral contraceptive use and in up to 50% cases associated with pregnancy. The condition is marked by the presence of small nodules arising from the visceral and parietal peritoneal surfaces, and treatment is usually by surgical excision, although hormonal manipulation may be effective.

KEY POINTS

1. The overall 5-year survival is only 65.1% and, stage for stage, is similar to that of carcinoma of the cervix.
2. The incidence of corpus cancer varies markedly, not only from country to country, but between different racial groups in the one geographical area.
3. Most of the known risk factors for the development of this cancer share a common basis — excessive, unopposed oestrogen stimulation of the endometrium.
4. Postmenopausal bleeding is the most common presenting symptom as 75–80% of women with the disease are in this age group.
5. Over one-third of premenopausal patients present with heavy but regular periods.
6. Patients with endometrial tumour involving the cervix have a survival rate about 25% less than those with tumour confined to the corpus.
7. Clear cell tumours, serous papillary carcinomas and grade 3 tumours all have a poor prognosis.
8. The depth of myometrial invasion is an important prognostic indicator.
9. A surgical and pathological staging scheme has replaced the clinical classification.
10. Total abdominal hysterectomy and bilateral salpingo-oophorectomy is the treatment of choice for stage I disease.
11. Vault irradiation reduces the incidence of vault recurrence and is omitted only in superficial, well differentiated tumours.
12. External beam therapy is reserved for women with poor prognostic factors such as poorly differentiated tumours or deep myometrial invasion.
13. Stage II disease may be treated with radical hysterectomy or radiotherapy and the treatment of more advanced disease is individualized.
14. Isolated vaginal recurrent disease in the non-irradiated patient has a fair prognosis if treated with radiotherapy.

15. The value of adjuvant progestin therapy is not established.

16. Progestins given for recurrent disease produce a response in 15–20% of cases.

REFERENCES

Bean H A, Bryant A J, Carmichael J A, Mallik A 1978 Carcinoma of the endometrium in Saskatchewan 1966–1971. Gynecological Oncology 6: 503–514

Bickenback W 1967 Factor analysis of endometrial cancer in relation to treatment. Obstetrics and Gynecology 29: 632–637

Bokhman J V 1983 Two pathogenetic types of endometrial carcinoma. Gynecological Oncology 15: 10–17

Christopherson W M, Connelly P J, Alberhasky R C 1983 Carcinoma of the endometrium. V. An analysis of prognosticators in patients with favourable subtypes and stage I disease. Cancer 51: 1705–1709

Cowles T A, Magrina J F, Masterson B J, Capen C V 1985 Comparison of clinical and surgical staging in patients with endometrial carcinoma. Obstetrics and Gynecology 66: 413–416

Creasman W T, Morrow P, Bundy B W, Homesley H D, Graham J E, Heller P B 1987 Surgical pathological spread patterns of endometrial cancer. A Gynaecologic Oncology Group study. Cancer 60: 2035–2041

FIGO 1988 Annual report on the results of treatment in gynaecological cancer, vol 20. International Federation of Gynaecology and Obstetrics, Stockholm

Fortune D W, Östör A G 1987 Mixed müllerian tumours of the uterus. In: Fox H (ed) Haines and Taylor: Obstetrical and gynaecological pathology, 3rd edn. Churchill Livingstone, Edinburgh, pp 457–478

Gallup D G, Gable D S, Talledo O E, Otken L B 1989 A clinical–pathologic study of mixed müllerian tumours of the uterus over a 16 year period — the Medical College of Georgia experience. American Journal of Obstetrics and Gynecology 161: 533–539

Gambrell R D, Massey F M, Castayeda T A, Ugenas A J, Ricci C A, Wright J M 1980 Use of the progestagen challenge test to reduce the risk of endometrial cancer. Obstetrics and Gynecology 55: 732–738

Graham J 1971 The value of preoperative or postoperative treatment by radium for carcinoma of the uterine body. Surgery, Gynecology and Obstetrics 132: 855–860

Greer B E, Hamberger A D 1983 Treatment of intraperitoneal metastatic adenocarcinoma of the endometrium by the whole-abdomen moving-strip technique and pelvic boost irradiation. Gynecologic Oncology 16: 365–373

Hanson M B, Van Nagell J R Jr, Powell D E et al 1985 The prognostic significance of lymph-vascular space invasion in stage I endometrial cancer. Cancer 55: 1753–1757

Hendrickson M R, Kempson R L 1897 Pure mesenchymal neoplasms of the uterine corpus. In: Fox H (ed) Haines and Taylor: Obstetrical and gynaecological pathology, 3rd edn. Churchill Livingstone, Edinburgh, pp 411–456

Iversen O E 1986 Cellular DNA and steroid receptors in endometrial and ovarian carcinomas: clinical and prognostic importance. University of Bergen, Landsforeningen Mot Kreft

Katn L, Merino M J, Sakamoto H, Schwartz P E 1987 Endometrial stromal sarcoma: a clinicopathological study of 11 cases with determination of estrogen and progestin receptor levels in three tumours. Gynecologic Oncology 26: 87–97

Kneale B L G 1986 Adjunctive and therapeutic progestins in endometrial cancer. Clinics in Obstetrics and Gynaecology 13: 789–809

Kohorn E I 1976 Gestagens and endometrial carcinoma. Gynecologic Oncology 4: 398–411

Koss L G, Schreiber K, Moussouris H, Oberlander S G 1982 Endometrial cancer and its precursors: detection and screening. Clinics in Obstetrics and Gynecology 25: 419–461

Piver M S, Rutledge F N, Copeland L, Walster K, Blumenson L, Suh O. 1984 Uterine endolymphatic stromal myosis: a collaborative study. Obstetrics and Gynecology 64: 173–178

Poulsen H E, Taylor C W, Sobin L H 1975 In: Histological typing of female genital tract tumours. International histological classification of tumours no 13. World Health Organization, Geneva, p 64

Quinn M A 1989 Endocrine aspects of human uterine sarcoma. American Journal of Obstetrics and Gynecology 159: 88

Quinn M A, Campbell J J 1989 Tamoxifen therapy in advanced or recurrent endometrial carcinoma. Gynecologic Oncology 32: 1–3

Quinn M A, Ruffe H, Brown J B, Ennis G 1981 Circulating gonadotrophins and urinary oestrogens in post-menopausal diabetic women. Australian and New Zealand Journal of Obstetrics and Gynaecology 21: 234–236

Quinn M A, Kneale B J, Fortune D W 1985a Endometrial carcinoma in premenopausal women: a clinicopathological study, Gynecologic Oncology 20: 298–306

Quinn M A, Cauchi M, Fortune D 1985b Endometrial carcinoma: steroid receptors and response to medroxyprogesterone acetate. Gynecologic Oncology 21: 314–319

Rendina G M, Donadio C, Fabri M, Mazzoni P, Nazzicone P 1984 Tamoxifen and medroxyprogesterone therapy for advanced endometrial carcinoma. European Journal of Obstetrics, Gynaecology and Reproduction 17: 285–291

Rome R, Fortune D W, Quinn M A, Brown J B 1981 Functioning ovarian tumours in postmenopausal women. Obstetrics and Gynecology 57: 705–710

Stratton J A, Maurel R S, Rettenmaier M A, Berman M L, Di Saia P J 1989 Treatment of advanced and recurrent endometrial carcinoma: correlation of patient response to hormonal and cytotoxic chemotherapy and the response predicted by the subrenal capsule chemosensitivity assay. Gynecologic Oncology 32: 55–59

Thigpen T, Vance R, Lambeth B et al 1987 Chemotherapy for advanced or recurrent gynaecological cancer. Cancer 60: 2104–2116

Voupala S 1977 Diagnostic accuracy and clinical applicability of cytological and histological methods for investigating endometrial carcinoma. Acta Obstetrica Gynecologica Scandinavica (suppl) 70

39. Malignant disease of the vulva and vagina

W. P. Soutter

CARCINOMA OF THE VULVA

INTRODUCTION

Invasive vulvar cancer is an uncommon and unpleasant but potentially curable disease even in elderly, unfit ladies if referred early and managed correctly from the outset. If mismanaged, the patient with vulvar cancer is condemned to a miserable, degrading death. The surgical treatment appears deceptively simple but few gynaecologists and their nursing colleagues acquire sufficient experience of this disease to offer the highest quality of care for these women. All too often, an initial attempt at surgery is made and the patient referred for specialist care only after recurrent disease is evident.

There are about 750 new cases of carcinoma of the vulva each year in England and Wales and the annual incidence is approximately 3.1/100 000, making it about five times less common than cervical cancer [Office of Population Censuses and Surveys (OPCS) 1985]. The majority of these women are elderly; only 7.5% are less than 55 years of age and 78% are over 65 (OPCS 1985). With increased life expectancy this cancer will be seen more frequently.

AETIOLOGY

Little is known of the aetiology of vulvar cancer. A viral factor has been suggested by the detection of antigens induced by herpes simplex virus type 2 (HSV2) and of DNA from type 16/18 human papillomavirus (HPV) in vulval intraepithelial neoplasia and also by the association of a history of genital warts with vulval cancer (Brinton et al 1990). The significance of this viral association remains uncertain. The majority of genital condylomata contain HPV 6/11, not now considered to have any oncogenic potential and very few contain HPV 16, the type found in invasive lesions (Bergeron et al 1987).

ANATOMY

The gross anatomy is discussed in Chapters 2 and 27.

Lymphatic drainage

The lymph drains from the vulva to the inguinal and femoral glands in the groin and then to the external iliac glands. Drainage to both groins occurs from midline structures — the perineum and the clitoris — but some contralateral spread may take place from other parts of the vulva (Iversen & Aas 1983). Direct spread to the pelvic nodes along the internal pudendal vessels occurs only very rarely and no direct pathway from the clitoris to pelvic nodes has been demonstrated consistently (Iversen & Aas 1983).

PATHOLOGY

Most invasive cancers (85%) are squamous. Some 5% are melanomas and the remainder are made up of carcinomas of Bartholin's gland, other adenocarcinomas, basal cell carcinomas, and the very rare verrucous carcinomas, rhabdomyosarcomas and leiomyosarcomas.

In a third of cases of Paget's disease, there is an adenocarcinoma in underlying apocrine glands; these carry an especially poor prognosis (Boehm & Morris 1971; Creasman et al 1975).

NATURAL HISTORY

Microinvasive disease

The definition of microinvasion of the vulva has proved extremely problematical. The purpose is to identify a group of women with invasive carcinoma who could safely be treated with a less mutilating procedure than radical vulvectomy. Although it was initially suggested that up to 5 mm invasion into the stroma might be acceptable (Rutledge et al 1970; Wharton et al 1974), subsequent reports have suggested lower limits. Some have suggested 2 mm (Friedrich & Wilkinson 1982), others preferred 1 mm (Iversen et al 1981), while further reports emphasize the importance of lymphatic or vascular invasion and the degree of differentiation (Parker et al 1975) or confluence (Hoffman et al 1983). It seems that the safest course is to perform radical vulvectomy and groin node dissection in all cases with more than 1 mm stromal invasion and not to attempt to differentiate between superficial and deep nodes (Hacker et al 1984a; Monaghan 1985a).

Frank invasion

Invasive disease involves the labia majora in about two-thirds of cases and the clitoris, labia minora or posterior fourchette and perineum in the remainder (Cavanagh et al 1985). The tumour usually spreads slowly, infiltrating local tissue before metastasizing to the groin nodes. Spread to the contralateral groin occurs in about 25% of those cases with positive groin nodes so bilateral groin node dissection is required in almost all cases (Monaghan 1985a). Pelvic node involvement is not common (1.4–16.1%; Cavanagh et al 1985) and haematogenous spread to bone or lung is rare. Death is a long unpleasant process and is often due to sepsis and inanition or haemorrhage. Uraemia from bilateral ureteric obstruction may supervene first. Such is the abject misery of this demise that all patients with resectable vulvar lesions should be offered surgery regardless of their age and general condition.

CLINICAL STAGING

The FIGO classification is shown in Table 39.1. In spite of the apparent limitations of this classification, it does give a reasonable guide to the prognosis. The main drawback was reliance on clinical palpation of the groin nodes which is notoriously inaccurate (Monaghan 1985a). Now that the surgical findings are incorporated in the staging evaluation the prognostic value of stage is greatly improved.

Table 39.1 The FIGO staging of vulvar cancer

Stage	Definition
Stage I	Confined to vulva and/or perineum, 2 cm or less maximum diameter. Groin nodes not palpable.
Stage II	Confined to vulva and/or perineum, more than 2 cm maximum diameter. Groin nodes not palpable.
Stage III	Extends beyond the vulva–vagina, lower urethra or anus; or unilateral regional lymph node metastasis.
Stage IVa	Involves the mucosa of rectum or bladder; upper urethra; or pelvic bone; and/or bilateral regional lymph node metastases.
IVb	Any distant metastasis including pelvic lymph node.

DIAGNOSIS AND ASSESSMENT

Most patients with invasive disease (71%) complain of irritation or pruritus and 57% note a vulvar mass or ulcer (Monaghan 1985a). It is usually not until the mass appears that medical advice is sought. Bleeding (28%) and discharge (23%) are less common presentations (Monaghan 1985a). One of the major problems in invasive vulvar cancer is the delay between the first appearance of symptoms and referral for a gynaecological opinion. This is only partly due to the patient's reluctance to attend. In many cases the doctor fails to recognize the gravity of the lesion and prescribes topical therapy, sometimes without examining the woman. Delays of over 12 months are common, occurring in 33% of a large series collected in Florida (Cavanagh et al 1985).

Because of the multicentric nature of female lower genital tract cancer (Hammond & Monaghan 1983), the investigation of a patient with vulvar cancer should include inspection of the cervix and cervical cytology. The groin nodes must be palpated carefully and any suspicious nodes sampled by fine-needle aspiration. A chest X-ray is always required but an intravenous pyelography or lymphangiography may sometimes be helpful. Thorough examination under anaesthesia and a full-thickness, generous biopsy are the most important investigations. The examination should note particularly the size and distribution of the primary lesion, especially the involvement of the urethra or anus, and secondary lesions in the vulval or perineal skin must be sought. The groin should be re-examined under general anaesthesia as previously undetected nodes may be palpated at that time.

TREATMENT

Surgery

With the uncertainty about the criteria for microinvasion already discussed, there is no general agreement as to the best line of management for early invasive disease. The groin node dissection may be omitted and surgery restricted to wide local excision in carefully selected cases with invasion less than 1 mm (Hacker et al 1984a).

In all other cases, a radical removal of the affected vulva with wide margins on both the skin and subcutaneous edges is required. This is combined with complete removal of the groin nodes by incising through the fascia covering the sartorius muscle and dissecting this off the femoral vessels from the inguinal ligament to the apex of the femoral triangle caudally and the aponeurosis of gracilis longus medially. There is little value in performing a pelvic node dissection as this probably has no therapeutic value (Shimm et al 1986) and as radiation therapy to the groins and pelvis gives superior results when the groin nodes are involved (Homesley et al 1986).

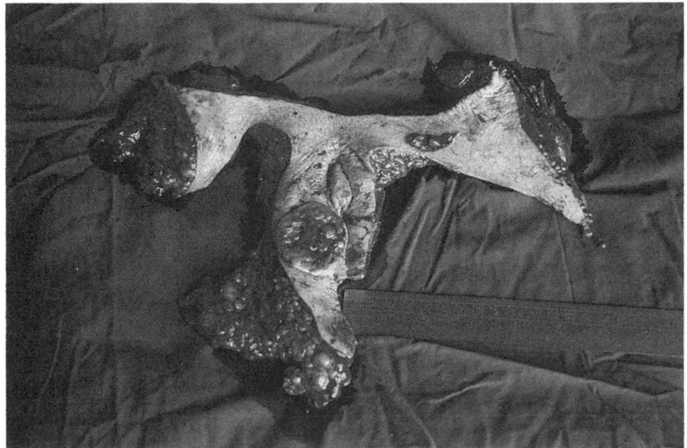

Fig. 39.1 A specimen from a radical vulvectomy and groin node dissection en bloc using a modified incision removing a minimum of skin from the groins. Note the large amount of subcutaneous tissue removed from the vulva seen on the right.

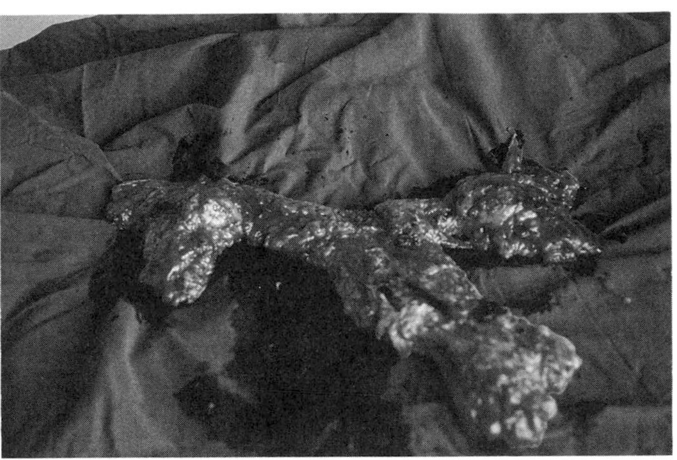

Fig. 39.2 The radical vulvectomy specimen seen from behind, showing the extent of subcutaneous tissue removed.

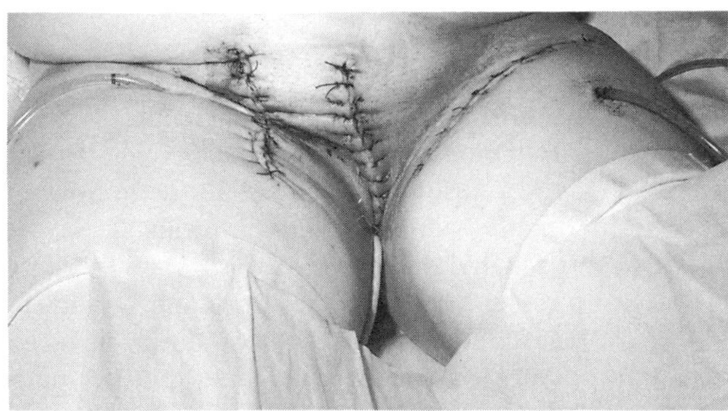

Fig. 39.3 In this patient, separate linear groin incisions were used. The incision in the left groin was made parallel to the inguinal ligament. In the right groin, a vertical incision was used to give better access. The patient was discharged on the 18th postoperative day with the wounds well healed.

Formerly, the groin nodes and vulva were removed en bloc with a wide excision of skin from the groin. The result was greatly delayed healing. By using a modified incision, the same objectives can be accomplished without the removal of large areas of normal skin and with the enormous benefit that primary closure can be achieved in nearly all cases (Figs 39.1 and 39.2; Monaghan 1985a, 1986). A further refinement aimed at reducing still further the problems of wound healing is the use of separate groin incisions for stage I–II cases (Fig. 39.3; Hacker et al 1981). However, care needs to be taken in undercutting the skin edges to leave sufficient subcutaneous fat to provide a blood supply for the skin without, on the other hand, leaving superficial nodes in situ.

Complications

The most common complication is wound breakdown and infection. With the modified surgical technique referred to above, this is seldom more than a minor problem. Conservative therapy with Eusol and liquid honey packs is all that is required. Osteitis pubis is a rare but very serious complication that requires intensive and prolonged antibiotic therapy. Thromboembolic disease is always a greatly feared complication of pelvic surgery for malignant disease but the combination of peroperative epidural analgesia to ensure good venous return with subcutaneous heparin begun post-operatively seems to reduce this risk (Monaghan 1985a). Secondary haemorrhage occurs from time to time. Leg oedema may be expected in about 30% of women (Hacker et al 1981). Numbness and paraesthesia over the anterior thigh are common due to the division of small cutaneous branches of the femoral nerve. Loss of body image and impaired sexual function undoubtedly occur but patients' responses to surgery are enormously variable and probably dependent on their upbringing and attitudes to life.

The role of radiotherapy

Radiotherapy is effective in the management of women with positive groin nodes. Homesley et al (1986) recommend 45–50 Gy in 1.8–2.0 Gy fractions to the midplane of the pelvis in opposed anterior and posterior fields. The dose is measured halfway between the superior border of the obturator foramen and the L5–S1 junction. In addition, 45–50 Gy, measured 2–3 cm from the anterior surface, is given to the centre of the inguinal and femoral nodes. Using this technique, both the time to recurrence and the survival were improved, especially when more than one node was involved. Radiotherapy may also have a role to play in shrinking large vulvar tumours prior to surgery that would otherwise require exenterative therapy (Acosta et al 1978; Hacker et al 1984b).

Interstitial therapy may have a small role in the palliation of recurrent disease. If a local recurrence is delayed for more than 2 years the prognosis is much better and a second surgical attempt may be valuable (Shimm et al 1986). Chemotherapy has little to offer in this situation (Thigpen et al 1986) but bleomycin may have some activity (Deppe et al 1979).

Results

With negative groin nodes, the 5-year survival rates for invasive cancer of the vulva range from 69 to 100% (Cavanagh et al 1985; Monaghan 1985a). When the groin nodes are positive the survival rates fall to 21–55% (Cavanagh et al 1985, Monaghan 1985a). Positive pelvic nodes, which are much less common, carry a much worse prognosis with a 5-year survival in the region of 20% (Cavanagh et al 1985).

UNCOMMON TUMOURS OF THE VULVA

Melanoma

Approximately 5% of melanomas in women occur on the vulva and it is the second most common carcinoma of the vulva (Monaghan & Hammond 1984; Morrow & DiSaia 1976). Melanin production is variable and the lesions range from black to completely amelanotic. The most usual presenting complaint is of a lump or an enlarging mole. Pruritus and bleeding are less common.

The prognosis is strongly related to the depth of invasion (Clark et al 1969; Breslow 1970; Podratz et al 1983). Because of the absence of a well defined papillary dermis in much of the vulvar skin, levels of invasion as defined by Clark and co-workers (1969) are unsuitable for use on vulvar skin (Chung et al 1975) and measurement of the thickness of the lesion as suggested by Breslow (1970) may be more reproducible. No patient from the Sloan–Kettering series died with a lesion with less than 1 mm penetration but thereafter the outlook was bleak (Chung et al 1975).

Local invasion occurs in an outward direction as well as downward so excision margins must be very wide, 3–5 cm being suggested for all but the most superficial lesions (White & Polk 1986). Approximately one-third of patients have inguinal lymph node metastases at presentation and 2.6% have distant spread (Morrow & DiSaia 1976). When the nodes are negative the 5-year survival is approximately 56%, falling to 14% when the nodes are positive (Morrow & DiSaia 1976). Involvement of urethra or vagina or the presence of satellite lesions all worsen the prognosis.

It is probable that the minimum therapy should be wide local excision — this usually requires a radical vulvectomy — without lymphadenectomy unless there is clinical evidence of groin disease (White & Polk 1986; Davidson et al 1987). If the groin nodes are removed, the operation should be performed en bloc rather than through separate incisions because of the melanoma's propensity to spread unseen by lateral intradermal infiltration (Karlen et al 1975). Radiation therapy is ineffective (White & Polk 1986) and adjuvant chemotherapy and immunotherapy have no proven value. Chemotherapy has not proved effective in the treatment of recurrent disease (Seeger et al 1986).

Verrucous carcinoma

This slowly growing neoplasm is seen rarely on the vulva (Gallousis 1972; Isaacs 1976). Both macroscopically and histologically it resembles condyloma acuminata and the diagnosis can be difficult. Generous biopsies are required to provide sufficient material for the pathologist. The treatment is surgery, usually a radical vulvectomy but very occasionally wide local excision. The place of lymph-adenectomy is debatable as lymph node metastases are uncommon. Radiotherapy is ineffective and may result in anaplastic transformation (Kraus & Perez-Mesa 1966).

Basal cell carcinoma

This tumour is rarely found on the vulva. Wide local excision gives excellent results.

Bartholin's gland carcinoma

Usually an adenocarcinoma, this tumour may be squamous, transitional cell type, or even mixed squamous and adenocarcinoma (Cavanagh et al 1985). It has often spread widely to pelvic and groin nodes before the diagnosis is made. It must be distinguished from adenoid cystic carcinoma which is similar to the tumour found in salivary glands and which seldom gives rise to metastatic disease (Webb et al 1984; Cavanagh et al 1985). The treatment is surgery but, because of its deep origin, part of the vagina, levatores ani and the ischiorectal fat must be removed.

Sarcoma

This is a particularly rare tumour. Leiomyosarcomata may be difficult to distinguish from their benign counterpart histologically but the presence of more than 10 mitoses per high power field serves to differentiate the two. These tumours tend to grow slowly and metastasize late. In contrast, rhabdomyosarcomata are rapidly growing, aggressive tumours. A radical vulvectomy and groin node dissection is the usual treatment but local recurrence is common and haematogenous spread is unaffected by this treatment (DiSaia et al 1971; Cavanagh et al 1985).

CONCLUSIONS

The main problems with carcinoma of the vulva are delay in presentation and diagnosis, and inadequate initial therapy. Surgery remains the cornerstone of treatment but, in carefully selected cases, this can be made less extensive than in the past. Even when radical surgery is necessary, new techniques have reduced the morbidity enormously. Radiotherapy has an important role to play in the treatment of patients with metastatic groin node disease.

CARCINOMA OF THE VAGINA

INTRODUCTION

Invasive vaginal cancer is rare. With 184 cases in England and Wales in 1981, the incidence was 0.7/100 000 women (OPCS 1985). However, like the cervix, the vagina has a range of premalignant lesions, many of which may be previously unrecognized extensions of cervical abnormalities. Coincident with the rise in prevalence of cervical intraepithelial neoplasia (CIN) is an increase in the frequency with which vaginal intraepithelial neoplasia (VAIN) is seen.

AETIOLOGY

Irritation, immunosuppression, infection

There is little firm evidence of aetiological agents. The irritation caused by procidentia and vaginal pessaries has been suggested but this is an infrequent association (Al-Kurdi & Monaghan 1981; Benedet et al 1983). A field effect in the lower genital tract has been suggested by the observation of multicentric neoplasia involving cervix, vagina and vulva (Hernandez-Linares et al 1980; Weed et al 1983) and both immunosuppression and infection with HPV have been impugned (Weed et al 1983; Carson et al 1986).

Radiation-induced vaginal cancer

The aetiological role of radiotherapy is hard to determine but is no longer simply a theoretical question in view of the proposal that preinvasive disease of the vaginal vault after hysterectomy should be treated by radiotherapy (Woodman et al 1988).

The evidence suggesting radiation induces vaginal cancers

Three studies have raised a concern that young women, less than 40 years old, treated with radiotherapy for cervical cancer may be at a high risk of subsequently developing vaginal cancer 10 to 40 years later. A high proportion of those women who developed a primary vaginal cancer after radiotherapy for cervical cancer were less than 40 years of age when treated for the first cancer (Barrie & Brunschwig 1970; Choo & Anderson 1982). Futoran & Nolan (1976) reported the appearance of a primary vaginal cancer in 8 of 42 women treated with radiotherapy for stage I cervical cancer when less than 40 years of age and followed for 10 years or more.

The evidence for the defence

However, only 50 (1.54%) of 3239 patients treated for cervical cancer, most with radiotherapy, subsequently developed a primary vaginal neoplasm and only 29 of these had invasive lesions (Choo & Anderson 1982). Furthermore, an international collaborative study of cancer registers recorded only 48 cancers of the vagina or vulva (ICD7-176) in 25 995 women treated with radiotherapy for cervical cancer and followed for 10 or more years (Boice et al 1985). The proportion of women treated with surgery and followed for 10 or more years and who were recorded as developing a vaginal or vulval cancer was similar (7 of 5125) to that seen following radiotherapy. These data suggest that if vaginal cancer is induced by radiotherapy it is a very rare event.

Diethylstilboestrol

For some time the prevalence of clear cell adenocarcinoma of the vagina was thought to be increased by intrauterine exposure to diethylstilboestrol (Herbst et al 1971). With the accrual of more information the risks now seem to be very low and lie between 0.1 and 1.0 per 1000 (Coppleson 1984; Herbst 1984). While vaginal adenosis and minor anatomical abnormalities of no significance (e.g. cervical cockscomb) are common following intrauterine diethylstilboestrol exposure the only lesion of any significance that is seen more commonly is CIN (Robboy et al 1984). Uterine malformations may be more common and may result in impaired fecundity in a small minority of cases.

ANATOMY

The anatomy of the vagina is described in Chapters 2 and 27.

PATHOLOGY

The great majority (92%) of primary vaginal cancers are squamous. Clear cell adenocarcinomas, malignant melanomas, embryonal rhabdomyosarcomas and endodermal sinus tumours are the commonest of the small number of other tumours seen very rarely in the vagina. These are discussed separately.

NATURAL HISTORY

Although the upper vagina is the commonest site for invasive disease, about 25–30% is confined to the lower vagina, usually the anterior wall (Pride et al 1979; Monaghan 1985b; Gallup et al 1987). Squamous vaginal cancer spreads by local invasion initially. Lymphatic spread occurs by tumour embolization to the pelvic nodes from the upper vagina and to both pelvic and inguinal nodes from the lower vagina (Monaghan 1985b). Haematogenous spread is unusual.

CLINICAL STAGING

The modified clinical staging suggested by Perez and colleagues (1973) has been widely adopted (Table 39.2).

Table 39.2 Modified FIGO staging of vaginal cancer

Stage	Definition
Stage 0	Intraepithelial neoplasia
Stage I	Invasive carcinoma confined to vaginal mucosa
Stage IIa	Subvaginal infiltration not extending to parametrium
Stage IIb	Parametrial infiltration not extending to pelvic wall
Stage III	Extends to pelvic wall
Stage IVa	Involves mucosa of bladder or rectum
Stage IVb	Spread beyond the pelvis

DIAGNOSIS AND ASSESSMENT

Before making a diagnosis of primary vaginal cancer, the following criteria must be satisfied: the primary site of growth must be in the vagina; the uterine cervix must not be involved; and there must be no clinical evidence that the vaginal tumour is metastatic disease (International Federation of Obstetrics and Gynaecology 1963). To this list, Murad and colleagues (1975) would add that the patient should not have had any antecedent genital cancer. Choo & Anderson (1982) dissent from this view which they regard as too restrictive. In their series, 11 of the 14 invasive vaginal cancers following radiation therapy for cervical cancer occurred after an interval of more than 10 years, and 3 were of a different histological type.

The most common presenting symptom is vaginal bleeding (53–65%), with vaginal discharge (11–16%) and pelvic pain (4–11%) being less common (Pride et al 1979; Gallup et al 1987). The rate of detection of asymptomatic cancer with vaginal cytology varies greatly (10–42%) depending on the patient population studied and most of the disease thus detected is at an early stage (Pride et al 1979; Choo & Anderson 1982; Gallup et al 1987).

The most important part of the pretreatment assessment of invasive cancer of the vagina is a careful examination under anaesthesia. Colposcopy will identify coexisting VAIN and help to define the location of the lesion. A combined vaginal and rectal examination will help to detect extravaginal spread. Cystoscopy and proctosigmoidoscopy are indicated if anterior or posterior spread is suspected. A generous, full-thickness biopsy is essential for adequate histological evaluation. A chest X-ray and an intravenous pyelogram are the only radiological investigations required routinely but lymphangiography can help occasionally in stage II cases to determine the need for teletherapy. Transrectal ultrasound and magnetic resonance imaging can be used to define the size and extent of the lesion.

TREATMENT AND COMPLICATIONS

Radiotherapy

Invasive vaginal cancer is usually treated with radiotherapy. Early cases, stage I–IIa, may be treated entirely with interstitial therapy with ^{192}iridium. In the Hammersmith Hospital this is after-loaded into three concentric rings of stainless steel guide needles located by a specially designed template (Branson et al 1985). The two outer rings of needles are located in the paravaginal space by being inserted through the perineum under general anaesthesia. The inner ring is located in grooves on a vaginal obturator. The objective is to achieve a tumour dose of 70–80 Gy in two fractions, each over 72 h, 2 weeks apart. Cases with parametrial involvement receive teletherapy to the pelvis as for carcinoma of the cervix with a tumour dose of 45 Gy followed by interstitial or intracavitary therapy to a total dose of 70–75 Gy. The field may be extended to include the groins if the tumour involves the lower half of the vagina.

Complications of radiotherapy

Vaginal stenosis may occur and is more likely when advanced tumours are treated (Puthawala et al 1983). The overall prevalence of vaginal stenosis is 25–32% (Pride et al 1979; Puthawala et al 1983; Gallup et al 1987) and is an undoubted problem for sexually active patients. Mucosal ulceration, either immediate or delayed, can be a distressing complication but conservative therapy, sometimes aided by grafts, is usually effective. Approximately 10% of patients develop a fistula or other serious complication (Pride et al 1979; Puthawala et al 1983; Gallup et al 1987) and these are almost invariably associated with teletherapy for advanced disease (Pride et al 1979). Vesicovaginal and rectovaginal fistulae, and small bowel complications are especially frequent if previously irradiated patients are treated with radiotherapy (Choo & Anderson 1982).

Surgery

A stage I lesion in the upper vagina can be adequately treated by radical hysterectomy (if the uterus is still present), radical vaginectomy and pelvic lymphadenectomy (Ball & Berman 1982; Johnston et al 1983). Exenteration is required for more advanced lesions and carries the problems of stomata. However, surgery may be the treatment of choice for women who have had prior pelvic radiotherapy (Choo & Anderson 1982).

Table 39.3 Five-year survival rates for vaginal cancer

Stage	Perez & Camel (1982)		Kucera et al (1985)	
	n	% alive	*n*	% alive
0	15	90		
I	39	90	67	75
IIa	39	58		
IIb	21	32		
II			120	46
III	12	40	191	29
IV	8	0	83	19

RESULTS

Probably as a result of the small numbers of cases in the reported series, the 5-year survival figures described for stage I range widely from 64 to 90% and for stage II from 29 to 66% (Monaghan 1985b). The results of therapy in more advanced disease are less satisfactory with 5-year figures for stage III of 17–49% (Monaghan 1985b). Some of the best results in a reasonably sized series are quoted by Perez & Camel (1982) and the largest series reported is by Kucera and colleagues (1985) (Table 39.3).

CONCLUSIONS

Invasive vaginal cancer is a rare tumour more often seen in association with an antecedent cervical malignancy. Radiotherapy is the main treatment method. Interstitial therapy offers good cure rates in stages I–IIa with only a small risk of seriously impairing vaginal function. Teletherapy is added for more advanced cases. Previous pelvic radiotherapy greatly increases the risk of serious complications and individualization of treatment regimens is essential for the best results.

UNCOMMON VAGINAL TUMOURS

Clear cell adenocarcinoma

The relation of this rare tumour to intrauterine exposure to diethylstilboestrol is discussed under aetiology. The histology is characterized by vacuolated or clear areas in the cytoplasm and a hobnail appearance of the nuclei of cells lining the lumen of glands. Radical surgery or radical radiotherapy is required for invasive lesions. As most are situated in the upper vagina they may be treated as cervical lesions. Lymph node metastases and 5-year survival figures are equivalent to cervical cancer (Herbst & Scully 1983).

Malignant melanoma

Vaginal melanoma has a 5-year survival rate of only 7% (Lee et al 1984). Vaginal bleeding and discharge are the commonest presenting symptoms. The prognosis depends upon the depth of epithelial invasion. Radical surgery and radiotherapy are of little value if the lesion is deeply invasive because of its propensity to metastasize early by the blood stream. There is at present no effective chemotherapy.

Rhabdomyosarcoma (sarcoma botryoides)

Some 90% of these rare tumours occur in children less than 5 years old. They present with vaginal bleeding and a grape-like mass in the vagina. The appearance of cross-striations in the rhabdomyoblasts is characteristic of this tumour. The results of radical surgery are poor (Huffman

1968) but chemotherapy alone with VAC (vincristine, actinomycin D and cyclophosphamide) now gives 'cures' in 82% of cases (Raney et al 1983). Indeed, Dewhurst (1985) reported 7 alive and well out of a small personal series of 9 children followed for 4–19 years.

Endodermal sinus tumour

These very rare tumours may resemble rhabdomyosarcomata but histology shows a primitive adenocarcinoma. Most occur in infants under the age of 2. Although surgery used to be the mainstay of treatment with an occasional long-term survivor (Dewhurst & Ferreira 1981), chemotherapy with regimens used for this tumour in other sites may offer a hope for more long-term cures (Wiltshaw 1985).

KEY POINTS

1. The prognosis for vulval cancer is good if the lesion is treated adequately at an early stage.
2. Even elderly and relatively unfit ladies should be treated surgically.
3. Cases suitable for local radical excision must be chosen with great care — most will need radical vulvectomy and bilateral groin node dissection.
4. Radiotherapy should be used to treat the pelvis and groins of women with positive groin nodes.
5. Radiotherapy may have a role in treating large tumours prior to surgery — but this remains an experimental approach.
6. Radiotherapy rarely, if ever, causes a vaginal carcinoma.
7. The risks to diethylstilboestrol exposed women of vaginal cancer now appear to be very low indeed.
8. Early vaginal cancer is probably best treated with interstitial brachytherapy as this is often effective and coital function may be preserved.

REFERENCES

Acosta A A, Given F T, Frazier A B, Cordoba R B, Luminari A 1978 Preoperative radiation therapy in the management of squamous cell carcinoma of the vulva: preliminary report. American Journal of Obstetrics and Gynecology 132: 198–206

Al-Kurdi M, Monaghan J M 1981 Thirty-two years experience in management of primary tumours of the vagina. British Journal of Obstetrics and Gynaecology 88: 1145–1150

Ball H G, Berman M L 1982 Management of primary vaginal carcinoma. Gynecologic Oncology 14: 154–163

Barrie J R, Brunschwig A 1970 Late second cancers of the cervix after apparent successful initial radiation therapy. American Journal of Roentgenology and Therapeutic Nuclear Medicine 108: 109–112

Benedet J L, Murphy K J, Fairey R N, Boyes D A 1983 Primary invasive carcinoma of the vagina. Obstetrics and Gynecology 62: 715–719

Bergeron C, Ferenczy A, Shah K, Naghashfar Z 1987 Multicentric human papillomavirus infections of the female genital tract: correlation of viral types with abnormal mitotic figures colposcopic presentation and location. Obstetrics and Gynecology 69: 736–742

Boehm F, Morris J M 1971 Paget's disease and apocrine gland carcinoma of the vulva. Obstetrics and Gynecology 38: 185–192

Boice J D, Day N E, Andersen A et al 1985 Second cancers following treatment for cervical cancer. An international collaboration among cancer registries. Journal of the National Cancer Institute 74: 955–975

Branson A N, Dunn P, Kam K C, Lambert H E 1985 A device for interstitial therapy of low pelvic tumours — the Hammersmith Perineal Hedgehog. British Journal of Radiology 58: 537–542

Breslow A 1970 Thickness, cross-sectional areas and depth of invasion in the prognosis of cutaneous melanoma. Annals of Surgery 172: 902–908

Brinton L A, Nasca P C, Mallin K, Baptiste M S, Willbanks G D, Richart R M 1990 Case control study of cancer of the vulva. Obstetrics and Gynecology 75: 859–866

Carson L F, Twiggs L B, Fukushima M, Ostrow R S, Faras A J, Okagaki T 1986 Human genital papilloma infections: an evaluation of immunologic competence in the genital neoplasia-papilloma syndrome. American Journal of Obstetrics and Gynecology 155: 784–789

Cavanagh D, Ruffolo E H, Marsden D E 1985 Cancer of the vulva. In: Cavanagh D, Ruffolo E H, Marsden D E (eds) Gynecologic cancer — a clinicopathological approach. Appleton-Century-Crofts, Connecticut, pp 1–40

Choo Y C, Anderson D G 1982 Neoplasms of the vagina following cervical carcinoma. Gynecologic Oncology 14: 125–132

Chung A F, Woodruff J M, Lewis J L 1975 Malignant melanoma of the vulva — a report of 44 cases. Obstetrics and Gynecology 45: 638–646

Clark W H, From L, Bernadino E A, Mihm M C 1969 The histogenesis and biologic behaviour of primary human malignant melanomas of the skin. Cancer Research 29: 705–726

Coppleson M 1984 The DES story. Medical Journal of Australia 141: 487–489

Creasman W T, Gallacher H S, Rutledge F 1975 Paget's disease of the vulva. Gynecologic Oncology 3: 133–148

Davidson T, Kissin M, Westbury G 1987 Vulvo-vaginal melanoma — should radical surgery be abandoned? British Journal of Obstetrics and Gynaecology 94: 473–476

Deppe G, Cohen C J, Bruckner H W 1979 Chemotherapy of squamous cell carcinoma of the vulva: a review. Gynecologic Oncology 7: 345–348

Dewhurst J 1985 Malignant disease of the genital organs in childhood. In: Shepherd J H, Monaghan J M (eds) Clinical gynaecological oncology. Blackwell, London, pp 270–85

Dewhurst J, Ferreira H P 1981 An endodermal sinus tumour of the vagina in an infant with 7-year survival. British Journal of Obstetrics and Gynaecology 88: 859–862

DiSaia P J, Rutledge F, Smith J P 1971 Sarcoma of the vulva. Obstetrics and Gynecology 38: 180–184

Friedrich E G, Wilkinson E J 1982 The vulva. In: Blaustein A (ed) Pathology of the female genital tract, 2nd edn. Springer-Verlag, New York, pp 13–58

Futoran R J, Nolan J F 1976 Stage I carcinoma of the uterine cervix in patients under 40 years of age. American Journal of Obstetrics and Gynecology 125: 790–797

Gallousis S 1972 Verrucous carcinoma — report of three vulvar cases and review of the literature. Obstetrics and Gynecology 40: 502–507

Gallup D G, Talledo O E, Shah K J, Hayes C 1987 Invasive squamous cell carcinoma of the vagina: a 14-year study. Obstetrics and Gynecology 69: 782–785

Hacker N F, Leuchter R S, Berek J S, Castaldo T W, Lagasse L D 1981 Radical vulvectomy and bilateral inguinal lymphadenectomy through separate groin incisions. Obstetrics and Gynecology 58: 574–579

Hacker N F, Berek J S, Lagasse L D, Neiberg R K, Leuchter R S 1984a Individualisation of treatment for stage I squamous cell vulvar carcinoma. Obstetrics and Gynecology 63: 155–162

Hacker N F, Berek J S, Juillard G J F, Lagasse L D 1984b Preoperative radiation therapy for locally advanced vulvar cancer. Cancer 54: 2056–2061

Hammond I G, Monaghan J M 1983 Multicentric carcinoma of the female genital tract. British Journal of Obstetrics and Gynaecology 90: 557–561

Herbst A L 1984 Diethylstilboestrol exposure — 1984. New England Journal of Medicine 22: 1433–1435

Herbst A L, Scully R E 1983 Newsletter — Registry for research on hormonal transplacental carcinogenesis

Herbst A L, Ulfelder H, Poskanzer D C 1971 Adenocarcinoma of the vagina: association of maternal stilbestrol therapy with tumour appearance in young women. New England Journal of Medicine 284: 878–881

Hernandez-Linares W, Puthawala A, Nolan J F, Jernstrom P H, Morrow C P 1980 Carcinoma in situ of the vagina: past and present management. Obstetrics and Gynecology 56: 356–360

Hoffman J S, Kumar N B, Morley G W 1983 Microinvasive squamous carcinoma of the vulva: search for a definition. Obstetrics and Gynecology 61: 615–618

Homesley H D, Bundy B N, Sedlis A, Adcock L 1986 Radiation therapy versus pelvic node resection for carcinoma of the vulva with positive groin nodes. Obstetrics and Gynecology 68: 733–740

Huffman J W 1968 The gynecology of childhood and adolescence. W B Saunders, Philadelphia

International Federation of Obstetrics and Gynaecology 1963 Annual report on the results of treatment in carcinoma of the uterus and vagina, vol 13. International Federation of Obstetrics and Gynaecology, Stockholm, pp 25–27

Isaacs J H 1976 Verrucous carcinoma of the female genital tract. Gynecologic Oncology 4: 259–269

Iversen T, Aas M 1983 Lymph drainage from the vulva. Gynecologic Oncology 16: 179–189

Iversen T, Abeler V, Aalders J 1981 Individualised treatment of stage I carcinoma of the vulva. Obstetrics and Gynecology 57: 85–89

Johnston G A, Klotz J, Boutselis J G 1983 Primary invasive carcinoma of the vagina. Surgery, Gynecology and Obstetrics 156: 34–40

Karlen J R, Piver M S, Barlow J J 1975 Melanoma of the vulva. Obstetrics and Gynecology 45: 181–185

Kraus F T, Perez-Mesa C 1966 Verrucous carcinoma — clinical and pathological study of 105 cases involving oral cavity larynx and genitalia. Cancer 19: 26–38

Kucera H, Langer M, Smekal G, Weghaupt K 1985 Radiotherapy of primary carcinoma of the vagina: management and results of different therapy schemes. Gynecologic Oncology 21: 87–93

Lee R B, Buttoni L, Dhru K, Tamimi H 1984 Malignant melanoma of the vagina: a case report of progression from preexisting melanosis. Gynecologic Oncology 19: 238–245

Monaghan J M 1985a Management of vulvar carcinoma. In: Shepherd J H, Monaghan J M (eds) Clinical gynaecological oncology. Blackwell, London, pp 133–153

Monaghan J M 1985b Management of vaginal carcinoma. In: Shepherd J H, Monaghan J M (eds) Clinical gynaecological oncology. Blackwell, London, pp 154–166

Monaghan J M 1986 Bonney's gynaecological surgery, 9th edn. Baillière Tindall, Eastbourne, pp 121–128

Monaghan J M, Hammond I G 1984 Pelvic node dissection in the treatment of vulvar carcinoma — is it necessary? British Journal of Obstetrics and Gynaecology 91: 270–274

Morrow C P, DiSaia P J 1976 Malignant melanoma of the female genitalia: a clinical analysis. Obstetrical and Gynecologic Survey 31: 233–271

Murad T M, Durant J R, Maddox W A et al 1975 The pathologic behaviour of primary vaginal carcinoma and its relationship to cervical cancer. Cancer 35: 787–794

Office of Population Censuses and Surveys 1985 Cancer statistics — registrations. Her Majesty's Stationery Office, London, pp 27, 39

Parker R T, Duncan I, Rampone J, Creasman W 1975 Operative management of early invasive epidermoid carcinoma of the vulva. American Journal of Obstetrics and Gynecology 123: 349–355

Perez C A, Camel H M 1982 Long term follow-up in radiation therapy of carcinoma of the vagina. Cancer 49: 1308–1315

Perez C A, Arneson A N, Galakatos A, Samanth H K 1973 Malignant tumours of the vagina. Cancer 31: 36–44

Podratz K C, Gaffey T A, Symmonds R E, Johansen K L, O'Brien P C 1983 Melanoma of the vulva: an update. Gynecological Oncology 16: 153–168

Pride G L, Schultz A E, Chuprevich T W, Buchler D A 1979 Primary invasive squamous carcinoma of the vagina. Obstetrics and Gynecology 53: 218–225

Puthawala A, Syed A M N, Nalick R, McNamara C, DiSaia P J 1983 Integrated external and interstitial radiation therapy for primary carcinoma of the vagina. Obstetrics and Gynecology 62: 367–372

Raney R B, Crist W M, Maurer H M, Foulkes M A 1983 Prognosis of children with soft tissue sarcoma who relapse after achieving a complete response. Cancer 52: 44–50

Robboy S J, Noller K L, O'Brien P et al 1984 Increased incidence of cervical and vaginal dysplasia in 3980 diethylstilbestrol-exposed young women. Journal of the American Medical Association 252: 2979–2983

Rutledge F N, Smith J P, Franklin E W 1970 Carcinoma of the vulva. American Journal of Obstetrics and Gynecology 106: 1117–1130

Seeger J, Richman S P, Allegra J C 1986 Systemic therapy of malignant melanoma. Medical Clinics of North America 70: 89–94

Shimm D S, Fuller A F, Orlow E L, Dosoretz D E, Aristizabal S A 1986 Prognostic variables in the treatment of squamous cell carcinoma of the vulva. Gynecologic Oncology 24: 343–358

Thigpen J T, Blessing J A, Homesley H D, Lewis G C 1986 Phase II trials of cisplatin and piperazinedione in advanced or recurrent squamous cell carcinoma of the vulva: a Gynecologic Oncology group study. Gynecologic Oncology 23: 358–363

Webb J B, Lott M, O'Sullivan J C, Azzopardi J G 1984 Combined adenoid cystic and squamous carcinoma of Bartholin's gland. British Journal of Obstetrics and Gynaecology 91: 291–295

Weed J C, Lozier C, Daniel S J 1983 Human papilloma virus in multifocal, invasive female genital tract malignancy. Obstetrics and Gynecology 62: 83–87S

Wharton J T, Gallagher S, Rutledge F N 1974 Microinvasive carcinoma of the vulva. American Journal of Obstetrics and Gynecology 118: 159–162

White M J, Polk H C 1986 Therapy of primary cutaneous melanoma. Medical Clinics of North America 70: 71–87

Wiltshaw E 1985 Chemotherapy of ovarian carcinoma and other gynaecological malignancies. In: Shepherd J H, Monaghan J M (eds) Clinical gynaecological oncology. Blackwell, London, pp 215–238

Woodman C B J, Mould J J, Jordan J A 1988 Radiotherapy in the management of vaginal intraepithelial neoplasia after hysterectomy. British Journal of Obstetrics and Gynaecology 95: 976–979

40. Trophoblastic diseases

G. J. S. Rustin

INTRODUCTION

The spectrum of trophoblastic diseases extends from benign hydatidiform moles which usually resolve spontaneously to life-threatening choriocarcinoma. Virtually all patients are now potentially curable provided they are correctly diagnosed and the appropriate therapy is administered early enough in the course of disease. Only doctors in specialist centres gain adequate experience in treating these rare tumours. However with the incidence of hydatidiform mole ranging from 0.5 to 2.5/1000 pregnancies most obstetric units will see at least one case per year. A woman who has had a hydatidiform mole has approximately a 1000-fold greater chance of developing choriocarcinoma than one who has had a live birth. Continued awareness and education are required not just about the optimal management and follow-up of molar pregnancy but also so that choriocarcinoma developing after non-molar pregnancy is detected as early as possible.

PATHOLOGY OF GESTATIONAL TROPHOBLASTIC DISEASE

A World Health Organization scientific group (1983) clarified the clinical and pathological definitions of the various conditions that make up gestational trophoblastic disease. This term includes the diseases detailed below as well as two conditions which are not followed by malignant sequelae. These are hydropic degeneration — an aborted conceptus containing excessive fluid or liquefaction of placental villous stroma without undue trophoblastic hyperplasia — and placental site reaction — the presence of trophoblastic cells and leukocytes in a placental bed.

Complete hydatidiform mole

This term is derived from the Greek word *hydatis* meaning a drop of water and the Latin word *mola* meaning a mass. It is defined as an abnormal conceptus without an embryo, with gross hydropic swelling of the placental villi and usually pronounced trophoblastic hyperplasia, having both cytotrophoblastic and syncytial elements. The villous swelling leads to central cistern formation with a concomitant compression of the maturing connective tissue that has lost its vascularity. A classical mole resembles a bunch of grapes.

Partial hydatidiform mole

This is an abnormal conceptus with an embryo or fetus that tends to die early, with a placenta subject to focal and villous swelling leading to cistern formation and focal trophoblastic hyperplasia, usually involving the syncytiotrophoblast only. The unaffected villi appear normal and vascularity of the villi disappears following fetal death. Unequivocal choriocarcinoma has never been recorded after partial hydatidiform mole but chemotherapy has been given to some women because of metastases or elevated human chorionic gonadotrophin (hCG levels). Most studies suggest that complete is more common than partial hydatidiform mole.

Invasive mole

This is a tumour invading the myometrium and is characterized by trophoblastic hyperplasia and persistence of placental villous structures. It commonly results from complete hydatidiform mole and may do so from partial hydatidiform mole. It does not often progress to choriocarcinoma. It may metastasize, but does not progress like a true cancer and may regress spontaneously.

Gestational choriocarcinoma

This is a carcinoma arising from the trophoblastic epithelium that shows both cytotrophoblastic and syncytiotrophoblastic elements. It may arise from conceptions that give rise to a live birth, a stillbirth, an abortion at any stage, an ectopic pregnancy, or a hydatidiform mole. The lack of villous structures distinguishes choriocarcinoma morphologically from invasive mole. Over 50% of cases of choriocarcinoma are preceded by hydatidiform mole in most series.

Placental site trophoblastic tumour

This tumour arises from the trophoblast of the placental bed and is composed mainly of cytotrophoblastic cells. This accounts for the relatively low level of hCG associated with this condition. About one case of this tumour is seen for every 100 cases of invasive mole and choriocarcinoma. Pathologists may initially consider it as atypical choriocarcinoma. It was earlier called trophoblast pseudotumour of the uterus but the term 'placental site trophoblastic tumour' is now preferred because of the malignant behaviour reported in some cases. Complete surgical excision is the preferred treatment are these tumours are not as chemosensitive as choriocarcinoma (Lathrop et al 1988).

Gestational trophoblastic tumours

This term is used to denote those conditions that require more active intervention, usually chemotherapy, and includes invasive mole, choriocarcinoma and placental site tumours. The reliance on persistently elevated hCG levels for diagnosis and the frequent absence of tissue for histology make it often impossible to differentiate between invasive mole and choriocarcinoma, so the term 'gestational trophoblastic tumour' covers both diseases.

EPIDEMIOLOGY

The very high incidence of hydatidiform mole in Asia, parts of Africa and South and Central America may have been exaggerated by many hospital-based studies due to selection bias (Bracken 1987). Japanese population studies report an average incidence of about 2.5/1000 pregnancies, compared to a nationwide Chinese incidence of 0.78/1000 pregnancies. Studies in the USA report incidence rates from 0.5 to 1.08/1000 pregnancies, whilst a recent study from England and Wales showed an incidence of 1.54/1000 live births. Large differences in incidence in different racial groups have not been confirmed.

Studies from many countries show that the risk of hydatidiform mole increases progressively in women aged over 40, reaching almost 1 in 3 live births in those aged over 50. The risk is also slightly higher in pregnancies of those aged less than 15 years.

Increasing gravidity does not appear to increase the risk of hydatidiform mole. However a woman who has had a hydatidiform mole has a greater than 20-fold increased chance of having a further one; the rate for a second hydatidiform mole is 0.8–2.9% and for a third 15–28% (Bagshawe et al 1986).

A recent case-control study has suggested that low oestrogen levels may be associated with a disruption of normal ovulation and predispose to choriocarcinoma. Other reported weak associations include prior miscarriages, artificial insemination by donor, longer duration of smoking and reduced carotene intake. Oral contraception appears to be unrelated.

Genetics

Complete hydatidiform mole appears to result from fertilization of an egg from which the nucleus has been lost or inactivated. The chromosomal complement arises by androgenesis and there are no maternal chromosomes, although the mitochondrial DNA is of maternal origin (Lawler & Fisher 1987). In most cases the paternal contribution stems from a duplication of a haploid sperm or from two different sperm. The 10% of hydatidiform mole that are heterozygous do not appear to have a higher chance of progressing to choriocarcinoma than the homozygous ones. Although both homozygous and heterozygous cases of choriocarcinoma have been reported one would expect all cases of gestational choriocarcinoma to be androgenetic whilst non-gestational tumours showing trophoblast differentiation would contain just maternal chromosomes.

Genetic studies show partial hydatidiform mole to be triploid with one maternal and two paternal chromosome sets. It is thought to arise by dispermy. This genetic distinction is important as choriocarcinoma has never been shown to develop from a partial mole. Flow cytometry on nuclei prepared from fresh or formalin-fixed paraffin-embedded tissue is very useful in confirming the triploid nature of partial hydatidiform mole. Twin pregnancies with a hydatidiform mole and normal fetus occasionally occur and some of these pregnancies result in a live birth.

PRESENTATION

Hydatidiform mole

The great majority of hydatidiform moles are detected between 8 and 24 weeks of gestation with a peak around 14 weeks. Vaginal bleeding is the most common presenting symptom. Many women pass molar tissue mixed with blood clot per vaginam. A fluid like prune juice, consisting of old blood, may be seen. This blood loss can lead to severe anaemia, especially in malnourished women. Acute life-threatening haemorrhage can occasionally occur. The uterus is large for dates in approximately half the patients at presentation. Theca lutein cysts are also common. These cysts may cause abdominal pain due to torsion or rupture and commonly take up to 4 months to regress following evacuation. Pre-eclampsia and hyperemesis gravidarum are seen in about a quarter of these patients.

Clinical hyperthyroidism is uncommon although increased thyroid function may be detected biochemically. This is probably due to the high levels of hCG which is thyrotropic in bioassays. There is a correlation between hCG levels and endogenous thyroid function but only those with hCG levels over 100 000 iu/l are overtly thyrotoxic. The possibility of thyrotoxicosis must be mentioned to an anaesthetist prior to evacuation because of the danger of precipitating a thyroid crisis.

Symptoms due to uterine perforation, pelvic sepsis and disseminated intravascular coagulopathy can occur. Severe symptoms due to trophoblastic pulmonary embolization sometimes develop after evacuation but these usually resolve with supportive care. The major long-term risk after molar pregnancy is the development of either invasive mole or choriocarcinoma. In the pre-chemotherapy era the risk of choriocarcinoma after hydatidiform mole was estimated to be less than 3%. The risk of developing invasive mole depends upon the criteria used for its identification, but probably 90% of hydatidiform moles resolve spontaneously.

There are several factors which have been shown to be associated with an increased risk of gestational trophoblastic tumour. (Table 40.1). There is little relationship between histological grading of hydatidiform mole and subsequent clinical course.

Table 40.1 Factors increasing the risk of chemotherapy after hydatidiform mole

Factor
Pre-evacuation hCG level >100 000 iu/1*
Uterine size >gestational age*
Large (>6 cm) theca lutein cysts*
Maternal age >40 years*
Medical induction hysterectomy or hysterotomy[†]
Oral contraceptive before hCG falls to undetectable levels[†]

Factors *plus previous molar pregnancy, hyperthyroidism, toxaemia, trophoblastic emboli and disseminated intravascular coagulation were considered high-risk by Goldstein et al (1989); [†]considered increased risk by Stone & Bagshawe 1979.

Invasive mole and choriocarcinoma

Invasive mole is seen in the early months following the evacuation of hydatidiform mole and is only rarely recognized in the absence of such a history. Some centres diagnose invasive mole if the hCG level is still elevated at 8–10 weeks, giving an incidence of about 25%. Using high levels at 6 months gives an incidence of about 7%. A few cases of metastatic invasive mole with characteristic villi on histology have been seen in deposits in the lungs, cervix, vagina, vulva and even brain. Apart from problems associated with these metastases, the symptoms of invasive mole are due to the invasive trophoblast. These include vaginal bleeding, amenorrhoea, infertility, abdominal pain and symptoms resulting from uterine perforation (Table 40.2).

Histology is the only way of differentiating invasive mole from choriocarcinoma. The symptoms may be identical but whilst all invasive moles are preceded by a hydatidiform mole only about 50% of choriocarcinomas have a history of prior molar pregnancy. The remainder follow a live birth, stillbirth, abortion or ectopic pregnancy, which may have occurred up to several years previously. Choriocarcinoma occasionally presents in postmenopausal women.

Table 40.2 Differential diagnosis and distinguishing features

Diagnosis	Investigation
Molar pregnancy	
Pregnancy	Ultrasound
Abortion	Ultrasound
Partial hydatidiform mole	Histology, genetics
Toxaemia of pregnancy	Ultrasound
Hyperemesis gravidarum	Ultrasound
Ovarian cysts	Ultrasound, hCG
Invasive mole Choriocarcinoma	
Abortion	Ultrasound
Menorrhagia	hCG
Amenorrhoea, infertility	hCG
Metastases from any tumour	hCG Colour if superficial; histology (if safe); distribution: vagina and lung, common; bone and lymph nodes, rare
Pulmonary hypertension	hCG

hCG = Human chorionic gonadotrophin.

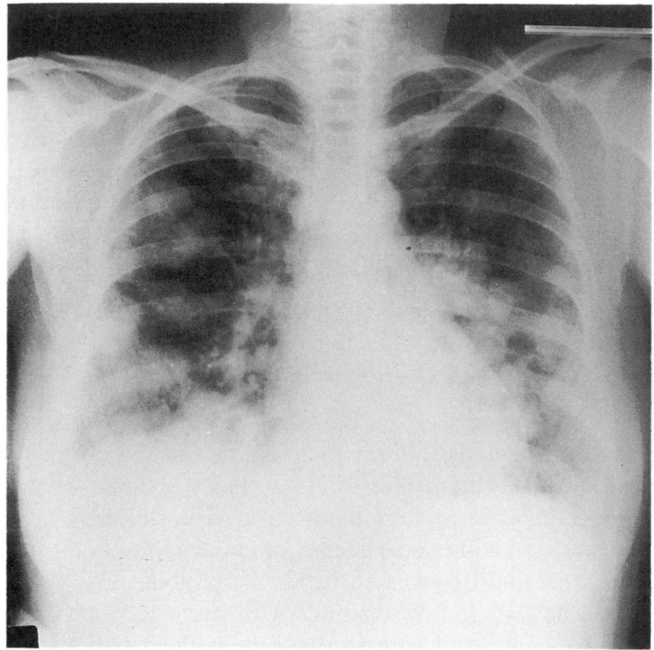

Fig. 40.1 Classical cannonball metastases in a woman with choriocarcinoma. Serum hCG should always be measured in a woman of reproductive age with such an X-ray.

Invasive mole can metastasize to virtually any part of the body. The commonest site is the lungs where it is usually asymptomatic (Fig. 40.1). Pleuritic pain and haemoptysis can occur due to tumour invasion or following pulmonary infarction. Dyspnoea is seen with more extensive metastases. Dyspnoea and signs of pulmonary hypertension can also result from the rare growth of choriocarcinoma in the pulmonary arterial bed.

The vagina is the next commonest site of metastases. Their great vascularity makes them appear densely reddened. They bleed easily and may be missed without careful visual inspection. Cerebral metastases may present suddenly as a cerebrovascular accident. Symptoms may be non-specific such as headache, fits or loss of consciousness or related to the site of neurological damage. Liver metastases are usually now discovered incidentally on scans. Purple skin deposits are sometimes seen. Lymph node and bone deposits are so rare that histological review is advisable.

INVESTIGATIONS

hCG estimation

In trophoblastic tumours hCG comes close to being the ideal tumour marker. It is a placental hormone that is secreted by the syncytiotrophoblast and serves to maintain corpus luteum function and preserve progesterone secretion during the early stages of gestation. In a normal pregnancy it can be detected about 5 days after conception and reaches its peak at 8–10 weeks of pregnancy. Although syncytiotrophoblast is the physiological source of hCG, an hCG-like substance has been detected in a wide variety of normal human tissues and low levels can be measured in normal human plasma.

The alpha subunit of hCG is nearly identical to the alpha units of thyroid-stimulating hormone, follicle-stimulating hormone and luteinizing hormone. The beta subunit shares many similarities with the beta subunits of other glycoprotein hormones, but the carboxyl terminal end contains unique amino acid sequences giving distinct antigenic characteristics. Immunoassays that utilize the intact hCG molecule as immunogen may be influenced by luteinizing hormone levels. A good assay detects down to 2 iu/l in serum.

Assays on urine are useful in the long-term follow-up of patients although the background noise on urine assays tends to be higher than in serum so that values up to the equivalent of 30 iu/l may not be significant. Urine estimations should be based on timed collections or be related to creatinine concentration. The preferred preservative for immunoassay is merthiolate (Thiomersal 100 mg per 24-h collection). Pregnancy tests will be positive in most patients with trophoblastic diseases but may miss some cases due to the lower sensitivity.

In an attempt to distinguish between normal placenta and trophoblastic tumours, many placental proteins have been investigated, including pregnancy-specific β_1 glycoprotein, human placental lactogen and inhibin. Their clinical value remains unclear.

Diagnosis and determining prognosis

Hydatidiform mole

In a woman thought to be pregnant, ultrasound scanning of the pelvis is the investigation most likely to confirm the presence of hydatidiform mole (Table 40.2). Hydatidiform

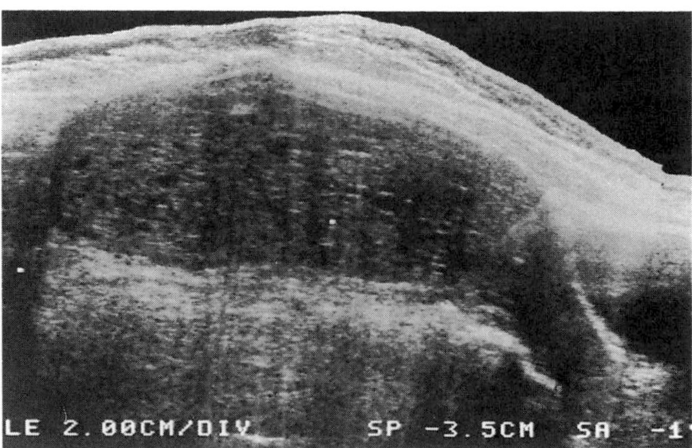

Fig. 40.2 Pelvic ultrasound of a woman with a hydatidiform mole showing the characteristic snowstorm pattern.

mole produces a characteristic pattern of echoes that appear like a snowstorm (Fig. 40.2). The presence of a live fetus must be excluded on ultrasound by carefully searching for a gestational sac and fetal heart. Large ovarian cysts are commonly visualized on the ultrasound and should be observed. It is advisable to demonstrate an elevated hCG level prior to evacuation. A chest X-ray should be performed to exclude trophoblastic emboli or metastases of invasive mole or choriocarcinoma. The products obtained at evacuation are usually the only tissue available for histology. Biopsy of vaginal metastases should not be performed as this frequently leads to profuse bleeding which may be difficult to control. A full blood count is required to check for anaemia and 2 units of blood should be cross-matched prior to evacuation. T3 and T4 should be measured prior to surgery if there is any suspicion of thyrotoxicosis.

Invasive mole and choriocarcinoma

Choriocarcinoma may be excluded by a normal serum hCG level (<2 iu/l). An elevated level could be due to pregnancy, residual placental elements, ovarian germ cell tumour, placental site tumour, trophoblast differentiation in a carcinoma (most frequently gastric), or ectopic production from a variety of different tumours. Non-trophoblastic tumours are rarely associated with hCG levels >1000 iu/l.

Histological confirmation of the diagnosis is not required if there is a history of a recent molar pregnancy, the hCG level is grossly elevated and the distribution of disease is typical of choriocarcinoma. Provided pregnancy has been excluded in patients with grossly elevated levels of hCG, even without a history of a mole, it is safer to treat them as choriocarcinoma than to risk biopsying a metastasis. Needle biopsies of the liver or other sites have resulted in fatal haemorrhage and delay in starting therapy whilst recovering from surgical biopsies allows the tumour to grow.

Clinical examination should include inspection of the vagina for metastases. The only routine staging investigations required are posteroanterior and lateral chest X-rays and pelvic ultrasound. Cerebrospinal fluid hCG should be measured if the patient fits into the high-risk prognostic group (see later) or has lung metastases and is in the middle-risk group. Cerebrospinal fluid levels of hCG that are more than 1/60 of the serum level indicate the presence of brain metastases, though a normal ratio does not exclude them.

A computerized tomography (CT) scan of the brain is only required if there is clinical suspicion of brain metastases or the hCG ratio is abnormal. Magnetic resonance imaging (MRI) should be performed if, despite suspicions of a cerebral metastasis, the CT scan is normal. MRI sometimes detects lesions missed on CT scan, especially in the posterior fossa. MRI is the investigation of choice if spinal metastases are suspected. CT scans of the chest will detect metastases missed on chest X-ray but in our experience have not led to a change in management and are not performed routinely. Scans of the abdomen are only performed if there is clinical suspicion of disease there. Pelvic arteriograms are rarely performed now except in patients who have severe vaginal haemorrhage after eradication of the mole. Radioimmunolocalization using radiolabelled antibody against hCG can locate drug-resistant deposits of tumour which may then be resected. This method of imaging can sometimes detect deposits missed on CT or ultrasound scans and may differentiate between viable and necrotic deposits (Begent et al 1987).

Prior to starting therapy a full blood count is required and renal and hepatic function must be assessed. Thyroid function should be measured. The blood group of the patient and her partner responsible for the most recent or molar pregnancy is required for the prognostic score (see later).

Staging

A staging system has been considered by the International Federation of Gynaecology and Obstetrics. This groups patients with a molar pregnancy as stage 0; lesions confined to the uterus without any metastases as stage I; lesions extending outside the uterus but confined to genital organs as stage II; lung metastases as stage III and other metastatic sites as stage IV. This staging system is not used by most major trophoblastic disease centres as it does not help in treatment planning.

Investigations for follow-up

Postmolar pregnancy

Following the diagnosis of a molar pregnancy, follow-up is essential to detect those women who require chemotherapy for invasive mole or choriocarcinoma. Follow-up relies upon measurement of hCG in serum or urine. The serum half-life of hCG is approximately 24–36 h. After a full-term normal delivery, serum and urine hCG become undetectable (<2 iu/l) within 10–20 days, but a small proportion of women have detectable hCG for longer periods. After a non-molar abortion, hCG takes a few days longer to become undetectable, partly because the level is higher early in pregnancy and possibly due to retained products of conception. Following evacuation of a hydatidiform mole in a series of patients who did not require chemotherapy, hCG levels were still detectable in 3% of women until 20–22 weeks following evacuation (Bagshawe et al 1986). However an early normalization of hCG suggests a shorter follow-up as, among 5124 patients, none of the 42% in whom the hCG level was undetectable by 7 weeks post evacuation required chemotherapy. Regular hCG estimations will detect a plateau or rise in hCG levels which would indicate persistence or growth of trophoblast.

A national follow-up service for hydatidiform mole patients has been in operation in the UK since 1972. Patients are registered centrally and then automatically sent boxes with prepaid returnable postage containing tubes and a letter requesting urine or serum samples be returned to one of three assay centres. It is recommended that hCG measurements be performed every 2 weeks until the limit of detection is reached, monthly during the first year after evacuation and 3-monthly during the second year. Measurements should continue for at least 6 months after the hCG has been undetectable because of the occasional late recrudescence. It is advisable to confirm that the hCG is undetectable for 6 months before starting another pregnancy.

hCG must be monitored after all further pregnancies because of the 2% chance of a second hydatidiform mole and the slightly increased risk of choriocarcinoma arising either from a subsequent mole or normal pregnancy. Follow-up is not necessary after hydropic degeneration because of the low risk of malignant sequelae, but when the diagnosis is in doubt, it is necessary to ensure that hCG remains undetectable in 3-monthly measurements.

Post chemotherapy

Our policy is to continue hCG follow-up for life because of the potential of choriocarcinoma to recur after several years.

Investigations for monitoring therapy

The close linear relationship between the number of choriocarcinoma cells present and the serum concentration of hCG allows for a more accurate assessment of response than for any other tumour. It is estimated that only 10^4–10^5 cells are required to produce a serum concentration of 1 iu/l. hCG levels can sometimes rise during the early days of drug therapy even though the tumour is chemosensitive. This is thought to be related to tumour lysis. Serum hCG levels should be monitored at least weekly during therapy.

A plateau above the normal range may be due to cross-reaction of the assay with luteinizing hormone if the patient has become menopausal. However a plateau or rising levels usually indicate drug resistance. Due to the accuracy of hCG monitoring repeat X-rays and scans are required only to confirm resolution of metastases or uterine or ovarian abnormalities at the end of treatment or to detect surgically resectable masses in patients with drug-resistant disease. Radiological abnormalities may persist for some time after the hCG has become normal before finally resolving.

TREATMENT

Evacuation of hydatidiform mole

Patients with clinical and ultrasound features suggestive of hydatidiform mole should have any significant blood loss replaced and the uterus evacuated by suction. Even a large hydatidiform mole can be evacuated with little blood loss. The need for chemotherapy after evacuation of hydatidiform mole is two- to threefold greater in patients who have undergone a medical induction, hysterectomy or hysterotomy compared with those whose hydatidiform mole has been evacuated by vacuum or surgical curettage or who have aborted spontaneously. If bleeding is severe after uterine evacuation, use of ergometrine is sometimes unavoidable. The single contraction produced by this agent appears to be less likely to produce embolization of trophoblast than repeated contractions induced by oxytocin or prostaglandin. Many gynaecologists perform a second dilatation and curettage routinely 2 weeks later or if there is persistent bleeding following the initial evacuation. Because curettage cannot remove invasive mole from the myometrium, further dilatation and curettages are of no value. Hysterectomy should be avoided because of the intense vascularity and high risk of uncontrollable bleeding.

We advise patients not to take oral contraceptives until hCG has been normal for 3 months after molar evacuation because of the increased chance of requiring chemotherapy found by us but not by some other investigators.

Prophylactic chemotherapy

Prophylactic chemotherapy following hydatidiform mole has been abandoned by certain centres because of unacceptable toxicity in women who had a high chance of never requiring chemotherapy. There is a suggestion from non-randomized studies that those patients who received prophylaxis had less chance of requiring subsequent chemotherapy than those patients not given prophylactic chemotherapy. Actinomycin D 12 μg/kg for 5 days following evacuation is advocated by the New England Trophoblastic Disease Centre for women who fit into their high-risk group following evacuation of hydatidiform mole (Table 40.1). The arguments for prophylactic chemotherapy are less persuasive in those centres which treat a considerably smaller percentage of their patients following a molar pregnancy. The major attraction of prophylactic chemotherapy is for those patients in whom follow-up is likely to be difficult.

Selection of cases for chemotherapy

Chemotherapy may be given because of persistence or complications of invasive mole; because choriocarcinoma has been diagnosed; or, in some centres, as prophylaxis to hydatidiform mole patients with the aim of preventing malignant sequelae. Criteria for treatment vary between different centres and it is often difficult to compare results between reported series. The World Health Organization Scientific group (1983) agreed that treatment should be started if any of the following applies after a hydatidiform mole:

1. High level of hCG more than 4 weeks after evacuation (serum level >20 000 iu/l; urine levels >30 000 iu/l).
2. Progressively increasing hCG values at any time after evacuation.
3. Histological identification of choriocarcinoma at any site or evidence of central nervous system, renal, hepatic, or gastrointestinal metastases, or pulmonary metastases >2 cm in diameter or >3 in number.

Persistent uterine haemorrhage with an elevated hCG is an indication for therapy in most centres. The major risk in delaying treatment in the patient with very high levels of hCG is uterine perforation. There is considerable disagreement about management of patients with persisting hCG levels. Some centres give chemotherapy to patients in whom hCG is detectable at a defined time, such as 8–10 weeks after evacuation. Others treat all patients who have a stationary hCG level for 2, 3 or more consecutive weeks. This results in approximately 27% of molar patients receiving chemotherapy. The policy at the Charing Cross Hospital since 1973 has been to allow the hCG to remain detectable for up to 4–6 months after evacuation as spontaneous disappearance of hCG can take that long. This results in less than 8% of molar patients requiring chemotherapy.

Surgery

Apart from evacuation of hydatidiform mole as discussed above, surgery has only a limited role. Uterine perforation is best managed by local resection of tumour and uterine repair. Hysterectomy may be required for persistent heavy bleeding but this usually settles on chemotherapy. Angiographic embolization may be used to control bleeding if uterine preservation is desired. Surgical removal of drug-resistant disease has a curative role in the rare patient in whom the disease is limited to resectable sites.

Elective hysterectomy has been used in the hope of reducing the need for or the duration of chemotherapy in patients not wishing to retain their reproductive potential. However, many such patients still require a full course of chemotherapy.

Prognostic scoring factors

The spectrum of gestational trophoblastic disease extends from persistence of a small focus of trophoblast in the uterus to widespread metastases. Obviously they do not all require the same intensity of treatment. Retrospective analysis has shown that various factors are related to survival (Table 40.3). To stratify treatment according to prognostic factors Bagshawe in 1976 devised a scoring system in which a weighting was applied for each factor. Each was assumed to act as an independent variable and their effects were assumed to be additive. This system, which defined low-medium- and high-risk groups, was used successfully in several centres. Over the years it has been simplified and Table 40.3 shows the system adopted by the World Health Organization. Between 1958 and 1982, of the 860 patients

Table 40.3 Scoring system based on prognostic factors

Prognostic factors	Score*			
	0	1	2	4
Age (years)	<39	>39		
Antecedent pregnancy	Hydatidiform mole	Abortion	Term	
Interval[†]	4	4–6	7–12	12
hCG (iu/l)	$<10^3$	10^3–10^4	10^4–10^5	$>10^5$
ABO groups (female × male)		O × A A × O	B AB	
Largest tumour, including uterine tumour		3–5 cm	>5 cm	
Site of metastases		Spleen, kidney	Gastrointestinal tract, liver	Brain
Number of metastases identified		1–4	4–8	>8
Prior chemotherapy			Single drug	2 or more

* The total score for a patient is obtained by adding the individual scores for each prognostic factor. Total score: <4 = low risk; 5–7 = middle risk; >8 = high risk.
[†] Interval time (in months) between end of antecedent pregnancy and start of chemotherapy.

treated for gestational trophoblastic tumours at the Charing Cross Hospital, 223 were in the high-risk group and 47% died; 232 fitted into the middle-risk group, of whom 1.3% died, and 405 fell into the low-risk group of whom 1 died from an intercurrent tumour.

Chemotherapy

Patients for whom chemotherapy is considered necessary require the care of a doctor well versed in the use of cytotoxic drugs, a subject which is beyond the scope of this chapter (see Ch. 33). The three drugs with the greatest activity against gestational trophoblastic tumours are methotrexate, actinomycin D and etoposide. 6-Mercaptopurine, vincristine, cyclophosphamide, cisplatin, and hydroxyurea also have proven activity. 5-Fluorouracil has been used successfully in China but not elsewhere (Song et al 1979). Primary drug resistance has been seen only rarely after methotrexate and actinomycin D but not yet after etoposide. Drug resistance developing during treatment is a problem, especially in patients with a high prognostic score (see above). The prognostic group must be determined so that patients at higher risk of developing drug resistance are given combination chemotherapy from the start.

Low-risk patients

There is general agreement that methotrexate followed by folinic acid is the preferred treatment for the low-risk group, provided renal and hepatic function are normal. The most proven regimen is given over 8 days (Table 40.4). To prevent relapse, treatment should be repeated every 14 days and continued until the hCG level has been undetectable (<2 iu/1) for about 6 weeks (Fig. 40.3). Provided patients drink at least 2 litres of fluid a day they are unlikely to develop mucositis. Apart from occasional cases of chemical pleurisy other side-effects are very uncommon. Of 347 low-risk patients treated at the Charing Cross Hospital between 1974 and 1986, all entered complete remission and only 1 died from intercurrent lymphoma (Bagshawe et al 1989). However 69 (20%) had to change treatment because of drug resistance and 23 (6%) needed to change treatment because of drug-induced toxicity.

Short infusions of higher doses of methotrexate are used in some centres but due to differences in patient selection it is impossible to compare results. Actinomycin D 1.25 mg/m^2 has been recommended but nausea, vomiting, alopecia, skin rashes and myelosuppression become problems with repeated courses. Etoposide cannot be recommended in this patient group as it invariably causes alopecia and its long-term carcinogenic properties are unknown.

Table 40.4 Low-risk regimen

Day	Treatment
1	Methotrexate (MTX) 50 mg i.m. at noon
2	Folinic acid (FA) 6 mg i.m. at 6.00 p.m. (30 h later)
3	MTX 50 mg i.m. at noon
4	FA 6 mg i.m. at 6.00 p.m.
5	MTX 50 mg i.m. at noon
6	FA 6 mg i.m. at 6.00 p.m.
7	MTX 50 mg i.m. at noon
8	FA 6 mg i.m. at 6.00 p.m.

Note: Courses are repeated after an interval of 6 days. Start each course on the same day of the week.

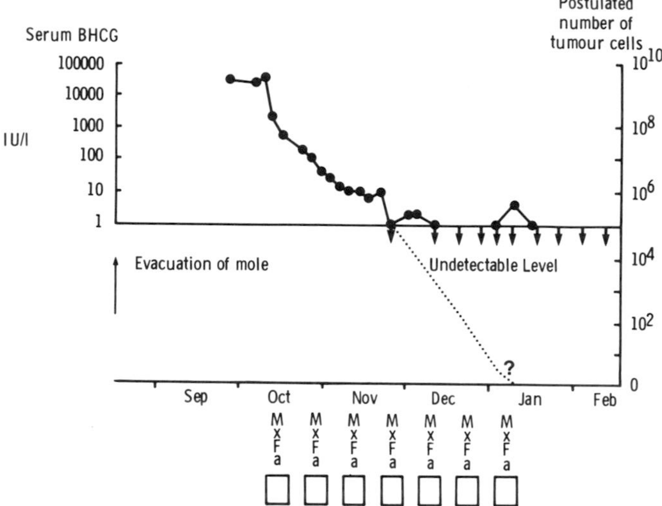

Fig. 40.3 Graph of hCG levels in a women who required low-risk chemotherapy with methotrexate (Mx) and folinic acid (Fa) because of high levels of hCG following evacuation of hydatidiform mole. If chemotherapy had been stopped when the serum hCG became undetectable, approximately 10^5 tumour cells were postulated to be still present. Cell numbers associated with the hCG level are shown on the right-hand vertical axis.

Medium-risk patients

This group was designed to introduce a range of drugs sequentially, reserving the more toxic high-risk regimens for patients with a higher score of adverse prognostic factors. Many centres divide their patients into only low- and high-risk groups and since the high-risk regimens have become less toxic this approach appears sensible. The middle-risk regimen is maintained at the Charing Cross Hospital because it allows for the introduction as a single agent of new drugs shown to be active in resistant patients. The

Table 40.5 Medium-risk patients: cycling regimen

Day	Drug	Dosage
Regimen A		
1 and 3	Etoposide	250 mg/m^2 in 500 ml 150 mmol NaCl i.v.
Regimen B		
1	Hydroxyurea	500 mg p.o. 12-hourly for 2 doses
2	Methotrexate (MTX)	50 mg i.m. at noon
3	Folinic acid (FA)	6 mg i.m. at 6.00 p.m.
	6-Mercaptopurine (6MP)	75 mg p.o.
4	MTX	50 mg i.m. at noon
5	FA	6 mg i.m. at 6.00 p.m.
	6MP	75 mg p.o.
6	MTX	50 mg i.m. at noon
7	FA	6 mg i.m. at 6.00 p.m.
	6MP	75 mg p.o.
8	MTX	50 mg i.m. at noon
9	FA	6 mg i.m. at 6.00 p.m.
	6MP	75 mg p.o.
Regimen C		
1–5	Actinomycin D	0.5 mg/day

Note: Courses are given in the sequence ABACA with intervals usually of 6 drug-free days between courses.

Table 40.6 EMA/CO regimen for high-risk patients

Course 1 EMA	
Day 1	Actinomycin D 0.5 mg i.v. stat Etoposide 100 mg/m^2 in 200 ml N/S over 30 min Methotrexate 300 mg/m^2 i.v. 12-h infusion
Day 2	Actinomycin D 0.5 mg stat Etoposide 100 mg/m^2 i.v. in 200 ml N/S over 30 min Folinic acid 15 mg p.o. or i.m. b.d. for 4 doses starting 24 h after the start of methotrexate 5 day drug-free interval to course 2
Course 2 CO	
Day 1	Vincristine 1.0 mg/m^2 i.v. stat (maximum 2.0 mg) Cyclophosphamide 600 mg/m^2 i.v. infusion over 20 min 6 day drug-free interval

If there is no mucositis, patients normally start each course on the same day of the week.
Note: Intervals between courses should not be increased unless white blood count $<1.5 \times 10^9$/l or platelets $<75 \times 10^9$/l or mucositis develops.
If mucositis develops, delay next course until it has healed. Continue alternating courses 1 and 2 until the patient is in complete remission or there is evidence of drug resistance.
N/S = 150 mmol NaCl.

medium-risk regimen, which is continued for 8–10 weeks after hCG has become undetectable, is shown in Table 40.5. At the Charing Cross Hospital 103 patients were treated in this group between 1973 and 1980. There have been 3 deaths, all due to drug resistance.

High-risk patients

Only 31% of patients in this group survived if given single-agent methotrexate (Bagshawe et al 1989). Several intensive multidrug regimens have been developed. These include CHAMOCA developed at the Charing Cross Hospital and MAC III used in Boston (Goldstein & Berkowitz 1982). Since 1979, patients in the high-risk group at the Charing Cross Hospital have received a weekly alternating regimen called EMA/CO (Table 40.6; Fig. 40.4). This regimen is given on the same day each week unless the total white cell count falls below 1.5×10^9/l or platelets below 75×10^9/l or mucosal ulceration develops. Of 27 patients who received EMA/CO as initial therapy, 93% survived and 1 patient relapsed; of 20 who received EMA/CO after prior therapy, 74% survived and 5 patients relapsed (Newlands et al 1986). In patients who develop drug resistance, cisplatin 75 mg/m^2 and etoposide 100 mg/m^2 can lead to a durable remission when substituted for the CO of EMA/CO.

In patients with extensive pulmonary metastases, deaths may occur due to respiratory failure, which can be exacerbated by too aggressive initial therapy. Ventilation or high-dose steroids have not been shown to be of any value in this situation so extracorporeal membrane oxygenation is now being assessed.

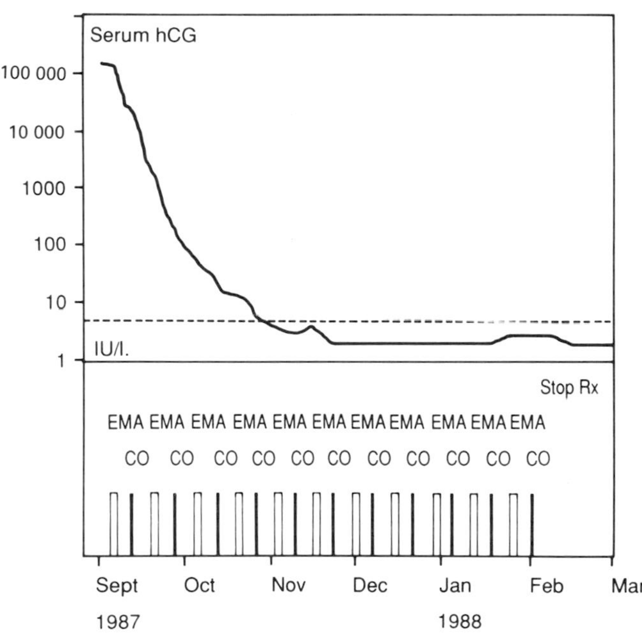

Fig. 40.4 Graph of hCG levels of a woman who required high-risk chemotherapy with EMA/CO for choriocarcinoma.

Central nervous system metastases

In countries without adequate hydatidiform mole follow-up and in patients presenting with choriocarcinoma following an abortion or term delivery there is an incidence of central nervous system metastases of 3–15%. Since 1980 we have used the EMA/CO regimen for these patients with the dose of methotrexate increased to 1 g/m^2 and 12.5 mg of methotrexate is given intrathecally with each course of CO. Of 18 patients who presented with central nervous system metastases 13 (72%) are surviving disease-free (Rustin et al 1989). Because of the vascular nature of these tumours and the 22% incidence of early deaths we now attempt early surgical excision to prevent intracerebral haemorrhage. Although radiotherapy has been used in other centres their reported results do not approach the 72% survival we obtained without radiotherapy.

LONG-TERM SIDE-EFFECTS OF THERAPY

Patients are advised against pregnancy for a year after chemotherapy to avoid confusing a further pregnancy with relapse and to reduce the risk of delayed teratogenicity. A study of 445 long-term survivors following chemotherapy showed that 86% of patients wishing to have a further pregnancy succeeded in having at least one live birth (Rustin et al 1984). The incidence of congenital abnormalities was not greater than expected.

The incidence of second-tumours has also been investigated. One case of myeloid leukaemia and one case of breast cancer were found in 457 long-term survivors followed for a mean period of 7.8 years (Rustin et al 1983). The expected number for this group of women would have been 3.5 second tumours.

ACKNOWLEDGEMENTS

The author wishes to thank Professor K D Bagshawe, Dr E S Newlands and Dr R H J Begent and his other colleagues at Charing Cross Hospital without whom this review would not have been possible. He is also indebted to the gynaecologists who have referred patients. The author is supported by the Cancer Research Campaign.

KEY POINTS

1. Virtually all patients with trophoblastic disease are curable.
2. Referral to specialist centres is essential.
3. The incidence is 1–2/1000 live births and is increased with increasing maternal age.
4. Hydatidiform mole usually presents with vaginal bleeding and amenorrhoea and the uterus is often large for dates.
5. Choriocarcinoma may present in a similar way but is notorious for its protean manifestations. Symptoms related to cerebral metastases may be the first sign of disease.
6. The diagnosis of gestational trophoblastic tumours is usually made by finding elevated hCG levels. Provided pregnancy is excluded, a histological diagnosis is not required.
7. Ultrasound is useful in the diagnosis of hydatidiform mole. A chest X-ray should be performed.
8. Cerebrospinal fluid hCG levels should be measured in high- risk cases and in medium-risk cases with lung metastases.
9. hCG levels should be monitored after every molar pregnancy for at least 6 months after they have become undetectable and again after every subsequent pregnancy.
10. Hydatidiform mole should be evacuated by suction and chemotherapy given if the hCG levels remain >20 000 iu/l more than 4 weeks after evacuation or if the hCG increases progressively.
11. Apart from evacuation of hydatidiform mole, surgery has only a limited role.
12. When chemotherapy is required, the regimen should be chosen according to the prognostic score.
13. Patients should avoid pregnancy for 1 year after chemotherapy. A large majority who wish to conceive again will be successful.

REFERENCES

Bagshawe K D 1976 Risk and prognostic factors in trophoblastic neoplasia. Cancer 38: 1373–1385

Bagshawe K D, Dent J, Webb J 1986 Hydatidiform mole in England and Wales 1973–83. Lancet ii: 673–677

Bagshawe K D, Dent J, Newlands E S, Begent R H J, Rustin G J S 1989 The role of low-dose methotrexate and folinic acid in gestational trophoblastic tumours (GTT). British Journal of Obstetrics and Gynaecology 96: 795–802

Begent R H J, Bagshawe K D, Green A J, Searle F 1987 The clinical value of imaging with antibody to human chorionic gonadotrophin in the detection of residual choriocarcinoma. British Journal of Cancer 55: 657–660

Bracken M B 1987 Incidence and aetiology of hydatidiform mole: an epidemiological review. British Journal of Obstetrics and Gynaecology 94: 1123–1135

Goldstein D P, Berkowitz R S 1982 Gestational trophoblastic neoplasms. W B Saunders, Philadelphia, p 143

Goldstein D P, Berkowitz R S, Bernstein M R 1981 Management of molar pregnancy. Journal of Reproductive Medicine 26: 208–212

Lathrop J C, Lauchlan S, Nayak R, Ambler M 1988 Clinical characteristics of placental site trophoblastic tumor. Gynecologic Oncology 31: 32–42

Lawler S D, Fisher A 1987 Genetic studies in hydatidiform mole with clinical correlations. Placenta 8: 77–88

Newlands E S, Bagshawe K D, Begent R H J, Rustin G J S, Holden L, Dent J 1986 Developments in chemotherapy for medium- and

high risk patients with gestational trophoblastic tumours (1979–1984). British Journal of Obstetrics and Gynaecology 93: 63–69
Rustin G J S, Rustin F, Dent J, Booth M A, Salt S, Bagshawe K D 1983 No increase in second tumours after cytotoxic chemotherapy for gestational trophoblastic tumours. New England Journal of Medicine 308: 473–477
Rustin G J S, Booth M, Dent J, Salt S, Rustin F, Bagshawe K D 1984 Pregnancy after cytotoxic chemotherapy for gestational trophoblastic tumours. British Medical Journal 288: 103–106
Rustin G J S, Newlands E S, Begent H J, Dent J, Bagshawe K D 1989 Weekly alternating chemotherapy (EMA/CO) for treatment of central nervous system metastases of choriocarcinoma. Journal of Clinical Oncology 7: 900–903
Song H, Z Xia, Wu B, Wang Y 1979 20 Years' experience in chemotherapy of choriocarcinoma and malignant mole. Chinese Medical Journal 92: 677–687
Stone M, Bagshawe K D 1979 An analysis of the influences of maternal age, gestational age, contraceptive method, and the mode of primary treatment of patients with hydatidiform moles on the incidence of subsequent chemotherapy. British Journal of Obstetrics and Gynaecology 86: 782–792
World Health Organization scientific group 1983 Gestational trophoblastic diseases. Technical Report Series 692. WHO, Geneva

FURTHER READING

Berkowitz R S, Goldstein D P, Bernstein M R 1984 Modified Triple Chemotherapy in the Management of High-Risk Metastatic Gestational Trophoblastic Tumours. Gynecologic Oncology 19: 173–181
Buckley J D, Henderson B E, Morrow C P, Hammond C B, Kohorn E I, Austin D F 1988 Case-Control Study of Gestational Choriocarcinoma. Cancer Research 48: 1004–1010
Rustin G J S, Bagshawe K D 1984 Gestational Trophoblastic Tumours. Critical Review in Oncology/Haematology CRC Press Inc. 3: 103–142

41. Supportive care for gynaecological cancer patients: psychosocial and emotional aspects

L. Goldie P. Robson W. P. Soutter

A woman suffering from cancer needs more than treatment for her disease if she is to avoid becoming a cancer cripple — a person whose life and personality are circumscribed by her disease. This applies equally to those who survive and to those whose life is shortened. Those who care for her must be prepared to stand by her in the mental and physical turmoil to come, helping her to tap those hidden resources that lie within us all. Such a prospect is bound to be painful for the carers but the rewards are great. This chapter aims to provide some guidance in the psychological support of women with cancer and their families, and in the control of symptoms in the seriously ill.

BEING TRUTHFUL

It is in the nature of gynaecological malignancies that the possibility of cancer is uppermost in patients' minds even before the investigations which confirm their worst fears. This is unlike cancer in other parts of the body where the patient can be unaware of the nature of her condition until told. Whether or not to be truthful in these circumstances is no longer an issue (Goldie 1982). The problem is how best to help the woman to cope with the knowledge of her disease and its implications. This should not be seen as a task that can be disposed of in one interview, nor should it be seen as the sole responsibility of one individual. Support will be required for an extended period of time, in a variety of different forms and from a number of different individuals, but the prime responsibility lies with the physician who is caring for her.

In order to deal effectively with this situation, a doctor must understand his or her own feelings and be aware of the natural devices he or she may use to avoid what is always a difficult duty and one for which no training has been given.

Until relatively recently it was common for patients not to be told that they had cancer. The diagnosis and prognosis were imparted to the nearest relative who was left with the unenviable responsibility of telling some, all or none of the truth to the patient and the rest of the family. This reluctance to inform the patient of the diagnosis may have stemmed from a genuine belief that she did not wish to be confronted with the truth. While that is the case for some, there are more who do want information about their illness (Hinton 1979). Indeed, it is almost impossible to administer cytotoxic chemotherapy or radiotherapy without the patient realizing the diagnosis. Not to talk openly about her illness with the woman denies her the opportunity of talking about her fears, many of which will be inappropriate anxieties about the possible effects of the cancer or the treatment.

More often the decision not to tell the truth (or totally to obscure it by euphemism) is a subconscious defence mechanism generated by the doctor. Firstly, he or she has no wish to provoke the emotional anguish that such grave news will bring and fears the outpouring of emotion which may follow. The doctor may feel in danger of being overcome if exposed to this emotional maelstrom. As a result, he or she tries to be emotionally detached. This carapace of cold professionalism prevents the doctor from responding to the patient's distress. By protecting ourselves from the possibility of failing or of saying the wrong thing, we doctors fail to discover our potential in such circumstances and do not grow as a person. Another mechanism for self-protection is to impart the bad news just before going to theatre or when late for a busy clinic. This provides an apparently valid excuse for not facing the inevitable emotional turmoil which ensues. These avoidance techniques may be subconscious or simply due to thoughtlessness.

This behaviour is entirely understandable. From the earliest years of their training student doctors are exhorted to know all the answers. Whilst they may be thoroughly trained in the various organic disease processes, little emphasis is given to the psychological and emotional dimensions of disease. Moreover, they may have little personal experience of tragedy because of their relative youth. When an operation or treatment has failed they may feel that they have failed personally.

BREAKING THE NEWS TO THE PATIENT

When there is a reasonable clinical suspicion of malignancy this possibility should be discussed as it is certainly uppermost in the mind of the patient. This is an opportunity to establish a relationship with the woman by talking about the potential diagnosis, the investigations needed and possible treatment. The majority of patients wish to know the truth and an honest, straightforward approach lays a basis of trust and openness from which the patient–doctor relationship can grow. Some women will wish to cope with this news by denial. They should not be assaulted with the truth but allowed to come to terms with the news in their own time.

Organizing the interview

It is important to allow sufficient time for these consultations. Although it is often difficult within the constraints of a busy clinic, arrangements should be made to prevent interruptions by bleeps, telephone calls or other people. When time has been allocated, the doctor will tend to indicate by body language that he or she has time to listen. No conversation of worth can be initiated by a doctor showing signs of impatience. Should it be impossible to provide a reasonable length of time (at least 20 minutes) then it is perhaps better to make a specific arrangement to see the patient again at the end of the clinic.

This may also be an opportunity to introduce the other member of the team who will be providing psychosocial help. This may be a specially trained counsellor, nurse, doctor or psychotherapist. Joint interviews can be helpful for the patient when the two staff members work in concert, but they are also useful for the staff who learn from one another.

Patients' frequent dissatisfaction with the explanations given to them may not be due solely to a failure of communication or lack of time. They may not retain the information or may even repress it when the content of the conversation is emotionally distressing. Hogbin & Fallowfield (1989) have suggested that tape-recording 'bad news' consultations and giving the tapes to the patients to take away with them may help in understanding the problem, in overcoming failures of recall and in explaining the diagnosis to their relatives. The fact that the consultation was recorded also had the effect that the doctor often attached more importance to the consultation than hitherto. However, this approach may prevent the interview from achieving the degree of privacy and intimacy which is necessary for a real interaction.

BACUP, the British Association of Cancer Patients (121-123 Charterhouse St, London EC1M 6AA; tel. 071-608-1661), provides a series of leaflets which explain simply the nature of different cancers and their modes of treatment. These are often very helpful for patients. Many areas also have local support groups to which patients can be referred.

Give the patient opportunities to ask

Simple questions such as 'Have I made myself clear?' or 'Is there anything I have not explained?' will give the patient a cue to speak. Clinicians should be conscious of their body language, avoid interposing large desks between themselves and the patient, and try to sit at the same level and maintain eye contact. If an authoritarian posture is avoided, patients will be more likely to express their fears and feelings.

Reply honestly to questions

The clinician should always be realistic and avoid giving false reassurance. At the same time, it is important not to deny the patient all hope. Encouraging a positive but realistic attitude will help. The importance of this stage cannot be emphasized too strongly. If the doctor forms an open and honest relationship when there is hope for cure, it will be far more acceptable and easier for the patient to accept his or her help if disease recurs or her condition becomes terminal.

Allow the expression of feelings

To do this effectively the doctor should empty the mind of any preconceptions about what may occur. This is difficult because a doctor is trained to deduce what will happen in a certain set of circumstances. A doctor may think that he or she knows what it feels like to be the patient and respond accordingly. The certainty with which misconceptions about the patient's state of mind are held is possibly the biggest obstacle to sensitivity. The nurse or doctor may be seeing only a reflection of themselves and may mistakenly attribute their own preconceptions and reactions to the patient. When doctors become ill themselves they often realise how mistaken they have been in their assumptions about how patients feel and their responses to treatment.

BREAKING THE NEWS TO THE FAMILY

The conspiracy of silence

Relatives often ask that the patient should not be told the diagnosis. This wish can sometimes be very strongly stated, occasionally amounting to an absolute veto. This view arises from a desire to protect the patient from this fearful news. Whilst doctors must always remember that their contract is with the patient rather than the relatives, some discussion will usually allow the relative to see the value of a more open approach.

Modern cancer treatment, involving radical surgery, chemotherapy and radiotherapy, can hardly be carried out without the patient realizing that she has cancer. Even if the medical and nursing staff collude with relatives to conceal the diagnosis, day-to-day discussion and comparison of treatments with other patients will usually result in her guessing the truth. If an open approach is not adopted it imposes an almost intolerable burden on the person who is fully informed. There is a tragic irony in the situation where the nearest relative has been told the diagnosis but tries to preserve a façade whilst the patient who has guessed the truth attempts to maintain a brave face for the benefit of her relatives. She then has to face alone the prospect of death and the relatives live separated from her by this conspiracy of silence. How much better to be able to discuss their fears with each other and to provide the close emotional support that they have shared in their relationship thus far.

Telling children

Children also need to be given information about their mother's condition to a degree which is dependent on their maturity. If she is frequently absent or not well enough to care for and play with them as she did before her illness, they may become excessively demanding, disobedient or show other signs of disturbance because they feel inexplicably rejected. Without reassurance, a child may feel responsible for its mother's illness and subsequent death. Many adults still bear feelings of guilt over how they treated their mother before her death. Frequently they were not told of the prognosis and now regret and resent the lost opportunities for giving her their time and love before her demise. Such unresolved guilt feelings often give rise to significant problems in personality and emotional adjustment in adolescents and adults. A child's understanding of illness and death, whilst not the same as an adult's, is often underestimated. Children can often accept the inevitable more easily than their elders.

PROBLEMS SPECIFIC TO WOMEN WITH GYNAECOLOGICAL CANCER

The gynaecologist should empathize with feminine attitudes to the menarche, menopause, menstruation and fertility. These attitudes will vary with age, social class and ethnic grouping. In younger women, gynaecological cancer may require treatment which produces sterility. Whilst an infertile woman may receive sympathy for her inability to conceive, a young woman who has had radical surgery or radiotherapy often receives no such consideration because survival from the malignant condition is considered paramount and her infertility may be disregarded as being relatively unimportant. Her sterility may affect her prospects of marriage or a current relationship. Women who have had children may not be unduly concerned about their reproductive abilities but still exhibit marked anxiety over their perceived loss of femininity and sexual function. The treatment of gynaecological cancer often produces a premature menopause and oestrogen replacement is sometimes mistakenly withheld.

The genital region is psychologically very special, being both exquisitely sensitive and primal in sexual arousal. A malignancy, literally something 'bad', in this area is especially disturbing and significantly different in its emotional effects from cancers in other parts of the body. Surgical and radiological treatments invade and expose these private parts. Reactions will vary according to the fantasies and feelings of the individual woman abut her genitalia prior to developing cancer. The over-publicized and greatly exaggerated association of cervical cancer with sexual promiscuity is a particularly potent source of unjustified and unnecessary guilt in some women.

PROBLEMS DURING AND AFTER TREATMENT

Simple questions such as 'What particularly worries you about the treatment?' provide an opportunity for the patient to express her fears. The exploration of these anxieties may be undertaken in a formal setting or informally when the time seems opportune, on a one-to-one basis or in group therapy. There is some evidence that support of this sort may prolong the survival of cancer patients (Spiegel et al 1989).

The patient's view of time

People who are ill and receiving treatment are abstracted from the world of arranged time. For a patient waiting for the results of histological examination, a week may seem an eternity. It is important to keep the patient informed at each stage of investigation and treatment and to explain the often mundane reasons for any delay. She will frequently assume that a delay in the results of a blood test, for example, means a serious turn for the worse rather than the more prosaic reason that the sample has been mislaid or not collected from the ward.

Fears about treatment and side-effects

Almost invariably a patient's fears about treatment and possible side-effects are worse than the reality. Surgery is often more easily understood but fears about anaesthesia are extremely common and often overlooked. Specific reassurance about premedication, the induction of anaesthesia and the management of postoperative pain should be given by the surgeon.

Chemotherapy and radiotherapy are potent sources of anxiety because in the public consciousness the frequency and severity of side-effects are usually exaggerated. For example, most women expect complete hair loss after chemotherapy and should be reassured when this will not occur. If alopecia is anticipated, a suitable wig should be chosen at the start of treatment so that it can be matched to the woman's natural colour and so that it will be available whenever necessary. Nausea and vomiting are a common problem but with the use of prophylactic antiemetics the treatment becomes more tolerable.

Sexual activity after treatment

When a sexually active woman undergoes radical gynaecological surgery or radiotherapy she will be concerned about her future ability to enjoy sexual activity and whether it will be as pleasurable for her partner as before her illness. However, she may be too embarrassed to ask about such matters and some may regard it as tasteless or inappropriate to discuss because of the gravity of her illness.

The quality of a woman's life has to be considered in relation to what it was before she became ill. An unsatisfactory relationship prior to the illness may be improved because of having to cope with cancer as a couple. Alternatively, a poor relationship may simply continue to be poor, devoid of intimacy and affection. A counsel of perfection is that the doctor should be experienced in dealing with sexual problems in both the male and female but this is seldom the case. However, simple enquiries and a willingness to listen are often all that is required. Occasionally a patient will not have resumed sexual intercourse because she was not told that a shortened vagina can stretch with coital activity. Atrophic vaginitis is another potential cause of coital difficulty.

Loss of libido is more difficult to treat. It may arise from an altered body image — 'I am not a real woman any more, — or there may be unresolved guilt about sexual activity because of the fear of an association between sexual intercourse and cancer. Frequently, all that is required is a sympathetic hearing, a full discussion and the removal of misconceptions. Occasionally, testosterone implants may be of value in the stimulation of libido. Whether this is a placebo effect or not remains undetermined.

The effect of the diagnosis on the male partner is often overlooked and close enquiry may be required to elicit an admission of difficulties. Almost invariably when the patient admits to sexual difficulties she will also quickly add that her partner is 'very understanding', whether he is or not. Some men become impotent. This may be due to fear on his part that he may damage his partner in some way; others may feel that they can catch cancer themselves. A cessation of normal sexual activity can make the patient feel unloved and fear that her partner is being unfaithful. Indeed, it is not uncommon for an affected male partner to regain his potency with another woman whom he regards as intact. To complicate matters further these motivations may be entirely subconscious.

It cannot be emphasized too strongly that preparation is better than avoidance and silence. Whilst the patient is in hospital undergoing treatment, simple explanations and reassurance, preferably to both the woman and her partner, can prevent problems arising. Sexual function should be enquired into at the early follow-up visits, so that if any problems have occurred they can be recognized and dealt with, before they become entrenched behaviour patterns. Sometimes this will require skilled psychotherapeutic help.

Returning to normal life

Prior to leaving hospital, the patient should be warned that some of her relatives and friends may show some degree of embarrassment, appear ill at ease, or even avoid her. They simply do not know what to say, or how to behave. This situation may be eased if she herself brings up the subject of her illness, in order to give her relatives and friends an opportunity to voice their fears and concerns about her health, both present and future.

The woman may have been the central supporting figure in a household of some complexity and may have provided the main economic support. The very act of returning to work is often a significant milestone in recovery. Although attitudes are changing rapidly, the diagnosis of cancer may mean the end of her previous employment. Apart from the obvious anxieties about her prognosis and family relationships, financial worries can be an immense source of stress for the patient. The follow-up appointment is a suitable occasion to explore this area with such questions as 'Are you back at work yet?' or 'The finances must be difficult with you not working'. Some employers and companies may discriminate against employees who have had cancer but who are to all intents and purposes cured. Often a letter from the doctor can help, or he or she may be able to facilitate the intervention of social services where the patient is unaware of financial assistance which may be available.

Review appointments provide an excellent opportunity for reassurance and the reduction of unnecessary anxiety. A patient who is in the seventh year of follow-up following a Wertheim hysterectomy may not be aware that the chances of recurrence are very small because she has not been told that simple fact. At each visit the patient should be told the outcome of any investigations or examinations and these should be presented in as optimistic and positive a fashion as honesty and the clinical situation permit. Women often put on weight because of comfort eating and lack of exercise. They should be encouraged to avoid this and to take a pride in their appearance, and to return to normal life.

WHEN DISEASE RECURS OR FAILS TO RESPOND

It is important at this stage to reassure the patient that she will not be abandoned. Her treatment will now be focused on her symptoms rather than on her tumour. It is vital to watch and listen with care and to respond to what is seen and heard. It is always possible to deal honestly with her without moving into stark truth (Saunders & Baines 1989). Now the patient has to face the more immediate prospect of death. The immediate reaction may be disbelief or denial. She may react with anger either immediately or at a later stage. Depression is common. These different emotions may occur at any time and daily alternation between one and another is possible.

Whilst most patients welcome the truth, it will take some time and much discussion on several occasions for the woman to face her situation fully. She needs to feel that she can survive as an integrated caring person, whatever length of time she has and whatever the disease or treatment do to her, until such time as she loses consciousness. She will require a considered, truthful answer to each of her questions. The doctor has to decide exactly what is meant by each question. 'Am I going to be all right, doctor?' could mean 'Is there any hope of a cure?', or 'Will my death be painful?', or 'Will you abandon me?'. It may be more appropriate, when faced with an ambiguous question to reply with: 'Tell me what you mean'. This provides the patient with a cue to express her fears and ask the questions she need to have answers to. Bland reassurance rarely provides more than transient comfort. It is only by giving the patient an opportunity to voice her hidden fears that her mental anguish can be relieved. She will find it difficult to talk about her impending death and will need gentle encouragement. The situation is obviously made easier if there has been an open, truthful relationship at an earlier stage of the disease.

During this time many patients ruminate over their past lives and ponder their mistakes and omissions. Essentially, the process is one of trying to find some order and meaning in their life and impending death. At this stage many personal and family quarrels can be resolved and reconciliations with estranged siblings and children may be achieved. The personal growth which can occur at this stage is substantial and personalities can be transformed as mental peace and acceptance of the inevitable are achieved.

MENTAL AND PHYSICAL PAIN

The depression which may follow the patient's realization of the severity of her illness should not be confused with an endogenous depression. When an individual is faced with the imminent prospect of death, depression and grief are appropriate, not pathological reactions. However, the patient's mental state will profoundly affect her symptomatology. Mental pain may present as a physical pain which is only poorly controlled by large doses of parenteral narcotics. When a better psychological adjustment is achieved the quantity of analgesia required may be markedly reduced. Saunders & Baines (1989) have stressed the role of symptom control but also point out that this requires time and close contact with the patient to give her the confidence to impart her deeper feelings, whether they be of anger, depression, guilt or regret. When a physician learns to accept mental pain as inevitable, he or she is freed from feelings of inadequacy and futility which inhibit the intimate discussion of the patient's hopes and fears.

PAIN CONTROL

This is dealt with in more detail elsewhere (Chapter 58). However, it is useful to emphasize some simple general rules here (Regnard & Mannix 1989).

Determine the cause of the pain

Obtain a detailed history and perform a clinical examination. An obvious factor which is often overlooked is that between 20 and 30% of the pain felt by cancer patients is not related to the cancer but to some other cause such as osteoarthritis. Patients find it reassuring to have the cause of their pain identified and dealt with. Where diagnosis is in doubt an educated guess at the cause of the pain is better than blind treatment.

Treatment goals

Treatment goals must be realistic. The aim is to free the

patient from the limitations imposed upon her life by pain or by the analgesics required. The pain must be attacked both with analgesics and with measures designed to improve her ability to endure her pain by restoring her sense of personal worth and by providing her with opportunities for creative and meaningful activity.

It is almost always possible to achieve a full night's sleep free from pain. The next step is to try to ensure that the patient is sufficiently comfortable to be able to continue to engage in social intercourse and to make arrangements for her life.

Route and frequency of drug administration

Whenever possible, analgesics should be given by mouth. Adequate analgesia is obtained only by the regular administration of an adequate dose of an appropriate drug at time intervals which take into account the compound's pharmacokinetics. This prevents breakthrough pain. Pethidine is not a useful drug for long-term pain control because of its short duration of action.

Choosing the correct analgesic

Analgesics can be divided into three major categories: simple analgesics, e.g. paracetamol, which may or may not have anti-inflammatory activity; mild opioids, e.g. dihydrocodeine, and strong opioids such as morphine. The initial choice of drug depends on the perceived severity of the pain, its putative cause and the success or failure of the medication which has been prescribed hitherto.

In severe pain morphine is prescribed 4-hourly and the dose escalated every 2–3 days until good pain relief is obtained. It may then be replaced by a slow-release preparation (MST) which can usually be given in a convenient, twice-daily dosage. In the early stages of treatment, nausea and vomiting are common and can be relieved by low doses of haloperidol, 1.5–3 mg at night (Regnard & Mannix 1989). Constipation is an almost invariable consequence of narcotic analgesia and prophylactic laxatives should be given routinely. A combination of stool softener (lactulose, docusate) with a stimulant (senna, danthron) is often needed. Co-danthrusate is a combination of danthron and docusate in capsule form.

Prostaglandins are involved in pain transmission and are especially implicated in the pain derived from secondary deposits in bone. Drugs which have prostaglandin synthetase-inhibiting activity (aspirin, naproxen) are often used in conjunction with mild or strong opioids. Corticosteroids may reduce the inflammatory response around a tumour and so relieve compression pain. They are of benefit where there is nerve compression, hepatosplenomegaly or raised intracranial pressure. Dysthetic symptoms may be ameliorated with the use of tricyclic drugs.

CONTROL OF NAUSEA, COLIC AND VOMITING

Local gastrointestinal causes are obstruction by tumour, mucosal irritation by drugs or delayed gastric emptying caused by opioids or other medication. The central chemoreceptor trigger zone may be stimulated by narcotics, disseminated carcinoma, uraemia, hypocalcaemia or raised intracranial pressure. Constipation can cause pseudo-obstruction. Drugs which increase gastrointestinal motility (e.g. metoclopramide or domperidone) may also cause colic.

Once the diagnosis of true obstruction has been made, parenteral hydration and nasogastric suction should be avoided unless definitive surgery is contemplated. Most patients find that persistent nausea is more debilitating than occasional vomiting. Cyclizine 50 mg 8-hourly plus haloperidol 1.5–3 mg at night if necessary will usually control nausea (Regnard & Mannix 1989). The patient may continue with oral fluids and even a low-residue diet. Most patients find this regime satisfactory even though they may vomit once or twice daily. Colicky abdominal pain can be eased by the administration of hyoscine butylbromide (Buscopan). This is not as effective by mouth. Hyoscine hydrobromide is effective sublingually but has greater anticholinergic effects.

COMBATING LONELINESS AND LOSS OF SELF-RESPECT

Towards the end of the illness the patient can no longer live a normal life and is relatively immobile. She remains mentally alert but is bored and may feel herself to be a burden. At such a time it is possible for occupational therapists and physiotherapists to find ways of encouraging the patient's creativity and making the best of her physical capacity. This allows her to use the time in a creative and fulfilling way. Feelings of loneliness and isolation are particularly difficult to endure and are not helped by the mere physical proximity of other people. These women need to be helped to retain a sense of their own personal worth. They need to feel that others want to share time with them — a joke, a chat or a moment of reflection — and that their opinions are still sought and valued.

FAMILY REACTIONS

The family and friends will often exhibit similar reactions of grief, anger or denial. They need time to express their feelings. Children need to be included. Any attempts to protect them are usually unhelpful. They need explanations of the disease and its treatment and, occasionally, they will need reassurance that the disease is not contagious or hereditary and that it is not their fault. There is no emotional or psychological advantage in shielding them from the situation, because they will have to face the inevitable traumatic reality of bereavement in the foreseeable future. Financial and social problems have to be considered. Relatives may wish to protect the patient from these worries but avoiding discussion of these matters increases the patient's feelings of isolation.

ALTERNATIVE CARE SPECIALISTS

In the past these have been regarded sceptically by the medical establishment, with just cause in some cases. The desperation of those unfortunate individuals with terminal malignant disease leads them to grasp at any hope of treatment, however unlikely its provenance. Naturopathy and homeopathy have their advocates and reported successes but unlike some conventional medical therapy they have not been subjected to scientific evaluation. Recent studies have attempted to evaluate alternative therapies as adjuncts to conventional treatment, with apparently discouraging results (Bagenal et al 1990).

The burgeoning interest in alternative medicine is probably an expression of the desire of patients to be treated as individuals rather than have their care focused solely on the disease process. The organic model of disease which is implicit in modern scientific treatment excludes consideration of the mental or psychological dimension of illness. The success of the organic model hitherto has probably reinforced the neglect of psychological aspects which are not so amenable to study by scientific methods. That the mind has profound effects on bodily function and vice versa is demonstrated both in common parlance ('she lost the will to live') and by profound effects of hysterical disturbance on the motor and sensory nervous systems as described by Breuer & Freud at the turn of the century. The Cartesian dichotomy between mind and body has permeated western thought for centuries and, possibly because of this, the mental process has been regarded as qualitatively a different form of existential activity from physical function. This assumption has perhaps mitigated against efforts to search for a mechanism linking the two. That the two are interdependent is becoming more firmly established. Intensive counselling and supportive therapy significantly improved the mean survival time of women with breast cancer (Spiegel et al 1989). It is not unreasonable to surmise that there may be some mechanism whereby the immune system is activated or depressed by the mental state and that this may influence tumour growth.

COMMUNITY CARE

The general practitioner

Good communication with the general practitioner is important from the outset. He or she should have detailed information about the initial problem and prognosis. The general practitioner's knowledge of the family setting may be extremely helpful where there are problems with the patient's adjustment to the diagnosis, family pressures, or her return to work. He or she can play a central role in mobilizing help for the patient and family from local services and organizations at all stages of the disease.

The social services

The diagnosis of malignant disease may have social effects far beyond loss and bereavement. The economic effects of loss of income may have disastrous consequences for family finances. More importantly, the patient may be a single parent, the prime carer of an elderly infirm parent or of a disabled husband. The patient, who has to face the prospect of death, may be even more distressed by concern over her family's welfare. The social worker should be involved, not only to enlist what help social services can offer but also to contact other members of the family and close friends to try to solve what the patient may regard as insurmountable problems.

Domiciliary nursing services and hospice care

Domiciliary terminal-care teams have been an important development of the hospice movement. These may be community-based, hospice-based or located in a general hospital. The Douglas MacMillan & Marie Curie Foundation nurses have had special training in terminal care and bereavement counselling. Selection ensures that these nurses do not have family commitments which would prevent them from being available 24 hours a day and 7 days a week. This availability and support is greatly appreciated by families and makes a home death possible where it would not otherwise be feasible. Only a small percentage of patients die in a hospice. Hospices will continue as centres for research, for the training of staff to work in home-care teams, and for those patients with problems considered too intractable for home care.

Support organizations

There are often local branches of BACUP, CancerLink (17 Brittania St, London WC1; tel. 071-833-2451) or other local organizations which run support groups. These offer a range of services from group therapy to leaflets and advice phone lines. These can often be very helpful, not only to the patient but also to the family, both during her illness and afterwards during the period of bereavement.

BEREAVEMENT

Family and friends

Bereavement is the complex of emotions felt by those close

to the patient who has died. This painful condition takes many months or years to heal. Numbness, shock and disbelief are common. The best preparation for bereavement is sympathetic handling of the patient's and family's problems throughout her illness.

There may be displaced anger, which may be directed towards the staff but is subconsciously felt towards the deceased because she has left the bereaved. Anger may be directed inappropriately at the staff, especially if there appear to have been delays in diagnosis or problems with treatment. Feelings of guilt may be because of unresolved family disputes or failure to be present at the time of death or because they did not feel able to look after the patient at home. Time and opportunities should be allowed for the family to express their feelings. If anger is displayed, a confrontational or authoritarian approach should be avoided. Questions should be answered honestly and often the real cause of the anger will then become apparent.

Immediate expressions of grief may vary. Certain ethnic groups have a cultural necessity to express their grief in a noisy and demonstrative fashion and every effort should be made to allow this without disturbing other patients. An apparent absence of emotion commonly indicates that an abnormal grief reaction will develop. Abnormal grief reactions should be noted so that early intervention by the medical team, general practitioner or bereavement counsellors can avert significant psychological disturbance. CRUSE (126 Sheen Rd, Richmond, Surrey TW9 1UR; tel. 081-940-4818) is an organization which specializes in the care of widows and widowers. Attempts to obliterate grief reactions by the use of psychotropic drugs are usually unhelpful and occasionally bring about dependence in the vulnerable personality. If an abnormal grief reaction is established, the help of a skilled psychotherapist should be sought sooner rather than later.

The staff

Saunders & Baines (1989) use the concept of 'staff pain'. They emphasize that the staff also need to grieve the loss of the patient and highlight the importance of group support for staff to allow opportunities for expression of these feelings. In the context of the general gynaecological ward, group meetings are probably not appropriate but all members of staff in close contact with dying patients should offer each other support, if only in an informal way. Needs will vary. It may be a junior nurse who does not understand the need for, and hence disapproves of, a radical and possibly mutilating operation or chemotherapy, or she may feel that she acted ineptly or inadequately at the time of death (Goldie 1990). The gynaecological surgeon or oncologist may become imperceptibly more depressed with every treatment failure or may seek refuge by adopting a cold, impersonal attitude, avoiding non-professional contact with patients and family. He or she may try to deal with these feelings of loss and sadness by denial or repression. Exhaustion, frustration and despair can overtake the doctor or nurse. Recognition of these feelings and acceptance of help in coming to terms with them is the only way to retain the resilience and humanity required for the task.

KEY POINTS

1. Most patients prefer to be told the truth about their condition.
2. Supportive care is not the sole responsibility of one person; nevertheless, the prime onus lies with the patient's doctor.
3. Staff need to be aware of their own feelings and attitudes to illness and death.
4. Staff must watch and listen carefully and respond to what they observe rather than have any preconceived ideas about the woman's feelings and needs.
5. Time with the patient must be protected from interruption and adequate time must be allocated.
6. Accepting the inevitability of mental pain in the patient frees the physician from feelings of inadequacy.
7. There must be no conspiracy of silence in the family and children need to be included.
8. Many sexual problems can be avoided by simple discussion and reassurance.
9. Analgesia should be given orally in regular doses.
10. Cyclizine and haloperidol are very useful for controlling nausea in obstruction.
11. The general practitioner can play a central role in mobilizing local help.
12. Bereavement affects both family and staff. Both need to mourn.

REFERENCES AND FURTHER READING

Bagenal F S, Easton D F, Harris E, Chilvers C E D, McElwain T J 1990 Survival of patients with breast cancer attending Bristol Cancer Help Centre. Lancet 336: 606–610

Goldie L 1982 Ethics of telling the patient. Journal of Medical Ethics 8: 128–133

Goldie L 1983 Doctors in training and the dying patient. Journal of the Royal Society of Medicine 76: 995

Goldie L 1984 Psychoanalysis in the NHS general hospital. Psychoanalytic Psychotherapy 1: 23–24

Goldie L 1988 The interdisciplinary treatment of cancer: cooperation or competition. In: Psychiatric oncology — Proceedings of the 2nd and 3rd Meetings of the British Psychosocial Oncology Group 1985 and 1986. London, Pergamon Press

Goldie L 1990 The ethical and emotional problems of nurses. Psychoanalytic psychotherapy. London, Association for Psychoanalytic Psychotherapy in the National Health Service

Hinton J 1979 Comparison of places and policies for terminal care. Lancet i: 29–32
Hogbin B, Fallowfield L 1989 Getting it taped: the 'bad news' consultation with cancer patients. British Journal of Hospital Medicine 41: 330–333
Regnard C, Mannix K 1989 Pain relief in advanced cancer. Manchester, Haigh and Hochland
Saunders C, Baines M 1989 Living with dying. Oxford, Medical Publications
Spiegel D, Bloom J R, Kraemer H C, Gottheh E 1989 Effect of psychosocial treatment on survival of patients with metastatic breast cancer. Lancet ii: 888–891

SECTION 5

Urogynaecology

42. The mechanism of continence

P. Hilton

INTRODUCTION

Urinary incontinence may be defined as 'a condition in which involuntary loss of urine is a social or hygienic problem, and is objectively demonstrable'. Continence then, by inference, might be considered as the ability to retain urine within the bladder between voluntary acts of micturition. In order to comprehend fully the pathological processes which lead to the development of urinary incontinence, a clear understanding of the normal mechanisms for the maintenance of continence is of course fundamental; this in turn must be based on a knowledge of the morphology and physiology of the bladder and urethra, and their supporting structures.

ANATOMY OF THE LOWER URINARY TRACT

The bladder

Detrusor

The bladder muscle or detrusor is often described as consisting of three distinct smooth muscle layers, the outer being oriented longitudinally, the middle circularly, and the inner longitudinally. More recent studies, however, suggest that there is frequent interchange of fibres between bundles, and separate layers are not easily defined. Moreover, from a functional point of view, the detrusor appears to be constructed so as to contract as a single syncytial mass. With the exception of the muscle fibres of the superficial trigone, all areas of the detrusor show similar histological and histochemical characteristics. In distinction from other smooth muscle cells within the urinary tract, those of the detrusor are shown to contain significant amounts of acetylcholinesterase, in keeping with their abundant cholinergic parasympathetic nerve supply.

Trigone

The smooth muscle of the trigone, in contrast to that of the rest of the bladder, is easily visualized as two distinct layers (Fig. 42.1a). The deep trigonal muscle is in all respects similar to the detrusor; the superficial muscle in this region, however, has several distinguishing features. It is relatively thin, and consists of small muscle bundles; the

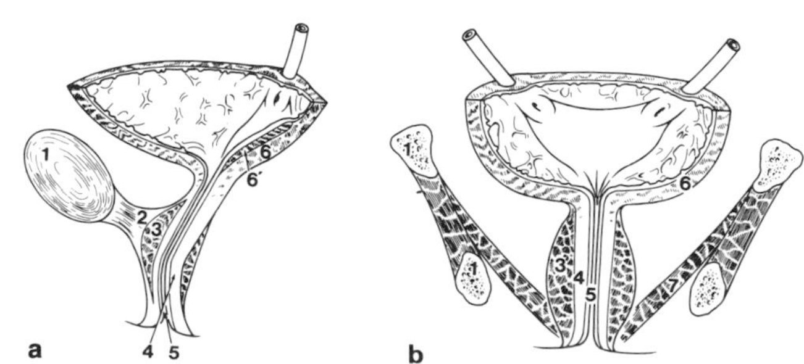

Fig. 42.1 Schematic diagrams of female bladder and urethra in (**a**) sagittal and (**b**) coronal sections. 1, Pubic symphysis/rami; 2, posterior pubourethral ligaments; 3, intrinsic striated muscle (rhabdosphincter urethrae); 4, intrinsic smooth muscle; 5, mucosa and submucosal vascular tissues; 6, smooth muscle of detrusor/deep trigone; 6^1, smooth muscle of superficial trigone; 7, extrinsic striated muscle/levator ani. From Hilton (1986) with permission.

cells themselves are devoid of acetylcholinesterase and have a more sparse cholinergic nerve supply. It may be traced distally where it fades out in the proximal urethra, forming a low crest on the posterior wall, and proximally, where it is continuous with the ureteric smooth muscle. Indeed it has been suggested that whilst the bulk of this muscle is too small for it to be of any relevance to bladder neck or urethral function, it may have significance in the control of the ureterovesical junction during voiding, thereby preventing ureteric reflux.

Bladder neck

The smooth muscle of the bladder neck is also distinct from that of the detrusor. In the male a well defined preprostatic smooth muscle sphincter is present, consisting of small diameter muscle bundles. In the female, however, whilst the smooth muscle is similarly distinct from the detrusor in terms of muscle bundle size, the orientation of bundles is largely oblique or longitudinal and they appear to have little or no sphincter action.

Urothelium

The mucosal lining of the bladder is consistent in appearance in all regions in the distended state, and is made up of two or three layers of transitional cells. When empty, however, except over the trigone, the bladder lining is thrown up into extensive rugae and the urothelium may be up to six cells thick.

The urethra

The normal female urethra is between 30 and 50 mm in length from internal to external meatus. Its structure, in particular that of the smooth and striated muscle components, has been the subject of considerable debate.

Urethral smooth muscle

It was previously held by many workers that the smooth muscle of the bladder and that of the urethra were distinct; others, however, have suggested that they are in direct continuity and that inner longitudinal and outer oblique layers of urethral muscle are continuous with the inner and outer longitudinal layers of the detrusor. More recent work, however, has indicated a return to the concept of bladder and urethral smooth muscle being separate entities. Whilst morphologically they may appear continuous, histochemically they are different in that the urethral smooth muscle cells are devoid of the acetylcholinesterase which is found in profusion within the cells of the detrusor.

Urethral and periurethral striated muscle

Controversy has also surrounded the striated muscle components of the urethra. It was previously considered that the external striated urethral sphincter and the periurethral striated muscle of levator ani were in continuity. There is now increasing evidence that they are distinct. The intrinsic striated portion of the urethral sphincter mechanism (the external sphincter or rhabdosphincter urethrae) consists of bundles of circularly arranged fibres maximum in bulk at the midurethral level anteriorly, thinning laterally, and being almost totally deficient posteriorly (Fig. 42.1). The extrinsic periurethral muscle of levator ani has no direct contiguity with the urethra, being separated from it by a distinct connective tissue septum. Its muscle bundles lie in general terms lateral to the urethra, the most medial fibres being inserted into the anterolateral vaginal walls, and their bulk is maximal at the junction of middle and lower thirds of the urethra, i.e. at a somewhat lower level than the intrinsic striated muscle. It has also been demonstrated that these muscles are histochemically distinct, and of different functional specialization. The intrinsic striated muscle is made up of small-diameter muscle fibres, rich in acid stable myosin adenosine triphosphatase, and possessing numerous mitochondria; they are therefore classified as slow twitch fibres, and are thought to be responsible for the striated muscle contribution to urethral closure at rest. By contrast, the extrinsic periurethral striated muscles are made up of a heterogeneous population of fibres, some of which show the above characteristics of slow twitch muscle, while others are rich in alkaline stable adenosine triphosphatase, characteristic of fast twitch muscle. The latter fibres are suspected to contribute an additional reflex component to aid urethral closure on stress.

Mucosa and submucosa

The epithelial lining of the urethra is of two types, proximally it is continuous with that of the bladder and consists of pseudostratified transitional cells, while distally it is continuous with introital skin, and consists of non-keratinized stratified squamous cells. The junction between the two varies with age and oestrogen status and may be of significance with regard to the prevention of ascending infection.

Within the submucosa of the female urethra two prominent venous plexi have been identified: a distal one whose structure varies little with age, and a proximal one beneath the bladder neck, where marked age-related changes are seen. In women of reproductive age the vessels are highly folded, thin-walled and with numerous arteriovenous anastomoses, giving a cavernous appearance to the submucosa not seen in postmenopausal women.

These findings have been interpreted as indicating that the urethral vascular system plays a major role in the closure of the urethra in young women. The role of mucosal softness in the effective occlusion of the urethral lumen has been emphasized (see below) and it is perhaps in this context that the vascularity of the urethra has its significance.

The pubourethral ligaments

The pubourethral ligaments form an important suspensory mechanism for the female urethra. They are described as consisting of a single anterior and paired posterior ligaments, the latter being of much greater functional significance. Three anatomical expansions of the posterior ligaments have been described: posteriorly to the paraurethral tissues, laterally to the levator fascia, and recurrently, beneath the subpubic arch towards the anterior ligament, forming the so-called intermediate ligament. These ligaments contain large numbers of smooth muscle bundles, which extend upwards towards the lower fibres of the bladder, and indeed have been shown to be histologically identical with the detrusor, possessing an abundant presumptive cholinergic nerve supply. It is possible therefore that these ligaments provide both active and passive components to the maintenance of the normal spatial relationships of urethra, bladder and pelvis.

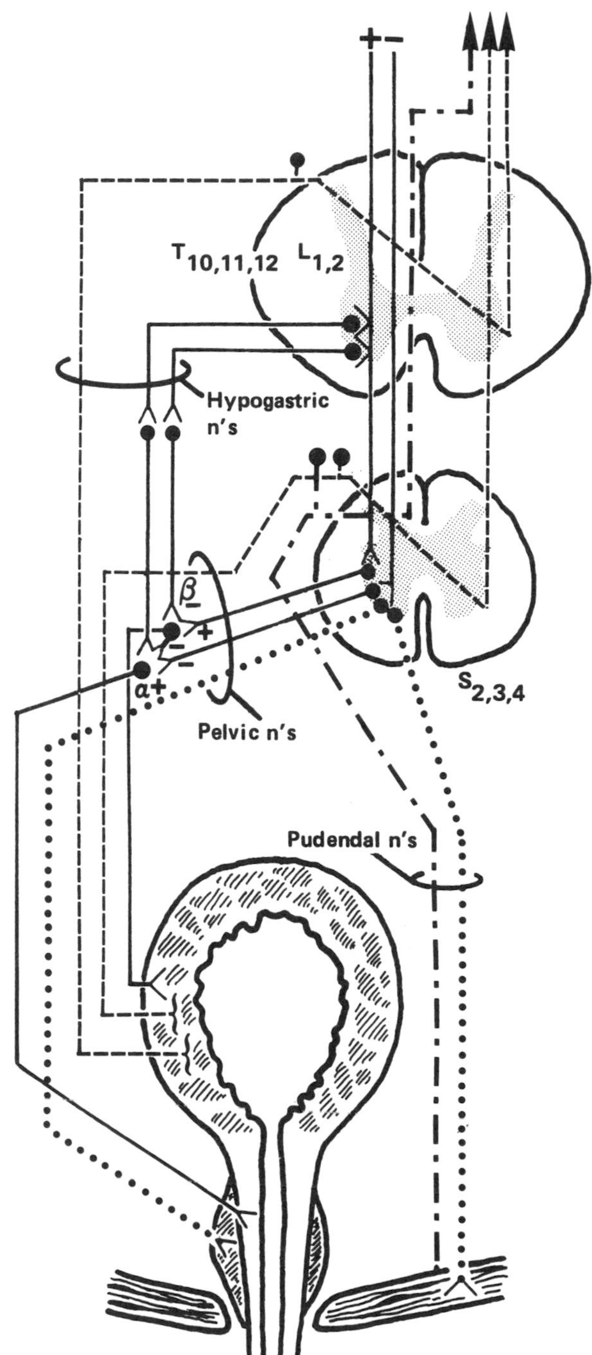

Fig. 42.2 Peripheral nerve supply to the lower urinary tract. — Visceral efferents (parasympathetic and sympathetic); — — — visceral efferents; . . . . somatic efferents; — · — somatic afferents.

NEUROLOGICAL CONTROL OF MICTURITION

The main function of the bladder is to convert the continuous excretory process of the kidneys into a more convenient intermittent process of evacuation. In order to achieve this the bladder must serve firstly as an efficient — i.e. continent — low-pressure reservoir whose function interferes minimally with an individual's other activities, and secondly it must allow the intermittent voluntary relinquishment of that former function, within socially acceptable limits with respect to time and place, to allow voiding. These two requirements call for an extraordinarily complex neural control to co-ordinate sensory input from and motor output to bladder and urethra in reciprocal fashion (Fig. 42.2).

Innervation of the detrusor

Parasympathetic supply

The bladder muscle is diffusely and richly supplied with cholinergic nerve fibres, to the extent that each individual muscle cell may be supplied by one or more cholinergic nerves. The cell bodies of these fibres lie either within the pelvic plexus or within the bladder wall itself. These postganglionic fibres are supplied by preganglionic fibres with cell bodies in the intermediolateral grey columns of the sacral segments S2 to S4.

Sympathetic supply

Several authors have reported noradrenergic terminals to

be present throughout the bladder in small numbers, and in greater concentration in the bladder neck. Others, however, found such terminals to be surprisingly sparse, and have suggested that those fibres that are present in the bladder wall are associated with blood vessels. The preganglionic fibres terminating on these postganglionic noradrenergic fibres have their cell bodies in the intermediolateral grey areas of the thoracic and lumbar segments T10 to L2. They travel in the sympathetic chain and then via the lumbar splanchnic nerves to the superior hypogastric plexus. From there the right and left hypogastric nerves ramify within the pelvic plexus. It is suggested that sympathetically mediated inhibition of the bladder depends not on direct effects from noradrenergic fibres on the detrusor but indirectly, by inhibition of the excitatory parasympathetic supply within the ganglia of the pelvic plexus.

There is clear evidence that acetylcholine, acting as transmitter from the parasympathetic efferents, is responsible for the detrusor contraction during micturition. Noradrenaline, however, may be either excitatory or inhibitory depending on the predominant receptor type. In several mammalian species alpha receptor sites, producing contraction in response to noradrenaline binding, have been shown to predominate in the bladder base, whilst beta receptors, producing relaxation, are predominant in the vault.

Visceral afferent supply

Visceral afferent fibres may be identified travelling with both sacral and thoracolumbar visceral efferent nerves. Sacral afferents have been shown to be evenly distributed between muscle and submucosa throughout the bladder; they appear to convey the sensations of touch, pain, and bladder distension, and are essential to complete normal micturition. Afferents in the thoracolumbar nerves become activated only during marked bladder distension and their transection seems to have little effect on voiding.

All the above findings conform to the hypothesis that the sympathetic innervation of the bladder, along with the associated thoracolumbar visceral afferent supply, is concerned mainly with the filling and storage phases of the micturition cycle, whereas the parasympathetic supply and accompanying sacral afferent fibres are important for normal voiding.

Innervation of the urethral smooth muscle

Sympathetic and parasympathetic efferent and associated visceral afferent fibres from the vesical plexus also innervate the urethra. Parasympathetic efferents terminate in the urethral smooth muscle, and cholinergic stimulation produces contraction. The functional significance of this muscle, however, remains in some doubt. The orientation of its fibres suggests little sphincteric action, and its parasympathetic innervation suggests importance with respect to voiding function; contraction produces shortening and widening of the urethra along with detrusor contraction during micturition.

Sympathetic efferents also innervate the intrinsic smooth muscle which possesses predominantly alpha adrenoreceptor sites. Whilst there are no sex differences in adrenergic innervation of the bladder body, the sympathetic innervation of the bladder neck and urethra in the female is much less dense than in the male, where it has been suggested to have a genital rather than urinary function.

Innervation of striated muscle

Intrinsic urethral striated muscle

It was long held that the rhabdosphincter urethrae was supplied by somatic efferent fibres via the pudendal nerves, but it has now been shown that this muscle is supplied via the pelvic splanchnic nerves travelling with the parasympathetic fibres to the intrinsic smooth muscle of the urethra.

Extrinsic periurethral striated muscle

In contrast to the intrinsic striated muscle sphincter, the levator ani is innervated by motor fibres from the pudendal nerves. The above findings have clinical significance in that firstly pudendal blockade might not reduce urethral resistance to a major extent, since the intrinsic striated sphincter will be unaffected, and secondly in that electromyogram activity recorded from the pelvic floor does not necessarily correlate with activity of the external sphincter.

Associated somatic afferent fibres also travel with the pudendal nerves; they ascend via the dorsal columns to convey proprioception from the pelvic floor.

Central nervous connections

The connections of the lower urinary tract within the central nervous system are extraordinarily complex, and many discrete centres with influences on micturition have been identified: within the cerebral cortex, in the superior frontal and anterior cingulate gyri of the frontal lobe, and the paracentral lobule; within the cerebellum, in the anterior vermis and fastigial nucleus; and within subcortical areas including the thalamus, the basal ganglia, the limbic system, the hypothalamus, and discrete areas of the mesencephalic pontine medullary reticular formation. The full function and interactions of these various areas are incompletely understood, although the effects of ablation and tumour growth in humans and stimulation studies in animals have given some insights.

The centres within the cerebral cortex are important in the perception of sensation from the lower urinary tract and the inhibition and subsequent initiation of voiding. Lesions of the superior frontal or anterior cingulate gyri impair conscious and subconscious inhibition of the micturition reflex, and are therefore associated with symptoms of urgency and incontinence. The paracentral lobule appears to be more concerned with sphincteric function, and lesions are likely to result in urinary retention resulting from impaired sensation and spasticity of the pelvic floor.

The thalamus is the principal relay centre for pathways projecting to the cerebral cortex, and ascending pathways activated by bladder and urethral receptors synapse on neurones in specific thalamic nuclei which have reciprocal connections with the cortex. Electrical stimulation of the basal ganglia in animals leads to suppression of the detrusor reflex, whereas ablation has resulted in detrusor hyperreflexia; patients with parkinsonism commonly are shown to have detrusor instability on cystometric examination.

Within the pontine reticular formation are two closely related areas with inhibitory and excitatory effects on the sacral micturition centre in the conus medullaris. Lesions of the cord below this always lead to inco-ordinate voiding with failure of urethral relaxation during detrusor contraction; lesions above this level may be associated with normal though involuntary micturition.

PHYSIOLOGY OF THE LOWER URINARY TRACT

From the definitions given above it is self-evident that continence is dependent on 'the powers of urethral resistance exceeding the forces of urinary expulsion', that is to say that continence is maintained when the maximum urethral pressure exceeds the bladder pressure or when the urethral closure pressure is positive. Normal micturition may be said to result from the controlled reversal of this equilibrium, and incontinence from its uncontrolled reversal. The important aspects of the control of continence therefore are firstly those factors which maintain low intravesical pressure and secondly those which ensure that the urethral pressure remains high — or at least higher than intravesical pressure — at all times during the filling and storage phases of the micturition cycle.

Behaviour of the bladder

The intravesical pressure is dependent upon a number of factors (Fig. 42.3) including the following.

The hydrostatic pressure at the bladder neck

Liquid in the bladder, when in hydrostatic equilibrium, has a vertical gravitational pressure gradient, and the measured pressure must therefore be referred to a standard level. For clinical practice the intravesical pressure is defined as the pressure in the bladder with respect to atmospheric pressure measured at the level of the upper border of the symphysis pubis. In terms of the maintenance of continence, the critical pressure is that acting at the bladder neck, tending to work against the closure forces of the urethra; this has a hydrostatic element dependent on the head of fluid above it; this, of course, increases with increasing bladder volume, though rarely amounts to more than 10 cm H_2O.

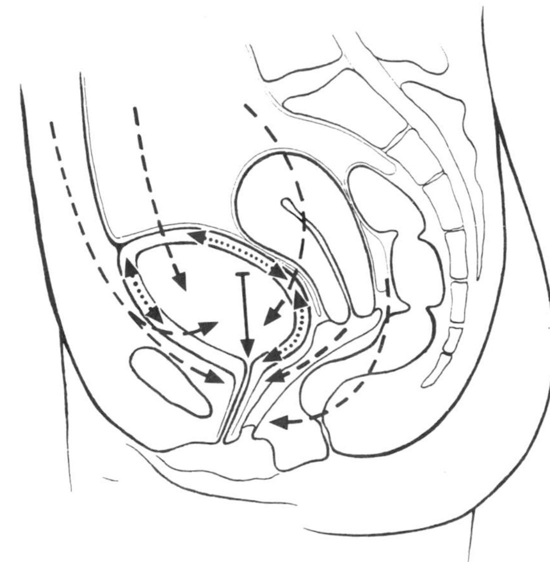

Fig. 42.3 Factors determining the intravesical pressure, and which are therefore of relevance to the maintenance of urethral closure pressure. Hydrostatic pressure at the bladder neck ——►; transmission of intra-abdominal pressure – – ►; passive and active tension in the bladder wall ······►. From Hilton (1992) with permission.

The transmission of intra-abdominal pressure

The bladder is normally an intra-abdominal organ, and is therefore subject to pressures transmitted from adjacent viscera and elsewhere within the abdominal cavity. This is not of great importance in the resting situation since pressures transmitted to the bladder are low and generally are transmitted equally to bladder neck and proximal urethra; this effect may, however, be critical in the maintenance of continence in the face of stress (see below).

The tension in the bladder wall itself

This is in part a passive phenomenon related to the distensibility or viscoelastic properties of the bladder wall itself, and in part an active phenomenon due to the contractility of the detrusor muscle and its neurological control.

Viscoelasticity of the bladder. During rapid stepwise filling of the bladder the detrusor pressure rises rapidly and afterwards decays exponentially with time (Fig. 42.4a); this

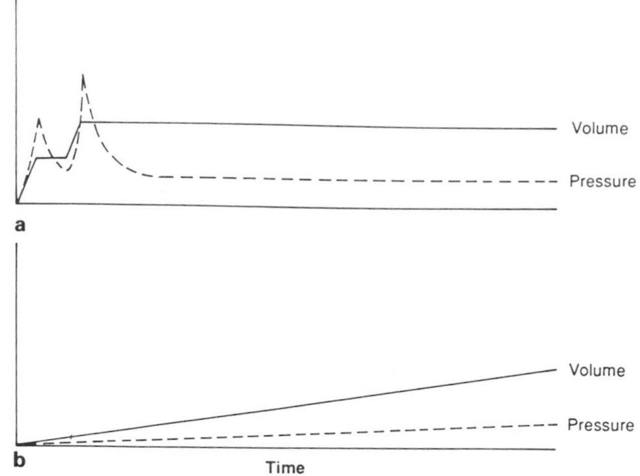

Fig. 42.4 The behaviour of the bladder in terms of pressure and volume changes with time during (**a**) rapid stepwise filling and (**b**) slow continuous (physiological) filling. From Hilton (1992) with permission.

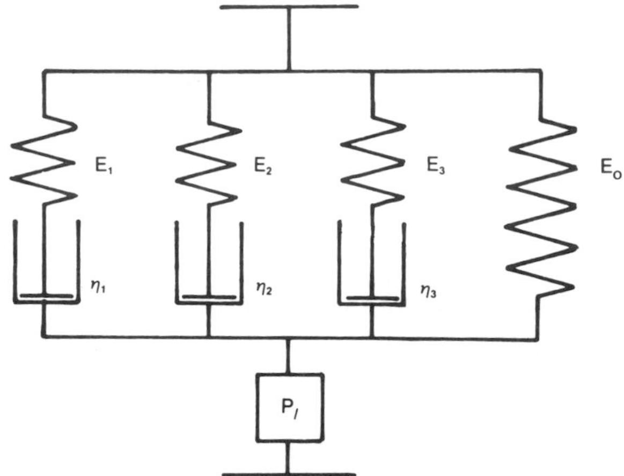

Fig. 42.5 Mechanical model representing the behaviour of the bladder wall (after Griffiths 1980). The springs E_1, E_2, E_3 and E_0 represent elastic properties, and dashpots η_1, η_2 and η_3 viscous properties; E_0 represents the force remaining when no more time-dependent phenomena are involved; P_l represents a plastic element, or extension when the force exceeds a critical value (the unstretched length increasing after stretching).

time dependence is similar to that expected of a passive viscoelastic solid. However, under the near static conditions of physiological filling, the detrusor's behaviour is more accurately described as elastic. That is to say, the detrusor pressure rises little as the bladder volume increases from zero to functional capacity (Fig. 42.4b).

The relationship between the volume in the bladder and the strain (or deformation) of its walls, between the strain and stress (or wall tension), and between the stress and intravesical pressure, have been investigated in vitro and the contractility of the bladder has thus been modelled mathematically in the following terms:

$$\sigma = A.e^{-\alpha t} + B.e^{-\beta t} + C.e^{-\gamma t} + \mathrm{K}$$

where σ represents stress or force per unit area, coefficients A, B, C and K the elastic length-dependent properties, and decay constants α, β and γ the time-dependent properties. This mathematical model may be represented by a mechanical model (Fig. 42.5) in which a series of Maxwell elements each consisting of a spring (elastic properties) and a dashpot (viscous properties); the constant K is represented by the parallel elastic element E_0. An additional characteristic of the bladder wall is that its unstretched length increases after stretching; to allow for this a plastic element is incorporated into the model in series with the other elements.

From an examination of this model it becomes clear why there is little or no increase in intravesical pressure as the bladder fills physiologically. Time dependence is not relevant under these circumstances so the Maxwell elements produce no force; the dashpots have time to follow the elongation, and thus the springs, which would otherwise generate force, are not elongated. The force in the model and the stress in the bladder wall will thus be

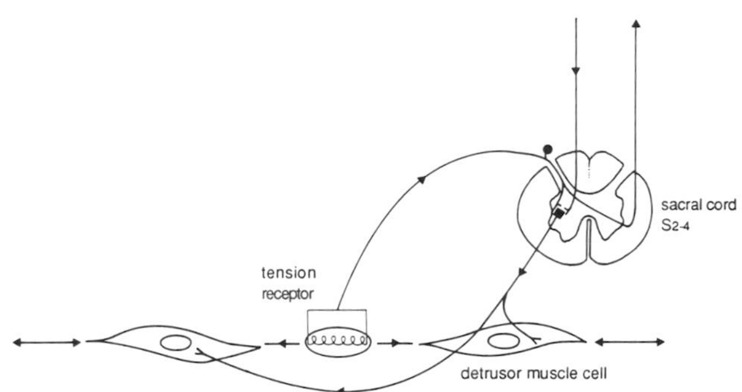

Fig. 42.6 The basic visceral reflex arc concerned in detrusor contractility. From Hilton (1992) with permission.

determined only by the parallel elastic element E_0; in practice this means that at physiological rates of bladder-filling the normal cystometrogram is essentially flat.

Contractility of the bladder and its neural control. The neurological control of detrusor contractility is dependent upon a sacral spinal reflex under control of several higher centres, as considered earlier in this chapter. This basic reflex arc is best considered as a loop (Fig. 42.6) extending from sensory receptors within the bladder wall, through the pelvic plexus and via visceral afferent fibres travelling with the pelvic splanchnic nerves, to enter the spinal cord in the S2 to S4 level, via internuncial neurones within the cord synapsing with cell bodies in the intermediolateral grey area of the same sacral levels, and thence via parasympathetic fibres in the pelvic splanchnic nerves through the pelvic plexus to the smooth muscle cells of the detrusor. The stretch receptors or proprioceptors within the bladder wall are in effect connected in series with muscle cells and are therefore stimulated by both passive stretch and by active contraction of the detrusor. Once a critical level of stretch is achieved impulses pass in the afferent limb of the reflex arc, and the resultant efferent discharge leads to a detrusor contraction.

The higher control over the basic visceral reflex arc is mediated through descending pathways from the pontine reticular formation. Although both excitatory and inhibitory centres have been located in this region, their net effect is primarily an inhibitory one, and their normal influence is therefore to prevent contraction of the detrusor, and thus to encourage the maintenance of a low intravesical pressure during the filling phase of the micturition cycle.

Urethra

In order to maintain continence it is vital not only that the intravesical pressure should remain low during the storage phase of the micturition cycle, but also that the urethral lumen should seal completely. Three components of urethral function are necessary to achieve this hermetic property:

1 Urethral inner wall softness.
2 Inner urethral compression.
3 Outer wall tension.

Whilst the closure of any elastic tube can be obtained if sufficient compression is applied to it, the efficiency of closure is dramatically increased if its lining possesses the property of plasticity, or the ability to mould into a watertight seal.

There has been much debate over the morphological components which contribute to the functional characteristics of softness, compression and tension in the urethra. Several authors have commented on the vascularity of the urethra and pointed out that the submucosal vascular plexi far exceed the requirements of a blood supply for the organ. Some have suggested a significant vascular contribution to urethral closure, although others have found no specific features to suggest an important occlusive role for the urethral vascular supply. Nevertheless, whatever the contribution of the urethral blood supply to the measured intraluminal pressure, it is likely to be of significance as regards the plasticity of the urothelium and submucosa.

The structures leading to inner wall compression by virtue of their contribution to outer wall tension can be and have been quantified in terms of the urethral pressure profile (Fig. 42.7). These structures may include the intramural elastic fibres, the intrinsic smooth and striated muscle and the extrinsic or periurethral striated muscle. From urethral pressure studies in animals it has been suggested that approximately 50% of the resting pressure was due to striated muscle components; it has, however, been demonstrated that it is possible to remain continent following complete striated muscle blockade. Perhaps the best work carried out in this regard in human subjects was a series of elegant peroperative studies undertaken at various stages during radical pelvic surgery; these showed that approximately one-third of the resting urethral pressure is due to striated muscle effects, one-third to smooth muscle effects, and one-third to its vascular supply.

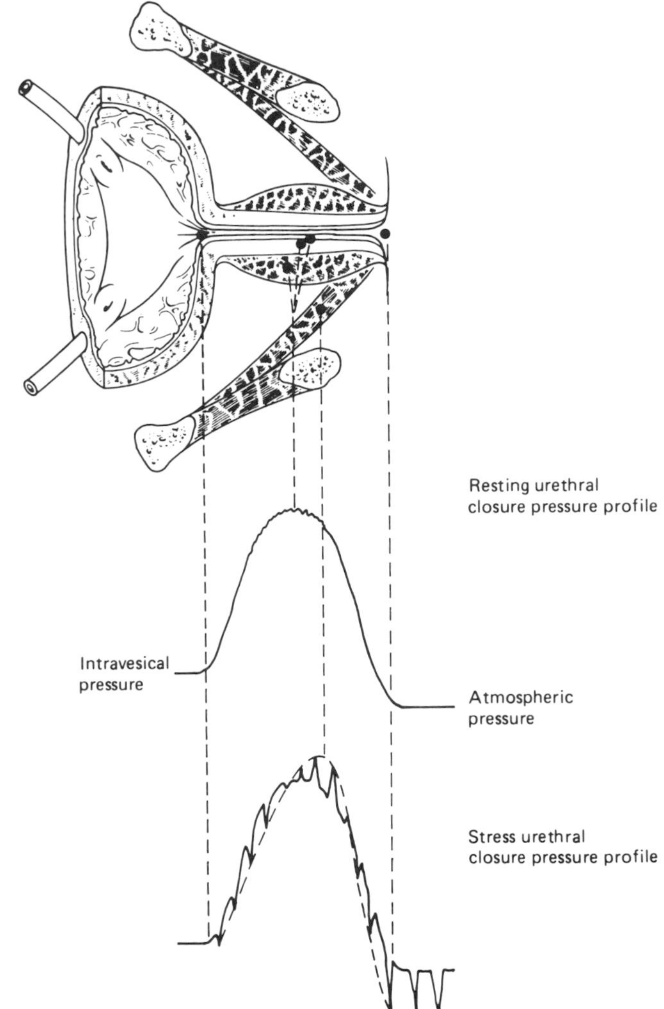

Fig. 42.7 **Top** Schematic drawing of the female bladder and urethra in coronal section. Below are shown urethral closure pressure profiles at rest (**middle**) and on stress (**bottom**) to demonstrate the morphological and functional correlation. From Hilton (1990) with permission.

Whatever the relative importance of the above factors to active wall tension, it should be remembered that these same structures also contribute a passive or elastic tension, together with the supporting elements of collagen and elastin.

The usual level of continence in the female is not, as one might expect, in the mid-urethra at the level of maximum resting pressure, but at the bladder neck. This region in the female has no sphincteric circular smooth muscle and is virtually devoid of striated muscle; it would therefore seem that the passive elastic tension is the most important factor leading to closure at the bladder neck and proximal urethra (Fig. 42.7). In mid-urethra the most prominent structural feature is the intrinsic striated muscle or rhabdosphincter. Electron microscopic and histochemical evidence suggests that this may be responsible for the bulk of active urethral tone at rest. Electromyographic studies, histochemical evidence and urethral pressure measurements all suggest that the periurethral striated muscles have their maximum effect at a level slightly distal to that of the resting urethral pressure profile (Fig. 42.7) and do not contribute greatly to the maintenance of continence at rest. It is likely, however, that these muscles play a significant role in the maintenance of urethral closure in the face of increased intra-abdominal pressure (see below).

THE NORMAL MICTURITION CYCLE

From the background information contained in previous sections of this chapter it is now possible to discuss the mechanisms whereby urine is retained within the bladder during the filling and storage phases and evacuated during the voiding phase of the normal micturition cycle (Fig. 42.8).

Filling and storage phase

The bladder normally fills with urine by a series of peristaltic contractions at a rate of between 0.5 and 5 ml/min; under these conditions the bladder pressure increases only minimally. Even during the course of cystometry at rapid filling rates, in normal individuals the pressure rises by no more than 15 cm H_2O from empty to cystometric capacity.

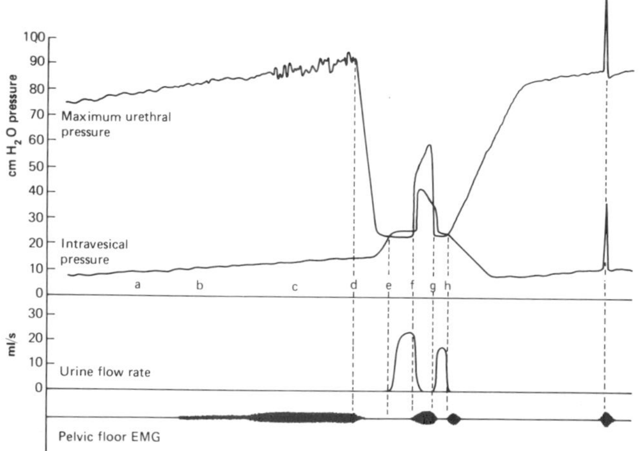

Fig 42.8 The normal micturition cycle showing changes in urethral and intravesical pressure, urine flow rate and pelvic floor electromyogram (EMG). a, Phase of subconscious inhibition; b, phase of conscious (suppressible) inhibition; c, phase of reinforced (unsuppressible) inhibition; d, initiation or transition; e, voiding; f, interruption of micturition by pelvic floor contraction; g, resumption of micturition; h, end of void; i, increase in intra-abdominal pressure due to a cough. From Hilton (1986) with permission.

Urethral closure meanwhile is maintained by the combined passive and active effects of its smooth and striated muscle components, its elastic content, and its blood supply. The hermetic efficiency is accentuated by the softness of its mucosa.

During the early stages of bladder filling, proprioceptive afferent impulses from stretch receptors within the bladder wall pass via the pelvic nerves to sacral dorsal roots S2–S4. These impulses ascend in the cord via the lateral spinothalamic tracts and a detrusor motor response is subconsciously inhibited by descending impulses from the subcortical micturition centres (Fig. 42.8a).

As the bladder volume increases, further afferent impulses ascend to the cerebral cortex, and the sensation of bladder filling associated with the desire to micturate is first consciously appreciated usually at between 200 and 300 ml or half the functional bladder capacity. The inhibition of detrusor contraction is now cortically mediated, although the desire to void may be further suppressed to subconscious levels again, given sufficient distracting afferent stimuli. Whilst descending impulses inhibit preganglionic parasympathetic cell bodies in the sacral cord, there may also be excitatory effects on the sympathetic neurones in the thoracolumbar region, causing increased efferent discharge to the beta-adrenoreceptors within the bladder (and/or further inhibition within the pelvic plexus of parasympathetic fibres to the bladder), leading to its relaxation, and to alpha-adrenoreceptors in the proximal urethra (and/or further excitation within the pelvic plexus of postganglionic parasympathetic fibres to the urethra), leading to a slight increase in urethral pressure (Fig. 42.8b).

With further filling, impulses within the visceral afferent fibres accompanying the sympathetic efferents to thoracolumber roots T10 to L2 ascend to the cerebral cortex, and a further desire to void is appreciated; reinforced conscious inhibition of micturition then occurs whilst a suitable site and posture for micturition are sought. During this time, in addition to the cortical suppression of detrusor activity, there may also be a voluntary pelvic floor contraction in an attempt to maintain urethral closure; this may be evidenced by a further increase in urethral closure pressure and by marked fluctuations in urethral pressure as the sensation of urgency becomes increasingly severe (Fig. 42.8c).

Initiation phase

When a suitable time, site and posture for micturition are selected the process of voiding commences. This may be considered in two phases — the initiation or transition from the non-voiding state and micturition itself. Several theories have been propounded to explain the transition phase. The earliest proposed a reciprocal functional relationship between bladder neck and detrusor, the former undergoing active relaxation as the latter contracts. It has, however, been suggested that smooth muscle relaxation alone was not sufficient to account for the initiation of voiding, and that the muscles of the pelvic floor relax in concert with the urethral smooth muscle in response to detrusor contraction. Others, however, have proposed that transition to the voiding state occurs not by relaxation of urethral smooth muscle fibres but rather by an increase in their tension consequent upon detrusor contraction, resulting in shortening and widening of the urethra. This is of course not incompatible with the relaxation theories, since relaxation of the urethral and periurethral striated muscle may occur coincident with detrusor and urethral smooth muscle contraction, and by virtue of the continuity of the longitudinal smooth muscle fibres of the detrusor and urethra, funnelling of the bladder neck would be encouraged as the detrusor contracts.

The process of initiation is perhaps best viewed as combining features of each of the above theories. Relaxation of the pelvic floor may be shown to occur early in the process, both radiologically and electromyographically; it is likely that simultaneous relaxation of the intrinsic striated muscle also occurs, since a marked fall in intraurethral pressure is seen before the intravesical pressure rises, during both voluntary and provoked voiding, and the same has been shown in response to sacral nerve stimulation (Fig. 42.8d).

A few seconds later the descending inhibitory influences from the cerebral cortex acting on the sacral micturition centre are suppressed, allowing a rapid discharge of efferent parasympathetic impulses via the pelvic nerves, to cause contraction of the detrusor, and probably also to pull open the bladder neck and shorten the urethra; simultaneous inhibition of the efferent sympathetic discharges via the thoracolumbar outflow to the pelvic plexus probably also occurs, encouraging detrusor contraction and urethral relaxation. Depending on the relationship between the force of detrusor contraction and the residual urethral resistance, the intravesical pressure may rise to a variable extent (usually less than 60 cm H_2O). When the falling urethral and increasing intravesical pressures equate, urine flow will commence (Fig. 42.8e).

Voiding phase

The application of physical laws to explain the mechanism of continence is often considered inappropriate and misleading. In considering the bladder during micturition, however, the law of Laplace may be useful. It states that the pressure (P) in a vessel varies directly with the mural tension (T), and inversely with the radius (R). Since the bladder at the initiation of micturition takes on a nearly spherical shape, and has walls which are thin in comparison to its radius, its behaviour may be usefully expressed by the basic formula of the law as applied to a sphere: $P = 2T/R$. As the mural tension rises in the absence of voiding the intravesical pressure also rises. When a critical opening pressure is achieved, urine will start to flow and the bladder radius will fall. The pressure, however, usually remains constant during voiding, and the mural tension therefore must fall. Once initiated therefore, the process of micturion requires little to sustain it. Whilst active tension is required throughout, the effectiveness of detrusor contraction increases as the muscle fibres shorten and therefore decreasing forces are required as micturition proceeds.

If micturition is voluntarily interrupted midstream, this is usually achieved by a contraction of the periurethral striated muscle of the pelvic floor. In association with this contraction the urethral pressure rises rapidly to exceed the intravesical pressure and therefore urine flow stops. The detrusor, being a smooth muscle, is much slower to relax, and therefore goes on contracting against the closed sphincter. That is to say, an isometric contraction occurs, and again applying the law of Laplace, the intravesical pressure rises (Fig. 42.8f). If micturition is resumed by relaxation of the pelvic floor, both urethral and intravesical pressures will return to their previous voiding state (Fig. 42.8g).

At the end of micturition the intravesical pressure gradually falls as urinary flow diminishes (Fig. 42.8h). The pelvic floor and intrinsic striated muscle are contracted and flow is interrupted in mid-urethra; the few drops of urine left in the proximal urethra are milked back into the bladder by the intrinsic mechanisms discussed above which contribute to the hermetic closure of the urethra and bladder neck competence. Simultaneously the subconscious inhibition of the sacral micturition centre is reapplied as the filling phase of the cycle recurs.

Mechanism of stress continence

The above discussion of the normal micturition cycle relates to the events occurring in a patient essentially at rest, and assumes that intravesical pressure is unaffected by extravesical influences. Acute intra-abdominal pressure rises due to coughing or more sustained pressure variations due to straining or movement would easily exceed the normal resting maximum urethral closure pressure and result in incontinence unless additional influences were brought to bear on the mechanism of continence.

The factors which maintain the positive urethral pressure at rest (i.e. which ensure that the urethral pressure exceeds the bladder pressure) have been considered above. This positive closure pressure is also maintained in symptom-free women in the face of intra-abdominal pressure rises (see Fig. 42.8i) by at least two mechanisms.

Firstly there is a passive or direct mechanical transmission of the intra-abdominal increase to the proximal urethra (Fig. 42.9). This effect is dependent upon the normal spatial relationships between the bladder and urethra, and on their fixation in a retropubic position by the posterior pubourethral ligaments. The extent of this trans-

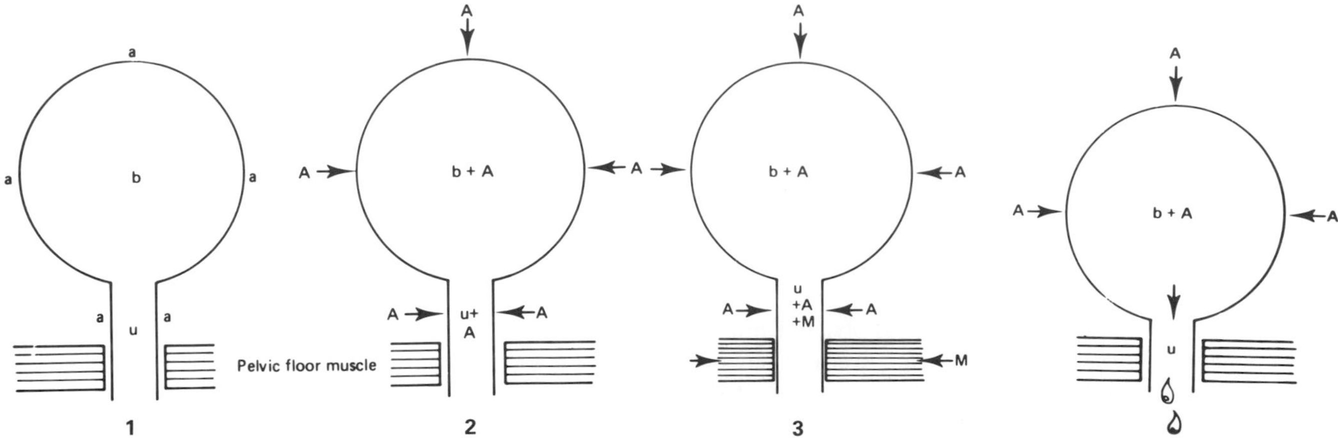

Fig. 42.9 Diagram to show the relationship between bladder, urethra and pelvic floor in (**1**) the resting state and on stress, to illustrate the passive (**2**) and (**3**) active components of pressure transmission to the proximal urethra aiding stress continence. When these components are ineffective (**4**) stress incontinence results. a = resting intra-abdominal pressure; A = intra-abdominal pressure when straining; b = intravesical pressure; u = intra-urethral pressure, M = pressure exerted by the pelvic floor muscles. From Hilton (1987) with permission.

mission of intra-abdominal pressure to the urethra may be quantified by means of urethral pressure profiles recorded during stress (Fig. 42.7). The pressure transmission ratio is defined as the increment in urethral pressure as a percentage of the simultaneously recorded increment in intra-abdominal pressure; this parameter may be recorded at several points along the urethra, and a pressure transmission profile can be constructed which details the transmission of intra-abdominal pressure rises from bladder neck to external urethral meatus. Using this technique it has been shown that in normal women transmission of intra-abdominal pressure rises is effective throughout the proximal three-quarters of the urethral length, i.e. throughout that portion of the urethra lying above the urogenital diaphragm (Fig. 42.10).

Secondly, an active or neuromuscular effect on transmission may be important in stress continence. It may also be shown by simultaneous bladder and urethral pressure measurements that in a region around the third quarter of the functional urethral length, pressure transmission ratios often exceed 100% (Figs 42.7 and 42.10). It has been suggested that this may reflect a reflex pelvic floor contraction in response to stress, augmenting urethral closure

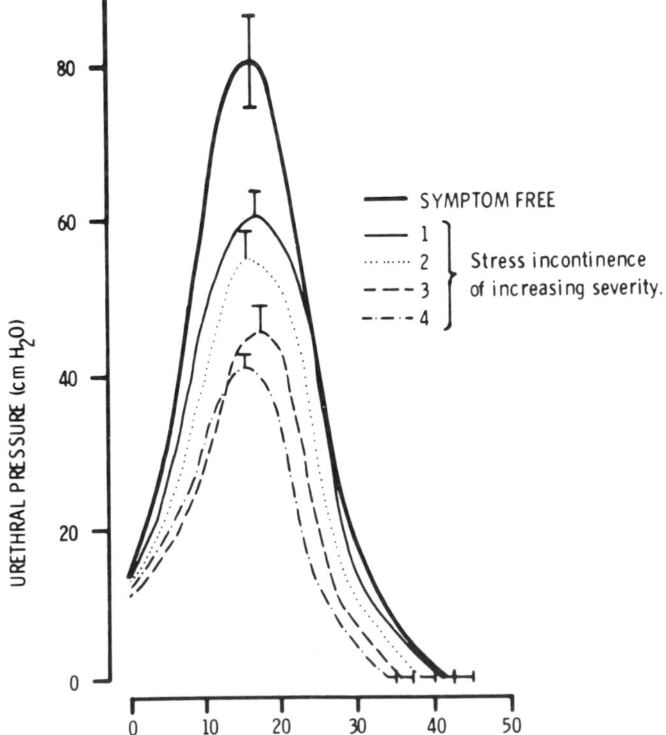

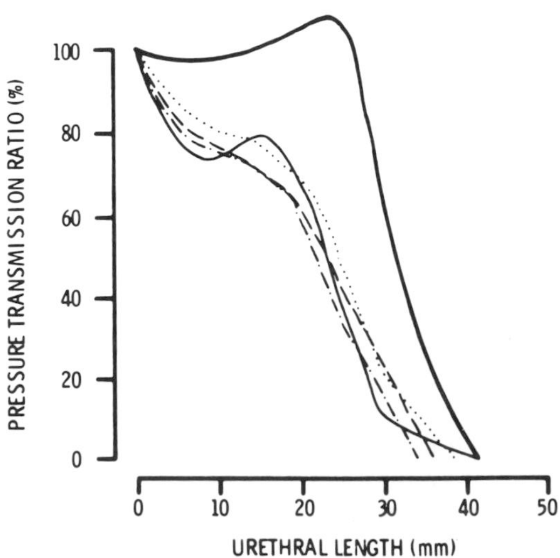

Fig. 42.10 **Left** Average resting urethral pressure profiles and **right** pressure transmission profiles in a group of symptom-free women and four groups with stress incontinence of varying severity. From Hilton & Stanton (1983) with permission.

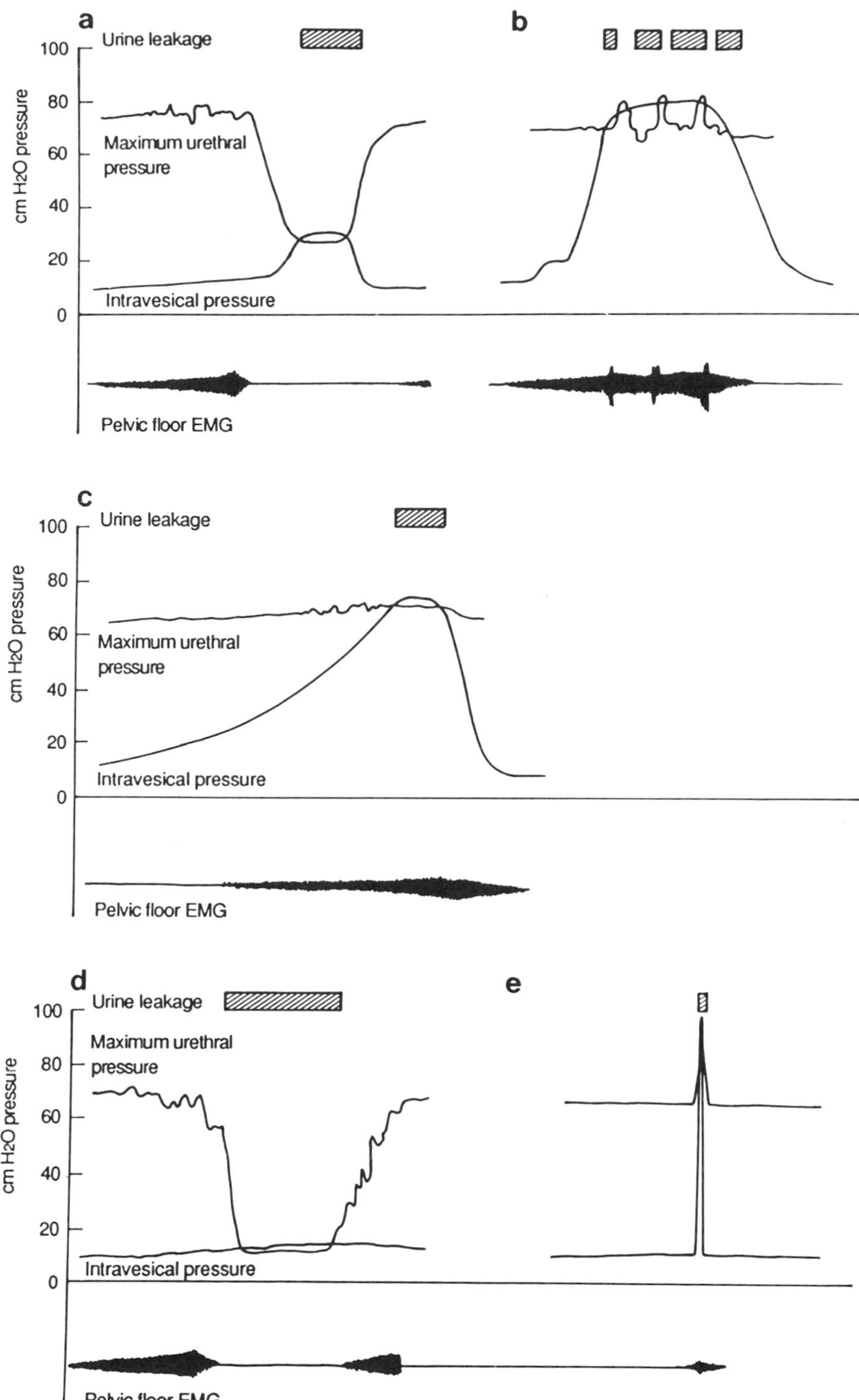

Fig. 42.11 Mechanisms of urinary incontinence showing changes in urethral and intravesical pressure and pelvic floor electromyogram (EMG) at various stages of bladder filling, in different types of incontinence. **a** Normal voiding or detrusor instability; **b** detrusor instability with detrusor–sphincter dyssynergia; **c** impaired bladder compliance; **d** urethral instability; **e** genuine stress incontinence. From Hilton (1992) with permission.

(Fig. 42.9). Certainly the observed pressure changes do fit closely with the current concepts of the anatomy of the region, and an active neuromuscular element in the maintenance of normal stress continence is accepted by many authors.

PATHOPHYSIOLOGY OF URINARY INCONTINENCE

General considerations

The pathophysiology of several causes of incontinence is

considered in greater detail in this volume in chapters relating to individual conditions; here general comments are made in so far as the pathophysiology relates to abnormalities of the micturition cycle as described above.

Assuming an intact lower urinary tract, urine flow occurs only when the intravesical pressure exceeds the maximum urethral pressure, or when the maximum urethral closure pressure becomes zero or negative. In general terms this may occur as a result of:

1 A fall in urethral pressure associated with an increase in intravesical pressure (Fig. 42.11a) — as in normal voiding or in many cases of detrusor instability, primarily those of idiopathic or psychosomatic origin, or those resulting from neurological lesions above the level of the pontine micturition centre.
2 An increase in intravesical pressure associated with an increase in urethral pressure, the latter being insufficient to maintain a positive closure pressure (Fig. 42.11b) — as in detrusor instability with associated detrusor sphincter dyssynergia, resulting from neurological lesions above the sacral but below the pontine micturition centre.
3 An abnormally high increase in detrusor pressure during bladder filling (Fig. 42.11c) — a situation considered by some workers to be analogous to detrusor instability, but perhaps better considered as impaired bladder compliance. This may be seen in chronic inflammatory conditions such as tuberculosis or interstitial cystitis and also following pelvic irradiation; a similar situation also accounts for the incontinence in chronic urinary retention, where the bladder pressure rises acutely at the end of filling.
4 A loss of urethral pressure alone, without any coincident change in intravesical pressure (Fig. 42.11d) — as in urethral instability.
5 Where on stress the intravesical pressure rises to a greater extent than the intraurethral pressure (Fig. 42.11e) — as in genuine stress incontinence.

EFFECTS OF CONTINENCE SURGERY ON MECHANISMS OF CONTINENCE

Well over 100 different operations have been described for the treatment of genuine stress incontinence, reflecting not merely the inadequacy of any single procedure to deal satisfactorily with all cases, but also uncertainties about the nature of the problem, and the mechanism of its cure.

The aims of incontinence surgery have been variously defined as tightening of the pubocervical fascia, elevation of the bladder neck, restoration of the posterior urethrovesical angle, increasing urethral pressure, increasing functional urethral length, and increasing urethral resistance. There is, however, little information as to the extent to which these aims are achieved by the various surgical techniques. Cure rates between 40 and 97% have been reported, but which aspects of the procedures, or of urethral function, determine success or failure is still poorly understood.

Urethral pressure profiles have been recorded at rest and on stress, before and after a variety incontinence operations, including the anterior colporrhaphy, Burch colposuspension, Marshall–Marchetti–Krantz, suburethral sling, and Stamey endoscopic bladder neck suspension procedures. Whilst marked changes are noted in the resting urethral profile peroperatively, these are short-lived, and could not account for the success of surgery. In stress profiles, however, improvements in pressure transmission in mid-urethra are consistently found following successful surgical treatment (Figs 42.12 and 42.13). Whilst the results of these various studies are qualitatively similar, there are considerable quantitative differences — improvements in transmission vary from only a few per cent with the anterior repair to well over 100% with the colposuspension.

The nature of the improvement in urethral pressure transmission following surgery is uncertain. It has previously been suggested that it is simply due to elevation of the bladder neck and proximal urethra into the abdo-

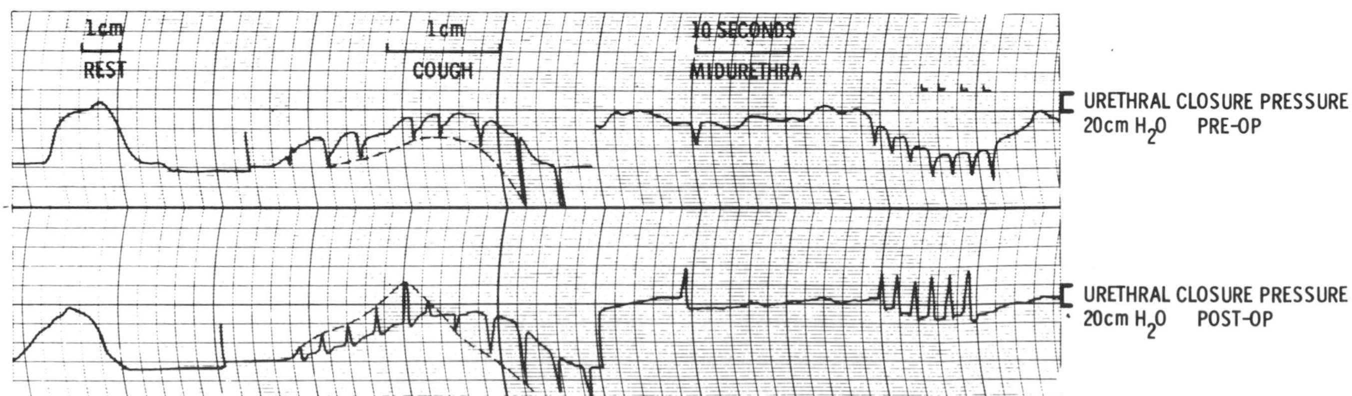

Fig. 42.12 Example of pre- and postoperative urethral closure pressure recordings in a patient undergoing successful Burch colposuspension. L = demonstrated urinary leakage during preoperative trace. From Hilton & Stanton (1983b) with permission.

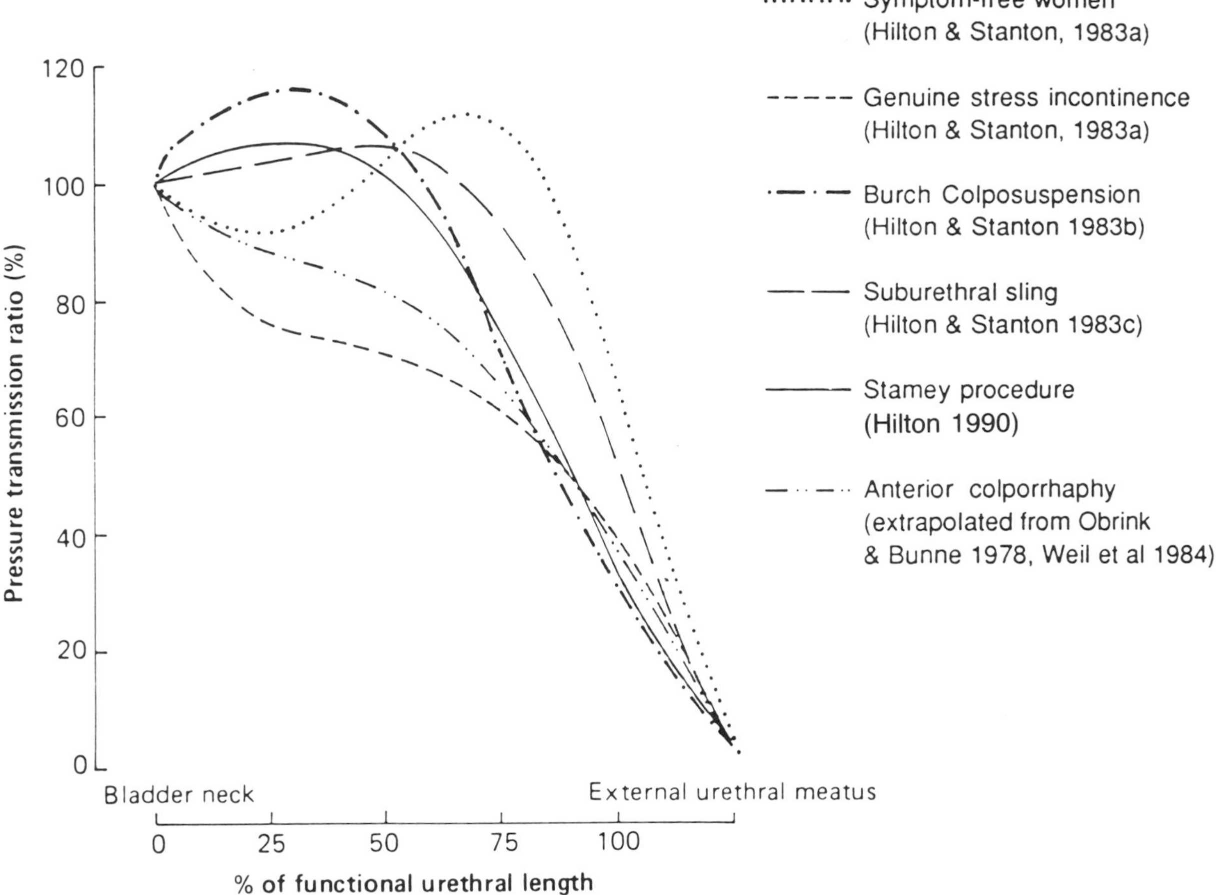

Fig. 42.13 Average pressure transmission profiles for symptom-free women, those with genuine stress incontinence, and patients undergoing successful treatment for stress incontinence using a variety of surgical procedures.

minal pressure zone, thereby allowing improved passive transmission to the region. Whilst this would explain transmission ratios approaching 100%, it clearly could not explain ratios over 100%, as noted above. It is possible that the elevation of the bladder neck not only allows improved passive transmission, but also promotes greater efficiency of the pelvic floor reflex with accentuation of urethral closure by active means. The distribution of pressure transmission along the urethra following successful suprapubic surgery is quite different from that seen in healthy women (Fig. 42.13), and the delay between intravesical and urethral pressure rises on coughing — around 10 ms — is too short to involve a neuromuscular reflex.

It would seem more likely therefore that the improved transmission has a mechanical rather than neuromuscular basis. The most obvious anatomical change following successful suprapubic incontinence surgery is the relocation of the urethra in a high retropubic position, and it is possible that downward pressure from abdominal viscera on coughing compresses the urethra against the posterior surface of the symphysis accentuating urethral closure.

It appears that those operations which give the best

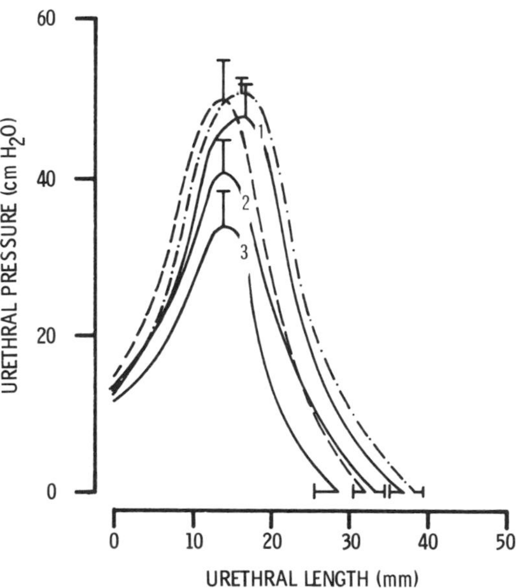

Fig. 42.14 Average resting urethral pressure profiles for stress incontinent patients according to previous surgical history. —·— No pelvic surgery (n = 58); — one (n = 25), two (n = 14), and three or more (n = 7) previous unsuccessful incontinence operations; — — — previous pelvic surgery other than for incontinence (n = 16). From Hilton & Stanton (1983a) with permission.

results in terms of cure of stress incontinence are those which produce maximum urethral and bladder neck elevation — and at the same time the greatest enhancements in pressure transmission — but are also those with the greatest risk of increasing urethral resistance; operations which produce lesser degrees of elevation may cause less postoperative voiding difficulties, but are also less likely to cure stress incontinence. This principle has been proven for the colposuspension in particular, and seems likely to apply to incontinence surgery in general.

Little research has been done into the effects of unsuccessful incontinence surgery on bladder and urethral function. It has, however, been shown that the improvements in pressure transmission noted following successful surgery are not found following unsuccessful surgery. It has also been shown that following some failed procedures a reduction in urethral closure pressure may ensue, and that the more unsuccessful procedures a patient has undergone, the less efficient her urethral closure is likely to be (Fig. 42.14).

CONCLUSIONS

If dysfunction of the urinary tract is to be effectively managed, the choice of treatment must be optimal. This choice must be based on a firm knowledge of the normal mechanisms of continence, and of the mechanisms whereby this normal control may break down. Only in the light of this knowledge can the meaningful investigation of the individual incontinent patient be carried out.

The results of this investigation, taken in conjunction with a knowledge of the effects of various treatment modalities, should allow the selection of a rational and specific therapy for each patient.

KEY POINTS

1. The urethral sphincter contains slow and fast twitch muscle fibres to produce continuous closure at rest and additional closure on effort respectively.
2. The epithelial lining of mucosa and submucosal venous plexuses of the urethra are important in its hermetic closure.
3. The bladder and urethra have complex coordinated sympathetic and parasympathetic innervation.
4. Continence is maintained by direct mechanical transmission of intra-abdominal pressure to the proximal urethra by reflex pelvic floor contraction.
5. Successful continence surgery is related to elevation of the bladder neck and to improvement in abdominal pressure transmission to the proximal urethra. In some patients, the increase in bladder neck elevation may lead to voiding difficulty.

SUGGESTED READING

Definitions and terminology

Abrams P, Blaivas J, Stanton S L, Andersen J 1990 The standardisation of terminology of lower urinary tract function. British Journal of Obstetrics and Gynaecology 97: suppl 6

Anatomy of the lower urinary tract

DeLancey J 0 1988 Structural aspects of the extrinsic continence mechanism. American Journal of Obstetrics and Gynecology 72: 296–301

Gosling J A, Dixon J, Critchley H O D, Thompson S A 1981 A comparative study of human external sphincter and periurethral levator ani muscle. British Journal of Urology 53: 35–41

Gosling J A, Dixon J, Humpherson J R 1983 Functional anatomy of the urinary tract. Churchill Livingstone, Edinburgh

Huisman A B 1983 Aspects of the anatomy of the female urethra with special relation to urinary continence. Contributions to Gynaecology and Obstetrics, vol 10: Female stress incontinence. Ulmsten U (ed) Karger, Basel, pp 1–31

Neurological control of micturition

Bradley W E, Timm T W, Scott F B 1974 Innervation of the detrusor muscle and urethra. Urological Clinics of North America 1: 3–27

Fletcher T F, Bradley W E 1978 Neuroanatomy of the bladder–urethra. Journal of Urology 119: 153–160

Torrens M 1984 Neurophysiology. In: Clinical gynecological urology Stanton S L (ed) C V Mosby, St Louis, pp 13–21

Physiology of the lower urinary tract

Asmussen M, Ulmsten U 1983 On the physiology of continence and pathaphysiology of stress incontinence in the female. Contributions to Gynaecology and Obstetrics, vol 10: Female stress incontinence Ulmsten U (ed) Karger, Basel, pp 32–50

Constantinou C E 1985 Resting and stress urethral pressures as a clinical guide to the mechanism of continence. Clinics in Obstetrics and Gynaecology 12: 343–356

Rud T 1980 The urethral pressure profile in continent women from childhood to old age. Acta Obstetricia et Gynaecologica Scandinavica 59: 331–335

Rud T, Andersson K-E, Asmussen M, Hunting A, Ulmsten U 1980 Factors maintaining the intraurethral pressure in women Investigative Urology 17: 343–347

Wein A 1986 Physiology of micturition. Clinics in Geriatric Medicine 2(4): 689–699

The mechanics and hydrodynamics of bladder and urethra

Coolsaet B L R A 1984 Cystometry. In: Stanton S L (ed) Clinical gynecological urology C V Mosby, St Louis, pp 59–81

Griffiths D J 1980 Urodynamics. Adam Hilger, Bristol

Hilton P 1981 Urethral pressure measurement by microtransducer: observations on the methodology, the pathophysiology of genuine stress incontinence and the effects of its treatment in the female. MD Thesis, University of Newcastle-upon-Tyne.

Hilton P 1990 Urethral pressure profilometry in the female. In: George N, O'Reilly P, Weiss R (eds) Diagnostic techniques in urology. WB Saunders, Philadelphia, pp 309–335

Zinner N R, Ritter R C, Sterling A M 1976 The mechanism of micturition. In: Williams D I, Chisholm G D (eds) Scientific foundations of urology. Heinemann, London, pp 39–51

Pathophysiology of urinary incontinence

Anderson R S 1984 A neurogenic element to urinary genuine stress incontinence. British Journal of Obstetrics and Gynaecology 91: 41–46

Enhorning G E 1961 Simultaneous recording of the intravesical and intraurethral pressure. Acta Chirurgica Scandinavica (suppl) 276: 1–68

Hilton P 1988 Clinical algorithms. Urinary incontinence in women. British Medical Journal 295: 426–432

Hilton P, Stanton S L 1983a Urethral pressure by microtransducer: the results in symptom-free women and in those with genuine stress incontinence. British Journal of Obstetrics and Gynaecology 90: 919–933

The effects of incontinence surgery on continence mechanisms

Hertogs K, Stanton S L 1985 Mechanism of urinary continence after colposuspension: barrier studies. British Journal of Obstetrics and Gynaecology 92: 1184–1188

Hilton P, Stanton S L 1983b A clinical and urodynamic assessment of the Burch colposuspension for genuine stress incontinence. British Journal of Obstetrics and Gynaecology 90: 934–939

Hilton P 1987 Surgery for urinary stress incontinence. In: Monaghan J M (ed) Operative surgery: gynaecology and obstetrics, 4th edition. Butterworths, London, pp 105–126

Hilton P 1989 A clinical and urodynamic comparison of the abdomino-vaginal sub-urethral sling and Stamey endoscopic bladder neck suspension in the treatment of genuine stress incontinence. British Journal of Obstetrics and Gynaecology 96: 213–220

Obrink A, Bunne G 1978 The margin to incontinence after three types of operation for stress incontinence. Scandinavian Journal of Urology and Nephrology 12: 209–214

Weil A, Reyes H, Bischof P, Rottenberg R D, Krauer F 1984 Modifications of the urethral resting and stress profiles after different types of surgery for urinary stress incontinence. British Journal of Obstetrics and Gynaecology 91: 46–55

Hilton P 1986 The mechanism of continence. In: Tanagho E A (eds) Stanton S L, Surgery for female incontinence. Springer Verlag, Berlin, pp 1–21

Hilton P 1990 Urethral pressure profilometry in the female. In: George N, O'Reilly P, Weiss R (eds) Diagnostic techniques in urology. WB Saunders, Philadelphia, pp 309–335

Hilton P 1992 The mechanism of continence. In: Stanton S L (ed) Clinical gynaecological urology, 2nd edn. Churchill Livingstone, Edinburgh (in press)

43. History and examination

S. L. Stanton

Early description of disease relied much on the ability of the clinician to record accurately the history and clinical examination; confirmatory investigations were rudimentary, most information being provided by histological specimens removed at operation or at post-mortem. Complex and sophisticated investigations have gradually evolved but we still rely on the history and examination to provide the framework for diagnosis.

HISTORY

Most history-taking still uses the patient's own words and is written in prose (usually neither as lengthy nor as literate as in the past). More use is made now both of the structured questionnaire (designed for the condition being studied and computer-coded for easy data collation and analysis) and the facility of entering data from the patient immediately on to the computer. These methods have the following advantages:

1. Questioning is consistent without omission of data. This is especially important before an operation, since frequently the patient's later recall of symptoms is incomplete.
2. Different doctors can produce similar data, ensuring consistency of recording within the department.
3. The history is legible and is an efficient and rapid method of dealing with a large patient throughput (Cardozo et al 1978).

A variety of questionnaires have been developed (Hodgkinson 1963; Robertson 1974). Reliance on simple questions and examination is nowadays considered too inaccurate because the bladder is an unreliable witness. Bates et al (1973) studied a group of patients following bladder repair and demonstrated that 50% of those with detrusor instability complained of stress incontinence. Jarvis et al (1980) showed that clinical diagnosis was accurate in only 65% of cases. Symptom analysis or the use of symptom complexes where groups of symptoms are linked is more accurate, reaching 96% accuracy in the diagnosis of some conditions (Farrar et al 1975). Our own questionnaire (Cardozo et al 1978) has now been updated. In redesigning the questionnaire, we took note of the findings of Norton et al (1988) who surveyed patients attending the urodynamic unit: 25% of patients waited more than 5 years before seeking advice because of embarrassment or they felt their symptoms were normal. More than 50% said their symptoms adversely affected their work and nearly half said they felt 'odd' or 'different' from other people. Some two-thirds of patients avoided sexual intercourse because of their urinary problems.

The questionnaire provides a note of the order of symptom importance, the reason why the patient presented now, the amount of interference of symptoms with life-style, the occurrence of symptoms at intercourse and a quantitative measure of severity as well as frequency of symptoms. Under the examination section, mobility and dementia scores are included.

There is an initial space for the patient's history in her own words and then a series of questions with graded answers. The questionnaire is printed on self-carbonating paper, so that one copy is filed in the patient's hospital notes and the other is retained in the unit; this is invaluable for retrieving research data as the notes never leave the department. Alternatively, answers can be entered directly on to a computer and stored on disk, with speedy retrieval for insertion of additional information as the patient's investigations and treatment proceed.

In some hospitals, the history is completed by the patient alone or aided by the nurse. We think this is disadvantageous and prefer a doctor to be responsible for history taking so that ambiguous questions can be clarified.

The history is divided into urological, neurological, gynaecological and medical sections, followed by psychiatric, drug and past history sections.

Urological

Incontinence

The most common initial symptom is incontinence and it needs careful evaluation. Stress incontinence is a symptom and a sign, *not* a diagnosis. It must be distinguished from urgency leading to urge incontinence. The following qualifying questions should be asked: is it intermittent or continuous? Is it precipitated by effort or is it present at rest or on physical stress, giggling, seeing running water, putting the key in the door, intercourse or orgasm? Does it occur after micturition as the patient stands up (postmicturition dribble)? How severe is the incontinence, how often does it require a change of pants or pads and does incontinence occur at night?

Urethral sphincter incompetence is likely to cause stress incontinence alone but sometimes there is accompanying urge incontinence. Detrusor instability usually causes urge incontinence but some patients also have stress incontinence, incontinence on giggling or seeing running water or putting the key in the front door. Both conditions can cause nocturnal enuresis; stress incontinence due to urethral sphincter incompetence is usually associated with some physical effort whereas detrusor instability may present as nocturnal enuresis. Postmicturition dribble may be due to a urethral diverticulum. Continuous incontinence may be associated with a congenital anomaly (e.g. ectopic ureter or epispadias), a urinary fistula or retention with overflow. Frontal lobe lesions produce lack of social awareness and lead to incontinence at any time and without any apparent precipitating cause.

Table 43.1 Causes of urgency, urge incontinence and frequency

Urgency/urge incontinence and frequency	Additional causes of frequency
Urinary tract infection	Increased fluid intake
Upper motor neurone lesion	Impaired renal function
Irritative mucosal lesion	Reduced bladder capacity
Urethral syndrome	Pelvic mass
Detrusor instability	Chronic residual urine
Habit	Diabetes insipidus
	Diabetes mellitus
	Increased age
	Diuretic therapy
	Hypothyroidism
	Hypercalcaemia
	Hyperkalaemia

Urgency

Sudden desire to void, if uncontrolled or unfulfilled, may result in urge incontinence. Urgency on its own is a commonplace symptom. Bungay et al (1980) surveyed fit women between 30 and 64 years of age and found that approximately 20% had urgency. The common causes are shown in Table 43.1.

Frequency

Voiding more than seven times a day or being woken twice or more at night whilst asleep is defined as frequency. Its common causes are also shown in Table 43.1. Urgency and frequency are often linked, and it is tempting to think that sometimes a vicious circle of frequency → urgency → frequency exists. We have shown that an operative cure of one is associated with cure of another (Stanton et al 1976). The incidence can be charted by a patient using a urinary diary or frequency/volume chart, recording input and output volumes and permitting a subjective assessment of the volume of urine lost together with episodes of urgency and leakage.

Voiding difficulty

Most women are completely unaware of their voiding ability and potential; they have little concept of stream velocity or cast distance. They are aware of hesitancy, difficulty in voiding, poor stream, having to stand to void and incomplete emptying but these symptoms are uncommon. Acute retention, which is the most serious symptom, may need to be defined. It may or may not be painful and catheterization is required for its relief. The volume removed should be at least 75% of the functional bladder capacity. Catheterization is sometimes carried out in the mistaken belief that retention is present and amounts much less than this are removed.

The prevalence of symptoms of confirmed voiding disorders in new attenders at a urodynamic unit is 12%; however a further 2% of patients attending had asymptomatic voiding difficulties (Stanton et al 1983). No one symptom seemed to accord more accurately with the clinical situation, but poor stream was the most common. Hesitancy is an uncommon symptom, but its postpartum prevalence in a group of healthy women without previous urological abnormality was between 8 and 10% (Stanton et al 1980).

Neurological

The frequent occurrence of bladder disturbances associated with neurological disease makes it imperative that a neurological history and examination be completed. Evidence of general neurological disease should be sought and questions directed towards motor and sensory abnormalities, particularly those affecting sacral roots S2 to S4. The common neurological diseases that may appear are multiple sclerosis, peripheral neuropathy associated with diabetes mellitus, cerebral vascular accident, parkinsonism and autonomic dysreflexia (with symptoms of sweating, palpitations and headaches). It is important to question the patient about visual changes (e.g. blurred or double vision), back pain, disturbance of balance, alteration in bowel control and in lower limb sensation and motor power.

Gynaecological

Because of the close embryological, anatomical and physiological relationship between the urological and genital tracts, lesions of either may affect both. The urothelium is oestrogen-sensitive and dependent. Changes in functional urethral length but not pressure have been correlated with E_2 levels (Van Geelen et al 1981). However Hilton (1981) studied patients with urological symptoms and found significantly higher maximum urethral closure pressure in the early luteal phase than at any other time in the menstrual cycle. Smith (1972) has demonstrated the symptomatic and psychological changes associated with postmenopausal oestrogen deficiency and the benefits of oestrogen therapy. Thus the relationship of the menstrual cycle and menopause to urethral function is important. Most women whose symptoms are affected by their menstrual cycle claim they are worse in the week preceding their period.

The association of genital prolapse with stress incontinence is established. About 40% of patients with urethral sphincter incompetence have significant anterior vaginal wall descent (Cardozo & Stanton 1980).

The relationship between urological symptoms and gynaecological surgery is important. Occasionally repair of uncomplicated prolapse may cause postoperative urethral sphincter incompetence, resulting from interference with the urethral sphincter mechanism. In a pre- and postoperative study of anterior colporrhaphy and vaginal hysterectomy for prolapse with or without stress incontinence, we could find no evidence of increase in symptoms of urgency and frequency postoperatively (Stanton et al 1982). Jequier (1976) studied patients' symptoms before and after total abdominal hysterectomy and found no overall increase in urological symptoms. The colposuspension operation for urethral sphincter incompetence can lead to initial postoperative dyspareunia and symptoms and signs of enterocele. Usually, urgency and frequency are decreased following colposuspension, but sometimes symptoms arise de novo, with or without detrusor instability.

Ovarian and uterine enlargement may cause symptoms of frequency and sometimes, if impaction occurs, urinary retention can result. Endometriosis involving the bladder can lead to frequency, urgency and cyclical haematuria. Frequency and urgency may also be associated with pelvic inflammatory disease. Oral contraception (either combined oestrogen and progestogen or progestogen alone) is not found to cause specific urological symptoms.

Medical

Any condition increasing abdominal pressure, for example constipation or chronic cough, may induce stress incontinence caused by urethral sphincter incompetence by altering the pressure gradient between bladder and proximal urethra. Cardiac and renal failure will also produce frequency, and diabetes mellitus and insipidus should be considered when polydipsia and polyuria or frequency appear.

Psychiatric

For an elderly patient who may suffer from dementia, a dementia score to determine the awareness and degree of understanding and co-operation is helpful in her assessment. The patient's appearance and behaviour at the interview, mood state (e.g. sad or elated), form and content of 'talk' and intelligence and orientation are important. Various self-administered psychiatric questionnaires are available for patient assessment; however these are usually research tools and are not widely used in routine clinical practice. Examples include the Wakefield Self-Assessment of Depression Inventory (WDI) to detect depression, Middlesex Hospital Questionnaire (MHQ) to detect neuroticism and the Minnesota Multiphasic Personality Inventory (MMPI) to detect personality change. Referral to a psychiatric colleague is advisable if psychiatric disease is suspected.

Drug history

The current drug regimen is important. Drugs taken directly for gynaecological or urological symptoms and drugs taken for other conditions that might indirectly affect the lower urinary tracts should be noted. It is relevant to confirm that the patient is taking her drugs at the correct time; a common cause for nocturia is late administration of diuretic therapy.

Past history

The obstetrical history should include parity, method of

delivery and weight of the largest infant (which may suggest late-onset diabetes mellitus if over 4.5 kg). Details of the length of labour are often incorrectly recalled by the patient and are not helpful.

All past major surgery should be recorded. Pelvic surgery is of particular importance, especially if the bladder or urethra was involved. Full operative and postoperative data are required and any resultant side-effects and complications should be detailed. Often a patient with a current voiding disorder has had a troublesome past surgical history requiring recurrent catheterization and a prolonged time before the catheter could be removed. Surgery involving the spine (e.g. laminectomy) should be included because of a potential for damage to the nerve supply of the bladder, urethra and pelvic floor.

Urinary tract infection and its treatment should be enquired about; the frequency of episodes over the past 2 years and whether or not a positive bacterial culture was obtained before treatment should be recorded.

A history of past enuresis may indicate the possibility of ongoing detrusor instability. Retention of urine, its antecedent causes such as surgery or childbirth and its subsequent treatment should be enquired about. Finally, a note should be made of drug allergy and of any drug treatment for lower urinary tract disorders and the outcome.

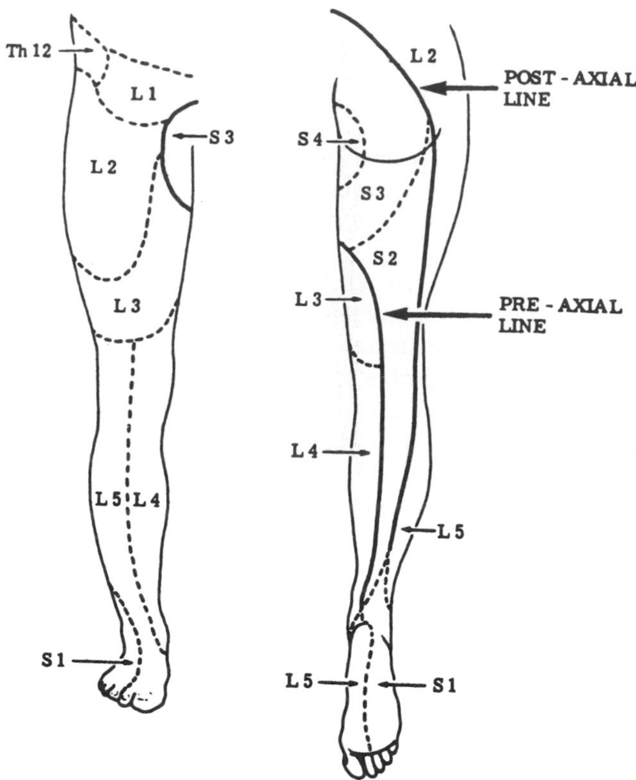

Fig. 43.1 Cutaneous distribution of sacral nerve roots S2 to S4.

EXAMINATION

Before commencing, it is important to place the patient at ease by reassuring her that no embarrassment should be felt if she loses urine during the course of the examination. The attitude and demeanour of the patient and any obvious personality or mental disorders should be noted. The height and weight of the patient is recorded and a simple score made of her mobility. Similarly a dementia score is compiled. General, neurological and gynaecological examinations are performed.

Neurological

A simplified neurological examination should be performed to screen all patients. Referral to a neurologist is advised if the neurological history and examination are abnormal or if cystometry suggests an upper or lower motor neurone lesion.

The pupils are tested for pupillary reflex and nystagmus. Limbs are tested for tone, power, reflex and sensation. Particular attention is paid to sensation over the sacral dermatomes S2 to S4 (Fig. 43.1). The back is examined for lesions such as spina bifida (overt or occult; Fig. 43.2) and prolapsed intervertebral disc or spondylosis. A Rhomberg test is used to confirm whether balance is normal. A rectal examination is carried out to check anal sphincter tone.

Special neurological tests to confirm an intact sacral reflex include stroking the skin lateral to the anus to elicit contraction of the external anal sphincter and tapping or squeezing the clitoris which will produce a contraction of the ischio- and bulbocavernosus muscles (the bulbo-

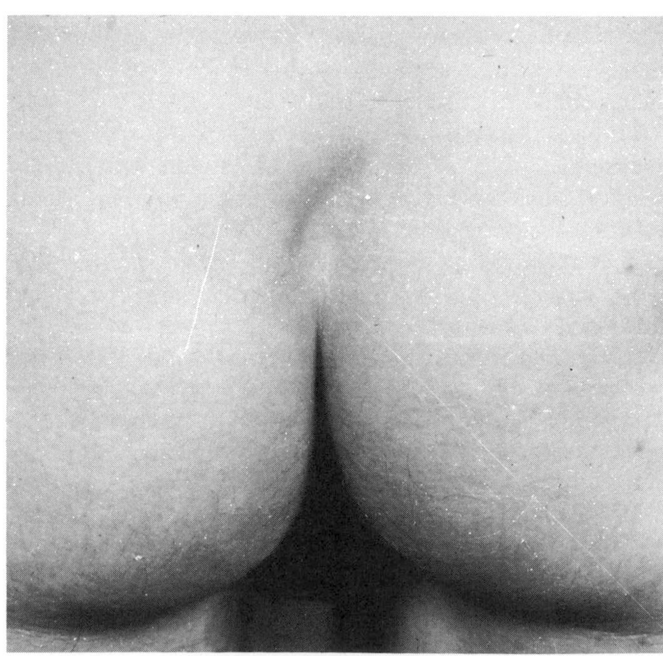

Fig. 43.2a Sacral hollow overlying spina bifida occulta of S2 to S4.

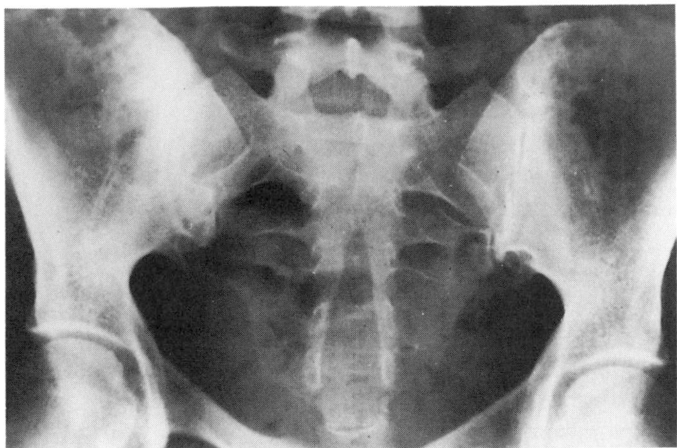

Fig. 43.2b Radiograph showing spina bifida occulta of S2 to S4.

cavernosus reflex) which can also be elicited by pulling on a suprapubic or foley catheter.

Gynaecological

As part of the abdominal examination, renal enlargement or a palpable bladder should be detected; the latter may be difficult in the obese patient, but a bimanual examination may enable ballottement of the bladder by the vaginal hand; a crude assessment can be made of the residual urine. The external appearance of the vulva should be noted to detect congenital anomalies such as epispadias (Fig. 43.3) or an opening of an ectopic ureter which may be difficult to detect. Vulval excoriation will give some indication of the severity of incontinence. The presence of stress incontinence may be detected in the supine or erect position but is most noticeable when the patient has a comfortably full bladder (Robinson & Stanton 1981). Wetness within or around the vagina needs differentiation from healthy vaginal discharge (which is clear or opalescent and without symptoms) and pathological vaginal discharge (which may be white or yellow and associated with symptoms of discomfort, presence of vaginitis and an offensive odour). After drying the vagina with a swab, the doctor should observe the patient for a while with a speculum in place and ask her to cough. Provided urine has not leaked from the external urethral meatus, any fresh appearance of urine suggests a fistula.

The presence of atrophic genital change should be noted and the capacity and mobility of the vagina determined; these may have been compromised by previous pelvic surgery, and certainly affect the choice of a subsequent incontinence operation. The vagina should normally accommodate two fingers which should be able to be separated. If a colposuspension is to be performed, the fingers should be able to elevate the lateral vaginal fornices to the ipisilateral ileopectineal ligament. The urethra is examined for discharge, tenderness, inflammation, rigidity

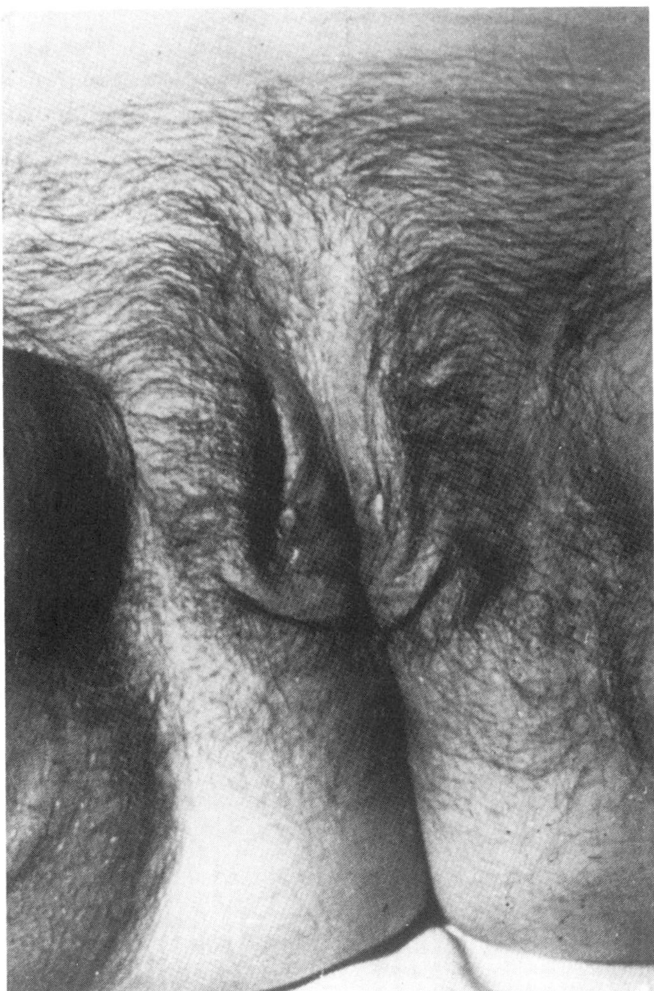

Fig. 43.3a Female epispadias showing separation of clitoris.

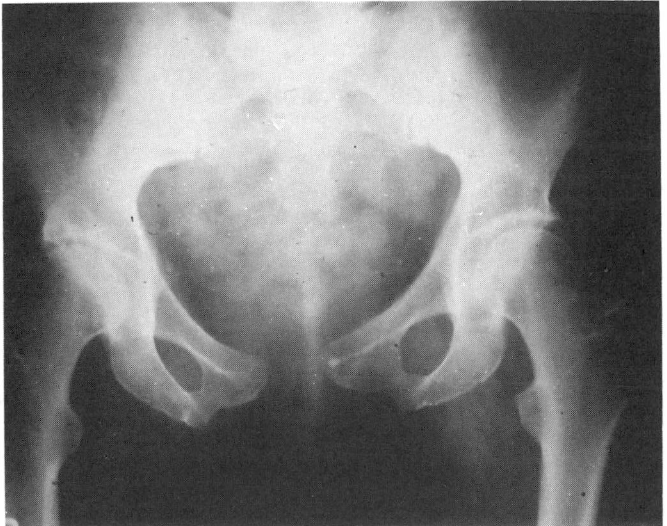

Fig. 43.3b Underlying symphyseal separation.

or fixation. An anterior vaginal wall mass may be either a urethral diverticulum or a paraurethral or vaginal cyst.

Bimanual examination will confirm the presence of normal or abnormal pelvic organs and detect any bladder enlargement caused by residual urine or neoplasm. Genital prolapse, comprising descent of the anterior and posterior vaginal wall and uterus, may be detected on coughing and straining with the use of a Sims' or similar speculum. Some clinical grading of prolapse is helpful: I differentiate between anterior wall descent and a cystocele and a cysto-urethrocele; a urethrocele on its own is rare. Descent may be slight (within the vagina) or marked (descent to or beyond the introitus). Uterine descent is graded as first-degree (descent within the vagina), second-degree (descent to the introitus) and third-degree or procidentia (descent beyond the introitus).

Posterior vaginal wall prolapse comprises enterocele (pouch of Douglas descent usually containing small bowel and rectocele and is graded similarly to anterior vaginal wall prolapse.

The examination is concluded by a rectal examination to detect rectal or anal pathology, and in particularly faecal impaction. The integrity of the pelvic floor and anal sphincter innervation is confirmed by asking the patient to squeeze on the examining finger.

KEY NOTES

1. Symptoms and signs may not accurately reflect the underlying pathophysiology of the bladder and urethra.
2. It is important that history should include urological, neurological, psychiatric and drug information.
3. Neurological examination, particularly of sacral roots 2, 3, and 4, is important where symptomatology is complex.

REFERENCES

Bates C P, Loose H, Stanton S L, 1973 Objective study of incontinence after repair operations. Surgery, Gynecology and Obstetrics 136: 17–22

Bungay G T, Vessey M P, McPherson C K 1980 Study of symptoms in middle life with special reference to the menopause. British Medical Journal 281: 181–183

Cardozo L, Stanton S L 1980 Genuine stress incontinence and detrusor instability: a review of 200 patients. British Journal Obstetrics and Gynaecology 87: 184–190

Cardozo L, Stanton S L, Bennett A E 1978 Design of a urodynamic questionnaire. British Journal Urology 50: 269–274

Farrar D J, Whiteside C G, Osborne J L, Turner-Warwick R T 1975 A urodynamic analysis of micturition symptoms in the female. Surgery Gynecology and Obstetrics 141: 875–881

Hilton P 1981 Urethral pressure measurement by microtransducers: observations on methodology, the pathophysiology of genuine stress incontinence and the effects of its treatment in the female. MD thesis, University of Newcastle-upon-Tyne

Hodgkinson C P 1963 Urinary stress incontinence in the female: a programme of preoperative investigations. Clinics in Obstetrics and Gynecology 6: 154–177

Jarvis G J, Hall S, Stamp S, Millar D R, Johnson A, 1980 An assessment of urodynamic examination in the incontinent woman. British Journal of Obstetrics and Gynaecology 87: 893–896

Jequier A 1976 Urinary symptoms and total hysterectomy. British Journal of Urology 48: 437–441

Norton P, MacDonald L, Sedgwick P, Stanton S L 1988 Distress and delay associated with urinary incontinence, frequency and urgency in women. British Medical Journal 297: 1187–1189

Robertson J, 1974 Ambulatory gynecologic urology. Clinics in Obstetrics and Gynecology 17: 255–275

Robinson H, Stanton S L 1981 Detection of urinary incontinence. British Journal of Obstetrics and Gynaecology 88: 59–61

Smith P 1972 Age changes in the female urethra. British Journal of Urology 44: 667–676

Stanton S L, Williams J E, Ritchie D 1976 The colposuspension operation for urinary incontinence. British Journal of Obstetrics and Gynaecology 83: 890–895

Stanton S L, Kerr-Wilson R, Harris V G 1980 Incidence of urological symptoms in normal pregnancy. British Journal of Obstetrics and Gynaecology 87: 897–900

Stanton S L, Hilton P, Norton C, Cardozo L 1982 Clinical and urodynamic effects of anterior colporrhaphy and vaginal by sterectomy for prolapse with and without incontinence. British Journal of Obstetrics and Gynaecology 89: 459–463

Stanton S L, Ozsoy C, Hilton P 1983 Voiding difficulties in the female: prevalence, clinical and urodynamic review. Obstetrics and Gynecology 61: 144–147

Van Geelen J M, Doesburg W H, Thomas C M G, Marin C B 1981 Urodynamic studies in the normal menstrual cycle: the relationships between hormonal changes during the menstrual cycle and the urethral pressure profile. American Journal of Obstetrics and Gynecology 141: 384–392

44. Urodynamic investigations

S. M. Creighton

INTRODUCTION

Lower urinary tract symptoms are common and objective assessment of patients is important. An accurate and detailed history and examination provide a framework for the diagnosis but there is often a discrepancy between the patient's symptoms and the urodynamic findings. Jarvis et al (1980) found the clinical diagnosis to be accurate in only 65% of cases. Cardozo & Stanton (1980) reviewed 200 patients and found 55% of patients with genuine stress incontinence on cystometry; 35% of those patients with detrusor instability on cystometry actually complained of mixed symptoms of urge and stress incontinence. As the results of surgery are jeopardized by pre-existing detrusor instability, urodynamic studies on patients with symptoms of both urge and stress incontinence would seem, from these studies, to be necessary.

When stress incontinence is the sole symptom, Farrar et al (1975) found that the clinical and cystometric diagnoses agreed in 96% of patients and concluded that urodynamic investigations were superfluous in these patients. The poor predictive value of symptoms in those patients with a mixed clinical picture was again confirmed.

In patients with neurological disorders the symptoms may be even less likely to correlate with the urodynamic findings. Blaivas et al (1979) showed a 27% improvement in patients with multiple sclerosis treated empirically but an 81% improvement when the treatment was based on the urodynamic findings.

Urodynamic studies are also important to exclude voiding disorders (which can be asymptomatic) and in the evaluation of the success or failure of surgical or conservative treatment. Bates et al (1973) studied patients with recurrent incontinence following bladder neck surgery and found that 50% of those patients complaining of stress incontinence postoperatively had a urodynamic diagnosis of detrusor instability.

BASIC TESTS

Midstream urine specimen

A midstream urine specimen must be taken from all patients presenting with urinary symptoms. A urine infection may be responsible for some or all of their symptoms and if present must be treated before invasive urodynamic studies are performed as it will deteriorate.

A significant bacteriuria is considered to be 100 000

organisms per millilitre of urine and is usually associated with pyuria. The presence of epithelial cells, erythrocytes and casts is also noted.

Invasive urodynamic studies, if performed competently and cleanly, have a less than 2% risk of urinary tract infection (Walter & Vejlsgaard 1978).

Urinary diary

A urinary diary is a simple record of the patient's fluid intake and output (Fig. 44.1). It should be completed by all patients for 1 week. It also records episodes of leakage, whether or not these were precipitated by urgency or activities. These diaries aid diagnosis and are more accurate than attempted recall by the patient. An idea of the functional capacity of the bladder is obtained and the diary can also be used as a baseline for bladder retraining.

DAY: Monday.

TIME	INTAKE (ml)	OUTPUT (ml)	LEAKAGE: ACTIVITY	LEAKAGE: Amount	LEAKAGE: Urge	LEAKAGE: Wet Bed
07.00		350	Getting out of bed	Soaked Pad.	Yes	
08.00	200	75			Yes	
08.30	200	50			Yes	
08.50	.	100			Yes	
09.30	240	75			Yes	
10.20		50			Yes	
11.30	120	100			Yes	
12.30		100			Yes	
1.15	240	75			Yes	
1.50	240	50			Yes	
2.30		50			Yes	
3.50	240	120	Getting to toilet.	Few Drops	Yes	
4.40		100			Yes	
5.15	240	50			Yes	
6.00		50			Yes	
7.10	100	100	Washing up	Soaked Pad.	Yes	
8.20	120	100			Yes	
9.30		75			Yes	
10.15		50			Yes	
11.00	240	75			Yes	
2.00		100			–	
4.30	100	150			–	
TOTAL	2280	2045				

Fig. 44.1 Urinary diary showing the input and output for each day. The patient records timing and amount of leakage and precipitating events.

Pad test

Two types of pad test are in common use. A simple pad test can be performed on all patients presenting with incontinence and also as an easy follow-up measure for incontinence surgery. The patient, with a comfortably full bladder, wears a sanitary towel and performs some simple exercises including coughing, sitting and standing, bending to pick objects from the floor and hand-washing for 5–10 minutes. The test is positive if the pad becomes damp.

The extended pad test is a more lengthy and objective measurement of leakage and can be used to confirm or refute leakage in those patients complaining of stress incontinence which has not been demonstrated on cystometry. The International Continence Society pad test takes 1 hour. The patient wears a preweighed sanitary towel, drinks 500 ml of water and rests for 15 minutes. She then performs half an hour of gentle exercise such as walking and climbing stairs. She then performs 15 minutes of more provocative exercise including bending, standing and sitting, coughing, hand-washing and running if possible. The sanitary towel is removed and reweighed. An increase in weight of greater than 1 g is considered a significant loss.

UROFLOWMETRY

Uroflowmetry is a simple non-invasive investigation and can be easily performed in an outpatient department. Flowmeters are relatively inexpensive and give a permanent graphic record.

Indications

Measurement of the flow rate is indicated in women with complaints or hesitancy or difficulty in voiding, with neuropathy or a past history of urinary retention. It can also be used to evaluate patients before incontinence surgery to exclude voiding difficulties which may be aggravated by bladder neck surgery.

Measurements

The flow rate is defined as the volume of urine (in ml) expelled from the bladder each second (Fig. 44.2). The flow time is the total duration of micturition and includes interruptions in a non-continuous flow. The maximum flow rate is the maximum measured rate of flow and the average flow is the volume voided divided by the flow time. The total volume voided is therefore the area under the curve. The two most useful parameters are the maximum flow rate and the voided volume. In patients with intermittent flow the same parameters can be used but time intervals between flow episodes must be discounted.

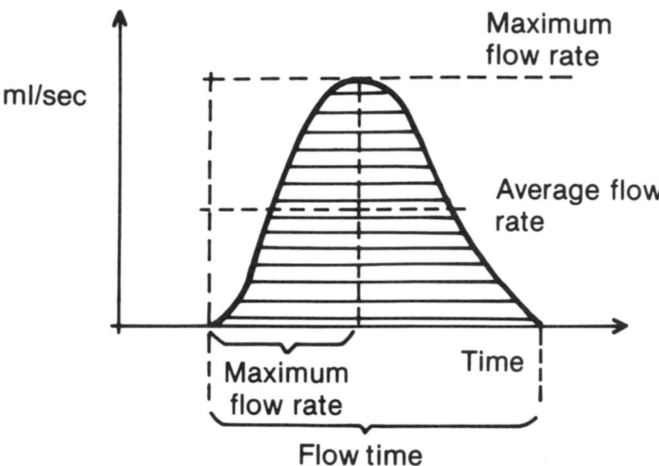

Fig. 44.2 Diagrammatic representation of a urinary flow rate. The shaded area represents voided volume.

Equipment

There are three main types of flow meter (Abrams et al 1983). The earliest models used a strain-weighing transducer which measured the rate of change of the weight of urine voided which was converted into a flow rate.

The rotating disc flowmeter has a disc which is spun at a constant speed. As the patient voids on to the disc the inertia of the urine reduces its speed. The flow rate can be calculated from the amount of power needed to maintain the disc spinning at a constant speed. This is a simple and relatively inexpensive system but is more fragile and more liable to mechanical failure.

The capacitance flowmeter has a metal strip capacitor attached to a plastic dipstick inserted vertically into the jug containing the voided urine (Fig. 44.3). The rate and volume changes are measured by a change in electrical conductance across the capacitor. This is the most expensive type of flowmeter but is robust and very reliable.

Abnormal flow rates

Nomograms for peak and average urine flow rates in women have been constructed from flow rates of 249 normal women (Haylen et al 1988). These allow comparison of a single value with a standard flow rate. A flow rate below 15 ml/s on more than one occasion is taken as abnormal in female patients. The voided volume should be above 150 ml as flow rates on smaller volumes than this are not reliable.

A low peak flow rate and a prolonged voiding time suggest a voiding disorder (Fig. 44.4). Straining can give abnormal flow patterns with interrupted flow (Fig. 44.5). More useful detailed information is obtained by the addition of simultaneous voiding pressure measurements.

CYSTOMETRY

Cystometry involves the measurement of the pressure/volume relationship of the bladder during filling and voiding and is the most useful test of bladder function. It is a simple and accurate investigation and is easy to perform, taking between 15 and 20 minutes per patient.

Indications

Cystometry is indicated in the investigation of the following bladder disorders:

1. Multiple symptoms, i.e. urge incontinence, stress incontinence and frequency.
2. Voiding disorder.
3. Previous unsuccessful incontinence surgery.
4. Neuropathic bladder disorders.

When there is difficulty of access to urodynamic investigations, it is reasonable to operate on patients with the sole symptom of stress incontinence without prior investigation. Discretion should be exercised where symptomatology is multiple or complex.

Equipment

Modern twin-channel cystometry requires a transducer, a recorder and an amplifying unit (Fig. 44.6).

Bladder pressure is measured using a fluid-filled line or a solid microtip pressure catheter. For the former, a 1 mm fluid-filled catheter (such as an epidural cannula) is inserted into the bladder with a filling line and connected to an external pressure transducer. To measure abdominal pressure, a rectal catheter is required; a fluid-filled 2 mm diameter catheter covered with a rubber finger cot to

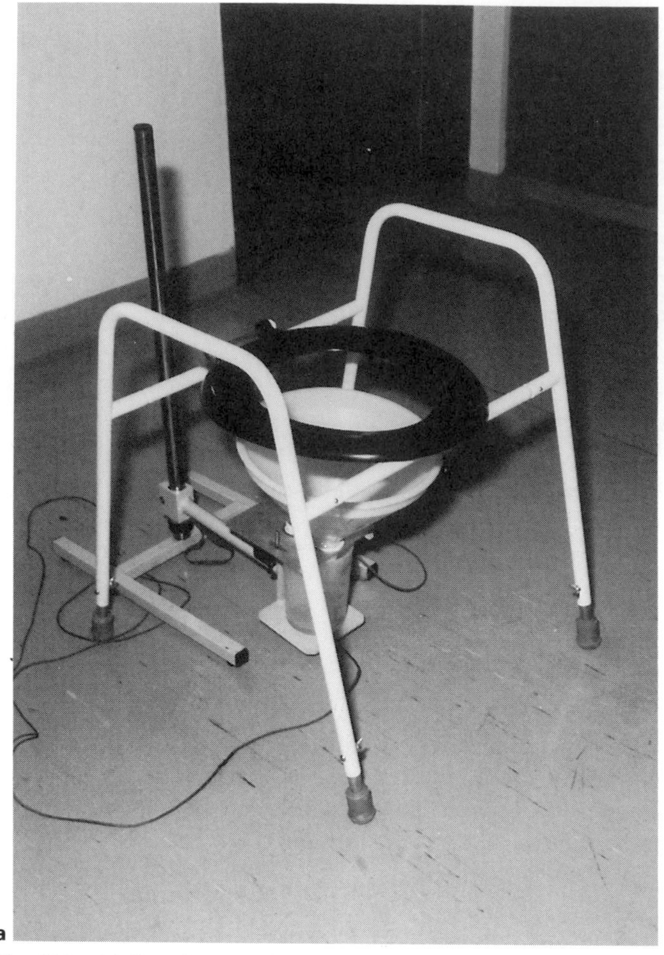

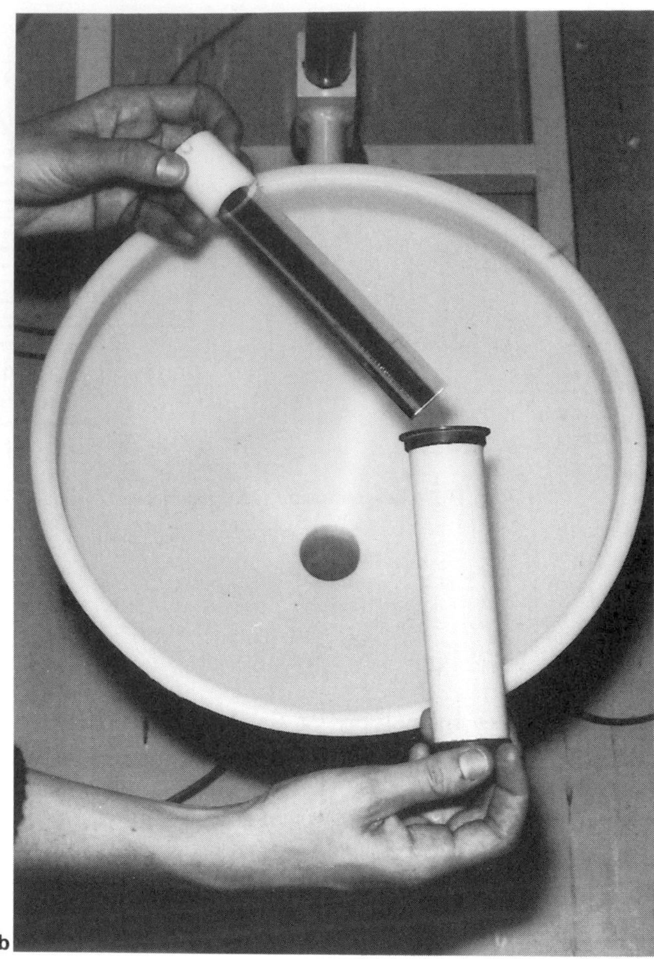

Fig. 44.3 (a) Capacitance urinary flow meter; (b) the capacitance strip.

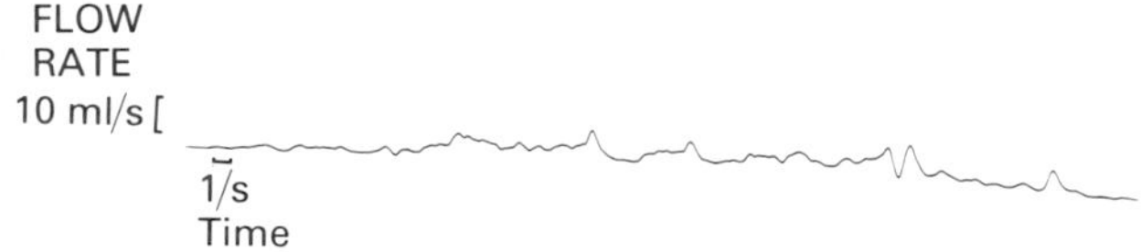

Fig. 44.4 Urinary flow rate showing a prolonged flow with a low maximum peak flow rate suggestive of a voiding disorder.

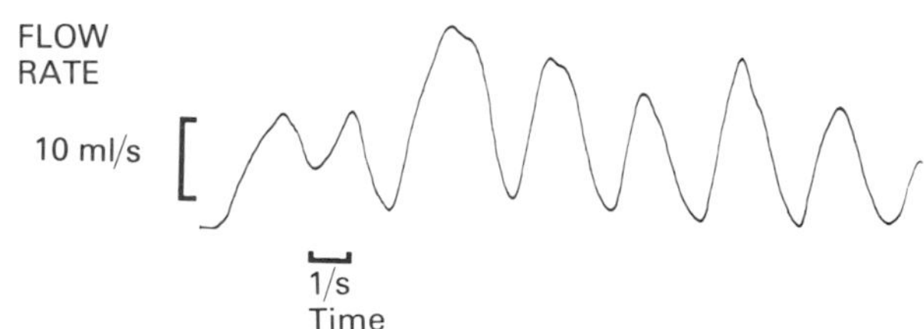

Fig. 44.5 A straining flow rate also suggestive of a voiding disorder.

prevent blockage with faeces is inserted into the rectum (Fig. 44.7). The microtip transducer catheter has a transducer mounted on the tip of a solid catheter and has a diameter of about 7 French gauge. It is inserted into the bladder and the level of the bladder neck is taken as approximately level with the upper edge of the pubic symphysis: this is the zero reference for all measurements which are made in centimetres of water.

The external transducer is cheaper and less fragile but the microtip transducer is more accurate as it eliminates error due to the column of water in the connecting catheter; it is more expensive and more easily damaged.

The bladder is filled using a 12 FG catheter with a continuous infusion of normal saline at room temperature. The standard filling rate is between 10 and 100 ml/min and is provocative for detrusor instability. Slow-fill cystometry at a rate of below 10 ml/min is indicated in patients with neuropathic bladders. Rapid fill of over 100 ml/min is rarely used but can be a further provocative test for detrusor instability.

Measurements

The parameters measured are the intravesical pressure

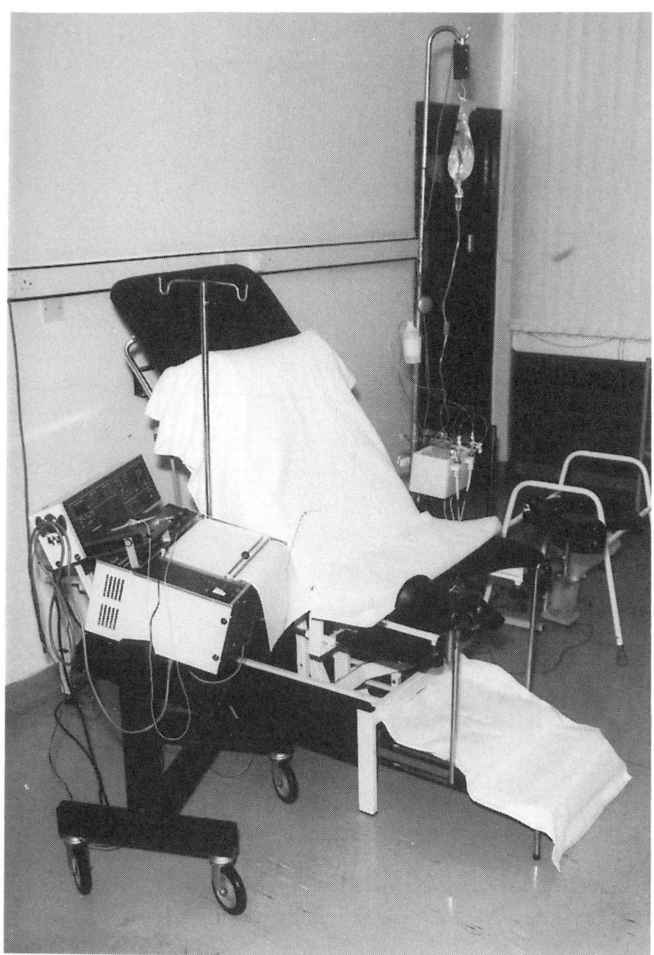

Fig. 44.6 Urodynamic equipment. From left to right: a twin channel cystometry unit, patient couch, patient unit with transducer and uroflowmeter.

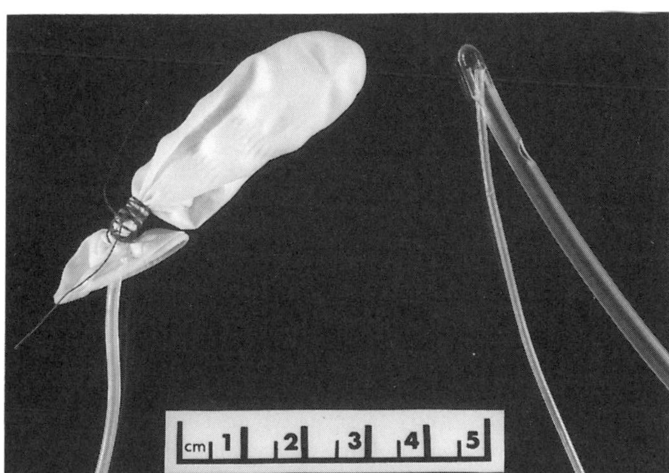

Fig. 44.7 Pressure lines for cystometry. From left to right: bladder and rectal filling lines.

(P_{ves}; measured with the bladder transducer) and the intra-abdominal pressure (P_{abd}) measured with the rectal line. The detrusor pressure (P_{det}) is obtained by subtracting the abdominal pressure from the intravesical pressure and if twin-channel cystometry is used this subtracted value is displayed concomitantly. The filling and voided volumes are also displayed.

Method

Prior to performing the cystometry, the patient voids on the flowmeter. Any residual urine on subsequent catheterization of the patient is noted. During filling the patient is asked to indicate her first desire to void and the maximal desire to void and these volumes are noted. The presence of systolic detrusor contractions and whether associated with urgency is observed. Any precipitating factors such as coughing or running water are also noted. Any detrusor pressure rise during filling and on standing is again recorded.

At the end of filling, the filling line is removed and the patient stands. She is asked to cough and leakage is noted. Provocative tests for detrusor instability such as listening to running water and hand-washing are performed at this stage. The patient then transfers to the commode and voids with the pressure transducer still in place. Once urinary flow is established she is asked to interrupt the flow if possible.

Normal cystometry

The following are parameters of normal bladder function:

1. Residual urine of less than 50 ml.
2. First desire to void between 150 and 200 ml.
3. Capacity (taken as strong desire to void) of greater than 400 ml.
4. Detrusor pressure rise on filling which does not return to the baseline when filling stops.
5. Absence of systolic detrusor contractions.
6. No leakage on coughing.
7. A detrusor pressure rise on voiding (maximum voiding pressure) of less than 70 cm H_2O with a peak flow rate of greater than 15 ml/s for a volume over 150 ml.
8. The patient should be able to interrupt her urine flow on command; failure to do so is not necessarily abnormal.

Abnormal cystometry

If leakage on coughing occurs in the absence of a rise in detrusor pressure, genuine stress incontinence is diagnosed (Fig. 44.8). It is therefore a diagnosis of exclusion as cystometry by itself cannot indicate bladder neck or urethral function; radiographic imaging or the addition of urethral function tests is required.

Detrusor instability is diagnosed if during the filling

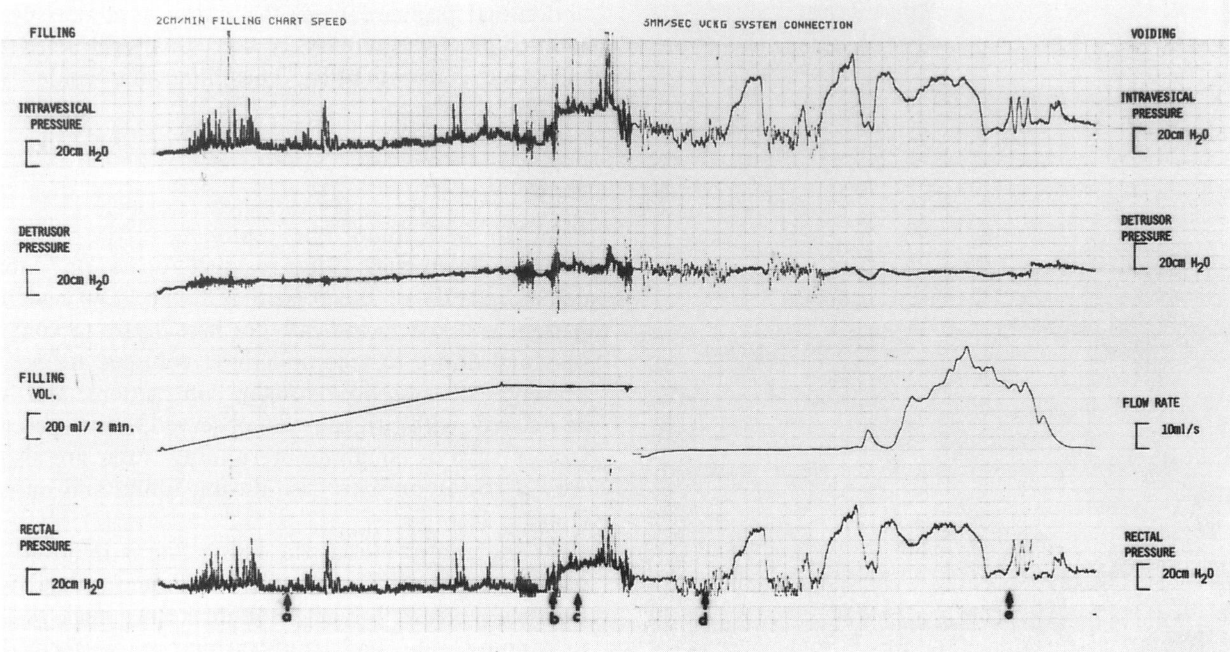

Fig. 44.8 Cystometric trace showing genuine stress incontinence. The detrusor line remains flats. Each arrows (a–e) indicates a cough, when leakage occurred. The voiding phase shows voiding by abdominal straining and a peak flow rate of 40 ml/s.

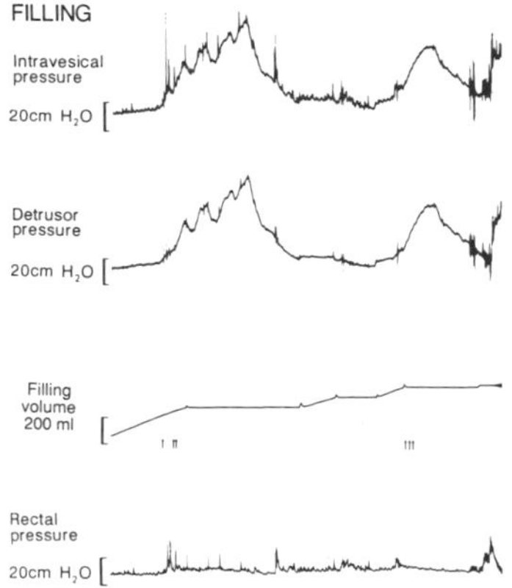

Fig. 44.9 Cystometric trace showing detrusor instability. The arrows indicate where the patient complained of urgency and leakage occurred.

phase spontaneous or provoked detrusor contractions occur which the patient cannot suppress (Fig. 44.9). Systolic detrusor instability is shown by phasic contractions whilst low compliant detrusor instability is diagnosed when the pressure rise on filling is greater than 15 cm H_2O and it does not settle after filling is stopped.

RADIOLOGY

General radiology

A plain abdominal X-ray is useful when symptoms suggest bladder calculi. Osteitis pubis is a rare complication of the Marshall–Marchetti–Krantz procedure presenting with suprapubic pain and is diagnosed on an anteroposterior pelvic X-ray. Sacral and lumbar spine X-rays are indicated if a congenital abnormality is suspected, e.g. spina bifida and meningomyelocele which are important causes of neuropathic bladder disorders in children. Spinal cord trauma and tumours can also cause disturbances of micturition. Disc prolapse is common and is demonstrated on a myelogram.

Intravenous urography

Intravenous urography is not indicated in most women with lower urinary tract symptoms. It is however indicated in patients with neuropathic bladders, suspected uretero-vaginal fistulae or haematuria.

Videocystourethrography

Videocystourethrography (VCU) is radiological screening of the bladder synchronized with pressure studies of the bladder recorded with a sound commentary on video (Fig. 44.10). This study is regarded in some centres as a fundamental investigation but Stanton et al (1988) reviewed 200 cases of urinary incontinence following failed surgery and concluded that VCU was shown to have an advantage over a cystometrogram in only a few selected groups of patients. VCU is indicated in patients complaining of postmicturition dribble which may be due to diverticula (Fig. 44.11), where incontinence occurs on standing up, where ureteric reflux may be a cause of urinary symptoms

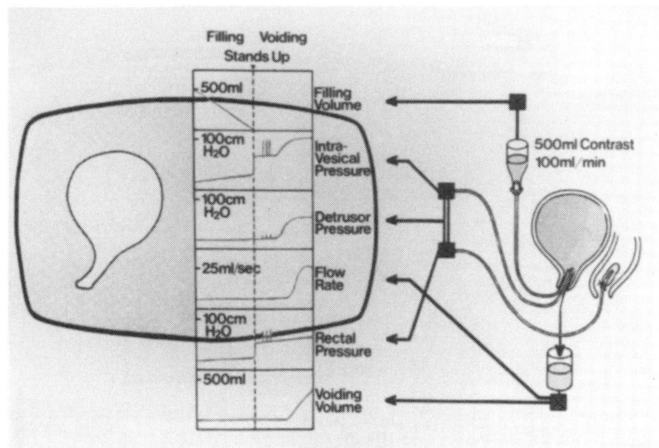

Fig. 44.10 Diagrammatic representation of a videocystourethrogram.

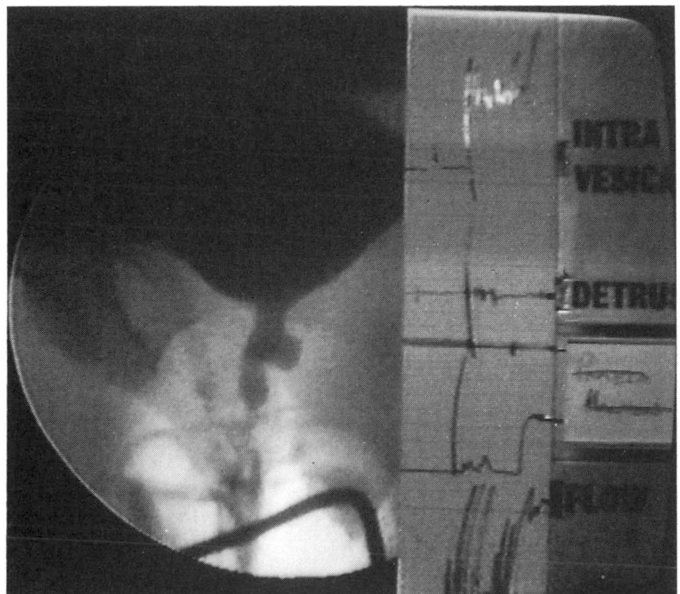

Fig. 44.11 VCU showing a urethral diverticulum.

associated with pain, or in the investigation of a neuropathic bladder. It is not necessary in the routine evaluation of female incontinence.

Technique

On arrival the patient voids into a flowmeter and then lies on a tilting X-ray table. Routine filling cystometry is performed using a contrast medium such as Urografin 35% to fill the bladder. At the maximum desire to void, the filling line is removed and the patient tilted upright and positioned in the erect lateral oblique position. She is asked to cough and strain. Leakage, bladder neck opening and bladder base descent are all noted. Any ureteric reflux and detrusor contractions are also noted. The patient then commences voiding and once the flow is established, she is asked to interrupt the flow. The ability to milk back urine from the urethra is noted.

All data are recorded on a twin-channel recorder and displayed at the same time as the bladder image (Fig. 44.11). A sound commentary can also be recorded.

Micturating cystogram

This investigation also involves radiological screening of the bladder but without pressure or flow measurements and is therefore less useful in the investigation of incontinence. Its main value is to demonstrate vesicoureteric reflux, abnormalities of bladder and urethral anatomy, e.g. diverticula and bladder and urethral fistulae. It is not however useful in incontinence.

Lateral chain X-rays

A lateral pelvic X-ray with a metallic bead chain can be used to outline the urethra and bladder neck. Downward and backward displacement of the bladder neck during coughing and straining can be demonstrated (Hodgkinson et al 1958). Lateral chain X-rays have been advocated in the assessment of patients with failed incontinence surgery. This use is based on the premise that if the bladder neck has not been moved upwards and forward compared with the preoperative position, the operation is a technical failure (Stamey 1983). Radiographic evaluation of the posterior urethral angle has however proved neither reliable nor consistent in clinical practice. Wall et al (1991) examined lateral chain X-rays on 98 women undergoing one of four different bladder procedures and confirmed that no useful information was obtained regarding the dynamics of incontinence or its surgical cure. This technique has since been discontinued in some units.

INVESTIGATIONS OF URETHRAL FUNCTION

Urethral pressure measurement

To maintain continence, the urethral pressure must remain higher than the intravesical pressure and various methods of measuring the urethral pressure have been devised. It

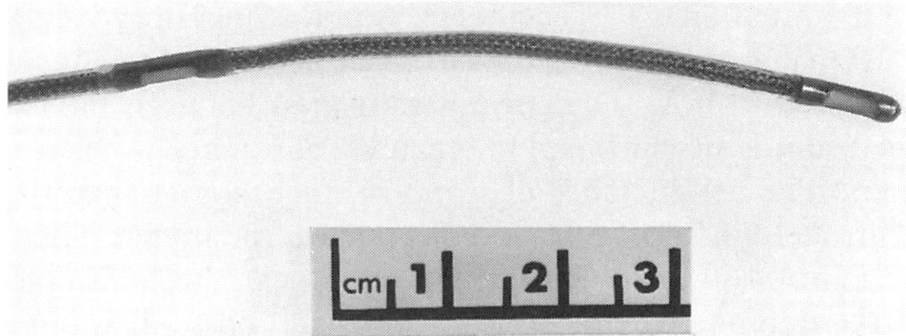

Fig. 44.12 Gaeltec urethral pressure catheter.

is usually measured with a catheter tip dual sensor microtransducer, although in the past resistance to fluid or gas and intraluminal balloons have all been used. The two transducers are 12 mm long and 1.6–2.3 mm in diameter, mounted on a 7 FG catheter at the tip and 6 cm along the catheter (Fig. 44.12). The microtip transducer is easy to use but fragile and expensive.

Technique

The bladder is filled with 250 ml of physiological saline and the catheter passed so that both sensors are within the bladder. The catheter is then connected to a catheter withdrawal mechanism set at a standard speed of 5–15 cm/min and also to a chart recorder. The *static urethral pressure* is the urethral intraluminal pressure along its length with the bladder at rest. The *dynamic urethral pressure* (the urethral closure pressure) is the difference between the maximal urethral pressure and the intravesical pressure, whilst the patient gives a series of coughs. Women with stress incontinence have a lower urethral closure pressure than continent women and this is directly proportional to the severity of their incontinence (Hilton 1984).

Urethral pressure measurements are useful in defining the physical properties; however, their value in clinical practice is not certain. The static urethral pressure profile is of no clinical value. The dynamic urethral pressure profile more closely approximates to the clinical problem but there is a large overlap for both the functional urethral length and the urethral closure pressure between normal and stress-incontinent women and it may not be possible to separate the two groups on urethral pressure profile alone. The urethral pressure profile also may not be reproducible when repeated in the same patient. Richardson (1980) studied 144 patients and found a 92% specificity but only a 41% sensitivity in the evaluation of stress-incontinent women. Versi et al (1986) compared the urethral pressure profile with VCU as the 'gold standard' investigation and found that accurate diagnosis was not possible with the urethral pressure profile alone.

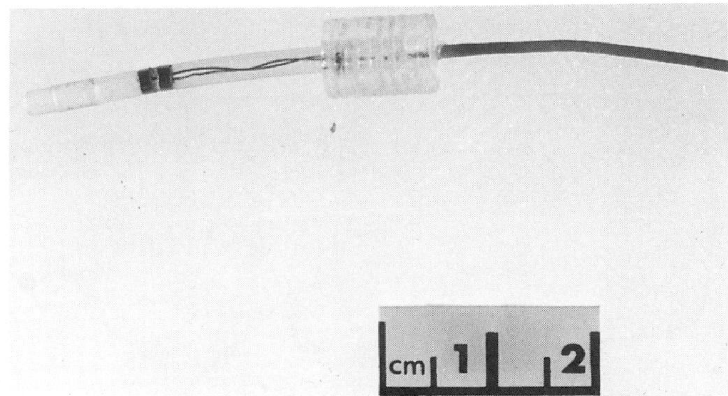

Fig. 44.13 DUEC catheter. The two gold-plated brass electrodes can be seen mounted towards the tip of the catheter.

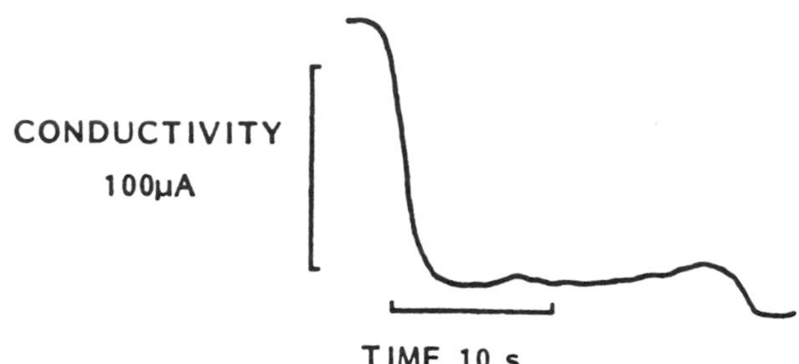

Fig. 44.14 Urethral electrical conductance profile.

Urethral electrical conductance

This is a relatively new technique using changes in electrical conductance to detect movement of urine along the urethra (Plevnik et al 1985). Two gold-plated electrodes are mounted on a 7 FG catheter. A non-stimulatory voltage of 20 mV is applied and the electrode connected to a meter calibrated in mA. The current measured between the two electrodes is proportional to whatever substance is between them. The conductance of urine is much higher than that of urothelium and causes a deflection on the meter. Therefore entry of urine into the urethra can be sensitively detected. The catheter is either short and positioned in the distal urethra (distal urethral electrical conductance; DUEC; Fig. 44.13) or long and lies at the bladder neck (bladder neck electrical conductance; BNEC). Urethral electrical conductance profiles can be measured by withdrawing the BNEC catheter at a fixed speed from the bladder to the external meatus (Fig. 44.14).

DUEC measurement is used during cystometry following removal of the filling line, to detect stress incontinence more accurately than just by observation. Three different patterns of DUEC have been shown. Types 1 and 2 patterns (deflections of greater than 8 mA with a quick return to the baseline; Fig. 44.15a) are associated with a cystometric diagnosis of stress incontinence and type 3 (deflections of greater than 8 mA lasting longer than 3 s; Fig. 44.15b) is associated with a cystometric diagnosis of detrusor instability (Peattie et al 1988a). Any reduction in urethral pressure is invariably associated with an increase in urethral electrical conductance if the two parameters are measured simultaneously in women with genuine stress incontinence (Hilton & Mayne 1988). DUEC may be an alternative screening test to cystometry for detection of incontinence.

BNEC is performed in the investigation and treatment of patients with detrusor instability and sensory urgency. Both of these conditions can demonstrate bladder neck opening associated with urgency and, if this occurs, it can be used for biofeedback (Peattie et al 1988b).

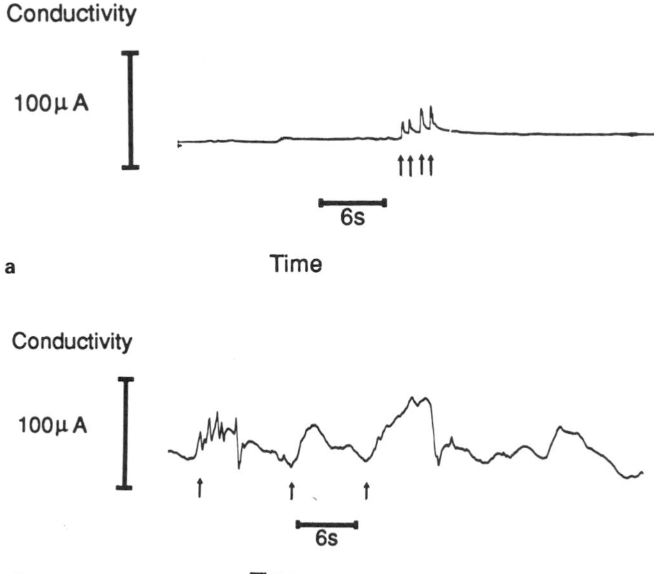

Fig. 44.15a Type 1 DUEC pattern. At each cough a spike of increase in conductance demonstrates leakage. (**b**) Type 3 DUEC pattern. In this pattern the coughs provoke a more sustained rise in urethral electrical conductance.

CYSTOURETHROSCOPY

Cystoscopy establishes the presence of disease in the bladder or urethra. It is indicated in a small group of women with incontinence but is not a part of the routine investigation of incontinence as it gives little information about the function of the bladder neck.

Cystoscopy is indicated where there is:

1. A reduced bladder capacity at cystometry.
2. Recent (<2 years) history of urinary symptoms, e.g. frequency and urgency.
3. A suspected urethrovaginal or vesicovaginal fistula.
4. Suspicion of interstitial cystitis.
5. Haematuria not related to urinary tract infection.
6. To exclude neoplasm in the presence of persistent urinary infection.

Cystoscopy also comprises part of the operative technique in needle suspension operations for incontinence, such as the Stamey and Raz procedures, to ensure no sutures have passed through the bladder or urethra and that the sutures are correctly placed at the bladder neck.

Technique

Cystoscopy is a sterile technique and can be performed under general or local anaesthetic. If performed to assess reduced bladder capacity during urodynamic studies, it must be performed under a general anaesthetic. The urethra is difficult to examine in women and is best done on withdrawing the cystoscope and using a urethroscope sheath. Residual urine should be noted, although it is not always accurate if the patient has not recently voided. Bladder capacity is the volume at which filling usually stops using a litre bag under gravity feed. The mucosa should be inspected for abnormalities such as signs of infection, and tumour. A note is made on the state of the bladder and urethral mucosa and the presence of normally situated ureteric orifices. Interstitial cystitis may be suspected by the presence of linear splits which bleed on decompression and a reduced capacity. If diverticula are present an attempt must be made to see inside to exclude carcinoma and calculi. Bladder calculi may be present, particularly in patients with neuropathic bladder and/or indwelling catheters. Abnormal areas must be biopsied.

Most makes of cystoscope are similar and as they are often not interchangeable it is preferable to stick to one kind. A standard set should include a cystoscope, urethroscope sheath, 0°, 30° and 70° telescopes, a catheterizing bridge and a fibreoptic light. A biopsy forceps is essential, as is a method for dilating the urethra such as an Otis urethrotome or a set of Hegar dilators. Flexible cystoscopes are available and can be more suitable for cystoscopy under local anaesthetic but have the disadvantage that instrumentation such as biopsy is not feasible.

ULTRASOUND

Ultrasound is becoming more widely used in gynaecological urology. Its most simple use is in the estimation of postmicturition residual urine volume and to assess the bladder neck and surrounding area.

Postmicturition urine estimation

This useful technique obviates the need for urethral catheterization with its risk of infection. It is indicated in the investigation of patients with voiding difficulties — either idiopathic or preoperative, and also occasionally following postoperative catheter removal. The bladder is scanned in two planes and three diameters are measured. As the bladder only approaches a spherical shape when it is full, a correction factor has to be applied. Several different formulae have been devised; the most common is to multiply the product of three diameters (height × width × depth) by a figure of 0.625 (Hakenberg et al 1983). This has an error rate of 21%, which is acceptable.

Urethra

Urethral cysts and diverticula can be examined using ultrasound. The disadvantage of this method is that unless the opening of the diverticulum is seen directly, the two cannot be differentiated.

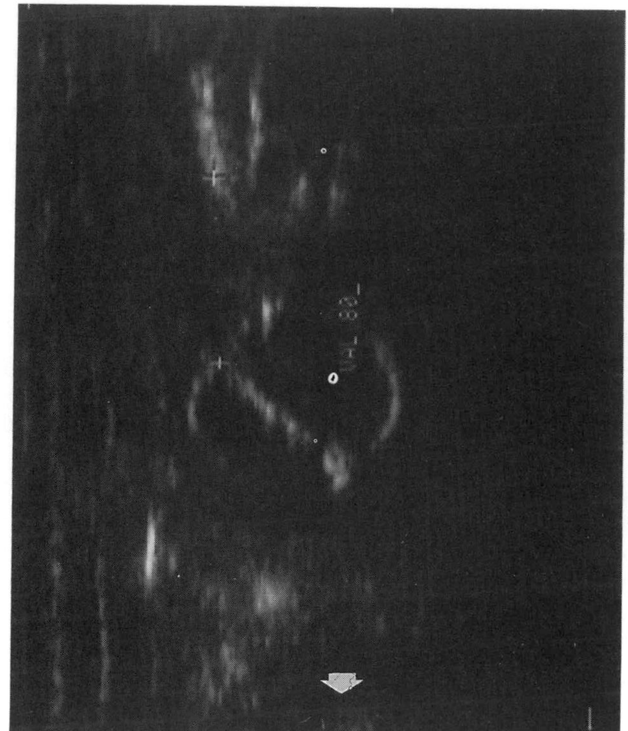

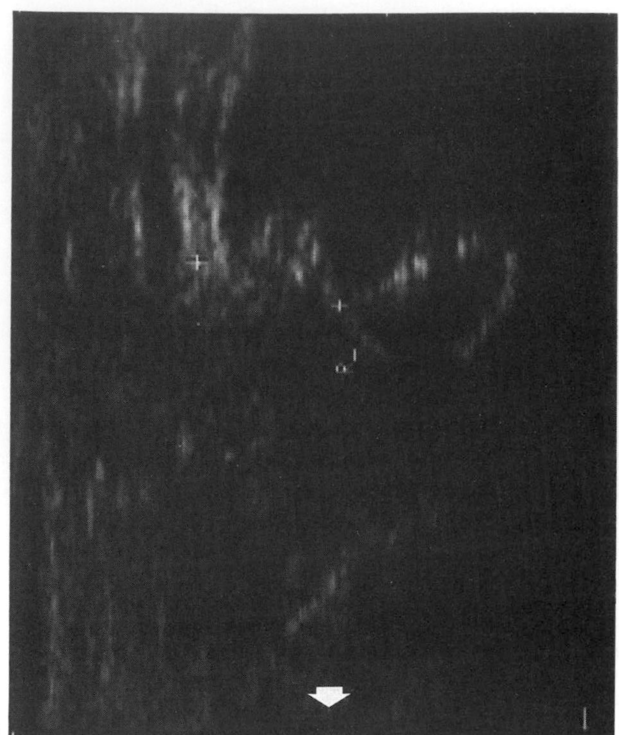

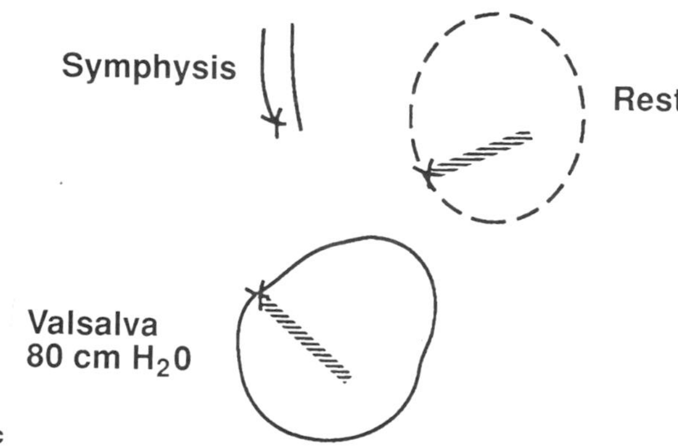

Fig. 44.16 Perineal ultrasound of bladder neck. (**a**) Bladder at rest. Crosses mark the inferior border of the pubic symphysis and the bladder neck, which is demarcated by a foley catheter. (**b**) Valsalva manoeuvre. (**c**) Diagrammatic representation of the two scans showing downward and forward movement of the bladder neck on Valsalva manoeuvre.

Bladder neck

Ultrasound scanning of the bladder neck is used as an alternative to radiological screening (with its radiation hazard) but is undergoing evaluation. It obviates the need for contrast and catheterization, avoids irradiation and provides good visualization of structures around the bladder neck.

Ultrasound of the bladder neck has been performed using the transabdominal approach (White et al 1980); recently rectal, vaginal and perineal probes have also been used. Transabdominal scanning is more difficult in the obese patient and does not utilize a fixed reference point when assessing bladder neck descent. This means any movement of the patient or the transducer will introduce artefact into the measurements.

Vaginal, rectal and perineal probes use the pubic symphysis as a fixed reference. The rectal probe is less acceptable to patients and difficulties arise with rotation of the probe, causing loss of the image. The vaginal probe has been used successfully to investigate the bladder neck. Descent of the bladder base together with bladder neck opening has been demonstrated in a majority of patients with stress incontinence but not in controls (Quinn et al 1988). However bladder neck opening also occurs with detrusor instability and this may be difficult to distinguish from stress incontinence unless there is concomitant bladder pressure recording. The potential for distortion of the bladder neck by the probe has not been fully assessed.

Perineal scanning is the most readily available and least expensive technique as standard equipment which is already available can be used. It is less likely to cause pelvic distortion, is more acceptable to the patient and is feasible in the obese patient (Fig. 44.16). It has been shown to be as accurate as lateral chain urethrocystography in assessment of patients with failed incontinence surgery and has the advantages, listed above, of no radiation risk. The equipment is accurate, portable and available in most departments of gynaecology (Gordon et al 1989).

ELECTROPHYSIOLOGICAL TESTS

Electromyography

Electromyography is the study of bioelectrical potentials generated by smooth and striated muscles and can be used to evaluate pelvic floor damage in women with urinary or faecal incontinence and prolapse. A motor unit comprises a motor nerve and the fibres it innervates. The potential it generates during contraction is called the motor nerve unit potential and this can be measured using electromyography. If denervation occurs, the remaining nerves sprout collaterals to reinnervate the muscle fibres, thus increasing the dispersion of the motor unit so that more fibres of a particular unit will fire together at one time. This is seen on electromyography as an increase in the amplitude, duration and number of phases of the action potential. If reinnervation is present, polyphasic potentials are seen.

Partial denervation has been proposed as the mechanism by which childbirth contributes to the aetiology of stress incontinence. Allen & Warrell (1987) performed transvaginal electromyography on primiparous women before and after delivery and detected a highly significant increase in mean motor unit potential duration which was positively associated with birth weight and length of second stage of labour. Smith & Warrell (1984) studied anal sphincter density in patients with stress incontinence and/or prolapse and found an increased fibre density in all groups compared with normal controls.

Electromyography can be performed using surface electrodes such as anal or vaginal plugs and ring electrodes mounted on a urethral catheter, or it can be performed using needle electrodes inserted into the external anal sphincter or periurethral muscles (Fig. 44.17). Surface recordings are easier to perform and pain-free but as they only record overall changes in muscle electrical activity, they do not allow accurate assessment of motor unit potentials and may record movement of the patient. Electromyography of the anal sphincter has been previously assumed to be similar to electromyography recordings of the urethral sphincter recordings; however, the innervation of these two sphincters has been demonstrated to be different (Gosling et al 1983). Urethral ring electrodes provide direct recordings from the urethral sphincter but are not able to record during voiding. Vaginal plug electrodes may be difficult to insert in the older patient with vaginal atrophy and give poor recordings during voiding. Anal plug electrodes can also be uncomfortable and difficult to retain.

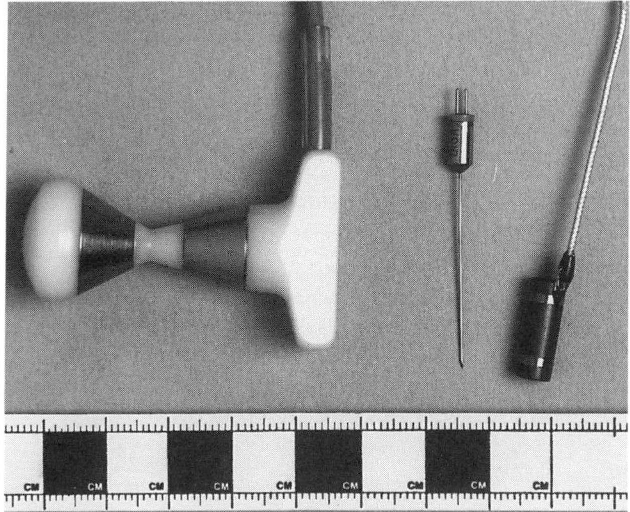

Fig. 44.17 Electrodes for electromyography. From left to right: anal plug electrode, concentric needle electrode and urethral ring electrode.

Needle electrodes directly record activity of motor units by insertion into the muscle bulk. Needles can be either single-fibre or concentric. Single-fibre needles give a more selective recording and allow measurement of motor unit fibre density. A single-fibre reading is more difficult to obtain than concentric needle signals — 55% of patients were successfully sampled in the former compared with 85% in the latter (Krieger 1990).

Technique

To assess the urethral sphincter, a needle is inserted 1 cm lateral to the external urethral meatus and advanced until sphincter activity is heard. The position of the needle can then be adjusted until the discharge of a single unit is heard and then recorded. The action potential can then be assessed for the duration of the potential, the shape or number of phases and the amplitude of the motor unit potential.

Electromyography is a useful research tool but its routine use in clinical investigation is restricted. It also causes mild discomfort to the patient, particularly if the lengthy procedure of attempting to obtain single-fibre recordings is undertaken. It is useful in evaluating the site of pathology in patients with clinical neuropathy but at present is not used in the evaluation of women with lower urinary tract dysfunction.

Sacral evoked responses

Sacral evoked responses indicate the integrity of the sacral reflex arc by measuring the conduction time between a stimulus and an evoked muscle contraction. Electrical stimuli can be applied to the skin over the clitoris or, using a fingerstall surface electrode, to the perineal nerve. An electromyography needle is inserted into the levator ani muscle or the urethral sphincter. Weak responses with an increased latency have been observed in women with urethral sphincter incompetence. Snooks et al (1984) studied electromyography of the external anal sphincter in this manner and found an increased pudendal nerve latency in women following a vaginal delivery as compared with women following caesarean section. Terminal motor latency is more difficult to record as the response is decreased in the abnormal patient. It is also a less sensitive measure of pelvic floor damage than electromyography.

KEY POINTS

1. Clinical history is often not a good predictor of urodynamic findings.
2. Urinary infection must be excluded before any urodynamic investigation takes place.
3. Peak urinary flow rate is indicated in all women with voiding difficulty, particularly prior to incontinence surgery, which may aggravate this.
4. Stress incontinence diagnosed on cystometry is a diagnosis of exclusion; it is assessed by leakage in the absence of detrusor contractions.
5. Cough-induced detrusor instability may clinically mimic genuine stress incontinence.
6. All patients undergoing repeat continence surgery must have urodynamic studies performed.
7. Intravenous urography is not indicated in the routine investigation of incontinent women.
8. Cystoscopy must be performed in the case of recurrent urinary tract infections to exclude malignancy.
9. Ultrasound is becoming more widely used in the assessment of the incontinent patient with the advantage that radiological screening can be avoided.
10. Partial denervation of the pelvic floor following childbirth contributes to the development of both incontinence and prolapse.

REFERENCES

Abrams P, Feneley R, Torrens M 1983 Urodynamics. Springer-Verlag, Berlin, pp 31–40

Allen R E, Warrell D W 1987 The role of pregnancy and childbirth in partial denervation of the pelvic floor. Neurourology and Urodynamics 6: 183–184

Bates C P, Loose H, Stanton S L 1973 Objective study of incontinence after repair operations. Surgery, Gynecology and Obstetrics 136: 17–22

Blaivas J G, Bhimani G, Labib K B 1979 Vesicourethral dysfunction in multiple sclerosis. Journal of Urology 122: 342–345

Cardozo L D, Stanton S L 1980 Genuine stress incontinence and detrusor instability; a review of 200 patients. British Journal of Obstetrics and Gynaecology 87: 184–190

Farrar D J, Whiteside C G, Osbourne J L, Turner Warwick R T 1975 A urodynamic analysis of micturition symptoms in the female. Surgery, Gynecology and Obstetrics 141: 875–881

Gordon D, Pearce J M, Norton P, Stanton S L 1989 Comparison of ultrasound and lateral chain urethrocystography in the determination of bladder neck descent. American Journal of Obstetrics and Gynecology 160: 182–185

Gosling J, Dixon J, Humpherson J 1983 Functional anatomy of the female urinary tract. Churchill Livingstone, Edinburgh

Hakenberg O W, Ryall R L, Langlois S L, Marshall V R 1983 The estimation of bladder volume by sonocystography. Journal of Urology 130: 249–251

Haylen B T, Ashby D, Frazer M I, Sutherst J R, West C 1988 Peak and average urine flow rates in a normal female population — the Liverpool nomograms. Neurourology and Urodynamics 7: 176–178

Hilton P 1984 Urethral pressure measurement. In: Stanton S L (ed) Clinical gynecologic urology. C V Mosby, St Louis, pp 110–126

Hilton P, Mayne C J 1988 Urethral pressure variations; the correlation between pressure measurement and electrical conductance in genuine stress incontinence. Neurourology and Urodynamics 7: 175–176

Hodgkinson C P, Doub H, Keely W 1958 Urethrocystograms: metallic bead technique. Clinics in Obstetrics and Gynecology 1: 668–677

Jarvis G J, Hall S, Stamp S, Millar D R, Johnson A 1980 An assessment of urodynamic examination in the incontinent woman. British Journal of Obstetrics and Gynaecology 87: 893–896

Krieger M S 1990 M D Thesis. Sydney University, Australia

Peattie A B, Plevnik S, Stanton S L 1988a Distal urethral electric conductance (DUEC) test: a screening test for female urinary incontinence? Neurourology and Urodynamics 7: 173–174

Peattie A B, Plevnik S, Stanton S L 1988b The use of bladder neck electrical conductance (BNEC) in the investigation and management of sensory urge incontinence in the female. Journal of the Royal Society of Medicine 81: 442–444

Plevnik S, Holmes D M, Janez J, Mundy A R, Vrtacnik P 1985 Urethral electrical conductance (UEC) — a new parameter for the evaluation of urethral and bladder function: methodology of the assessment of its clinical potential. Proceedings of the 15th International Continence Society, London

Quinn M J, Beynon J, Mortenson N J, McSmith P J B 1988 Transvaginal endosonography: a new method to study the anatomy of the lower urinary tract in urinary stress incontinence. British Journal of Urology 62: 414–418

Richardson D A 1980 Value of the cough pressure profile in the evaluation of patients with stress incontinence. American Journal of Obstetrics and Gynecology 155: 808–811

Smith A R B, Warrell D W 1984 A neurogenic aetiology of stress urinary incontinence and uterovaginal prolapse. Proceedings of the 14th International Continence Society, Innsbruck pp 485–487

Snooks S J, Setchell M, Swash M, Henry M M 1984 Injury to innervation of pelvic floor sphincter musculature in childbirth. Lancet ii 2: 546–550

Stamey T A 1983 Endoscopic suspension of the vesical neck. In: Raz S (ed) female urology. W B Saunders, Philadelphia, pp 267–268

Stanton S L, Krieger M S, Ziv E 1988 Videocystourethrography: its role in the assessment of incontinence in the female. Neurourology and Urodynamics 7: 172–173

Versi E, Cardozo L D, Studd J, Cooper D 1986 Evaluation of urethral pressure profilometry for the diagnosis of genuine stress incontinence. World Journal of Urology 4: 6–9

Wall L L, Helms M, Peattie A, Pearce M, Stanton S L 1991 Bladder neck mobility and the outcome of surgery for genuine stress urinary incontinence. Submitted for publication.

Walter G J, Vejlsgaard R 1978 Diagnostic catheterization and bacteriuria in women with urinary incontinence. British Journal of Urology 50: 106–108

White R D, McQuown D, McCarthy T A, Ostergard D R 1980 Real time ultrasonography in the evaluation of urinary stress incontinence. American Journal of Obstetrics and Gynecology 138: 235–237

45. Applied pharmacology

D. M. Holmes

INTRODUCTION

The more widespread recognition of the problems of incontinence in our society has led to considerable research into the dynamics of the lower urinary tract. Much of this has been directed not only towards recognizing pathology, but also towards gaining a better picture of the normal physiology. This new knowledge has allowed a more logical approach to the pharmacological manipulation of the bladder and urethra, thus sparing many women (and gynaecologists) the indignity of failed treatment of lower urinary tract symptoms.

NEUROPHYSIOLOGY

The autonomic nerve supply of the lower urinary tract has both parasympathetic and sympathetic elements. The sympathetic arises from the 10th thoracic to the second lumbar roots, whilst the parasympathetic arises from the second to fourth sacral roots. Both run in the pelvic nerves with the vesical arteries to be distributed to the base and sides of the bladder.

In the bulk of the detrusor muscle the preganglionic parasympathetic fibres terminate in the small ganglia spread through the bladder wall (Gosling 1979). The majority of the postganglionic fibres are presumed to be cholinergic, because of their rich content of acetylcholinesterase. They form a dense plexus among, and are probably motor to, the detrusor muscle bundles, since stimulation of the parasympathetic fibres in the sacral nerves produces a sustained detrusor contraction (Torrens 1978). There is evidence that some cholinergic fibres have a sensory function (Dixon et al 1984). There is a less dense cholinergic nerve supply to the urethra (Ek et al 1977).

A sparse supply of sympathetic noradrenergic fibres has been identified in the detrusor muscle, but this runs predominantly with the blood vessels and does not terminate on the detrusor muscle bundles (Sundin et al 1977). Some terminate on the parasympathetic intramural ganglia and may be inhibitory (Torrens 1984). In the trigonal area sympathetic fibres predominate. In the bulk of the detrusor muscle, beta receptors are the most common sympathetic receptors, whilst in the trigone and bladder neck area alpha receptors predominate (Awad et al 1974). Alpha-adrenergic receptors seem to be stimulatory, whilst beta-adrenergic receptors seem to be inhibitory. The alpha and beta receptors are divided into subtypes 1 and 2. The distinction between these subgroups has not been shown to have any clinical significance in the pharmacological manipulation of the lower urinary tract. Increased maximum urethral closure pressure should result from alpha-adrenergic stimulation or beta-adrenergic blockade. Conversely alpha-adrenergic blockage or beta-adrenergic stimulation should result in a decrease in the maximum urethral closure pressure.

A third type of nerve fibre, which is non-cholinergic and non-adrenergic, has been identified in the detrusor muscle of some animals (Ambache & Zar 1970). One of the mediators is thought to be vasoactive inhibitory polypeptide (Gu et al 1983a; Klarskov et al 1983) which has been shown to inhibit spontaneous contractions of detrusor muscle in vitro (Kinder & Mundy 1985). The role of this peptidergic transmission has been investigated in stable and unstable bladders and shown to be significantly reduced in the latter (Gu et al 1983b). Other mediators suggested are

5-hydroxytryptamine, adenosine-5-triphosphate (Burnstock et al 1972) and prostaglandins.

The parasympathetic and sympathetic nervous systems interact under the control of the central nervous system, which in turn acts through the corticospinal and reticulospinal tracts, with reflex centres at the spinal and brainstem levels. Theoretically transection of the spinal cord above S2 level should still allow for reflex micturition but in practice the co-ordination between urethral relaxation and detrusor contraction is lost (detrusor–sphincter dyssynergia), resulting in inefficient, incomplete voiding (Siroky & Krane 1981).

Bladder afferent (sensory) fibres are transmitted through the posterior spinal columns and the spinothalamic tract to the thalamus and sensory cortex.

The somatic supply to the lower urinary tract is confined to the urethral sphincter mechanism. The female urethra is surrounded by the striated muscle fibres which comprise the rhabdosphincter. These fibres are predominantly of the slow-twitch variety and are under somatic control via the pudendal nerve (S2–4). The slow-twitch fibres are tonically contracted, compressing the urethra to give rise to the resting urethral pressure. Activation of the pudendal nerve, found during a sudden rise in the intra-abdominal (and therefore intravesical) pressure, gives a rise in the urethral pressure, presumably due to recruitment of the fast-twitch fibres also found in the sphincter. If recruitment is ineffective, due to damage to either the sphincter or its innervation (Snooks & Swash 1984) then there may be insufficient pressure reserve to maintain continence, particularly if there is inefficient transmission of intra-abdominal pressure to the proximal urethra.

Many different drugs are used to control the symptoms of urinary dysfunction, because no one drug exists which effectively improves the storage or the expulsive powers of the bladder. The complex neurophysiology of bladder control is relatively poorly understood, and so it is not surprising to find that the theoretical actions of a particular compound do not always concur with what is found in practice.

DRUGS WHICH FACILITATE BLADDER EMPTYING

Theoretically bladder emptying may be improved by either improving detrusor muscle contractility or by decreasing urethral outflow resistance. A normal void involves a drop in urethral resistance with a sustained detrusor contraction. Since these actions occur by different — though co-ordinated — mechanisms it is unlikely that a single drug acting peripherally will effect a normal void. Currently available drugs are mainly directed towards improving detrusor contractions, although some interesting results seem to be obtained by reducing outflow resistance and helping the initiation of a contraction with alpha-adrenergic blocking agents.

Bethanechol

Method of action

The detrusor muscle is stimulated to contract by the action of acetylcholine on muscarinic receptors. Any compound which has an acetylcholine-like structure may stimulate the smooth muscle to contract. Acetylcholine is not itself active orally, but bethanechol is. Its actions are not limited to the bladder, indicating that the bladder parasympathetic receptors function no differently from those elsewhere in the body.

The half-life of the drug is short, and a 6-hourly oral dose of 25 mg is required to maintain the serum levels; the dose is increased by 25 mg until either satisfactory voiding is achieved or side-effects supervene. Doses of 5–10 mg given subcutaneously are also effective. Bethanechol should be used in gradually increasing doses, particularly in women whose bladders are denervated, since receptor proliferation will theoretically cause hypersensitivity to acetylcholine-like substances.

Information on the clinical usefulness of bethanechol is limited. The administration of bethanechol to 6 women who had stress incontinence gave a statistically significant increase in intravesical pressure, but with no change in the maximum urethral pressure (Ek et al 1978a). Unfortunately the statistical significance of the decrease in closure pressure does not seem to be clinically significant in terms of increased flow rates or decreased residual urine volumes (Wein et al 1979).

Side-effects

The side-effects of bethanechol are related to its action on muscarinic receptors, particularly in the gastrointestinal tract. Nausea and vomiting with lower abdominal cramps are the most frequently reported. Excess salivation may also occur.

Distigmine, neostigmine and pyridostigmine

Method of action

All anti-cholinesterase drugs act to potentiate the release of acetylcholine from parasympathetic (and somatic) nerve endings by blocking the action of acetylcholinesterase, the enzyme which degrades acetylcholine in the synapse. All are active either orally or parenterally; the differences between the three drugs are the lengths of time over which they act. Distigmine has a long action of at least 24 h, requiring a once-daily dose. Pyridostigmine has a shorter action than distigmine, and may have a weaker cholinergic action than the shorter-acting neostigmine.

Clinical efficacy trials of these compounds are sparse, and clinical experience with them indicates a mixed response.

Side-effects

The side-effects of anti-cholinesterase administration are predominantly those of excess cholinergic activity. Nausea, vomiting, diarrhoea and excess salivation are frequently encountered, indicating the relatively non-specific action of these compounds. Extreme caution should be exercised when administering these compounds to patients who have bronchial asthma. Bradycardia and hypotension occur with overdosage.

Prostaglandins

Method of action

Prostaglandins of the E_2 and $F_{2\alpha}$ groups have been shown in vitro to increase spontaneous detrusor muscle contractions. This phenomenon is dose-related, and the instillation of known prostaglandin synthetase inhibitors reduces both spontaneous detrusor muscle contractions and prostaglandin-induced contractions in vitro (Bultitude et al 1976). The mechanism by which this is achieved is not known, but prostaglandins have been postulated to be neurotransmitters for the non-cholinergic, non-adrenergic nerve fibres found in the bladder. The finding has been investigated clinically to establish the clinical efficacy of intravesical administration of prostaglandin E_2 to a group of 36 women with a proven voiding difficulty (Desmond et al 1980). The results were encouraging, although the study was uncontrolled. They also noted that the effects sometimes continued long after the initial administration of the prostaglandins if the patients had an intact reflex arc. The findings were unfortunately not reproducible by other workers investigating women with voiding disorders (Anderson et al 1976; Delaere et al 1981).

Intravesical instillation of prostaglandins was found to be of no value in the routine postoperative management of colposuspension (Stanton et al 1979). This study found that diazepam given at night was more effective, probably because of its striated muscle relaxation effect on the sphincter and pelvic floor muscle.

The use of postoperative prostaglandin E_2 to relieve urinary retention following anterior colporrhaphy has been investigated in a double-blind placebo-controlled study (Wagner et al 1984). This failed to show any dose-related response to intravesical administration of prostaglandin E_2 at doses of up to 2.25 mg in women who had retention following anterior colporrhaphy. The use of prostaglandin $F_{2\alpha}$ following vaginal hysterectomy has been reported both to reduce the length of hospital stay and the incidence of postoperative urine retention (Jaschevatsky et al 1985). This much larger study involved 102 women randomly allocated to receive either 16 mg of prostaglandin $F_{2\alpha}$ in saline or saline only instilled into the bladder 24 h postoperatively. These two studies used different criteria for inclusion, different prostaglandins (which have been reported to have different efficacies; Abrams & Feneley 1976) and also markedly different doses of prostaglandins and cannot therefore be compared.

Side-effects

Prostaglandin is instilled intravesically and therefore systemic absorption is low. The commonest side-effect is a burning pain in the perineum, with an increased sensation of urgency. Occasional systemic effects more characteristic of systemic prostaglandin usage have been noted. Most of these reports indicate an absence of side-effects.

In summary, the literature indicates that at present neither prostaglandin E_2 nor prostaglandin $F_{2\alpha}$ has a major therapeutic role in the management of voiding disorders in the female. The author's clinical experience concurs with this.

Phenoxybenzamine and prazosin

Method of action

Phenozybenzamine and prazosin are reversible alpha-blocking agents. Prazosin is a selective α_1 blocker, whilst phenoxybenzamine blocks both α_1 and α_2 receptors. Their administration relaxes the smooth muscle where these receptors exist. It has been recognized that the trigone, bladder neck and proximal urethra have a rich supply of alpha-adrenergic receptors both in the male and the female. Relaxation of the circumferentially arranged muscle bundles will open the bladder neck and urethra. The symptoms of bladder neck obstruction in the male have been shown to improve with alpha-blockade, with a concomitant increase in the radiologically measured bladder neck diameter during micturition (Waterfall 1982). Whilst it is recognized that the male and female bladder neck anatomy is functionally different, it is also realized that the proximal urethra and bladder neck open prior to the genesis of a detrusor pressure rise in both the male and female. Theoretically, phenoxybenzamine or prazosin should have the same effect in the female, and either aid the initiation of a detrusor contraction or reduce the outflow resistance by increasing the diameter of the bladder neck. Both of these actions would improve the efficiency of a void. These drugs have been shown to be effective in both the neuropathic and non-neuropathic bladder in the male. In the female, phenoxybenzamine has been studied in a randomized controlled trial to determine its usefulness as a prophylactic to prevent postoperative retention of urine following both vaginal (56 women) and abdominal

(99 women) hysterectomy (Livne et al 1983). The number of women in each treated group who required postoperative catheterization was significantly less than the corresponding control group. The dose of phenoxybenzamine used was 10 mg/day, which is a relatively low dose, avoiding the recognized side effects of alpha-blockade.

Phenoxybenzamine has also been investigated in women undergoing elective caesarean section as a measure to prevent postepidural retention of urine (Evron et al 1984). Sixty women were randomly allocated to receive either four 10 mg doses of phenoxybenzamine or no treatment. They all had 4 mg morphine instilled through the epidural cannula at the end of the procedure, and were not electively catheterized. The mean volumes of the first two voids and the mean delay to the first void were all significantly better in the treated than the untreated group. The number of women who required catheterization was significantly less in the phenoxybenzamine-treated group (3 versus 16).

Side-effects

The side-effects of alpha-blockade are predominantly related to cardiovascular regulation failure. Postural hypotension with a compensatory tachycardia is the commonest manifestation. Caution should be exercised in the selection of women for treatment with phenoxybenzamine since it has been shown to be carcinogenic to rats.

In summary, both phenoxybenzamine and prazosin are clinically useful in the male. As yet there are scanty published data on their use in women. In the author's experience they do occasionally seem to be effective in the short-term management of postcolposuspension voiding difficulties. Gradual increases in the dose are required; the maximum dose is limited by the severity of the side-effects.

DRUGS WHICH FACILITATE URINE STORAGE

Involuntary leakage of urine from the urethra can only occur if the intravesical pressure exceeds the maximum urethral closure pressure. Urethral sphincter contraction and detrusor relaxation are achieved by different mechanisms and so it is not surprising that no single drug will effectively achieve both.

Drugs may act in several different ways to relax the detrusor muscle. The classical anti-cholinergic drug, atropine, acts to block muscarinic receptors, rendering the detrusor muscle immune to the actions of acetylcholine and acetylcholine-like drugs. Other drugs act to block the flow of calcium in the sarcoplasmic reticulum thus inhibiting the smooth muscle contraction. Some drugs are reputed to act as local anaesthetics in the bladder, raising the threshold for stimulation of the sensory fibres, presumably thereby raising the bladder volume at which reflex micturition is triggered.

In practice the agents used do not have such clear-cut mechanisms of action. The complex higher control mechanisms which govern urethral and detrusor activity confuse the pharmacological manipulation of the end organs, making interpretation of their actions difficult in vivo. The assumption that it is only the cholinergic fibres which generate a detrusor contraction may be wrong, since the non-cholinergic, non-adrenergic fibres which have been described may also have a motor function. Two conditions where the bladder contracts in an uninhibited manner have been recognized by the International Continence Society. These are detrusor instability which occurs in a neurologically normal woman and detrusor hyper-reflexia which occurs when there is a co-existent neurological abnormality. The hyper-reflexic bladder may be exquisitely sensitive to anti-cholinergics, particularly if there has been any denervation of the bladder.

The urethra and bladder neck must open to allow urine to pass. There is no evidence to suggest a sphincteric action of the bladder neck in the female. Its function in the maintenance of continence may be to dampen the intraluminal transmission of intravesical pressure to the distal sphincter mechanism.

Propantheline bromide

Method of action

Propantheline has been reported as being used in the management of incontinence since 1953 (Draper et al 1953) and nocturnal enuresis since 1956 (Braithwaite 1956). Its action is almost completely anti-cholinergic, acting to block muscarinic receptors at the postganglionic level with little evidence of direct smooth muscle action. Its effects are therefore not specific to the detrusor muscle and this is reflected in its side-effects. The suppression of involuntary detrusor contractions may be achieved by an oral dose of 15 mg t.d.s. The action is not predictable, presumably because of variable absorption, and it may be necessary to increase the dose incrementally up to 45 mg t.d.s, or until side-effects supervene.

Relaxation of smooth muscle will decrease the detrusor pressure, without a decrease in the maximum urethral pressure (since this is mediated through nicotinic receptors which are not blocked by propantheline). Several controlled and uncontrolled trials have shown its symptomatic and urodynamic effects on the bladder. It undoubtably increases the volume at which the first desire to void occurs. This does not seem to be a local anaesthetic effect, inferring the trigger for this sensation is probably mediated through pressure rather than stretch receptors. The relaxing effect on the detrusor muscle is also demonstrated by a reduction in the maximum detrusor pressure rise found during filling cystometry when the drug is given.

Side-effects

The actions of propantheline are predominantly anti-cholinergic. It is used clinically to control irritable bowel syndrome, so it is not surprising that constipation is one of the main side-effects. It also inhibits saliva and sweat production and can precipitate narrow-angle glaucoma by its relaxing action on the smooth muscle of the iris which blocks the canal of Schlemm.

Oxybutynin hydrochloride

Method of action

Oxybutynin is a potent orally active anti-cholinergic agent. It is also reputed to have local anaesthetic effects on the bladder (Diokno & Lapides 1972) and to have a direct effect on smooth muscle similar to papaverine.

Oxybutynin has been found by many clinicians to be a useful and effective drug in the management of symptoms due to detrusor instability (Moisey et al 1984; Cardozo et al 1987) and detrusor hyper-reflexia (Hennessey et al 1988). Objective urodynamic studies in a double-blind trial confirm these benefits, although Meyhoff et al (1981) found that a placebo in this trial could produce up to 47% improvement in symptoms.

Direct comparison of oxybutynin with propantheline in the management of idiopathic detrusor instability has not shown a clear difference between the two drugs (Holmes et al 1989), though oxybutynin is reported to be more effective in patients with detrusor hyper-reflexia (Gajewski & Awad 1986).

Side-effects

Despite the extra actions which oxybutynin is reported to have compared with propantheline, the side-effects are remarkably similar. Urinary retention can occur, especially when treating detrusor hyper-reflexia. In the management of idiopathic detrusor instability, an increased residual urine is found when compared with propantheline, though the clinical significance of this is doubtful. Oxybutynin undoubtably has a therapeutically useful action in suppressing involuntary detrusor contractions.

Terodiline

Method of action

Terodiline acts mainly as an anti-cholinergic and has a calcium antagonist action. As such it is a powerful spasmolytic with reduced side-effects compared to a pure anti-cholinergic. Animal models indicate that it is also a local anaesthetic, and that its action is selective for bladder rather than cardiac muscle. Clinical trials have been undertaken which demonstrate its efficacy in decreasing involuntary detrusor pressure rises and improving their associated symptoms (Ekman et al 1980; Rud et al 1980; Peters 1984; Kinn et al 1988). A larger multicentre trial used a placebo (Tapp et al 1987). Placebo gave an overall subjective improvement rate of 42% compared with 62% for the active group. Both placebo and active groups experienced similar side-effects. There was significantly greater improvement in frequency, nocturia and number of incontinence episodes in the active group. Treatment has been monitored for up to 3–5 years, and the therapeutic effects have been maintained (Ulmsten et al 1985). The very elderly seem to tolerate the drug well (Beisland & Fossberg 1985) and overall there is a low treatment withdrawal rate, because of side-effects. The drug has been found to be as effective as oxybutynin in a single-blind trial of 40 patients with detrusor hyper-reflexia associated with multiple sclerosis. Side-effects were reported to be less than oxybutynin (Hennessey et al 1988).

Side-effects

The side-effects of terodiline are predominantly anti-cholinergic at low doses. As the dose is increased to toxic levels the calcium antagonist effects on the cardiovascular system predominate, with hypotension and collapse. Terodiline has been found to be associated with arrhythmias and it is wise to avoid using it in patients over 75 years of age, or with ischaemic heart disease or cardiac arrhythmia, or where cardio-active drugs, diuretics, tricyclic anti-depressants or anti-psychotic drugs are taken or where hypokalaemia exists.

In summary, terodiline has been extensively investigated, and the results indicate that it has a major role to play in the suppression of involuntary detrusor activity.

Imipramine

Method of action

Tricyclic anti-depressants, of which imipramine is an example, act centrally to potentiate the sympathetic outflow by blocking the re-uptake of noradrenaline. They also have powerful peripheral anti-cholinergic and local anaesthetic actions. The predominant site of action has always been presumed to be peripheral, but this cannot be assumed, since its central action may have profound effects on the higher control mechanisms. Imipramine also has a sedative action which, subjectively, seems to have a shorter action than its therapeutic action. A small dose such as 25 mg nocte increasing to 50 mg nocte alleviates urinary symptoms, whilst the sedative action occurs during sleep.

Imipramine has been used since 1960 in the treatment of nocturnal enuresis in children (MacLean 1960). Although its use has been predominantly in nocturnal enuresis, it has also been used both as a single agent (Castleden et al 1986) and in conjunction with propantheline (Barker & Glenning 1987) in the treatment of idiopathic detrusor instability. This latter combination seems to have a synergistic action, and is particularly effective in the elderly.

Imipramine may also have peripheral action at the bladder neck. Its action here would be to potentiate the sympathetic effects and increase the functional urethral length. An uncontrolled study of 30 women showed significant increases in the maximum urethral closure pressure (Gilja et al 1984). The authors claim a 71% 'cure' rate for the symptom of stress incontinence, but the findings are unsubstantiated by other workers.

Side-effects

The anti-cholinergic actions of imipramine contribute most of the side-effects. Dry mouth, blurred vision and constipation are common. There may be significant postural hypotension in the elderly, and the drug is contraindicated in those who have recently had a myocardial infarction. Myelosuppression has also been reported. Confusion may be precipitated in the elderly.

Flavoxate

Method of action

Flavoxate is a tertiary amine chromone and was first formulated in 1960. It is a smooth muscle anti-spasmodic with selective action on pelvic organs and is reported to be a calcium antagonist which also has direct or papaverine-like actions on detrusor muscle. It is also reported to have a local anaesthetic action (Cazzulanni et al 1984). Clinical studies on the drug have indicated a mixed degree of success in treating involuntary detrusor contractions. In a small study of 6 elderly patients (4 women) with detrusor instability neither intravenous nor oral flavoxate produced a cystometric or clinical improvement (Briggs et al 1980). A higher dosage regimen of either 600 or 1200 mg/day is however reported to give significant improvement in symptoms of detrusor instability in a younger group of women. Whereas there was no dose relation to the symptom improvement, the cystometric measurements did show a dose-related trend (Milani et al 1988). Other investigators have shown that flavoxate will give a symptomatic improvement rate of 83% (Stanton 1973) which is similar to the 87% improvement found in a Chinese series of 361 patients (Gu Fang-lui et al 1987). This series was unfortunately unblinded and uncontrolled, but carefully reported. Side-effects were minimal. Other authors are less enthusiastic, finding flavoxate to be no different from placebo (Zeegers et al 1987).

Side-effects

The anti-cholinergic side-effects of flavoxate are few, but dry mouth and blurred vision are reported. Other non-specific effects of headache, intestinal upset and fatigue occur, but are rare.

Phenylpropanolamine and ephedrine

Method of action

Alpha-adrenergic stimulation by phenylpropanolamine, and alpha- and beta-stimulation by ephedrine or its stereo-isomer pseudoephedrine is postulated to result in closure of the bladder neck with a concomitant increase in the functional urethral length.

The use of phenylpropanolamine in women with stress incontinence has been shown to increase the maximum urethral and closure pressure with a significant improvement in symptomatology (Ek et al 1978b). Similar symptomatic improvement has been found with the use of ephedrine (Diokno & Taub 1975), but properly controlled trials have not been carried out. The consensus of opinion, however, seems to be that improvement in measurements has a clinical effect only on women with mild symptoms of incontinence, and that tachyphylaxis limits its long-term usage.

Side-effects

All sympathomimetics will cause tachycardia with peripheral vasoconstriction and subsequent increase in blood pressure. Phenylpropanolamine (50 mg) is only available in the UK in a slow-release combination with diphenylpyraline (5 mg), an antihistamine. The effects of the preparation are therefore prolonged. Initially the drug should be used with caution at a dose of one tablet twice a day, increasing to three times a day after a few days if neither cure nor side-effects are apparent.

Oestrogens

Method of action

Oestrogens have long been reported to have a beneficial effect on the symptoms of stress incontinence (Salmon et al 1941). Several studies since then have shown increases in maximum urethral pressure measurements in post-menopausal women with improvement in not only the symptom of stress incontinence, but also other lower urinary tract symptoms (Caine & Raz 1973; Rud 1980; Hilton & Stanton 1983). Changes in skin collagen content which correlate with changes in urethral pressure measurements have also been found, but the hypothesis that increases in urethral pressure following oestrogen administration are a result of increased urethral collagen has not yet been proven (Versi et al 1988).

Desmopressin (DDAVP)

Method of action

Arginine vasopressin reduces urine production dramatically and is effective in controlling nocturia when taken at night. There must be a compensatory diuresis during the day but in general it has a good therapeutic effect, with no significant side-effects (Hilton & Stanton 1982). It has been used in women with detrusor hyper-reflexia to control nocturia effectively (Hilton et al 1983). It is taken intranasally at a dose of 20 μg nocte and should not be used in the presence of hypertension.

Placebo

Method of action

The beneficial effects of the placebo in placebo-controlled trials are well recognized in the treatment of detrusor instability. Symptomatic improvement rates of 42 and 47% have been reported with minimal side-effects (Meyhoff et al 1981; Tapp et al 1987). Any therapeutic effect of a drug must be compared against this placebo effect, taking into account the side-effects of the active drug.

KEY POINTS

1. The nerve supply to the bladder is parasympathetic and sympathetic: a third nerve supply is believed to be non-cholinergic and non-adrenergic and remains unidentified.
2. The alpha-1-adrenergic blocking agents are probably the most effective drugs in promoting bladder emptying.
3. Anti-cholinergic drugs will reduce uninhibited bladder activity but in doses which often produce parasympathetic side-effects.
4. Placebo treatment of detrusor instability has been shown to produce improvement rates of up to 47%.

REFERENCES

Abrams P, Feneley R C L 1976 The actions of prostaglandins on the smooth muscle of the human urinary tract in vitro. British Journal of Urology 47: 909–915

Ambache N, Zar M A 1970 Non-cholinergic transmission by post ganglionic motor neurons in the mammalian bladder. Journal of Physiology 210: 761–783

Anderson K E, Hendricksson L, Ulmsten U 1976 Effects of prostaglandin E_2 applied locally on intravesical and intra-urethral pressures in women. European Urology 4: 366–369

Awad S A, Bruce A W, Carro-Ciampi G, Downie J W, Lin M, Marks G S 1974 Distribution of alpha- and beta-adrenoreceptors in human urinary bladder. British Journal of Pharmacology 50: 525–529

Barker G, Glenning P P 1987 Treatment of the unstable bladder with propantheline and imipramine. Australia and New Zealand Journal of Obstetrics and Gynaecology 27: 152–154

Beisland H, Fossberg E 1985 The effects of terodiline and meladrazine on severe motor urge incontinence in geriatric patients. Journal of the American Geriatric Society 33: 29–32

Braithwaite J V 1956 Some problems connected with enuresis. Proceedings of the Royal Society of Medicine 49: 33–38

Briggs R S, Castelden C M, Asher M J 1980 The effect of flavoxate on uninhibited detrusor contractions and urinary incontinence in the elderly. Journal of Urology 123: 665–666

Bultitude M I, Hills N H, Shuttleworth K E D 1976 Clinical and experimental studies on the action of prostaglandins and their synthetase inhibitors on detrusor muscle in vitro and in vivo. British Journal of Urology 48: 631–637

Burnstock G, Dunsday B, Smythe A 1972 Atropine resistant excitation of the urinary bladder: the possibility of transmission via nerves releasing a purine nucleotide. British Journal of Pharmacology 44: 451–461

Caine M, Raz S 1973 The role of female hormones in stress incontinence. Proceedings of the 16th Congress of Société Internationale d'Urologie, Amsterdam

Cardozo L D, Cooper D, Versi E 1987 Oxybutinin in the management of idiopathic detrusor instability. Neurourology and Urodynamics 6: 256–257

Castleden C M, Duffin H M, Gulati R S 1986 Double blind study of imipramine and placebo for incontinence due to detrusor instability. Age and Aging 15: 299–303

Cazzulanni P, Panzarasa R, Luca C, Oliva D, Graziani G 1984 Pharmacological studies on the mode of action of flaxovate. Archives of International Pharmacodynamic Therapy 268: 301–312

Delaere K P J, Thomas C M G, Moonen W A, Debruyne F M J 1981 The value of intravesical prostaglandin E_2 and F_2 in women with abnormalities of bladder emptying. British Journal of Urology 53: 306–309

Desmond A D, Bultitude M I, Hills N H, Shuttleworth K E D 1980 Clinical experience with intravesical prostaglandin E_2: A prospective study of 36 patients. British Journal of Urology 52: 357–366

Diokno A C, Lapides J 1972 Oxybutinin: a new drug with analgesic and anti-cholinergic properties. Journal of Urology 108: 307–309

Diokno A C, Taub M 1975 Ephedrine in treatment of urinary incontinence. Urology 5: 624–625

Dixon J S, Gilpin S A, Gilpin C J, Gosling J A 1984 Presumptive sensory nerves in the human urinary bladder. Proceedings of the 14th Meeting of the International Continence Society 272–273

Draper J W, Wolf S, Murphy J F, Kravetz H 1953 The effect of Banthene in the treatment of genito-urinary disorders. Journal of Urology 69: 632–640

Ek A, Andersson K E, Persson C G A 1977 Adrenergic and cholinergic nerves of human urethra and urinary bladder. Acta Physiologica Scandinavica 99: 345–357

Ek A, Andersson K E, Ulmsten V 1978a The effects of norephedrine and bethanechol on the human urethral closure pressure. Scandinavian Journal of Urology and Nephrology 12: 97–104

Ek A, Andersson K-E, Gullberg B, Ulmsten V 1978b The effects of long-term treatment with norephedrine on stress incontinence and urethral closure pressure profile. Scandinavian Journal of Urology and Nephrology 12: 105–110

Ekman G, Andersson K E, Rud T, Ulmsten U 1980 A double-blind cross-over study of the effects of terodiline in women with unstable bladder. Acta Pharmacologica et Toxicologica (suppl) 46: 39–43

Evron S, Magora F, Sadovsky E 1984 Prevention of urinary retention with phenoxybenzamine during epidural morphine. British Medical Journal 288: 190

Gajewski J B, Awad S A 1986 Oxybutinin versus propantheline in patients with detrusor hyper-reflexia. Journal of Urology 135: 966–968

Gilja I, Radej M, Kovacic M, Parazajder J 1984 Conservative treatment of female stress incontinence with imipramine. Journal of Urology 132: 909–911

Gosling J A 1979 The structure of the bladder and urethra in relation to function. Urology Clinics of North America 6: 31–38
Gu Fang-lui, Reng Zong-ying, Shang Gang-zhi et al 1987 Treatment of urgency and urge incontinence with flavoxate in the People's Republic of China. Journal of International Medical Research 15: 312–318
Gu J, Restorick J M, Blank M A et al 1983a Regulatory peptides in the normal and unstable bladder. Proceedings of the 13th Meeting of the International Continence Society, Aachen 66–77
Gu J, Restorick J M, Blank M A et al 1983b Vasoactive intestinal polypeptide in the normal and unstable bladder. British Journal of Urology 55: 645–647
Hennessey A, Robinson L Q, Weston P, Ford M, Stephenson T P, Compston A 1988 A comparison between oxybutinin and terodilene in patients with multiple sclerosis. Neurourology and Urodynamics 7: 195–196
Hilton P, Stanton S L 1982 The use of desmopressin (DDAVP) in nocturnal urinary frequency in the female. British Journal of Urology 54: 252–255
Hilton P, Stanton S L 1983 The use of intra-vaginal oestrogen cream in genuine stress incontinence. British Journal of Obstetrics and Gynaecology 90: 940–944
Hilton P, Hertogs K, Stanton S L 1983 The use of desmopressin (DDAVP) for nocturia in women with multiple sclerosis. Journal of Neurology, Neurosurgery and Psychiatry 46: 854–855
Holmes D M, Montz F J, Stanton S L 1989 Oxybutinin versus propantheline in the treatment of detrusor instability: a patient regulated variable dose trial. British Journal of Obstetrics and Gynaecology 96: 607–612
Jaschevatsky O E, Anderman S, Shalit A, Ellenbogen A, Grunstein S 1985 Prostaglandin F_2 for prevention of urinary retention after vaginal hysterectomy. Obstetrics and Gynecology 66: 244–246
Kinder R B, Mundy A R 1985 Inhibition of spontaneous contractile activity in isolated human detrusor muscle strips by vasoactive intestinal polypeptide. British Journal of Urology 57: 20–23
Kinn A C, Brekkan E, Jansson A et al 1988 Terodiline for patients with urinary incontinence in neurogenic bladder disorders — efficacy and tolerance. Neurourology and Urodynamics 7: 196–197
Klarskov P, Gerstenberg T C, Hald T 1983 Vasoactive intestinal polypeptide (VIP) influence on lower urinary tract smooth muscle from human and pig. Proceedings of the 13th Meeting of the International Continence Society, Aachen 59–62
Livne P M, Kaplan B, Ovadia Y, Servadio C 1983 Prevention of post operative urinary retention by alpha-adrenergic blocker. Acta Obstetrica of Gynecologica Scandinavica 62: 337–340
MacLean R E G 1960 Impramine hydrochloride and enuresis. American Journal of Psychiatry 117: 551
Meyhoff H H, Gerstenberg T, Nordling J 1981 Placebo — the drug of choice in female urge incontinence. Proceedings of the Meeting of the International Continence Society, Lund p. 49
Milani R, Scalambrino S, Carrera S, Pezzoli P, Ruffmann R 1988 Comparison of flavoxate hydrochloride in daily dosages of 600 versus 1200 mg for the treatment of urgency and urge incontinence. Journal of International Medical Research 16: 244–248
Moisey C, Stephenson T, Brendler C 1984 The urodynamic and subjective results of treatment of detrusor instability with oxybutinin chloride. British Journal of Urology 52: 472–475
Peters D 1984 Terodiline in the treatment of urinary frequency and motor urge incontinence. A controlled multicentre trial. Scandinavian Journal of Urology and Nephrology (suppl) 87: 21–33
Rud T 1980 The effects of estrogens and gestogens on the urethral pressure profile in urinary continent and stress incontinent women. Acta Obstetrica et Gynecologicaca Scandinavica 59: 265–270
Rud T, Andersson K-E, Boye N, Ulmsten U 1980 Terodiline inhibition of human bladder contraction. Effects in vitro and in women with unstable bladder. Acta Pharmacologica et Toxicologica (suppl) 46: 31–38
Salmon V J, Walter R J, Geist S H 1941 The use of estrogen in the treatment of dysuria and incontinence in postmenopausal women. American Journal of Obstetrics and Gynecology 42: 845–851
Siroky M B, Krane R J 1981 Neurological aspects of detrusor–sphincter dyssynergia with special reference to the guarding reflex. Journal of Urology 127: 953–957
Snooks J, Swash M 1984 Abnormalities of the innervation of the urethral sphincter musclature in incontinence. British Journal of Urology 56: 401–405
Stanton S L 1973 A comparison of emepromium bromide and flavoxate hydrochloride in the treatment of urinary incontinence. Journal of Urology 110: 529–532
Stanton S L, Cardozo L D, Kerr-Wilson R 1979 Treatment of delayed onset of spontaneous voiding after surgery for incontinence. Urology 13: 494–496
Sundin T, Dahlstrom A, Norlen L, Svedmayr N 1977 The sympathetic innervation and adrenoreceptor function of the human lower urinary tract in the normal state and after parasympathetic denervation. Investigative Urology 14: 322–328
Tapp A, Fall M, Norgaard J 1987 A dose-titrated, multicentre study of terodiline in the treatment of detrusor instability. Proceedings of the 17th Meeting of the International Continence Society, Bristol, pp 254–255
Torrens M J 1978 Urethral sphincteric responses to stimulation of the sacral nerves in the human female. Urology Internationalis 33: 22–26
Torrens M J 1984 Neurophysiology. In: Stanton S L (ed) Clinical Gynecologic Urology. CV Mosby, St Louis, pp 13–21
Ulmsten U, Ekman G, Andersson K-E 1985 Treatment of women with motor urge incontinence with terodiline — a drug with combined anticholinergic and calcium blocking effects. American Journal of Obstetrics and Gynecology 153: 619
Versi E, Cardozo L, Brincat M, Cooper D, Montgomery J, Studd J 1988 Correlation of urethral physiology and skin collagen in post menopausal women. British Journal of Obstetrics and Gynaecology 95: 147–152
Wagner G, Husslein P, Enzelberger H 1984 Is prostaglandin E_2 really of therapeutic value for post operative urinary retention? Results of a prospectively randomised double blind study. American Journal of Obstetrics and Gynecology 151: 375–379
Waterfall N B 1982 The effect of phenoxybenzamine on bladder neck opening. In: Yeates W K (ed) Phenoxybenzamine in disorders of micturition. Smith Klein & French, pp 67–70
Wein A J, Malloy T R, Shofer F, Raezer D M 1979 The effects of bethanechol chloride on urodynamic parameters in normal women and in women with significant urine volumes. Journal of Urology 124: 397–399
Zeegers A G M, Kiesswetter H, Kramer A E, Jonas U 1987 Conservative therapy of frequency, urgency and urge incontinence: a double-blind clinical trial of flavoxate hydrochloride, oxybutinin chloride, emepronium bromide and placebo. World Journal of Urology 5: 57–61

46. Classification of urogynaecological disorders

S. L. Stanton

If the body were sometimes divided into specialties by physiological rather than anatomical boundaries, there would be no need for an explanation of urogynaecology. As it is, this specialty represents an interface between gynaecologist and urologist. Physiological events or disease affecting gynaecological organs invariably affect the urinary tract, as they will also sometimes affect the adjacent alimentary system.

Following introduction of subspecialization by the American College of Obstetricians and Gynecologists, the Royal College of Obstetricians and Gynaecologists considered and then recommended subspecialization in 1982. Four subspecialties were created, amongst them urogynaecology. It comprised the following disorders: congenital anomalies, incontinence, voiding difficulties, urinary fistulae, bladder neuropathy, genital prolapse, urgency and frequency and urinary tract infection. By common consent, all 'supravesical' conditions and neoplasia arising anywhere in the urinary tract belong to the realm of urology.

TERMINOLOGY

Like any developing branch of medicine and science, old terms and definitions have become inadequate. To provide a common language for both clinician and researcher the International Continence Society (ICS) formed a standardization committee in 1973 to draw up and revise standards of terminology of lower urinary tract function. Five reports have appeared; the latest supersedes the others (Abrams et al 1988).

The term 'stress incontinence' was coined by Sir Eardley Holland in 1928 and meant the loss of urine during physical effort. It came to be used not only as a symptom and sign, but also as a diagnostic term. As the pathophysiology of urinary incontinence became more clearly understood, it was apparent that the term 'stress incontinence' was ambiguous as it could be applied to a symptom, a sign and a diagnosis — indeed the symptom and sign of stress incontinence can be found in most types of incontinence.

Nowadays the term 'stress incontinence' is retained for the symptom of involuntary loss of urine on physical exertion and the sign of urine loss from the urethra immediately on increase in abdominal pressure. The term 'genuine stress incontinence' was proposed by the ICS in 1976 (Bates et al 1976) to mean the condition of involuntary loss of urine when the intravesical pressure exceeds the maximum urethral pressure in the absence of a detrusor contraction. This condition has a number of synonyms — urethral sphincter incompetence, stress urinary incontinence, anatomical stress incontinence and pressure equalization incontinence. I prefer the term 'urethral sphincter incompetence' because this accurately describes the pathophysiology of this condition.

In a similar way, the term 'dyssynergic detrusor dysfunction' was introduced by Hodgkinson et al in 1963 and other synonyms followed — urge incontinence, uninhibited bladder, bladder instability/unstable bladder. In 1979, the ICS defined an unstable bladder as one 'shown objectively to contract, spontaneously or on provocation during the filling phase, while the patient is attempting to inhibit micturition. Unstable contractions may be asymptomatic and do not necessarily imply a neurological disorder'. The contractions are phasic. Another term, 'low compliance', is used to mean a gradual increase in detrusor pressure without a subsequent decrease during bladder filling. The term 'detrusor hyper-reflexia' is used for phasic uninhibited contractions when there is objective evidence of a relevant neurological disorder. Terms to be avoided include 'hypertonic', 'spastic' and 'automatic'.

CLASSIFICATION

Congenital anomalies (see Ch. 1)

The subject of congenital anomalies reaffirms the principle that a lesion affects multiple systems. Often these present to the urologist as a primary urological problem (e.g. bladder exstrophy, horseshoe kidney) The gynaecologist's expertise lies in the area of diagnosis and management of dubious sexuality or later, when reconstructive surgery may be required for epispadias or haematocolpos.

Incontinence

Urinary incontinence forms the major proportion of urogynaecology. It is defined by the ICS as 'an involuntary loss of urine which is objectively demonstrable and a social or hygienic problem'.

Incontinence is considered to be involuntary; for two categories of patients further explanation is needed. In a child under 3 years of age, control of continence has not yet developed; however careful observation shows that the normal child is dry between involuntary voids whilst the incontinent child is wet the whole time. On the other hand, the mentally incompetent patient may be incontinent because she has lost her social consciousness and appreciation of the need to be dry.

The social isolation caused by incontinence is demonstrated by 25% of patients delaying for more than 5 years before seeking advice, due to embarrassment (Norton et al 1988). Ostracism and rejection by relatives may lead to an elderly patient being institutionalized solely because of incontinence; paradoxically, some allegedly 'caring' institutions will not accept an elderly patient if she is incontinent.

There is a growing awareness that incontinence should be objectively demonstrable using urodynamic studies which will define the cause and detect other conditions such as voiding disorders.

The hygienic aspect of incontinence occupies some 25% of nursing time in hospitals and unless managed, urinary odour is offensive to both patient and relatives alike.

Incontinence may be divided into urethral and extra-urethral conditions (Fig. 46.1).

Urethral conditions

1. The commonest form is *genuine stress incontinence* (urethral sphincter incompetence) presenting from the teens onwards (see Ch. 47). This condition may have one of several causes and is eminently treatable by surgery.
2. *Detrusor instability* (see Ch. 48): Depending on its cause, this may be subdivided into neuropathic (hyper-reflexia) or non-neuropathic (idiopathic). Some patients with instability and a competent sphincter mechanism may remain dry. If however there is any coexistent sphincteric incompetence, the patient may complain of stress incontinence or urge incontinence.
3. *Urinary retention and overflow* (see Ch. 49): This may be acute or chronic; the former is usually sudden in onset and painful. There may be an obvious cause such as an impacted pelvic mass. Chronic retention,

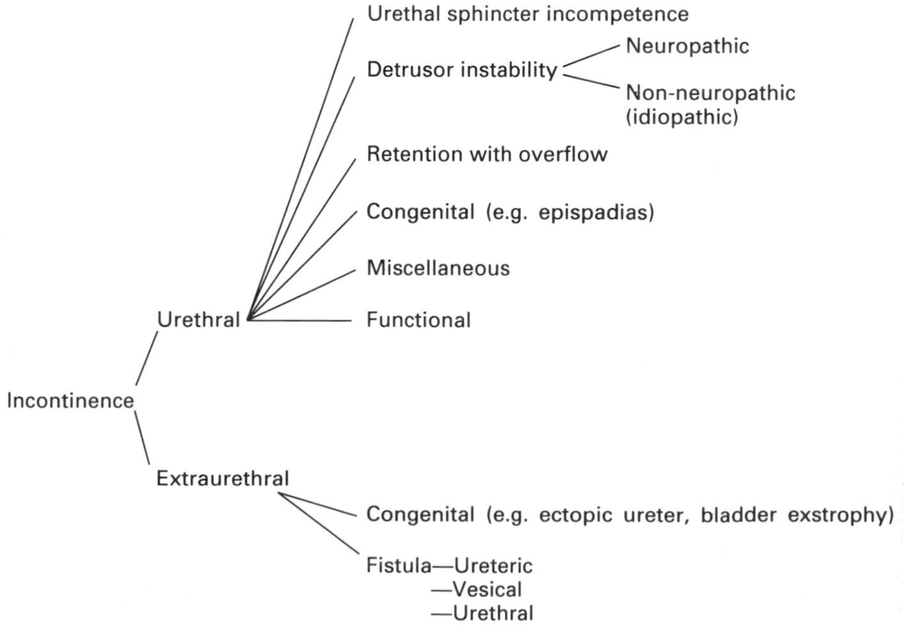

Fig. 46.1 Classification of incontinence.

on the other hand, is often painless and insidious and frequently undetected, so errors in diagnosis are often made. It occurs more commonly in the elderly as a result of neuropathy, e.g. peripheral diabetic neuropathy or stenosis of the lumbar spinal canal.

4. *Congenital disorders*: Epispadias is usually detected during childhood, but occasionally it is not diagnosed until adult life.
5. *Miscellaneous*: These causes include urethral diverticulum, urinary tract infection (temporary and commonest in the elderly) and drugs (such as alpha-adrenergic blocking agents).
6. *Functional disorders*: These are rare and the patient should be fully investigated and all the above causes excluded before this diagnosis is made. The loss of social awareness of the need to be continent is usually associated with dementia or a space-occupying lesion of the frontal cortex.

Extraurethral conditions

These are distinguished from urethral conditions by the symptom of continuous incontinence. The congenital disorders include ectopic ureter and bladder exstrophy. Urinary fistulae in the western world are largely iatrogenic, the majority occurring after abdominal hysterectomy for benign conditions (Ch. 53). Other causes include pelvic carcinoma and its attendant surgery or radiotherapy. In the developing world, obstetrical causes such as obstructed labour with an impacted vertex are commoner. If the fistula is small, skill and patience are required to detect it.

Voiding difficulties (see Ch. 49)

These are uncommon in the female and are frequently undiagnosed. If untreated, they can lead to recurrent urinary tract infection or retention following otherwise successful bladder neck surgery for incontinence.

Urinary fistulae

These have already been referred to and are dealt with at length in Chapter 53.

Bladder neuropathy

This is rightfully dealt with by the urologist but it is important for the gynaecologist to be aware of and recognize these disorders (see Ch. 50).

Genital prolapse (see Ch. 31)

Prolapse should not be considered in isolation as it is sometimes associated with genuine stress incontinence or with perineal descent and faecal incontinence (see Ch. 61). The latter conditions represent an important interface with the rectal surgeon, due to the common antecedent aetiology of childbirth (Snooks et al 1984).

Urgency and frequency

These symptoms can of course be part of a urinary disease process, viz, urinary tract infection or detrusor instability, but can often present as single or combined symptoms in the absence of an obvious pathology (see Ch. 52).

Urinary tract infection (see Ch. 51)

This is of common interest to the obstetrician-and-gynaecologist, urologist and nephrologist, and the experience of all three may be required for difficult cases. However the majority of patients are treated by the general practitioner without referral to hospital, albeit urinary tract infection is frequently unproven. Inadequate treatment during pregnancy can lead to acute pyelonephritis and abortion and, if neglected in later life, can lead to chronic pyelonephritis, hypertension and later renal failure.

CONCLUSION

This classification is an introduction to urogynaecology and the ensuing chapters will cover more depth. For more specialized reading, a list of selected books is given after the references.

KEY POINTS

1. It is important to recognize and use the internationally agreed terminology as agreed by the International Continence Society.
2. Incontinence has a variety of causes which may need urodynamic studies to diagnose them.
3. Stress incontinence means a symptom and a sign and not a diagnosis.

REFERENCES

Abrams P, Blaivas J, Stanton S L, Andersen J 1988 Standardization of terminology of lower urinary tract function. International Continence Society. Scandinavian Journal of Urology and Nephrology (suppl) 114: 5–19

Bates P, Bradley W, Glen E et al 1976 First report on standardization of terminology of lower urinary tract function. International Continence Society. British Journal of Urology 48: 39–42

Hodgkinson C P, Ayers M, Drukker B 1963 Dyssynergic detrusor dysfunction in the apparently normal female. American Journal of Obstetrics and Gynecology 87: 717–730

Norton P, MacDonald L, Sedgwick P, Stanton S L 1988 Distress and delay associated with urinary incontinence, frequency and urgency in women. British Medical Journal 297: 1187–1189

Snooks S, Swash M, Henry M, Setchell M 1984 Injury to innervation of pelvic floor sphincter musculature in childbirth. Lancet ii: 546–550

FURTHER READING

Buchsbaum H, Schmidt J 1982 Gynecologic and obstetric urology, 2nd edn. W B Saunders, Philadelphia

Freeman R, Malvern J 1989 The unstable bladder. Butterworth Scientific, London

Mundy A, Stephenson T, Wein A 1984 Urodynamics; principles, practice and application. Churchill Livingstone, Edinburgh

Ostergard D, Bent A 1991 Urogynecology and urodynamics: theory and practice, 3rd edn. Williams & Wilkins, Baltimore

Stanton S L 1992 Clinical gynaecological urology, 2nd edn. Churchill Livingstone, London (in press)

Stanton S L, Tanagho E 1986 Surgery of female incontinence, 2nd edn. Springer-Verlag, Heidelberg

Zacharin R F 1988 Obstetric fistula. Springer-Verlag, Vienna

47. Urethral sphincter incompetence

S. L. Stanton

DEFINITIONS

When a woman coughs and loses urine, the condition used to be called stress incontinence, a term coined by Sir Eardley Holland in 1928. Today, investigations have shown that many conditions can cause stress incontinence and therefore it is preferable to use the term to refer only to symptoms and signs. In 1976, the International Continence Society (ICS) adopted the term 'genuine stress incontinence' for the condition, which was defined as involuntary urethral loss of urine when the intravesical pressure exceeds the maximum urethral pressure in the absence of detrusor activity (Abrams et al 1988). I prefer the term 'urethral sphincter incompetence', which conveys more precisely the pathophysiology. In the USA, the term 'stress urinary incontinence' or 'anatomic stress incontinence' is still commonly used.

We retain the symptom to indicate the patient's statement of involuntary urine loss on physical effort and the sign to denote observation of urine loss from the urethra synchronous with physical exertion.

AETIOLOGY

The mechanism of continence is dealt with in Chapter 42.

Urethral sphincter incompetence is due to two causes: descent of the bladder neck and proximal urethra, so that there is failure of equal transmission of intra-abdominal pressure to the proximal urethra, leading to reversal of the normal pressure gradient between the bladder and urethra and resulting in a negative urethral closure pressure. Alternatively, the intraurethral pressure at rest is below the intravesical pressure. The factors responsible for this are:

1. Congenital weakness of the bladder neck, e.g. epispadias (see Fig. 43.3). The urethra and bladder neck are imperfectly formed owing to faulty migration and midline fusion of mesoderm, resulting in a widened bladder neck, a short urethra and defective smooth and striated musculature. The symphysis and clitoris are split.

   Less obvious congenital weakness presents in the early teens, when healthy nulliparous girls exercise and find that they are incontinent. Nemir & Middleton (1954) and Thomas et al (1980) have shown that 5–10% of young girls have regular troublesome stress incontinence. In the evolutionary change from the horizontal to the vertical position, women have come to rely on a poorly constructed pelvic floor to support the bladder neck; it may fail to do so adequately during times of physical effort (Fig. 47.1). In addition, there may be genetic variations in collagen and other connective tissue, predisposing the bladder neck to excess descent even without childbearing.

   Weakness and malformation of the bladder neck found in epispadias produces incontinence resistant to conventional bladder neck elevating procedures and is corrected by increasing the urethral resistance, i.e. using an artificial urinary sphincter.
2. Childbirth, leading to denervation of smooth and striated components of the sphincter mechanism and

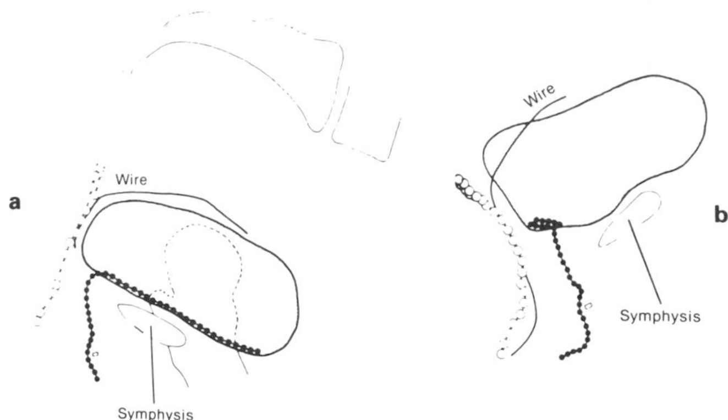

Fig. 47.1 (**a**) Chain urethrocystogram with patient in the non-straining lateral position on all fours showing urethra exiting from a high position in the bladder and supported by the symphysis. (**b**) Patient erect, showing bladder neck junction at lowest level of bladder and without symphysial support. From Hodgkinson (1970).

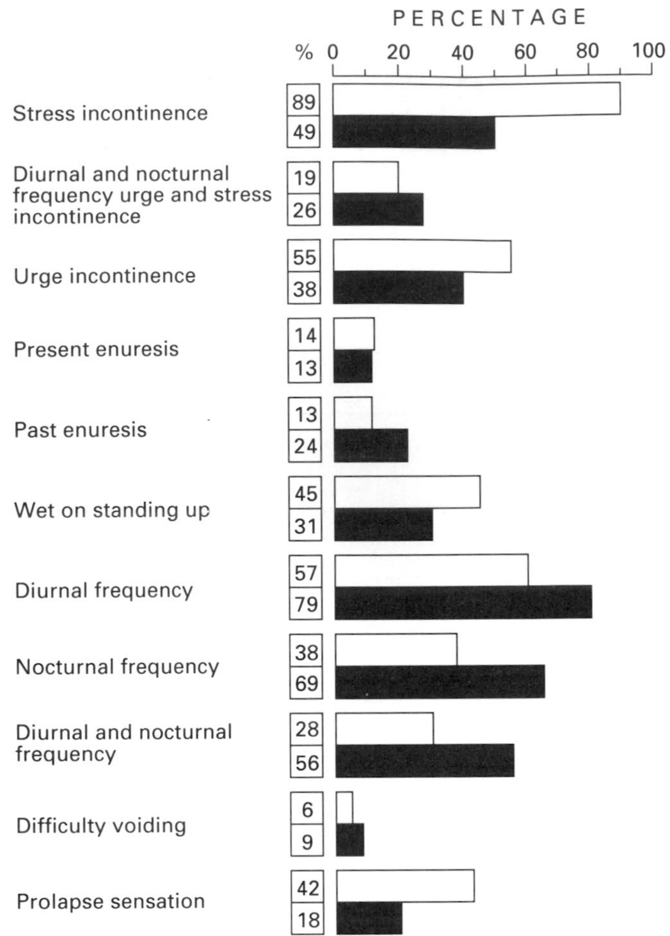

Fig. 47.2 Prevalence of symptoms associated with urethral sphincter incompetence and detrusor instability. From Cardozo & Stanton (1980). □ = Genuine stress incontinence; ■ = detrusor instability. *Stress incontinence is dominant; other symptoms include urgency, diurnal and nocturnal frequency.

pelvic floor and pubocervical fascia (Snooks et al 1984; Sayer et al 1989).
3. Menopause: oestrogen deficiency may lead to further weakness of bladder neck supports and loss of hermetic sealing of the urothelium.
4. Trauma: fracture of the pelvic ring and symphysial diastasis with avulsion of the bladder neck from its attachment to the back of the symphysis by the pubourethral ligaments (Stanton et al 1981).
5. Fibrosis of the urethra and urethral musculature secondary to bladder neck surgery, either for continence or prolapse.

PRESENTATION

Symptoms

The classical symptom of urethral sphincter incompetence is stress incontinence; however frequency, urge incontinence and incontinence on standing are also complained of by many patients (Cardozo & Stanton 1980; Fig. 47.2). Usually stress incontinence is worse in the week preceding the menstrual period. Interruption of the urinary stream can be confirmed objectively in about 83% of patients with sphincter incompetence and 87% in patients with detrusor instability so the symptom is of no use in differentiating between the two.

The patients are usually multiparous and symptoms commonly occur in pregnancy and deteriorate in the postnatal period and in successive pregnancies (Francis 1960; Stanton et al 1980).

Signs

There are no special general or neurological features on clinical examination.

Epispadias will be readily recognized. Anterior vaginal wall descent (cystourethrocele) will be present in about 50% of women with sphincter incompetence.

It is helpful to assess whether other genital prolapse is present and to detect pathology such as uterine or ovarian enlargement, so that surgery for that can be carried out at the same time as continent surgery.

The vaginal capacity and mobility (indicators of vaginal scarring) need to be assessed, as these may be relevant in determining the choice of any continence surgery.

INVESTIGATIONS

The bladder is not a reliable witness. Many clinicians have demonstrated the discrepancy between clinical findings and urodynamic studies (Haylen & Frazer 1987; Ng & Murray 1989). The difficulty lies in the complexity of the history. Stress incontinence alone is likely to indicate sphincter incompetence and a combination of stress incontinence, urge incontinence and frequency are more likely to suggest detrusor instability. In a consecutive group of 800 women attending the urodynamic clinic, approximately 50% were diagnosed by urodynamic studies as having urethral sphincter incompetence. Of these only 3% had the symptom and sign of stress incontinence and only 1.5% (6) had the sole symptom of stress incontinence (Haylen & Frazer 1987). Of the total group, 85% had urgency, urge incontinence and stress incontinence but only 25% had detrusor instability on testing. It was similar with voiding disorders: 53% had two symptoms suggestive of voiding disorder, which was confirmed in only 10% on testing. The aims of urodynamic studies are:

1. To confirm the symptoms (e.g. incontinence or voiding difficulty.
2. To make a diagnosis.
3. To detect other abnormalities, e.g. detrusor instability.
4. To refine the course of treatment.
5. To confirm the cure.

A full description of urodynamic studies is given in Chapter 44; the following tests are useful to make investigate a diagnosis of sphincter incompetence.

A negative midstream urine specimen should precede all urodynamic studies to avoid risk of invasive procedures aggravating urinary tract infection and because the subsequent results will be unreliable.

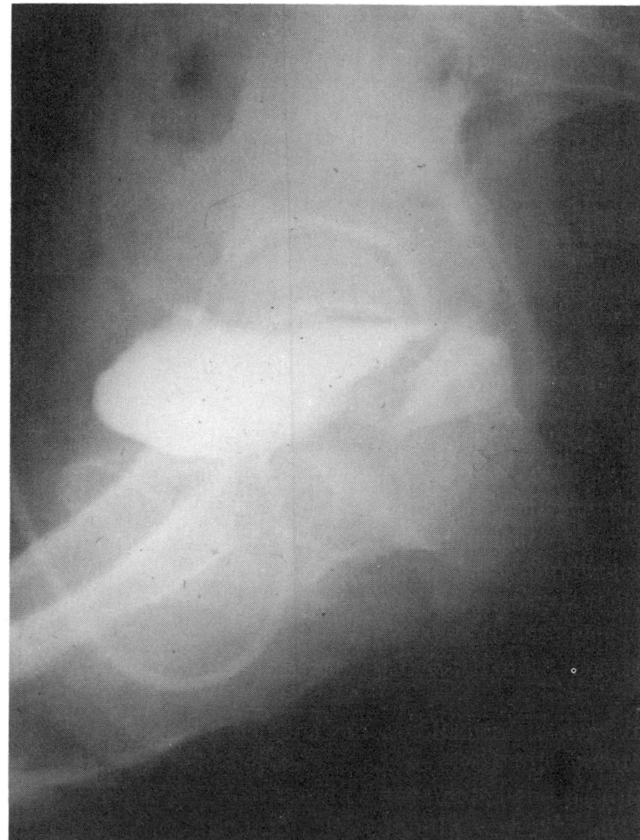

Fig. 47.3 Vesicovaginal fistula.

Pad test

A pad test is a simple inexpensive and non-invasive method of demonstrating urinary loss when this is unproven on a clinical examination or cystometry or videocystourethrography. Of the many varieties, a 1-hour test as recommended by the ICS (Abrams et al 1988) is probably the most reliable (Mayne & Hilton 1988). However the pad test does not confirm the cause of leakage.

Urethral electric conductance

Measurement of change in distal urethral electric conductance will confirm urinary leakage and may indicate whether this is due to sphincter incompetence, urethral or detrusor instability (Peattie et al 1989).

Cystometry and videocystourethrography

The cystometric diagnosis of urinary leakage will indicate the presence of detrusor instability or voiding difficulty; only if detrusor instability is absent is the diagnosis of urethral sphincter incompetence made by exclusion.

The combination of cystometry and radiological screening with recording on video tape together with sound commentary allows other diagnoses to be made, including the course of incontinence on assuming the upright position, the presence of a urethral diverticula (see Fig. 44.11) and occasionally the presence of a urinary fistula (Fig. 47.3). It otherwise adds little to the assessment of straightforward urethral sphincter incompetence (Stanton et al 1988).

Radiology

A plain anteroposterior pelvic radiograph will detect symphysial diastasis when associated with a pelvic fracture (Fig. 47.4) or a full bladder associated with chronic retention and overflow (Fig. 47.5), although the latter can be detected without irradiation using ultrasonography.

Intravenous urography would demonstrate an ectopic ureter, necessary when incontinence is present from birth, or when continuous incontinence follows pelvic surgery in order to exclude a ureteric fistula.

Uroflowmetry

The measurement of urine flow is simple and non-invasive and whilst it is not directly necessary for the diagnosis of sphincter incompetence, it will detect unsuspected voiding difficulty (which may compromise any intended bladder neck surgery). On its own, it serves only as a screening

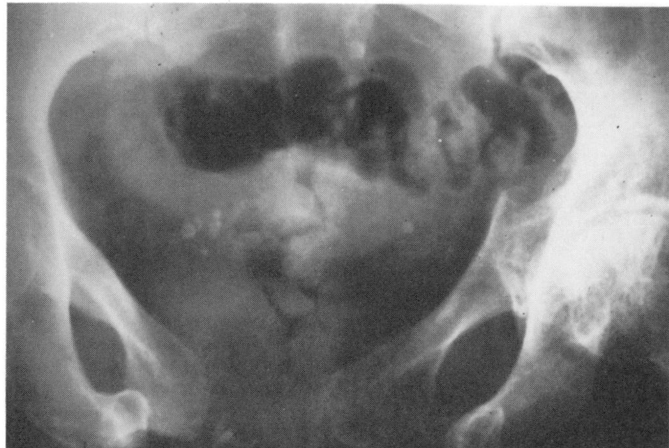

Fig. 47.4 Traumatic diastasis of symphysis and fractures of internal ring.

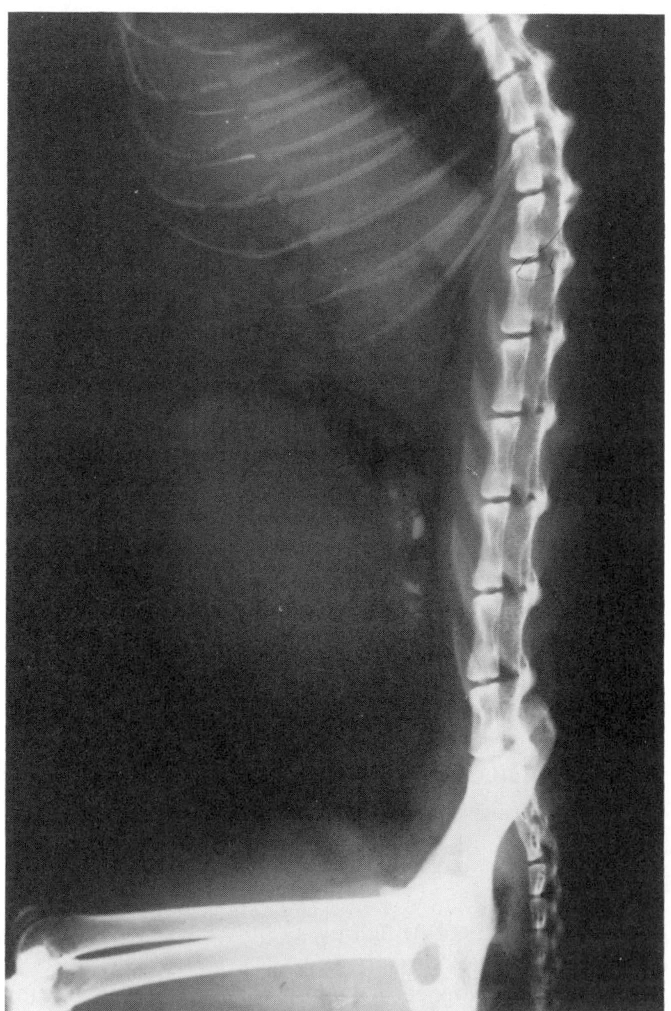

Fig. 47.5 Lateral radiograph showing full bladder associated with chronic retention and overflow. (Courtesy of Victor E. Travis.)

test and gives more information when combined with intravesical pressure measurement.

Urethral pressure profilometry

The role of urethral pressure profilometry in the diagnosis of urethral sphincter incompetence remains controversial and undecided. Versi et al (1986) declared that 'the overlap between normal and GSI [USI] was so great as to make accurate diagnosis impossible'. Sand and colleagues (1987) measured the urethral closure pressure and took a cut-off of 20 cm water to detect the problem of the low-pressure urethra which they said was a significant feature of failed continent surgery. Hilton (1988) reviewed the concept of the unstable urethra as a cause of sphincter incompetence, and found a relative change of 30% of maximum urethral closure pressure was the best discriminant to detect this.

The main disadvantages of the urethral pressure are the relative inflexibility of the catheter leading to artefact, and the marked overlap in results between continent and incontinent patients.

Ultrasonography

Ultrasound will detect incomplete bladder emptying which may be responsible for stress incontinence. It will also allow estimation of the position and excursion of the bladder neck which is relevant to the diagnosis of urethral sphincter incompetence and may help in the analysis of failure of conventional surgery and in the definitive choice of surgery (Creighton et al 1991). Examples of bladder neck position and excursion are shown in Figure 44.16.

Electrophysiological studies

Snooks et al (1984) demonstrated denervation of the sphincter mechanism and pelvic floor after childbirth. In complex cases of sphincter incompetence, especially where multiple bladder neck surgery is being performed and further surgery is contemplated, it may be worthwhile measuring electromyographic activity of these structures using a single fibre electrode (Krieger et al 1988) and terminal motor latencies in the perineal branch of the pudendal nerve.

TREATMENT

Conservative and surgical treatments are used depending on the patient's condition and urodynamic diagnosis. Conservative therapy is indicated when:

1. The patient refuses or is undecided about surgery.
2. The patient is mentally or physically unfit.
3. Childbearing continues.

4. There is uncontrolled detrusor instability or voiding difficulty.

Conservative treatment

1. The continuous indwelling catheter remains a simple method of managing urinary incontinence. However it predisposes to urinary tract infection and may be uncomfortable to wear. For long-term use, suprapubic insertion is preferable and the 'add-a cath' method of insertion (Bard) using a Foley silastic catheter (either 12 or 16 French gauge) is recommended (Lawrence et al 1989; Fig. 47.6). If there is urethral leakage, urethral closure may be performed.

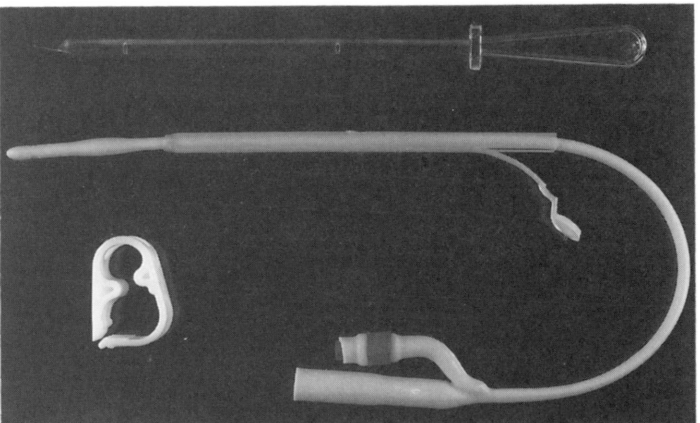

Fig. 47.6 'Add-a' suprapubic catheter showing the trocar and sheath containing foley catheter (Bard).

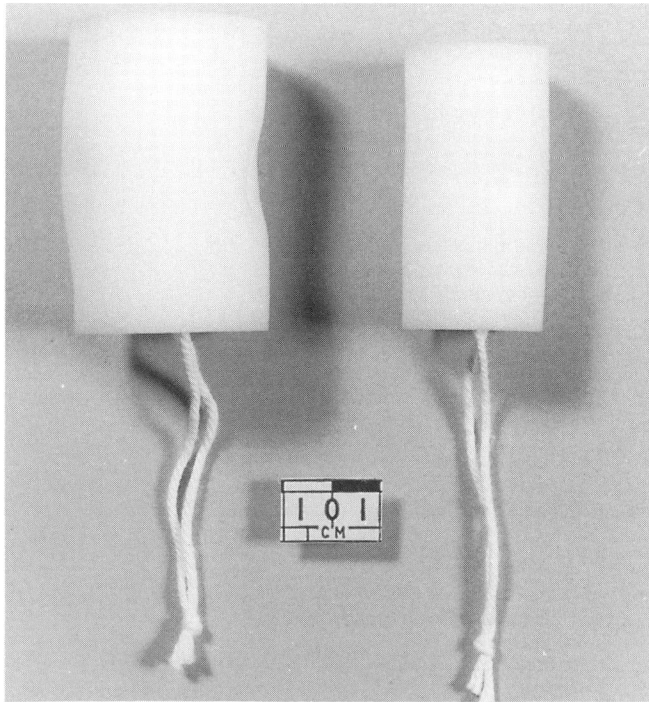

Fig. 47.7 Foam pessary (Rocket).

2. For mild sphincter incompetence, wearing a tampon or a re-usable foam pessary may temporarily cure incontinence by elevating the bladder neck (Fig. 47.7). This is recommended for patients who are incontinent at known times.
3. Absorbent pads are useful when incontinence is mild. The latest are made of a gel substance which absorbs many times its volume of water. The pads have a water-repellent backing and absorb urine without it leaking back to the patient's skin (to make damp) or forward, so making the patient's clothing wet. Good examples are the pads manufactured by Conveen.
4. The use of electronic vaginal devices to cure sphincter incompetence has had a variable popularity over the past 20 years. At present, the technique of using short-term electrical stimulation via vaginal or anal electrodes with daily treatments of 20 min over a period of 30 days has been found effective (Plevnik et al 1986). The current used was up to 90 mA with a frequency of 20 Hz and pulse duration of 0.75 ms.
5. There are a variety of exercises to enhance pelvic floor tone and control incontinence. However the exercise regimes are rarely objectively tested and often carried out for inadequate periods of time, so improvement in incontinence is unsatisfactory. Tapp et al (1989) found that about 50% of women awaiting surgery for urethral sphincter incompetence were improved with 6 months of physiotherapy alone. Marginally more were improved when faradism was added.

   At least 1 h of exercise a day for 3 months is required to show any improvement and of course it lasts only whilst the exercises are being carried out. The easiest one to teach is to interrupt the urinary stream and then to practice this at other times.

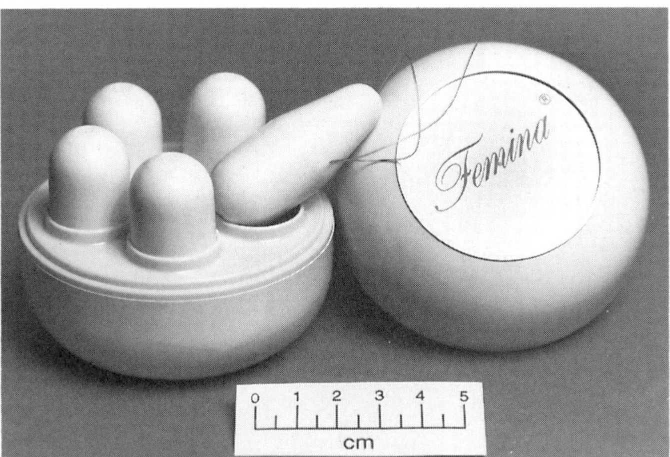

Fig. 47.8 A set of vaginal cones (Colgate Medical).

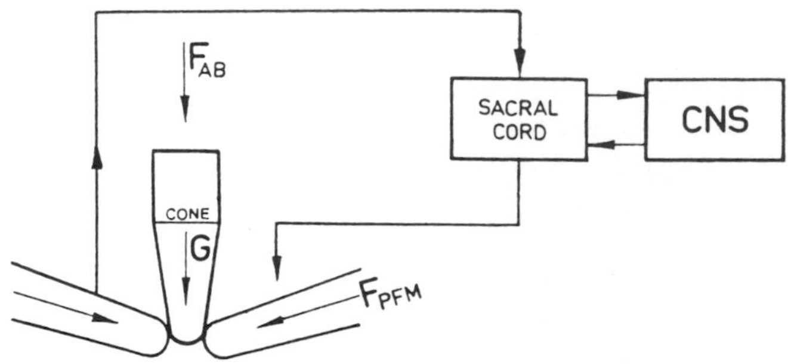

Fig. 47.9 Diagramatic representation of forces on the cones when in situ. G = weight of cone; F_{AB} = force due to abdominal pressure; F_{PFM} = force developed by pelvic floor muscle; CNS = central nervous system.

Interferential therapy can also be used to improve pelvic floor tone (Bridges et al 1988).

6. Vaginal cones were designed by Plevnik (1985), an engineer from Yugoslavia, as a method of actively and passively exercising the pelvic floor (Figs. 47.8 and 47.9). Since the patient knows the weight of the cone she is able to retain with her pelvic floor muscles, she can monitor her progress. Upwards of 70% of patients are cured or improved and 90% find it an acceptable method of treatment (Bridges et al 1988; Peattie et al 1988).

Surgical treatment

Continent surgery is indicated when conservative measures have failed or the patient wants definitive treatment now. If detrusor instability and voiding difficulty are present, the patient should be warned that surgery may make either condition worse. If the patient has not completed her family, bladder neck surgery can be performed but if she subsequently conceives and is dry, a caesarean section should be performed to avoid further pelvic floor trauma.

She should be counselled following any urethrovesical suspension operation that it is wise to avoid heavy lifting, certainly for at least 2 months.

Choice of operation

The choice of operation is influenced by the clinical fea-

Table 47.1 Clinical and urodynamic features

Access	Operation	Mechanism	Clinical indications	Urodynamic effects/ complications
Vaginal	Anterior colporrhaphy	Elevates bladder neck from below	Elderly; physically frail	Minimal recurrence of stress incontinence
	Periurethral injection (e.g. GAX collagen)	Increases urethral resistance	Mild urethral sphincter incompetence — primary and failed surgery; physically frail	Urinary retention
Vaginal and suprapubic	Endoscopic bladder neck suspension (Raz and Stamey)	Elevates from above; enhances pressure transmission in proximal urethra	Elderly; physically frail	Suture can pull through causing recurrence
Suprapubic	Marshall–Marchetti–Krantz	Elevates bladder neck from above	Urethral sphincter incompetence without cystocele	Osteitis pubis
	Colposuspension	Elevates bladder neck	Primary or secondary urethral sphincter incompetence with or without cystocele	Voiding difficulty; detrusor instability
	Sling	Elevates bladder neck from above; supports proximal urethra	Proximal urethra needs support; contracted vagina	Voiding difficulty and urinary tract infection; sling erosion; detrusor instability
	Artificial urinary sphincter	Increases urethral resistance	Neurogenic reconstructive surgery; failed conventional bladder neck surgery	Erosion, mechanical failure

GAX collagen = gluteraldehyde cross-linked bovine collagen.

tures and urodynamic data. An elderly or frail patient is less likely to make energetic demands on the site of operation and will benefit from a shorter operation of 20–30 min with a relatively pain-free postoperative period to aid mobilization. A younger and fitter patient will require more extensive surgery as she is more likely to be more physically active and will cope better with the pain of a major operation. In general, vaginal operations and endoscopic bladder neck suspensions are quicker and less painful but may not be as durable as the urethrovesical suspension operations.

Urodynamic studies will indicate whether surgery is required to correct bladder neck descent and support the bladder neck, or whether urethral resistance has to be enhanced, or whether both are necessary. The flow rate and maximum voiding pressure will suggest whether there is need for caution with an operation likely to produce obstruction.

To choose the operation, the clinical and urodynamic features of the patient and characteristics of each operation have to be matched (Table 47.1).

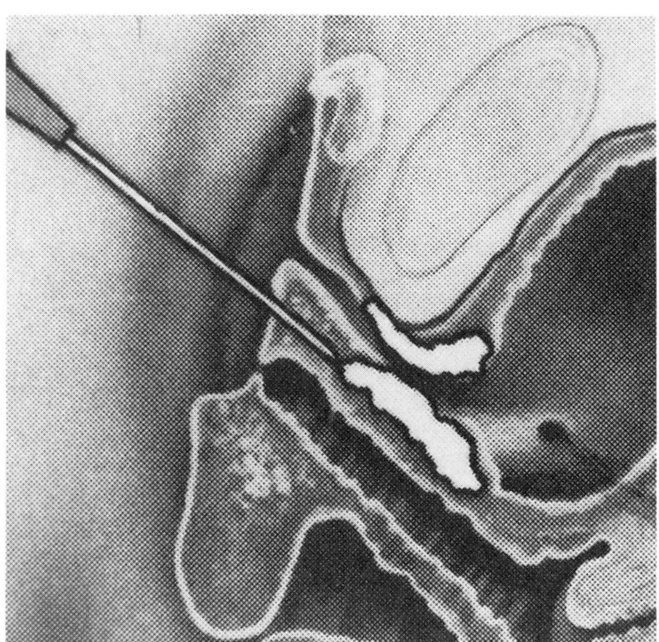

Fig. 47.10 Periurethral injection of material under the submucosa.

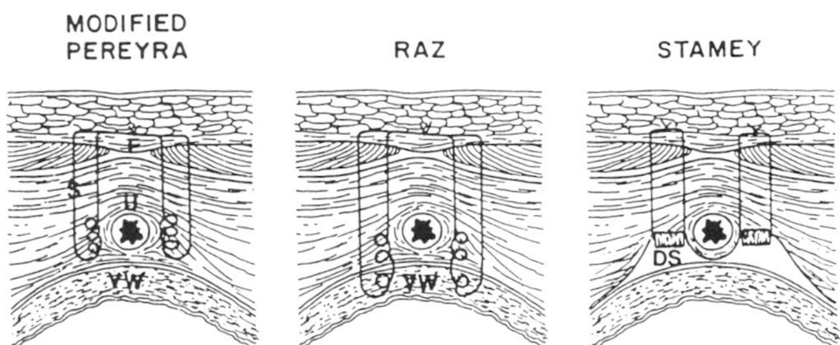

Fig. 47.11 Comparison of modified Pereyra, Raz and Stamey operations: coronal section of bladder neck and surrounding tissues. VW = Vaginal wall; U = urethra; S = suture; DS = dacron support; F = fascia.

Continence operations

Anterior colporrhaphy. A number of clinicians have now demonstrated that the anterior colporrhaphy has a lower success rate for cure of urethral sphincter incompetence than suprapubic operations (Bergman et al 1989). In our own study on 26 patients at the end of 2 years, 6 no longer complained of stress incontinence but only 14 (54%) were cured objectively (Stanton et al 1991). The advantage of an anterior colporrhaphy is that it will correct coexistent anterior vaginal wall prolapse and is unlikely to cause either voiding difficulty or detrusor instability. Apart from a low cure rate of urethral sphincter incompetence, the operation may produce narrowing and scarring of the vaginal tissues, which may render further bladder neck surgery more difficult.

In comparing results for anterior colporrhaphy, it is obvious that different surgical techniques exist. Some surgeons claim that the pubocervical fascia is found on the vaginal aspect of the bladder and plicate that, whilst others take the pubocervical fascia as being adherent to the undersurface of the anterior vaginal wall flap and use that for plication.

Periurethral injection. Periurethral injection of teflon and now GAX collagen (gluteraldehyde cross-linked bovine collagen) is a simple method of restoring continence by increasing urethral resistance, which may be satisfactory for mild incontinence (Fig. 47.10; Appell et al 1989).

Endoscopic bladder neck suspension operation. The Stamey (1973) operation consists of a needle insertion of a suture either side of the bladder neck anchored by a buffer below the pubocervical fascia and tied above, on top of the rectus sheath at a tension sufficient to close the bladder neck. Raz (1981) modified it to include a wider blunt dissection to free the endopelvic fascia from the back of the pubis and inserted helical sutures into the deep endopelvic fascia including part of the vaginal wall (Fig. 47.11).

I prefer the Raz technique and use it for the elderly woman. I use a number 2 prolene suture on a small 4 trocar pointed Mayo needle and a 15° angle Stamey needle to retrieve the suture. I tighten sufficiently to elevate the bladder neck and support it. A small vertical vaginal incision is used on either side of the bladder neck to insert the suture and a small suprapubic incision is placed in each iliac fossa, to retrieve and tie the suture on to the rectus sheath.

Whichever technique is used, it is essential to cystoscope the patient after all needle passes have been completed to ensure that no suture has passed through the bladder and that the sutures are at the level of the bladder neck.

Marshall–Marchetti–Krantz (MMK) operation. The MMK is probably the most widely used suprapubic procedure. The sutures are inserted between paraurethral tissue along the proximal half of the urethra and the periosteum or perichondrium of the symphysis pubis. Krantz (1986) prefers one suture of 2.0 braided Mersilene and uses a double bite and anchors this to the perichondrium. The main complications are osteitis pubis (0.5–5% of cases) and sometimes difficulty in finding tissue behind the symphysis in which to anchor the suture. The procedure will not correct a cystocele.

Colposuspension. The original description by Burch in 1961 has changed little apart from a more specific direction as to where to place the supporting sutures (Stanton 1986).

Before commencing, it is important to ensure that the vagina has adequate capacity and mobility so that the lateral fornices can be elevated towards each ipsilateral iliopectineal ligament. If not, the operation is unlikely to be technically feasible and an alternative procedure should be considered. If an enterocele or rectocele is present, they are likely to be made worse by this operation and ought to be corrected at the same time.

The abdomen and perineum are prepared in a sterile fashion and a urological drape (3 M-1071) is used to allow the operator to dissect with one finger in the vagina. A foley catheter is inserted and a low pfannenstiel incision or a combination of a pfannenstiel and cherney incision is used, if a previous lower abdominal incision is present; this avoids a tedious dissection and sometimes inadvertent opening of the peritoneum. After having dissected the base of the bladder medially, 2–3 Ethibond number 1 sutures (polybutylate-coated polyethylene; Ethicon) are inserted, 1 cm apart and starting as cephalad as possible, between endopelvic fascia (incorporating the whole thickness of the anterior vaginal wall if the fascia is thin) and the ipsilateral iliopectineal ligament (Fig. 47.12). To avoid the suture sliding through the fascia when later tied to the iliopectineal ligament and to aid haemostasis, the suture is tied on the endopelvic fascia. I try and avoid placing sutures distal to the bladder neck because of their tendency to produce voiding disorders. To do this, I gently pull on the foley catheter and determine by feel whether there is place for a further suture more distally. The procedure is repeated on the other side. After completing haemostasis, the sutures are tied, a vacuum drain is left in the retropubic space and a suprapubic catheter inserted.

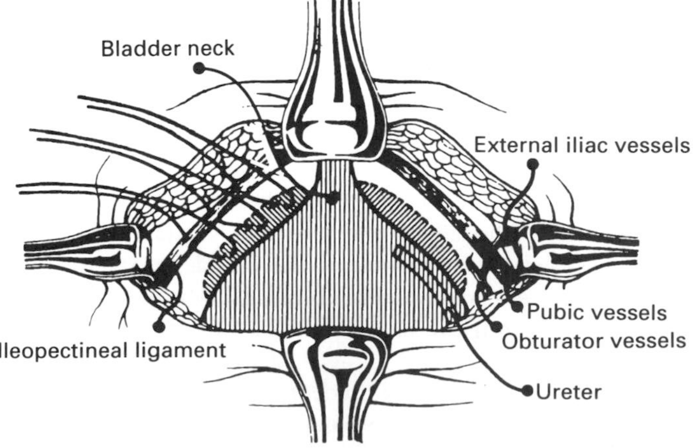

Fig. 47.12 Schema of colposuspension as exposed by a Pfannenstiel incision.

I would suggest the following order for additional procedures. If an enterocele repair is required, the uterosacral ligaments should be coapted at the beginning of the operation. If a hysterectomy is necessary, this should be carried out as an abdominal procedure, with careful attention to vault haemostasis and support. The colposuspension is then performed and finally, if a posterior repair is required, this is carried out as the last procedure.

Sling procedures. There are many varieties, depending on routes of access, type of material used and sling tension.

Most gynaecologists prefer a synchronous vaginal and suprapubic approach. This has the advantage of seeing exactly where the sling is placed and anchoring it at the bladder neck if required. It may be more effective in producing haemostasis and in avoiding sling erosions than the suprapubic approach alone. The disadvantage is the potential of the vaginal incision for infection, which is relevant when inorganic tissue is used. I prefer the single abdominal incision and use a 'blind tunnel' technique to insert the sling under the bladder neck, and then anchor it to each iliopectineal ligament.

Sling materials are either organic or inorganic. The former is either autogenous (from rectus fascia or if unavailable, fascia lata), or from animal tissues, e.g. porcine dermis. Cadaverous dural sling material may transmit Creutzfeldt–Jakob disease and should be used with caution. Inorganic materials are stronger, more consistent and readily available. However if infection occurs, the sling may have to be removed. Meshes such as Marlex (polypropylene) allow fibroblasts to grow into them and become inextricably bound with body tissues and are difficult to subsequently remove.

I prefer silastic bonded to Dacron which is strong, does not bond to body tissues but causes a fibrous sheath to form around the sling (Stanton et al 1985). The silastic sling must be sutured using a non-absorbable suture and to avoid obstruction, I place the sling under minimal tension, just sufficient to support the bladder neck and produce some elevation.

The cure rates for stress incontinence vary between 75 and 95%, depending on whether it is a primary or secondary procedure and whether subjective or objective evaluation is used. Slings often produce complications, including urinary retention and voiding difficulty and sling erosion. The intention is to provide proximal support to the bladder neck and sometimes bladder neck elevation. It is used both as a primary and secondary procedure, particularly where vaginal capacity and mobility are decreased.

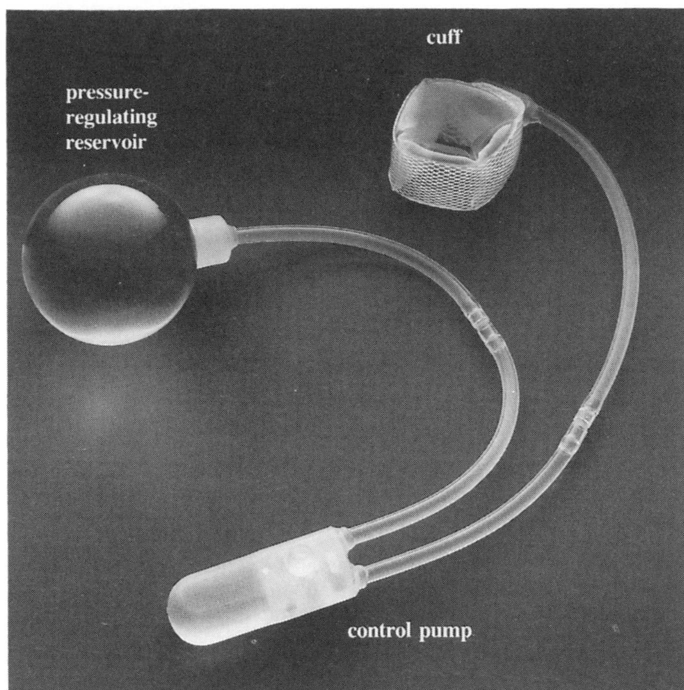

Fig. 47.13 Artificial urinary sphincter 800 showing cuff, reservoir and pump.

Artificial urinary sphincter (Fig. 47.13) . The artificial urinary sphincter has been used since 1973. It is indicated in the female for resistant urethral sphincter incompetence where conventional surgery has failed and the options of continued incontinence, catheter drainage or a diversion are not acceptable. The indications therefore are persistent incontinence with a patient who is mentally alert and manually dexterous. There should be no urinary infection, a bladder capacity greater than 250 ml, controlled detrusor instability and no voiding difficulty or upper urinary tract dilatation.

I have now implanted 30 sphincters and have an objective overall cure or improvement rate of 66%.

Postoperative catheter regime

I usually use a suprapubic catheter (e.g. Bonanno) as this allows the patient to void spontaneously without removal of the catheter. It is clamped on the second day and removed once the patient is able to void in excess of 150–200 ml and the evening and early morning residual urines are less than 150–200 ml respectively.

MANAGEMENT OF RECURRENT INCONTINENCE

The management will depend on the cause, which is likely to be one of the following:

1. Persistent urethral sphincter incompetence because the procedure was either incorrectly chosen or inadequately performed.
2. Occurrence of detrusor instability.
3. Overflow retention.
4. A fistula — ureteric, vesical or urethral.

Clinical and urodynamic assessments will differentiate between them and the management depends upon the cause. If urethral sphincter incompetence persists, either further elevation or an increase in urethral resistance is required and if the latter, an artificial urinary sphincter may be chosen. The alternative is a continent diversion, such as a Mitrofanoff (Woodhouse et al 1989).

CONCLUSION

The precise mechanism of urethral sphincter incompetence has not yet been fully explained. Improved investigation, particularly of urethral function, is required. The balance between invasiveness and information must be carefully assessed. Conservative methods are usually without long-term side-effects and should be tried first unless the patient wishes immediate and surgical correction. The many operations again demonstrate that no operation is supreme. The surgical operation is chosen by considering both clinical and urodynamic features. Recurrent incontinence is managed according to its cause and urodynamic assessment is essential for that.

KEY POINTS

1. Urethral sphincter incompetence is due to either descent of the bladder neck or decrease in urethral resistance or pressure.
2. Vaginal delivery is the commonest cause of urethral sphincter incompetence.
3. 50% of patients will have some cystourethrocele present when urethral sphincter incompetence exists.
4. If the sole symptom of stress incontinence is chosen to diagnose urethral sphincter incompetence, only 1.5% of patients attending with incontinence will present like this.
5. Most patients with sphincter incompetence will present with stress incontinence and urge incontinence and urodynamic studies are usually required to make an exact diagnosis.
6. Urodynamic studies are equally necessary to detect detrusor instability and voiding difficulty as well as to diagnose the cause of incontinence.
7. A battery of tests rather than one single test may be required to diagnose urethral sphincter incompetence.
8. Conservative measures will cure or improve 50% of patients but exercises have to be maintained.
9. The choice of surgery depends upon the patient's characteristics and particularly the position of the bladder neck and urethral resistance. Each continent operation also has its own characteristics.
10. Elderly or frail patients need an operation with a brief operating time, low postoperative morbidity and a quick recovery.

REFERENCES

Abrams P, Blaivas G, Stanton S L, Andersen J 1988 Standardisation of terminology of lower urinary tract function. Scandinavian Journal of Urology and Nephrology (Suppl) 114: 5–19

Appell R, Goodman J, McGuire E et al 1989 Multicenter study of periurethral and transurethral GAX collagen for urinary incontinence. Proceedings of the 19th Annual Meeting of the International Continence Society Ljubljana. Neurourology Urodynamics 8: 339–340

Bergman A, Ballard C, Cooning P 1989 Primary stress incontinence and pelvic relaxation: prospective randomised comparison of three different operations. 19th Annual Meeting of the International Continence Society, Ljubljana. Neurourology Urodynamics 8: 334–335

Bridges N, Denning J, Ollah K, Farrar D 1988 A prospective trial comparing interferential therapy and treatment using cones in patients with symptoms of stress incontinence. Proceedings of the 18th Annual Meeting of the International Continence Society, Oslo. Neurourology Urodynamics 7: 267–268

Burch J 1961 Urethrovaginal fixation to Cooper's ligament for correction of stress incontinence, cystocele and prolapse. American Journal of Obstetrics and Gynecology 81: 281–290

Cardozo L, Stanton S L 1980 Genuine stress incontinence and detrusor instability: a review of 200 patients. British Journal of Obstetrics and Gynaecology 87: 184–190

Creighton S M, Clark A, Pearce J M, Stanton S L 1991 Perineal bladder neck ultrasound: appearances before and after continence surgery. Submitted for publication.

Francis W 1960 The onset of stress incontinence. Journal of Obstetrics and Gynaecology British Empire 67: 899–903

Haylen B T, Frazer M I 1987 Is the investigation of most stress incontinence really necessary? Proceedings of 17th Annual Meeting of ICS. Neurourology and Urodynamics 6: 188–189

Hilton P 1988 Unstable urethral pressure: towards a more relevant definition. Neurourology Urodynamics 6: 411–418

Hodgkinson C P 1970 American Journal of Obstetrics and Gynecology 108: 1141–1168

Holland E. 1928 Cited in Jeffcoate T N 1967 Principles of gynaecology, 3rd edn. Butterworth, London

Krantz K 1986 Marshall–Marchetti–Krantz. In: Stanton S L, Tanagho E (eds) Surgery: female incontinence, 2nd edn. Springer-Verlag, Heidelberg pp 87–93

Krieger M, Gordon D, Stanton S L 1988 Single fibre EMG: a sensitive tool for evaluation of the urethral sphincter. Proceedings of the 18th Annual Meeting of the International Continence Society, Oslo. Neurourology Urodynamics. 7: 239–240

Lawrence W, McQuilkin P, Mann D 1989 Suprapubic catheterisation. British Journal of Urology 63: 443

Mayne C J, Hilton P 1988 The short pad test: standardization of method and comparison with the one hour test. Neurourology and Urodynamics 7: 443

Nemir A, Middleton R 1954 Stress incontinence in nulliparous women. American Journal of Obstetrics and Gynecology 68: 1166–1168

Ng R, Murray A 1989 Place of routine urodynamics in the management of female GSI. Neurourology and Urology 8: 307–308

Peattie A, Plevnik S, Stanton S L 1988 Vaginal cones: a conservative method of treating genuine stress incontinence. British Journal of Obstetrics and Gynaecology 95: 1049–1053

Peattie A, Plevnik S, Stanton S L 1989 Is the bladder really an unreliable witness? Proceedings of the 19th Annual Meeting of the International Continence Society, Ljubljana. Neurourology Urodynamics 8: 303–304

Plevnik S 1985 New method for testing and strengthening of pelvic floor muscles. Proceedings of the 15th Annual Meeting of the International Continence Society, London: 267–268

Plevnik S, Janez J, Vrtacnik P, Trsinar B, Vodusek D 1986 Short term electrical stimulation: home treatment for urinary incontinence. World Journal of Urology 4: 24–26

Raz S 1981 Modified bladder neck suspension for female stress incontinence. Urology 17: 82–85

Sand P, Bower L, Panganibani R, Ostergard D 1987 The low pressure urethra as a factor in failed retropubic urethropexy. Obstetrics and Gynecology 69: 399–402

Sayer T, Dixon J, Hosker G, Warrell D 1989 Histological study of pubo-cervical fascia in women with stress incontinence of urine. International Urogynaecology Journal 1: 18

Snooks S, Swash M, Setchell M, Henry M 1984 Injury to innervation of the pelvic floor and sphincter musculature in childbirth. Lancet ii: 546–550

Stamey T 1973 Cystoscopic suspension of the vesical neck for urinary incontinence. Surgery, Gynecology and Obstetrics 136: 547–554

Stanton S L 1986 Colposuspension. In: Stanton S L, Tanagho E (eds) Surgery of female incontinence, 2nd edn. Springer-Verlag Heidelberg, pp 95–103

Stanton S L, Kerr Wilson R, Harris V G 1980 Incidence of urological symptoms in normal pregnancy. British Journal of Obstetrics and Gynaecology 87: 897–900

Stanton S L, Cardozo L, Riddle P 1981 Urological complications of traumatic diastasis of the symphysis pubis. British Journal of Urology 53: 453–454

Stanton S L, Brindley G S, Holmes D 1985 Silastic sling for urethral sphincter incompetence in women. British Journal of Obstetrics and Gynaecology 92: 747–750

Stanton S L, Chamberlain G V P, Holmes D 1991 Comparison between anterior colporrhaphy and colposuspension in the correction of genuine stress incontinence. Submitted for publication.

Stanton S L, Krieger M, Ziv E 1988 Videocystourethrography: its role in the assessment of incontinence in the female. Proceedings of the 18th Annual Meeting of the International Continence Society, Oslo. Neurourology Urodynamics 7: 172–173

Tapp A, Hills B, Cardozo L 1989 Randomised study comparing pelvic floor physiotherapy with the Burch colposuspension. 19th Annual Meeting of the International Continence Society, Ljubljana. Neurourology Urodynamics 8: 356–357

Thomas T M, Plymat K, Blannin J, Meade T 1980 Prevalence of urinary incontinence. British Medical Journal 281: 1243–1245

Versi E, Cardozo L, Studd J, Cooper D 1986 Evaluation of urethral pressure profilometry for diagnosis of genuine stress incontinence. World Journal of Urology 4: 6–9

Woodhouse C R J, Malone P, Curry J, Reilly T 1989 The Mitrofanoff principle for continent urinary diversions. British Journal of Urology 63: 53–57

48. Detrusor instability

L. Cardozo

INTRODUCTION

The normal human adult bladder is stable and does not contract during micturition except under voluntary control. Conversely, an unstable bladder is one which contracts involuntarily or can be provoked to do so. Raised bladder pressure was first noticed in certain neurological conditions around 60 years ago (Rose 1931; Langworthy et al 1936) but its clinical significance was not appreciated until 1963 when Hodgkinson et al demonstrated urinary incontinence as a result of detrusor contractions in 64 neurologically normal women. They called this condition 'dyssynergic detrusor dysfunction'. Various other names have been used, including uninhibited detrusor and detrusor hyper-reflexia — the latter is now reserved for abnormal detrusor activity due to a neuropathy. The term 'detrusor instability' was coined by Bates et al (1970) as 'the objectively measured loss of ability to inhibit detrusor contractions even when it is provoked to contract by filling, change of posture, coughing etc.' More recently the International Continence Society (Bates et al 1981) have defined an unstable bladder as one that is shown objectively to contract, spontaneously or on provocation, during the filling phase while the patient is attempting to inhibit micturition.

INCIDENCE

It has been argued that detrusor instability is a variant of normal, occurring in about 10% of the population who have not learnt bladder control at the appropriate age (Frewen 1978). We have found that 10% of postmenopausal women complaining of climacteric symptoms but without urological complaints have unstable bladders (Versi & Cardozo 1988). In the adult female population detrusor instability is the second commonest cause of urinary incontinence, after genuine stress incontinence, accounting for 30–50% of cases investigated (Moolgaoker et al 1972; Torrens & Griffiths 1974). However, amongst the elderly population and those who have persistent symptoms after incontinence surgery, the incidence of detrusor instability is even higher.

AETIOLOGY

The causes of detrusor instability are listed below:

1. Idiopathic.
2. Psychosomatic.
3. Neuropathic (hyper-reflexia).
4. Incontinence surgery.
5. Outflow obstruction (men).

During infancy, prior to potty training it is normal for the bladder to contract uninhibitedly at a critical volume, and an unstable bladder may be the result of poorly learnt bladder control. In the majority of women who suffer from detrusor instability no cause can be found, although some have neurotic personality traits (Freeman et al 1985), and they may respond well to psychotherapy. Neurological lesions such as multiple sclerosis and spinal injuries may cause uninhibited bladder contractions but play an aetiological role in only a small group of women with detrusor hyper-reflexia. Following incontinence surgery there is an increased incidence of detrusor instability (Cardozo et al 1979; Steel et al 1985) for which no specific cause has been found, but it may be due to extensive dissection around the bladder neck as it is more commonly seen after multiple previous operations. Alternatively, the problem in some women may be the failure to diagnose the abnormality prior to surgery. Outflow obstruction is rare in women and does not seem to cause detrusor instability in the same way that prostatic hypertrophy does in men. The increased incidence of detrusor instability in the elderly may be due to the onset of occult neuropathy, e.g. senile atherosclerosis or dementia.

PATHOPHYSIOLOGY

The pathophysiology of the unstable bladder remains a mystery. In vitro studies have shown that the detrusor muscle in idiopathic detrusor instability contracts more than normal detrusor muscle. These detrusor contractions are not nerve-mediated and can be inhibited by the neuropeptide vasoactive intestinal polypeptide (Kinder & Mundy 1987). Other studies have shown that increased alpha-adrenergic activity causes increased detrusor contractility (Eaton & Bates 1982). There is evidence to suggest that the pathophysiology of idiopathic and obstructive detrusor instability is different. From animal and human studies on obstructive instability, it would seem that the detrusor develops postjunctional supersensitivity, with reduced sensitivity to electrical stimulation of its nerve supply but a greater sensitivity to stimulation with acetylcholine (Sibley 1985).

If outflow obstruction is relieved the detrusor can return to normal behaviour and re-innervation may occur (Speakman et al 1987).

CLINICAL PRESENTATION

Detrusor instability usually presents with a multiplicity of symptoms. Those seen most commonly are listed below:

1. Frequency (>7 times per day).
2. Nocturia (>1 time per night).
3. Urgency.
4. Urge incontinence.
5. Stress incontinence.
6. Nocturnal enuresis.
7. Coital incontinence.

The most common symptoms are urgency and frequency of micturition which occur in about 80% of patients (Cardozo & Stanton 1980). However, there are numerous other causes of urgency and frequency (Table 48.1).

Some women void frequently because they drink numerous cups of tea or coffee each day and this polyuria should be differentiated from small volumes voided frequently, by means of a frequency/volume chart. Most women who are incontinent develop frequency, which is voluntary, initially in order to try to leak less. Nocturia is also a common symptom in detrusor instability occurring in almost 70% of cases (Cardozo & Stanton 1980). However, being woken from sleep for some other reason and voiding because one is awake does not constitute nocturia. With increasing age there is an increasing incidence of nocturia and it is normal over the age of 70 years to void twice, and over the age of 80 years to void three times during the night.

Table 48.1 Common causes of frequency and urgency of micturition

Classification	Cause
Psychosocial	Excessive drinking, habit, anxiety
Urological	Urinary tract infection, detrusor instability, small-capacity bladder, interstitial cystitis, chronic urinary retention/residual, bladder mucosal lesion, e.g. papilloma, bladder calculus, urethral syndrome, urethritis, urethral diverticulum
Gynaecological	Pregnancy, cystocele, pelvic mass, e.g. fibroids, previous pelvic surgery, radiation cystitis/fibrosis, urethral caruncle, postmenopausal urogenital atrophy
Sexual	Coitus, sexually transmitted disease
Medical	Diuretic therapy, upper motor neurone lesion, impaired renal function, congestive cardiac failure (nocturia), hypokalaemia
Endocrine	Diabetes mellitus, diabetes insipidus, hypothyroidism

Urge incontinence is usually preceeded by urgency (a strong and sudden desire to void) and is due to an involuntary detrusor contraction. However, some women are unaware of any sensation associated with their detrusor contractions and just notice that they are wet. There seems to be a strong correlation between nocturnal enuresis, either childhood or current, and idiopathic detrusor instability (Whiteside & Arnold 1975). Some women complain of incontinence during sexual intercourse and they can be broadly divided into two groups: those who leak during penetration, who tend to have genuine stress incontinence, and those who wet themselves at orgasm. The most common pathology amongst the latter is detrusor instability (Hilton 1988).

The most noticeable feature of the symptomatology of detrusor instability is the infinite variability. Some patients may be severely incapacitated when at work but virtually asymptomatic when they go on holiday; others complain of severe urgency and frequency in the mornings but void normally during the rest of the day and others say that they wet themselves when they do the washing up, or put the door key in the lock.

There are usually no clinical signs in patients with detrusor instability but it is always worth looking for vulval excoriation and stress incontinence. Occasionally an underlying neurological lesion such as multiple sclerosis will be discovered by examining the cranial nerves and S2, 3 and 4 outflow.

INVESTIGATIONS

Urine culture

A midstream specimen of urine should be sent for culture and sensitivity in all cases of incontinence. An infection may contribute to the symptomatology, and urodynamic investigations, which are mainly invasive, may exacerbate any infection. These are certainly uncomfortable under such circumstances and the results may be inaccurate.

Frequency/volume chart

It is our practice to send all patients a frequency/volume chart with their appointment for urodynamic investigations, so that when they arrive we can evaluate their fluid intake and voiding pattern. They are asked to complete the chart (Fig. 48.1) every day for 1 week but are told that they need not measure their voided volumes when at work. Some women find that this is a useful exercise and it works as a kind of home bladder drill.

Uroflowmetry

Although voiding difficulties are uncommon in women, a large chronic urinary residual may present with the symptoms of urgency and frequency of micturition, so it is relevant to measure the urine flow rate prior to urodynamic assessment. Usually, in uncomplicated idiopathic detrusor instability the flow rate is high and the voiding time short, with only a small volume being passed each time.

KINGS COLLEGE HOSPITAL
FREQUENCY VOLUME CHART

	Day 1			Day 2			Day 3			Day 4			Day 5		
Time	In	Out	W	In	Out	W	In	Out	W	In	Out	W	In	Out	W
6, am		75		180	50		180	125					240	500	w
7 am	180									125	225	w			
8 am	180	150	✓	360	125		360	125			100		360	125	
9 am		100					180	350	✓	320	100			100	
10am	360	75		180	250	✓					100 75	w		125	w
11am							180	200	✓	180	50		180	100	w
12	180	225	✓	180	325	✓		100							
1 pm		100		180			180	75		180	300 75	w	180	125	✓
2 pm	100	50			100						200				
3 pm		25 75		180	25 75		220	220	✓	360	100	w	240		
4 pm	240	100	✓				75	90		75			180	320	✓
5 pm				220	200	✓					100			100	
6 pm	180	220	w	220	50		100	125		120			180	100	
7 pm	180				50			200			100	w			
8 pm		225					200			240				75	
9 pm				180	100			150	✓				360		
10pm	180	100		180	75		180	100		180	225	✓		150	
11pm								75		180	150		180	200	✓
12	240	100		180	150	✓	240	25			100		180	225	
1 am								100	✓						
2 am				180	125	✓				180	100			350	✓
3 am	180	300	w				180						220		
4 am					300	w		225	✓	180	100			100	✓
5 am													180		

Fig. 48.1 Frequency volume chart from a woman with detrusor instability.

Cystometry

The diagnosis of detrusor instability is made when detrusor contractions are seen on a cystometrogram. The original definition (International Continence Society) required a detrusor pressure rise greater than 15 cm of water during bladder filling or on provocative testing. It is now generally accepted that any uninhibitable detrusor contraction (even if less than 15 cm of water) constitutes an unstable bladder.

The detrusor pressure rise may take different forms on the cystometrogram trace. Most commonly, uninhibited systolic contractions occur during bladder filling (Fig. 48.2). Not all cases of detrusor instability will be diagnosed on supine filling alone (Turner-Warwick 1975). Some show an abnormal detrusor pressure rise on a change of posture and may void precipitately on standing (Fig. 48.3) or there may be detrusor contractions provoked by coughing which manifest as stress incontinence (Fig. 48.4). Sometimes a steep detrusor pressure rise occurs during bladder filling (Fig. 48.5). This usually represents low compliance of the detrusor but may be due to involuntary detrusor activity

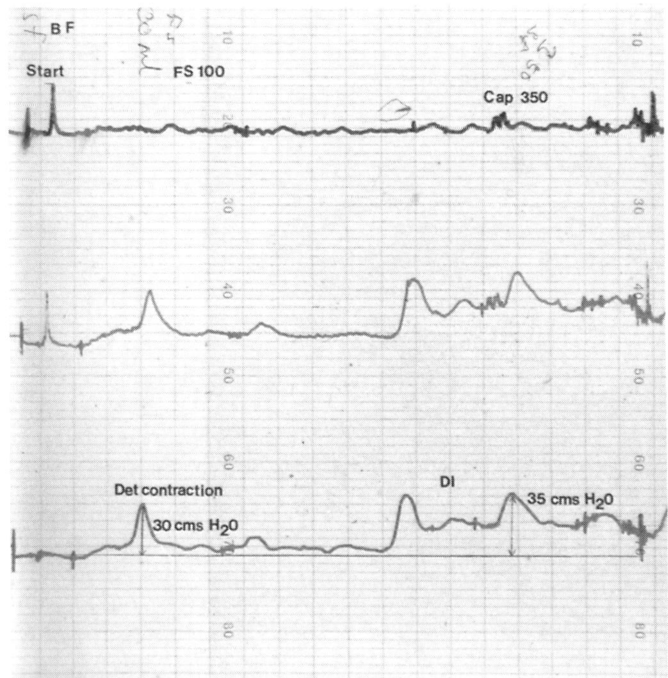

Fig. 48.2 Cystometrogram showing systolic detrusor contractions during bladder filling. FS100 = first sensation 100 ml; DI = detrusor instability.

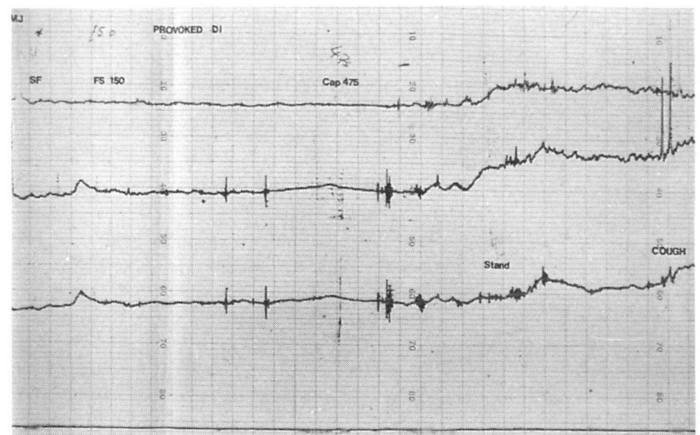

Fig. 48.3 Cystometrogram showing an uninhibited detrusor contraction on standing. SF = Start filling; FS150 = first sensation 150 ml; DI = detrusor instability.

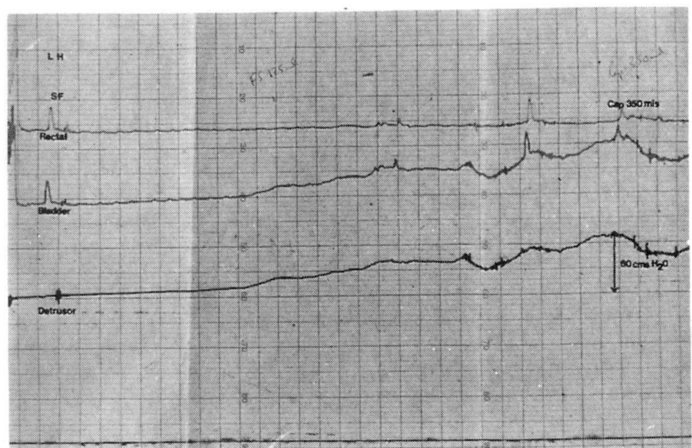

Fig. 48.5 Cystometrogram showing a low compliance bladder. SF = start filling.

in some cases. It can be difficult to differentiate between systolic (phasic) detrusor instability and low compliance, which may coexist. Both conditions usually produce the same symptoms.

During the cystometrogram it is important to ask the patient about her symptoms and relate them to the changes. Most patients will complain of urgency when a detrusor contraction occurs, or urge incontinence if the detrusor pressure exceeds the urethral pressure. Thus in order to diagnose or exclude detrusor instability subtracted provocative cystometry must be employed. Other common, though not universal, features of the cystometrogram in women with detrusor instability are early first sensation, small bladder capacity and inability or difficulty in interrupting the urinary stream. The latter may be associated with a high isometric detrusor contraction (Fig. 48.6), or if videocystourethrography is performed, slow or absent milkback of contrast medium from the proximal urethra into the bladder.

Cystourethroscopy

Endoscopy is not helpful in detrusor instability but may be used to exclude other causes of the patient's symptoms such as a bladder tumour or calculus. Coarse trabeculation of the bladder may be noted in long-standing cases of detrusor instability. This can also be seen during videocystourethrography (Fig. 48.7).

Other urodynamic tests are of limited benefit in detrusor instability. Urethral pressure profilometry (Hilton & Stanton 1983) may reveal coexistent urethral instability but its clinical significance is uncertain. A positive bladder neck electric conductance test (Holmes et al 1989) has been

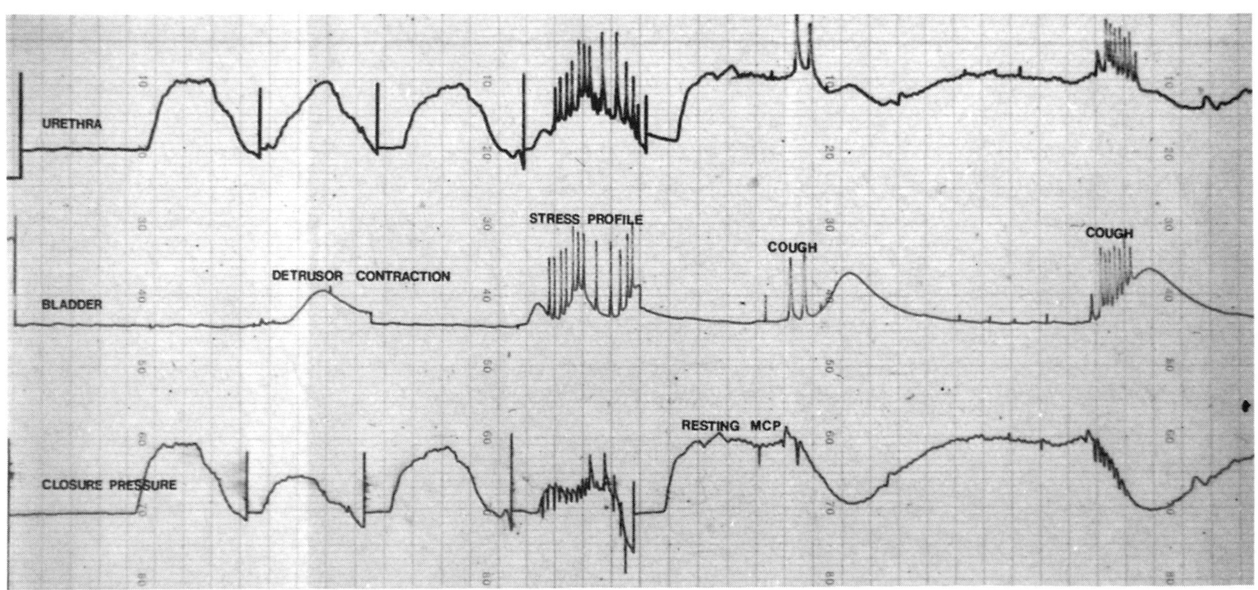

Fig. 48.4 Urethral pressure profile trace showing detrusor contractors in response to coughing. MCP = Maximum closure pressure.

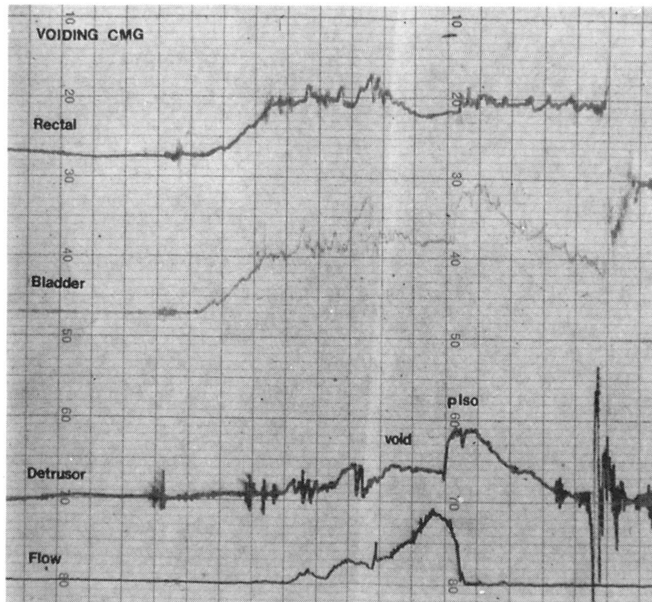

Fig. 48.6 Cystometrogram showing a large isometric detrusor contraction. PISO = Isometric contraction pressure.

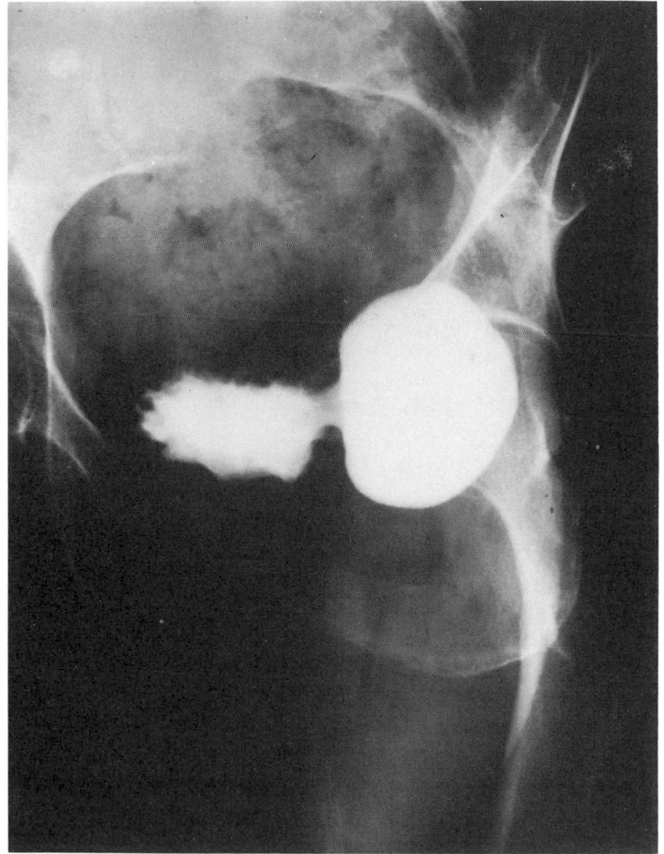

Fig. 48.7 Trabeculated bladder secondary to long-standing detrusor instability, with a large diverticulum on the left.

found to correlate well with the symptom of urgency, but this test is still fairly new and requires further evaluation.

TREATMENT

Not all patients with detrusor instability require treatment. Once the problem has been explained to them some women are able to control their symptoms by behaviour modification such as drinking less and avoiding tea, coffee and alcohol. However, most women with detrusor instability request treatment and although many different therapies have been tried, none has proven universally satisfactory. The currently employed methods are listed below:

1. Drugs.
2. Bladder retraining.
3. Phenol injections.
4. Augmentation cystoplasty.

Other types of treatment which have been tried include vaginal denervation (Hodgkinson and Drukker 1977; Warrell 1977; Ingelman-Sundberg 1978), caecocystoplasty, selective sacral neurectomy (Torrens & Griffiths 1974), cystodistension (Ramsden et al 1976; Higson et al 1978; Pengelly et al 1978), and bladder transection (Mundy 1983). They all give some short-term benefit in carefully selected cases, but may produce significant morbidity, and none has stood the test of time.

Drugs

Drugs which may be useful in the treatment of detrusor instability fall into three categories:

1. Those which inhibit bladder contractility.
2. Those which increase outlet resistance.
3. Those which decrease urine production.

In practice, only the first group are prescribed regularly. Neurotransmission in the detrusor is cholinergic so most of the agents used to treat detrusor instability have some anti-cholinergic properties. Unfortunately, it is very difficult to assess the clinical benefit of the drugs prescribed for this condition because they may act at more than one site, have different effects in vitro and in vivo and may have different short- and long-term effects. Many different drugs have been tried but few are in regular clinical use (Wein 1986).

The following types of drugs inhibit bladder contractility (the effectiveness of the drugs in brackets is uncertain):

1. Anti-cholinergic agents.
2. Musculotropic relaxants.
3. Tricyclic antidepressants.
4. Calcium channel blockers.
5. (Beta-adrenergic agonists.)
6. (Alpha-adrenergic antagonists.)
7. (Prostaglandin inhibitors.)

Anti-cholinergic agents, e.g. propantheline

These drugs produce competitive blockade of acetylcholine receptors at postganglionic parasympathetic receptor sites. They have typical side-effects of dry mouth, blurred vision, tachycardia, drowsiness and constipation. Virtually all the drugs which are truly beneficial in the management of detrusor instability produce these unwanted side-effects to a greater or lesser extent.

Propantheline bromide is relatively inexpensive and if prescribed in a high dose (for example 60 mg four times daily — twice the recommended dose) it can be effective. Introducing the drug slowly minimized side-effects. Propantheline is particularly useful for the symptom of frequency of micturition.

Musculotropic relaxants, e.g. oxybutynin chloride

These drugs are smooth muscle relaxants which act predominantly on the bladder. Their side-effects are anti-cholinergic.

Oxybutynin, a tertiary amine, is one of the most effective drugs currently available for the treatment of detrusor instability. Given in the maximum recommended dose of 5 mg three times daily many women find the side-effects less tolerable than the symptoms of detrusor instability. The worst problem seems to be a very dry mouth and throat and a lingering bad taste. However, oxybutynin does cause significant improvement in the symptom of urgency but this may be at the expense of an increased urinary residual volume (Cardozo et al 1987). In those patients who can tolerate this drug a 70% improvement rate can be expected.

Tricyclic antidepressants, e.g. imipramine hydrochloride

These drugs have a complex pharmacological action. Imipramine has anti-cholinergic, antihistamine and local anaesthetic properties. It may increase outlet resistance due to peripheral blockage of noradrenaline uptake and it also acts as a sedative. The side-effects are anti-cholinergic together with tremor and fatigue. Imipramine is particularly useful for the treatment of nocturia and nocturnal enuresis (Castleden et al 1981). Imipramine together with propantheline may be used to treat the combined symptoms of diurnal frequency and nocturia.

Calcium channel blockers, e.g. terodiline

These drugs limit the availability of calcium ions which are required for the contractile process. They all have some anti-cholinergic action as well. The side-effects are not usually severe but may include hypotension, headache, dizziness, constipation, nausea and palpitations. Terodiline is currently a very popular drug which has been shown to be effective in treating the symptoms of detrusor instability (Ulmsten et al 1985; Tapp et al 1987).

The best drugs to try first in the treatment of detrusor instability are probably oxybutynin and terodiline. The advantage of oxybutynin is that it can be given intermittently and still be effective whereas terodiline requires regular usage in order to reach its maximum efficacy. On the other hand, the side-effects of terodiline are less severe than those of oxybutynin.

Other drugs

Antidiuretic hormone analogues. Synthetic vasopressin (DDAVP) has been shown to reduce nocturnal urine production by up to 50%. It can be used for children or adults with nocturia or nocturnal enuresis but has to be avoided in patients with hypertension, ischaemic heart disease or congestive cardiac failure (Hilton & Stanton 1982). Recent evidence suggests that it is safe to use in the long term (Rew & Rundle 1989).

Oestrogens. There are abundant oestrogen receptors in the urethra and bladder and although many authors have shown that oestrogen deprivation following the menopause causes functional changes in the lower urinary tract (Tapp & Cardozo 1986) few studies have shown that oestrogens produce a cure in cases of urinary incontinence due to detrusor instability. However sensory urgency, which may be due to atrophic changes, does respond to oestrogen replacement therapy.

Bladder retraining

As continence is normally learned during infancy it is logical to suppose that it can be relearned during adult life. Various different forms of bladder re-education have been tried, including:

1. Bladder drill.
2. Biofeedback.
3. Hypnotherapy.

Bladder discipline was first described as a method of treating urgency incontinence by Jeffcoate & Francis (1966) in the belief that this type of incontinence was exacberbated or even caused by underlying psychological factors. Since then Frewen (1970, 1978) has shown that many women with detrusor instability 'are able to correlate the onset of their symptoms to some untoward event' which can be identified by taking a careful history. He has shown that both inpatient and outpatient bladder drill are effective forms of treatment for many such women.

The technique for performing inpatient bladder drill has been established by Jarvis (1989) and is shown below.

Techniques for inpatient bladder drill

1. Exclude pathology and admit to hospital.
2. Explain rationale to patient.
3. Instruct the patient to void every $1\frac{1}{2}$ h during the day (either she waits or is incontinent).
4. When $1\frac{1}{2}$ h is achieved, increase by $\frac{1}{2}$ h and continue with 2-hourly voiding etc.
5. Allow a normal fluid intake.
6. The patient keeps a fluid balance chart.
7. She meets a successful patient.
8. She receives encouragement from patients, nurses and doctors.

Jarvis & Millar (1980) performed a controlled trial of bladder drill in 60 consecutive incontinent women with idiopathic detrusor instability. They showed that following inpatient treatment 90% of the bladder drill group were continent and 83.3% remained symptom-free after 6 months. In the control group 23.2% were continent and symptom-free due to the placebo effect. Despite the excellent early results it has been shown that up to 40% of patients relapse within 3 years (Holmes et al 1983).

Biofeedback

Biofeedback is a form of learning or re-education in which the patient is given information about a normally unconscious physiological process in the form of an auditory, visual or tactile signal. The objective effects of biofeedback in the treatment of detrusor instability can be recorded on a polygraph trace, but the subjective changes may be difficult to separate from the placebo effect.

This technique was originally described by Cardozo et al (1978a). Biofeedback was performed for 4–8 1 h sessions during which the patient's detrusor pressure was measured cystometrically and converted into auditory and visual signals from which she could appreciate changes in her detrusor pressure. The efficacy of biofeedback was assessed by means of a urinary diary that the patient completed each week, and objectively by cystometry. Thirty women aged between 16 and 65 years suffering from idiopathic detrusor instability which was resistant to conventional therapy were treated in two centres (Cardozo et al 1978b). Some 80% of the women were cured or significantly improved subjectively and 60% were cured or improved objectively. Six patients failed to improve at all and these women had severe detrusor instability with detrusor contractions greater than 60 cm of water and cystometric bladder capacities of less than 200 ml. They found it impossible to inhibit their abnormal detrusor activity and one of them was later found to have multiple sclerosis.

Long-term follow-up of these women proved difficult, but of 11 who were initially cured or improved only 4 remained so 5 years later. Two of the others had undergone surgery and were symptom-free but the remaining 5 had relapsed (Cardozo & Stanton 1984). Biofeedback helps by giving the patient a better understanding of the mechanism of bladder function and of her particular bladder abnormality. The overall improvement rate is much the same as that achieved by Frewen (1984) or Jarvis (1989) using bladder drill but does not require hospital admission, although trained personnel are required to give the training.

Millard & Oldenberg (1983) used bladder training and/or biofeedback to treat 59 women with detrusor instability or sensory urgency. In addition they employed supportive psychotherapy or drugs. Their cure and significant improvement rate was 74 and 92% in detrusor instability and sensory urgency respectively. They stated that 'biofeedback was undoubtedly the most useful of the techniques'. Combined behavioural treatment with biofeedback has been used in 39 elderly outpatients, of whom 19 had stress incontinence, 12 detrusor instability and 8 sensory urgency (Burgio et al 1986). All patients showed an average of at least 80% improvement, 13 achieved total continence and 19 had fewer than one accident per week after treatment. Recently the successful use of bladder neck electric conductivity with biofeedback has been reported in a smaller series of women with detrusor instability (Holmes et al 1989).

Hypnotherapy

Hypnotherapy can be used in one of two ways — either symptom removal by suggestion alone or by attempting to help the patient disclose hidden emotions or memories which may be pathogenic. Freeman & Baxby (1982) treated 61 women with idiopathic detrusor instability using 12 sessions of hypnosis over a period of 1 month. Twenty-two women with genuine stress incontinence were managed similarly to act as controls.

Unfortunately 10 patients defaulted during treatment but of the remaining 51, 58% were symptom-free, 28% improved and 14% were unchanged. These results are similar to those for other methods of behavioural intervention. Three months after treatment 50% of the 44 women who underwent repeat urodynamics were shown to have converted from unstable to stable cystometrograms. Unfortunately at 2-year follow-up when 30 of the patients were contacted only 9 were symptom-free compared to 18 at 3 months following treatment (Freeman 1989). This high relapse rate is also in keeping with other forms of behavioural intervention (Holmes et al 1983; Cardozo & Stanton 1984).

Other types of non-surgical, non-pharmacological intervention may be helpful in the treatment of detrusor instability, but newer techniques require thorough evaluation before they can be recommended for routine clinical practice. Electric stimulation applied anally or vaginally may inhibit spontaneous detrusor contractions and thus represents a therapeutic alternative for the management of detrusor instability (Plevnik et al 1986). The neurophysiological basis for the resulting prolonged bladder inhibition remains unclear.

The technique is safe and inexpensive and can be performed by specialist nurses. A success rate (cure or significant improvement) of 77% on objective follow-up at 1 year after an average initial treatment regime of seven sessions has recently been reported (Eriksen et al 1989).

Acupuncture has also been tried in the management of detrusor instability or sensory urgency. Philp et al (1988) showed that 69% of 16 patients with idiopathic detrusor instability were cured or improved after treatment, but only one converted to stability.

All forms of bladder retraining in the treatment of detrusor instability are advantageous because there are few unpleasant side-effects and no patient is ever made worse.

Mild to moderate detrusor instability can be cured or significantly improved by re-educating the bladder. However, the relapse rate is very high and although this type of treatment avoids the morbidity associated with surgery and the side-effects of drug therapy, it requires skilled personnel and is time-consuming for both the patient and the operator.

Transvesical phenol

Originally described for the treatment of detrusor hyperreflexia (Ewing et al 1982), this treatment has since been used for women with idiopathic detrusor instability also. Through a 30° cystoscope a 35 cm semi-rigid needle is inserted under the bladder epithelium mid-way between the ureteric orifice and the bladder neck, and 10 ml of 6% aqueous phenol is injected on each side. In the largest published series, Blackford et al (1984) reported improvement for at least 1 year in 88 of the 116 women treated. They found that the response to treatment was best in those women over the age of 55 years. A number of side-effects and complications were recorded, of which transient postoperative haematuria was the most common. However they said that there was no significant morbidity. Other workers in the field have been less enthusiastic about the long-term result of transvesical phenol and more concerned about the incidence of significant complications (Rosenbaum et al 1988).

Surgery

Various different surgical techniques have been described for the treatment of detrusor instability but currently the most commonly performed operation is the 'clam' cystoplasty (Mundy & Stephenson 1985). The bladder is bisected almost completely and a patch of gut (usually ileum) equal in length to the circumference of the bisected bladder (about 25 cm) is sewn in place. This operation often cures the symptoms of detrusor instability but inefficient voiding usually results. Patients have to learn to strain to void or may have to resort to clean intermittent self-catheterization, sometimes permanently. In addition mucus retention in the bladder may be a problem.

As a last resort for those women with severe detrusor instability or hyper-reflexia who cannot manage clean intermittent self-catheterization it may be more appropriate to perform an ileal conduit urinary diversion. This is particularly useful in young disabled women as it is often easier for them or their carers to empty a bag rather than change wet underclothes or incontinence pads.

General management

All incontinent women benefit from advice regarding simple measures which they can take to help alleviate their symptoms. Many women drink far too much and they should be told to limit their fluid intake to 1 litre a day and to avoid tea, coffee and alcohol if these exacerbate their problem. The use of drugs which affect bladder function such as diuretics should be reviewed and if possible stopped. If there is coexistent genuine stress incontinence then pelvic floor exercises with or without electrical treatment such as faradism may be helpful.

It is usually preferable, in cases of mixed incontinence, to treat the detrusor instability prior to resorting to surgery for the urethral sphincter incompetence. Such treatment may obviate the need for surgery (Karram & Bhatia 1989). In addition there is always the risk that the incontinence operation may exacerbate the detrusor instability.

For younger women who leak only when exercising, a tampon in the vagina during sporting activities may be helpful. For peri- or postmenopausal women hormone replacement is unlikely to cure the problem but may increase the sensory threshold of the bladder and may also make the urinary symptoms easier for her to deal with. The most degrading aspect of urinary incontinence for many patients is the odour and staining of their clothes and this can be helped by good advice regarding incontinence pads and garments.

CONCLUSION

Detrusor instability is a common condition affecting people of all ages and characterized by multiple symptoms. It is not a life-threatening condition but may cause much embarrassment and a very restricted lifestyle. Our lack of understanding of the underlying pathology of detrusor instability is reflected in the numerous methods of treatment which are currently employed, none of them wholly satisfactory. Conventional bladder neck surgery is not useful in the treatment of detrusor instability unless there is concomitant genuine stress incontinence and therefore it is important to make an accurate diagnosis before treatment is commenced.

Surgical procedures are reserved for women with severe symptoms in whom other forms of treatment have been tried and failed. Behavioural intervention seems to be the best type of treatment for idiopathic detrusor instability because it may produce a permanent cure without any significant morbidity or side-effects.

However, the majority of patients are still treated with drug therapy which they may need to take indefinitely, as symptoms usually return once the tablets are discontinued. Fortunately, detrusor instability is a disease of spontaneous exacerbation and remissions and therefore short courses of drug therapy when the symptoms are worst may be sufficient for the sufferer to maintain a normal lifestyle.

Although it is rare to cure a patient completely with any form of treatment, most can have their symptoms significantly reduced. The elucidation of the patient's main complaints is therefore of great importance. As the pathophysiology of the condition becomes clearer we can expect significant advances in the management of detrusor instability.

KEY POINTS

1. Detrusor instability is a disease of spontaneous exacerbations and remissions.
2. Detrusor instability may occur in 10% of the normal population and be asymptomatic.
3. It is the second commonest cause of incontinence in the young and middle aged woman but the commonest cause in the elderly.
4. The cause of idiopathic detrusor instability is unknown but many patients have a neurotic personality trait.
5. The diagnosis of detrusor instability can be suggested by symptoms but confirmed only on cystometry.
6. Bladder retraining and behaviour modification are important treatments which can be augmented by anti-cholinergic drug therapy.
7. Most anti-cholinergic drugs require to be given at dosage which will produce parasympathetic side effects.
8. Mild instability can be cured or improved by bladder retraining but the relapse rate is high.
9. Where instability and genuine stress incontinence coexist, it is preferable to treat the instability first.

REFERENCES

Bates C P, Whiteside C G, Turner-Warwick R T 1970 Synchronous cine-pressure-flow cystourethography with special reference to stress and urge incontinence. British Journal of Urology 50: 714–723

Bates C P, Bradley W, Glen E et al 1981 International Continence Society: Fourth report of the standardisation of terminology of lower urinary tract function. British Journal of Urology 53: 333–335

Blackford W, Murray K, Stephenson T P, Mundy A R 1984 Results of transvesical infiltration of the pelvic plexus with phenol in 116 patients. British Journal of Urology 56: 647–649

Burgio K L, Robinson J C, Engel B T 1986 The role of biofeedback in Kegel exercise training for stress urinary incontinence. American Journal of Obstetrics and Gynecology 154: 64–88

Cardozo L D, Stanton S L 1980 Genuine stress incontinence and detrusor instability: a review of 200 cases. British Journal of Obstetrics and Gynaecology 87: 184–190

Cardozo L D, Stanton S L 1984 Biofeedback: a five year review. British Journal of Urology 56: 220

Cardozo L D, Abrams P H, Stanton S L, Feneley R C L 1978a Idiopathic detrusor instability treated by biofeedback. British Journal of Urology 50: 521–523

Cardozo L D, Stanton S L, Allan V 1978b Biofeedback in the treatment of detrusor instability. British Journal of Urology 50: 250–254

Cardozo L D, Stanton S L, Williams J E 1979 Detrusor instability following surgery for genuine stress incontinence. British Journal of Urology 51: 204–207

Cardozo L D, Cooper D, Versi E 1987 Oxybutynin chloride in the management of idiopathic detrusor instability. Neurourology and Urodynamics 6: 256–257

Castleden C M, George C F, Renwick A G, Asher M J 1981 Imipramine — a possible alternative to current therapy for urinary incontinence in the elderly. Journal of Urology 125: 318–320

Eaton A C, Bates C P 1982 An in vitro physiological study of normal and unstable human detrusor muscle. British Journal of Urology 54: 653–657

Eriksen B C, Bergmann S, Eik-Nes S H 1989 Maximal electrostimulation of the pelvic floor in female idiopathic detrusor instability and urge incontinence. Neurourology and Urodynamics 8: 219–230

Ewing R, Bultitude M E, Shuttleworth K G D 1982 Subtrigonal phenol injection for urge incontinence secondary to detrusor instability in females. British Journal of Urology 54: 689–692

Freeman R M 1989 Hypnosis and psychomedical treatment. In: Freeman R M, Malvern J (eds) the unstable bladder. Wright, Bristol, pp 73–80

Freeman R M, Baxby K 1982 Hypnotherapy for incontinence caused by the unstable detrusor. British Medical Journal 284: 1831–1834

Freeman R M, McPherson F M, Baxby K 1985 Psychological features of women with idiopathic detrusor instability. Urologia Internationalis 40: 247–259

Frewen W K 1970 Urge and stress incontinence; fact and fiction. Journal of Obstetrics and Gynaecology of the British Commonwealth 1977: 932–934

Frewen W K 1978 An objective assessment of the unstable bladder of psychological origin. British Journal of Urology 50: 246–249

Frewen W K 1984 The significance of the psychosomatic factor in urge incontinence. British Journal of Urology 56: 330

Higson R H, Smith J C, Whelan P 1978 Bladder rupture: an acceptable complication of distension therapy? British Journal of Urology 50: 529–534

Hilton P 1988 Urinary incontinence during sexual intercourse: a common but rarely volunteered symptom. British Journal of Obstetrics and Gynaecology 95: 377–381

Hilton P, Stanton S L 1982 Use of desmopressin (DDAVP) in nocturnal urinary frequency in the female. British Journal of Urology 54: 252–255

Hilton P, Stanton S L 1983 Urethral pressure measurement by microtransducer: the results in symptom-free women and those with genuine stress incontinence. British Journal of Obstetrics and Gynaecology 90: 919–933

Hodgkinson C P, Drukker B H 1977 Infravesical nerve resection for detrusor dyssynergia (the Ingleman–Sundberg operation). Acta Obstetrica Gynecologica Scandinavica 56: 401–408

Hodgkinson C P, Ayers M A, Drukker B H 1963 Dyssynergic

detrusor dysfunction in the apparently normal female. American Journal of Obstetrics and Gynecology 87: 717–730
Holmes D M, Stone A R, Barry P R, Richards C J, Stephenson T P 1983 Bladder training — 3 years on. British Journal of Urology 55: 660–664
Holmes D, Plevnick S, Stanton S L 1989 Bladder neck electric conductivity in female urinary urgency and urge incontinence. British Journal of Obstetrics and Gynaecology 96: 816–820
Ingelman-Sundberg A 1978 Partial bladder denervation for detrusor dyssynergia Clinical Obstetrics and Gynaecology 21: 797–805
Jarvis G T 1989 Bladder drill. In: Freeman R, Malvern J (eds) The unstable bladder. Wright, Bristol, pp 55–60
Jarvis G T, Millar D R 1980 Controlled trial of bladder drill for detrusor instability. British Medical Journal 281: 1322–1323
Jeffcoate T N A, Francis W J A 1966 Urgency incontinence in the female. American Journal of Obstetrics and Gynecology 94: 604–618
Karram M M, Bhatia N W 1989 Management of coexistent stress and urge urinary incontinence. Obstetrics and Gynecology 73: 4–7
Kinder R B, Mundy A R 1985 Pathophysiology of idiopathic detrusor instability and detrusor hyperreflexia - an 'in vitro' study of human detrusor muscle. British Journal of Urology 60: 509–515
Langworthy D R, Kolb L G, Dees J E 1936 Behaviour of the human bladder freed from cerebral control. Journal of Urology 36: 577–597
Millard R J, Oldenberg B F 1983 The symptomatic, urodynamic and psychodynamic results of bladder re-education programmes. Journal of Urology 130: 717–719
Moolgaoker A S, Ardran G M, Smith J C, Stallworthy J A 1972 The diagnosis and management of urinary incontinence in the female. British Journal of Obstetrics and Gynaecology 79: 481–497
Mundy A R 1983 The long term results of bladder transection for urge incontinence. British Journal of Urology 55: 642–644
Mundy A R, Stephenson T P 1985 Clam ileocystoplasty for the treatment of refractory urge incontinence. British Journal of Urology 57:647–651
Pengelly A W, Stephenson T P, Milroy E J G, Whiteside C G, Turner Warwick R 1978 Results of prolonged bladder distension as treatment for detrusor instability. British Journal of Urology 50: 243–245
Philp T, Shah P J R, Worth P H L 1988 Acupuncture in the treatment of bladder instability. British Journal of Urology 61: 490–493
Plevnik S, Janez J, Vrtacnik P, Trsinar B, Vodusek D B 1986 Short term electrical stimulation: home treatment for urinary incontinence. World Journal of Urology 4: 24–26
Ramsden P D, Smith J C, Dunn M, Ardran G M 1976 Distension therapy for the unstable bladder: late results including an assessment of repeat distensions. Journal of Urology 48: 623–629
Rew D A, Rundle J S H 1989 Assessment of the safety of regular DDAVP therapy in primary nocturnal enuresis. British Journal of Urology 63: 352–353
Rose D K 1931 Clinical application of bladder physiology. Journal of Urology 26: 91–105
Rosenbaum T P, Shah P J R, Worth P H L 1988 Transtrigonal phenol — the end of an era? Neurology and Urodynamics 7: 294–295
Sibley G N A 1985 An experimental model of detrusor instability in the obstructed pig. British Journal of Urology 57: 292–298
Speakman M J, Bradwing A F, Gilping C J, Dixon J S, Gilping S A, Gosling J A 1987 Bladder outflow obstruction — a cause of denervation supersensitivity. Journal of Urology 138: 1461–1466
Steel S A, Cox C, Stanton S L 1985 Long-term follow-up of detrusor instability following the colposuspension operation. British Journal of Urology 58: 138–142
Tapp A J S, Cardozo L D 1986 The postmenopausal bladder. British Journal of Hospital Medicine 35: 20–23
Tapp A J S, Fall M, Massey A et al 1987 A dose titrated multicentre study of terodiline in the treatment of detrusor instability. Neurology and Urodynamics 6: 254–255
Torrens M J, Griffiths H B 1974 The control of the uninhibited bladder by selective sacral neurectomy. British Journal of Urology 46: 639–644
Turner-Warwick R T 1975 Some clinical aspects of detrusor dysfunction. Journal of Urology 113: 539–544
Ulmsten U, Ekman G, Anderson K E 1985 The effect of terodiline treatment in women with motor urge incontinence. American Journal of Obstetrics and Gynecology 193: 619–622
Versi E, Cardozo L D 1988 Oestrogens and lower urinary tract function. In: Studd J W W, Whitehead M (eds) The menopause. Blackwell Scientific Publications Oxford, pp 76–84
Warrell D W 1977 Vaginal denervation of the bladder nerve supply. Urology International 32: 114–116
Wein A J 1986 Pharmacology of the bladder and urethra. In: Stanton S L, Tanagho E (eds) Surgery of female incontinence, 2nd edn. Springer-Verlag, Heidelberg, pp 229–250
Whiteside C G, Arnold G P 1975 Persistent primary enuresis: a urodynamical assessment. British Medical Journal 1: 364–369

49. Voiding difficulties

S. L. Stanton

INTRODUCTION

Voiding disorders in the female are important: they are frequently underdiagnosed and often badly managed. In the male, high bladder pressures lead to back pressure effects on the kidney with the development of hydronephrosis. Fortunately these rarely occur in the female; none the less she may be left with disturbing symptoms of difficulty in bladder emptying, recurrent urinary tract infections and a chronically overdistended bladder.

There is a spectrum of disease. Voiding disorders can be asymptomatic or may commence with symptoms of poor stream, hesitancy, incomplete emptying and straining to void. This may lead to chronic retention, or chronic retention can develop de novo. Acute retention can also occur de novo, and may either resolve or lead to chronic retention.

DEFINITIONS

Voiding disorders in the female are rarely defined in textbooks of either urology or gynaecology and have not yet been included in the standardization of terminology of lower urinary tract function, published by the International Continence Society (Appendix II). I would suggest the following working definitions:

1. *Acute retention* — the sudden onset of painful or painless inability to void over 12 h, requiring catheterization with removal of a volume equal to or greater than normal bladder capacity. Acute retention is usually painful but in the presence of a neurological lesion or following an epidural anaesthetic it may be painless. It seems reasonable to set a time limit and to state that it needs catheterization as this should provide confirmation of retention. Finally the volume should be at least equal to normal bladder capacity; sometimes the patient is catheterized unnecessarily and a volume very much less than bladder capacity is removed. That patient may be falsely labelled as having acute retention.
2. *Chronic retention* — insidious and painless failure of bladder emptying where catheterization yields a volume equal to at least 50% of normal bladder capacity. This can include the presence of residual urine after bladder neck surgery. Otherwise the cause of chronic retention is often obscure.

PATHOPHYSIOLOGY

Voiding in the female can occur by one of three mechanisms. These are a detrusor contraction, an increase in abdominal pressure generated by abdominal wall muscles and diaphragm, or relaxation of the pelvic floor and urethral sphincter mechanism. Voiding disorders therefore result when these mechanisms fail, i.e. when the detrusor is unable to contract or maintain an effective contraction, when the urethral sphincter mechanism fails to relax or when there is a combination of both. In suprasacral neurological lesions there is synchronous failure of detrusor contraction and urethral sphincter relaxation (detrusor sphincter dyssynergia), resulting in voiding disorder.

Acute and chronic retention can occur following a variety of causes. Acute retention may be recognized as a well defined entity, but chronic retention may be less readily recognized.

AETIOLOGY

Voiding disorders and urinary retention may be classified in the following way.

Neurological

Three main levels of neurological lesion are recognized: above the pons (suprapontine lesions), between the pons and parasympathetic outflow (cord lesions) and distal to the sacral parasympathetic outflow (peripheral lesions). All can produce voiding disorders. Suprapontine disorders (e.g. cerebrovascular accidents and Parkinson's disease) will cause voiding disorder but detrusor sphincter dyssynergia does not occur. Cord lesions (e.g. spinal cord injury or multiple sclerosis) frequently cause voiding difficulties and retention is present in the early phases of spinal cord injury. About 25% of multiple sclerosis patients will present with acute retention. Detrusor sphincter dyssynergia will occur in this group. Peripheral lesions (e.g. prolapsed intervertebral disc, diabetic autonomic neuropathy and other peripheral autonomic neuropathies) cause acontractile failure of the detrusor.

Painful conditions of the vulva and perineum (e.g. following posterior repair or with prolapsed haemorrhoids) will reflexly inhibit micturition.

Pharmacological

Epidural anaesthesia (especially in labour) and certain drugs, e.g. tricyclic antidepressants, anticholinergic agents, alpha-adrenergic stimulants and ganglion-blocking drugs, may all predispose to voiding disorder. The epidural in labour is the most commonly encountered pharmacological cause. Following delivery under epidural, nursing or medical staff fail to enquire about voiding and painless retention develops. In neglected cases, up to 4 litres of urine can be withdrawn. This produces a grossly overdistended bladder which may fail to function and leave the patient with retention for up to 3 months or more. Some patients will have permanent voiding disorders.

Inflammatory

Painful inflammatory lesions around the anogenital region such as genital herpes, acute vulvovaginitis, urethritis or cystitis can all precipitate acute retention of urine.

Obstructive

Postoperative urethral oedema (e.g. following anterior colporrhaphy) frequently causes voiding difficulties and up to 50% of patients fail to void spontaneously on the day following bladder neck surgery, hence conventional use of either a urethral or suprapubic catheter. As most operations for continence will produce some urethral obstruction, it is a sensible prophylaxis to catheterize patients at operation until they are able to void spontaneously.

Other causes of obstruction include an impacted pelvic mass (e.g. retroverted gravid uterus, uterine fibroids or an ovarian cyst), foreign bodies in the urethra, an ectopic ureterocele, and a bladder polyp or a carcinoma occluding the internal urethral meatus. Rarely, urethral distortion associated with a cystocele causes retention.

Bladder overdistension

Overdistension after failure to catheterize for retention develops insidiously, is much more common in the female than in the male and is difficult to treat effectively. Denervation, ischaemia of the detrusor muscle fibres and distraction of the detrusor syncytium are likely sequelae of overdistension and responsible for the continuation of voiding difficulty.

Psychogenic

This group should only be diagnosed after the above organic conditions can be excluded.

INCIDENCE

In a population attending a urodynamic clinic for a wide variety of gynaecological urology disorders, up to 2% may have asymptomatic voiding difficulty and up to 25% may have symptomatic proven voiding difficulty.

PRESENTATION

Voiding disorders are associated with symptoms of poor flow, intermittent stream, incomplete emptying, straining to void and hesitancy. Hilton & Laor (1989) reviewed these symptoms and compared them with urodynamic findings in a group of women attending a urodynamic clinic. Symptoms of poor urinary stream or intermittent stream correlated best with urodynamic evidence of voiding difficulty. When acute retention has developed, the patient has not voided and may be in pain. Chronic retention presents with frequency and then overflow incontinence. All of these may be associated with symptoms of a primary cause. Urine infection may occur with the residual urine, and these symptoms will be present as well.

Clinical examination will disclose a palpable bladder and there may be signs of the primary cause. A neurological examination should be carried out, including inspection of the back for stigmata of underlying neurological lesion, e.g. spina bifida occulta.

INVESTIGATION

Urine culture and sensitivity

A midstream sample of urine should be sent for analysis on all patients with voiding difficulty, as urinary infection may occasionally produce acute retention and infection is often a sequel to incomplete bladder emptying.

Urinary diary

An accurate record of fluid intake and output is important and a urinary diary can be easily maintained by the patient. When catheterization is carried out for acute retention, it is essential to note the amount of urine removed. Not only does this confirm acute retention but it may give some guide as to the severity of bladder distension and therefore a prognosis as to when spontaneous voiding may resume.

Uroflowmetry

Measurement of free urine flow rate is a good guide to voiding function. Flow rates consistently below 15 ml/s for a volume of >150 ml indicate impaired voiding and this may be a precursor of retention. However a flow rate of >15 ml/s may still be associated with voiding disorder if accompanied by a high maximum voiding pressure. The shape of the curve is also important. Compare the normal bell-shape cone (Fig. 49.1) with the attenuated and intermittent flow rate of the patient with voiding difficulty (Fig. 49.2).

Cystometry

The combination of uroflowmetry and cystometry provides the best information about bladder function. Both the filling and voiding phases will help establish whether there is

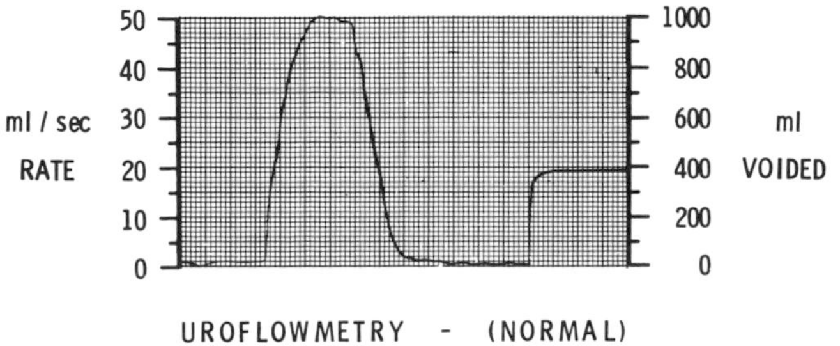

Fig. 49.1 Normal flow rate.

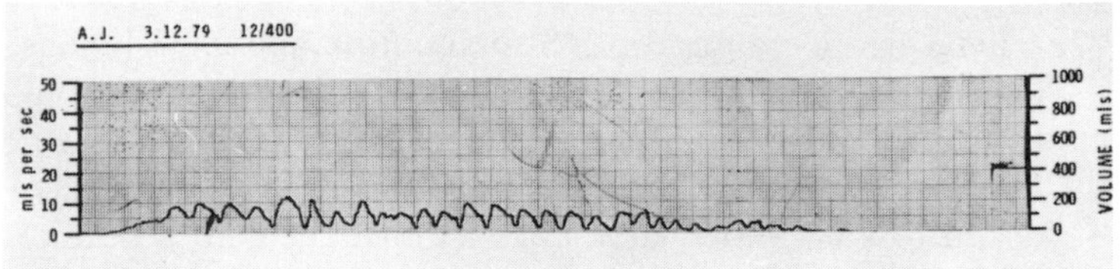

Fig. 49.2 Flow rate showing voiding difficulty with an attenuated flow, not exceeding 15 ml/s.

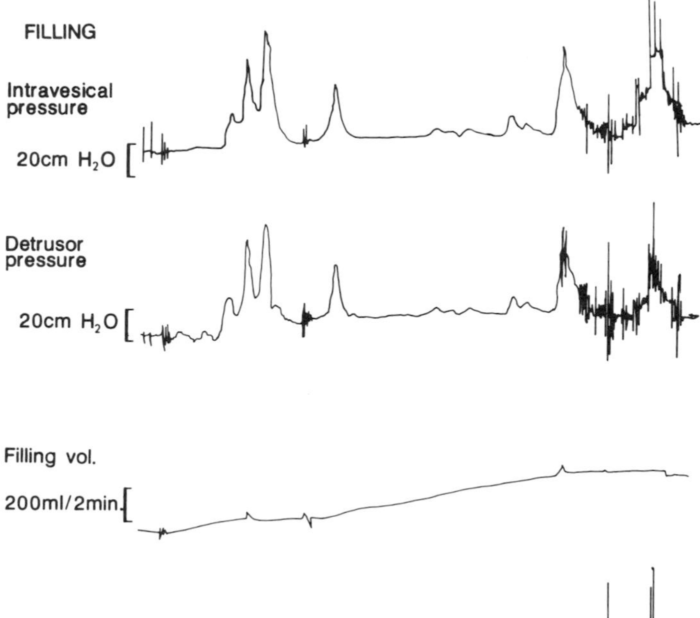

Fig. 49.3 Cystometry showing systolic detrusor contractions.

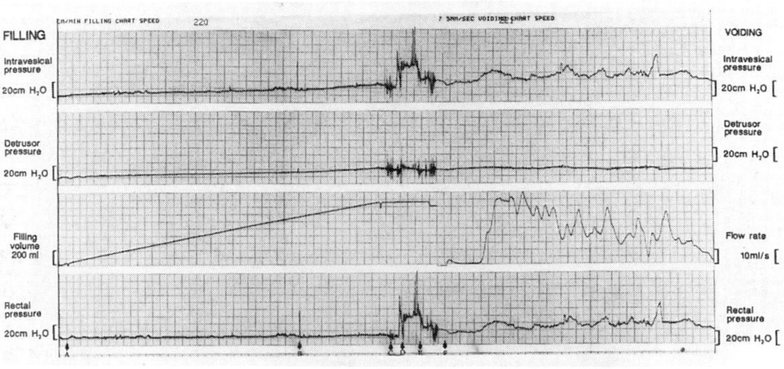

Fig. 49.4 Cystometry showing a peripheral (lower motor neurone) lesion with a residual urine, delayed desire to void and a large-capacity bladder. A = start; B = first desire to void; C = stop filling; D = stand; E = cough; F = start to void.

a neuropathic component. Suprapontine and cord lesions above S2, 3 and 4 may show systolic (phasic) detrusor contractions and a reduced bladder capacity (Fig. 49.3). Peripheral lesions of the cord will show residual urine, late desire to void and a large-capacity bladder with a normal pressure rise (Fig. 49.4). Both may show an inability to produce a voluntary and sustained detrusor contraction.

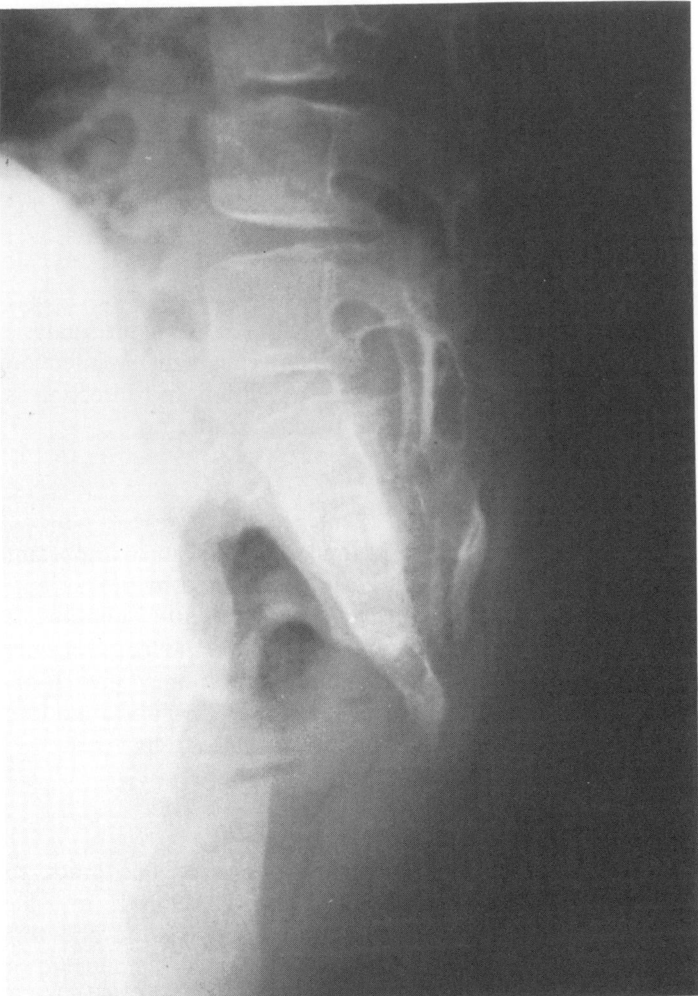

Fig. 49.6 Lumbosacral spine X-ray showing sacral agenesis.

Radiology

A plain abdominal X-ray will disclose a large residual urine (Fig. 49.5). A lumbosacral spine X-ray is important to exclude congenital (e.g. sacral agenesis; Fig. 49.6) or acquired (prolapsed intervertebral disc) lesions. Both will produce a peripheral neurological disorder.

Intravenous urography is less useful than it was before as ultrasound now produces comparable information on back pressure effects on the ureter and kidney.

Videocystourethrography (the combination of cystometry, uroflowmetry and radiological screening during bladder filling and voiding, recorded with sound on a video tape) provides a comprehensive study of bladder function, but whether this is necessary in all cases of voiding difficulty is debatable. In addition to the information provided by cystometry, it will also show abnormal bladder morphology secondary to voiding difficulty, e.g. sacculation and diverticulum formation, and the presence of vesicoureteric reflux (Fig. 49.7).

Ultrasonography

Abdominal ultrasound scanning will provide an estimate of residual urine to within 20%, which is sufficiently ac-

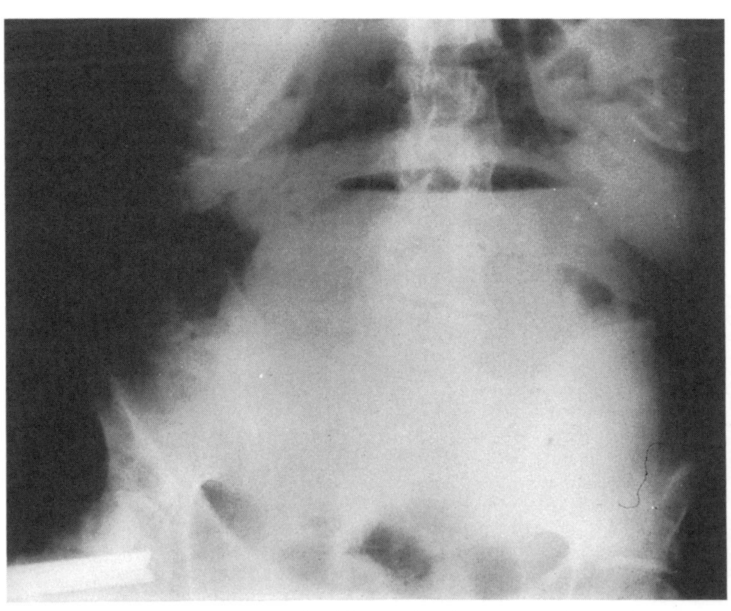

Fig. 49.5 Plain abdominal X-ray showing large residual urine.

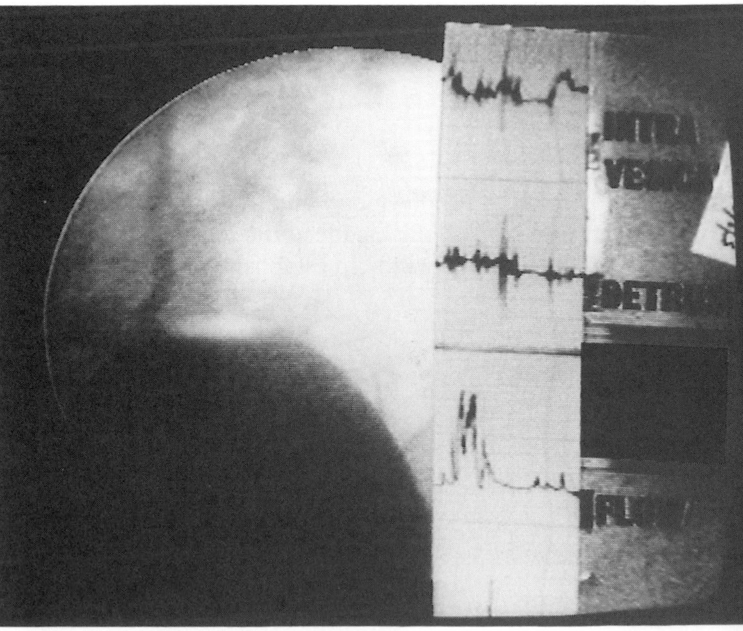

Fig. 49.7 Videocystourethrogram image showing vesicoureteric reflux.

curate. Intravesical lesions such as an ectopic ureterocele can be demonstrated.

Cystourethroscopy

Difficulty in instrumentation of the urethra will show if there is significant urethral narrowing (e.g. distal urethral stenosis). Cystoscopy demonstrates whether there is any intravesical pathology and whether or not trabeculation, sacculation and diverticulum formation have occurred. These indicate long-standing obstruction but not its cause.

Electrophysiological tests

Concentric or single-fibre electromyography of the pelvic floor and urethral sphincter mechanism with terminal motor latency studies of the perineal branch of the pudendal nerve will indicate whether denervation or nerve damage to these structures has occurred.

TREATMENT

Principles of therapy

Both the primary condition and its effects on the bladder may need treatment and in the case of acute retention, these may be simultaneous.

Catheterization is either urethral or suprapubic: urethral is quickest and simplest. The disadvantages are that this is an uncomfortable method of catheterization. If maintained for longer than 24 h, it is associated with a higher incidence of urinary tract infection than a suprapubic catheter and it is impossible to see whether a patient can resume spontaneous voiding with a urethral catheter in place. However it is ideal for short-term catheterization.

Clean intermittent self-catheterization is a clean (and not sterile) technique to enable the patient (or her partner) to catheterize herself intermittently for the management of chronic urinary retention. The catheters are disposable and are changed once a week (Fig. 49.8). A suprapubic catheter is ideal if the catheter is required for more than 24–48 h. Its main use is following pelvic and especially bladder neck surgery. Its disadvantages include the requirement of a doctor for its insertion; caution must be taken during insertion to avoid bowel injury.

Drugs may be used either to treat symptoms of voiding difficulty or as an adjunct to catheterization; they are often ineffective. They may either relax the sphincter mechanism or stimulate the detrusor to contract.

Alpha adrenergic blocking agents (phenoxybenzamine 10 mg (b.d.) are non-selective alpha-blocking agents, with the unwanted side-effects of tachycardia and fainting due to alpha$_2$ stimulation. Prazosin (0.5–3 mg daily in divided doses) and indoramin (50–200 mg daily in divided doses) are selective alpha$_1$-blocking agents. Baclofen (5 mg t.d.s.–25 mg q.d.s.) is a striated muscle relaxant used to treat spasticity and diazepam (10–15 mg nocte) acts centrally as a muscle relaxant and has an anxiolytic effect; both may be used for sphincteric relaxation.

Muscarinic agents (e.g. bethanechol chloride 20–100 mg q.d.s.) should be used with caution in the elderly, in asthmatic patients and those with cardiovascular disease or parkinsonism. Anticholinesterase agents such as distigmine bromide (5 mg/day) have been tried but have little proven effect. The E_2 and $F_{2\alpha}$ prostaglandins will cause detrusor contractions in vitro, but have an inconsistent effect when administered intravesically to patients in retention.

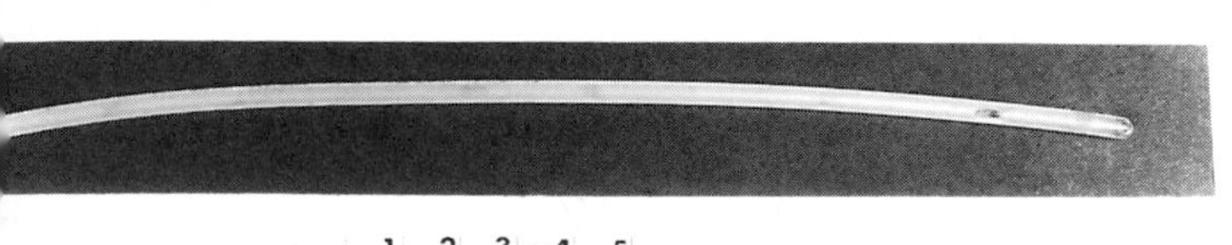

Fig. 49.8 Disposable female self-catheter.

Prophylaxis

It is a simple and wise precaution to measure the free urine flow rate in any patient who is to have continence surgery; most of these procedures are obstructive and any predisposition to a voiding difficulty will result in retention.

Asymptomatic voiding difficulty

These patients need supervision to avoid urinary tract infection. Upper tract dilatation rarely occurs in the female unless associated with a neuropathy.

Symptoms only

Patients with only symptoms of voiding difficulty may be treated with alpha adrenergic blocking agents in the dosages detailed above. Lying and standing blood pressures and an electrocardiogram should be taken beforehand. The dosage will often be limited by the side-effects of hypotension.

Retention

Acute retention

Where the cause is likely to recur, simply relieving retention and then removing the catheter is likely to lead to retention again. Equally, if the amount withdrawn is greater than 1 litre, the bladder is unlikely to recover immediately. In these situations it is sensible to use a suprapubic catheter and this will ensure that spontaneous voiding can be easily re-established.

When there is not an obvious cause and an amount of less than 1 litre is removed, a Foley catheter can be left in place for 24–48 hours.

Chronic retention

This includes conditions without an obvious cause as well as postoperative and postpartum retention.

Postoperative and postpartum retention are best managed by a suprapubic catheter or the use of clean intermittent self-catheterization. For the latter, the patient should be manually dexterous and able to carry out self-catheterization 3–4 times a day, depending on the amounts of urine removed. Most patients develop a subclinical urinary tract infection and antibiotics are only required if symptoms of urinary infection are present.

For some causes of chronic retention, an Otis urethrotomy may be helpful.

A suprapubic catheter can remain in place for many months and is ideal for the patient who is not manually dexterous. Once the patient is voiding amounts of greater than 150–200 ml and the evening and early morning residual urines are less than 200 ml the catheter can be removed.

Some conditions (e.g. distal urethral stenosis) will benefit from an Otis urethrotomy. The epithelium and submucosa of the urethra is cut in three longitudinal incisions at 4, 7 and 12 o'clock and a large Foley catheter (26 French gauge) is left in place for 5–7 days.

CONCLUSION

Voiding difficulties form a spectrum of disorders ranging from symptoms only to established retention. Often these are poorly recognized and inadequately treated. Prevention, early diagnosis and treatment with catheterization, where indicated, are key points.

KEY POINTS

1. Voiding disorders may be asymptomatic and occasionally lead to upper tract dilatation.
2. Normal voiding in the female occurs by detrusor contraction or pelvic floor relaxation or abdominal straining. Failure or incoordination of the first two may lead to voiding difficulty.
3. The epidural in labour is a potent cause of undiagnosed urinary retention and subsequent voiding difficulty.
4. Symptoms of poor urinary stream or intermittent stream are the best markers of voiding difficulty.
5. Uroflowmetry is the simplest screening test: when combined with cystometry this will be sufficient to diagnose most voiding disorders.
6. Treatment is directed towards bladder emptying and management of the primary cause.
7. Drug therapy has little proven clinical effect.

REFERENCE

Hilton P, Laor D 1989 Voiding symptoms in the female: the correlation with urodynamic voiding characteristics. Neurourology and Urodynamics 8: 308–310

FURTHER READING

Hilton P 1990 Bladder drainage. In: Stanton S L (ed) Clinical uro-gynaecology, 2nd edn. Churchill Livingstone, London

Shaw P J R 1992 Voiding difficulties and retention. In: Stanton S L (ed) Clinical uro-gynaecology, 2nd edn. Churchill Livingstone, Edinburgh (in press)

Snooks S J, Swash M 1984 Abnormalities of the innervation of the urethral striated musculature in incontinence. British Journal of Urology 56: 401–405

Stanton S L, Ozsoy C, Hilton P 1983 Voiding difficulties in the female: prevalence, clinical and urodynamic review. Obstetrics and Gynecology 61: 144–147

Worth P 1986 Urethrotomy. In: Stanton S L, Tanagho. (eds) Surgery of female incontinence, 2nd edn. Springer-Verlag, Heidelberg

50. Neuropathic bladder

A. R. Mundy

INTRODUCTION

Compared with stress incontinence, detrusor instability, dysfunctional voiding and other non-neuropathic continence problems in women, the neuropathic bladder is not very common. It is none the less a fairly common problem and an almost inevitable consequence of certain spinal cord problems, notably spina bifida, multiple sclerosis and spinal cord injury. It is rare for patients with these problems not to suffer bladder dysfunction. Indeed in multiple sclerosis and other spastic paraplegias, urinary incontinence is the main cause for admission to hospital (Miller et al 1965), and in spina bifida and spinal cord injury, urinary tract-related problems are the commonest causes of death after the initial neurological/neurosurgical problem has stabilized (Bors & Comarr 1971).

The term 'neuropathic bladder' is in fact misleading because in the vast majority of patients with neurological disease and bladder dysfunction there is simultaneous urethral dysfunction which may be pathophysiologically more important than the bladder abnormality (Mundy et al 1985). Thus the commonest cause of long-term morbidity and mortality in spinal cord lesions is bladder outflow obstruction due to urethral sphincteric obstruction. In neurological disease one should always expect there to be both bladder and urethral dysfunction and it is this factor more than anything else that distinguishes neuropathic from non-neuropathic lower urinary tract problems. This is not to say that detrusor instability or simple stress incontinence does not have a neurological component as an aetiological factor; indeed this may well be the case. The importance in distinguishing between the bladder and urethral dysfunction seen in neurological disease from that seen in the absence of overt neuropathy is that in the absence of overt neuropathy bladder outflow obstruction, poor bladder compliance (see below) and secondary obstructive nephropathy are extremely rare whereas in neuropathic abnormalities, particularly in spina bifida and spinal cord injury, they are common and must be looked for in every patient. This factor together with the almost universal existence of dual bladder and urethral pathology in neuropathy, as distinct from the usual single pathology in non-neuropathic problems, are the two important reasons for distinguishing between these two types of lower urinary tract dysfunction.

It is always important to remember that patients with neuropathic lower urinary tract dysfunction commonly have other problems as well. Abnormalities of bowel function, neurological problems affecting the lower limbs and sexual dysfunction are all common. Sexual dysfunction in female patients is unlikely to be a major concern, either to the patient or to her medical attendants, but in men it is likely to be a particular concern. Bowel and lower limb abnormalities are not only important in their own right but because they also affect the approach to management. Many patients with neuropathic lower urinary tract dysfunction therefore require attention not only to their lower urinary tract but also to other organ systems — there is thus considerable 'horizontal' care. There is also considerable 'longitudinal' care as most patients require long-term follow-up.

Until recently, the management of lower urinary tract dysfunction in neurological disease received little attention, partly because diagnostic ability was limited and partly because there was little to be offered in the way of treatment.

This has changed in recent years for several reasons. Firstly urodynamic investigation has given far greater diagnostic accuracy and this in turn has lead to improved understanding of pathophysiology and improved application of available treatment modalities. Secondly, there has been the development of alternatives to the three traditional conservative methods of treatment — external appliances (in men); long-term urethral catheterization and ileal conduit urinary diversion. The most important recent development in this respect has been clean intermittent self-catheterization (CISC; Lapides et al 1972). There has also been an improvement in the anti-cholinergic drugs available for the treatment of detrusor overactivity. Finally there has been the development of specific surgical treatment modalities such as cystoplasty (Mundy 1988) and artificial sphincter implantation (Mundy 1986a) for the specific treatment of certain urodynamic abnormalities. Finally there has been the development of undiversion for the salvage and corrective treatment of patients previously palliated by ileal conduit urinary diversion (Mundy 1987).

It is possible these days to correct almost all types of neuropathic lower urinary tract dysfunction by surgical or non-surgical means. The question now arises not how to treat a specific pattern of lower urinary tract abnormalities but in whom these therapeutic modalities should be used. This is because not all patients warrant surgical intervention on the sort of scale that might be necessary. Thus whereas one would have no doubt as to the advisability of performing cystoplasty and artificial sphincter implantation, for example, in a patient whose only abnormality is lower urinary tract dysfunction, one might — indeed should — have serious doubts about performing the same procedure in a youngster with hydrocephalus, gross kyphoscoliosis and a complete paraplegia who has a low IQ, leads a wheelchair existence and is entirely dependent upon others for her care.

PATHOPHYSIOLOGY

Outline of normal lower urinary tract function

(For more detailed reviews and specific references to individual points mentioned here the reader is referred to Gosling et al (1983) and Gosling & Chilton (1984) for a discussion of the anatomical issues, and to Mundy (1984) and Torrens & Morrison (1987) for the physiological issues.)

The bladder fills at a rate of about 1–2 ml/min from the ureters. At first there is no sensation of bladder filling. When about 150–200 ml has entered the bladder, the subject will normally be aware of a full bladder if she thinks about it but not otherwise. As bladder filling progresses, the sensation of fullness impedes more and more upon consciousness until finally, when about 500 ml is in the bladder, the subject is constantly aware of it and will usually wish to empty her bladder. If however this is not convenient, she can hold the urine until it is convenient to void. If bladder filling reaches 600 ml or more, the desire to void will be urgent.

During this filling phase there is little or no rise in intravesical pressure. This is because the bladder is readily distensible (it is said to have normal compliance) and because detrusor contraction does not occur. Throughout bladder filling there is a rise in urethral resistance and the bladder neck above the urethral sphincter mechanism remains closed. When the subject decides that she wishes to empty her bladder she goes to an appropriate place and then, under voluntary control, urethral relaxation occurs, and this is rapidly followed by detrusor contraction and bladder neck opening. The detrusor contraction is of a sufficient amplitude and duration to empty the bladder completely, at which time the detrusor contraction will have dissipated, the bladder neck will close and urethral resistance will return to normal.

The anatomical basis for this sequence of events lies in the distinction between three separate zones of the lower urinary tract — the bladder, the bladder neck and the sphincter-active urethra, which in females includes all of the urethra below bladder neck level. The detrusor layer of the bladder consists of a relatively large amount of detrusor smooth muscle embedded in a relatively small amount of connective tissue. The muscle bundles themselves are large. There is no specific muscle fibre or muscle bundle orientation. The detrusor layer as a whole, all the way down to the bladder neck, is homogeneous and should be considered as a single functioning unit.

At bladder neck level the muscle bundles become much smaller. There is a considerable relative increase in the amount of connective tissue around the muscle bundles and the orientation of muscle bundles becomes more or less longitudinal. There is no anatomically definable sphincter mechanism in the region of the bladder neck although urodynamically the bladder neck behaves as a sphincter in that it does not open except when the detrusor contracts.

This longitudinally oriented smooth muscle pattern continues down the urethra until it becomes dissipated in the region of the external meatus. In the lower half of the urethra there is, in addition, a collar of striated muscle surrounding the smooth muscle component which is maximal anteriorly and relatively deficient posteriorly. This striated muscle collar within the wall of the urethra consists of small-diameter muscle bundles consisting, in turn, of small-diameter fibres which show several other factors that distinguish them from typical striated muscle fibres. Physiologically they are characterized as slow-twitch fibres which are capable of maintaining their tone for a long time and are therefore well suited to a sphincteric role. This intramural striated muscle component is commonly referred to as the intrinsic rhabdosphincter. Thus in the mid to lower urethra there is an internal smooth muscle component surrounded by a collar — the intrinsic rhabdosphincter — of striated muscle, both within the urethral wall. There is in addition an effect on the urethra from the sling muscles of the levator ani. These are fairly remote from the urethra anatomically but by their contraction they tend to elevate the whole of the pelvic viscera upwards and anteriorly toward the pubic symphysis; the part of levator ani most closely related to the urethra is considered to be a third component of the urethral sphincter mechanism. There are therefore two sphincter mechanisms — the bladder neck or proximal sphincter mechanism, and the urethral or distal sphincter mechanism which has three components, of which the most important appears to be the intrinsic rhabdosphincter.

Physiologically, the detrusor is a phasic smooth muscle; it spends most of its time relaxed but on stimulation will contract in a co-ordinated fashion to produce bladder emptying. The smooth muscle of the bladder neck and urethra is tonic by contrast and exerts a sustained contractile force which if anything is relaxed by neural activity. The intrinsic rhabdosphincter, as has already been mentioned, is specifically designed for sustained tonic activity.

The motor innervation of the detrusor is predominantly excitatory. In human beings this excitatory innervation is exclusively parasympathetic and cholinergic but this is not the case in all animal species; in some animals there is a non-cholinergic excitatory nerve supply whose effect seems to be mediated by adenosine triphosphate. This is called purinergic innervation. There is, in addition, an inhibitory nerve supply to the bladder but this is poorly understood and thought to be mediated by neurotransmitters called neuropeptides, of which vasoactive intestinal polypeptide is the best known example. These neuropeptides do not seem to have their own nerves as such, but are released as co-transmitters from other nerve terminals. Thus vasoactive intestinal polypeptide is thought to be a co-transmitter in cholinergic nerve terminals where it acts to modulate the effects of released acetylcholine.

There is also a cholinergic innervation to the urethra but the physiology of this is poorly understood.

The cholinergic parasympathetic innervation of the bladder and urethra is derived from the pelvic plexuses and ultimately from cell bodies in the intermediolateral grey column of the second, third and fourth sacral segments of the spinal cord.

There is also a sympathetic innervation to the lower urinary tract which, in the bladder, is almost exclusively to the blood vessels and to the extension of ureteric smooth muscle which constitutes the superficial trigone. There is no significant adrenergic innervation of the detrusor muscle proper. There is a more dense adrenergic innervation of the urethral smooth muscle which is predominantly alpha in type. Again this is poorly understood.

The innervation of the intrinsic rhabdosphincter is from a particular group of anterior horn cells that constitute what is known as Onuf's nucleus which also innervates the anal sphincter mechanism. Thus the muscle fibres that constitute the intrinsic rhabdosphincter are different from normal striated muscle, as is the innervation. The nerve fibres to the intrinsic rhabdosphincter run with the parasympathetic fibres through the pelvic plexuses to reach the urethra. The nerve fibres to levator ani, by contrast, are typical alpha motor neurones with typical cell bodies in the anterior horn which run in the pudendal nerve. Sensory nerves from both the lamina propria underneath the urothelium and from the muscle layer of the bladder and urethra run with the sympathetic and parasympathetic nerves to reach the spinal cord.

Although there is some interaction between afferent and efferent fibres within the sacral spinal cord, the most and by far the most important interactions occur at the level of the pons. It is in the pons that afferent fibres registering bladder sensation subtend upon efferent fibres that initiate and co-ordinate detrusor contraction with urethral relaxation so that the two occur synchronously. It should be stressed that by far and the most important co-ordinating centre of lower urinary tract function is in the pons, not the sacral spinal cord.

There are various neurological areas that may affect the pontine micturition centre, as it is called, notably the hypothalamus, concerned with autonomic regulation in general; the septal and preoptic nuclei which correlate bladder function, bowel function and coitus and are also responsible for the associated activities that occur with voiding (more marked in lower animals such as the cat); and the frontal lobe areas responsible for the voluntary initiation of voiding. The most important area, however, is the pons because that is where detrusor contractions and urethral relaxation during voiding are initiated and where these two events are co-ordinated.

Outline of the pathophysiology of neuropathic lower urinary tract dysfunction

Almost everything outlined in the last section may be deranged in neuropathy. Bladder and urethral sensation may be deranged or absent. There may be a steady rise in pressure associated with bladder filling — poor compliance. There may be abnormal contractility, either overactivity — detrusor hyper-reflexia — or underactivity — detrusor areflexia. There may be abnormal urethral contractility producing either overactivity and obstruction or underactivity and sphincter weakness incontinence. Finally there may be loss of co-ordination between detrusor contractile and sphincteric relaxant activity. In theory then, any number of patterns of abnormal lower urinary tract function may be found but in practice there are only three — contractile, intermediate and acontractile (Rickwood et

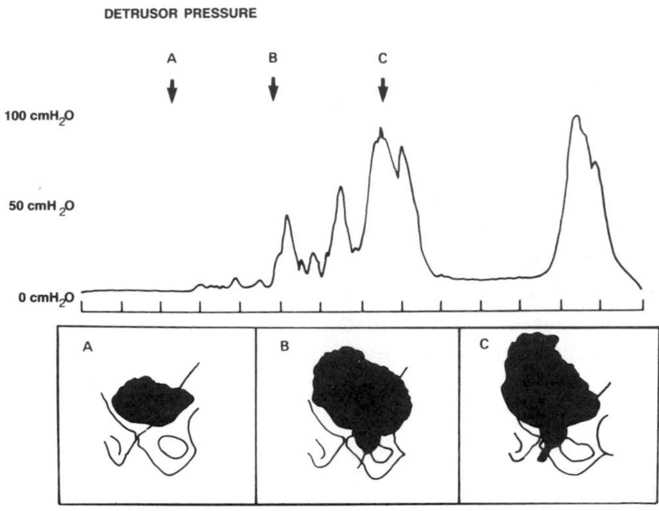

Fig. 50.1 Contractile dysfunction — videourodynamic features. (In this and Fig 50.2 and 50.3 only the detrusor pressure trace is shown.) Detrusor pressure trace shows high-amplitude swings in pressure (detrusor hyper-reflexia). Synchronous video micturating cystourethrogram shows (**A**) initial bladder neck competence and trabeculation (**B**) opening of the bladder neck with a detrusor contraction but (**C**) failure of opening of the distal sphincter mechanism due to detrusor sphincter dyssynergia (from Mundy 1986b).

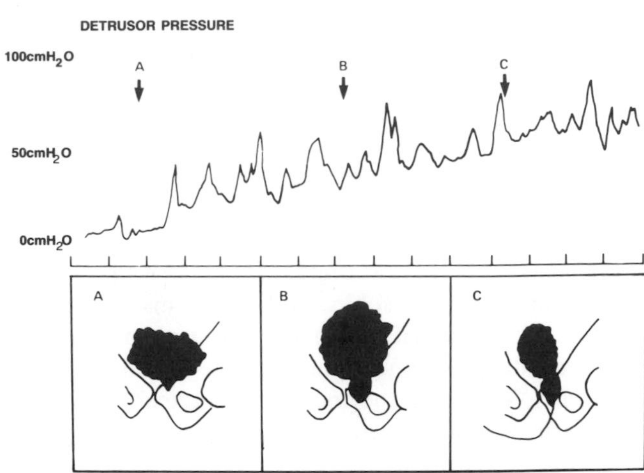

Fig. 50.2 Intermediate dysfunction. Detrusor pressure trace shows a steady rise in baseline pressure (low compliance) and constant detrusor activity of varying amplitude. However, as distinct from Figure 50.1 this activity is poorly sustained and therefore ineffective; it is sufficient to restrict filling but insufficient to produce voiding. Synchronous video-micturating shows (**A**) bladder neck incompetence which (**B**) gets progressively worse with sphincteric obstruction allowing filling of the urethra only when (**C**) intravesical pressure exceeds urethral resistance (from Mundy 1986b).

al 1982; Mundy et al, 1985; Mundy 1986b; Parry et al 1990).

In contractile bladder dysfunction (Fig. 50.1), detrusor contractile activity is retained although voluntary control of the contractile activity may be and commonly is lost. None the less, detrusor contractions when they occur are of sufficient amplitude and duration to give a useful degree of bladder emptying, assuming that any associated urethral obstruction (which is commonly present; see below) is eliminated. This is called detrusor hyper-reflexia. Between detrusor contractions, detrusor pressure returns to normal; in other words the detrusor relaxes normally and therefore baseline pressures with bladder filling are normal; there is normal compliance. When the detrusor is not contracting the bladder neck is often but by no means always competent. During bladder filling urethral sphincteric resistance rises as in normal subjects but at the onset of detrusor contraction there may be (but not always) a rise rather a fall in urethral resistance due to contraction of the intrinsic rhabdosphincter because of loss of detrusor–sphincter co-ordination. This is called detrusor–sphincter dyssynergia, and causes high-pressure bladder outflow obstruction and impaired emptying. This may be sufficient to cause large residual urine volumes, secondary vesicoureteric reflux and secondary obstructive changes in the upper urinary tract.

In the intermediate bladder (Fig. 50.2), contractile activity is retained in both the bladder and the urethra but this is no longer useful. Detrusor contractions tend to be of high frequency, short duration and relatively low amplitude so that bladder filling is restricted but useful bladder emptying does not occur. Detrusor pressure never returns to normal so that there is a constant rise in bladder pressure during filling; there is poor compliance. Bladder neck incompetence is the rule at normal bladder volumes, and because the urethra behaves like the bladder there is no true relaxation. Therefore sphincteric obstruction is present and may cause similar changes proximally to those seen in detrusor–sphincter dyssynergia. On the other hand, because urethral sphincteric resistance fluctuates around a rather fixed level, unlike the surges of pressure seen in detrusor–sphincter dyssynergia, sphincter weakness incontinence may occur when detrusor or perivesical pressure rises above the level of the urethral resistance. Thus the sphincter may be both obstructive, causing residual urine, and incompetent, allowing sphincter weakness incontinence to occur. It is important to understand this apparent paradox of obstruction on the one hand, causing residual urine and potential upper tract problems, and sphincteric incompetence on the other hand, causing sphincter weakness incontinence.

In the acontractile bladder (Figure 50.3) there is no detrusor activity, bladder pressure never rises, no detrusor contractions occur, the bladder neck is always incompetent and sphincter weakness incontinence occurs because of similar changes in urethral physiology. There is, however, a degree of intrinsic tone to the urethra which may cause residual urine. Thus the pattern of sphincter behaviour is similar to the intermediate type; however, in the intermediate type the obstructive effect is more important than

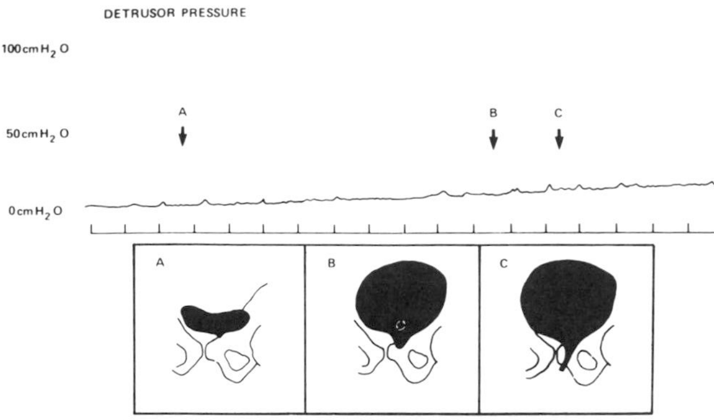

Fig. 50.3 Acontractile dysfunction. Detrusor pressure trace shows no evidence of detrusor contractility. Synchronous video-micturating cystourethrogram shows bladder neck incompetence with (**A**) early 'beaking' of the bladder neck, which becomes marked (**B**) with filling. On coughing or attempted voiding by straining, sphincter weakness incontinence occurs (**C**) but the urethra in the region of the distal sphincter mechanism fails to open adequately because of static distal sphincter obstruction (from Mundy (1986b).

the sphincter weakness effect whereas in the acontractile type the sphincter weakness effect usually predominates. The important distinction between intermediate and acontractile types is that bladder pressures are low in the acontractile type so upper tract changes do not occur, whereas they commonly occur in the intermediate type because of elevated intravesical pressure.

Patterns of bladder behaviour according to level of neurological lesion

Above the level of the efferent outflow from the sacral spinal cord the lower urinary tract will have contractile activity of either contractile or intermediate types. Distal to the cord the lower urinary tract will be acontractile. Between the sacral parasympathetic outflow and the pons, detrusor–sphincter co-ordination may be disturbed; above the level of the pons it will not. Thus three main levels of neurological lesion can be defined: above the pons (suprapontine lesions), between the pons and the parasympathetic outflow (cord lesions) and distal to the sacral parasympathetic outflow (peripheral lesions).

The commonest causes of suprapontine lesions are cerebrovascular accidents, Parkinson's disease and some instances of multiple sclerosis. The commonest causes of cord lesions are spina bifida, spinal cord injury and most cases of multiple sclerosis. The commonest causes of peripheral lesions are diabetes and trauma, although the majority of instances of peripheral autonomic neuropathy are idiopathic.

Suprapontine lesions cause contractile dysfunction without detrusor sphincter dyssynergia because they are above the level of the co-ordinating centre of the pons. Cord lesions may cause contractile, intermediate or acontractile dysfunction. Because these lesions are below the level of the pontine co-ordinating centre, contractile dysfunction may be associated with detrusor–sphincter dyssynergia. Peripheral lesions cause acontractile dysfunction.

In cord lesions, contractile dysfunction is usually seen in localized, discrete and high lesions whereas intermediate dysfunction is usually found in extensive, diffuse thoracolumbar lesions. Discrete lesions causing contractile dysfunction may be complete or incomplete. The pattern of complete lesions has already been described — detrusor hyper-reflexia, loss of sensation, normal compliance, bladder neck incompetence (usually) and detrusor sphincter dyssynergia. In incomplete lesions, bladder neck function and sensation may be preserved and there may be control of pelvic floor function if the spinal cord pathway responsible for the innervation of levator ani is preserved. For these reasons the patient may be aware of lower urinary tract function because of preserved sensation, and therefore have the symptoms of urge incontinence rather than insensible or total incontinence; because of preservation of pelvic floor function, she may be able to resist the urge incontinence to a degree. This may mean she has frequency and urgency rather than frank incontinence. This situation does occur but is not common in spina bifida and spinal cord injury and generally correlates with well preserved lower limb function; it is common in multiple sclerosis.

Secondary effects on the upper urinary tract

The three serious factors in neuropathic lower urinary tract dysfunction are the detrusor–sphincter dyssynergia and consequent high-pressure outflow obstruction seen in the contractile group, and the sphincteric obstruction and poor compliance causing persistently elevated intravesical pressures seen in the intermediate group. All three may cause obstructive effects on the upper urinary tract which may be compounded by the presence of vesicoureteric reflux and recurrent urinary tract infection. Occasionally the bladder is so thick-walled that it nips the intramural ureters causing vesicoureteric junction obstruction. There are therefore four causes of hydroureteronephrosis and consequently of impaired renal function in neuropathic dysfunction — bladder outflow obstruction, high intravesical pressures associated with poor compliance, vesicoureteric reflux and vesicoureteric junction obstruction.

ASSESSMENT OF PATIENTS WITH NEUROPATHY

Physical examination of patients with neuropathic dysfunction is important more from a general and neurological than from a urological point of view. It is rare to find a urological abnormality other than a distended bladder. A description of neurological assessment is beyond the scope of this chapter but it is worth mentioning the cardinal signs of sacral nerve function. These are perianal sensation, anal sphincter tone and the response of the anal sphincter to cutaneous stimulation alongside the anal margin. In general it may be said that if there is anal sensation there will be urethral and bladder sensation, and if anal tone and the anocutaneous reflex are preserved then bladder contractile activity will be preserved with a high likelihood of urethral sphincteric obstruction. The negative correlation of absent sensation, a patulous anus and absent anocutaneous reflex with an acontractile detrusor and sphincter weakness incontinence is not so good.

The best screening investigation for the urinary tract as a whole is an intravenous urogram. A good-quality ultrasound scan is perfectly adequate for follow-up. The other general screening investigations are midstream urine specimen to look for urinary infection and an ultrasound scan of the bladder to assess bladder emptying. If the upper urinary tracts are distended, a serum creatinine study will show the presence of significant impairment of renal function and if this is significant, a Cr^{51} ethylenediaminetetraacetic acid-estimated glomerular filtration rate should be ordered. A ^{99m}Tc diethylenetriamine pentoacetic acid renal scan will distinguish between obstructed and non-obstructed ureters and can be adapted to show the presence of vesicoureteric reflux without the need for a micturating cystogram (see below). If there is significant reflux nephropathy a ^{99m}Tc dimercaptosuccinate scan will show differential renal function and differential loss of function within each individual renal unit.

For a definitive urodynamic diagnosis of the type of lower urinary tract dysfunction a videourodynamic study will be required. If specific treatment is not to be instigated, whether at that time or ever, then a micturating cystogram to look for reflux (if upper urinary tract dilatation is present on ultrasound) is all that is required although, as mentioned, a DTPA scan can be modified to show reflux if required. If a videourodynamic study is to be performed then there is no need for this modified DTPA scan.

The patterns of urodynamic dysfunction have been described in detail above and will not be reiterated here. Suffice it to say that assessment has two roles: firstly to look for those with evidence of impaired renal function or at risk of deterioration of renal function and secondly — and only secondly — to make a definitive urodynamic diagnosis for the purposes of treating incontinence.

Associated problems

Several other factors common in neurological problems should be enquired about or looked for. The patient's intelligence should be noted, bearing in mind that intelligence and motivation — much the more important factor with respect to treatment — do not necessarily correlate. Many individuals, particularly those with hydrocephalus in association with spina bifida, may appear intelligent and articulate but lack sustained interest, motivation and concentration. All of these may be important to sustain the individual through protracted periods of intense medical care, particularly when surgery is required.

It is important to decide whether the patient has a static or a progressive neurological lesion, particularly if progression is liable to lead to loss of the patient's to care for herself, loss of mobility, or loss of manipulative skills. Mobility is important because the demands for continence (or controlled incontinence) are much greater in those with restricted mobility. Manipulative skills are obviously important if the patient may at any time become dependent upon techniques such as CISC or the manipulation of an artificial urinary sphincter (AUS).

Severe physical deformity in the form of spinal kyphoscoliosis usually correlates with a wheelchair existence and reduced mobility as a result. Kyphoscoliosis commonly causes distortion and deformity of the abdominal wall making surgery difficult, if not impossible.

The importance of bowel and sexual function has already been mentioned, particularly bowel problems in females, since sexual problems, as has been noted, are rarely a problem. Minor urinary incontinence, for example, is not really a problem if a patient already has to wear pads or nappies for faecal incontinence. However severe constipation as in non-neuropathic patients can make bladder problems worse.

MANAGEMENT

Management may be specific or non-specific. In specific management the patient's urodynamic disorder is accurately diagnosed and each abnormal parameter is treated with an agent or surgical technique specifically designed to correct it. In non-specific management surgical or non-surgical palliative measures designed to contain or control incontinence are used to bypass the specific urodynamic disorder.

Non-specific measures include the use of urethral or suprapubic catheters, absorptive pads with appropriately designed underwear, conduit or continent urinary diversion and in male patients the use of external appliances such as condom drainage devices. These techniques are appropriate when the patient's general condition does not warrant selective specific treatment and under certain special circumstances. Thus in infants it is perfectly appropriate (assuming that there is no impairment of renal function) to use nappies as in normal children of the same age. Likewise in patients of grossly restricted mobility who are totally dependent on others for their care, indwelling catheters, by whatever route, are a perfectly reasonable form of treatment. When these are ineffective such patients are best considered for ileal conduit urinary diversion. The use of such containment techniques does not require extensive assessment, nor is neurological diagnosis or prognosis important.

For those less affected neurologically, particularly those who can care for themselves, with a static neurological lesion, with normal intelligence and manipulative skills, specific corrective treatment is indicated. In such circumstances, full videourodynamic assessment and investigation of upper urinary tract function become mandatory. The specific neurological diagnosis and likely prognosis, particularly the likelihood of progression, are also important.

As mentioned above the first question to ask is whether or not there is any secondary effect of lower urinary tract dysfunction on the upper urinary tracts or whether the patient is at risk of this in the future. If this is the case it is treated by the appropriate means, as described below. If there is no impairment of upper tract function and no likelihood of this occurring, the only question that remains is that of incontinence. The next question therefore is: does the patient have a degree of incontinence that warrants treatment and does she want treatment? If significant incontinence is present and the patient wants treatment, then videourodynamic diagnosis is the next step. A videourodynamic study will allow a decision as to whether the patient has a contractile, intermediate or acontractile type of dysfunction.

Contractile dysfunction

Most patients with contractile dysfunction and a lesion above the level of the pons will either have had a cerebrovascular accident or have Parkinson's disease. A few will have multiple sclerosis, although this has only recently been recognized as a cause with the introduction of nuclear magnetic resonance imaging (Eardley et al 1989). A few others will have cerebral tumours or vascular malformations or will have had surgery to correct these or surgery for cerebral trauma.

These patients will have detrusor hyper-reflexia but no obstructive detrusor sphincter dyssynergia. Some, by virtue of their age, may have a coexisting but incidental problem such as genuine stress incontinence, which may confuse the picture.

The treatment for detrusor hyper-reflexia in such situations, if the patient needs and wants treatment, is with anti-cholinergic medication. The best form of anti-cholinergic treatment currently available is with oxybutynin 5 mg q.d.s (Moisey et al 1980). Terodiline 25 mg b.d is an alternative. Other alternatives include propantheline and imipramine; the latter has the theoretical additional advantage of an alpha-sympathetic effect on the urethra which may possibly eliminate minor forms of associated sphincter weakness. The limiting factor with all anti-cholinergic medication is the side-effect of dryness of the mouth and throat. In hot weather there is also loss of sweating and in a few patients there is some loss of visual focusing. As a general rule the dose of oxybutynin or any other anti-cholinergic medication that produces a beneficial effect on the bladder will also cause side-effects, except in children. There is no way of avoiding this but some patients are more sensitive to the side-effects of one drug than to the others in this group, so if the patient has a beneficial effect with oxybutynin but severe side-effects, it is worth trying one of the other agents. As a general rule, if oxybutynin fails to produce a beneficial effect on the bladder, irrespective of side-effects, then no other anti-cholinergic medication will help.

Most patients with contractile dysfunction due to a cord lesion will either have multiple sclerosis or a relatively high and discrete spinal cord injury or spina bifida. In these patients, detrusor–sphincter dyssynergia may be present in addition to detrusor hyper-reflexia. This very rarely causes problems in women with multiple sclerosis or spinal cord injury but commonly causes upper tract problems in spina bifida for reasons that are not clear. Anti-cholinergic medication is again the first line of treatment for the detrusor hyper-reflexia but if there is detrusor sphincter–dyssynergia then acute or chronic retention may result. If this happens then CISC may be required to achieve bladder emptying. Most patients are quite happy with a regime of anti-cholinergic medication plus CISC, assuming they have the necessary manipulative skills.

In those patients with spinal cord injury who have a complete spinal cord transection but with preservation of an intact spinal cord and nerve roots below the level of the lesion, implantation of a sacral anterior root stimulator as designed by Professor Brindley (Brindley et al 1986) may be appropriate and should be considered.

Most patients with detrusor hyper-reflexia respond to anti-cholinergic medication with or without CISC as required. Some 78% of patients are satisfactorily treated in this way. The least satisfactory group to treat is Parkinson's disease which seems to be peculiarly refractory to all forms of treatment. If anti-cholinergic medication fails then for the majority of patients with suprapontine lesions containment is the best option available — surgery is rarely if ever indicated because of associated infirmities.

For those with cord lesions who are generally younger and fitter and with a stable neurological problem, then surgery should be considered if non-surgical methods fail to achieve continence. Surgery in such circumstances means 'clam' ileocystoplasty (Mundy 1988). The bladder is almost completely bisected in the coronal plane leaving just an intact bridge on either side of the bladder neck about 1–2 cm wide (Fig. 50.4). The bladder circumference is then measured and a segment of ileum equal in length to the measured bladder circumference is mobilized on its vascular pedicle, isolated, opened along its antimesenteric border to form a patch (Fig. 50.5) and then sewn into the

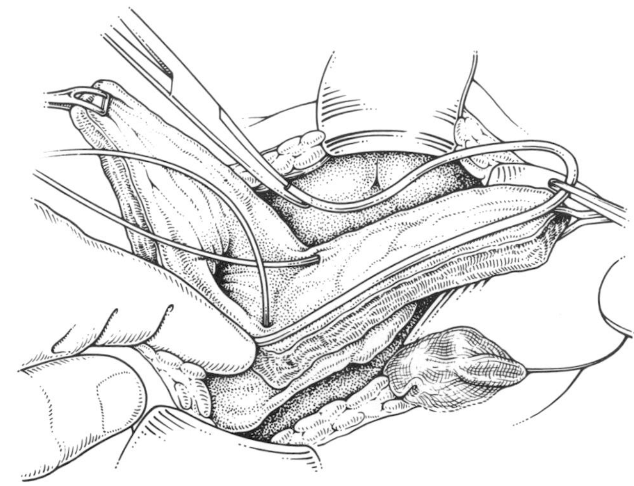

Fig. 50.4 'Clam' ileocystoplasty: the bladder is bisected in the coronal plane and the bladder circumference is measured.

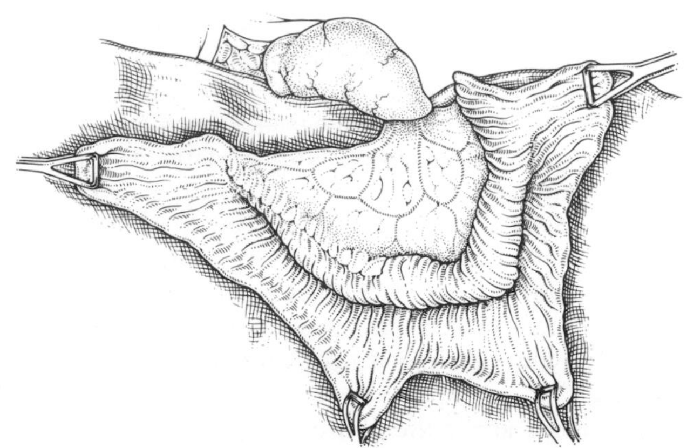

Fig. 50.5 'Clam' ileocystoplasty: a section of ileum equal in length to the measured bladder circumference is isolated on its vascular pedicle and opened to form a patch.

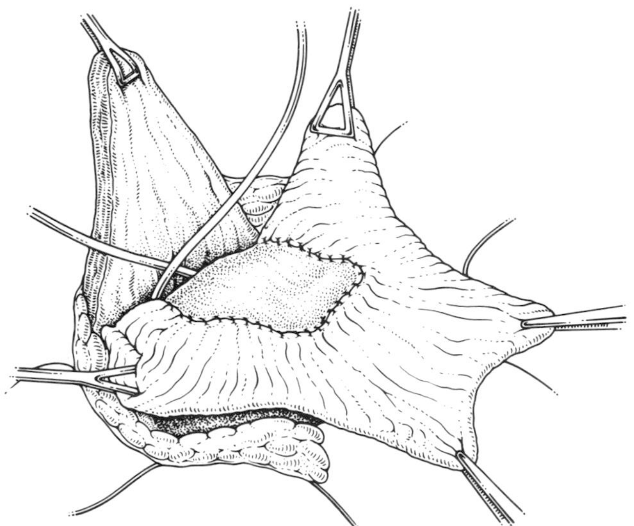

Fig. 50.6 'Clam' ileocystoplasty: the ileal patch has been sewn on to the posterior bladder wall.

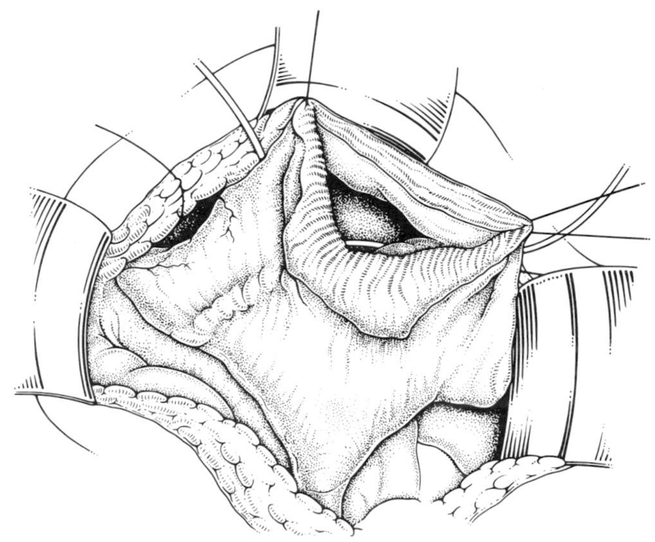

Fig. 50.7 'Clam' ileocystoplasty: the ileal patch has been flipped over and tacked to the anterior bladder wall with stay sutures prior to completing the anastomosis.

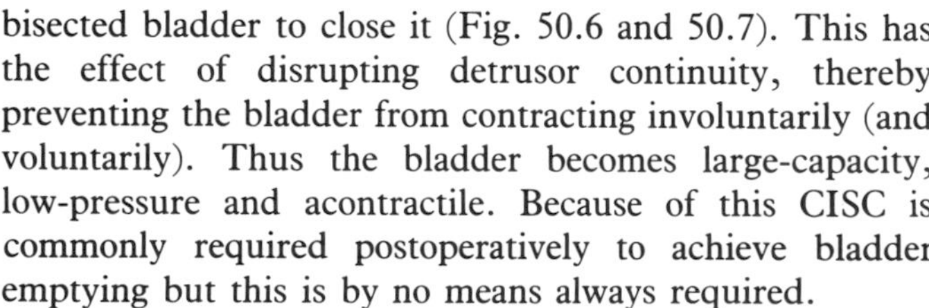

bisected bladder to close it (Fig. 50.6 and 50.7). This has the effect of disrupting detrusor continuity, thereby preventing the bladder from contracting involuntarily (and voluntarily). Thus the bladder becomes large-capacity, low-pressure and acontractile. Because of this CISC is commonly required postoperatively to achieve bladder emptying but this is by no means always required.

Intermediate dysfunction

Most patients in this group will either have spinal cord injury or spina bifida. As with contractile dysfunction, patients with complete spinal cord transection as a result of spinal injury who satisfy the relevant criteria should be considered for the Brindley sacral anterior root stimulator. If this is inappropriate, or in spina bifida where it is rarely applicable because of anatomical deformity, then medical or surgical treatment depends upon the exact nature of the problem. Although all patients will have high-frequency, low-amplitude, short-duration detrusor overactivity, poor compliance, bladder neck incompetence and a distal urethral sphincter mechanism that is both obstructive and incompetent, the end-result of these effects may be variable. At one extreme there is the grossly overactive bladder giving a markedly reduced bladder capacity but at the other extreme, intravesical pressure may be much lower, sphincteric resistance may be much higher and residual urine may be considerable. Anti-cholinergic medication with oxybutynin sometimes helps to reduce detrusor contractility in intermediate dysfunction but not nearly so often as it does in contractile dysfunction. Equally there is little in the way of pharmacological treatment of sphincter weakness in an attempt to improve bladder capacity.

The cornerstone of non-surgical treatment in this group is CISC in those who have a substantial residual urine volume. If there is a substantial residual urine volume then CISC will not only give bladder emptying but will also give continence for the time it takes for the bladder to fill to the volume at which it usually begins to overflow and cause incontinence. If CISC produces some benefit but response is restricted by detrusor contractile activity and the patient fails to show any benefit from oxybutynin then a 'clam' ileocystoplasty should be considered to reduce intravesical pressure, increase bladder capacity and thereby give a larger residual urine volume which will in turn give greater continence and for a longer period of time, with CISC to provide bladder emptying. If in addition to the detrusor dysfunction there is significant sphincter weakness incontinence, then the patient should be considered for implantation of an artificial urinary sphincter in addition to the cystoplasty (Parry et al 1990).

The combination of a cystoplasty to increase bladder capacity and reduce intravesical pressure and an AUS to produce adequate bladder outflow resistance is an extremely effective way of producing continence in this group of patients, as would be expected on theoretical grounds. There is the theoretical risk that simultaneous bowel surgery at the time of implantation of an AUS may increase the prosthesis infection rate but in practice experience shows that this is not the case (Nurse & Mundy 1988). This combined surgical manoeuvre does not however reduce the requirement for CISC to produce adequate bladder emptying. The AUS produces continence; it cannot be expected on its own to produce good bladder emptying.

Acontractile dysfunction

About 10% of patients with spinal cord injury and spina bifida have acontractile dysfunction but the majority of patients with acontractile dysfunction have a peripheral autonomic neuropathy due to diabetes, pelvic trauma (including surgery) or most commonly an idiopathic autonomic neuropathy. When acontractile dysfunction is due to spina bifida or spinal cord injury, sphincter weakness incontinence is the predominant urodynamic problem and significant sphincteric obstruction is uncommon. In peripheral autonomic neuropathy, particularly in patients with diabetes, the obstructive element of sphincter dysfunction causing a high residual urine is often much more important and commonly the predominant factor. In such patients CISC is often effective in giving good bladder emptying and, as a result, improved continence. Techniques designed to reduce bladder outflow resistance and thereby improve bladder emptying, such as urethral dilatation or urethrotomy, should not be used except in very selected patients because they usually improve bladder emptying at the expense of increasing stress incontinence. If given the option, many patients find the idea of dilatation or urethrotomy attractive because it seems like a simple, quick and easy 'cure' for their problem when compared with the prospect of lifelong self-catheterization. They will however be much less satisfied should they become grossly stress incontinent as a result, so CISC should always be presented as the best option for them.

In those with acontractile dysfunction who have gross sphincter weakness incontinence, CISC will obviously not help and sympathetic stimulant drugs such as ephedrine or phenylpropanolamine are unlikely to help either. In some patients a standard bladder neck or urethral suspension procedure as used for non-neuropathic genuine stress incontinence will help but the results are not nearly as satisfactory in neuropathy as in non-neuropathic conditions. If they are successful then it is usually by causing complete bladder outflow obstruction and CISC will then be required to achieve bladder emptying thereafter (Lawrence & Thomas 1987). The alternative is implantation of an AUS (Fig. 50.8 and 50.9). This is extremely effective at

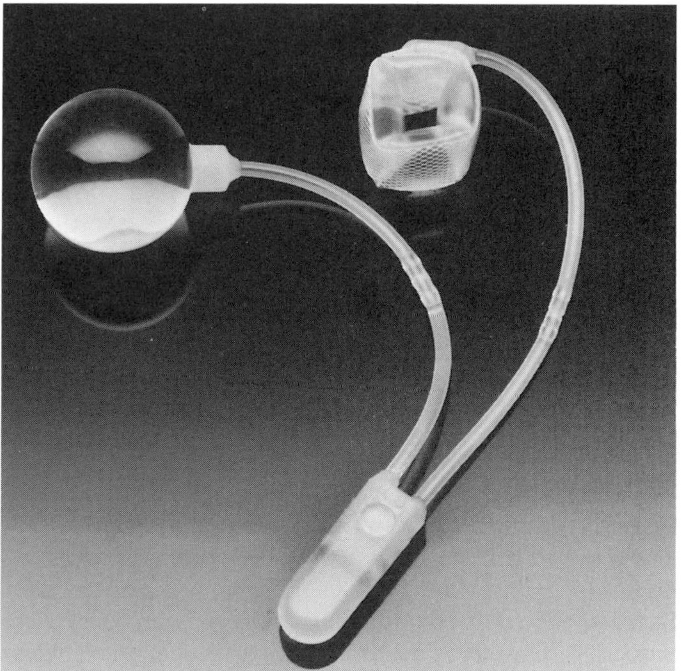

Fig. 50.8 The Brantley Scott artificial urinary sphincter (AUS) — the AS 800 model. This consists of a circumferential cuff that is placed around the bladder neck or (in males) the bulbar urethra, a pressure-regulating balloon that lies extraperitoneally in the pelvis or iliac fossa and a control pump which lies subcutaneously in either a labium majus or (in males) the scrotum, all of which are fluid-filled and interconnected via the control pump. The pressure inside the system is controlled by the pressure-regulating balloon and this is predetermined during manufacture. This pressure is transmitted to the cuff which thereby occludes the bladder neck (or bulbar urethra) constantly, unless the pump is squeezed.

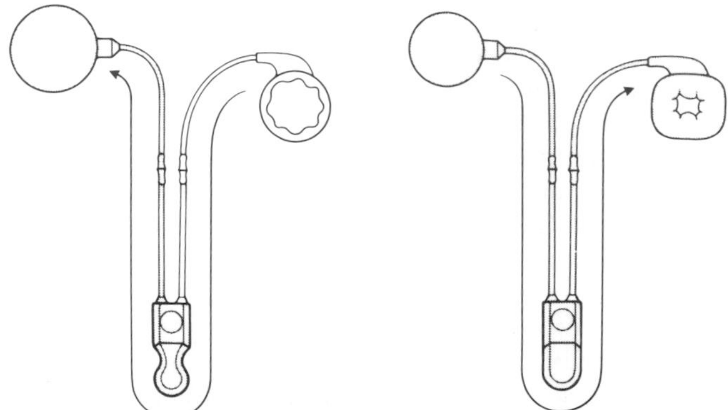

Fig. 50.9 The Brantley Scott artificial urinary sphincter (AUS). When the pump is squeezed 2–3 times, fluid is rapidly transmitted from the cuff through the control assembly part of the control pump to the balloon, allowing the patient to void. The fluid then slowly returns from the balloon to the cuff through a series of delay-resistors in the control assembly until the occlusive pressure of the cuff is fully restored. This allows about 3–4 min for the patient to void.

controlling sphincter weakness incontinence, whatever the cause, but carries all of the complications of an implanted prosthesis, specifically infection, urethral erosion and a major financial outlay (Mundy 1986a; Nurse & Mundy 1988). These devices currently cost £2677 and for this reason are not generally available. In practice they are rarely required for peripheral autonomic neuropathy and are only needed for occasional patient who fails to respond to more standard bladder neck or urethral suspension procedures. They are much more commonly required in acontractile dysfunction due to spinal cord injury and spina bifida.

Undiversion

A full discussion of undiversion of the previously diverted urinary tract in patients with neuropathic bladder dysfunction is beyond the scope of this chapter (see Mundy 1987). Suffice it to say that many patients who were diverted in childhood may be candidates for undiversion in later life if they satisfy the criteria given above for primary corrective treatment of their lower urinary tract dysfunction. As a general rule, it is probably not a good idea to suggest undiversion in a patient with normal upper urinary tract function and a satisfactory diversion unless they themselves request it. On the other hand if the patient has a problem with the diversion that requires surgical correction then undiversion should be suggested as an alternative to revision of the diversion.

The principles of undiversion are to restore urinary tract continuity and at the same time to correct the lower urinary tract abnormalities, either by cystoplasty or implantation of an artificial sphincter or both. Upper-to-lower urinary tract continuity is most commonly restored by mobilizing the bladder and bringing it up by means of a psoas hitch or a Boari flap or, more usually, a combination of the two, to reach the proximal ureters after separation of the ureters from the ileal conduit. Usually one ureter — the one on the side of the psoas hitch/Boari flap — is reimplanted into the bladder and the contralateral ureter is then drained into the ipsilateral reimplanted ureter by means of transureteroureterostomy. Occasionally substitution cystoplasty will be required if the defunctioned neuropathic bladder is too small to allow the mobilization procedures described above. Occasionally also the length of ureters above the ileal conduit will be too short to reach the bladder, however well it is mobilized, and the ileal conduit will need to be tailored to form a substitute ureter which can then be reimplanted into the mobilized bladder.

Dialysis and transplantation in patients with neurophatic bladder dysfunction

More and more patients with neuropathic bladder dysfunction who have developed end-stage renal failure as a result of neuropathic bladder dysfunction affecting the upper urinary tracts are being considered for renal substitution, usually by renal transplantation. Many of these patients have an ileal conduit as a result of earlier attempts to arrest the progression of renal failure and many of these are transplanted into their ileal conduit to provide urine drainage. The same considerations should be given to these patients however as to those with urinary diversions (discussed in the last section); corrective surgical intervention should be considered first if they are otherwise suitable.

If it is decided that the patient warrants corrective surgery to the lower urinary tract then this is best performed prior to transplantation before she is subjected to the immunosuppressive regime that goes with transplantation. It is more important however, that the patient should be reconstructed at a time when she has a good urine output, so if she is on dialysis and the urinary tract is essentially 'dry' then reconstructive surgery should be postponed until after the transplant has stabilized to ensure an adequate urine flow.

CONCLUSION

With currently available non-surgical treatment modalities and surgical techniques it is possible to reconstruct the entire urinary tract from the renal pelvis onwards and, by adding renal transplantation, the kidney as well. Proper management therefore consists not of selecting the treatment for the patient but, in the first instance at least, the patient for the treatment. In general, treatment depends more on the patient's general condition and other factors related to the neurological diagnosis than to the state of the lower urinary tract and urodynamic diagnosis. It is utterly pointless to subject a patient to all of the pain and inconvenience of major surgical reconstruction when she lacks the motivation to see it through, the intelligence to understand what is going on or the manipulative skills to use CISC or manipulate an AUS if these are a necessary part of the treatment. In such circumstances containment of the incontinence is much more suitable for the patient. On the other hand, in properly selected patients almost any urinary tract can be salvaged in the expectation of a satisfactory result.

KEY POINTS

1. The commonest cause of morbidity and mortality in spinal cord lesions is bladder outflow obstruction.
2. Any neuropathy affecting the lower urinary tract will usually also affect the bowel, lower limbs and sexual function.
3. Assessment has two objectives — firstly to determine the extent of renal impairment or deterioration, and secondly to make a definitive urodynamic diagnosis for the purpose of treating incontinence.
4. The pattern of bladder dysfunction is dictated by the level of neurological lesion which may be suprapontine, cord or peripheral.
5. In practice, there are only three patterns of abnormal bladder function — contractile, intermediate and acontractile.
6. Obstructive nephropathy may develop in contractile and intermediate forms of bladder dysfunction.
7. For the whole urinary tract, intravenous urography is the best screening investigation although ultrasound is adequate for follow-up.
8. Nephropathy comprises hydroureteronephrosis and recurrent urinary tract infection.
9. Renal function is preserved by the appropriate use of anti-cholinergic drugs, clean intermittent self-catheterization (CISC) or renal substitution if renal failure has developed.
10. Urinary incontinence is managed by techniques which include anti-cholinergic drugs, clean intermittent self-catheterization, ileal conduit, calm cystoplasty, Brindley sacral anterior route stimulator and the artificial urinary sphincter.

REFERENCES

Bors E, Comarr A E 1971 Neurological urology. S. Karger, Basel, pp 346–357

Brindley G S, Polkey C E , Rushton D N, Cardozo L 1986 Sacral anterior root stimulators for bladder control in paraplegia: the first 50 cases. Journal of Neurology, Neurosurgery and Psychiatry 49: 1104–1114

Eardley I, Kirby R S, Nagendran C et al 1989 Where are the lesions that cause the neurogenic bladder in multiple sclerosis? Neurourology and Urodynamics 8: 310–311

Gosling J A, Dixon J S, Humpherson J A 1983 Functional anatomy of the urinary tract: an integrated text and colour atlas. Churchill Livingstone, Edinburgh

Gosling J A, Chilton C P 1984 The anatomy of the bladder, urethra and pelvic floor. In: Mundy A R, Stephenson T P, Wein A J (eds) Urodyamics: principles, practice and application. Churchill Livingstone, Edinburgh, pp 3–13

Lapides J, Diokno A C, Silber S J, Lome B S 1972 Clean intermittent self-catheterisation in the treatment of urinary tract disease. Journal of Urology 107: 458–461

Lawrence W T, Thomas D G (1987) The Stamey bladder neck suspension operation for stress incontinence and neurovesical dysfunction. British Journal of Urology 59: 305–510

Miller H, Simpson C A, Yeates W K 1965 Bladder dysfunction in multiple sclerosis. British Medical Journal 1: 1265–1269

Moisey C U, Stephenson T P, Brendler C B 1980 The urodymamic and subjective results of treatment of detrusor instability with oxybutynin chloride. British Journal of Urology 52: 472–475

Mundy A R 1984 Clinical physiology of the bladder, urethra and pelvic floor. In: Mundy A R, Stephenson T P, Wein A J (eds) Urodynamics: principles, practice and application. Churchill Livingstone, Edinburgh, pp 14–25

Mundy A R 1986a Artificial urinary sphincters. Archives of Disease in Childhood 61: 1–3

Mundy A R 1986b The neuropathic bladder. In: Postlethwaite R J (ed) Clinical paediatric nephrology. John Wright, Bristol, pp 312–328

Mundy A R 1987 Refunctional urinary tract surgery with particular reference to undiversion. In: Hendry W F (ed) Recent advances in urology/andrology. Churchill Livingstone, Edinburgh, pp 147–168

Mundy A R 1988 Current operative surgery — urology. Baillière Tindall, London, pp 140–159

Mundy A R, Shah P J, Borzyskowski M, Saxton H M 1985 Sphincter behaviour in myelomeningocele. British Journal of Urology 57: 647–651

Nurse D E, Mundy A R 1988 One hundred artificial sphincters. British Journal of Urology 61: 318–325

Parry J R W, Nurse D E, Boucaut H A P, Murray K H A, Mundy A R 1990 The surgical management of the congenital neuropathic bladder. British Journal of Urology 65: 164–167

Rickwood A M K, Thomas D G, Philp N H, Spicer R D 1982 Assessment of congenital neuropathic bladder by combined urodynamic and radiological studies. British Journal of Urology 54: 512–518

Torrens M, Morrison J F B (1987) The physiology of the lower urinary tract. Spinger-Verlag, Heidelberg

51. Urinary tract infections

A. J. France   R. P. Brettle   J. A. Gray

INTRODUCTION

Urinary tract infections (UTIs) are important because 20% of women aged 20–65 years suffer one attack per year, approximately 50% of women develop a UTI during their lives and there is a prevalence rate of 5% per year of asymptomatic or covert bacteriuria in non-pregnant women between the ages of 21 and 65 years. UTI is a common reason for visiting a general practitioner, accounting for between 1–6% of consultations. Amongst working women, days lost from work as a result of UTIs account for about 1/10th of those due to respiratory infections. Depending upon the survey, between 12 and 25% of cases of chronic renal failure are attributed to chronic pyelonephritis. Before the antibiotic era febrile UTIs, especially in children, were life-threatening with a mortality of 20% and a morbidity of 20%, mostly from hypertension and renal failure. Whilst 60% healed spontaneously the patient was often seriously ill for 6–8 weeks.

Many women however are frustrated by a lack of interest and knowledge of the problem shown by doctors. They are even more confused by the profession's inability to find a 'cure' for this apparently simple disorder.

TERMINOLOGY

UTIs are defined by the presence of viable microorganisms within the urinary tract, although it may be difficult to distinguish between contamination, colonization or infection. The term 'bacteriuria' is used to define the presence of living bacteria in freshly voided urine or urine obtained via suprapubic aspiration. In 1956 Kass proposed that the isolation of more than 100 000 colony-forming units (cfu) or organisms per millilitre of midstream voided urine should be used to differentiate probable contamination from covert infection or asymptomatic bacteriuria (ASB). The use of this simple technique enabled detection of significant bacteriuria to be made in the healthy population as well as allowing the determination of the natural history of covert bacteriuria. Unfortunately this statistical probability has been extended to acute UTIs, which is inappropriate since Stamey and others have shown that symptomatic UTIs are associated with a pure growth of an organism, often at levels of only 100 to 1000 organisms per millilitre of urine. In addition, even in the presence of sterile urine it is possible to grow bacteria from bladder biopsies, suggesting that in the presence of sterile urine, the classical symptoms of a UTI may still be caused by bacteria.

UTIs are described by many confusing terms. The term 'cystitis' indicates inflammation of the bladder but is often used by patients to indicate any UTI. The term 'bacterial cystitis' should technically be used where bladder inflammation is caused by bacterial infection. However the symptoms of bacterial cystitis also occur without bacteriuria, which suggests that the patients have urethritis. Another term that is often used is the 'frequency dysuria syndrome' or FDS, which describes symptoms such as frequency and/or urgency of micturition, dysuria, strangury and nocturia, without attributing an exact cause. Another term, 'the urethral syndrome', has a variety of meanings depending upon the author. It may mean the FDS with or without bacteriuria, FDS as a consequence of oestrogen withdrawal or FDS secondary to a urethritis due to an organism such as *Chlamydia*.

The term 'acute bacterial pyelonephritis' indicates acute infection of the kidneys. There is usually fever, loin pain, pyuria ($>10^6$ white cells per litre of uncentrifuged urine), bacteriuria and possibly bacteraemia. More confusion occurs over the term 'chronic pyelonephritis'. This consists of chronic inflammation of renal and tubular tissue with scarring and shrinkage secondary to interstitial fibrosis. There is accompanying reduction in the glomerular filtration rate, tubular function and ability to concentrate urine. Causes of chronic pyelonephritis include bacterial infection together with vesicoureteric reflux (VUR) and/or intrarenal reflux (IRR), analgesics, X-rays, formation of crystals within the urine and drugs. The characteristic appearances comprise clubbing of calyces, focal scars overlying the clubbing, polar scars and loss of renal size.

BACTERIOLOGY

UTIs are usually caused by Gram-negative aerobic organisms originating from the gut flora. In 80–90% of first infections, *Escherichia coli* is usually isolated. The outer genital and periurethral bacterial flora usually reflect the gut flora, e.g. *Pseudomonas klebsiella*. With subsequent infections *E. coli* are seen in around 70% of cases, although more unusual organisms occur after antibiotic therapy, surgery, or the presence of obstruction or stones. *Proteus* species are often associated with renal calculi.

Many bacteriology laboratories merely report the presence of coliform bacteria in the culture. In doing so, they adopt the pragmatic view that antibiotic sensitivities are a more important part of the result than precise species identification. In our experience *E. coli* is the most commonly isolated organism. *Klebsiella*, *Proteus* and enterococci are less commonly encountered. It is our experience that staphylococcal UTI is very rare. We believe the high isolation rate in other studies may reflect contamination with staphylococci which normally reside on the skin.

AETIOLOGY

In acute pyelonephritis the bacteria not only attach to the mucosal surfaces but also penetrate the tissues, causing an inflammatory response. In lower UTIs penetration of submucosal tissue can also occur. It is obvious from everyday clinical practice that some women suffer repeated attacks of bacteriuria whilst others do not. Up to 80% of recurrent infections are reinfections and occur despite treatment with antibacterial agents with excellent in vitro efficacy. These two facts suggest a failure of host defences which is currently poorly understood. UTIs may occur because of the *virulence* of the organisms, the *susceptibility* of the host or a *combination* of both factors.

The normal urinary tract is resistant to colonization by bacteria and the integrity of the urinary tract is a balance between host defences and the virulence of the organism. These factors are not yet completely understood.

Virulence factors

Certain organisms are more virulent than others; for instance some strains of *E. coli* are spontaneously eliminated after their introduction into the urinary tract whilst others cause persistent infection. Bacteria causing acute pyelonephritis are more resistant to the bactericidal action of human serum than those organisms causing ASB. By comparison, *Proteus mirabilis* rarely causes a UTI in persons with a normal urinary tract. *P. mirabilis* is less efficient than *E. coli* in its adherence to uroepithelial cells and does not have a lipopolysaccharide capsule. The structures thought to be involved in pathogenicity are:

1. *Fimbriae* — proteinaceous rigid hair-like extensions from bacterial cells which recognize various specific chemical receptors, usually carbohydrates, glycolipids or glycoproteins.
2. *Glycocalyx* — the term used to describe capsules, sheaths, slime layers. These are composed of polysaccharides and glycoproteins which are exterior to the cell wall. They facilitate adhesion to epithelial cells, reduce adhesion to phagocytes and reduce penetration of antibiotics. They have a high component of sialic acid which prevents activation of complement and is poorly immunogenic.
3. *Outer membrane constituents* — the lipopolysaccharides of the outer membrane prevent complement activation and inhibit adhesion to phagocytes. Five different K antigens account for 70% of the *E. coli* involved in acute pyelonephritis in children and the K1 antigen is involved in 39% of the infections. In all, 80% of the *E. coli* causing acute pyelonephritis belong to eight common O antigenic groups whilst 45% of the *E. coli* strains causing ASB had incomplete lipopolysaccharide (endotoxin) of the cell membrane and were spontaneously agglutinating.

The ability of organisms to adhere to cell surfaces is an important virulence factor in itself and applies to many organisms beside urinary tract pathogens, including streptococci, enteropathogenic *E. coli*, *Neisseria* species and *Bordetella*. Adhesion to cell surfaces is important for the normal flora as well and appears to be mediated by non-specific factors like electrostatic forces and hydrophobic interactions. There are also specific interactions, usually between bacterial proteins (ligands) and cell carbohydrates (receptors). The forces involved in these specific interactions are however still a mixture of electrostatic and hydrophobic interactions. There is a correlation between the severity of infection and ability to adhere; for instance, those strains causing pyelonephritis adhere better than those causing cystitis.

Currently the best characterized receptors are associated with fimbriae. Fimbriae are characterized by their ability to agglutinate red cells. Two broad types of agglutination have been described, that inhibited by the sugar mannose, called mannose-sensitive, MS or type 1, and that resistant to mannose, called mannose-resistant or MR. The MS fimbriae recognize alpha D mannopyranosyl, agglutinate guinea pig red cells, yeast cells and Tamm–Horsfall protein of urinary mucus. One common MR receptor in urinary *E. coli* is D galactose-1-4-alpha D galactose-1-beta, which agglutinates human red cells carrying the ubiquitous P blood group antigens and binds to human uroepithelial cells. Agglutination of red cells is proportionate to the ability to adhere to uroepithelial cells. Another term commonly used is therefore 'P fimbriae'. Other as yet poorly described ligands are the M fimbriae, neuraminyl 2–3 galactoside fimbriae and X fimbriae.

Some 85% of urinary *E. coli* express MS receptors and *E. coli* of this type can elicit degranulation of polymorphs and initiate a respiratory burst. They might therefore cause tissue damage. The *E. coli* associated with pyelonephritis however usually are MR or P fimbriate, the P blood group antigen acts as a receptor for these organisms and they have improved binding to uroepithelial cells. Animal experiments show these organisms to cause acute pyelonephritis by the ascending route of infection against urine flow. There is however controversy over the clinical importance of these receptors, even whether these fimbriae are expressed in vivo or only after culture. The use of receptor analogues supports the importance of adhesion as a virulence factor. For instance, the instillation of mannose into the bladders of mice reduces bacteraemia with type 1 or MS *E. coli*. Similar work with globotetraose (a P blood group antigen analogue) protected mice against MR *E. coli*. Lastly, the active vaccination of animals with highly purified P fimbriae conferred protection against acute or chronic pyelonephritis.

Clinical studies also suggest a role for receptors. For instance, 97% of children with a first episode of acute febrile non-obstructed pyelonephritis are infected with a P fimbriate *E. coli*, compared to only 19% for cystitis and only 14% for covert bacteriuria. Similarly, in adults with acute non-obstructed pyelonephritis, 90% are P fimbriate. Intestinal colonization with P fimbriate *E. coli* predisposes to acute pyelonephritis and nosocomial spread of acute pyelonephritis in neonates has been documented.

Host factors

The bacteria causing UTIs interact with the host at two levels, namely at the mucous surfaces lining the urinary tract and in the tissues of the kidney or bladder. Several host factors predispose towards a UTI, such as an abnormal flow with urethral valves, foreign bodies, including renal calculi, and instrumentation with catheters which obviously bypass the usual host defences. The continuous flow of urine through the bladder presumably eliminates those organisms with poor adhesion. The establishment of a UTI is related to the presence of a residual volume and the frequency of micturition. Common examples are obstruction, spastic or dysfunctional bladders, urethral obstruction in males or females, reflux or duplex systems. In females the shorter urethra and abnormal positions of the urethral opening have been suggested as one reason for the increased susceptibility to UTIs for women.

Vaginal intercourse also has an effect on susceptibility to UTIs, although the exact mechanisms remain unknown. Episodes of FDS are often associated with the onset of sexual intercourse. Women having regular intercourse have 3–4 times as many episodes of infection per year compared to women not having intercourse. Those women not having intercourse still suffer infections but at a reduced frequency. The act of vaginal intercourse is thought to massage organisms into the bladder but in most individuals these organisms are washed out over about 24 h without symptoms.

The mechanical cleansing action of the flow of urine is potentiated by ureteric peristalsis or bladder contractions and it has been suggested that smooth muscle activity may be reduced by the release of bacterial endotoxin.

The mucosa of the urinary tract is similar in organization and function to other mucosal surfaces. There is a folded multilayered epithelium of transitional or squamous type overlain with mucus or urinary slime. The transitional epithelium of the bladder is three or four cell layers deep, helps to avoid non-specific binding and has a bactericidal action which is poorly understood. The basal cells are relatively small and undifferentiated whilst the surface cells are larger and are highly differentiated. The surface cells are arranged with tight junctions and are covered with microvilli. In the presence of an acute UTI there is widening of the junctions and extensive exfoliation of surface cells to expose the underlying undifferentiated cells which lack microvilli. Organisms in these deeper exposed areas seem to be more resistant to the activity of antibiotics compared to bacteria within urine. Bacteria in urine were lysed by an antibiotic but those organisms below the surface uroepithelium survived and became filamented. This is one explanation for the common clinical problem of failure of apparently effective antibiotic regimes.

Patients with chronic UTIs have grossly disturbed bladder uroepithelium. There is extensive widening of the junctions, exfoliation and resulting exposure of underlying cells to which greater numbers of bacteria are able to attach. Thus adherence of organisms to uroepithelium is not uniform; the majority adhere to the altered surfaces. The persistence of exposed surfaces in patients with recurrent UTIs is one explanation of increased susceptibility.

The normal uroepithelium of patients known to be susceptible to UTIs binds more organisms and becomes more easily colonized. This appears to be due to a higher density of receptors. For instance, those individuals with the P1 phenotype of the P blood group antigen have a higher density of glycolipid receptors on their erythrocytes and presumably on their uroepithelium than individuals with the P2 phenotype. Receptor binding seems to be more important in those individuals with a normal urinary tract and less important in individuals with VUR. The presence of VUR or residual urine presumably allows organisms with poorer virulence factors to gain access to the urinary tract.

The host response to acute pyelonephritis involves the production of serum antibodies, commonly to O antigens and occasionally to K antigens and type 1 fimbriae. These antibodies have been shown in animals to be protective against haematogenous or ascending infection. Local production of immunoglobulins (IgG and secretory or dimeric IgA) occurs at an increased level in response to infection such as acute pyelonephritis but their importance is not fully understood. A similar but less striking increase in urinary antibodies occurs in an acute lower UTI. These urinary immunoglobulins do possess antibody activity, as seen by bacterial agglutination. The bladder and urethra are sites of antibody production either by active secretion for dimeric IgA or by transudation from serum for IgG. These antibodies are excreted continuously but increase in response to an antigenic stimulus.

The presence of ammonia in urine suggests that, in the fluid phase at least, complement is less effective. Whilst phagocytosis is impaired because of the osmotic variability of urine it does occur and is one other important host defence mechanism which takes place on the uroepithelial surface.

Susceptibility to infections has been linked to particular ABO blood groups. Patients with blood group B had a 50% greater chance of contracting a UTI with *E. coli* in one study and patients who were B or AB and non-secretors were three times as likely to suffer recurrent UTIs than controls in another study. In a third study patients with blood group B or AB had a 55% increased chance of an *E. coli* enteric infection, a 131% increased chance of a *salmonella* enteric infection and a 300–400% increased chance of an *E. coli* meningitis, pyelonephritis or septicaemia. Blood group B antigens are found on many *E. coli* but the reason for the increased susceptibility does not appear to be the absence of anti-B antibodies. The non-secretion of ABO blood group antigens is a stable host marker associated with susceptibility of non-immune hosts to meningococcal and pneumococcal infections. There is also a higher incidence of non-secretors in adult women with recurrent UTIs and non-secretion appears to predispose the host to kidney scarring, associated with pyelonephritic infection. Non-secretors with recurrent UTIs who improved over 20 years had significantly higher levels of serum IgA, suggesting that non-secretors were more dependent on specific immune responses to infection. Soluble blood group substances found in secretions may have a role in reducing adhesion and this would explain the even greater susceptibility of non-secretors to infection. There is as yet no convincing association of UTIs with any specific human leukocyte antigen haplotype but a number of animal studies do suggest that several genes are responsible for resistance to infection.

The mechanism responsible for the development of renal scars is still poorly understood. It is known that scars are initiated in infancy following acute pyelonephritis. There is a poor correlation between bacterial growth in the kidney and the extent of the pathological damage. Persistent renal infection is not required and scarring from VUR and bacteriuria can only be prevented if treatment is started within 24 h. This time coincides with the appearance of neutrophils and monocytes and scarring depends on the inflammatory response. This suggests that tissue damage may be caused by toxic products from inflammatory cells and it has been postulated that the release of active oxygen radicals and/or granulocytic enzymes are responsible. This hypothesis is supported by the fact that only organisms that are able to stimulate neutrophils are associated with renal scarring.

NATURAL HISTORY

The prevalence of UTIs varies with age and sex. The risk for boys is greater than girls in the first month of life but by 6 months of age the risk for girls is greater than boys. Estimates of the prevalence of UTIs up to 11 years suggests a figure of around 1% for boys and 3% for girls. There is a 10-fold increase in incidence for older girls compared to boys and this continues through adult life until around 55 years when the incidence of UTIs in men and women is equal, mostly as a consequence of prostatic problems in men.

It is difficult to attribute primary mortality to UTIs, although they often complicate other illnesses and conditions, and approximately 12% of cases of chronic renal failure are now attributed to chronic pyelonephritis.

The complications and effects of UTIs are confounded by the fact that many infections are asymptomatic and in describing natural history it is important to specify whether bacteriuria is overt or covert. There is a prevalence rate of 5% per year of covert bacteriuria in non-pregnant women between the ages of 21 and 65 years and some 10–25% of these infected subjects annually clear the infection. There is as yet no convincing explanation for why covert infections are asymptomatic but clinical experience shows that treatment of ASB may strangely initiate the onset of symptoms. In adults ASB is not associated with decline in renal function but this is not the case for the young or old. For instance, UTIs are associated with a 20% decline in renal function in those over 70 years compared to only 5% in those uninfected.

On average 5% of women at their first antenatal clinic have ASB and unlike the non-pregnant state, only 3% of these individuals lose their bacteriuria over the course of the pregnancy. The prevalence of ASB increases with parity and in women with prior ASB, 40% had infection documented during pregnancy. Several studies have shown ASB does have an effect on maternal health. Between 10 and 30% of women with ASB developed acute pyelonephritis during the pregnancy; they have lower haemoglobins which improve with eradication of the ASB and hypertension is commoner, especially in association with renal scars. There is no significant effect on renal function but a significant number of patients with ASB have chronic renal disease. Some studies suggest greater risks of prematurity, an increase in perinatal mortality and a higher incidence of mental retardation. However most studies have not been large enough to investigate these problems effectively.

The prevalence of ASB in children is around 1–2% between the ages of 4 and 11 years and *E. coli* is the organism in 97% of cases. Of children with ASB, 47% have radiological abnormalities, 26% renal scars and 33% VUR (50% associated with renal scars). In 60% of patients with scarred kidneys infection was detected over a 10-year period. The majority of scars had developed by the age of 4 years and the glomerular filtration rate on average was reduced by 50% in those with scarred kidneys.

In the absence of obstruction, VUR alone or symptomatic bacteriuria alone did not initiate renal scarring but VUR and bacteriuria — whether symptomatic or asymptomatic — can initiate renal scarring. VUR and symptomatic bacteriuria carry a continuing risk of renal scarring throughout childhood, particularly in younger age groups. In children with renal scars detected by the presence of ASB, progressive renal scarring was observed in 27% of those with scars over 4 years and in 50% over 10 years.

The commonest age to present with UTI symptoms as an adult is around the mid 20s, although 28–60% of patients with renal scars have symptoms dating back to childhood compared to only 10% of patients without scars. Recurrent UTIs are common in the presence or absence of renal scars: 36% of women suffered a recurrence of symptoms within 1 year and 75% within 2 years. In 80% of cases the recurrence is due to a reinfection. Renal scars are present in around 0.25% of the female population and may predispose an individual to recurrent UTIs. Symptomatic UTIs however tend to occur in clusters and there may be long periods free of infection followed by further infection. Many symptomatic infections disappear rapidly with minimal treatment and over 70% of these recurrent UTIs are due to *E. coli*.

Adult patients with recurrent symptomatic bacteriuria do not develop new renal scars if the urinary tract is normal and renal function does not decline significantly over time. The development of new renal scars is also a rare event in adult patients with pre-existing renal scars, and decline in renal function is unrelated to the frequency of bacteriuria. The presence of renal scars predisposes the patient to a rise in blood pressure later in life especially during pregnancy and with the use of the oral contraceptive pill. The development of hypertension in patients with symptomatic UTIs correlates with age however rather than renal scarring.

The decline in renal function in those patients with renal scars is associated with proteinuria and hypertension. Pathologically focal glomerulosclerosis develops in the normal kidney. The underlying pathogenesis of these changes is unclear but autoimmune attack against Tamm-Horsfall proteins deposited in the mesangium and hyperfiltration have been suggested. In the latter case it is suggested that the healthy glomeruli between the scarred tissue undergo hyperfiltration such that they are in constant use instead of intermittent use, resulting in faster wearing out. Irrespective of the presence or absence of renal scars the frequency of UTIs decreased in two-thirds of patients and remained unchanged in one-third. This decrease in frequency of bacteriuria occurred across all age groups, suggesting it was unrelated to declining sexual activity and was more indicative of some form of immunization process.

Whilst UTIs in adult life have little influence on renal function this cannot be said for the elderly where bacteriuric individuals have a mean glomerular filtration rate 20% less than non-bacteriuric controls. In addition over a 2-year follow-up period the glomerular filtration rate declined four to six times as much in the bacteriuric individuals. It would thus appear that the nephrosclerotic changes associated with ageing are accelerated by UTIs.

The prevalence of bacteriuria is estimated to increase by 1% per decade for women. In those over 70 years the prevalence of bacteriuria increases by more than 1% per decade. Bacteriuric and non-bacteriuric states are relatively constant in adult women but in the elderly bacteriuria can be induced by diuresis and is a marker of unsuspected upper renal infection. Whilst the incidence of new UTIs is normally estimated at 1% per year, over the age of 70 years it is 23% for women and 11% for men. In geriatric hospitals this can rise to 50% per year and is associated with loss of mobility although at present it is not known whether this is cause or effect.

Patients in hospital with incontinence have a 50% incidence of bacteriuria whilst those with dementia have a

70% incidence of bacteriuria. There appears to be no obvious excess of dementia or loss of psychomotor function developing in patients with bacteriuria. There is however an association between bacteriuria and increased mortality. In men and women aged 70–79 years the respective mean survival for bacteriurics was 33 and 34 months compared to 53 and 75 months for non-bacteriurics. Thus an individual with a covert bacteriuria has a life expectancy of less than 3 years. The acquisition or conversion to bacteriuric state from a previously negative state is a marker of impending death, with 100% of 15 subjects dying within 2 months.

PRESENTATION

The patient's reasons for consulting her doctor are for the relief of symptoms and the prevention of their recurrence. These aims are most readily achieved by establishing an accurate diagnosis with a careful assessment of the predisposing factors and prompt recognition of the complications.

Symptoms

In adult women the archetypal attack of acute cystitis is heralded by the abrupt onset of one or more of the following symptoms: urinary frequency, dysuria, nocturia, urgency, haematuria, malodorous urine, suprapubic pain, nausea. In some cases the patient recognizes that sexual intercourse may be the precipitating factor. In acute pyelonephritis, loin pain and fever are more common although the symptoms of cystitis may coexist. In children the symptoms of urinary tract infection may be non-specific abdominal pain or simply failure to thrive. In elderly patients the classical symptoms are usually absent. UTI is a common cause of confusion or loss of mobility in a previously fit elderly woman. Thus the clinician should have no difficulty recognizing UTI in young and middle-aged adults but must be aware of the paucity of classical symptoms at the two extremes of life. It must be remembered that urethral strictures can occur in women and that the symptoms of poor flow rate may not be apparent to the patient.

The complete history should include an enquiry about previous UTIs, particularly during childhood and pregnancy. Contraceptive practice may influence advice regarding treatment (see below). A family history of tuberculosis should alert the clinician to this chronic but treatable condition.

Not all patients are good witnesses. In some patients with recurrent urinary symptoms it is often enlightening to have the patient keep a record of the time of day and the volume every time she passes urine. This introduces an objective measurement which is useful when assessing the severity of her symptoms and monitoring the response to treatment.

Predisposing factors

These are discussed in detail above. In summary the clinician should enquire about:

1. Diabetes mellitus which may cause glycosuria — an enriched culture medium.
2. The presence of foreign bodies such as stones or catheters.
3. Recent instrumentation of the urinary tract.
4. Neurological disorders or anticholinergic drugs which may cause incomplete bladder emptying.
5. Coexisting pelvic disease including tumours and inflammatory bowel disease which may directly invade the bladder or alter its mechanical properties.

Physical signs

In acute cystitis/urethritis, suprapubic tenderness is often present; alternatively palpation in this region will provoke a desire to pass urine. The patient may be restless. Fever is unusual. In acute pyelonephritis the patient looks ill. She is usually pyrexial — temperature >38°C — and has a tachycardia. Loin tenderness is a common finding and is bilateral if both kidneys are infected. Septicaemia must be suspected when hypotension accompanies the tachycardia. In young adults with septicaemia the supine blood pressure may be normal but postural hypotension is invariable.

In children and in the elderly the physical signs may be misleading by their atypical nature. The absence of the common physical findings does not exclude significant UTI in these age groups.

If a neuropathic bladder is suspected then the skin over the buttocks must be examined for sensory loss. Spinal cord lesions and damage to the sacral nerve roots may be detected in this manner.

INVESTIGATIONS

These are performed to confirm the diagnosis and to look for complications. The clinician must bear in mind the risks to the patient and to her future offspring which accompany certain investigations. This section includes an account of the commonly used investigations and discusses their relative merits.

Urine microscopy and culture

This is mandatory in all cases of suspected UTI. The microbiologist will report the results of culturing the specimen delivered to the laboratory. However, this may not reflect the microbiology of the urine in the patient's bladder. The principal reasons for this discrepancy are contamination of the specimen at the time of collection and delay in transporting the sample to the laboratory. When a woman passes urine a perineal lavage is an almost inevitable event. It is a consequence of normal female anatomy. Thus the midstream or clean-catch specimen of urine will be contaminated by vulval and vaginal flora. This may be minimized by asking the patient to wash her perineum and then spread her labia apart before collecting the urine sample. There is, of course, great variability in compliance with these instructions so it is preferable to collect a clean-catch specimen of urine, accepting that it may be contaminated at source. Prompt delivery to the laboratory will minimize the growth of contaminant organisms. In young children a midline suprapubic fine-needle aspiration of bladder urine is the preferred method of collection because it avoids all the problems of contamination mentioned above.

Microscopy of a fresh specimen of urine from a patient with a UTI will detect bacteria and pus cells in abundance. The presence of casts indicates renal disease. The presence of pus cells and subsequent failure to isolate a pathogen is called sterile pyuria and alerts the clinician to the possibility of tuberculosis. The presence of haematuria in the absence of pus cells or bacteria suggests pathologies other than infection.

The urine is cultured on selective media such as MacKonkey or CLED. This helps to restrict the growth of contaminants but allows recognition of most pathogens after 24 h culture. Identification and antibiotic sensitivity testing complete the microbiological report. If tuberculosis is suspected then at least three early-morning urine samples must be collected and cultured for mycobacteria. The patient is asked to collect the whole of her early-morning urine sample and deliver it for culture. The laboratories have techniques for concentrating the sample by centrifugation, thus improving the detection rate.

If there is a significant delay between collecting a sample of urine and plating it on culture media, then the final culture result may be misleading, because it will not be a true reflection of urinary tract flora. The inevitable contamination of the sample with skin flora during collection can lead to an overgrowth of these organisms on the culture medium. In an attempt to overcome this problem, some clinicians use a dipslide system. Briefly, a slide coated with solid culture media is dipped into the urine specimen and then transported to the laboratory in a sealed container. The resulting colonies remain fixed in one place and do not mix, as happens in liquid media. This system has a number of disadvantages: first there is no microscopy, thus red cells, white cells, casts and crystals will not be detected. Second, the technique has a false-positive rate of up to 10% and a false-negative up to 3%. Thus a negative dipslide result does not mean the urinary tract is healthy.

If a sexually transmitted disease is suspected then the reader is referred to Chapter 56 for further details.

Imaging

Ultrasound examination

Ultrasound examination is a well tolerated investigation with no recognized hazard. It is used to measure the dimensions of the kidneys and to detect obstruction of their drainage. It will not assess renal function at all and is best regarded as an adjunct to other imaging techniques.

Isotope renograms

Isotope renograms are performed by giving an intravenous injection of ^{99}TC-labelled mercapto-acetyl-triglycine (MAG3) and then detecting radioactivity with a gamma camera placed over the urinary tract. TcMAG3 is secreted by the proximal tubules. It is superior to ^{99}Tc-labelled diethylenetriaminepentaacetic acid because it produces better quality images with a lower dose of radiation. The information gained from this examination includes:

1. The relative contribution made by each kidney to total renal function.
2. The presence of obstructed drainage of each kidney.
3. VUR while voiding urine. Merrick et al (1977) showed that isotope techniques were at least as good as conventional micturating cystourethrography at detecting VUR in children with UTI. They pointed out that the isotope method was cheaper, did not require catheterization and involved a lower dose of radiation.

Renal scintigraphy

Renal scintigraphy with ^{99}Tc-labelled dimercaptosuccinic acid (DMSA) detects functioning proximal tubular cells. Its application in patients with UTI is the demonstration of renal scars. Monsour et al (1987) showed that renal scintigraphy was superior to ultrasound or intravenous urography when searching for early renal scars in children under the age of 5 years. Over this age the three examinations were equally sensitive. A further application of DMSA scintigraphy is the sequential measurement of renal function in patients without severe renal impairment. Nimmo et al (1987) reported serial studies with this isotope-labelled compound and showed that differences in relative function of >5% indicated a high probability that a change in renal function had occurred.

The radiation dose of a ^{99}TcMAG3 study is approximately 0.1–1 mSv. This compares with 4 mSv from an intravenous urography without tomography. Conventional voiding studies contribute a dose of 1–10 mSv, depending on the duration of X-ray screening.

Intravenous urography

Intravenous urography now has limited application in the investigation of the urinary tract. Ultrasound and isotope studies are superior to or equally as sensitive as intravenous urography. A further disadvantage is the relatively high dose of radiation of intravenous urograms. The one area where it is superior is in the demonstration of precise anatomical relations of the ureter. This may be helpful when planning surgical operations involving the ureters.

Blood tests

Plasma creatinine and urea concentrations are important measurements of renal function which should be performed in all cases, other than solitary episodes of cystitis in adult women. The fasting plasma glucose concentration and oral glucose tolerance test are superior to tests for glycosuria when considering diabetes mellitus.

MANAGEMENT

General principles

The management and the prevention of UTIs are closely related subjects. Often the patient's management should include advice as to how further infections can be avoided. The opportunity to educate a patient or a parent about the aetiology and prevention of infection should never be missed.

Many women and girls can be saved from the needless prescription of antibacterial agents if they are given and abide by some simple instructions. These can be either verbal or written in the form of a hand-out (ideally, both). They should include basic information about the source of the bacteria that invade the urinary tract from the patient's own bowel and how important it is to wipe the perineum from front to back to avoid faecal contamination of the urethra, especially during an episode of diarrhoea. Potentially irritant vaginal deodorants and bubble baths should be avoided and a high standard of perineal hygiene maintained.

The adult patient with recurrent UTI should drink a minimum of 2 litres of fluid daily — more if exercising strenuously or staying in a warm climate. This should be increased to 3 litres or more daily if symptoms of UTI are suspected, irrespective of the degree of urgency and frequency of micturition or painful dysuria. Keeping a bladder chart may be the best way of reinforcing this advice. Regular and complete bladder emptying must be taught and the concept of double micturition emphasized to those with residual bladder urine after voiding. Women working on assembly lines and girls who abhor unhygienic school lavatories are very prone to acquire overstretched bladders and a tendency to VUR if they are unable to void regularly.

The complaint of post-coital UTI symptoms provides the ideal opportunity to review contraceptive methods, perhaps advising the oral contraceptive rather than the condom if there is much irritation with the latter and asking the patient to be sure to void as soon as decently possible after intercourse.

The place of alkalinizing agents in relieving symptoms of UTI and the urethral syndrome is highly individual, some getting much comfort, others none at all from agents like mixture of potassium citrate and effervescent potassium citrate.

The patient educated in this simple way by her doctor will derive a lot of satisfaction from being largely in control of her own urinary symptoms. In addition to keeping healthier, she will also be less dependent on her medical advisers when she feels symptoms coming on. Like a well trained diabetic, she should be in command of her illness most of the time.

Sometimes, however, antibacterial drugs must be given. Their use where appropriate will be discussed in the following sections.

Asymptomatic bacteriuria

Most women with ASB do not require antibacterial treatment. There are, however, certain well defined groups of female patients who do need treatment for ASB. These include babies with proven urinary tract infection, especially if failing to thrive or shown to have already scarred kidneys or a predisposition to scarring from the combination of bacteriuria and VUR. Both these infants and older girls with damaged kidneys or reflux in the context of bacteriuria should have treatment for ASB and probably also be considered for long-term prophylactic antibiotic chemotherapy. It is important to manage these young patients correctly to reduce the risk of pyelonephritic scarring.

Kass found ASB in 4% of the female population when assessed by the midstream culture method. In pregnancy this figure rises to between 6 and 7%. At least 30–40% of expectant mothers with ASB or symptomatic lower UTI will develop upper UTI during pregnancy if left untreated. The possible sequel of bacteraemia and endotoxin shock with their potential for abortion makes it mandatory to screen pregnant women regularly for UTI and to treat those found positive whether they have symptoms or not. If they are shown to have bacteriuria again when checked a few weeks later, long-term prophylaxis may be indicated using a non-teratogenic and fetus-friendly antibacterial agent.

Female patients of any age with kidneys already damaged by previous infections are particularly prone to further infection and liable to additional scarring resulting from new infections. They should therefore always have bacteriuria promptly treated with antibacterial agents whether they have symptoms or not. This applies particularly to patients whose pyelonephritis has induced renal failure, when care must be taken to avoid using nephrotoxic antibiotics. The dose and interval between doses of the antibiotic chosen must be carefully monitored.

Ideally the sensitivity of the infecting organism should be known before treatment is instituted and an appropriate drug chosen to which the patient is likely to respond without developing hypersensitivity or other known side-effects. A 7–10-day course of treatment should be given and the possibility considered of using long-term prophylaxis thereafter. A follow-up midstream urine should be cultured 2–3 weeks after the end of treatment.

Symptomatic lower urinary tract infections

Seven days' treatment should be given to all the high-risk patients described above — infants, children with VUR, pregnant women, those with already scarred kidneys and those with established renal failure — when they have symptoms of bacterial cystitis or urethritis. Many others can be managed — or can manage themselves — by increasing their fluid intake and alkalinizing their urine so that by the time the sensitivity results are available they may be so much better as not to warrant antibacterial therapy.

The cause of abacteriurial urethritis, the urethral syndrome, is not yet firmly established. Despite the use of sometimes inappropriate antibiotics, symptoms may persist for months or years. Inspection of the external genitalia may help to identify non-infective causes amenable to treatment. *Chlamydia* should be excluded using appropriate media or immunofluorescent methods on slides smeared with freshly taken urethral and/or vaginal and cervical swabs. If *chlamydia* are demonstrated, tetracyclines may help to relieve the discomfort and, even when the swabs yield negative results, an empirical course of antichlamydial treatment may be justified.

Some doctors advocate single large-dose therapy for lower urinary tract symptoms thought to be due to bacteriuria whilst awaiting the outcome of urine culture. This acts as a therapeutic–diagnostic test. If significant bacteriuria is demonstrated and the patient does not respond clinically and bacteriologically to this treatment — assuming the bacteria isolated were sensitive to the drug chosen — intravenous urography or an ultrasound scan may be indicated to find out if there is an underlying anatomical reason for the failure to respond. A typical regimen would be 3 g amoxycillin morning and night for 1 day.

All patients in this group should be encouraged to drink plenty of fluid, and empty their bladders regularly and completely, even if this is initially painful. A follow-up urine culture should be taken in 2–3 weeks' time.

Acute pyelonephritis

Acute pyelonephritis is a medical emergency especially in pregnancy; Gram-negative bacteraemia, endotoxin shock and disseminated intravascular coagulation can occur. There should be no delay in taking blood and urine cultures and in instituting antibacterial therapy. It is important to choose an antibiotic which will achieve bactericidal concentrations in the blood as well as in the urine. As chemotherapy must start before the results of these cultures are known, the 'best-guess' antibiotic will have to be selected and this will partly depend on the prescriber's knowledge of the antibiotic sensitivity of the locally prevalent microbial flora.

The patient must be asked about previous hypersensitivity reactions to avoid the disaster of adding acute drug toxicity to the already hazardous situation. If she has already had a succession of oral antimicrobial agents, has been hospitalized for a long time, has had recent instrumentation of the bladder or an indwelling catheter, she is likely to be infected with organisms resistant to the commonly used antibiotics. This may also apply to the immunocompromised patient with malignant disease or who is being treated with radiotherapy, corticosteroids or other immunosuppressive agents. Pathogens like *Pseudomonas aeruginosa*, *Klebsiella pneumoniae* and *Serratia marcescens* may be found.

Under these circumstances a broad-spectrum agent such as a third-generation cephalosporin, an aminoglycoside or a combination of agents is indicated until the sensitivity results of the pathogens are reported. The patient with a known or suspected obstruction to the urinary tract or with previously scarred kidneys also falls into this category. Urease-producing *Proteus* spp. are common in the high-pH urine of patients with calculus disease of the urinary tract. Here ampicillin might be the 'best-guess' choice. In other circumstances intravenous Augmentin, co-trimoxazole or ciprofloxacin could be used until the sensitivity results were known. After that therapy should be rationalized taking into account the efficacy, toxicity, ease and comfort of administration and, not least, the cost of the antibiotics being used, assuming that the patient has weathered the bacteraemia.

Antibiotics are initially given intravenously to ensure bactericidal concentrations in the blood. After a few days of intravenous antibiotics, oral therapy is usually substituted as the patient responds. Treatment should be for at least 10 days and the patient carefully followed up thereafter, investigated to find if there was an underlying anatomical cause and the urine cultured 3 and 6 weeks later to exclude relapse or recurrence. Consideration is then given to the possibility of preventing further infections with long-term suppressive antibiotics.

If an aminoglycoside like gentamicin is used intravenously to treat acute pyelonephritis its potential for toxicity to the eighth nerve and the kidneys must be remembered. Gentamicin is excreted unchanged in the urine. In a patient with bacteraemic shock the blood pressure drops suddenly, reducing the renal artery pressure which leads to diminished glomerular filtration and oliguria. Gentamicin is then poorly excreted and its serum concentration rises dangerously.

It is important therefore to monitor the blood pressure every hour or so initially and to keep an accurate record of the urine output during treatment. Hypotension, oliguria or a rising blood urea would suggest that the dose of gentamicin be reduced and/or the interval between doses increased. Monitoring of the peak-and-trough serum concentrations of the antibiotic gives two valuable bits of information — ensuring that the serum concentration exceeds the MIC of the pathogen and that an oto- or nephrotoxic level is not reached. For example, a patient may receive 3–5 mg/kg body weight gentamicin daily in divided doses when in normal renal function but will need a much reduced dose if she becomes oliguric. Peak serum levels of gentamicin should not exceed 10 mg/l and trough levels should not exceed 1.5–2 mg/l. Netilmicin is a newer aminoglycoside which is less toxic than earlier aminoglycosides. It is, however, considerably more expensive and peak-and-trough serum levels are still required.

Safer alternatives to aminoglycosides are the third-generation cephalosporins like cefotaxime and the expensive but highly effective ceftazidime. They have the merit of not requiring such strict monitoring as aminoglycosides — but all renally excreted drugs need dose reduction if the patient's urine output falls.

Augmentin, ureidopenicillins, co-trimoxazole and more recently ciprofloxacin have been used successfully in potentially bacteraemic patients with acute pyelonephritis.

When endotoxin shock occurs, the most important therapy not to delay is the administration of an intravenous bactericidal antibiotic. Even in a patient with negligible renal function a single initial intravenous dose of 80 mg gentamicin or 2 g cefotaxime may be life-saving whilst arranging monitoring and other aspects of intensive care. The place of intravenous corticosteroids in Gram-negative septicaemia has recently been challenged and there is clear evidence that they offer no benefit.

A central venous pressure line will help in the decision of how much fluid or plasma expander to give without overload. Vasoactive drugs like dopamine may be required to dilate renal blood vessels and to support cardiac function. Regular frequent monitoring of temperature, pulse, arterial blood pressure, respiration rate, urine output (with a temporary urinary catheter if necessary) and state of consciousness is mandatory. Urgent estimation of blood urea, electrolytes and creatinine should be requested. Knowledge of the peak-and-trough levels of any aminoglycoside given becomes an important consideration.

A 'clotting screen' to measure the concentrations of platelets, prothrombin, fibrinogen and fibrin split products will assist in deciding whether disseminated intravascular coagulation has occurred. Expert haematological help is advised if this is diagnosed to decide if heparin should be given to all but the pregnant patient.

Chronic pyelonephritis

When bacteriuria is diagnosed in a patient with chronic pyelonephritis, antibacterial therapy should be given irrespective of whether the patient is asymptomatic or symptomatic. Failure to do so may lead to worsening of renal scarring. This applies particularly to infants and small children who have a greater tendency to VUR and consequently more easily convert a lower into an upper urinary tract infection. A 10-day course of oral antibacterial treatment is needed.

The choice of antibacterial agent depends on the sensitivity of the urinary isolate, any past history of hypersensitivity reactions in the patient, the use of a drug that is largely excreted in the urine and one that will not accumulate dangerously and cause toxicity if the patient has chronic renal failure.

If it is decided to use long-term suppressive therapy, it is very important to avoid drugs like nitrofurantoin. This can cause peripheral neuropathy, eosinophilic lung infiltrates or irreversible pulmonary fibrosis when given to a patient with only marginal renal decompensation.

Long-term suppressive therapy

Absolute indications for long-term suppressive therapy include the infant or young child certainly up to the age of 5 years who has had recurrent infections, a serious upper UTI with pyelonephritis or who is known to have VUR and bacteriuria. The pregnant woman with recurrent infection also requires suppressive antibiotics.

Relative indications include a patient at any age who has both recurrent bacteriuria and VUR or chronic pyelonephritis. Occasionally patients with an obstructive uropathy which for some reason cannot be corrected surgically may benefit from long-term therapy. There are also patients with recurrent or relapsing bacteriuria whose urinary tracts are anatomically normal who may require long-term treatment. There may be justification sometimes to give suppressive antibiotics for a month or two to ease the problem of genuine post-coital cystitis if self-help measures have failed. An alternative regimen, much used in the USA, is for the patient to take the antibiotic only after each act of intercourse.

Patients with neuropathic bladders, indwelling catheters,

a reduced bladder volume from radiotherapy or interstitial cystitis or those with ileal conduits should not receive long-term suppressive chemotherapy but be treated only when they have symptoms highly suggestive of urinary infection together with proven bacteriuria.

The suppressive dose usually employed is one-quarter (or occasionally one-half) of that given for the management of an acute episode. Thus the patient whose acute infection might be treated with 500 mg ampicillin every 6 h should receive a long-term dose of 500 mg ampicillin daily. The drug is best given in the late evening before retiring so that, in the patient without nocturia at least, a high antibacterial concentration remains in the urine for a prolonged period.

The question of how long is long-term? is best answered by considering the reason why the long-term medication was originally supplied. For example, when the infant has grown up to be a 4–5-year-old, when the expectant mother has delivered or when the patient put on suppressive treatment because of recurrent infections has been symptom- and bacteriuria-free for some months or years, then treatment may be discontinued. The patient should however be encouraged to attend regular follow-up appointments for urine culture. In some individuals long-term suppressive therapy may be given almost indefinitely, again providing careful follow-up arrangements are made. Monitoring for antibacterial agent toxicity during follow-up is very important when suppressive therapy is supplied.

Long-term oral cephalosporin treatment often causes vaginal thrush. More serious are the neurological and pulmonary complications of nitrofurantoin, the psychogenic problems with cycloserine and the solar sensitivity and subjective ocular symptoms with long-term quinolones like nalidixic acid.

Individual antibacterial agents

Only a selection of the many possible drugs can be given (Tables 51.1 and 51.2). Which one to choose depends on individual circumstances. In women of child-bearing potential it is better to use drugs known to be safe in pregnancy. In women taking a low-dose oestrogen contraceptive, the interaction with drugs like rifampicin must be remembered and also in a few there may be a possible reduction in the contraceptive effect of the pill with high doses of ampicillin.

Table 51.1 Antibacterial agents for intravenous use in acute pyelonephritis (doses for adults with normal renal function)

Drug	Dose	Dose interval (h)
Gentamicin	1–1.7 mg/kg	8
Co-trimoxazole	960 mg	12
Cefotaxime	1–2 g	8–12
Ceftazidime	1–2 g	8
Augmentin	1.2 g	6–8
Ciprofloxacin	100 mg	12

Table 51.2 Oral antibacterial agents for acute lower urinary tract infection and chronic pyelonephritis. The doses are for adults with normal renal function. For long-term suppressive therapy the stated dose is given once only at night

Drug	Treatment course		Suppressive dose
	Dose (mg)	Frequency (times daily)	(mg nocte)
Ampicillin	500	4	500
Amoxycillin	500	3	250
Augmentin	375	3	375
Trimethoprim	200	2	200
Co-trimoxazole	960	2	480
Cephalexin	500	4	500
Cephradine	500	4	500
Nitrofurantoin	50–100	3	50
Nalidixic acid	500	4	500
Ciprofloxacin	250–500	2	250

URINARY TRACT TUBERCULOSIS

There may occasionally be an underlying tuberculous infection of the urinary tract in patients who also show significant bacteriuria with expected urinary tract pathogens like *E. coli*, *Proteus* spp. or enterococci. Diagnostic suspicion should be high in immigrant families who have come from a country where there is still much tuberculosis; any patient with a suspect chest X-ray; so-called 'sterile' pyuria or frank haematuria, or a strongly positive tuberculin test outside the context of a recent BCG immunization.

In addition to an abnormal chest X-ray, there is usually a characteristic appearance on intravenous urography, often showing hydronephrosis and/or a small bladder with a straight or stretched-looking ureter in between. An autonephrectomy may already have taken place with loss of function on one side. Calcium often lies over the renal shadow. Six early-morning urine cultures should be taken for acid-fast bacilli and a tuberculin test performed.

Apart from possible surgical relief of obstruction or insertion of a stent in the lower ureter to prevent obliteration by fibrosis, antituberculous chemotherapy should start as soon as the diagnosis is reasonably certain. A 3-week course of prednisolone 20 mg daily at the start of antituberculous chemotherapy helps to keep the lower ureter patent.

Four-drug treatment is usually recommended, with modification to two-drug treatment in 2 months when the results of the sensitivity of the tubercle bacilli are known. A total of 9 months' chemotherapy is given providing that one of the drugs used is rifampicin. Depending on the patient's weight, standard once-daily doses of isoniazid, rifampicin, ethambutol and pyrazinamide should be given initially. Because of the teratogenic potential of antituberculous drugs, expert advice should be sought in the choice of chemotherapy for a pregnant patient with urinary tract tuberculosis. Isoniazid and ethambutol are probably the least likely to upset the fetus. A radiographic check of the patency of the urinary collecting system should be made after a few weeks of treatment to ensure free drainage. Surgical intervention will be necessary if obstruction occurs.

Tuberculosis is a notifiable infectious disease in the UK. Although renal tuberculosis is rarely infectious to the patient's contacts it is important to notify the community medicine specialist so that other members of the family can be screened for occult infection.

URINARY TRACT SCHISTOSOMIASIS (BILHARZIA)

As with urinary tract tuberculosis, routine coliform pathogens may also be found in the urine of a patient with underlying schistosomiasis. This helmintic infestation is contracted from washing or bathing in fresh water harbouring the cercerial stage of the life cycle of *Schistosoma haematobium*. The cercaria penetrate the skin, migrate to the liver where the sexual forms copulate and the gravid female then moves to the venous plexuses around the bladder or rectum. There she lays her eggs whose tiny spines erode through the bladder wall and enter the urine to be shed during micturition. The life cycle of the worm is completed by the rupture of the ova in fresh water, releasing a ciliated miracidium which finds its way into a fresh-water snail. There it undergoes asexual reproduction and emerges as a free swimming cercaria ready to invade another human being.

This disease cannot spread in the UK. It is usually acquired in the Near East, East Africa and South America. Early symptoms which may be ignored by the patient are of 'swimmer's itch' at the site of entry of the cercaria. Months or years later terminal haematuria may be noted, especially by the male. Damage with chronic inflammation, calcification and fibrosis can take place throughout the urinary tract leading to obstructive uropathy, a tiny non-distensible bladder and renal failure. At the same time the worm load in the liver may cause chronic cirrhosis with portal hypertension.

Diagnosis is made by finding schistosomal ova in terminal specimens of urine or in a biopsy taken at proctoscopy from what may appear to be a healthy rectal mucosa. A characteristic heaped-up appearance may be seen on the inflamed bladder lining at cystoscopy and again biopsy may reveal ova. There is usually but not invariably an eosinophilia. A schistosomal enzyme-linked immunosorbent assay test should be positive within a few months of contracting the infestation.

If treatment is given promptly and the worm load is not huge, cure can be effected with a single oral dose of praziquantel. Assuming that the individual is not re-exposed to the infestation, a second dose of praziquantel is rarely needed.

KEY POINTS

1. Urinary infections are a significant cause of morbidity in women aged 20–65 years.
2. Infections can present with only 10^2 or 10^3 organisms per ml of urine, and even in the presence of sterile urine.
3. Up to 80% of recurrent infections are re-infection.
4. Between 10–30% of women with asymptomatic bacteriuria develop acute pyelonephritis during pregnancy.
5. Pre-disposing factors include diabetes mellitus, foreign body, instrumentation of the urinary tract and incomplete bladder emptying.
6. Prevention entails a high standard of perineal hygiene, avoidance of vaginal deodorants and bubble baths.
7. Management includes drinking at least 2 litres of fluid a day, regular and complete bladder emptying and voiding after intercourse.
8. Asymptomatic bacteriuria may not require treatment unless there is vesico-ureteric reflux, renal scarring or in a failing to thrive infant.
9. Symptomatic lower urinary infection requires at least a 7 day course of antibiotic and follow-up within 2–3 weeks.
10. Urinary tract infection in a patient with a neuropathic bladder, indwelling catheter or ileal conduit, should only be treated when it is symptomatic or there is proven bacteriuria.
11. Note that certain antibiotics may reduce the effectiveness of the oral contraceptive pill.

FURTHER READING

Ascher A W, Brumfitt W (eds) 1986 Microbial diseases in nephrology. John Wiley, Chichester

Maskell R 1988 Urinary tract infection in clinical and laboratory practice. Edward Arnold, London

Merrick M V, Uttley W S, Wild. 1977 A comparison of two techniques of detecting vesico-ureteric reflux. British Journal of Radiology 50: 792–795

Monsour M, Azmy A F, MacKenzie J R 1987 Renal scarring secondary to vesico-ureteric reflux. Critical assessment and new grading. British Journal of Urology 70: 320–324

Nimmo M J, Merrick M V, Allan P L 1987 Measurement of relative renal function. A comparison of methods and assessment of reproducibility. British Journal of Radiology 60: 861–864

Smith C C, Morris L, Wallace E T, Gray J A 1973 Comparison of two commercially available dipinocula with standard bacteriological assessment of bacteriuria. British Journal of Urology 45: 323–326

52. Frequency and urgency in the female

A. Peattie

INTRODUCTION

Frequency and urgency are symptoms of urinary disease that may be attributable to a number of situations. It is important to be aware of the differing possible causes when planning investigation and treatment. Frequency is defined as the passage of urine more than seven times during the waking hours and/or being awoken from sleep twice or more to micturate, whilst urgency is a sudden, strong desire to micturate which if not relieved may lead to urge incontinence.

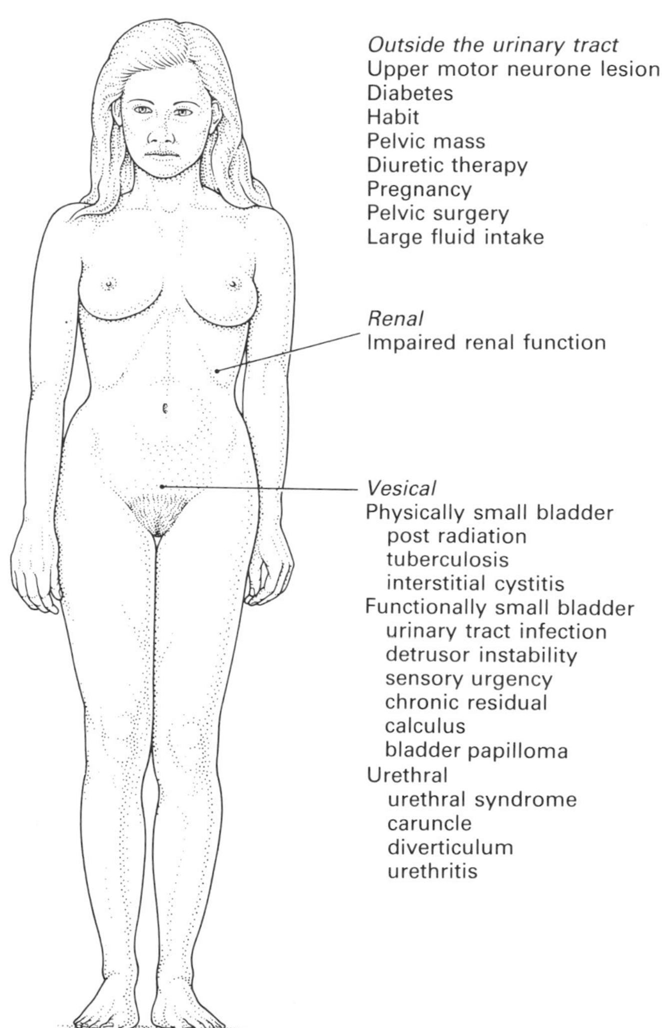

Fig. 52.1 Aetiology of frequency and urgency.

Prevalence

In 1980, Bungay et al conducted an epidemiological study of 1120 women and reported that about 20% complained of frequency whilst 15% reported urgency; neither symptom altered significantly with increasing age. It is probable that the size of the problem is at present underestimated as Norton and colleagues (1988) found that embarrassment prevents many women seeking help despite severe urinary symptoms.

Aetiology

The problem may arise from the bladder, the urethra or disease outside the urinary tract (Fig. 52.1). The bladder may be physically or functionally small due to a number of causes. The urethral syndrome or a urethral diverticulum may give rise to these symptoms as may diabetes mellitus or insipidus.

DISEASE OUTSIDE THE URINARY TRACT

Many conditions affecting the urinary tract do not seem directly related to it but produce their effect by a variety of ways. The pregnant patient may well complain of urinary frequency as one of her first indicators of pregnancy. A pelvic mass produces symptoms by filling the pelvis, leaving little room for the bladder; the amount of urine produced will affect the number of times the bladder needs to be emptied. Diuretic therapy increases urinary output and is therefore best taken in the morning. Diabetes mellitus and insipidus will be associated with urinary frequency due to increased urinary output. Similarly an excessive fluid intake will produce frequency: some patients drink large quantities by habit or have a psychiatric disorder. The usual daily fluid intake is around 2 litres which varies according to climate and social circumstances. A daily intake of greater than 3 litres will automatically lead to greater urinary production and apparent frequency.

Fluid charting is of great value in determining this problem. The patient records her fluid intake and urinary production over a period of 7 days. Figure 52.2 illustrates a typical case of excessive intake leading to urinary frequency. The treatment involves an explanation to the patient of why she has frequency and if she feels unable to drink less often, she should drink smaller amounts to keep fluid intake to approximately 2 litres every 24 hours.

DAY: TUES 24 MARCH

TIME	INTAKE (ml)	OUTPUT (ml)	LEAKAGE ACTIVITY	Amount	Urge	Wet Bed
7^{30}		350				
7^{40}	100					
8^{00}		100				
8^{00}	240					
8^{40}		250				
9^{00}	150		SNEEZING	1	NO	
10^{00}	180					
10^{15}		275				
10^{30}	180					
11^{00}	240					
11^{30}		250				
12^{00}	240					
12^{30}	80					
13^{15}		180				
14^{00}	150					
15^{00}	150		RUNNING	1	NO	
15^{15}		250				
16^{30}	80					
18^{00}	150					
19^{00}		300				
19^{30}	300					
20^{00}	300					
20^{15}		180				
20^{30}	300					
21^{00}	100					
21^{30}		400				
21^{40}	100					
22^{10}		200				
23^{00}		200				
03^{00}		250ml				
TOTAL	3040	3185				

Fig. 52.2 Urinary diary showing excess intake of fluid.

Post surgery

Radical hysterectomy is known to cause bladder and urethral dysfunction possibly due to disruption of the pelvic plexus of nerves supplying the lower urinary tract. Reports of the incidence of bladder disturbance vary from 16 to 80% but the range of problems is wide and includes genuine stress incontinence, frequency and urgency, detrusor instability, voiding disorders and disturbed urethral function. When frequency and urgency are the main problems, infection, detrusor instability and urethral instability must all be considered so urine culture and urodynamic studies will be necessary before appropriate treatment can be carried out.

RENAL DISEASE

Polyuria is one of the signs of chronic renal failure and if suspected, measurement of the blood urea and electrolyte concentration and creatinine clearance will indicate the degree of renal dysfunction. A midstream urine specimen (MSU) may reveal bacterial infection and granular casts and urine osmolality should be noted.

VESICAL DISEASE

The physically small bladder

Chronic inflammation

Tuberculosis. Bladder lesions are always secondary to

renal tuberculosis with infection starting around the ureteric orifice. There is inflammation with granulation and ulceration of the mucous membrane. Fibrous tissue forms in the bladder wall leading to contraction of the bladder and a reduced capacity. An intravenous urogram is appropriate as bladder changes are never present without changes in the radiological appearances of the pelvicaliceal system. By this stage treatment will not be able to reverse the changes in the bladder; a small contracted bladder may need an augmentation procedure to treat the frequency.

Interstitial cystitis. This chronic condition presents with severe frequency, urgency, lower abdominal pain, dysuria and haematuria in the absence of bacterial cystitis. It was originally described by Hunner (1914, 1915) in a group of women with prolonged symptoms of cystitis: At cystoscopy Hunner found ulcers with a granulomatous base and surrounding hyperaemia. He also reported white scars of the bladder urothelium, again surrounded by a hyperaemic area which bled when touched. Some authors consider the cystoscopic findings to be characteristic (Editorial 1972) but Hunner felt the most characteristic feature was the discrepancy between the severity of symptoms and the relatively minor findings at cystoscopy. The lack of agreement in the reports of prevalence suggest that diagnostic criteria may vary — from 5% (Hand 1949) to 50% prevalence in patients with recurrent cystitis (Hanash & Pool 1970). Biopsy of the lesion shows chronic non-specific ulceration but a number of authors have reported a prominent infiltration with mast cells (Larsen et al 1982). Unfortunately this finding has not led to improved results with treatment and a recent study could find no evidence to support the diagnosis of interstitial cystitis as an autoimmune disorder but proposed that the findings were probably an immunological response to the disease (Anderson et al 1989).

Many different treatments have been tried but with singularly little success. Hunner (1930) tried surgical removal of the affected portion of the bladder but recurrence was common and made surgery unacceptable. Instillations of silver nitrate or dimethylsulphoxide have given some relief but again recurrence of symptoms is common. As pain is a feature, denervation of the bladder or bilateral sacral neurectomy has been reported but again with poor results. Cystodistension seemed to show promise but again symptomatic relief was only transient (Badenoch 1971). Psychiatric therapy has been tried as many patients were found to have high emotional or neurotic symptom scores but the chronicity and severity of symptoms may account for this finding. This chronic condition is notoriously difficult to manage and patients usually become long-term attenders at clinics.

Post radiation

Pelvic irradiation is the treatment of choice in the later stages of carcinoma of the cervix and although the dose and method of administration are planned to minimize the dose received by the bladder, radiation cystitis is a not infrequent complication of therapy. The patient has frequency, urgency and suprapubic pain, which usually settle with symptomatic treatment. In more severe cases haematuria may be noted but with a high fluid throughput this should settle spontaneously. Fibrosis may result causing a physically small bladder with decreased bladder wall compliance, resulting in frequency of micturition which in severe cases may need urinary diversion or bladder augmentation. Cystoscopy reveals a whitened bladder mucosa with telangiectasia characteristic of the irradiated bladder. If the bladder capacity at cystoscopy is 300 ml or greater then by adjustment of fluid load the patient should be able to achieve a frequency of micturition that is acceptable.

The functionally smaller bladder

Acute inflammation

The patient commonly presents with frequency, dysuria, suprapubic pain and hesitancy. She may also have a fever, loin pain and haematuria but symptoms alone are not enough for a diagnosis of cystitis due to urinary tract infection. Bacteriological examination of the urine reveals pus cells indicative of inflammation and significant bacteriuria ($>10^5$ organisms/ml). Treatment initially is a high fluid intake (approx 3 l/day) and appropriate antibiotics. Once an MSU has been sent for culture and sensitivity it is appropriate to treat the symptomatic patient with trimethoprim, amoxycillin or nitrofurantoin. Symptomatic relief may be obtained with potassium citrate or sodium bicarbonate. For women with recurrent problems advice about perineal toilet and advice to void before and after sexual intercourse are simple measures that may be helpful.

Detrusor instability

Detrusor instability or motor urge incontinence is characterized by involuntary detrusor contractions which the patient cannot completely suppress. The commonest presenting symptoms are frequency and urgency. The diagnosis is made by subtracted cystometry. This topic is discussed further in Chapter 48.

Sensory urgency

This condition has to date received scant attention in urodynamic texts, despite being a management problem. The patient complains of urgency but on cystometric testing no abnormality is detected — more specifically, detrusor instability is absent. The incidence is difficult to determine as presumably the condition is often managed and therefore also classed with motor urge incontinence or detrusor instability. In our urodynamic unit we found an incidence of 6% sensory urgency compared to 31% detrusor instability. It is difficult to justify treating these patients similarly as it is recognized that anticholinergic medication for detrusor instability has troublesome side-effects and poor results.

Neither cystometry nor urethral pressure measurement provides helpful information about bladder neck activity. Recently, a new method of investigation, urethral electric conductance (UEC), has shown bladder neck opening to correlate well with the patient's symptoms (Peattie et al 1988). UEC takes advantage of the fact that urothelium and urine have different electric impedance and with a specially designed conductivity catheter, this difference can be used to detect opening of the bladder neck. We employed the new technique of UEC to investigate bladder neck movements in our patients. In sensory urgency the recording obtained showed marked variation associated with the sensation of urgency.

A positive diagnosis becomes useful if we have an appropriate treatment for the problem and by using the recording as a form of biofeedback good results have been obtained.

URETHRAL CONDITIONS

Urethral syndrome

This term has been applied to symptoms of frequency, urgency, dysuria and voiding disorder where no cause can be found and symptoms persist despite all attempts at treatment. At initial presentation, the patient is often misdiagnosed as having a urinary tract infection. Treatment with antibiotics may give symptomatic relief but the symptoms always return and may become refractory to antibiotic therapy. The other common feature is pain suprapubically, often described as a feeling of pressure and relieved by micturition. Sometimes the pain is more localized in the vagina or the urethra and relief of pain is thought to be associated with relaxation of the urethral sphincter. The spectrum of symptoms includes hesitancy, dribbling and an intermittent stream during voiding so it was proposed that dysfunction of the urethral sphincter may be causative. Urethral swabs for *Chlamydia* are negative.

Urodynamic investigation has revealed a high urethral pressure in some of these patients (Raz & Smith 1976; McGuire 1978) which may be associated with increased anal sphincter tone. On passage of a urethral catheter, resistance will be noted and movement of the catheter may replicate the patient's symptoms. Palpation of the levatores ani may also produce symptoms which the patient can learn to control by relaxing the levatores. Not all patients with urethral syndrome have urodynamic evidence of sphincter dysfunction. Other investigators have assessed the sensitivity of the urethral mucosa and demonstrated hypersensitivity in patients with frequency, dysuria and associated suprapubic discomfort (Powell et al 1981). They propose that treatment should be directed towards reducing this urethral hypersensitivity by surgical or pharmacological means.

Urethral diverticulum

A urethral diverticulum can cause frequency and urgency. It is believed to arise from inflammation in the paraurethral glands and is found mainly in parous patients. The diverticulum is found on the posterior wall and may be tender on vaginal examination. Pus can sometimes be milked out of the urethra and appropriate antibiotic therapy should be started before surgical excision.

HISTORY

Patients presenting with urinary frequency and urgency need to be questioned about associated incontinence which may imply the presence of detrusor instability. Dysuria can be found with urinary tract infection, urethral syndrome or a urethral caruncle and if haematuria is present then bladder carcinoma, calculus, urinary tract infection or interstitial cystitis must be excluded. There may be predisposing factors to urinary tract infection that can be elicited from the history, e.g. first intercourse ('honeymoon cystitis'), use of the contraceptive diaphragm and recurrent episodes of infection possibly associated with bladder calculus or renal disease. A voiding disorder due to bladder or pelvic floor dysfunction may be suspected with complaints of hesitancy, poor stream and incomplete bladder emptying, though a pelvic mass must also be ruled out.

From the gynaecological history the last menstrual period must be ascertained as pregnancy is a well recognized cause of urinary frequency. The past medical history will reveal any previous pelvic surgery as a cause for the complaint and a history of diuretic intake may explain diurnal frequency.

EXAMINATION

A general abdominal examination should rule out a full bladder, pelvic mass or pregnancy whilst a brief neurological assessment is essential to exclude an upper motor neurone lesion with special attention to the S2–4 dermatomes which inform about innervation of the bladder.

Pelvic examination may reveal a urethral caruncle whilst the sight of pus at the external urethral meatus after examination may suggest a urethral diverticulum. Tenderness on bimanual palpation of the bladder may be found with interstitial cystitis whilst tenderness on palpation of the pelvic floor muscles has been found in the urethral syndrome. A large fibroid uterus, ovarian cyst or pregnancy may produce symptoms by pressure on the bladder.

INVESTIGATIONS

MSU

This should be the first test to exclude any infection.

Urinary diary

Each patient should be asked to bring this with her before she attends for investigation. It is simple to complete and gives useful information. The patient records her fluid intake and output over the course of a week along with any episodes of urgency (Fig. 52.2). The record gives information on the frequency, volumes voided and average daily intake and output. It is a simple matter to correct any patient's bad habit by pointing out to her the excessive intake causing her urinary frequency.

Miscellaneous

Blood tests for renal function and urine osmolality may be appropriate. If acute urethritis is suspected then a urethral swab will be needed and in patients with a history of having delivered an infant over 4.5 kg, a glucose tolerance test may be indicated.

Subtracted cystometry

Having ruled out infection or the more obvious causes of symptoms, urodynamic tests are necessary. Subtracted cystometry will make a diagnosis of detrusor instability or genuine stress incontinence.

Urethral electric conductance

This test may be performed at the same time as cystometry and detects movement of fluid around the catheter. If the catheter is placed to record at the bladder neck in cases of sensory urgency or detrusor instability then distinct movements can be detected during times when the patient experiences urgency. In Figure 52.3 the arrows denote when the patient experiences urgency. This may imply that these two conditions are part of the same disease process; however, all cases of sensory urgency do not progress to detrusor instability.

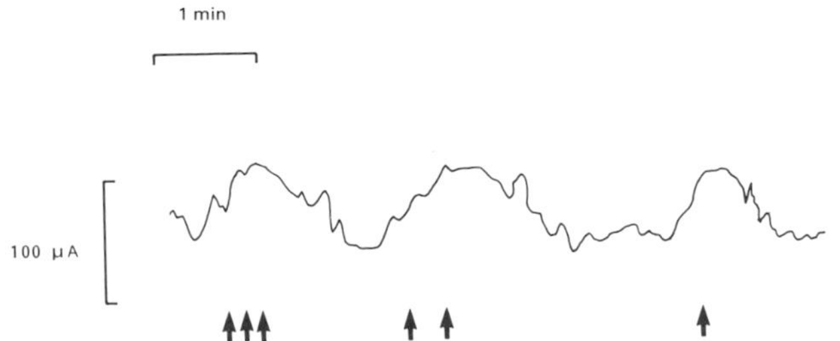

Fig. 52.3 Bladder neck urethral electric conductance, showing bladder neck opening on experiencing urgency.

Cystoscopy

This will be necessary in cases of recurrent urinary tract infection, suspected urethral syndrome, urethral diverticulum and interstitial cystitis.

TREATMENT

Treatment must be directed towards the cause with antibiotics for infection, restriction of fluid intake in renal failure, adjustment of diuretic therapy and neurological referral as appropriate.

Bladder training has been successfully employed in the management of urinary urgency. The patient uses timed voiding to overcome her urgency and by slowly increasing the time intervals between voids she can work up to an acceptable daily frequency. Jarvis (1982) reported that more than 50% of his group with sensory urgency were symptom-free and objectively dry 6 months after treatment with bladder drill. Frewen (1980) felt that voluntary frequency may be a factor in the genesis of detrusor instability and advocated bladder training in all cases of frequency and urgency, whether due to sensory urgency or detrusor instability.

Biofeedback is the process of providing visual or auditory evidence of the status of an autonomic bodily function so that the patient may exert control over that function. It has been in use for a number of years in the management of detrusor instability; the patient learns to control detrusor pressure rises (Cardozo et al 1978). The rises in electrical conductivity associated with urgency are due to movement of urine around the catheter as a result of opening of the bladder neck; this may be a very early stage in the genesis of a detrusor contraction. If patients could be taught to close the bladder neck this reduced the conductivity reading and was associated with the abolition of the sensation of urgency. After a course of biofeedback therapy using bladder neck conductivity all patients who became asymptomatic returned to normal variation in the conductivity recording and 93% were cured of symptoms.

Drug therapy for urgency is the same as that employed in cases of detrusor instability and centres around the anticholinergics, though often if no abnormality is found on investigation imipramine is used as first-line therapy for its anticholinergic and specific bladder effect. Oxybutynin or propantheline may have a place in the treatment of these patients, as may the newer terodiline which employs synergism between calcium blocking and anticholinergic effects to achieve a greater action on the bladder for fewer side-effects.

SUMMARY

The causes of urinary frequency and urgency in the female are numerous. Some conditions are readily amenable to treatment but others have a chronic course where only symptomatic relief is available. It is essential in all patients with frequency and urgency, to elicit from the history and examination the most likely causes of their symptoms and then to investigate accordingly. Success in alleviating symptoms depends on appropriate treatment or, in cases where a cause cannot be found, a detailed explanation with symptomatic treatment.

KEY POINTS

1. Frequency and urgency are common symptoms but embarrassment or a feeling that these symptoms are normal prevents many women seeking advice.
2. Frequency and urgency can be caused by many lesions outside the urinary tract.
3. The urinary diary is a simple and inexpensive investigation and also serves as a basis for treatment.
4. Simple treatment measures such as antibiotics for urinary tract infection, flow restriction and adjustment of diuretic therapy may be all that is required.

REFERENCES

Anderson J B, Parivar F, Lee G et al 1989 The enigma of interstitial cystitis — an autoimmune disease? British Journal of Urology 63: 58–63

Badenoch A W 1971 Chronic interstitial cystitis. British Journal of Urology 43: 718–720

Bungay G T, Vessey M P, McPherson C K 1980 Study of symptoms in middle life with special reference to the menopause. British Medical Journal 281: 181–183

Cardozo L D, Stanton S L, Hafner J, Allan V 1978 Biofeedback in the treatment of detrusor instability. British Journal of Urology 50: 250–254

Editorial 1972 Interstitial cystitis. British Medical Journal 1: 644

Frewen R K 1980 The management of urgency and frequency of micturition. British Journal of Urology 52: 367–369

Hanash K A, Pool T L 1970 Interstitial and haemorrhagic cystitis: viral, bacterial and fungal studies. Journal of Urology 104: 705–706

Hand J R 1949 Interstitial cystitis: report of 223 cases. Journal of Urology 61: 291–292

Hunner G L 1914 A rare bladder ulcer in women. Transactions of the Southern Surgical and Gynecological Association 27: 247

Hunner G L 1915 A rare type of bladder ulcer in women: report of cases. Boston Medical and Surgical Journal 172: 660

Hunner G L 1930 Neurosis of the bladder. Journal of Urology 24: 567

Jarvis G J 1982 The management of urinary incontinence due to primary vesical sensory urgency by bladder drill. British Journal of Urology 54: 374–376

Larsen S, Thompson S A, Hald T 1982 Mast cells in interstitial cystitis. British Journal of Urology 54: 283–286

McGuire E J 1978 Reflex urethral instability. British Journal of Urology 50: 200–204

Norton P A, MacDonald L D, Sedgwick P M, Stanton S L 1988 Distress and delay associated with urinary incontinence, frequency and urgency in women. British Medical Journal 297: 1187–1189

Peattie A B, Plevnik S, Stanton S L 1988 What is the current needed to close the gate? Journal of the Royal Society of Medicine 81: 442–444

Powell P H, George N J R, Smith P J B, Feneley R C L 1981 The hypersensitive female urethra — a cause of recurrent frequency and dysuria. Proceedings of the International Continence Society 11th AGM, Lund pp 81–82

Raz S, Smith R B 1976 External sphincter spasticity syndrome in females. Journal of Urology 115: 443–446

53. Fistulae

C. Hudson

DEFINITION

Abnormal communications between viscera lined by epithelium are known as fistulae. Fistulous communications wherever they occur throughout the body are liable to give rise to pathological disturbance of function and are frequently associated with unpleasant symptoms. Before epithelialization is complete an abnormal communication between viscera will generally tend to close provided that the natural passages are unobstructed. Unfortunately for the genital tract, the process of continence involves the physiological intermittent obstruction of the natural passages, with intermittent rises in intraluminal pressure due to peristalsis or other mural muscular activity (e.g. contraction of the detrusor muscle). As a result only a small number of relatively insignificant genital fistulae will close spontaneously.

ANATOMY

Fistulae to the genital tract can occur from any adjacent viscus (bladder, ureter, urethra, rectum, anal canal). They may also involve any mobile loop of intestine — most commonly, terminal ileum or rectosigmoid colon; rarely other loops may be involved including stomach. Fistulae may enter any part of the genital tract from the vulva to the oviduct; those of clinical significance due to defective continence almost always involve the vagina and in some instances the level of the fistula may be critical.

Other fistulae, although rare, are important as sources of diagnostic confusion and therapeutic difficulty. For instance, adnexal inflammatory conditions are unlikely to be cured by medical means alone if associated with an unrecognized salpingocolic fistula, such as may occur with chronic specific infection due to actinomycosis or tuberculosis.

Fistulae may be multiple with several tracks, particularly after attempts at surgical repair. They may also be complex involving an intervening cavity so that the fistulous nature of the inflammatory mass may not be immediately obvious. Such fistulae may also have additional external communications, such as a sinus to an abdominal wound. Finally multi-organ fistulae are quite common. Dual involvement of the bowel and urinary tract is regularly seen and concurrent involvement of both the ureter and bladder in certain strategically placed or large urinary fistulae occurs.

AETIOLOGY

Apart from differential diagnosis, congenital fistulae are

outside the scope of this chapter. They involve maldevelopment of the metanephric system or the proctodeum. Some examples of ectopic ureter may discharge into the vagina (the vaginal ectopic ureter). This abnormality may represent reduplication of the pelvicalyceal system on one or both sides, or ectopy of a single ureter on one side. Curiously the diagnosis may be delayed until adult life if the abnormal ureter is draining only a small pyelonephritic portion of kidney tissue. The diagnosis may be extremely elusive because such tissue may be insufficient to show up as a soft tissue shadow and so poorly functional that contrast will not be sufficiently concentrated for visualization. A high index of clinical suspicion is required if the appropriate esoteric investigations are to be requested. There is in fact little substitute for careful and painstaking examination under anaesthesia using a probe to explore every possible crevice in the lower genital tract.

Abnormal communication between the bowel and the vagina associated with congenital malformation of the anorectal region is, however, rather more common. The investigation and management of most of these lesions lie within the realm of the paediatric surgeon and some require initial surgery in the early neonatal period. Clinical obstetricians and gynaecologists will need to be aware of the elements of this complex subject as they may well find themselves the first point of reference in the diagnosis and assessment of a newborn infant with an obvious anogenital malformation. The critical factor is usually the presence or absence of the rectum (rectal agenesis). Complete rectal agenesis is associated with a high stenotic rectovaginal fistula and early diversion is required. By contrast the simplest and most distal lesion amounting to no more than a covered anus may respond to simple dilatation. Clinicians should be aware that an ill considered 'cut-back' operation can seriously jeopardize future continence. This procedure should only be undertaken after full local evaluation with assessment of concealed anal sphincter function. In practice an anteriorly displaced anus even involving the navicular fossa may need no intervention until after puberty as satisfactory toilet control is usually achievable.

ACQUIRED FISTULAE

Acquired fistulae may arise from pathological conditions in either of the two viscera concerned or from external events common to both. The recognized divisions are given below:

1. Obstetric
   a. Necrosis.
   b. Laceration.
2. Trauma
   a. Surgical.
   b. Other.
3. Inflammatory
   a. Genital.
   b. Intestinal.
4. Malignancy
   a. Intestinal.
   b. Genital.
   c. Metastatic.
5. Irradiation.
6. Combinations.

MECHANISM OF FISTULA FORMATION

Direct trauma may be acute, such as inadvertent surgical penetration, or chronic from ulceration, for instance due to a foreign body. Acute trauma may be penetrating or associated with a stripping injury of the adjacent viscus. It is the latter type of injury which, even though recognized and repaired at the time, is more likely to result in fistula formation as there is an indeterminate degree of damage to the adjacent hitherto healthy tissue. The fistulae resulting from penetrating trauma are usually small, short and relatively unscarred. Fibrosis will to some extent depend upon extravasation of the contents of the adjacent viscus. For instance, if at hysterectomy the bladder is inadvertently injured at some distance from the vaginal vault, extravasation of urine into the intraperitoneal space will occur and discharge from the vaginal vault may be delayed. Extravasation of urine provokes an extreme inflammatory response and the walls of the 'urinoma' may take some time to settle down. This situation would be in direct contrast to the natural history of a direct leak from trauma discovered in the immediate recovery phase.

Much more difficult, however, are fistulae associated with tissue loss. Such loss may arise from the genital tract or the adjacent viscus or both. The major cause of tissue loss is ischaemia commonly compounded by infection. The most obvious example is the pressure necrosis which is the mechanism of the majority of obstetric fistulae. This results from neglected obstructed labour with compression of vulnerable soft parts between the advancing fetal head and the bony pelvis. Irradiation injury is another cause of fistula formation by ischaemia. The periarteritis associated with ionizing irradiation in therapeutic dosage proceeds over many years and may be aetiological in fistula formation years after the primary malignancy has been treated. Not only does this ischaemia produce the fistulae, it also causes significant damage in the adjacent tissues so that ordinary surgical repair is not only doomed to failure but stands a significant risk of making the fistula worse.

Tissue loss may also be occasioned by destruction with malignant disease arising from any of the adjacent viscera, usually cervix, vagina or rectum — rarely bladder. Local tissue destruction occurs with inflammatory fistulae, but these are rarely of great size; the major problem is the existence of infective granulations, which will never heal while the basic inflammatory process is uncontrolled.

In all situations, therefore, in which a fistula has been caused by anything other than simple trauma, including obstetric fistulae and tissue loss, the pathology of the tissues involved is of paramount importance. Quite commonly more than one pathological condition may be present and it can be extremely difficult to elucidate the situation.

The common pathologies associated with genital fistula are listed below:

1. Malignant disease.
2. Prior irradiation
3. Schistosomiasis
4. Lymphogranuloma venereum (lymphopathia venereum).
5. Tuberculosis.
6. Actinomycosis.
7. Crohn's disease of ileum, colon or anorectum.
8. Ulcerative colitis.
9. Diverticular disease.

EPIDEMIOLOGY

In countries where deficient maternity services continue to produce a significant number of genital fistulae following neglected obstructed labour, there are ethnic variations in pelvic shape which increase the likelihood of obstructed labour. The situation is aggravated if the practice of childhood pregnancy is prevalent. Injuries to the urinary tract (vesicovaginal fistulae) are much more common than obstetric injuries to the anorectum. However, in the worst cases dual fistulae may be present.

In developed countries, traumatic fistulae are the most common; surgery is the prime cause. Any pelvic specialty may be involved, but the majority tend to following gynaecological operations, both abdominal and vaginal. Other trauma is rare, but penetrating injuries in children should not be overlooked. Coital injury following genital surgery may sometimes result in fistula formation. In parts of the world where female circumcision is still a practice, this barbarous habit can result in fistulae.

Of the inflammatory fistulae, Crohn's disease is by far the most important underlying cause. Crohn's disease is a disorder of the western world and appears to be increasing. A total fistula rate approaching 40% has been reported and in females the involvement of the genital tract may be 7%. Ulcerative colitis has a small incidence of low rectovaginal fistulae. Diverticular disease can produce colovaginal fistulae and rarely colouterine fistulae with surprisingly few symptoms attributable to the intestinal pathology. The possibility should not be overlooked if an elderly woman becomes incontinent without concomitant urinary problems. Schistosomiasis and tuberculosis would be very rare causes of genital fistula formation, exceptionally so in the western world. Genital actinomycosis has seen an increase in prevalence associated with the use of the intrauterine contraceptive device. It may be associated with multiple and complicated fistulae.

PRESENTATION

Most fistulae present with incontinence of urine or intestinal content. The diagnosis is then made by finding the orifice through which the efflux is detectable. Difficulty arises if either the history is atypical or the orifice is small, elusive or occasionally completely invisible.

History

With urinary fistulae, the history is less likely to be misleading. Small high vesicovaginal fistulae may only leak when the bladder is full, and ureteric fistulae, one would suppose, would not drain more than half the total volume of voided urine. Even this can be misleading because if the ureter has been partly occluded before the obstruction breaks down to form a fistula, there will have been impairment of renal function and in the recovery phase an increased volume of dilute urine will be lost which can be well in excess of 50% of the urine output. In rare instances ureteric injury can occur without obstruction as a side leak from the ureteric tube. This can be very difficult to diagnose as excretion urography may be entirely normal. Moreover the loss through the fistula may be confined to a time when the bladder is full with compression of the distal intramural ureter. Finally vesicouterine fistula — an uncommon complication of caesarean section — may produce no incontinence at all; such cases may however present with cyclical haematuria at the time of menstruation.

Sometimes a very watery discharge, even one with small bowel contents, has been mistaken for a urinary leak. Biochemical analysis of the fluid will disclose whether the urea content is compatible with urine or of fluid derived from serum.

With intestinal fistulae the history may be much more misleading. A small communication with the large bowel may cause only an offensive discharge. This is particularly likely to be the case if there is an intervening abscess cavity when all that may be seen is pus. Even traumatic fistulae of obstetric origin may be rendered symptomless by the cicatrization of the vagina which occurs following sloughing. A small high posterior horseshoe-shaped fistula may only become apparent during division of constricting bands for the repair of a vesicovaginal fistula. Regrettably some have only been diagnosed following ureteric diversion and ureterosigmoid anastomosis; faecal urine then leaks from the vagina where only uncontaminated urine has previously leaked. The moral is that investigation of a patient with a fistula must always be pursued bearing in mind the possibility of a dual or complex fistula being present.

INVESTIGATIONS

Careful examination, if necessary under anaesthetic, may be required to determine the presence of a fistula. A malleable silver probe is invaluable for the exploration of nooks and crannies, often marked by the presence of a granulation, which can be the mouth of the fistula. If such a probe passes directly into the adjacent viscus such as the rectum, where it may be felt or seen via the proctoscope, or the bladder or urethra where it may be seen by a cystoscope the diagnosis is then obvious. With fistulous communications with a ureter or a more proximal loop of bowel (ileum, caecum, sigmoid colon) the end of the probe will not easily be detected by simple clinical examination. A sigmoid colonic loop, which is adherent in the pouch of Douglas and the seat of a fistula, is not amenable to inspection by a rigid sigmoidoscope and the proximal orifice may only be viewed by an appropriate flexible instrument. Imaging studies are therefore required. The same situation will obtain when a fistula to the uterus is suspected.

Imaging

Colpography

If a large foley catheter with a big balloon is distended in the lower vagina, injection of a non-viscous opaque medium under pressure may outline a fistulous track to an adjacent organ. However, failure to demonstrate a fistula by this means does not exclude its presence.

Fistulography

This is a special example of the X-ray technique commonly referred to as sinography. For small fistulae a ureteric catheter is a suitable vehicle through which to deliver the radiopaque dye; if the hole is large enough a small foley catheter may be used. This is particularly of value for fistulae for which there is an intervening abscess cavity, when the process is an extension of that already described for colpography. If a ureteric catheter will pass through a small vaginal aperture into an adjacent loop of bowel its nature may become apparent from the appearance of the mucous membranes and haustrations. Although the fistula may be demonstrated in this way, further imaging studies are required to demonstrate the underlying pathology.

Cystography

Cystography is not particularly helpful in the basic diagnosis of small fistulae, as a dye test carried out under direct vision is likely to be more sensitive. A cystogram is, however, occasionally useful in achieving a diagnosis of vesicouterine fistula, as a lateral view may show the cavity of the uterus filled with radiopaque dye behind the bladder.

Hysterography

If a patient with a vesicouterine fistula has no history of incontinence but rather tells of cyclical haematuria, contrast studies carried out through the uterus (hysterotrachelogram) may be more rewarding than cystography. Once again a lateral view is necessary to detect the anterior leak.

Excretion urography

This is an essential investigation for any urinary fistula, and indeed for any major fistula, whatever its site. Dilatation of an ureter may provide suspicion of a dual fistula involving the ureter in the wall of, say, a vesicovaginal fistula. Furthermore embarrassment of ureteric function is a common sequel to the underlying pathology present whenever a fistula occurs in relation to malignant disease or its treatment (irradiation or surgery). Knowledge of upper urinary tract status can have a profound influence on treatment measures to be adopted. Intravenous urography is essential for the diagnosis of ureteric fistula but, as indicated above, is not completely sensitive. Ureteric dilatation commonly indicates the side of an ureteric injury but this observation may be misleading in two situations. First, where a bilateral obstruction has arisen a fistula may allow its ureter to be decompressed and therefore be less dilated than its still obstructed fellow on the other side. Secondly, where a fistula occurs but nevertheless ureteric patency through to the bladder is maintained, there may well be no ureteric dilatation at all. However, the presence of a periureteric flare around the ureter is highly suggestive of extravasation at this site.

Intravenous urography is also an important part of the investigation where a congenital fistula (ectopic ureter) is suspected. It is essential, however, for radiologists to be aware of the potential diagnosis, as the clues suggesting an ectopic ureter may be very subtle indeed (see above).

Small bowel enema, barium enema and computerized tomography scan

Any or all of these may be required for the evaluation of the intestinal condition when an intestinal fistula above the anal canal or lowest part of the rectum is present. Evidence of Crohn's disease, neoplasia, diverticular disease or ulcerative colitis may be forthcoming.

Dye studies

Instillation of coloured dye (methylene blue) into the adjacent viscus is an important way of diagnosing small fistulae, particularly after an attempt at repair of a known fistula. The traditional 'three-swab test' has its limitations and the examination is best carried out with direct inspection, with or without prior cystography. It is important to be alert for leakage around the catheter which may spill back into the vagina creating the illusion of a fistula. It is also important to ensure that adequate distension of the bladder occurs as some fistulae do not leak until at least 200 ml of fluid has been instilled. Dye tests are less useful for intestinal fistulae and rectal distension via sigmoidoscope may be of more value if a patient is kept in a slight Trendelenburg position with clear fluid in the vagina through which bubbling can be detected.

For the detection of ureteric fistulae it is necessary to produce systemic discoloration of the urine by intravenous or oral ingestion of an appropriate agent (phenoxypyridine, methylene blue or indigo carmine). It is important that the patient should empty her bladder immediately before ingesting the dye and that an appropriate time should elapse to allow for the ureteric efflux to be discoloured before careful visual examination of the vagina is undertaken. This must be achieved before spontaneous micturition is permitted otherwise staining of the introitus and lower vagina may occur, thus vitiating the test.

Endoscopy

Cystoscopy

Cystoscopy has little role in the evaluation of any but the smallest of fistulae. For obvious reasons bladder distension without obturation of the fistula may be virtually impossible. The principal purpose of this investigation would be to establish the relationship of a known fistula to ureteric orifices and thus assess the likelihood of inclusion in the fistula wall or damage during a subsequent repair.

Cystoscopy should always be carried out before a dye test. Indeed distension of the bladder with clear fluid may well give the diagnosis in uncertain cases even before dye is instilled. With juxtaurethral fistulae the failure to pass a cystoscope or sound up the distal urethra may indicate that there has been circumferential loss of the proximal urethra, a circumstance which is of considerable importance in determining the appropriate surgical technique and the likelihood of urethral incompetence. Similar considerations may apply to investigation of the lower bowel following major obstetric injuries in which segmental circumferential loss of the upper rectum may have occurred.

Sigmoidoscopy and proctoscopy

On rare occasions the distal anus may end in a blind pouch, if there has been segmental loss of the rectum. Lesser degrees of this situation result in severe stricture formation after closure. These examinations are very important for the diagnosis of inflammatory bowel disease, which may well not have been suspected before the occurrence of a fistula. Biopsies of the fistula edge or any unhealthy-looking area should always be obtained.

Histological

In addition to endoscopically obtained biopsies Tru-cut samples of indurated areas are essential where irradiation damage and malignant disease form the differential diagnosis. Studies which are negative for active malignancy should always be treated with some reserve; regrettably subsequent events all too often prove that such results are false negatives.

Microbiological

Schistosomiasis or tuberculosis may become apparent in biopsy material. Urine culture is not easily obtained when a fistula produces severe incontinence. Rather surprisingly urine may not be obviously infected in those situations where there is no longer any stasis. A pipette may be used to obtain a small intravesical sample for study.

GENERAL TREATMENT

Surgical correction of a genital fistula is usually possible for a communication of traumatic origin, whether due to surgery or obstetric pressure necrosis. Circumferential loss of the bladder neck and proximal urethra may turn successful closure of such a juxtaurethral fistula into a pyrrhic victory. The unfortunate patient may be as incontinent through her urethral stump as she was through the fistula, there being no sphincter mechanism at all.

For fistulae of malignant origin treatment of the cancer clearly takes priority, although the effect on the quality of life due to the malignant fistula means that this complication should not be ignored. The choice of management will then lie between some form of exenterative procedure or the use of radical radiotherapy with subsequent treatment of the fistula in the immediate aftermath. In the interim, faecal diversion by temporary colostomy is feasible and usually desirable. Urinary diversion is not necessarily required and its eventual use may even be avoided by colpocleisis (see below). Inflammatory fistulae require the source of infection to be treated or removed.

Conservative surgery when there is intrinsic inflammatory bowel disease tends to be unrewarding. In cases of Crohn's disease, successful surgical closure has only been achieved when the inflammatory process has been rendered completely quiescent by adequate medical therapy, usually with temporary faecal diversion by ileostomy.

A fistula is the ultimate expression of local tissue damage. It is almost axiomatic that a fistula will be surrounded by tissue which is substandard in terms of mobility and healing capability. It is essential, therefore, that the general health of the patient should be optimal.

Because of social ostracism individuals with entirely benign obstetric fistulae may have been rejected and deprived, and be suffering from malnutrition, the effects of prolonged sepsis and other infections. In tropical countries the treatment of malaria, typhoid, tuberculosis and parasitic infections should be rigorously undertaken before elective surgery. Where human immunodeficiency virus is prevalent, appropriate serological and immunological studies may be required. In all cases attention to nutrition in the preoperative phase is worthwhile. Where there is severe inflammatory bowel disease the question of utilization of total parenteral nutrition will have been considered by the gastroenterologist involved.

Local

Calculi and foreign bodies

Calculi in the bladder, vaginal vault or diverticula may be detected by plain radiography or clinical examination. Their removal prior to any attempt at correction is essential.

Often synchronous with the examination outlined in the previous section on diagnosis and evaluation, preliminary examination under anaesthesia is commonly utilized to assess the feasibility of the various surgical approaches which may be adopted for genital fistulae. Access will need to be determined and this may require alteration of the position of the anaesthetized patient. For instance, adoption of the knee–elbow (jack knife) or prone lithotomy positions may be required for transanal surgery or procedures on juxtaurethral fistulae adherent to the posterior aspect of the symphysis pubis.

It is essential also to assess the quiescence of local tissue. Signs of infection and induration may be obvious and a further period of healing may be desirable. The length of time required before surgical intervention will vary with the aetiology, site and previous intervention. In general, abdominal surgery may be undertaken earlier than repairs via the vaginal route and intervention on the ureter earlier than for injury to the bladder.

Haematological

Anaemia obviously has to be corrected and any associated haemoglobinopathy should be recognized. Antibody screening is essential and should be complete as blood transfusion may be required. Fistula surgery is quite often unpredictable in its extent and rarely may be associated with major intraoperative haemorrhage.

Chemoprophylaxis

Opinions differ on the desirability of prophylactic antibiotic cover. The author's preference is to avoid this other than in the treatment of specific infection. However, transperitoneal incision of the alimentary canal is usually covered by peroperative use of broad-spectrum antibiotics (e.g. imidazole and gentamicin or a cephalosporin).

Mechanical cleansing

It is very important that calculi and faecoliths be removed. Mechanical irrigation of the bowel is required and because inspissated faeces may not be removed by this method, endoscopic evaluation prior to surgery may be necessary, particularly if temporary faecal diversion has been instituted. In order to achieve distal intestinal wash-out, plugging of the vagina will be required, otherwise enemas and irrigations are immediately returned through the fistula.

Physiotherapy

Obstetric fistulae may be associated with foot-drop and limb contracture. Early involvement of the physiotherapist in perioperative management and rehabilitation is desirable.

Counselling

Many of these individuals will have been seriously demoralized by their plight. Confident but honest counselling by the surgeon is essential. Because of the need for reinforcement, the involvement of senior trained nursing staff in this process is also highly desirable and, as is increasingly recognized in many fields of medicine, involvement of patient self-help organizations is of great importance. The support given by previously treated sufferers is one of the most critical features in this process, particularly if there is an initial setback.

SURGICAL

No treatment

Small true urethral fistulae do not usually give rise to incontinence and there may be no pressing need for intervention. A vesicouterine fistula whose only symptoms are cyclical haematuria and amenorrhoea is sometimes perceived by the patient as an improvement on nature in terms of the toilet of menstruation and offers of surgical intervention may be rejected. Small low rectal fistulae may give rise to few symptoms except when associated with diarrhoea; the risks of making the situation worse in inflammatory bowel disease may suggest that it is prudent for those with minimal symptoms to be managed expectantly.

Lay open

Low inflammatory bowel fistulae are merely a special example of fistula-in-ano and can be treated by laying open. If this procedure is adopted for anterior fistulae to the vagina there is a significant risk of inducing incontinence from sphincter damage; the procedure is really only feasible for an anovestibular fistula.

Transvaginal repair

For mid vaginal fistulae a straightforward flap-splitting procedure with repair in layers using interrupted sutures, usually of fine high-polymer absorbable material, is the standard practice. There are advocates of extra chromic catgut and monofilament nylon for the vagina (which is removable) and interrupted wire sutures which may be left in the intestinal canal. Anterior fistulae close to the cervix require mobilization of the bladder from uterus and subsequent rolling of the vesical suture line away from the anterior fornix. For the posterior high rectal fistula, opening of the pouch of Douglas allows mobilization of peritoneal covered rectum for closure. The vaginal defect may then be left open.

Bladder neck fistulae with tissue loss adherent to the back of the symphysis pubis are often best placed in the prone position for surgery. They require careful mobilization of the angles of the fistulae from its bone. If circumferential loss has occurred, closure of the bladder defect requires creation of a spout-like aperture compatible in size with the distal urethral stump to which an entrance is made. Total destruction of the urethra involves more intricate plastic reconstruction.

Saucerization

Historically the first method of fistula repair, saucerization still has a place for small fistulae, particularly those which follow previous attempts at surgery. For small rectovaginal fistulae this approach is usually accompanied by the insertion of a pursestring suture and inversion of the fistula track into the anal canal.

Episiotomy

Episiotomy is applicable only to low rectal fistulae. Division of an anterior band of scar tissue and conversion to a so-called 'third-degree' tear is a recognized form of management. Closure in layers with excision of scar tissue and reconstruction of the anal sphincter is required.

Transanal repair

A similar technique may be used for access to low rectal fistulae through the anal canal. This may be achieved with the use of an anal speculum (peranal repair) — a Parke's or Eisenhammer speculum would give the necessary access. Even better access can be achieved by incision of the anal sphincter posteriorly, together with the posterior rectal wall (transanal, trans-sphincteric approach), which is an adaptation of a surgical approach devised for rectoprostatic fistulae. It is particularly apposite following colpocleisis if an attempt is to be made to close a resultant rectovesical fistula.

Transabdominal operations

A retropubic cystotomy may be used to obtain access to most relatively high vesicovaginal fistulae. By preference such a fistula should be situated above the trigone as access to the bladder neck by this route is limited, especially in small women with a narrow fore-pelvis who tend to develop a vesicovaginal fistula in the juxtourethral situation. An intravesical repair may be facilitated by preliminary packing of the vagina to elevate the fistula site; stragetically placed traction sutures are also helpful. Otherwise the repair is carried out by flap-splitting and closure in layers, the only difference being that when operating via this route, the use of a continuous suture for the bladder layer is not only permitted but recommended, as haemostasis is particularly important.

Combined transvesical transperitoneal approach (Swift Joley operation)

A median fissure of the bladder extended as a racquet-shaped incision to encompass the fistula provides excellent exposure, particularly if the space behind the bladder is obscured by adhesions. This approach is useful for the posthysterectomy fistula and for vesicouterine fistulae.

In any abdominal repair, interposition of a pedicled graft of omentum is a useful measure, and indeed essential if the blood supply has been compromised, for example by prior radiation. The vascular pedicle used is usually the left or right gastroepiploic artery.

Transperitoneal fistula closure

Separation of the viscera and closure with sutures is rarely adequate for bladder fistulae. It may be used for simple fistulae involving mobile loops of bowel (colon, ileum), although resection and anastomosis may be easier (see below).

Sometimes hysterectomy is carried out to allow access to the inferior margin of a high fistula, particularly a rectal fistula. Where there is considerable fibrosis in the pelvis, subtotal hysterectomy followed by sagittal fissure of the cervix may provide the safest access (Lawson operation).

Resection and anastomosis

This procedure is required for colovaginal or ileovaginal fistulae when there is intrinsic disease or damage to the intestine. It is not essential to close the vagina, as the anastomotic areas can usually be well separated. An extension of this technique may be necessary for high rectal fistulae with circumferential loss. Under such circumstances there may even be a blind distal anorectal pouch. A re-anastomosis requires retrorectal mobilization comparable to that employed in radical oophorectomy and the procedure is akin to the restoration of continuity after a Hartmann's operation. The end-to-end anastomosis staple gun is particularly useful for such a repair, as it reduces the amount of preparation needed for the distal stump.

Colostomy

An end colostomy of the sigmoid or descending colon is much easier to manage than one raised in the transverse colon. However, as a temporary measure transverse colostomy is to be preferred as this will not disturb the site and blood supply of the distal colon if a complex restorative procedure is contemplated at a later date.

Diversion

On rare occasions diversion of urine or faeces (or both) may be required. This is a particularly serious move in the presence of fistulae due to benign disease. It really should only be undertaken if an expert assessment of the possibility of more involved repeat surgery has been obtained. Relative indications will be destruction of the distal sphincter apparatus and a frozen pelvis. Restoration of continuity of a small contracted non-compliant bladder may confer no benefit even if successful.

Ureterocolic anastomosis has the attraction of avoiding an external appliance which has some appeal in those communities where there are cultural objections to abdominal stoma formation. However, the operation has a bad reputation from leakage and subsequent upper renal tract deterioration together with metabolic disturbance. Modern reflux-preventing techniques have improved the situation greatly and the possibility of this procedure should be borne in mind especially when life expectancy is limited. More usual is the creation of an intestinal conduit with a separate stoma. Traditionally the terminal ileum is used for such a conduit but this may be difficult or imprudent after pelvic irradiation. Under such circumstances an isolated segment of tranverse colon may be preferred, but of course it does produce a significant mucus discharge.

For the management of double fistulae the use of sigmoid colon may be considered if an end colostomy is also contemplated. This has the advantage that it dispenses with any intestinal anastomosis. The ureters may be joined to the isolated conduit independently or joined together in spatulate form to become a double-barrelled ureterointestinal end-to-end anastomosis. More complex continent conduits dealt with by intermittent self-catheterization can now be constructed and this possibility should always be considered in an elective situation.

Colpocleisis

If diversion is considered the possibility of vaginal obliteration as an alternative should be addressed. This is particularly appropriate for the older patient, particularly for a fistula due to the treatment of malignant disease — even occasionally when malignancy is still active. Total colpocleisis involves denuding the vagina of epithelium and obliterating the dead space beneath the fistula. Partial colpocleisis may be more appropriate. Upper partial colpocleisis is obliteration of the vaginal vault and this is a technique which may be used for the repair of benign post-hysterectomy fistulae when other methods of repair are difficult or contraindicated. Lower partial colpocleisis is a technique particularly suited for the management of post-irradiation fistulae, including the double rectovesico-vaginal fistula. In this technique a sleeve of lower vagina is removed and the upper cuff is closed as a 'diverticulum' of the bladder or as a bridge between the bladder and rectum. It is usually necessary to fill the dead space below this sealed-off cuff with fresh tissue brought from outside and either a pedicle of fat from the vulva (Martius operation) or the gracilis muscle of the thigh (Ingelmann–Sundberg operation) is utilized.

It is particularly important when this procedure is used for a double fistula to determine whether the intestinal component is rectal rather than colonic. A colovaginal fistula from the apex of the sigmoid loop is almost always associated with distal stenosis and vaginal obliteration will inevitably be 'blown apart' if this is not relieved. Under such circumstances it would be desirable to create a high rectovaginal fistula before carrying out colpocleisis; this will allow faeces and pus to discharge per rectum from the isolated upper vaginal cuff.

URETERIC FISTULAE

In general an established ureteric fistula is best dealt with by section of the ureter at a convenient site just above the fistula where the tissues are healthy and the blood supply is apparent. There are several techniques for ureteroneocystostomy; that which is chosen will depend upon local conditions and the nature of the antecedent pathology. The most generally available techniques are direct re-implantation using a psoas hitch, creation of a flap of bladder muscle (Boari–Ockerblad) and interposition of a loop of bowel. Whichever is chosen it is preferable to use a reflux-preventing form of anastomosis (Leadbetter–Politano). An alternative procedure which is commonly favoured is transabdominal ureteroureterostomy. This involves an end-to-side anastomosis between the injured ureter and the good contralateral ureter. There are few lesions which are too high for this to be applicable, but use of this technique does depend upon the certainty that the contralateral ureter has not been compromised in the pelvis by the same circumstances which gave rise to the original fistula.

The management of acute ureteric injury is beyond the scope of this chapter.

POSTOPERATIVE MANAGEMENT

Nursing care of patients who have undergone a fistula repair is of critical importance. Failure of haemostasis and secondary haemorrhage will almost always presage failure. Prophylactic measures include careful obliteration of dead space as well as attention to haemostasis. Free urinary drainage will normally be maintained for longer than would be usual for uncomplicated bladder surgery and likewise, if catheter blockage occurs and is not recognized, disruption of the suture line and failure of the operation are almost inevitable.

Opinion is divided on whether ureteric anastomosis is best performed over a splint. What is clear is that if a splint has insufficient side-holes and becomes blocked, diversion of the urine flow entirely to the outside of the splint is an obvious method of disrupting an ureteric anastomosis. It is important that the urine should be kept clear of infection; Gram-negative septicaemia is a rare but serious sequel.

PROGNOSIS

It is desirable to carry out a test of closure using dye some 2–3 weeks after an apparently successful operation. Small residual fistulae may be difficult to detect until later. The results of urinary fistula surgery are in general not quite as good as those involving the alimentary canal. What is quite clear is that there is a law of diminishing returns and with every repeat repair the prospect of success is reduced. The gynaecologist is the specialist common denominator for all genital fistulae, but complex reconstructive techniques may require considerable urological or proctological experience.

The average generalist gynaecologist will probably lack experience in this rather specialized area. What is quite clear also is that the combination of an inexperienced gynaecologist and an inexperienced urologist is no solution to the problem of a difficult fistula.

For gynaecologists in developing countries, regrettably the repair of obstetric fistula still remains a major feature of clinical practice. This situation will remain until the World Health Organization objective of safe motherhood for all is achieved.

KEY POINTS

1. Obstetric fistulae are usually due to pressure necrosis.
2. When a fistula is due to anything other than simple trauma, it is important to treat the underlying pathology as well as correct the fistula.
3. A fistula should always be regarded as potentially dual or complex and investigation must be orientated towards this.
4. In developed countries, the commonest kinds of fistulae are those due to traumatic cause, usually secondary to surgery.
5. Of the inflammatory causes, Crohn's disease is the most important.
6. With both urinary and faecal fistulae, the history may be misleading.
7. Biopsy of the fistula edge or unhealthy looking local tissue is mandatory.
8. Successful correction of a urinary fistula may leave behind an incompetent sphincter mechanism.
9. Use of a pedicled fat graft in fistula closure is an important source of a new blood supply.
10. With malignant fistulae, treatment of the cause is the first priority.
11. Malnutrition, anaemia and infection should be treated before attempting surgical closure.
12. On rare occasions urinary or faecal diversion may be required.
13. The type of fistula closure would depend on the site and nature of the fistula.
14. Haemostasis, avoidance of tension on the suture line, obliteration of dead space and closure in layers are important technical points for successful closure.

FURTHER READING

Bentley R J 1973 Abdominal repair of high recto-vaginal fistula. Journal of Obstetrics and Gynaecology of the British Commonwealth 80: 364–367

Blandy J, Anderson J D 1977 Management of the injured ureter. Proceedings of the Royal Society of Medicine 70: 187–190

Diricuta I, Goldstein A M B 1972 The repair of extensive vesico-vaginal fistulas with pedicled omentum: a review of 27 cases. Journal of Urology 108: 724–727

Hamlin R H J, Nicholson E C 1969 Reconstruction of urethra totally destroyed in labour. British Medical Journal 1: 147–150

Harrison K A 1983 Obstetric fistula: one social calamity too many. British Journal of Obstetrics and Gynaecology 90: 385–386

Hendry W F 1977 The pelvic ureter. Proceedings of the Royal Society of Medicine 70: 183–186

Hudson C N 1962 Vesico-uterine fistula following Caesarean section. Journal of Obstetrics and Gynaecology of the British Commonwealth 69: 121–124

Hudson C N 1970 Acquired fistula between the intestine and the vagina. Annals of the Royal College of Surgeons 46: 20–40

Javadpour N, John T, Wilson M R et al 1973 Transperitoneal vesical bivalve in repair of recurrent vesico-vaginal fistula. Obstetrics and Gynecology 41: 469–473

Lawson J B 1972 Vesical fistulae in to the vaginal vault British Journal of Urology 44: 623–631

Lawson J B 1978 The management of genito-urinary fistulae Clinics in Obstetrics and Gynaecology 5: 209–236
Lawson J B 1985 The vesico-vaginal fistula — a continuing problem. J Y Simpson oration. Royal College of Obstetrics and Gynaecology, London
Mahfouz N 1934 A new technique in dealing with superior rectovaginal fistulae. Journal of Obstetrics and Gynaecology of the British Empire 41: 579–587
Moir J C 1964 Reconstruction of the urethra. Journal of Obstetrics and Gynaecology of the British Commonwealth 71: 349–359
Moir J C 1969 The vesico-vaginal fistula, 2nd edn. Baillière, London
Moir J C 1973 Vesico-vaginal fistulae as seen in Britain. Journal of Obstetrics and Gynaecology of the British Commonwealth 80: 598–602
Shaw W 1949 The Martius bulbocavernosus interposition operation. British Medical Journal 2: 1261–1264
Stephens F S, Smith E D 1971 Ano-rectal malformation in children. Year Book Medical Publishers, Chicago
Turner-Warwick R T 1976 The use of the omental pedicle graft in urinary tract reconstruction. Journal of Urology 116: 341–347
Zacharin R F 1988 Obstetric Fistula. Springer-Verlag, Vienna

SECTION 6

Infections

54. Principles of antibiotic therapy, prophylaxis and treatment of postoperative infection

E. Houang W. P. Soutter

INTRODUCTION

This chapter outlines the principles of antimicrobial therapy and prophylaxis. It describes briefly the vaginal microbial flora in health and disease as well as other microbes commonly involved in gynaecological infection. It gives guidelines to the treatment of postoperative and postabortal infections. Urinary tract infections, pelvic inflammatory disease and sexually transmitted diseases are all discussed elsewhere.

BACTERIOLOGICAL DIAGNOSIS

The place of bacteriological diagnosis

Generally speaking, to treat patients on the basis of a bacteriological report alone is an unsound practice. On the other hand, treatment given to an ill patient with unexplained pyrexia without searching for the bacterial cause usually leads to further difficulty in establishing the diagnosis. In everyday clinical practice, antimicrobial therapy can often be withheld until the result of bacteriological investigation is known and therefore the best choice of treatment can be made. Exceptionally, antibiotics are given on epidemiological grounds, for example in the treatment of asymptomatic female contacts of male patients suffering from non-specific urethritis because the laboratory facility for diagnosing chlamydial infection is not widely available.

When a patient is seriously ill treatment may have to be started before the result of bacteriological culture is available. Simple and rapid laboratory techniques such as Gram-stains of the urine sediment, sputum or pus will provide initial guidance to the selection of antibiotics. Immunological methods for antigen detection such as enzyme-linked immunoabsorbent assay (ELISA) or latex agglutination are being developed and can also provide clues for the rapid identification of the infecting pathogens. Nevertheless, final and definitive identification of the causative pathogen or pathogens and their antimicrobial susceptibility requires culture. Therefore, specimens of urine, sputum and blood, together with those from appropriate operative sites, should always be obtained for culture before the commencement of therapy. It is important to remember to obtain cervical specimens (and uterine specimens if possible) in all cases of suspected pelvic sepsis.

Obtaining good samples for bacteriological testing

The information obtained from bacteriological investigation depends upon the quality and appropriateness of the samples sent to the laboratory. An immunofluorescent test (ELISA) or a culture method for *Chlamydia trachomatis* is essential in the investigation of pelvic inflammatory disease. Anaerobic organisms are common pathogens in infections in obstetric and gynaecological patients. The optimal condition for the isolation of these fastidious organisms requires an oxygen-free transport system for the specimen (preferably the pus rather than a swab of it) and a minimal transit time to the laboratory. Suitable transport media with added reducing agents such as sodium thioglycollate include Stuart's transport medium and Amies' transport medium. Although this method is simple, the chance of isolating gonococci or anaerobes is reduced if there is a delay of more than 24 hours.

Outside normal working hours, agar plates may be inoculated in the theatre or by the bedside and incubated in an anaerobic jar using Gas Pak system if proper laboratory facilities are not available. Similarly, a carbon dioxide Generation Pak or a lidded candle jar offers the correct conditions for the isolation of *Neisseria gonorrhoeae*. These simple systems require little technical skill but achieve the optimal conditions for the isolation of fastidious organisms and should be considered seriously in centres where transport to the laboratory may incur delay.

Blood culture

Blood culture is invaluable for the diagnosis of infection when the primary site is not accessible to the clinician. Although it is readily performed in patients with evidence of septicaemia, its value in suspected pelvic infection is underestimated. Thadepalli et al (1973) surveyed the blood culture results from their hospital and found that the Gynaecology Ward had the highest incidence of positive anaerobic isolates. The isolation of microaerophilic or anaerobic organisms from blood culture may suggest the presence of pelvic abscesses.

It is therefore important to use culture media which support the wide range of bacteria likely to be encountered in pelvic infection — including the genital mycoplasmas, *N. gonorrhoeae* and the anaerobes. In the UK, the commonly used routine blood culture set consists of three bottles: a nutrient broth with 0.05% liquoid, a brain–heart infusion broth with 0.05% cysteine and a 0.1% glucose broth with 0.05% liquoid. Whenever possible at least two separate sets should be collected before the start of antibiotic therapy.

High vaginal swab

The high vaginal swab is a common test performed for the investigation of gynaecological infection but it is of limited value in the management of upper genital tract infection, such as endometritis, salpingitis, pyosalpinx and tubo-ovarian abscess. These may have been caused by sexually transmitted bacteria that can be identified in the vaginal swab but when infection is due to bacteria endogenous to the lower genital tract it is very difficult to determine which organism grown from the vagina is responsible. A sound understanding of the vaginal microbial flora in health and disease and of the organisms commonly involved in gynaecological infections is necessary in the interpretation of the culture results and in choosing an antibiotic before bacteriological confirmation is available

NORMAL VAGINAL FLORA

The indigenous microflora appear to be a major host defence mechanism against invading pathogens. In addition, some organisms normally found in the healthy vagina may become pathogenic under certain circumstances.

Menarchal women

There are about 10^8–10^9 anaerobes/ml and about 10^7–10^8 aerobes/ml of vaginal secretion. The most frequent isolates in numbers exceeding 10^5/ml are facultative and obligate anaerobic lactobacilli, peptostreptococci and peptococci. The carrier rate for bacteroides organisms may be 55–65%. Over two-thirds of the bacteroides isolates belong to the *Bacteroides melaninogenicus/oralis* group. The commonest species identified in this group include those of the *B. bivius/disiens* complex. About 10% of healthy vaginas harbour *B. fragilis* and Enterobacteriaceae including *Escherichia coli* usually in low concentrations ($<10^6$/ml). Other commonly found anaerobes include *Eubacterium* spp. and fusobacteria. *Gardnerella vaginalis* has been found in 20–70% of asymptomatic women in some studies, *Candida* spp. in 12–16% of studies of single samples and in sequential studies with multiple specimens/yeasts (mainly *C. albicans*) were found in more than 33% of subjects. T-strain mycoplasmas were found in 30–60% and *Mycoplasma hominis* in 10–22% of vaginal specimens.

Children and postmenopausal women

The organisms found in the vagina of healthy children are shown in Table 54.1 (Hammerschlag et al 1978). *E. coli* and other enterobacteria are found mainly in children under 4 years of age. *B. fragilis* and *B. melaninogenicus* are more common in children than in adult women.

Although there are lower average numbers of aerobes and anaerobes in the vaginal or cervical flora of postmenopausal than premenopausal women, the differences are not statistically significant. Among postmenopausal women,

Table 54.1 The prevalence of bacteria in the vagina of healthy children (Hammerschlag et al 1978)

Organism	Prevalence (%)
Staphylococcus epidermidis	84%
Diphtheroids	80%
Bacteroides fragilis	24%
Bacteroides melaninogenicus	56%
Clostridium perfringens	32%
Gardnerella vaginalis	13%
Yeasts	28%

lactobacilli and diphtheroids occur more frequently and anaerobes less frequently in those treated with oestrogen.

Other factors affecting the vaginal flora

The presence of *E. coli* is associated with the phase of the menstrual cycle, prior use of antibiotics, use of diaphragm or cervical cap for contraception and a history of previous urinary tract infection (Chow et al 1986).

POSTOPERATIVE SEPSIS

Infection following a surgical procedure is common and may result in serious long-term morbidity. Criminal abortion in particular is associated with substantial morbidity and mortality. The organisms associated with gynaecological postoperative infections and recommended antibiotics are listed in Table 54.2.

Source of infecting organisms

The traditional view of a single-species pathogen for postoperative sepsis has been replaced with the realization that several species of bacteria are often involved. The source of bacteria recovered postoperatively from a wound infection is most commonly the patient herself: from the cervicovaginal flora, the skin, the respiratory or the gastrointestinal tract. In comparison, contamination by members of the surgical team is less common. The majority of Gram-negative bacilli, haemolytic streptococci and staphylococci can survive for 20 minutes or longer on the hands of hospital staff and the hands are the most important means of spreading infection from one patient to another in hospital wards.

General causes of postoperative pyrexia

Not all patients with a raised temperature have an infection. A mild self-limiting pyrexia is common after major surgery and blood transfusion may also provoke a febrile response. A degree of pulmonary atelectasis is very common postoperatively. This will settle with physiotherapy.

Established pulmonary infection will result in a productive cough, purulent sputum and dyspnoea. *Streptococcus pneumoniae* is a common cause of postoperative pneumonia. If the dyspnoea is out of proportion with the other signs, pulmonary embolism must be excluded. Deep venous thrombosis may present with pyrexia.

Septic pelvic thrombophlebitis is an uncommon cause of postoperative fever and dull lower abdominal pain. It should be considered in an ill patient with no localized signs of infection who fails to respond to antibiotic therapy. A therapeutic trial of heparin should produce a response within 48 hours.

Urinary tract infection is one of the most common postoperative infections in gynaecology. It is associated with catheterization or instrumentation of the bladder. *E. coli* is the commonest organism found but other Gram-negative aerobes, such as *Klebsiella* spp. or *Proteus* spp. are involved occasionally. Highly resistant Gram-negative aerobes such as *Pseudomonas aeruginosa* and *Serratia marcescens* are uncommon.

Infections in skin wounds

An infected wound is painful and tender. It becomes red and oedematous when the infection involves the superficial layers of the wound but often looks normal in the early stages if the infection began deep in the incision. Wound infections often start in a haematoma but may originate around the sutures especially in the region of a bulky knot. If pus collects it will usually discharge through the skin. This is made more difficult if a continuous suture of non-absorbable material has been used. The organisms found in wound infections are listed in Table 54.2; *Staphylococcus aureus* is most common of the Gram-positive organisms.

Most wound infections settle spontaneously but, if an obvious collection of pus is present, this should be drained. This can usually be accomplished in the ward but will require general anaesthesia if the abscess is very large or deeply situated. Small areas of necrotic tissue should be excised in the ward as part of daily wound toilet. This may be assisted by hydrogen peroxide. An old and effective remedy for a gaping, infected wound is to soak the cavity with honey and pack with gauze. A more modern (and more expensive) equivalent is Debrisan. Antibiotic therapy is only of value in the more severe wound infections with systemic symptoms.

Necrotizing fasciitis

Necrotizing fasciitis is a rare but serious clinical entity which presents like a subcutaneous infection. Most of the patients are diabetic or have some other chronic disease. It presents as an area of subcutaneous induration and oedema from which a discharge like dirty dishwater may exude. It may originate from a surgical incision or, more usually,

Table 54.2 Guidelines for the use of antimicrobial agents for some conditions in gynaecology*

Clinical condition	Likely causative organism(s)	Recommended antimicrobial(s)	Comments
Chest infections			
Aspiration -pneumonia	Mouth organisms, including anaerobes	Penicillin & metronidazole	Cover for aerobic Gram-negative rods, e.g. gentamicin may be required.
Broncho-pneumonia	*Streptococcus pneumoniae*, *Haemophilus influenzae*, less frequently, *Staphylococcus aureus*, coliforms, *Pseudomonas*	Trimethoprim, clavulanic acid + amoxycillin	Results of culture and sensitivity tests required for unresponsive patients
Wound infections	*Staphylococcus aureus*, *Escherichia coli*, *Streptococcus pyogenes*, *Streptococcus agalactiae*, *Bacteroides fragilis*, microaerophilic and anaerobic streptococci; occasionally, other coliforms	Amoxycillin & clavulanic acid or cephradine + metronidazole or cefuroxime + metronidazole	Await culture result if possible; severe infections require intravenous therapy
Actinomycosis	*Actinomyces israelii*	Amoxycillin for oral therapy; intravenous penicillin G for severe infection (erythromycin**)	Prolonged therapy required; Remove foreign body, e.g. IUCD, if present
Severe infection e.g. septicaemia	Unknown	Metronidazole plus gentamicin + ampicillin or metronidazole + cefuroxime	Intravenous therapy essential; culture and sensitivity required for adjustment of therapy
	Staphylococcus aureus	Flucloxacillin (erythromycin) + fusidic acid	Intravenous therapy essential; remove infected cannula if present
	Streptococcus pyogenes	Penicillin G (erythromycin)	Intravenous therapy essential
	Escherichia coli, *Proteus* spp., *Klebsiella* spp.	Ampicillin + gentamicin or gentamicin or cefuroxime	
	Pseudomonas spp.	Ceftazidime or gentamicin + carbenicillin	
e.g. septic — abortion	if *Clostridium perfringens* suspected	Penicillin G (erythromycin) + metronidazole	Large doses required

* For urinary tract infection, sexually transmitted diseases and pelvic inflammatory diseases, see individual chapters in this book.
** For patient with penicillin allergy.

Prophylaxis for hysterectomies
Metronidazole suppository 1 g is given at premedication and cephradine 500 mg or ampicillin 500 mg is given intravenously at the induction of anaesthesia.
In patients with penicillin allergy, metronidazole alone is given.

Prevention of endocarditis in patients with heart-valve abnormalities undergoing genitourinary surgery
Intramuscular amoxycillin 1 g & intramuscular gentamicin 1.5 mg/kg immediately before induction of anaesthesia, then oral or intramuscular amoxycillin 500 mg 6 hours later or, if the patient is penicillin-allergic, intravenous vancomycin 1 g over 60 minutes then intravenous gentamicin 1.5 mg/kg immediately before induction; metronidazole may also be added.

from a minor injury to the skin. It is seen most commonly in the vulval, perineal or gluteal skin or in the skin of the thigh. As the condition progresses, signs of toxicity worsen and are often out of proportion to the apparent extent of the lesion which may look relatively minor. However, the subcutaneous infection spreads widely under apparently normal looking skin.

All of the first 20 cases were attributed to 'haemolytic streptococci' but, since then, a variety of combinations of aerobic and anaerobic organisms has been recorded when appropriate culture techniques have been employed. It is likely that these infections are polymicrobial and that bacterial synergism is a key factor in the pathogenesis.

The importance of early diagnosis and radical excision of affected skin cannot be over-emphasized. Treatment with antibiotics alone or with antibiotics plus incision and drainage is associated with 100% mortality. Any tissue that is indurated, oedematous, crepitant to palpation, or does not bleed readily when incised should be removed (Allen Addison et al 1984).

Postoperative pelvic infection

Postoperative pelvic infection tends to arise in an area of devascularized, damaged tissue or in a haematoma. In addition to the general symptoms of fever and tachycardia, the patient will complain of pelvic or perineal pain. Pressure on the rectum from an enlarging abscess will give a sensation of needing to defecate. Pressure symptoms on the bladder are less common. An area of pelvic tenderness is felt vaginally and it may be possible to palpate a mass. Pelvic ultrasound can be useful in identifying a haematoma or abscess. When the abscess discharges through the vagina or rectum some bleeding may also occur. This is mostly old blood, but there is often some fresh bleeding too. Occasionally, pelvic infection is responsible for massive postoperative haemorrhage.

The exact bacteriology in pelvic cellulitis is difficult to determine because of inaccessibility of the infected site. The examination of a high vaginal swab may be helpful but is unlikely to reveal the complete picture. Blood culture should be performed and will sometimes help to identify one of the organisms responsible. Using fastidious anaerobic technique, Thadepalli et al (1973) carried out a detailed bacteriological study of the pus obtained in the operating theatre in 27 patients and of the blood cultures of a further 6 patients who had been admitted with a variety of severe infections such as pelvic abscesses, septic abortions, puerperal sepsis, tubo-ovarian abscesses, and endometritis after dilation and curettage. Anaerobic bacteria were cultured from all patients and aerobes from 21. The commonest aerobic and facultative bacteria were *E. coli*, followed by streptococci and *Staphylococcus epidermidis*. By far the commonest anaerobe was *Bacteroides fragilis*, followed by *Peptostreptococcus*. Lactobacilli, the most common constituent of the normal vaginal flora, were recovered in only 4 patients. This study emphasizes the importance of anaerobic organisms in pelvic infections.

Because of the difficulties in making a bacteriological diagnosis and the polymicrobial nature of most of these infections, antibiotic therapy is usually started after bacteriological samples have been obtained but before the results are available. The choice of agents will be determined by the severity of the infection and the sensitivity of the most likely organisms in that hospital. Some suggestions are listed in Table 54.2.

Most cases of postoperative pelvic sepsis settle with antibiotics and conservative therapy. If a foreign body such as an intrauterine contraceptive device is present, it should be removed. A pelvic abscess that shows no signs of draining spontaneously should be incised and drained under general anaesthesia, through either the vagina or the rectum depending upon which is closest to the abscess.

A laparotomy is required in patients who fail to respond to standard therapy or who develop signs of peritonitis. The abdomen should be explored carefully to rule out unsuspected damage to bowel or urinary tract. The subdiaphragmatic spaces and the entire intestinal tract should be examined to exclude multiloculated abscesses. Tubo-ovarian masses are better removed. The uterus may be conserved in young women if menstruation induced by hormone replacement therapy is important to the patient. Drains should be inserted into the pelvis, the paracolic gutters and the subdiaphragmatic space.

Following severe postoperative pelvic infection, many patients continue to experience chronic pelvic pain. If adhesions involving bowel have formed, intermittent subacute obstruction may result. In women whose pelvic organs were not removed in the primary surgery nor in the treatment of the infection, fertility is likely to be severely impaired by tubo-ovarian damage.

Infection following legal or criminal abortion

Patients who become infected after abortion can be critically ill, especially after criminal abortion. In addition to the systemic signs of infection, these patients complain of abdominal pain and a purulent vaginal discharge. They often present with vaginal bleeding.

The cervix may be open and products of conception palpable. The uterus is often enlarged, boggy and tender. Tender masses may be felt in the adnexae. There may be evidence of trauma to the vagina or cervix. If septicaemia is well established, the pulse will be rapid and thready and the patient's hands and feet deathly cold.

The bacteriology of infected abortion is comparable to that of pelvic infection. It is usually a polymicrobial infection resulting from a mixed flora of aerobic and anaerobic streptococci, *Bacteroides* spp. *E. coli* and other enteric organisms as well as microaerophilic organisms.

Dehydration, anaemia and hypovolaemia should be corrected rapidly. Broad-spectrum antimicrobial therapy with bactericidal effects should be initiated immediately. A combination of amoxycillin, an aminoglycoside and metronidazole or a third-generation cephalosporin such as cefuroxime may be used.

Successful management of these patients requires evacuation of the uterus after antimicrobial therapy has been commenced. Lacerations of the lower genital tract can be debrided and repaired but perforation of the uterus with criminal abortion usually results in hysterectomy being required. Even in the absence of perforation, hysterectomy may be required for neglected endometritis.

Clostridium perfringens is usually a saprophyte but it is a rare cause of lethal infections in patients with septic abortions. The alpha-toxin it produces causes shock and peripheral circulatory failure. Hysterectomy may be required, since the myometrium is the nidus from which the alpha-toxin is released into the blood stream. High doses of penicillin G are required and should be started before surgery and continued for the first 5 postoperative days.

Fertility is greatly reduced by postabortal sepsis largely because of tubo-ovarian damage. Many of these women continue to suffer from chronic pelvic pain often accompanied by irregular, heavy menses. Intrauterine adhesions are more common than is usually appreciated and contribute to reduced fertility. This is not always associated with diminished menstruation.

ANTIMICROBIAL SENSITIVITY OF INFECTING ORGANISMS

Once the pathogen has been isolated, a number of methods are available for determining sensitivity to antibiotics. The commonly used disk-diffusion method is simple to perform, is relatively inexpensive but gives a very approximate measure of the degree of sensitivity. Nonetheless, it provides data that are clinically useful.

Quantitative data are provided by methods that incorporate serial dilutions of antimicrobials in agar-containing or broth culture media. The lowest concentration of the antimicrobial agent that prevents visible growth after an 18–24-hour incubation period is known as the minimum inhibitory concentration (MIC). These more precise tests are carried out only for serious infections where optimal antimicrobial therapy is essential. It may be performed for some bacteria causing septicaemia in immunosuppressed patients or in patients with infective endocarditis.

ANTIBIOTIC RESISTANCE

Some bacterial species have remained largely sensitive to the same antimicrobial agents. For example, all group A streptococci remain sensitive to penicillins and cephalosporins, and virtually all anaerobes except *B. fragilis* are sensitive to ampicillin and chloramphenicol. However, this is uncommon and antibiotic resistance is a serious clinical problem.

Innate and acquired resistance

Some bacteria have always been innately resistant to certain agents. Examples are the resistance of staphylococci to polymyxins, of streptococci to gentamicin and of the aerobic Gram-negative rods to erythromycin and clindamycin. The widespread clinical and agricultural use of antibiotics in the past three decades has resulted in the emergence of many strains of bacteria resistant to one or more antimicrobial agents. Antibiotic sensitivity testing is particularly important for these organisms.

Mechanisms of resistance

Several mechanisms of resistance have been found. Some organisms produce beta-lactamases which hydrolyse the beta-lactam ring of various penicillins and cephalosporins. The resistance to some aminoglycosides by Gram-negative rods may also be mediated by the production of phosphotransferases, acetyltransferases and adenyltransferases. Resistance may result from the development of permeability barriers to drugs such as tetracycline or from alteration of the previous susceptible target site in the bacterium such as altered ribosome binding sites for streptomycin in resistant *E. coli*.

Resistance by spontaneous mutation

The frequency of spontaneous mutation of genes that control the susceptibility to a drug can be between 10^{-6} and 10^{-12} per generation. For some antimicrobial agents such as rifampicin or streptomycin, drug-resistant mutants may occur relatively often. Once these mutants appear, they become the surviving strains in the presence of the antibiotic. Chromosomal resistance is of particular clinical importance in the treatment of tuberculosis which requires the use of at least two effective drugs together to reduce the likelihood of insensitivity developing.

Plasmid-mediated resistance

Acquired drug resistance may be mediated by the 'R' factor (plasmid). Plasmids are extrachromosomal DNA which may code for antibiotic resistance and can be transferred from a resistant to a sensitive strain, thereby causing the sensitive strain to become antibiotic-resistant. Transfer of plasmids may occur between different genera of bacteria or between the flora of man and animals. By acquiring two or more different plasmids, the organism may become resistant to a wide range of antibiotics.

The incidence of plasmids is probably higher in environments where antibiotics are much used and the selective advantage for the resistant strains is therefore maintained. In the absence of any antibiotic prescribing, many of the bacteria lose the plasmid spontaneously. Sensitivity patterns vary between hospitals and the community or among hospitals, or between countries.

HOST FACTORS

There are several host factors which may influence the efficacy and toxicity of antimicrobial agents. A history of previous adverse reactions should always be sought. Pregnancy and breast-feeding pose problems in the selection of appropriate agents that will not affect the fetus or neonate adversely.

Drug absorption and excretion

The pH of gastric secretions may affect the absorption of some agents. It is higher in young children than in adults and there is also a decline in gastric acidity with the advance of age. Up to a third of people over the age of 60 may have achlorhydria. Penicillin G can be given to young children or elderly patients who have achlorhydria, as its absorption is markedly enhanced by the high gastric pH. Alteration in pH in the urine may have an important effect on the local activity of a number of antimicrobials. By the addition of acidifying or alkalinizing agents, the urine pH may be decreased to enhance the activity of methenamine, nitrofurantoin, and chlortetracycline, whereas increased pH enhances the activity of erythromycin, clindamycin and the aminoglycosidic aminocyclitol antibiotics.

Renal excretion is the most important route of elimination for the majority of antimicrobial agents but agents such as erythromycin and chloramphenicol are excreted by the hepatobiliary system and should not be used in patients with impaired hepatic function (Mandell et al 1985). It is important to remember that creatinine clearance may be significantly reduced in elderly patients even though they have a normal blood urea. Impaired renal excretion of aminoglycosides may result in raised serum concentrations and an increasing incidence of ototoxicity and nephrotoxicity.

Metabolism of antibiotics

Genetic or metabolic abnormalities may affect toxicity. The rate of inactivation of isoniazid by hepatic acetylation is genetically determined and polyneuritis as a complication of isoniazid therapy is seen more frequency in slow than in rapid acetylators. Patients with glucose-6-phosphate dehydrogenase (G6PD) deficiency may develop haemolysis when treated with sulphonamides, nitrofurantoin or chloramphenicol.

Interactions with other drugs

The patient may be taking other drugs which interact with the antimicrobial agent by the induction of enzymes. The result is increased metabolism of some drugs and endogenous hormones eliminated by the liver. This reduces the serum concentration and attenuates the pharmacological effects. Of the antimicrobials, the most potent enzyme inducer is rifampicin which reduces the effect of oral anticoagulants, oral contraceptives and barbiturates.

Another mechanism of drug interaction is enzyme inhibition. Lipid-soluble drugs such as warfarin, phenytoin and theophylline can have their hepatic metabolism inhibited by enzyme inhibitors such as metronidazole, chloramphenicol, erythromycin, isoniazid and sulphonamides. The degree of interaction and extent of the clinical effect varies between individual patients and is therefore unpredictable.

Some combinations of antibiotics may increase the toxicity of individual drugs. For example, nephrotoxicity is increased when gentamicin is used with cephalothin and ototoxicity when used with vancomycin. Information on possible drug interactions is readily available in the latest issue of the British National Formulary.

PHARMACOLOGY OF ANTIMICROBIAL AGENTS

Knowledge of the basic clinical pharmacokinetics and pharmacodynamics of a drug should help when choosing the optimal agent in a given condition. Pharmacokinetics refers to the time course of drug absorption, distribution, metabolism and excretion with the aim of relating these to the therapeutic and adverse effects of drugs. Pharmacodynamics refers to the relationship between drug concentration and effect with particular relevance to the time course of that effect. Detailed discussion of the pharmacokinetics and pharmacodynamics of antimicrobial agents is outside the scope of this chapter and only a general consideration is presented here.

Pharmacokinetics of oral agents

A rapidly achieved high peak concentration is important for antibiotics. For oral preparations, the time to peak plasma concentration is usually around 1 hour unless gastric emptying time is slowed and the drug's arrival in the jejunum is delayed. This may occur physiologically following a heavy meal, pathologically during severe pain such as migraine and pharmacologically due to opiate analgesics, tricyclic antidepressants or antihistamines. Extensive small bowel pathology such as coeliac disease or Crohn's disease has little effect on total bioavailability of most drugs as compensatory absorption occurs further down the gastrointestinal tract.

A number of beta-lactam drugs, for example, ampicillin, mecillinam and cloxacillin have been modified, as talampicillin or pivampicillin, pimecillinam, and flucloxacillin, to improve their absorption. Amoxycillin is twice as well absorbed as ampicillin and therefore should be used as the oral form of the latter. Similarly, cephradine is absorbed better than cephalexin. Cephradine and chloramphenicol are so well absorbed orally that their serum levels are higher than when the same drug is given by the intramuscular route.

Tissue distribution of antibiotics

The exact pattern of distribution of the drug in the body depends largely on the physicochemical and other properties of the drug including its lipid-solubility; protein and tissue-binding affinities; its ability to cross cell membranes and penetrate cells, and to cross the blood–brain barrier. The volume of distribution (V_d) of a drug is defined as that volume in which the total amount of drug in the body (A) would have to be uniformly distributed in order to give the observed plasma concentration (C_p). It is usually expressed in terms of the body weight as l/kg. Since $V_d = A/C_p$, the dose necessary to produce any desired plasma concentration can be calculated with a drug whose volume of distribution is known. Most antimicrobial agents have volumes of distribution between 0.15 and 0.40 l/kg.

In general, the lipid-soluble antibiotics like chloramphenicol and trimethoprim have large volumes of distribution, suggesting that most of the drug leaves the plasma and is bound in the tissues. The important clinical use of the V_d is that it allows the calculation of a loading dose that promptly provides a therapeutic plasma concentration. The V_d is also useful in calculating subsequent doses to maintain therapeutic and yet safe plasma concentrations.

Half-life of antibiotics

The half-life ($T_{\frac{1}{2}}$) of a drug is the time required for the plasma concentration to fall to one-half its former value. With regular, repetitive dosing the peak and trough plasma concentrations (C_{max} and C_{min}) rise to a steady state. The rate at which this plateau is attained is a function of the drug's $T_{\frac{1}{2}}$ and is independent of the rate of drug administration. To achieve the desired therapeutic levels quickly, a loading dose of the drug should be given whenever $T_{\frac{1}{2}}$ is estimated to be longer than 3 hours, and a delay of more than 12 hours in achieving therapeutic levels is unacceptable.

The half-lives of antimicrobial agents vary considerably. The usually quoted figures are applicable as a generalization to young, healthy adults. The first- and second-generation cephalosporins and penicillins have short $T_{\frac{1}{2}}$, usually less than 1.5 hours, whereas the $T_{\frac{1}{2}}$ of aminoglycosides is 2–3 hours; that of vancomycin is 3–6 hours and of tetracycline and trimethoprim 6–12 hours. Renal dysfunction may prolong $T_{\frac{1}{2}}$, but rational dosing adjustments can be calculated. For drugs eliminated mainly by the liver, there are no clear correlations between liver function tests and the rate of drug elimination. Patients with liver dysfunction should be monitored closely.

SELECTION OF APPROPRIATE ANTIBIOTICS

Spectrum of antimicrobial activity

The pathogens commonly encountered in gynaecological infections and their likely sensitivity patterns are listed in Table 54.2. These recommendations should be viewed as guidelines only. For urinary tract infection, pelvic inflammatory disease and sexually transmitted infections, the reader should consult the relevant chapters of this book.

It is a sound principle that a drug with a narrow spectrum of antibacterial activity is preferred to one with a broad spectrum and that combinations of two or more antibiotics should be avoided. Disadvantages of antibiotic combinations include increased likelihood of side-effects, superinfection with antibiotic-resistant bacterial strains, antagonism between the drugs and increased cost. However, in gynaecology, combination therapy is often required to cover the likely pathogens in pelvic infection or in septicaemia but a single antibiotic is usually adequate in uncomplicated wound or urinary tract infections as these are usually caused by a single bacterial species.

Some antibiotics have wide spectra of activity and are available in oral and injectable forms. Augmentin is a combination of amoxycillin with clavulanic acid to inhibit the degradation of amoxycillin by bacterial beta-lactamase. The combination is active against beta-lactamase-producing strains of *Staphylococcus aureus* and some Gram-negative aerobic rods, as well as *Bacteroides* spp.; it is therefore a reasonable first-line choice in patients with postoperative wound or pelvic infection (Houang et al 1987). It is not active against organisms which produce class 1 chromosomally mediated beta-lactamase, notably *Pseudomonas aeruginosa*, *Enterobacter cloacae* and some strains of *E. coli*. Ciprofloxacin (Ciproxin), a synthetic 4-quinolone derivative, inhibits the bacterial topoisomerase enzyme. It is active against a wide spectrum of aerobic Gram-positive cocci and Gram-negative rods including *P. aeruginosa* but has little activity against anaerobes.

However, the in vitro activity of a new antibiotic must be confirmed in clinical practice and possible side-effects must be considered. Pseudomembranous colitis has been reported not only in association with lincomycin and clindamycin but also after the use of almost all other antibiotics (except vancomycin).

Failure of response to antibiotic therapy

Occasionally, the patient may fail to respond to the treatment. In gynaecology, this often is associated with the presence of a substantial collection of pus which needs to be located and surgically drained. Septic pelvic thrombophlebitis, an uncommon diagnosis, may be responsible for the unabating fever in spite of the adequate antimicrobial treatment and absence of a collection.

Other possible causes of a failure of treatment include incorrect clinical or microbiological diagnoses. The fever may be due not to a bacterial infection but to viral infection, a drug reaction or to another systemic condition. Incorrect bacteriological diagnosis may result from inappropriate specimen collection or transport, or from failure to obtain a suitable specimen from the infected site. The laboratory may fail to recognize the causative organisms or to report correctly its antimicrobial susceptibility.

Incorrect choice or use of antibiotics would also lead to treatment failure. Antibiotics such as nitrofurantoin, commonly used to treat local infections, may not be suitable for systemic infection. The patient may have been treated with inadequate doses or duration of the correct antibiotics. In osteomyelitis pubis, treatment for 4–6 weeks is required with debridement if necessary. Increased drug elimination as a result of improved renal function may result in inadequate plasma concentrations of the drug. It is therefore important to monitor regularly the plasma levels of agents such as aminoglycosides or vancomycin, especially when the patient's condition is changing. Mixed infection may be present and the therapy may be active against only some of the pathogens.

When the condition of a patient deteriorates after a satisfactory initial response to antimicrobial therapy, superinfection with a resistant organism should be suspected. Opportunistic infection caused by microbes such as resistant aerobic Gram-negative rods, fungi or protozoa may occur in patients treated with corticosteroids, immunosuppressants, amino acid or lipid infusions, or a parenteral iron preparation.

ANTIBIOTIC PROPHYLAXIS IN GYNAECOLOGY

Prophylactic antibiotic therapy is usually valuable in operations involving clean contaminated wounds. A hysterectomy is a good example as microbial contamination from the vagina invariably takes place.

Mechanism of action of antibiotic prophylaxis

The mechanism by which chemoprophylaxis works is unclear, although it is generally believed that the antibiotic present during the operation reduces the number of contaminating organisms and also renders tissue fluid less suitable as a culture medium. In abdominal hysterectomy, contamination by skin organisms occurs in most patients upon entering the peritoneal cavity, when the bacterial count of the fluid in the pouch of Douglas may contain $10–10^4$ colony-forming units (cfu)/ml of skin organisms. After opening the vault, bacterial contamination by vaginal organisms increases markedly, maybe $>10^5$ cfu/ml (Helm et al 1986). Administering intravenous antibiotics during induction of anaesthesia substantially reduces the number of organisms. The magnitude of the contamination is likely to be determined by many factors, including the technical difficulty of the procedure, the surgeon's skill and the duration of the operation.

Antibiotic prophylaxis in hysterectomy

Vaginal hysterectomy

In vaginal hysterectomy, reduction in pelvic infection and febrile morbidity in the treated group has been reported from nearly all centres. The wide variation in infection rates in the placebo groups (12–57%) may be related to local factors and the well-recognized difficulty in defining and diagnosing pelvic infection. Significant reduction in postoperative urinary tract infection by perioperative chemoprophylaxis is more difficult to achieve. The overall cost-effectiveness is also evident in the significant reduction in the subsequent use of antibiotics and in the duration of hospital stay. For these reasons, it is generally agreed that chemoprophylaxis should be used in vaginal hysterectomy (Hirsch 1985).

Abdominal hysterectomy

The benefit of chemoprophylaxis in abdominal hysterectomy has been less uniformly demonstrated. A significant reduction in wound and pelvic infections has been observed in those studies in which the infection rate in the placebo-treated group was relatively high (>15%). Other benefits reported by some studies included significant reduction in postoperative urinary tract infection or in the febrile morbidity and a shorter duration of hospital stay. The decision to use chemoprophylaxis for abdominal hysterectomy should be made only after carrying out controlled studies at one's own centre.

Choice of antibiotics for prophylaxis during hysterectomy

In placebo-controlled studies, antibiotics with narrow spectra of activities, as well as those with broad spectra, have been used successfully. In comparative studies, it is often difficult to demonstrate a significant difference between the regimens used because the infection rate is low in patients who receive any form of chemoprophylaxis. Many more patients need to be studied to demonstrate reliably that differences between the two regimens do not exist. However, metronidazole plus cephradine or amoxycillin–clavulanic acid is superior to metronidazole alone.

Single-dose prophylaxis given at the induction of anaesthesia is as effective as multiple-dose regimens. If the surgical procedure is prolonged, a further dose may be given at the end of the operation if the half-life of the agent used is short. Otherwise, single-dose regimens reduce the cost, the toxicity and the likelihood of resistant organisms emerging. The newer cephalosporins with a longer half-life, such as cefoxitin, cefotetan and ceftriaxone, have been reported to cause increased colonization of vagina or bowel by resistant organisms such as *Streptococcus faecalis*, *Enterobacter* and yeasts (Faro et al 1988). It is not certain whether postoperative sepsis following use of these prophylactic agents would be caused by the resistant organisms.

Antibiotic prophylaxis and therapeutic abortion

Infection, frequently related to retained tissue, is an important complication after therapeutic abortion. Because of the lack of uniform definitions and diagnostic criteria, the incidence rates for chorioamnionitis, endometritis, salpingitis, and peritonitis are difficult to interpret. Furthermore, it is difficult to complete postoperative follow-up.

Uncertainty of the case for antibiotic prophylaxis with therapeutic abortion

The question of preventing infection after therapeutic abortion has been addressed by several placebo-controlled studies. Although benefits were reported in some of these studies, the wisdom of the use of antibiotic prophylaxis in all women was questioned (McGregor 1985). Apart from the problems of side-effects and emergence of resistant organisms, MacKenzie & Fry (1981) pointed out that the incidence of suspected postabortion infection and secondary subfertility in therapeutic abortion was similar to that following spontaneous abortion and full-term delivery. Furthermore, the regimens used for prophylaxis may be inadequate for treatment of existing infections. Qvigstad et al (1983) found that a single dose of tetracycline given at the time of therapeutic abortion did not protect against the development of pelvic inflammatory disease in women who had positive cervical culture for *Chlamydia trachomatis*.

Screening for sexually transmitted diseases

Endometritis after therapeutic abortion is three times more common in women with untreated gonorrhoea; the presence of *Chlamydia* in the cervix at the time of therapeutic abortion is associated with a high incidence of postoperative pelvic inflammatory disease, particularly among women under 20 years of age. An alternative approach to prophylaxis is to screen for established infection in women with risk factors such as a history of previous pelvic inflammatory or sexually transmitted disease. Preoperative screening for gonorrhoea or *Chlamydia* would allow treatment to be started before the termination.

Prophylaxis for endocarditis in gynaecology

Patients and procedures at risk

Bacterial endocarditis has been reported following hysterectomy; insertion of a ring pessary or intrauterine contraceptive device; vaginal repair or genitourinary tract instrumentation (Bayliss et al 1984). It is still a serious condition — around 15% of patients die despite treatment. Antibacterial prophylaxis has long been recommended when a procedure likely to be accompanied by bacteraemia is undertaken in a patient known to be at risk from endocarditis. The patients at risk include those with degenerative or rheumatic heart disease, patent ductus, ventricular (not atrial) septal defect and some other forms of congenital heart disease, incompetent 'floppy' mitral valve, and prosthetic heart valves (Editorial 1985).

Not infrequently, transient symptomless bacteraemia may follow alimentary and genitourinary surgery or investigation. Considering the enormous number of operations and investigations involving the alimentary and genitourinary tracts, the risk of infective endocarditis arising from these must be very small indeed. Among the factors influencing its development are the magnitude of the bacteraemia, the virulence of the organism and the susceptibility of the host. Whether or not antibiotic prophylaxis is indeed effective is unknown but for logistic and ethical reasons it is unlikely ever to be determined.

Indications for prophylaxis

Patients who are at risk of developing endocarditis may not be identified prior to the procedure. In a report by the Working Party of the British Society for Antimicrobial Chemotherapy (1982), no cardiac abnormality was recognized prior to the development of endocarditis in 41% of 577 cases. Thus, the authors do not recommend routine antibiotic prophylaxis for minor procedures such as cervical dilatation and curettage of the uterus or the insertion or removal of intrauterine contraceptive devices, except for patients with prosthetic valves.

Others hold more conservative views. Bayliss et al (1984) stressed that because of the appreciable morbidity and mortality from endocarditis, patients with cardiac abnormalities should be given antibiotic cover for all surgical, alimentary and genitourinary procedures. Furthermore, in view of the high proportion of older patients with normal hearts who contract infective endocarditis, those over 60 years of age should also receive prophylactic cover.

Endocarditis and intrauterine contraceptive devices

In women with a history of heart disease, Sparks (1985) suggests that the decision to fit an intrauterine contraceptive device should be made between the cardiologist and gynaecologist. An absolute contraindication should be a history of pelvic inflammatory disease or infective endocarditis. Women with prosthetic heart valves or who have had previous cardiac surgery or are drug abusers would seem to have a greater risk of developing endocarditis. For women in these risk groups for whom no other form of contraception is possible, antibiotic cover for insertion of intrauterine contraceptive devices should be mandatory and follow-up performed at a hospital clinic where sterile instruments are available. Any case of endocarditis in intrauterine contraceptive device users should be reported to the Committee on Safety of Medicines.

Choice of antibiotics

In genitourinary surgery, any antibiotic regimen to prevent endocarditis should be effective against *Streptococcus faecalis*. Suitable regimens are suggested in Table 54.2. The details of administration of antibiotics are available in the latest issue of the British National Formulary.

Antibiotic prophylaxis — conclusions

There is little doubt of the value of prophylaxis in vaginal hysterectomy and it is a sensible precaution in women undergoing difficult pelvic surgery. A single dose of antibiotics is as effective as multiple-dose regimens and metronidazole plus cephradine or amoxycillin–clavulanic acid is better than metronidazole alone.

Routine prophylaxis for women undergoing termination of pregnancy is of less certain value. Screening for gonorrhoea and *Chlamydia* may be worthwhile, especially in high-risk women.

Most gynaecologists would feel that patients with cardiac abnormalities should receive prophylaxis against bacterial endocarditis. Possible regimens are described in Table 54.2.

KEY POINTS

1. Bacteriological samples should always be obtained before commencing antibiotic therapy.
2. A wide range of anaerobic and aerobic organisms are found in the vagina of healthy women.
3. Postoperative infection is often due to infection with several different organisms, both anaerobic and aerobic. *Escherichia coli* and *Bacteroides fragilis* are the most common.
4. Infected abortion is usually polymicrobial resulting from a mixed flora of aerobic and anaerobic strcptococci, *Bacteroides* spp.; *E. coli* and other enteric organisms.
5. In gynaecology, a single antibiotic is usually adequate in uncomplicated wound or urinary tract infections as these are generally caused by a single bacterial species. Combination therapy is often required in order to cover the likely pathogens in pelvic infection or in septicaemia.
6. Successful management of septic abortion requires evacuation of the uterus after antimicrobial therapy has been commenced.
7. Surgery is indicated in the management of postoperative infection if the patient fails to respond to antibiotic therapy or develops generalized peritonitis or has a pelvic abscess that show no signs of draining spontaneously.
8. Any infected foreign body must be removed.
9. Necrotizing fasciitis is rare but very serious. It often looks like a minor wound infection in the early stages but requires vigorous surgical excision of all involved tissue.
10. Resistance to antibiotics may be acquired by genetic mutation or by the incorporation of a plasmid from a resistant strain.
11 A rapidly achieved high peak concentration is important for antibiotics. Amoxycillin is twice as well absorbed as ampicillin and therefore should be used as the oral form of the latter.
12. A loading dose of the drug should be given whenever $T_{\frac{1}{2}}$ is estimated to be longer than 3 hours; a delay of more than 12 hours in achieving therapeutic levels is unacceptable.
13. Antibiotic prophylaxis is indicated in vaginal hysterectomy and it is a sensible precaution in women undergoing difficult pelvic surgery.
14. A single dose of antibiotics is as effective as multiple-dose regimens in prophylaxis.

REFERENCES

Allen Addison W, Livergood C H, Hill G B, Sutton G P, Fortier K J 1984 Necrotizing fasciitis of vulvar origin in diabetic patients. Obstetrics and Gynecology 63: 473–479

Bayliss R, Clarke C, Oakley C M, Somerville W, Whitefield A G W, Young S E J 1984 The bowel and genitourinary tract and infective endocarditis. British Heart Journal 51: 339–345

Chow A W, Percival-Smith R, Bartlett K H, Goldring A M, Morrison B J 1986 Vaginal colonization with *Escherichia coli* in healthy women. Determination of relative risks by quantitative culture and multivariate statistical analysis. American Journal of Obstetrics and Gynecology 154: 120–126

Editorial 1985 Prophylaxis for endocarditis. Drugs and Therapeutics Bulletin 23: 53–56

Faro S, Phillips L E, Martens M G 1988 Perspectives on the bacteriology of post-operative obstetric-gynecologic infections. American Journal of Obstetrics and Gynecology 158: 694–700

Hammerschlag M R, Alpert S, Onderdonk A B et al 1978 Anaerobic microflora of the vagina in children. American Journal of Obstetrics and Gynecology 131: 853–856

Helm C W, Macdonald C, Houang E T 1986 Bacterial contamination during abdominal hysterectomy. Journal of Obstetrics and Gynaecology 6: S64–66

Hirsch H A 1985 Prophylactic antibiotics in obstetrics and gynaecology. American Journal of Medicine 78 (suppl 6B): 170–176

Houang E T, Colley N, Chapman M 1987 Comparison of amoxycillin with clavulanate (Augmentin), with ampicillin and metronidazole, as the first line treatment for post-operative infections after gynaecological surgery. Journal of Obstetrics and Gynaecology 8: 156–160

Mackenzie I, Fry A 1981 Post abortion sepsis and antibiotic prophylaxis. British Medical Journal 282: 476–477

Mandell G L, Douglas R G, Bennett J E 1985 Anti-infective therapy. Churchill Livingstone, New York

McGregor J A 1985 Prophylactic antibiotics unjustified for unselected abortion patients. American Journal of Obstetrics and Gynecology 152: 722–724

Qvigstad E, Skang K, Jerve F, Fylling P, Ulstrup J C 1983 Pelvic inflammatory disease associated with therapeutic abortion. British Journal of Venereal Disease 59: 189–192

Sparks R A 1985 Endocarditis and the IUD. British Journal of Family Planning 11: 19–23

Thadepalli H, Gorback S L, Keith L 1973 Anaerobic infections of the female genital tract: bacteriologic and therapeutic aspects. American Journal of Obstetrics and Gynecology 117: 1034–1040

Working Party of the British Society of Antimicrobial Chemotherapy

1982 The antibiotic prophylaxis of infective endocarditis. Lancet ii: 1323–1326

FURTHER READING

Kucers A, Bennett N McK 1987 The use of antibiotics, 4th edn. A comprehensive review with clinical emphasis. Heinemann Medical Books, London

Ledger W J 1986 Infection in the female, 2nd edn. Lea & Febiger, Philadelphia

Shanson D C 1989 Microbiology in clinical practice. Wright/Butterworths, Bristol

55. Pelvic inflammatory disease

J. Moodley

INTRODUCTION

Pelvic inflammatory disease (PID) is a major health problem in both developing and affluent societies despite advances in defining its aetiology, pathogenesis and the availability of many powerful antimicrobial drugs. Treatment of this condition and its sequelae, in particular infertility, consumes a significant portion of the medical resources of numerous countries. Often, the infection rates are highest in areas where medical resources are most severely limited. Even in developed countries where large sums of money are spent in defining the cause of infertility and in treating it, success cannot be guaranteed.

A variety of organisms cause pelvic infection, and secondary infection readily occurs, so that the primary infecting agent is often not identified. In most cases the infection ascends from the vagina and cervix to the uterus and parametrial tissues, fallopian tubes, ovaries and pelvic peritoneum. Salpingitis may also result from infection spreading from adjacent pelvic organs, e.g. following appendicitis or diverticulitis. Haematogenous spread may also occur, e.g. tuberculosis. There may also be an obvious predisposing factor such as a recent abortion, delivery, gynaecological surgical procedure or insertion of an intrauterine contraceptive device.

TERMINOLOGY

The pelvic infections are often grouped together under the term pelvic inflammatory disease (PID). This term lacks precise definition and should be avoided (Keith et al 1986). The extent to which the pelvic organs are involved in an infectious process is better described using anatomical terminology such as endometritis, parametritis, salpingitis, salpingo-oophoritis, pelvic peritonitis, or pelvic (tubal, ovarian) abscess. Thus PID is defined as the clinical syndrome attributed to the ascending spread of microorganisms (unrelated to pregnancy and surgery) from the vagina and cervix to the endometrium, fallopian tube and/or contiguous structures. This chapter will therefore concentrate on infections unrelated to pregnancy and surgery.

EPIDEMIOLOGY

Because PID is not a notifiable disease in most countries, accurate statistics are unavailable, but there is no question that thousands of young women have salpingitis every year and their sheer numbers make it an important health problem. One publication in the USA estimates the rate to be at least 2% per year among sexually active women (Keith et al 1984). Sweet (1988) states that 1 million women are treated for PID (acute salpingitis) in the USA annually: 250 000–300 000 are admitted to hospital and 150 000 have surgery. More accurate figures are probably obtained from the UK and Scandinavian countries where most women with sexually transmitted diseases attend state clinics. A widely quoted Scandinavian report (Westrom 1980) suggests that the annual incidence of PID in modern western society is 1% among women aged 15–34; in the high-risk age group (from age 15 to 24 years), the incidence is 2%

and the incidence of PID among women aged 30 years or older is approximately one-third that among women younger than 25 years.

There are few data from developing countries on the incidence of PID but it seems to be a problem of great magnitude. Lithgow & Rubin (1972) state that pelvic sepsis is probably the commonest gynaecological disease afflicting African women. Pelvic infection comprised 15.8% of all gynaecological admissions to Baragwanath Hospital, Johannesburg, in 1970. In 1989, 7% of all gynaecological admissions to King Edward VIII Hospital, Durban, South Africa had severe PID (severe acute salpingitis). It should be noted that many hospitals in the African continent admit only patients with severe disease. There is no doubt therefore that PID constitutes a serious health problem in developing countries.

PATHOGENESIS

The classic concept of the pathogenesis of PID unrelated to pregnancy, surgery, gynaecological procedures or extension of infection emanating from the gastrointestinal tract is that lower genital tract infections ascend along the endocervical mucosa to reach the uterine cavity. An alternative pathway of ascent is provided by lymphatic drainage from the cervix. In the opinion of many authors this spread of infection also paves the way for secondary invasion of the upper genital tract by bacteria normally found in the vagina (Mardh et al 1983).

While these concepts remain valid, it is suggested that the ascent of bacteria from the lower to the upper genital tract is promoted by sexually transmitted vectors, e.g. sperm and trichomonads (Keith et al 1984). Sperm intimately associates with a variety of infectious agents and the attachment of *Escherichia coli* to sperm has been shown experimentally. In addition, fertile and infertile men without a history of infection have similar numbers of isolates of aerobic, facultative and anaerobic bacterial flora from their semen while a significantly higher number of bacterial isolates were obtained from the semen of infertile men with a past history of infection (Toth 1983). Four observations from this work are noteworthy. First, most men with bacteriospermia were asymptomatic. Second, the severity of the patient's bacteriospermia was related to the number of previous sexual partners. Third, women married to men with high bacterial counts in their seminal fluid had the greatest chance of developing pelvic infections. And fourth, wives of azoospermic men rarely developed PID. This study provides additional evidence that sperm may transport bacteria. Similar evidence suggests that the trichomonad may act as a vector but further research needs to be performed to evaluate the role of vectors in the pathogenesis of PID.

The route of spread of the infectious agents causing salpingitis is most often through the lumen of the genital tract. Ascent of an infection from the lower genital tract via the tissues of the broad ligament resulting in parametritis and a subsequent ectosalpingitis has been suggested as a mode of spread of mycoplasmal infections (Moller et al 1980). Parametritis as a clinical entity however is most often encountered as a complication of gynaecological operative procedures. Haematogenous spread of infection to the upper genital tract from extragenital sites is rare. The most common exceptions are salpingitis in tuberculosis and oophoritis in mumps.

Direct spread of an infection to the fallopian tubes from nearby pelvic structure is seen occasionally. Appendicitis spreading to the right fallopian tube is the usual example of this.

Factors related to the onset of PID

It is not always clear what causes the onset of PID at a given time in a given patient. The mere presence of potentially pathogenic micro-organisms in the lower or upper genital tract does not necessarily lead to clinically recognizable disease. Numerous endogenous and exogenous factors affect the progression of cervical infection to the fallopian tubes.

Endogenous factors include, amongst others, the anatomical configuration of the cervix, the quantity and quality of cervical mucus and the duration and quantity of menstrual flow. Exogenous factors include the age at onset of sexual activity, the frequency and nature of sexual activity, the number of sexual partners, the number of partners of the sexual partner(s) and the contraception used.

The cervix offers a functional barrier to the ascent of micro-organisms. The properties of this barrier are at their lowest at the time of ovulation and when the mucus plug is absent (i.e. during menstrual bleeding and after abortion and parturition).

Hormonal treatment can also cause changes in the properties of the functional barrier of the cervix. The administration of progesterone induces a mechanically resistant plug of cervical mucus and this seems to protect against ascending infection. The use of combined (oestrogen/progesterone) oral contraceptives inhibits the periovulatory local changes in the cervix. Women using this method of contraception are less likely to develop salpingitis than women not using contraceptives.

Uterine factors also play an important role in promoting ascending infections. The mechanical transport of particles upwards in the genital tract is thought to be due to the muscular activity of the myometrium. Coital (orgasmic) contractions of the myometrium are said to result in the deposition of spermatozoa in the fallopian tubes a few minutes after they are deposited in the vagina (i.e. sooner than would be expected from their own motility; Ahlgren 1975).

Operative procedures that open the cervical canal can pave the way for micro-organisms to enter the upper genital tract (e.g. legal abortion, insertion of intrauterine contraceptive device, curettage, hysterosalpingography).

PATHOLOGY

Much of the information on the macroscopic appearance of the tubes has been obtained from laparoscopic studies performed in patients with PID (Jacobsen & Westrom 1969; Hager et al 1983). In mild cases of salpingitis, the fallopian tubes are swollen and their serosal surface slightly reddened. The tubes are freely mobile, their abdominal ostia are open and the tubal mucosa that can be seen in the fimbriated end is congested and often covered by a sticky exudate. Slight pressure on the tube often causes a purulent or seropurulent exudate to appear.

In moderately severe disease, the serosal surfaces of the tube are generally covered by patchy fibrin deposits. The tubes are not freely mobile and tend to adhere to nearby structures such as the ovaries, the broad ligament and the bowel. The adhesions are loose and moist, the fimbriae adhere to one another or to the ovary and seal the infectious process in the tubes from the pelvic cavity.

In severe salpingitis and pelvic peritonitis the infectious process has spread to the pelvic peritoneum. The peritoneal surfaces show intense congestion. The pelvic organs adhere to one another and the entire pelvic cavity is occupied by an inflammatory mass in which the anatomical structures are difficult to define. The infectious process in the sealed tube can lead to the formation of a tubal or tubo-ovarian abscess. In some, the tubal ostia are not completely sealed and pus escapes into the pelvic cavity. Generalized peritonitis is uncommon but may result from rupture of a tubo-ovarian abscess.

The infectious process can be self-limiting, or appropriate treatment can interrupt its progress at any stage. A complete functional restitution may follow after mild and moderately severe infections. In other instances, the lumen of the fallopian tube remains open, but scarring and replacement of functional tissue by fibrous and collagen tissue give the oviduct a rigid appearance and cause functional impairment. In cases with occluded tubes the end result is usually that of a pale, club-shaped uterine tube with a closed tubal orifice. The 'loose' adhesions and fibrin deposits may be converted into dense, fibrous strands which restrict the mobility of the tubes, cover the ovaries and cause adjacent structures to adhere to each other and result in what is referred to as chronic salpingitis or frozen pelvis.

A pelvic abscess if not surgically drained may rupture spontaneously into the rectum or vagina. Rupture of a tubo-ovarian abscess into the peritoneal cavity results in generalized peritonitis. Sometimes the pus of an abscess is replaced by serous fluid, the wall of the tube becomes thinned and its mucosal folds flattened. This pale, closed, thin-walled tube filled with clear watery fluid is called a hydrosalpinx.

MICROBIOLOGY

Traditionally PID has been divided into gonococcal or non-gonococcal disease depending on whether *Neisseria gonorrhoeae* was found in the endocervix. Since this organism was found in 30–80% of cases, it was generally believed to be the primary pathogen. However, the organisms grown from endocervical samples are not necessarily the same as those grown from samples taken from the fallopian tube and peritoneal cavity (Westrom 1980; Mardh et al 1983; Keith et al 1984). In six studies, the prevalence of *N. gonorrhoeae* in the endocervix ranged from 39 to 94%, but it was often absent from the peritoneal cavity. It was the only organism in the peritoneal cavity less than one-third of the time. In one-third of patients, peritoneal cultures revealed gonococci plus anaerobic and aerobic bacteria.

Sweet (1988) believes that PID is caused by a mixture of pathogens. His group recovered an average of 6 micro-organisms per patient from the upper genital tract, predominantly anaerobes and facultative aerobes. *Chlamydia-trachomatis* was found in the upper genital tract in 25% of patients admitted with PID. Thus, when the diagnosis of PID is made, the presence of multiple organisms must be assumed. Depending on the population studied, 25–50% of patients with PID will have gonococci, 25–50% will have anaerobes, 20–30% will have *C. trachomatis* and 10% will have *Mycoplasma hominis* (Table 55.1).

Table 55.1 Organisms isolated from the upper genital tract of patients with PID

Organism
Neisseria gonorrhoeae
Chlamydia trachomatis
Bacteroides bivius
Bacteroides discens
Other *Bacteroides* species
Peptostreptococcus asaccharolyticus
Peptostreptococcus anaerobius
Gardnerella vaginalis
Escherichia coli
Group B streptococcus
Alpha-haemolytic streptococcus
Non-haemolytic streptococcus
Coagulase-negative staphylococcus
Mycoplasma hominis
Ureaplasma urealyticum

CLINICAL MANIFESTATIONS AND DIAGNOSIS

Acute salpingitis can vary from symptomless disease to a life-threatening condition. The lower genital tract infection preceding salpingitis may pass unnoticed or cause only mild and transient symptoms. The classic description of PID is lower abdominal pain and tenderness, purulent cervical discharge, adnexal tenderness, fever, elevated erythrocyte sedimentation rate (ESR) and leukocytosis. Other symptoms include dyspareunia, urinary tract symptoms and irregular intermenstrual bleeding.

History

The onset of bilateral, lower abdominal or pelvic pain which is dull in character is regarded as the first symptom of ascending infection. In gonorrhoea-associated salpingitis, the onset of pain is significantly more often (46%) correlated with menstrual bleeding than in non-gonococcal cases (23%; Jacobsen & Westrom 1969). Gonococcal-associated salpingitis also has a more rapid onset of abdominal pain (<3 days) than non-gonococcal cases (5–7 days).

One-third of patients with salpingitis complain of irregular heavy vaginal bleeding. This symptom is a sign of accompanying endometritis. In young women such bleeding should always arouse suspicion of a genital infection.

Only 50% of patients with salpingitis report an increased vaginal discharge. All women with sexually transmitted salpingitis should have an infection in the lower genital tract. The absence of leukocytes on a wet mount excludes an ascending infection. Nausea and vomiting are infrequent but when present they suggest peritonitis. Dyspareunia is a common symptom.

Pain and discomfort in the upper right abdominal quadrant are symptoms of a possible concomitant perihepatitis (Fitz–Hugh–Curtiss syndrome). This is reported in less than 5% of patients with salpingitis. These symptoms are important because they may be mistaken for a cholecystitis or pleurisy if they are dominant features in the history.

Examination

A temperature greater than 38°C is found in one-third of laparoscopically verified cases of salpingitis. Febrile illness is more common in patients with gonorrhoea-associated salpingitis and severe (anaerobic) pelvic peritonitis than in the usually more benign chlamydial infections.

A palpable adnexal mass is found in half the patients with acute salpingitis. In patients with pelvic pain, the results of a pelvic examination should be interpreted with caution because the presence of a mass is confirmed at laparoscopy in only three-quarters of cases of salpingitis.

The simple test of wet mount smear taken from a cervical discharge can be used to exclude infection of the lower genital tract. In no instance of salpingitis is a wet smear similar to that of a healthy women, i.e. there are few or no leukocytes, a predominance of Gram-positive lactobacilli, and vaginal epithelial cells covered by only a few bacteria.

Laboratory tests

Laboratory tests discriminate poorly between mild tubal infections and genital infections not involving the tubes. Increased numbers of white blood cells are seen in just under two-thirds of patients with salpingitis and in one-third of patients with infection confined to the lower genital tract. Similarly, an elevated ESR is seen in three out of four patients with salpingitis but also in half of the patients with lower genital tract infections. The results of both tests correlate with the severity of the inflammatory reactions of the fallopian tube as seen at laparoscopy.

Because ectopic pregnancy is so difficult to exclude in women presenting with symptoms suggestive of salpingitis, it is prudent to measure the serum or urine levels of beta-human chorionic gonadotrophin (Buck et al 1987). Other laboratory tests include measurement of C-reactive protein, antichymotrypsin orosomucoid and specific genital isoamylases. The last needs further evaluation in patients with salpingitis while the first three are raised in both upper and lower genital tract infections. Determination on serial serum samples of levels of IgG and IgM antibodies may indicate ongoing infection. This may not necessarily be salpingitis because cervicitis and endometritis can also cause an antibody response.

Microbiological investigations

To establish the microbial aetiology of tubal infection, ideally specimens should be obtained at the time of laparoscopy or laparotomy. This is not practical in every case. Therefore, although cultures from cervical specimens give no reliable information on the aetiology of the tubal infection, they do provide information about sexually transmitted diseases related to the tubal infection. This information should be used for contact tracing as well as for treatment. Analysis of specimens obtained by culdocentesis is also unreliable for establishing the microbial aetiology of salpingitis and in particular for detecting chlamydial infections (Sweet 1980).

Laparoscopy

Much of the current knowledge about acute salpingitis has been obtained with the use of laparoscopy. It is still indispensable for clinical research.

For routine clinical practice, the risks of the procedure, the expense and the workload of the hospital must be taken into account. Laparoscopy is probably mandatory in those cases in which the differential diagnosis includes salpingitis, appendicitis or ectopic pregnancy.

Clinical syndromes

In the individual case of salpingitis, the clinical picture gives no definite aetiological diagnosis but certain features may suggest a likely microbial aetiology.

In gonorrhoea-associated salpingitis, the typical patient is young and from the lower socioeconomic strata of the community. The history of abdominal pain is short (<3 days); she has a pyrexia (>38°C), urinary tract symptoms and a palpable mass. Often the symptoms occur at or immediately after a menstrual period.

Patients with chlamydial salpingitis are also younger but the duration of symptoms are longer, usually 7–10 days prior to presentation. Febrile illness is rare, clinical findings are minimal and the general condition is good. The ESR is elevated.

The patient with an aerobic infection is generally older. Often it is her second or third episode and she is probably using an intrauterine contraceptive device. The onset is acute and the patient is usually severely ill. Palpable adnexal swellings and febrile illness are the rule.

Diagnosis

There are no signs or symptoms which are pathognomonic for salpingitis. Adherence to the rigid criteria of the classic description of PID (see above) will result in the diagnosis being made too late to prevent sequelae or in not being made at all (Svensson et al 1983; Westrom 1983). In addition, laparoscopy confirmed PID in only 62% of patients with a clinical diagnosis in one study (Allen & Schoon 1983).

While it is generally accepted that laparoscopy greatly enhances objectivity in the diagnosis of acute PID, it is not practical for all patients suspected of having acute PID to undergo this diagnostic procedure. Several groups have suggested improved criteria for the diagnosis of PID to decrease the likelihood of missing or misdiagnosing PID (Hager et al 1983; Westrom 1983; Sweet 1988). A compilation of these suggestions is shown in Table 55.2.

Table 55.2 Amended criteria for the diagnosis of PID

All three of these subjective findings must be present:

Abdominal tenderness (with or without rebound)
Cervical motion tenderness
Adnexal tenderness

Plus at least one of these objective signs:

Temperature >38°C
Leukocytosis >10 000/mm^3
Pelvic abscess or inflammatory complex found on bimanual examination or sonography
Gram's stain of endocervix positive for Gram-negative intracellular diplococci
Purulent endocervical discharge with leukocytes on smear
Monoclonal smear positive for *Chlamydia trachomatis*
Purulent material on culdocentesis

TREATMENT

The goals of therapy in PID are to control the current infection and to prevent infertility and other chronic sequelae. Towards this end, conservative treatment with rest, analgesia and antibiotics is the rule and surgery the exception. Some authors are inclined to hospitalize all patients in whom the diagnosis is made (Sweet 1988). This is obviously not practical in most countries, especially non-industrialized societies. The indications that may be used for hospitalization are shown in Table 55.3 (Sweet 1988). Chapin (1987) and Hemsell (1988) add further criteria to this list: a patient too unreliable to return for evaluation in 48 h and a patient less than 21 years of age.

Table 55.3 Indications for hospitalization

Temperature >38°C
Adnexal mass
Coexisting pregnancy
Presence of an intrauterine contraceptive device
Uncertain diagnosis
Inability to tolerate oral medication
Failure to respond to outpatient therapy within 48 h

Antibiotic therapy

Outpatients

In most cases antimicrobial treatment has to be instituted before the microbial aetiology has been established. Outpatient therapy proposed by the Center for Disease Control (1985) for the treatment of uncomplicated acute disease associated with *Neisseria gonorhoeae* include consideration of the penicillin-allergic patient (Table 55.4). Prolonged oral therapy is recommended primarily for eradication of *Chlamydia trachomatis*.

Women must be monitored closely following initiation of outpatient therapy to ensure the lowest possible incidence of sequelae. The patient should be seen at least 48 h later and then weekly for pelvic examinations and ESR determinations. Wet smears can be used as a guide for cure. When a wet mount of vaginal contents is normal the infection can be regarded as eradicated. With correct antibiotic treatment this usually takes 14 days. Thus Sweet (1988) argues that Center for Disease Control outpatient oral antibiotic recommendations should be extended to 14 instead of 7 days.

Table 55.4 Outpatient drug therapy for PID

Non-penicillin-allergic patients
After 1 g probenecid orally:
Amoxycillin 3 g orally
Ampicillin 3.5 g orally
Aqueous procaine penicillin G 4.8 Mu i.m.
Cefoxitin 2 g i.m.
Ceftriaxone 250 mg i.m. (or equivalent)
Penicillin-allergic patients
Spectinomycin 2 g i.m.
Tetracycline 1 g loading dose
plus maintenance dose as indicated below
All patients also receive a 7-day course of:
Tetracycline 0.5 g q.i.d.
Doxycycline 0.1 g b.d.
Erythromycin 0.5 g q.i.d.

Inpatients

Regimens recommended by the Center for Disease Control (1985) for inpatient treatment of uncomplicated PID limited to tubes and ovaries with or without peritonitis are shown in Table 55.5. Intravenous therapy is recommended for at least 4 days or for 48 h after the patient improves. Justification for these recommendations is limited. Patients without adnexal masses become afebrile and essentially asymptomatic during the first 24–36 h of parenteral therapy. Intravenous therapy for another 3–4 days may not be beneficial (Thompson 1980).

If the patient has a tubo-ovarian mass that has not ruptured, drug therapy must include an agent effective against *Bacteroides fragilis* such as metronidazole 250–750 mg 8-hourly; clindamycin 600 mg i.v. 6-hourly; chloramphenicol 500 mg i.v. 6-hourly, or cefoxitin 2–3 g i.v. 6-hourly.

About 70% of patients with tubo-ovarian abscesses respond to medical management. However, if no response is evident in 48–72 h, surgery is warranted.

Preventing re-infection

To prevent re-infection, sexual partners should be treated as if they have non-gonococcal urethritis with tetracycline 500 mg 6-hourly or doxycycline 100 mg 12-hourly orally for 7 days. Many men are asymptomatic carriers of gonorrhoea or *Chlamydia*. Treatment is justified even if the male denies symptoms.

Education of the patient about avoiding re-infection and the potential sequelae of PID is essential. She must be warned of the increasing risk of serious sequelae with each infection. After one properly treated episode of PID there is an infertility rate of 12% compared with 3% in the control population, but after two episodes the infertility rate increases to 23%, and 54% after three infections (Westrom 1985). She should be advised against multiple sexual partners and told about the protective effects of barrier contraception against infection.

Table 55.5 Inpatient drug therapy for PID

Uncomplicated infection
Cefoxitin 2.0 g i.v. 6-hourly plus
Doxycycline hyclate 100 mg i.v. 12-hourly
Continue for 4 days or for 48 h after pyrexia settles
Thereafter:
Doxycycline 100 mg orally 12-hourly to complete 10–14 days of therapy or
Clindamycin HCl 600 mg i.v. 6-hourly plus
Aminoglycoside 2 mg/kg i.v. loading dose followed by 1.5 mg/kg maintenance i.v. 8-hourly
Continue for 4 days or for 48 h after pyrexia settles
Thereafter:
Clindamycin 450 mg orally 6-hourly to complete 10–14 days of therapy

Surgery

Surgery is generally limited to those patients with generalized peritonitis; those with a tubo-ovarian abscess which does not respond to antimicrobial therapy within 48 h, and those with a pelvic abscess that points into the vagina, rectum or through the abdominal wall.

In patients with generalized peritonitis, dehydration, anaemia and acidosis should be corrected rapidly before the laparotomy. Broad-spectrum antimicrobial therapy with bactericidal effects should be initiated immediately. At King Edward VIII Hospital in Durban a combination of penicillin, an aminoglycoside and metronidazole is used. Alternatively, a third-generation cephalosporin such as cefotaxime may be used with metronidazole.

Adequate exposure is essential at the time of laparotomy and the whole abdominal cavity, particularly the sub-diaphragmatic spaces and the entire intestinal tract, should be examined to exclude multiloculated abscesses. The type of surgery required varies. In the South African context, particularly in young women, the tubo-ovarian masses are removed, a lavage is performed and drains are inserted in the paracolic gutters. The uterus is conserved so that hormone replacement therapy can be instituted following recovery. Menstruation is important to the female psyche in the local population. In the older patient, hysterectomy together with removal of the tubo-ovarian masses is usually performed. The entire peritoneal cavity should be lavaged with an antibiotic solution before closure. Vaginal suction drainage and delayed primary closure are useful adjuncts to surgical management.

A significant proportion of women with tubo-ovarian infection have unilateral disease (Golde et al 1977). These probably result from a different mechanism than the ascending infection seen with bilateral disease. It seems likely that the infection is blood-borne in these cases in the same way as those patients who develop adnexal abscesses after vaginal hysterectomy (Niebyl et al 1978). In the vast majority of such patients, a unilateral tubo-ovarian abscess requires removal of only the affected adnexae even if the contralateral organs are inflamed. Over 90% will require no further surgery.

In neglected cases, septicaemic shock may intervene. In such circumstances prompt vigorous treatment in an intensive care unit will be required to provide close monitoring, ventilatory support and maintenance of blood pressure with inotropic drugs if necessary. Although women with neglected PID are uncommon in affluent societies they are still seen in developing countries. There is still a significant morbidity and mortality among such patients.

Pelvic thrombophlebitis

Infection of the pelvic organs or postoperative sepsis may extend to involve the major pelvic vessels. Thrombophlebitis is of late onset and presents like a resistant infection with tachycardia, fever and dull, low abdominal pain. Pelvic examination reveals tenderness along the lateral pelvic wall. The essential feature is the lack of localizing signs. A therapeutic test of heparin, 24 000 u daily, is a non-invasive way of corroborating the diagnosis. Fever and abdominal pain should respond within 48 h. Oral anticoagulation is continued for 3–4 weeks.

TREATMENT RESULTS

With correctly chosen antibiotic therapy for the patient and her partner, the current treatment effectively eradicates sexually transmitted agents from the cervix. Mortality is rare and is limited to patients with generalized peritonitis. In such cases the mortality remains at about 8%.

The late complications of salpingitis are chronic abdominal pain, infertility and an increased risk of ectopic pregnancy. Abdominal pain lasting for longer than 6 months occurs in about 18% of patients.

The only unequivocal proof of successful treatment after salpingitis is an intrauterine pregnancy. Infertility, even following the use of appropriate antibiotics, is still common. After one episode of salpingitis the rate is 11%; after two, 23%; and after three or more episodes, 54%. Post-infection tubal damage is one of the most common aetiological factors in ectopic pregnancy. In a prospective study, a ratio of 1 ectopic to every 16 intrauterine pregnancies was found in the first pregnancy after salpingitis while in the control population the ratio was 1:147 (Westrom et al 1982).

CONCLUSION

PID is a disease of increasing frequency responsible for a great deal of human misery. Much of that unhappiness could be avoided by health education and by prompt, effective treatment of sexually transmitted infections. The traditional view must be discarded that the gonococcus is the main aetiological agent and the use of single-dose therapy for PID must give way to more effective regimens that take into account the polymicrobial nature of the infection.

Laparoscopy and ultrasonography should be used more frequently in both the diagnosis and follow-up. A liberal admission policy and multiple drug therapy will decrease the frequency of sequelae.

Future strategies should include education of both laypersons and physicians; screening for genital infections before operative procedures; the use of oral contraceptives or depot progestogens for women at risk of PID; follow-up of partners of women with salpingitis, and the development of simple, safe and specific diagnostic procedures.

KEY POINTS

1. PID affects 1% of women aged 15–34 in western countries and is the commonest gynaecological condition in many Third World countries.
2. Most infections ascend the lumen of the genital tract.
3. Women married to men with high bacterial counts in their semen are at high risk of PID.
4. Bacterispermia is often asymptomatic.
5. Sperm may act as vectors of infection.
6. Infection is commonly due to multiple organisms.
7. Salpingitis may give only mild symptoms or may be life-threatening.
8. Lower abdominal pain is the usual presenting symptom.
9. Vaginal discharge and irregular vaginal bleeding are less constant symptoms.
10. In patients with pelvic pain, the results of a pelvic examination should be interpreted with caution because the presence of a mass is confirmed at laparoscopy in only three-quarters of cases of salpingitis.
11. Because ectopic pregnancy is so difficult to exclude in women presenting with symptoms suggestive of salpingitis, it is prudent to measure the serum or urine levels of beta-human chorionic gonadotrophin.
12. Culture of endocervical material does not give a reliable indication of the microbiology of tubal infection.
13. Outpatient antibiotic therapy is sufficient for most patients with uncomplicated PID.
14. Therapy should be continued for at least 7 and more usually 14 days to eradicate chlamydial infection.
15. Outpatient therapy should be reviewed first 48 h later.
16. In patients requiring hospital admission, intravenous therapy is recommended for 24–48 h after the temperature has settled.
17. Surgery may be required if no response is evident within 48–72 h.

18. To prevent re-infection, sexual partners should be treated with tetracycline 500 mg 6-hourly or doxycycline 100 mg 12-hourly orally for 7 days even if they deny symptoms.
19. After one properly treated episode of PID there is an infertility rate of 12% but after two episodes the infertility rate increases to 23%, and 54% after three infections.
20. If surgery is required, unilateral salpingo-oophorectomy will suffice for unilateral disease in young women.
21. Chronic abdominal pain may affect 18% of women after PID.
22. Ectopic pregnancy is 10 times more likely after salpingitis.

REFERENCES

Ahlgren M 1975 Sperm transport to, and survival in, the human fallopian tube. Gynecology Investigation 6: 206–207

Allen L A, Schoon M G 1983 Laparoscopic diagnosis of acute pelvic inflammatory disease. British Journal of Obstetrics and Gynaecology 90: 966–968

Buck R H, Pather N, Moodley J, Joubert S M, Norman R J 1987 Bedside application of an ultrasensitive urine test for hCG in patients with suspected ectopic pregnancy. Annals of Clinical Biochemistry 24: 268–272

Center for Disease Control 1985 Sexually transmitted disease guidelines. Morbidity and Mortality Weekly Reports 34 (suppl): 925–929

Chapin D S 1987 Pelvic inflammatory disease. Medical Times 115: 49–57

Golde S H, Israel R, Ledger W J 1977 Unilateral tubo-ovarian abscess: a distinct entity. American Journal of Obstetrics and Gynecology 127: 807–812

Hager W D, Eschenback D A, Spence M R, Sweet R L 1983 Criteria for diagnosis and grading of salpingitis. Obstetrics and Gynecology 61: 113–114

Hemsell D L 1988 Acute pelvic inflammatory disease — etiologic and therapeutic considerations. Journal of Reproductive Medicine 33 (suppl): 119–123

Jacobsen L, Westrom L 1969 Objectivized diagnosis of acute pelvic inflammatory disease. American Journal of Obstetrics and Gynecology 105: 1088–1097

Keith L G, Berger G S 1984 The aetiology of pelvic inflammatory disease. In: Zathuchni G I (ed) Research frontiers in fertility regulation, vol 3. Chicago, North Western University, p 88

Keith L G, Berger G S, Edelman D A et al 1984 On the causation of pelvic inflammatory disease. American Journal of Obstetrics and Gynecology 149: 215–224

Keith L G, Berger G S, Lopex-Zeno J 1986 New concepts on the causation of pelvic inflammatory disease. Current problems in Obstetrics, Gynaecology and Fertility IX: 17–45

Lithgow D M, Rubin A 1972 In: Charlewood G P (ed) Gynaecology in South Africa. Johannesburg, Witwatersrand University Press, p 177

Mardh P A, Westrom L, Ripa K T 1983 Pelvic inflammatory disease: clinical, etiologic and pathophysiologic studies. In: Holmes K K, March P A (eds) International perspectives on neglected sexually transmitted diseases. Washington D C, Hemisphere Publishing, p 128·

Moller B R, Freund T E, March P A 1980 Experimental infection of the genital tract of female grivet monkeys by Mycoplasma hominis. American Journal of Obstetrics and Gynecology 138: 990–995

Niebyl J R, Parmley T H, Spence M R et al 1978 Unilateral ovarian abscess associated with the intrauterine device. Obstetrics and Gynecology 52: 165–168

Svensson K, Mardh P A, Westrom L 1983 Infertility after acute salpingitis with special reference to *Chlamydia trachomatis*. Fertility and Sterility 40: 322—329

Sweet R L 1980 Microbiology and pathogenesis of acute salpingitis as determined by laparoscopy. What is the appropriate site to sample? American Journal of Obstetrics and Gynecology 138: 985–989

Sweet R L 1988 Pelvic inflammatory disease: prevention and treatment. Modern Medicine 6: 70–80

Thompson S E 1980 Treatment of pelvic inflammatory disease. American Journal of Obstetrics and Gynecology 138: 588–589

Toth A 1983 Alternate causes of pelvic inflammatory disease. Journal of Reproductive Medicine 28 (suppl): 699–702

Westrom L 1980 Incidence, prevalence and trends of acute pelvic inflammatory disease and its consequences in industrialised countries. American Journal of Obstetrics and Gynecology 138: 880–892

Westrom L, Bengtsson L P H, Mardh L A 1982 Incidence and risks of ectopic pregnancy in population of women. British Journal of Obstetrics and Gynaecology 282: 15–18

Westrom L 1983 Clinical manifestations and diagnosis of pelvic inflammatory disease. Journal of Reproductive Medicine 28 (suppl): 703–708

Westrom L 1985 Influence of sexually transmitted diseases on sterility and ectopic pregnancy. Acta Europaea Fertilitatis 16: 21–25

56. Sexually transmitted diseases

G. R. Kinghorn

INTRODUCTION

In the UK, the hospital service for treating sexually transmitted disease (STD) was first established by statute in 1917. The clinics allowed for open patient access without the necessity of preliminary general practitioner referral, confidentiality concerning attendance and diagnosis, and free treatment. This service has now evolved into the specialty of genitourinary medicine (GUM) whose major functions are:

1. The diagnosis and treatment of patients suffering from STD.
2. The control of STD within the community.

In order to achieve these objectives high degrees of clinic accessibility and patient acceptability are required. Integration of clinics within the outpatient department and close liaison with allied disciplines have aided other efforts to destigmatize attendance. Patient awareness of STD has been increased by health education.

Speed of diagnosis is vital to promote good control. GUM clinics provide immediate microscopy and have sophisticated laboratory support for diagnosis of genital infection by culture, antigen detection and serological tests. The predominantly outpatient approach permits diagnosis of early disease, the prevention of complications and transmission and is very cost-effective.

EPIDEMIOLOGICAL ASPECTS

Increasing incidence

There has been a dramatic increase in the reported incidence of STD during the past 25 years. The sexual revolution of the 1960s, facilitated by the wider availability of reliable contraception and changing sexual mores, was followed by a rising incidence of all STDs. This trend was augmented by the earlier sexual maturity amongst girls and earlier age of onset of sexual activity in both sexes. The change in sexual behaviour amongst young women is manifest as a falling ratio of male:female patients for most STDs that now approaches 1. In the UK, the importance of prostitutes as vectors of STD transmission has declined although they remain of major importance in disease transmission in developing countries.

Other sociological changes which contribute to the increased incidence of STD include urbanization, increased mobility amongst the young, and the greater ease of worldwide-travel. This last factor has also promoted the importation of unusual tropical STDs and antibiotic-resistant infections. It is a strange paradox that, despite the availability of effective treatment during the past 40 years, STDs have become more common in many countries.

Changing pattern

In the UK during the past decade the traditional bacterial venereal diseases have become less common whereas those infections caused by *Chlamydia*, viruses and other non-specific genital conditions have become more widespread. The reasons for this changing pattern are not fully understood but may partially reflect the effectiveness of control methods for bacterial infections contrasting with the difficulties encountered with diseases due to other micro-organisms. The changing pattern of STD is mirrored by the changed aetiology of STD complications, such as pelvic inflammatory disease and neonatal ophthalmia, where chlamydial infections now far outnumber gonococcal infections.

Impact of HIV/AIDS

The advent of acquired immune deficiency syndrome (AIDS) has focused attention upon sexual behaviour and emphasized the importance of STD control. On a world-wide basis the commonest method of human immuno-deficiency virus (HIV) transmission is by heterosexual intercourse. Already in urban areas of sub-Saharan Africa there is widespread infection amongst young women and consequent vertical transmission in pregnancy. In the UK, HIV infection is still relatively confined to well defined risk groups — homosexual or bisexual men; intravenous drug users; and haemophiliacs and their consorts. There is considerable uncertainty as to the extent to which it will spread to a wider heterosexual population. Attempts to understand and modify risky sexual behaviour are crucial in curbing the spread of HIV.

In addition, it is well recognized that STDs, particularly those causing genital ulceration, are important co-factors in HIV transmission. This knowledge must lead to redoubled efforts to control STD as an essential, attainable objective in AIDS prevention.

At-risk groups

These major risk groups show considerable overlap with those of other medical conditions, e.g. women requesting termination of pregnancy or with increased obstetric hazards (Table 56.1). Until recently, homosexuals have been particularly susceptible to infections such as syphilis and hepatitis B. Changed sexual behaviour as a consequence of the HIV threat has dramatically reduced the incidence of all STDs amongst gay men.

There has been far less of a change amongst heterosexuals. High rate of sexual partner change, which is the single most important factor in determining risk for STD, remains common in many groups of young people. It is not necessarily related to social class, to educational attainment or to standards of personal hygiene.

STD not infrequently occurs in apparently stable relationships where neither partner admits infidelity. It is important to recognize that many STDs have long latent phases and that there are asymptomatic carriers in both sexes.

Table 56.1 Markers for women at risk of STD

Age	15–34 years (maximal incidence 20–24)
Marital status	Single; separated of divorced Married before the age of 20
Occupation	Patient or consort with mobile job
Medical history	Previous STD Previous termination of pregnancy Multiple pregnancies before age 20 Previous parasuicide or drug abuse Previous abnormal cervical cytology
Social history	Newly living away from home Distributed family background Previously in care of local authority History of prostitution Late booking for antenatal care Tattoos

ROUTINE ASSESSMENT OF FEMALE PATIENTS

The history and examination are identical to the routine assessment of the gynaecological patient. A good history will contain details of the presenting symptoms, associated local or constitutional features, menstruation, and contraceptive practice. Parity, previous obstetric, medical and surgical history are noted; current drug therapy, including self-medication, and drug allergies are also recorded. A sexual history which includes detailed information about recent partner change, partner symptoms and their geographical origin is essential.

Routine examination will include inspection of the external anogenital area in a good light, most easily performed in the lithotomy position; palpation of the inguinal lymph glands and any vulval swelling; speculum examination of the vagina and cervix, and bimanual pelvic examination. Where indicated by the history or other findings a full physical examination may be required.

Precise details of routine microbiological investigations will vary between clinics but will usually include microscopy of a wet film preparation of vaginal secretions and Gram-stained smears from the urethra, cervix and vagina together with culture for gonococcus, *Chlamydia trachomatis* and for vaginal pathogens. If reliable results are to be obtained, specimens must be taken from the appropriate site, be inserted into appropriate transport media and be suitably stored and transported to the laboratory. Serological tests for syphilis are performed routinely in all new patients.

PRINCIPLES OF MANAGEMENT

Whilst the effective drug treatment of STD is often simple, there are also psychological and social consequences for each affected individual which require additional management. The principles of management are listed below:

1. Establish a firm diagnosis before treatment.
2. Investigate for multiple infections.
3. Use simple dosage regimens, preferably single-dose.
4. Confirm cure clinically and microbiologically.
5. Trace sexual contacts.
6. Educate patients and counsel them in a non-judgemental way.

STDs occur together so that, for example, in patients presenting with genital warts screening for other infections should be mandatory. This principle is more easily forgotten with other sexually transmitted conditions, such as unwanted pregnancy in young girls, in whom surgical intervention may inadvertently result in ascending complications of unsuspected accompanying cervical or vaginal infection.

Control of STD demands that a precise diagnosis is reached before treatment is commenced, that follow-up is completed to ensure that both clinical and microbiological cure is achieved, and that contact-tracing is routinely carried out. The last is most easily achieved by non-judgemental presentation of the facts in order to seek patient co-operation. In only a small proportion of cases will home visits by a health adviser be necessary.

BACTERIAL DISEASES

Syphilis

Syphilis is one of four human treponemal diseases whose causative organisms are morphologically indistinguishable and which cannot be differentiated by the results of serological tests. These organisms remain sensitive to penicillin. In developed countries, infectious syphilis has decreased markedly in incidence during the past decade and is now more common in homosexual men than in heterosexuals. The non-venereal treponematoses — yaws, pinta and endemic syphilis — may cause concern in immigrant populations, when detected by routine antenatal screening tests for syphilis. In the developing countries, syphilis remains a significant cause of morbidity and mortality amongst adults and neonates.

Clinical features

Syphilis is a chronic infectious disease caused by a systemic infection by *Treponema pallidum* in which periods of florid clinical manifestations are interspersed by periods of latency when the disease is detectable only by serological tests. Both sexually acquired and congenital syphilis are subdivided into early and late disease. With the possible exception of the pregnant woman, who may potentially transmit infection to the fetus at any stage of the disease,

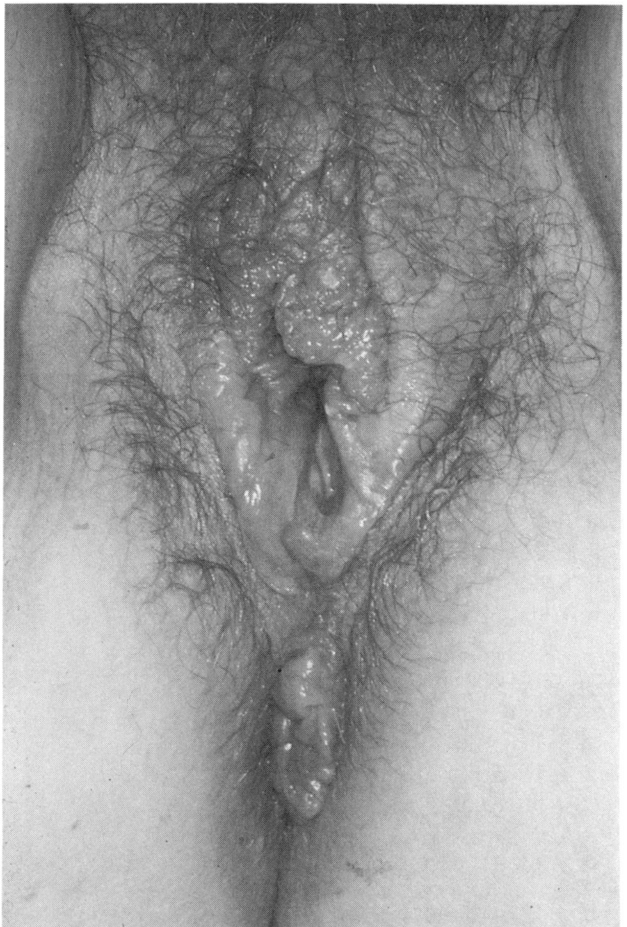

Fig. 56.1 Primary syphilis: this pregnant patient has a chancre at the fourchette with local oedema in the labia. She also has a trichomonal discharge.

those with late disease of longer than 2 years' duration are not infectious to others. Early syphilis includes the primary, secondary and early latent stages.

The primary chancre, a raised, round, indurated and usually painless ulcer, appears about 3 weeks after infection (Fig. 56.1). The incubation period can vary between 9 and 90 days. The chancre is usually single, sited on the external genitalia, and accompanied by bilateral, non-tender, rubbery inguinal lymphadenopathy. The untreated lesion will resolve spontaneously within 3–8 weeks. Presentation with secondary syphilis is more common in women when the primary lesion has been hidden in the vagina or on the cervix. Constitutional symptoms of fever, headache, bone and joint pains are accompanied by signs of a generalized non-irritant rash, most prominent on flexor surfaces and present on palms and soles. Initially the rash is macular but later becomes papular then nodular (Fig. 56.2). In moist areas — the genitals, the anus and beneath breasts — condylomata lata appear. These, like the erosive lesions on mucous membranes, are highly infectious. Generalized

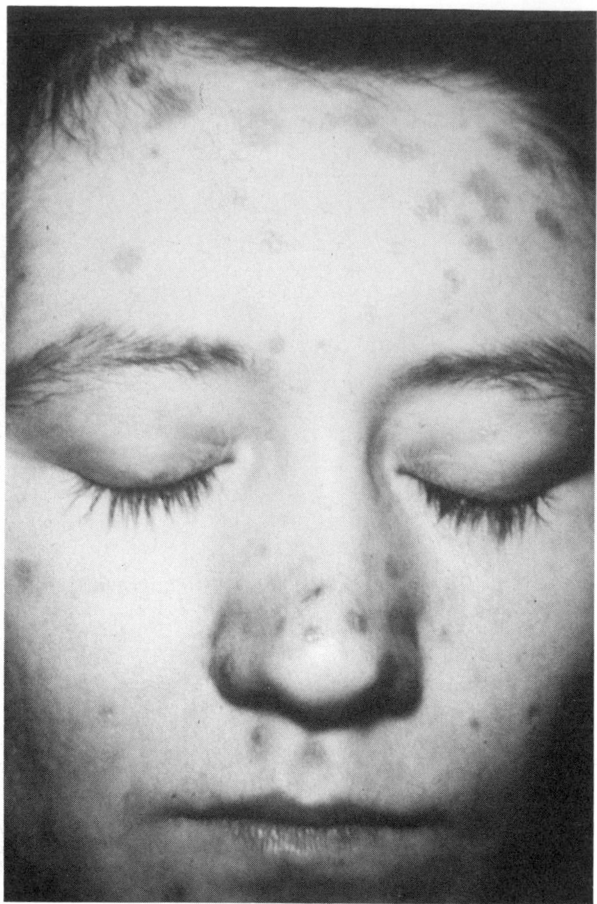

Fig. 56.2 Secondary syphilis: the maculopapular rash

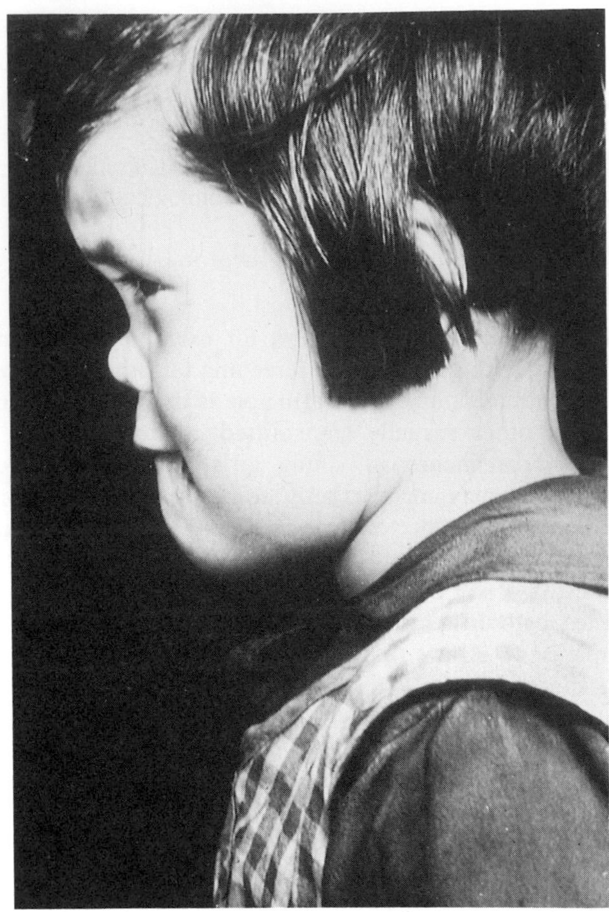

Fig. 56.3 Congenital syphilis: the typical facies has a depressed nasal bridge, frontal bossing and a prominent lower jaw.

painless lymphadenopathy is common; there may also be iritis, hepatitis or neurological manifestations.

Even without treatment all lesions will resolve and the patient will pass into the latent stage. The untreated patient may have persistent latent infection or may progress after several years to develop either tertiary gummatous syphilis, characterized by chronic inflammation of skin, bones, mucous membranes and, occasionally, viscera, or quaternary syphilis, typified by neurological and cardiovascular disease.

Congenital syphilis

Maternal syphilis often has an adverse effect on the pregnancy. *T. pallidum* can infect the fetus transplacentally at any time, typically leading to intrauterine death and mid-trimester abortion. In surviving fetuses, intrauterine growth retardation and prematurity are likely.

Congenital infection may be readily apparent at birth (Fig. 56.3). In less severely infected infants, clinical manifestations can be delayed for weeks, months or years. There is no primary stage as the blood-borne infection is systemic from the outset. Many of the early features are similar to those of acquired secondary syphilis, however skin rashes are often bullous, hepatosplenomegaly is common and nasopharyngitis with a highly infectious nasal discharge (the 'snuffles') occurs (Fig. 56.4a–c). With delayed presentation, bone involvement causing pseudoparesis appears during the first months after birth (Fig. 56.4d). Hutchinson's triad of interstitial keratitis leading to corneal scarring, nerve deafness and notched permanent incisor teeth may result when the diagnosis is not made until childhood.

Diagnosis

In primary and secondary syphilis the diagnosis is rapidly confirmed with dark-ground microscopy by demonstrating *T. pallidum* in serum from abraded lesions. Serological tests become positive in late primary disease, reach maximal titres in the secondary stage and decline slowly during the latent phase. Although the reagin tests, such as the Venereal Disease Research Laboratories (VDRL), may revert to negative spontaneously, it is unusual for the high-

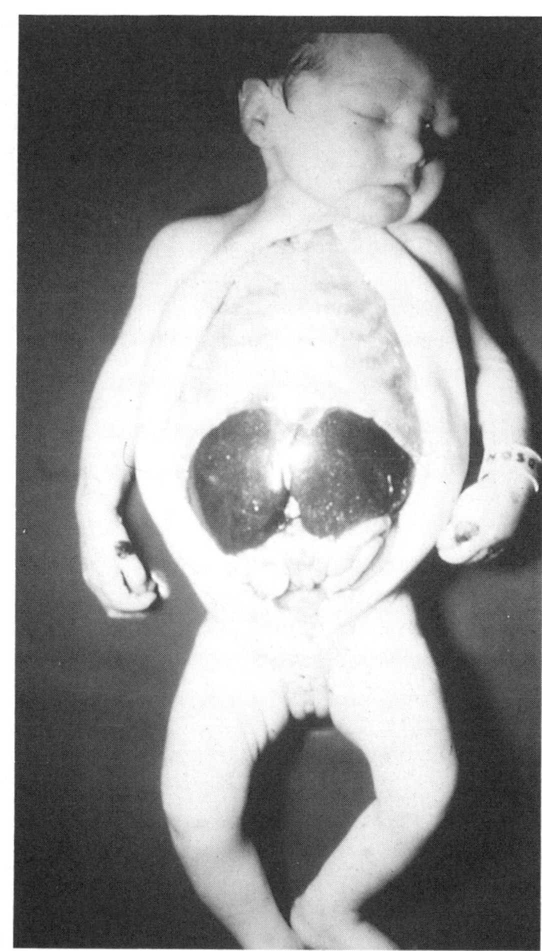

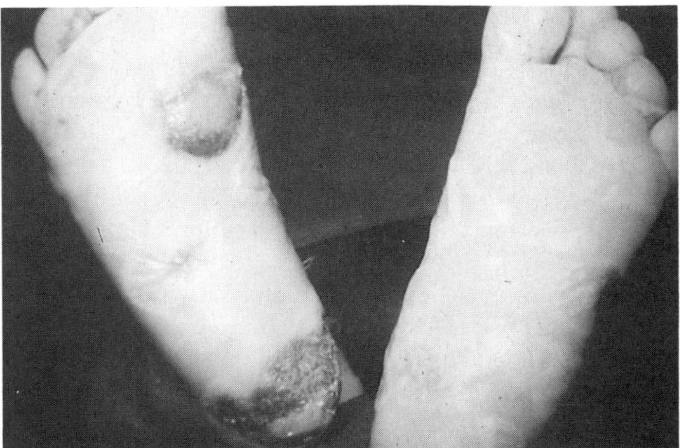

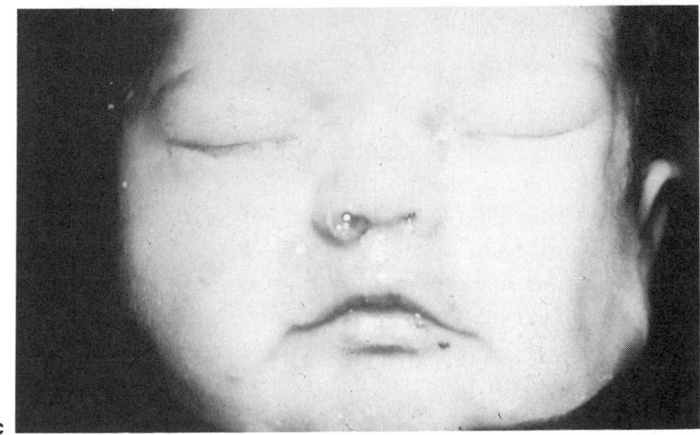

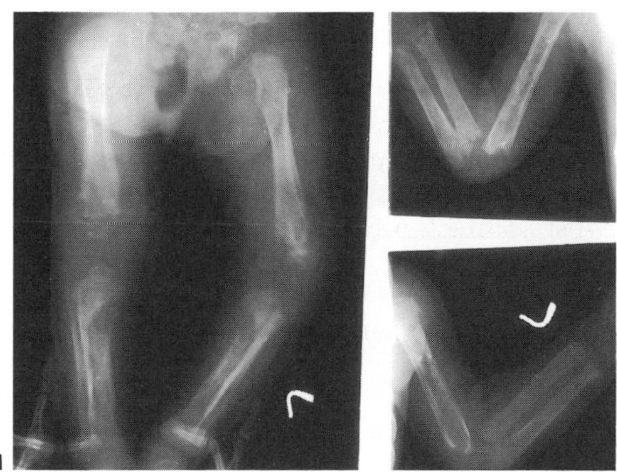

Fig. 56.4 Congenital syphilis: (**a**) stillbirth with hepatosplenomegaly; (**b**) bullous rash seen here on the feet; (**c**) serous discharge; (**d**) lytic bone lesions.

ly sensitive, specific treponemal antibody tests such as the TPHA and fluorescent treponemal antibody (FTA) (absorbed) to become completely negative, even after treatment.

Treatment

Penicillin remains the treatment of choice. Preparations which maintain treponemacidal serum levels for at least 7 days are used: for example, procaine penicillin G 600 000 iu i.m. daily for 10–14 days. In late disease, treatment is given for longer and repeated courses may be required. In penicillin-allergic patients either tetracycline or erythromycin 2 g daily for 15 days is used but treatment success is less assured.

Congenitally infected babies are treated with procaine penicillin 500 mg/kg i.m. daily for 10 days. Babies born to mothers treated at any stage of pregnancy with penicillin do not need additional therapy.

Prevention

A further fall in the incidence of acquired syphilis will depend upon adoption of safer sexual practices. Congenital syphilis is totally preventable and antenatal testing remains cost-effective despite the low prevalence of syphilis in developed countries. Some clinicians recommend additional insurance courses of penicillin treatment in all subsequent pregnancies.

Gonorrhoea

This infection, caused by *Neisseria gonorrhoeae*, reached a peak incidence in the UK during the mid 1970s and has since declined. In 1987, a total of 22 878 cases were reported from STD clinics. Gonorrhoea remains a common cause of morbidity in women and neonates worldwide and antibiotic resistance is increasingly encountered in developing countries.

The organism is highly infectious and is transmissible prior to the onset of symptoms. Gonorrhoea has a short incubation period, usually 2–5 days. Asymptomatic infections are common in women, especially during pregnancy, and also occur in men. This results in late presentation with complications and facilitates disease transmission.

Clinical features

At least half of all infected women have no symptoms and present as the result of contact-tracing procedures. When present, symptoms are similar to those of other lower genital tract infections and consist of excessive vaginal discharge and dysuria.

Examination may reveal no abnormality but there may be signs of cervicitis with a mucopurulent cervical discharge (Fig. 56.5). It is unusual to observe a urethral discharge in women. Rectal and pharyngeal infections are asymptomatic in the majority of cases and are more difficult to eradicate.

Complications

Complications may be local, ascending or distant. Acute local complications include skenitis, resulting in pain and swelling at the urinary meatus, and bartholinitis causing painful unilateral vulval swelling which is fluctuant if an abscess has formed. The major ascending complication is pelvic inflammatory disease which occurs in about 15% of infected women. Gonococcal pelvic inflammatory disease often starts at the time of menstruation.

Distant complications consist of perihepatitis and septicaemia. Gonococcal perihepatitis results from spread of infection to the liver capsule which may then form adhesions to the abdominal wall. Patients complain of pain in the right upper abdomen which is worse on coughing, deep breathing and on flexing the trunk. The pain may be referred to the right shoulder and may be accompanied by nausea and vomiting. Pyrexia, abdominal tenderness and signs of lower genital tract infection are usually present and pelvic inflammatory disease may coexist.

Septicaemia is most often due to gonococci with particular growth requirements; these organisms are very sensitive to penicillin. Pregnancy appears to be a predisposing factor. In the non-pregnant woman, menstruation may precede bacteraemia. This is usually a relatively benign illness, characterized by low-grade fever; asymmetrical arthralgia, tenosynovitis and arthritis affecting wrists, elbows, knees and small joints of the hand; a skin rash, occurring in crops which have a typical evolution through

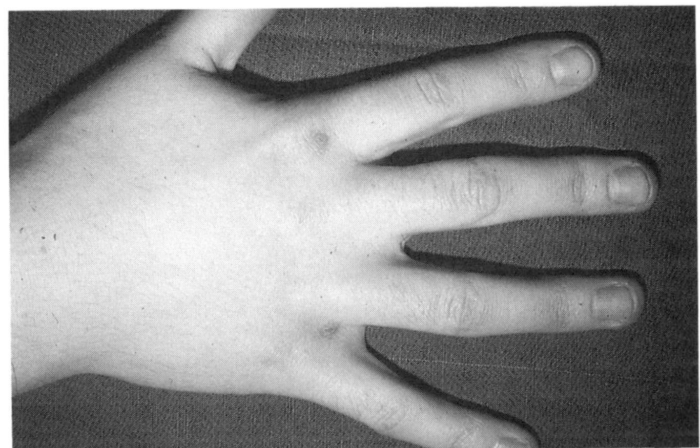

Fig. 56.6 Skin lesions caused by systemic gonococcal infection.

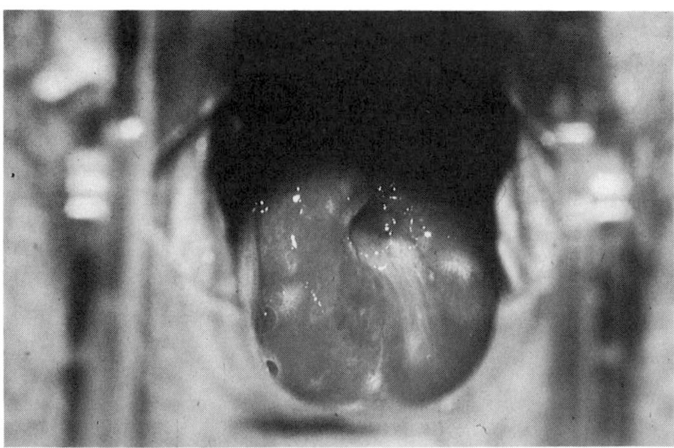

Fig. 56.5 Gonococcal cervicitis: the purulent endocervical discharge.

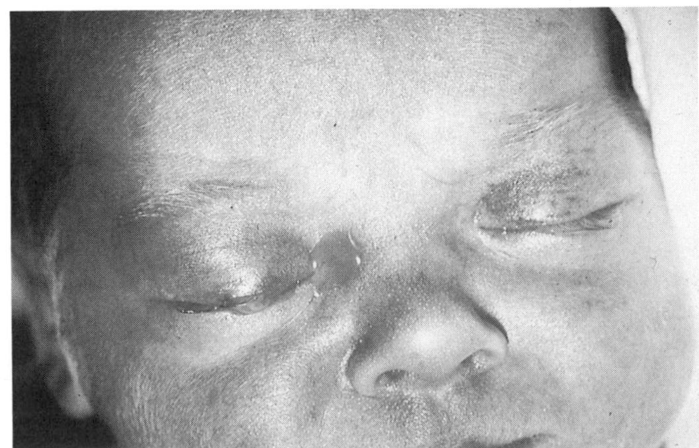

Fig. 56.7 Gonococcal ophthalmia neonatorum.

papular and pustular stages to leave a haemorrhagic lesion showing central necrosis sited over joints and the peripheral aspects of limbs (Fig. 56.6).

In pregnancy, gonorrhoea is associated with early abortion, intrauterine growth retardation, prematurity and postpartum sepsis. Gonococcal ophthalmia neonatorum usually begins 2–7 days after birth with severe bilateral conjunctivitis (Fig. 56.7). This can lead to keratitis and blindness unless promptly treated.

Although most men with gonorrhoea will develop an overt urethritis with dysuria and a urethral discharge, the male consorts of women with complicated gonorrhoea are often asymptomatic carriers of *N. gonorrhoeae*.

Diagnosis

Typically, the organism infects columnar epithelium. In women the appropriate sites to test for infection are the endocervix, the urethra, the rectum and the pharynx. If bacteraemia is suspected, blood cultures are also necessary. Microscopic identification of Gram-negative intracellular diplococci allows a presumptive diagnosis to be made and the treatment to be begun. Cultures are more sensitive, permit antibiotic sensitivity testing and are always desirable for confirmation.

Treatment

Gonorrhoea can usually be cured with a single dosage of a suitable antibiotic. In the UK, penicillin remains a mainstay of treatment. Elsewhere in the world, due to either plasmid-borne beta-lactamase production or chromosomally mediated factors, penicillin resistance is the rule, rendering it useless. This is often accompanied by resistance to aminoglycosides, tetracyclines, sulphonamides and other antibiotics.

Suitable single dosage regimens are shown in Table 56.2.

In complicated infections continuous therapy is given. In gonococcal pelvic inflammatory disease it is important to remember that concurrent infection with *Chlamydia*, mycoplasmas, anaerobes and other facultative pathogens is frequent. Thus, initial antibiotic regimes usually include metronidazole and will change from penicillin-based to tetracycline-based after the first 2–3 days.

Gonococcal ophthalmia is preventable and prophylaxis should continue in developing countries where infection rates remain high and antenatal maternal screening is not possible. Erythromycin (1%) or 1% tetracycline eye ointments can be used. Established neonatal disease is treated with a beta-lactam stable antibiotic such as cefotaxime 100 mg/kg/day i.m. or i.v. in three divided doses. It is probably unnecessary to use additional topical antibiotics although regular saline irrigation to remove inflammatory exudate from the eyes is required.

It is essential that contact-tracing is performed in all gonococcal infections and both parents of infected babies should be examined as a matter of urgency.

Table 56.3 Single-dose regimens for gonorrhoea

Medication	Dosage
Aqueous procaine penicillin with or without probenecid	2.4–4.8 Mu i.m. 1 g by mouth
Spectinomycin	2–4 g i.m.
Ampicillin with probenecid	3 g by mouth 1 g by mouth
Cefuroxime	1 g by mouth
Ciprofloxacin	250 mg by mouth
Doxycycline	300 mg by mouth
Minocycline	300 mg by mouth

Chlamydial infections

The commonest sexually transmitted pathogen in developed countries is *Chlamydia trachomatis*. This unusual bacterial pathogen has specific extracellular and intracellular forms and requires tissue culture techniques for its isolation.

It is responsible for at least half of all cases of non-specific genital infection, which includes non-specific urethritis in the male and related conditions in the female. In 1987 there were a total of 125 973 cases of non-specific genital infection reported from STD clinics in the UK.

Clinical features

In women, early chlamydial infections are often silent and may remain so for months and possibly years. Most women present as a consequence of symptoms in their partner. A wide variety of manifestations occur with symptomatic chlamydial infection. Urethral involvement may lead to

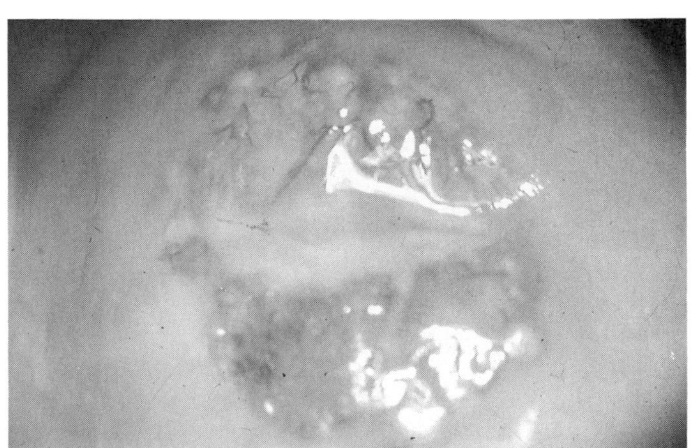

Fig. 56.8 Chlamydial cervicitis: a purulent discharge and inflamed follicles are seen.

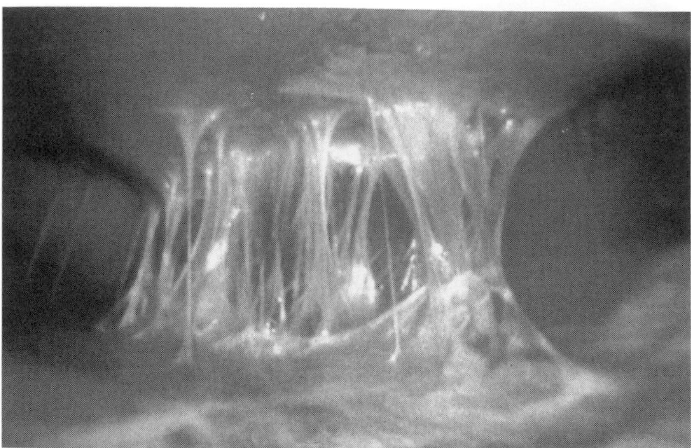

Fig. 56.9 Chlamydial perihepatitis: 'violin-string' adhesions are visible.

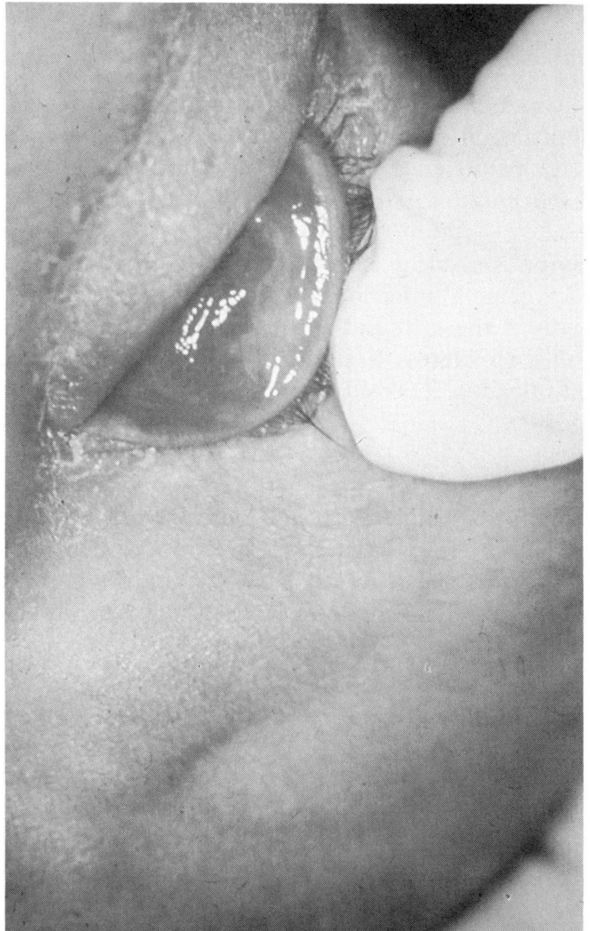

Fig. 56.10 Chlamydial ophthalmitis: the conjunctiva is swollen and inflamed.

dysuria and frequency; cervical infection is usually associated with an excessive discharge and postcoital bleeding. Examination may show congested, oedematous cervical ectopy with small follicles, or there may be unexpected contact bleeding from the endocervical canal (Fig. 56.8). Often there are no abnormal signs.

Complications of local infection include skenitis and bartholinitis. Ascending infection may cause endometritis and may manifest as painful and excessive menstrual loss. *Chlamydia* is now recognized to be associated with at least 50% of cases of acute and subacute pelvic inflammatory disease in developed countries. It is also a more common cause of perihepatitis than is the gonococcus (Fig. 56.9). Periappendicitis, in which inflammation begins in the serosal layer and adhesions form between the appendix and adjacent structures, is recognized as another chlamydial complication presenting as right iliac fossa pain in young sexually active women.

In those who are genetically predisposed, chlamydial infection is the usual precipitating cause of Reiter's syndrome in men. This syndrome is more common in women than was previously thought and should be considered as part of the differential diagnosis of arthropathy in young persons, especially if associated with dermatological, mucosal, conjunctival and genital symptoms.

In pregnancy, chlamydial infection has been associated with spontaneous abortion, intrauterine growth retardation and prematurity. It is also a common cause of neonatal disease. The associated conjunctival infection presents later than that due to the gonococcus — between 4 and 14 days — often after discharge from hospital (Fig. 56.10). Like all other chlamydial disease, this requires systemic antibiotic therapy to treat both the conjunctivitis and the accompanying nasopharyngeal infection which may later progress to afebrile pneumonitis and otitis media.

Diagnosis

Specimens should be taken from the urethra and cervix in uncomplicated disease. In salpingitis, tubal specimens are desirable. *Chlamydia* can be demonstrated in tissue culture, for which a special transport medium and prompt delivery to the laboratory are necessary. *Chlamydia* antigen can also be demonstrated in immunofluorescent-stained smears from the urethra, the endocervix and conjunctivae. Antigen detection using enzyme linked immunosorbent assay (ELISA) techniques is becoming more widely available and is most suitable for large-batch testing. *Chlamydia* serology to detect microimmunofluorescent antibody has no place in the diagnosis of lower genital tract infections but can be useful in the diagnosis of ascending infection and distant complications.

Treatment

C. trachomatis cannot be treated with single-dosage therapy and does not respond to penicillin or ampicillin. Systemic tetracycline or erythromycin 1–2 g daily for 7–14 days is the treatment of choice. Chlamydial disease of the neonate requires prolonged systemic therapy with oral erythromycin ethyl succinate suspension 50 mg/kg/day in four divided doses before feeds for 3 weeks. Both parents should be investigated.

VIRAL DISEASES

Genital warts

Genital warts (condylomata acuminata) are the commonest viral STD in the UK — annual incidence has increased threefold in the past decade to almost 75 000 cases in 1987. They are caused by human papillomaviruses (HPV): these are small, non-enveloped icosahedral DNA viruses which have a particular tropism for epithelial cells. At least 60 different types have been recognized. Genital warts are almost always associated with infection caused by HPV types 6 or 11 and occasionally 16, 18 or 31. Subclinical HPV infection is very common. Patients with clinical warts are merely a subgroup of the total population affected. The factors governing the appearance of warts are not known. The incubation period varies from a few weeks to 9 months, perhaps longer in some cases.

Clinical Features

Warts vary in their appearance according to their site and causative viral type. In women, they can occur anywhere in the anogenital region but most commonly appear on the vulva at sites of maximal trauma during intercourse (Fig. 56.11). In warm moist areas they are filiform but tend to be flatter upon keratinized skin. Although some women complain of an associated itch, this is usually the result of concomitant infections.

The growth of warts is favoured by warmth and moisture. They often proliferate in pregnant women, rarely posing obstetric problems, and regress spontaneously in the puerperium. Cervical warts are seen in less than 1 in 10 affected women although a third will have evidence of warty change on cervical cytology or colposcopy (Fig. 56.12). Warts in men may be equally difficult to visualize and show a wide variety of appearances and sites.

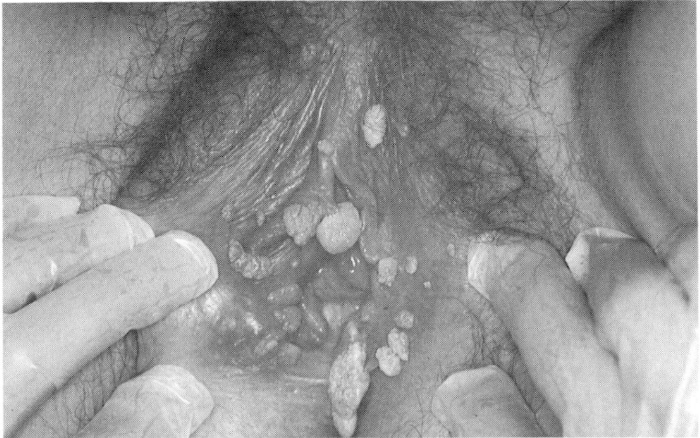

Fig. 56.11 Vulval warts.

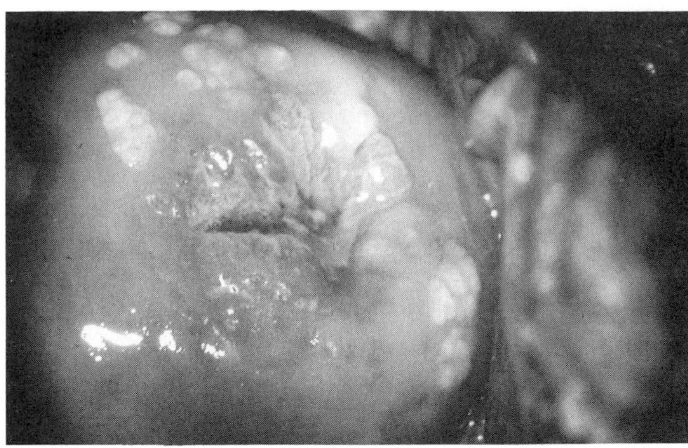

Fig. 56.12 Cervical warts.

Although warts are distinctive in appearance, biopsy is necessary if there is any suspicion about the nature of the lesion. This is especially true on the cervix. Warts characteristically show papillomatosis, acanthosis and koilocytotic changes.

Patients presenting with warts should be screened for other STDs, which will be present in 25%. A further 25% will have other genital infections such as candidiasis. Cervical cytology should be performed routinely. Colposcopic examination of the cervix and vagina is recommended if the smear is abnormal.

Complications

There may be an association between HPV infection and malignant epithelial transformation of the cervix, vagina, vulva and anus. It is usually associated with HPV types 16 or 18. In men, HPV 6 and 11 infections can rarely develop into a giant Buschke–Lowenstein tumour which is a locally aggressive non-metastasizing verrucous carcinoma prone to secondary bacterial infection.

Vertical transmission may cause anogenital warts to appear within the first year of life. Very rarely juvenile laryngeal papillomatosis may develop. The appearance of anogenital warts in older infants must raise the possibility of sexual abuse.

Treatment

There is a wide variety of local chemical and destructive treatment methods, each with its own practical limitations. Recurrence after apparent treatment successes is common.

Podophyllin. A plant extract prepared in ethanolic solution or in tincture of benzoin, podophyllin is applied to warts as a paint, left to dry, and then washed off 4 h later to prevent chemotrauma to healthy adjacent epithelium. It is best applied to women by medical or nursing staff but self-treatment of men is now possible with a 3% podophyllotoxin solution. Podophyllin should not be used in pregnancy. It is potentially teratogenic and systemic absorption has resulted in serious maternal toxicity affecting the liver, heart, kidneys and nervous system.

Trichloroacetic acid. In 90–100% saturated solution, this is a caustic agent which is useful to treat isolated, keratinized flat warts which respond poorly to podophyllin. Injudicious application can result in scarring.

Destructive methods. These include cryotherapy which can be administered either by closed systems containing nitrous oxide with variable-sized probes, or by liquid nitrogen applied directly to the wart on swabs. Curettage, diathermy, and laser therapy may be used. These methods often require anaesthesia and impatient admission.

Other chemical treatments. These include 5-fluorouracil, which has been used successfully to treat intraurethral warts. The α-and β-interferons given by subcutaneous or intramuscular injection have recently been studied intensively with variable reports on their efficacy. This is the only form of treatment with a potential action on the causative virus rather than merely on the resultant warts. Future treatment regimes may include interferon as an adjunct to existing chemical and destructive therapies in an attempt to reduce their relapse rates.

The partners of individuals with warts should always be examined, if necessary using a colposcope.

Genital herpes

All human herpes viruses have the capacity to cause latent infection and their subsequent reactivation results in repeated disease episodes. This can be of clinical importance in pregnant women.

Genital herpes is caused by herpes simplex virus (HSV), a large complex DNA virus of which there are two types. In the UK during the past decade there has been a large increase in the reported cases of genital herpes. This is partially a reflection of increased awareness and better diagnostic methods but is principally a true increase in in-

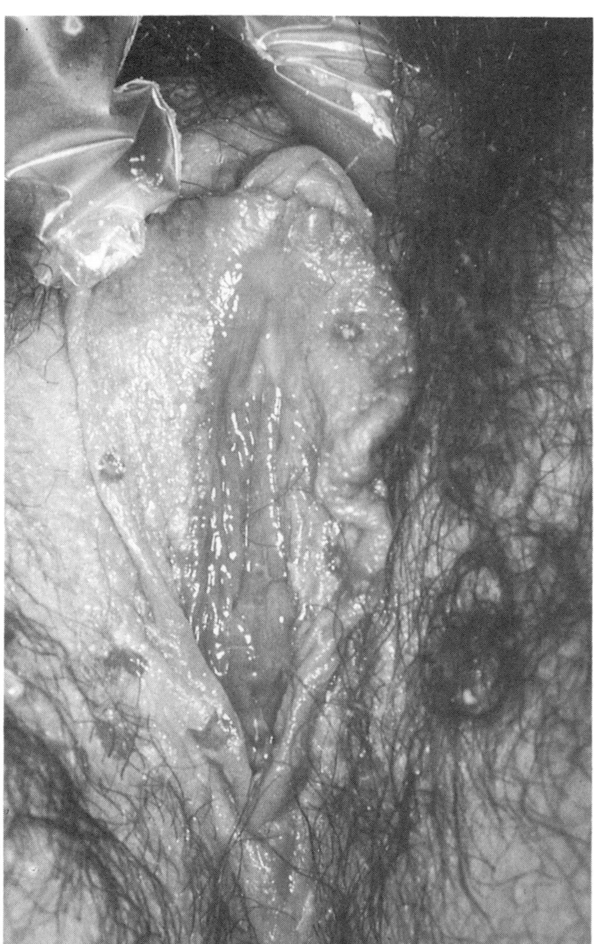

Fig. 56.13 Primary genital herpes: multiple, painful ulcers are present on the labia minora.

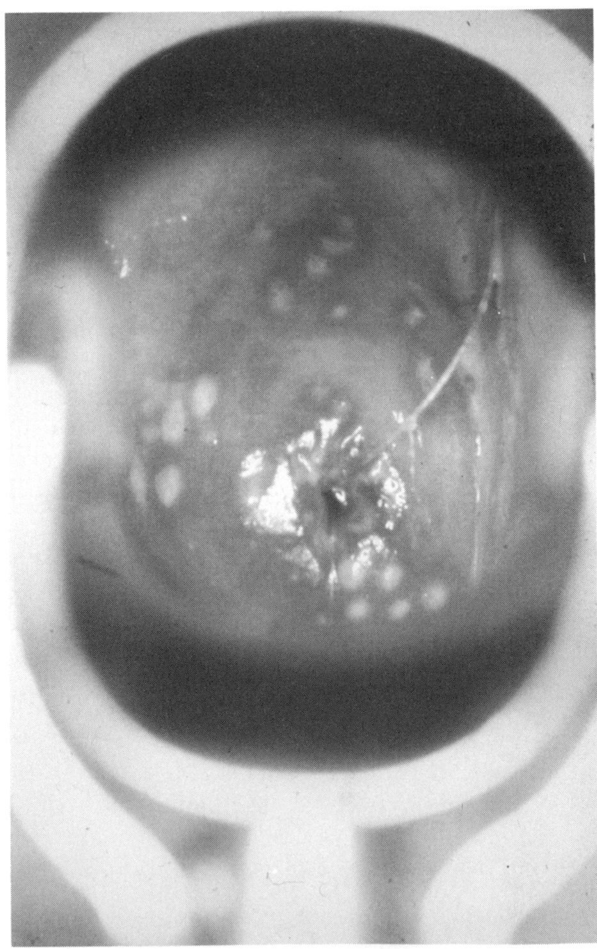

Fig. 56.14 Primary genital herpes: ulcers on the cervix.

cidence matching those of other STDs. In some parts of the UK, HSV 1 causes 50% of first episodes. This may reflect changes in sexual practices. Certainly HSV 1 may be transmitted in monogamous relationships from orolabial lesions to the genitals of the partner. HSV 1 is less likely to cause recurrent disease than HSV 2.

The incubation period of genital herpes is 2–14 days. Transmission may occur from asymptomatic individuals, though it is more commonly associated with unrecognized active lesions.

Clinical features

First attacks are often severe in women. They are less severe in those previously infected with orolabial herpes and may be mild in pregnancy. Symptoms are both local and constitutional. Pain, dysuria and discharge are commonly associated with flu-like symptoms.

The lesions begin as erythematous papules which vesiculate and then form extremely tender ulcers which possess an erythematous halo and a yellow or grey base. These are accompanied by bilateral inguinal lymphadenopathy. Lesions are widespread in women and affect the introitus, labia majora, perineum, vagina and cervix (Figs 56.13 and 56.14).

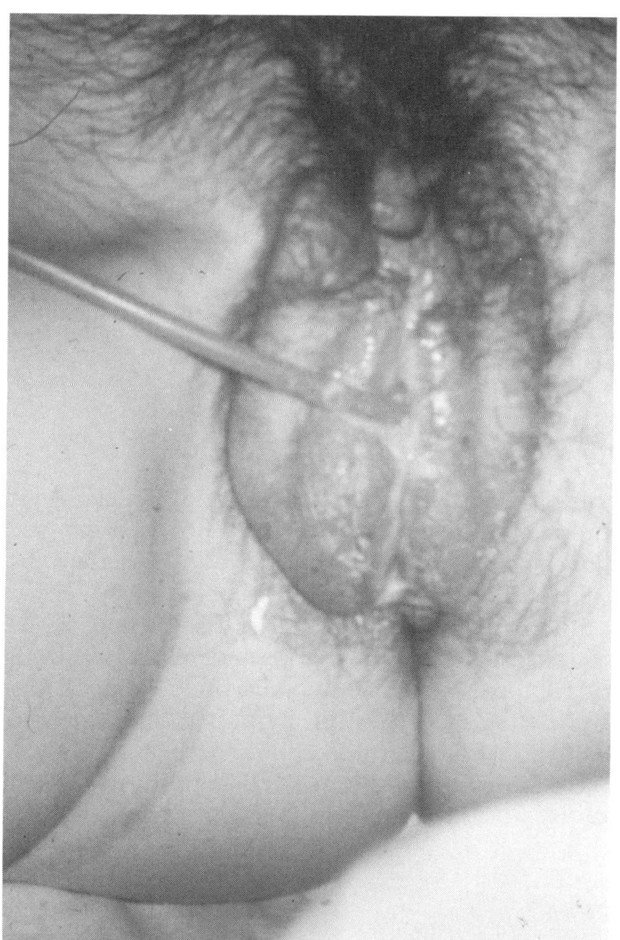

Fig. 56.15 Primary genital herpes: urinary retention and vulval oedema.

Complications of first episodes are common. There may be secondary bacterial infection of lesions. Autoinoculation to distant sites occurs, especially to the fingers and eyes. Local neurological complications include a sacral radiculomyelopathy causing self-limiting hyperaesthesiae in the buttocks, thighs or perineum, decrease in sensation over the sacral dermatomes and difficulty in bladder and bowel emptying (Fig. 56.15). A self-limiting meningitis is sometimes seen. Severe, potentially fatal encephalitis is an extremely rare complication more typical of immunosuppressed individuals. Untreated, a primary episode lasts for 3–4 weeks.

In contrast, recurrent episodes are shorter, lasting 5–10 days, less severe, and are usually unilateral. Prodromal symptoms preceding the outbreak by 1–2 days consist of neuralgic-type pain in the buttocks, ankles or groin, or hyperaesthesiae at the site of the lesion. Constitutional symptoms are less frequent. Psychological symptoms are often marked in those with frequent recurrences and may be accompanied by emotional and relationship difficulties. Recurrences may be precipitated by stress, dietary factors, menstruation and local trauma associated with intercourse.

Diagnosis

The diagnosis should be confirmed by isolation of the virus in tissue culture or by detection of virus antigen in immunofluorescent or ELISA assays. Serological tests are rarely useful. Screening tests for other STDs are essential but may have to be delayed in first episodes because of severe discomfort preventing adequate examination.

Treatment

The general management should be as for other STDs. Patients need counselling as well as both symptomatic and specific therapy. Bedrest, systemic and local analgesia are important. Antibiotics to control secondary bacterial infection may be required in first episodes although frequent saline bathing is not only soothing but also controls infection in most cases.

Specific therapy is with acyclovir, a potent antiviral drug administered either intravenously or preferably orally in first episodes within 6 days of the appearance of lesions. In recurrences the effect is less marked and acyclovir should be used within 1 day of onset. Topical 5% acyclovir cream is also useful in recurrent disease. In patients with very frequent attacks, long-term oral acyclovir, 800 mg daily, suppresses the disease. The need for such therapy should be re-evaluated after 6–12 months.

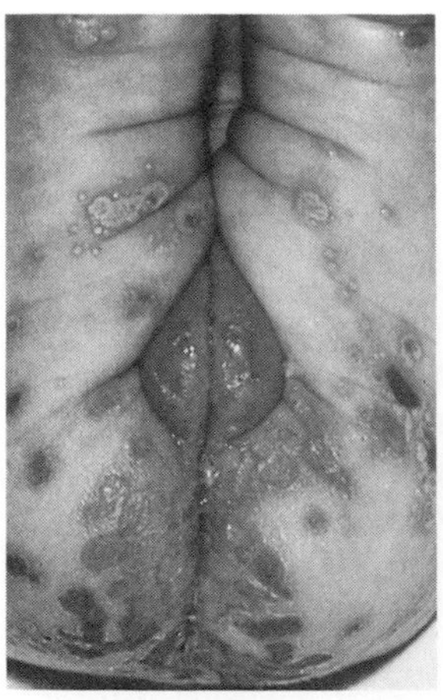
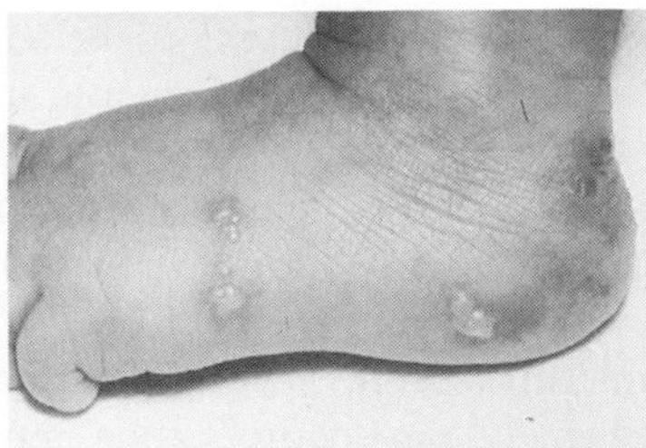

Fig. 56.16 Disseminated neonatal herpes: the lesions on the napkin area are haemorrhagic and ulcerated but vesicles are present on the foot.

Long-term complications

Apart from the risk of recurrences, which occur in about 50% of infected persons, women should be advised to have annual cervical cytology in view of the epidemiological association between HSV and cervical neoplasia. They should also be advised of the possibility of transmitting their infection to the fetus during delivery should there be either a clinical recurrence or asymptomatic shedding at term (Fig. 56.16). Neonatal transmission is more common with first episodes than with recurrences. Some women who have only experienced a first episode may develop a recurrence during the final trimester so many clinicians recommend weekly screening from about 36 weeks' gestation for clinical lesions and for asymptomatic viral shedding in all women with a history of genital herpes. Should either be found at term, caesarean section is recommended. In one survey, 25% of 197 consecutive women at risk required operative delivery because of active herpes at term (Woolley et al 1988).

Molluscum contagiosum

This is caused by a large pox virus. In young adults it occurs on the genitalia as a sexually transmitted infection although it can occur in children on the face, neck, upper limbs and trunk spread by non-sexual close contact. Lesions on the genitals are found particularly on the pubis, thigh and labia majora. They are easily mistaken for genital warts but close inspection of the small papular lesions shows a characteristic central umbilication. Expressed material shows myriads of inclusion bodies.

Treatment consists of disrupting the papule, expressing the core and applying phenol with a sharpened orangestick to the residual lesion. Cryotherapy is equally successful.

Viral hepatitis

Several viruses can cause hepatitis, including cytomegalovirus and Epstein–Barr virus. The major viral causes are hepatitis A, hepatitis B and non-A non-B viruses which are also capable of sexual transmission. Typically these are associated with homosexual men but they can also be heterosexually transmitted.

Hepatitis A is caused by a small RNA virus which is transmitted by the orofaecal route and can therefore be spread by oroanal sexual contact. With improving standards of hygiene, the majority of adults in the UK are susceptible to this infection.

Hepatitis B is caused by a DNA virus which is present in serum many weeks before the acute illness occurs. In tropical Africa and South-East Asia up to 20% of the population carry the virus and infection often occurs perinatally. In the UK, the carrier rate in the general population is low — about 1 in 1000 — and infection occurs in particular risk groups exposed to infected blood and genital secretions. Hepatitis B is an occupational hazard for medical and nursing staff.

Non-A non-B viruses also appear to be transmitted via percutaneous routes, blood and blood products. They affect the same risk groups as hepatitis B in developed countries and account for 15–30% of cases of sporadic acute hepatitis.

Clinical features

Acute hepatitis resulting in jaundice is the most typical manifestation although subclinical infections and anicteric pyrexial episodes are common. Fulminant hepatitis occurs in less than 1% of all cases. Although complete recovery after hepatitis is the rule, 5–10% of patients with hepatitis B develop a chronic infection and may develop chronic persistent and chronic active hepatitis, cirrhosis and primary hepatocellular carcinoma.

Diagnosis

Hepatitis A, Epstein–Barr virus and cytomegalovirus infections can be diagnosed by tests for specific serum immunoglobulin M antibodies. Hepatitis B surface and e antigens (HBsAg and HBeAg) appear early in acute hepatitis B. In some, HBsAg disappears before the onset of symptoms. During the illness, antibody to core antigen (anti-HBc) and subsequently anti-HBe appear. It is only with the later appearance of anti-HBs and disappearance of HBsAg that long-term immunity develops.

There are no specific serological tests for non-A non-B hepatitis, which remains a diagnosis of exclusion.

Treatment

Acute viral hepatitis is usually self-limiting and management is largely supportive with a low-fat, high-carbohydrate diet, bedrest and exclusion of alcohol until liver function tests return to normal. Patients who are carriers should be counselled about the risks of transmission and their condition should be monitored. In chronic hepatitis, systemic interferon has been successful in promoting seroconversion in some cases.

Prevention

Simple hygienic precautions and safe routine practice in the handling of blood and body fluids will reduce the occupational risk of transmission from infected patients. Passive immunization is possible with normal pooled immunoglobulin against hepatitis A and with hepatitis B immunoglobulin.

Active immunization against hepatitis B is now readily available with genetically engineered vaccine or with purified antigen derived from carriers. It should be offered to health care personnel; non-immune individuals whose sexual lifestyle places them at risk of such infection, and the newborn offspring of infected mothers.

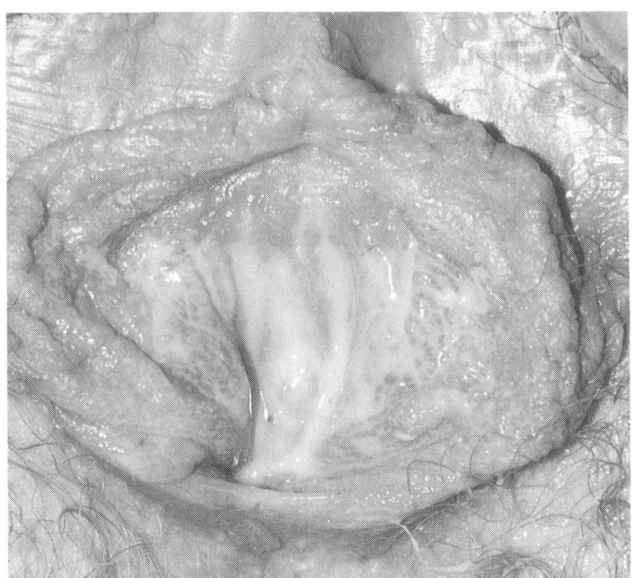

Fig. 56.17 Bacterial vaginosis.

VAGINITIS

Vaginal discharge may be due to a wide variety of physiological and pathological causes. It may also be the presenting complaint in women who suspect they may have been exposed to a STD. In these the true reason for seeking medical advice may only become apparent when a detailed sexual history is taken.

The infectious causes of vaginal discharge can be subdivided into those which are associated with a predominant cervicitis, such as *Chlamydia trachomatis*, *Neisseria gonorrhoeae* and HSV, and those associated with a predominant vaginitis. Although the latter group is not necessarily sexually acquired, it is more common in sexually active women, may cause symptoms in the male partner who can act as a source of reinfection, and may lead to accusations of infidelity. Careful sympathetic handling of both the woman and her partner is essential. The three commonest vaginal infections are associated with:

1. *Gardnerella vaginalis* (bacterial vaginosis).
2. *Candida albicans* ('thrush').
3. *Trichomonas vaginalis*.

Bacterial vaginosis

Bacterial or anaerobic vaginosis is not a specific, monobacterial infection but a synergic mixture of anaerobic and micro-aerophilic bacterial species normally present in small numbers in healthy women and in large numbers in bacterial vaginosis. This mixture includes *G. vaginalis*, various anaerobic species, and curved motile rods of *Mobiluncus* species. This polymicrobial vaginal flora replaces the normal predominant lactobacilli which promote the usual acid environment and their metabolism produces biologically active metabolites, including volatile amines which raise the vaginal pH and cause the characteristic smell of the condition.

Clinical features

The cardinal symptom of bacterial vaginosis is a smell, usually described as fishy. This is associated with a thin grey or white adherent vaginal discharge which is sometimes frothy (Fig. 56.17). It is seldom associated with mucosal inflammation or with irritation. Many women with bacterial vaginosis are asymptomatic.

Male partners are usually asymptomatic although some will complain of a subpreputial smell after intercourse. Others, especially uncircumcized men, may develop a florid erosive or punctate balanoposthitis.

Complications

Apart from the psychological distress and disruption to sexual activity suffered by some women with bacterial vaginosis there are few proven complications. It is suspected that infected women may be more susceptible to pelvic inflammatory disease and urinary tract infections. *G. vaginalis* has been reported to cause bacteraemia after instrumental vaginal delivery. Bacterial vaginosis is frequently associated with co-infection with *Ureaplasma urealyticum* and *Mycoplasma hominis* which are possible causes of preterm labour, prematurity, chorioamnionitis and puerperal fever.

Diagnosis

The clinical diagnosis of bacterial vaginosis can usually be confirmed by simple tests on the vaginal discharge. Typically the pH is elevated to 5.5. A drop of 10% potassium hydroxide added to a drop of secretion on a glass slide releases the fishy odour of volatile amines. Microscopy of a wet film shows active motility of *Mobiluncus* spp, and masses of small bacteria coating epithelial cells ('clue cells'). On a Gram stain preparation, the bacteria are Gram-variable. Lactobacilli and pus cells are usually absent.

Management

Metronidazole is the drug of choice. A single 2 g dose is effective although some prefer to repeat this dosage after 24–48 h. A longer 7-day course of 400 mg twice daily is often given to recurrent cases and may be combined with a course of tetracyclines to eradicate other vaginal pathogens. Metronidazole may cause nausea. Alcohol may precipitate a disulfiram reaction and should be avoided during a course of metronidazole. In pregnancy, metronidazole is best avoided in the first trimester when ampicillin 500 mg four times daily for 7 days is an alternative therapy.

There have been no controlled trials of the effect of treating the partner on relapse rates. In recurrent cases it is potentially worthwhile to see the partner, administer a similar single-dosage treatment, and to seek his co-operation in the temporary use of condoms to avoid semen in the vagina which undoubtedly precipitates recurrences in many women.

Trichomoniasis

This is caused by infection with the protozoan, *Trichomonas vaginalis*, which is actively motile by virtue of its four unipolar flagellae. The condition is usually sexually transmitted and may lie in a dormant state for months or years. Vertical transmission also occurs and although non-sexual transmission is theoretically possible owing to the organism's survival in moist secretions, mineral baths and toilets for several hours, it is likely to be an exceptional means of acquisition. Trichomoniasis is frequently associated with other STDs.

Unlike the other causes of vaginitis, the incidence of trichomoniasis has shown a slight fall in the past decade. *T. vaginalis* is more common in young sexually active girls, in women in their 40s and in users of non-hormonal, non-barrier methods of contraception.

Clinical features

The condition is typified by a foul-smelling, mucopurulent vaginal discharge with accompanying symptoms of dysuria and vulval soreness. Examination will often reveal a severe vulvovaginitis with perivulval intertrigo and petechial haemorrhage on the vaginal wall and ectocervix (Fig. 56.18).

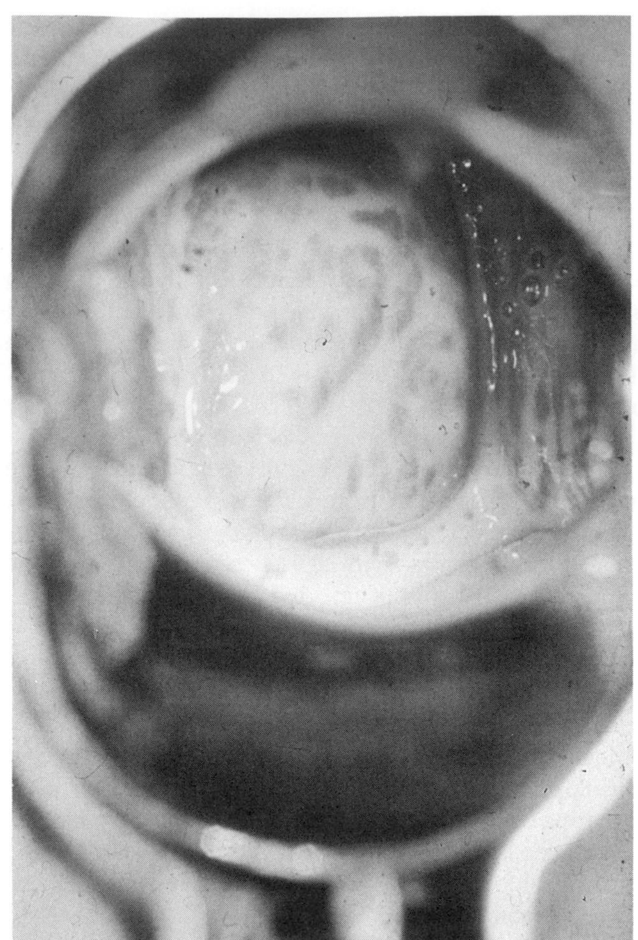

a

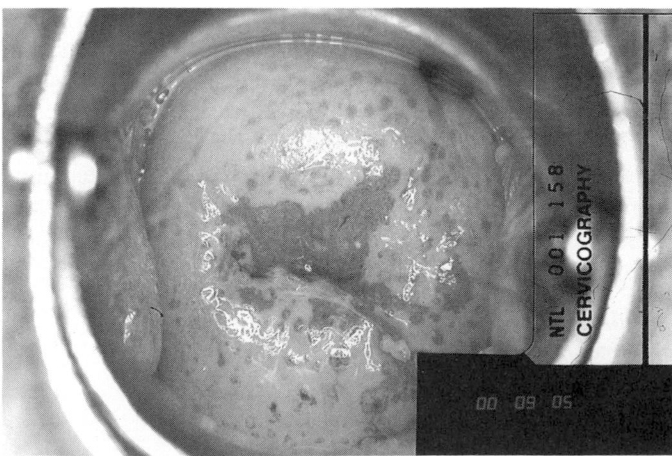

b

Fig. 56.18 Trichomoniasis:(**a**) grey, watery discharge and (**b**) 'strawberry cervix' with petechial haemorrhage.

Diagnosis

The diagnosis is most easily proven by the microscopic identification of the causative protozoan in a wet film. It can also readily be seen on cervical cytology. Swabs sent in a transport medium, such as Feinberg–Whittington, can also be cultured. Clinical diagnosis is unreliable in milder cases as the discharge can be mistaken for bacterial vaginosis, especially in intrauterine contraceptive device wearers.

Treatment

Metronidazole is the drug of choice using regimens similar to those in bacterial vaginosis. Other nitroimidazole drugs, such as nimorazole and tinidazole, are also successful in single- or multiple-dosage therapy. True metronidazole resistance in *T. vaginalis* is extremely rare. Failures are more often related to utilization and degradation of the drug by other vaginal bacteria or by failure to absorb the drug after oral administration, Combination broad-spectrum antibiotic–metronidazole regimes will usually eradicate the organism. Occasionally it proves necessary to give intravenous metronidazole on 5 consecutive days.

Most men have asymptomatic urethral infection with *T. vaginalis* but some develop urethritis or balanitis. Detailed investigations will reveal the organism in at least one-third of all sexual partners — hence the desirability of routinely treating the partner with metronidazole. A single 2 g dose is preferred as this minimizes the period of alcohol abstinence recommended.

Candidiasis

Vulvovaginal candidiasis occurs worldwide. About 75% of women will experience an episode at some time, usually in relation to pregnancy or following antibiotic therapy. About 1 in 10 of these will suffer recurrent attacks when the physical symptoms are often accompanied by profound psychological upset and sexual dysfunction. Although sexual acquisition probably plays only a small role in the aetiology of vulvovaginal candidiasis, the infection can be passed to male partners who may act as asymptomatic reservoirs of reinfection or may develop symptomatic balanitis. The commonest causative yeast is *Candida albicans*. Other *Candida* spp. and *Torulopsis glabrata* account for less than 10% of cases. About 20% of women attending STD clinics harbour vaginal yeasts. In most of these it represents asymptomatic carriage.

Predisposing causes

C. albicans is a secondary, opportunistic pathogen which requires an underlying deficit in host local or systemic immunity in order to invade the vagina and cause disease. Local immunity is compromised by the disturbance of commensal bacterial flora induced by broad-spectrum antibiotics; by other genital infections causing inflammation or ulceration of epithelial surfaces; by local trauma induced by intercourse or skin sensitizers, and by genital dermatoses.

Vulvovaginal candidiasis is a well recognized complication of the reduced cellular immunity in late pregnancy, and in all pathological states associated with immunosuppression. It is also more common in endocrine disorders such as diabetes mellitus and thyroid, parathyroid and adrenal disease. Although iron deficiency and other anaemias predispose to chronic mucocutaneous candidiasis, their association with vulvovaginal candidiasis is unproven.

The role of the male in reinfection has probably been over-emphasized. In less than one-quarter of cases is the consort the major source of reinfection. Other more common sources are the gastrointestinal tract and the deeper layers of the vagina itself which are penetrated by yeasts but which are relatively impervious to topical vaginal treatments.

Clinical features

The cardinal symptom is an intense vulval itch, worse with warmth and at night. This may be associated with external dysuria and dyspareunia. Excessive vaginal discharge is not a consistent feature. When present it is classically thick 'cottage cheese' in type but in some women can be thin and mucopurulent.

The physical signs vary widely — some women with disabling symptoms have little to see other than mild vulval erythema and a few introital fissures. In the most acute cases there is a pronounced vulvovaginitis with peripheral vulval satellite lesions, vulval oedema and vaginitis with adherent mycotic plaques on the vaginal wall and ectocervix (Figs 56.19 and 56.20).

Diagnosis

Clinical features should not be relied upon. The diagnosis should be confirmed and other pathogens excluded by

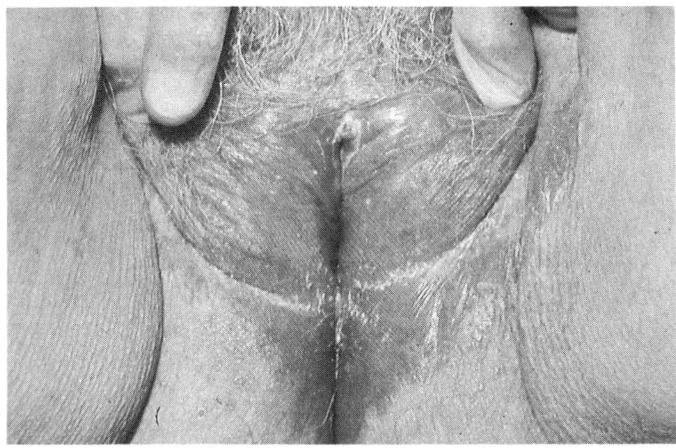

Fig. 56.19 Candida vulvitis.

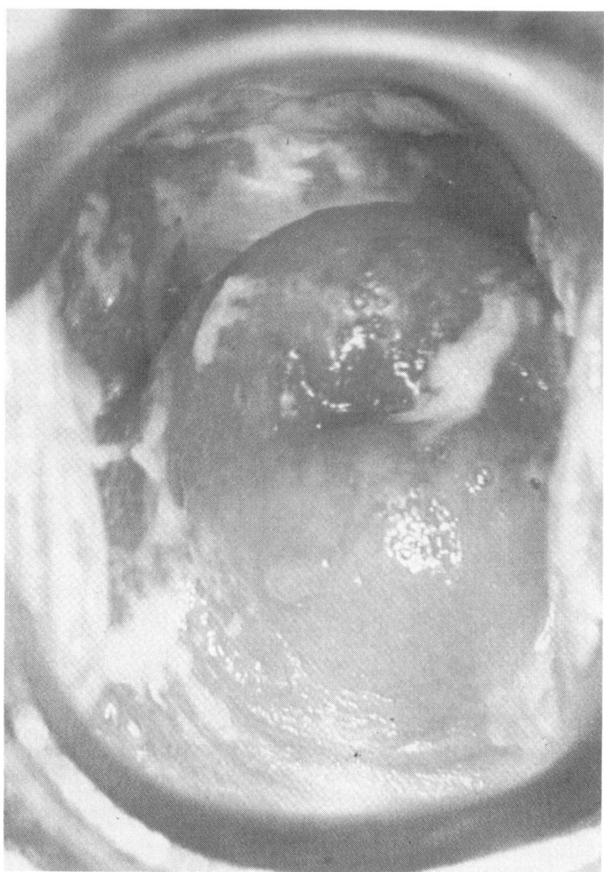

Fig. 56.20 Candida vaginitis: note the thick adherent discharge.

thorough microbiological investigation. Microscopy of the vaginal discharge shows fungal elements in either 10% potassium hydroxide or Gram stain. A high vaginal swab cultured for *Candida* will give a positive result in carriers as well as from women with symptomatic vulvovaginal candidiasis.

Treatment

Underlying causes should be corrected if possible. Drugs of the polyene group, such as nystatin, or of the imidazole group, such as clotrimazole, miconazole and econazole, are commonly employed as creams and pessaries in topical treatments lasting 1–14 days. Yeast resistance is virtually unknown to these drugs and topical sensitivity is rarely encountered. Acute isolated episodes are usually successfully treated in this way.

Chronic recurrent candidiasis is often a therapeutic problem, even after the consort has received concurrent penile treatment. Reinfection from underwear can be overcome by steam ironing or by prewash overnight soaks in candidacidal solutions. Eradication of gut and vaginal reservoirs is more difficult. Systemic antifungal therapy with orally absorbed drugs such as ketoconazole carries a risk of hepatotoxicity. A new oral triazole, fluconazole, is well absorbed and effective in single dosage for acute vulvovaginal candidiasis. It appears to be free of serious toxicity although continued caution is required. Good results have been obtained in recurrent vulvovaginal candidiasis by employing an initial 7-day course of fluconazole 50 mg daily followed by prophylactic treatment with 150 mg single doses at fortnightly or monthly intervals for 3–6 months.

ECTOPARASITIC INFESTATIONS

Both pediculosis pubis and scabies are common infestations in sexually active adults. Their presence should stimulate investigation for accompanying STD.

Pediculosis pubis

The pubic louse, *Phthirus pubis*, has greatly enlarged middle and hind legs with claws adapted to match the diameter of pubic and axillary hair. The louse has also been recovered from the beard area, eyelashes and eyebrows. Adult lice are sedentary, move slowly and survive up to 24 h when removed from their host. The adult female lays up to four eggs daily, cemented to hairs, and these eggs hatch within 5–10 days. Sexual transmission is usual although infestations acquired from shared beds and clothing are recorded.

Clinical features

Allergic sensitization to louse bites results in itching which develops within a week in some individuals while others remain asymptomatic for weeks or months. Characteristic blue spots occur at bite sites. Adult lice situated at the base of hairs are often mistaken for freckles or crusts. Nits on hair shafts are more obvious.

Treatment

Topical pediculocide preparations should kill both adults and their eggs. After application, the drug should remain in contact with eggs for at least 1 h. There are several proprietary preparations which, as lotions, creams or shampoos, usually have as their active constituents either gamma benzene hexachloride or malathion. Vaseline applied to the eyelashes and eyebrows will smother lice by obstructing their breathing apparatus.

Scabies

Scabies is caused by the itch mite, *Sarcoptes scabiei*. Adult females measure 400 μm in length, move rapidly, and burrow into the horny layer of the skin where they lay up to three eggs daily. These develop, via larval stages, into adult mites within 10 days.

Epidemiology

Scabies affects all age groups. Non-sexual transmission occurs in families and particularly affects children. Sexual transmission should be suspected in young adults, especially when genital lesions occur.

Clinical features

Although individuals may remain asymptomatic for months, the usual development of intense itching, worse at night, occurs 1–8 weeks after infestation. A rash develops symmetrically on the trunk and limbs. Lesions on the head and neck rarely occur. Thread-like linear burrows, crossing skin creases, most commonly affect the fingers, wrists, axillae and nipples. Characteristic excoriated papules occur on the genitals.

Complications include secondary bacterial infection of excoriated lesions. In the mentally retarded, steroid-treated or immunologically compromised individual, massive infestations resulting in a generalized psoriasiform dermatosis may occur. The diagnosis is readily confirmed by identification of the mite on microscopy of material removed from burrows.

Treatment

It is important to treat the patient and all close family and sexual contacts. Topical applications are applied with a paintbrush to all skin areas from the neck down and left for 24 h. Prior bathing should be avoided as it may increase the risk of systemic toxicity.

Gamma benzene hexachloride does not sting, can be used on eczematized skin, but should be avoided in children and pregnant women because of possible neurotoxicity. Malathion, in aqueous or alcoholic solution, has an unpleasant smell and stings on application to broken skin. Monosulfiram, 25% solution in methylated spirit, is diluted in 2–3 parts of water and applied on 3 successive nights. Alcohol should be avoided during treatment because of the risk of 'Antabuse-like' reactions.

Secondary bacterial infection will require appropriate antibiotics. Post-treatment pruritus will usually respond to topical hydrocortisone and reassurance.

KEY POINTS

1. STDs are not necessarily related to social class, to educational attainment or to standards of personal hygiene.
2. A patient with one STD is likely to have another — screening for other infections is essential.
3. Antenatal screening for syphilis remains cost-effective.
4. Gonorrhoea is often asymptomatic.
5. The commonest sexually transmitted pathogen in developed countries is *Chlamydia trachomatis.*
6. Early chlamydial infections are often silent in women and may remain so for months and possibly years.
7. Chlamydial infection can be diagnosed by culture or by antigen detection.
8. The treatment of choice is tetracycline or erythromycin for 7–14 days.
9. Subclinical HPV infection is very common.
10. Herpes genitalis can be recurrent but subsequent episodes are shorter and less severe.
11. Pregnant women with a history of genital herpes should be screened from 36 weeks and delivered by caesarean section if clinical lesions or asymptomatic viral disease are found.
12. The commonest vaginal infections are associated with *Gardnerella vaginalis* (bacterial vaginosis); *Candida albicans* ('thrush') and *Trichomonas vaginalis.*

REFERENCE

Woolley P D, Bowman C A, Hicks D A, Kinghorn G R 1988 Virological screening for herpes simplex virus during pregnancy. British Medical Journal 296: 1642–1643

FURTHER READING

Arya O P, Osoba A O, Bennett F J 1988 Tropical venereology, 2nd edn. Churchill Livingstone, Edinburgh

Center for Disease Control 1985 Sexually transmitted diseases treatment guidelines. Morbidity and Mortality Weekly Report 34 (suppl) : 4S

Corey L 1986 Genital herpes simplex virus infections: natural history and therapy. Recent Advances in Sexually Transmitted Diseases 3: 71–108

Mardh P A, Taylor Robinson D 1984 Bacterial vaginosis. Alinguist & Wiksell International, Stockholm

Oriel J D, Ridgeway G L 1983 Chlamydial trachomatis: genital infection in men. British Medical Bulletin 39: 133–137

Robertson D H H, McMillan A, Young H 1989 Clinical practice in sexually transmitted disease. Churchill Livingstone, Edinburgh

Thin R N 1982 Lecture notes on sexually transmitted diseases. Blackwell, London

Thin R H 1988 Management of genital herpes simplex infections. American Journal of Medicine 85: 3–6

Westrom L, Mardh P A 1983 Salpingitis. In: Holmes K K, Mardh P A, Sparking P F, Wiesner P J (eds) Sexually transmitted diseases. McGraw Hill, New York, pp 615–632

White T S, Coda F A, Ingram D L, Pearson A 1983 Sexually transmitted diseases in sexually abused children. Paediatrics 72: 16–20

Zurhausen H 1987 Papillomaviruses in human cancer. Cancer 15: 1692–1696

57. Human immunodeficiency viruses

C. Hudson

The human immunodeficiency viruses (HIVs) are micro-organisms which since the 1980s have emerged as one of the greatest threats to mankind within decades.

AIDS

The full clinical syndrome — acquired immune deficiency syndrome (AIDS) — is subject to international definition which is constantly being revised and updated to take account of rare circumstances and variations which are now being recognized. The original definition applies to the majority of cases. This requires:

1. The presence of reliably diagnosed disease at least moderately indicative of cellular immune deficiency.
2. The absence of an underlying cause for immune deficiency or indeed a defined cause for reduced resistance to disease.

CLINICAL MANIFESTATIONS

The final clinical manifestations of HIV infection are in the seroconversion illness (Pedersen et al 1987). Most of the features mimic glandular fever, recognizably protean in its manifestation. Noteworthy are the skin rash and symptoms of encephalitis which occasionally occur.

Many of the manifestations of AIDS are related to the occurrence of so-called opportunist infections. These are pathological states brought about by organisms which are only rarely if ever pathogenic in an individual with an intact immune system.

Malignant disease

Out of all proportion to its prevalence in the general population, Kaposi's sarcoma is a recognized and relatively common manifestation of the disease, especially in homosexual males. Other forms of malignancy particularly of the lymphoreticular system are described more commonly in individuals with HIV infection. An increased risk of cervical intraepithelial neoplasia or indeed invasive cervical cancer has not yet been described although this neoplasm associated with human papillomavirus infection is known to be more common in females who are immuno-compromised for other reasons.

Dementia

Direct involvement of the central nervous system is the probable cause of dementing symptoms, increasingly recognized as an important feature of the disease, and one which may rarely antedate other manifestations. This has important connotations for health care workers exposed to the virus.

AIDS-related complex (ARC)

In the presence of HIV seropositivity there are a number of non-specific clinical features which do not constitute the full syndrome but are likely to be evidence of disease activity. They include weight loss, diarrhoea, fever and lassitude.

Persistent generalized lymphadenopathy (PGL)

This is one of the earliest manifestations of HIV infection. Clearly this is a situation with several differential diagnoses. It is one of the first clinical situations in which the question of specific HIV testing may be raised. Even under such circumstances explicit consent to HIV testing is normally required.

AETIOLOGY

The first human immunodeficiency retrovirus was discovered in 1983 by Barré-Sinoussi and colleagues in Paris (Barré-Sinoussi et al 1985). There was a plethora of individually devised names. In 1986 under the auspices of the International Committee on the Taxonomy of Viruses, the basic term 'human immunodeficiency virus' was introduced to replace all the others. At the time of writing there are two described strains (HIV1, HIV2) both capable of producing the syndromes of AIDS and AIDS-related conditions.

The HIVs are examples of retroviruses, a group characterized by the ability to produce a particle-associated, enzyme-directed DNA polymerase or reverse transcriptase. This enzyme confers the particular ability to perform reverse transcription by which the RNA of the viruses is converted to a complementary DNA copy, which can then be inserted into the chromosomal DNA of an infected cell to create an integrated provirus. Although human T leukaemic viruses have been included with the C-type oncoviruses, HIV1 and HIV2 are now classed with the lentiviruses. Within this group are certain simian immunodeficiency viruses (SIVs), widespread in sub-Saharan Africa and apparently non-pathogenic in studies of the local primates, namely sooty mangabeys and vervets. SIV has caused immunodeficiency (simian AIDS) in captive macaques.

PATHOLOGY

The basic structure of the HIVs is common to the Retroviridae and a detailed description is beyond the scope of this chapter. In essence there is a viral core containing the viral RNA and the associated reverse transcriptase. There are various core antigens P18, P24 and P15, of which the P24 antigen is the most widely used for investigational study. The viral envelope is largely derived from the host cell. The emergence however of an envelope glycoprotein (gP120) has produced an affinity for a subset of T lymphocytes (helper cells) characterized by the expression on the cell membrane of the CD4 antigen. This antigen, which has been identified as the receptor for the virus, is also found on the cells of the macrophage series and in pulmonary and brain tissue. There is also some evidence of the possibility of direct involvement of the bowel. These features are all compatible with the known natural history of the developing clinical syndrome.

PATHOGENESIS

The mechanism whereby HIV1 infection produces progressive damage to the immune system is not fully understood. Aggregation occurs of both infected and uninfected cells and there may be the induction of an autoimmune process which can lead specifically to the destruction of CD4-bearing lymphocytes. There is a suggestion too that unintegrated viral DNA may have cytopathic effects which could be a feature of this type of infection.

INFECTIVITY

Viraemia occurs in the early stages after infection and persists, albeit at a lower level once antibody responses have developed. Because integrated proviral DNA remains within circulating lymphocytes, with the capability of being transcribed and producing virus particles, the continuing infectivity of blood and certain other body fluids remains beyond doubt. Infectivity is, however, fortunately low but may increase when the immune responses of a carrier fail and the clinical syndrome of AIDS and its related complexes begins to appear.

EPIDEMIOLOGY

The World Health Organization now recognizes three global patterns of AIDS and HIV infection (Chin 1988). The existence of these three patterns stems from the duration of significant local prevalence, the relative importance of the three main modes of transmission, and local variations in sexual and other high-risk behaviour in the population.

Pattern 1 is characteristic of western industrial society, including Australia, New Zealand and parts of Latin America. Extensive spread of this pattern probably began in the late 1970s, predominantly amongst homosexual males and intravenous drug abusers. Transmission due to blood and blood products followed but has virtually been eliminated since 1985. A small pool of persons transfused before that date remains. Within pattern 1 communities, population seroprevalence would generally be less than 1%, but has been found at or above 50% in some groups

Table 57.1 Estimation of the number of HIV-infected females in 1988 throughout the world. (After Chin 1988)

Geographic area	Estimated total HIV-infected persons	Observed male:female ratio of AIDS	Estimated total HIV-infected females
Pattern 1	2 500 000	9:1	250 000
Pattern 2	2 500 000	1:1	1 250 000
Pattern 3	10 000	1:1	5 000
Total	> 5 000 000		1 505 000

Table 57.2 Estimated number and age distribution of HIV-infected females in the UK in 1987 (After Chin 1988)

	Total	0–14 years	15–24 years	25–44 years	45–64 years	⩾ 65 years
Population ($\times 10^6$)	28.98	5.36	4.55	7.55	6.43	5.10
Number infected	1366	308	340	580	104	34
Number infected per 100 000	4.7*	5.8	7.5	7.7	1.6	0.7

* The estimated prevalence for the USA is 100/100 000.

of individuals practising high-risk behaviour. In these populations the male to female ratio is of the order of 10 to 1.

In pattern 2 areas the time-scale is roughly similar but the disease is mainly amongst heterosexuals. As a result the male:female ratio is approximately 1:1 and perinatal transmission is common. In a number of countries the overall population seroprevalence can be estimated to be little more than 1% but in localized urban areas may be as high as 25% in the sexually active reproductive age group. Transmission through contaminated blood products has been and remains a problem, and in the same context inadequate sterilization of needles in clinical practice poses a recognizable public health hazard.

In pattern 3 areas HIV appeared only from the second half of the 1980s with small numbers of cases. In many instances the infection is reasonably presumed to have been acquired abroad or has been produced by the import of contaminated blood products. Many Asian countries are pattern 3 areas. In some pattern 3 areas the sex ratio is 1:1 but curiously in others the figures suggest a proponderance of females. This may be a reporting bias due to selective study of cohorts of prostitutes (Table 57.1).

For the specialty of obstetrics and gynaecology it is the extent of the problem in the female population that is of prime importance, and with it the implications for a vertical transmission during pregnancy or possibly the perinatal period. Table 57.2 summarizes HIV seropositive cases in pregnant women in the UK in 1987. In the UK figures are collected and published through the Public Health Laboratory Service (Communicable Diseases Surveillance Centre) and the Home and Health Department

Table 57.3 Exposure categories of female AIDS cases, including visitors, and of female HIV1 antibody-positive reports: cumulative totals to 30 June 1989 in the UK (DHSS 1990).

Exposure category	AIDS	HIV1
Injecting drug user	17	529
Haemophiliac	2	6
Blood/component(s) recipient	19	47
Heterosexual contact		
Partner(s) with above risk factor	13	101
Others		
Known exposure abroad	24	127
No evidence of exposure abroad	2	13
Undetermined	—	86
Child of at-risk/infected parent(s)	13	47
Multiple risks	—	—
Other/undetermined	5	184
Total	95	1140

(Communicable Diseases Unit) in Scotland (Table 57.3). These record notifications of AIDS and also HIV seropositive tests. The first result of an anonymized population screen of pregnant patients in East London was published by Heath et al (1988): in that part of London a prevalence of infection of the order of 0.3% was noted.

The 1989 cumulative figures show marked regional differences between Scotland and England and significant variation in the sex ratio and seropositive rate amongst females in selected areas. This phenomenon is related to local conditions of drug use and in particular to an actual cult for needle-sharing as opposed to its sporadic and fortuitous use. It would appear that in the UK there is significant geographic variation which makes across-the-board prescription of universal policies and preventive measures inapplicable. There is a paramount need, therefore, for periodic sampling of selected populations in low-risk areas to monitor progress of the epidemic and to determine whether prevalence in any area is changing from low to high. Without such a study, logical and acceptable policies will be very difficult to obtain. Data collected by the Royal College of Obstetricians and Gynaecologists (Davison et al 1989) indicate that there is no region in the country in which HIV-seropositive pregnancies have not been reported.

PAEDIATRIC AIDS

The occurrence of HIV infection in children has added a new dimension to the significance of this epidemic. In pattern 2 countries the problem is already serious. In the UK over 400 pregnancies to seropositive women have been recorded (Davison et al 1989). Children may acquire HIV infection by being the recipients of an infected blood product or being injected with a dirty needle, by prenatal transfer from an infected mother, and possibly in the neonatal period by the ingestion of infected breast milk either from the infant's mother or perhaps from an infected wet nurse. Data on the impact of breast-feeding on the epidemic are scanty but those that are available do not at present suggest that breast-feeding is a major factor. It is quite clear that in developing countries interference with an accepted pattern of breast-feeding could create much greater morbidity and mortality than that occasioned by HIV transmission through this route. These considerations however may not apply in westernized communities where artificial feeding can be equally safe. The data from the European Collaborative Studies suggest that the vertical transmission rate of infection is of the order of 25%. Of 185 children older than 18 months, 41% were infected; the transmission rate was 22% and there was a 95% confidence interval in 16–28% (European Collaborative Study 1988).

Historical studies have not indicated that babies born by caesarean section are any less likely to have been infected than those which have traversed the birth canal for vaginal delivery. This may be because the face and mucous membranes of an infant delivered by caesarean section are more directly exposed to maternal blood than is the case with vaginal delivery.

TRANSMISSION IN THE HEALTH CARE SETTING

Ordinary clinical activity

Transmission between individuals in ordinary social or clinical activity has clearly been a matter of considerable concern both to the lay public and to members of the health care professions. Fortunately all the data suggest that the general infectivity of the immunodeficiency viruses is very low — substantially lower than that recognized for the hepatitis viruses. It is believed that ordinary social contact carries no definable risk and indeed this applies to more intimate contact between individuals short of penetrative intercourse. The use of communal toilet facilities has given rise to some concern but transmission via lavatory seats is most unlikely. However a special case has been made for care in the puerperium when there is concurrence of lochia and fresh incisions at the vulval introitus. In fact vaginal efflux very rarely contaminates a lavatory seat and incisions or lacerations of the perineum are not in the contact area when sitting. Meticulous ordinary hygiene would appear to be adequate in this situation although provision of dedicated toilet facilities in the puerperium for known HIV carriers is still recommended.

Other areas of public concern are activities such as contact sports, tattooing and barbering. The sharing of toothbrushes is obviously to be deprecated. The relevance of the above considerations to the female population is relatively low.

Invasive clinical practice

There remains concern about clinical situations where inadvertent blood-to-blood or blood-to-tissue contact could provide the basis for a transmission risk. The use of infected blood products has been considered above. There is no indication of a risk factor between patients except where inadequate sterilization of needles has been implicated.

In the reverse case of the infection of health care workers with HIV in the course of their professional activities, there is undoubtedly a small risk and the number of well documented cases is slowly increasing and at the time of writing exceeds 20. There is at least one other case within the UK which has excited considerable comment in which there was strong presumptive evidence that the infection acquired by a young surgeon was nosocomial. The importance of a small but avoidable risk under these circumstances cannot be overestimated. In the UK the General Medical Council (1987) and other similar professional bodies have given guidance which envisages the possibility that health care workers engaged in invasive clinical practice may have to modify or rarely cease practice if infected with HIV. Because in the health care setting the mechanism for transmission between patient and health care worker will be blood-to-blood or blood-to-tissue, certain measures in each area of clinical practice have been devised to minimize the risk (see below).

DIAGNOSIS

In the specialty of obstetrics and gynaecology, for reasons outlined above, the problem of HIV infection is almost entirely subclinical. At present, and for the foreseeable future, there is no test capable of identifying with absolute certainty all occult carriers of the virus.

In low prevalence areas the identification of HIV seropositive women in antenatal clinics must be achieved by the process of clinical case-finding. This is because universal antenatal testing would inevitably produce a number of false-positives on screening without the absolute certainty of identifying the very occasional true-positive in a population of thousands. Case-finding therefore must depend upon taking an adequate case history of factors which are known to engender a high risk. Collaboration with family practitioners who know the background of the individuals will be invaluable. Great tact and judgement are required as many women would be highly affronted to be questioned in depth about sexual practice when presenting for an antenatal booking. It is imperative therefore that all women at such a time be presented with documented information on the HIV problem and on the risk categories and risk behaviour which are likely to be relevant. They should be invited to declare themselves for further counselling and to accept blood testing if considered to be within such a category.

The problem of geographic risk factors gives rise to anxiety, resentment and claims of discrimination. It is less emotive to identify a risk behaviour rather than to categorize individuals on the basis of geographic origin or ethnic background. The risk behaviour in question is sexual intercourse within a high prevalence territory or sexual intercourse with an individual from a high prevalence territory. A history of prior blood transfusion is of course important, the time and the area in which the transfusion was given being vital to an assessment of the risk situation. In the case of drug abuse history is notoriously unreliable and the services of a skilled counsellor and background circumstantial evidence may be vital in forming a valid assessment of the risk situation.

When the background prevalence in the heterosexual population has reached a critical level the arguments against universal screening cease to be valid. This factor together with others such as feasibility and cost need evaluation before the introduction of voluntary universal testing.

As far as presentation in infants is concerned obstetricians should be aware that HIV infection may on occasions run an accelerated course and that the early manifestations are so non-specific that clinical diagnosis is very imprecise. The General Medical Council (1988, 1989) has ruled that it is not unethical for a doctor to arrange for the testing of a legally incompetent infant even against the specific wishes of the parent, in the knowledge that serotesting of an infant within the first year of life is effectively an oblique method of maternal testing. The ethical and legal constraints are complex and considerable, often involving dual responsibility which the doctor cannot shirk.

INVESTIGATIONS

HIV infection is most commonly diagnosed in the laboratory by the detection of relevant antibodies using enzyme immunoassay. A wide range of antigens are used in the several test systems. These include crude lysates of infected cells, genetically engineered surface glycoproteins of the virus and, more recently, synthetic peptides representative of these surface glycoproteins.

The individual immunoassays vary in their ability to detect antibodies induced by either or both of HIV1 and HIV2, and clearly a screening test should preferably detect both. In general the tests using engineered or synthetic peptides are highly specific and are therefore useful for confirmatory tests. However, test systems are now becoming available which contain appropriate genetically engineered antigens of both viruses and thus may be suited to screening purposes. Even so, the older tests using crude lysates are also used for screening purposes since at least those prepared from HIV1 will detect antibodies to HIV2 in the majority of individuals infected with this virus.

The disadvantage of all these immunoassays is that they are incapable of diagnosing recent infection because it takes time for antibodies to appear in detectable quantities after infection. This is the so-called 'window' which usually lasts 3 months or longer. Diagnosis in this early stage of infection can be made by virus isolation, a comparatively insensitive method, or by detecting the P24 core antigen in serum. However, in the future these methods will almost certainly be superseded by use of the ultrasensitive polymerase chain reaction method. At present its specificity is unproven, and reports of greatly lengthened window periods have not been confirmed.

CONFIRMATION

Because of the far-reaching unfortunate consequences of reporting false-positive results of screening tests, laboratories routinely request and take a further blood sample from the patient to exclude the possibility of transcription errors having occurred in the clinic or laboratory. Positive results are always confirmed by testing in at least one other immunoassay and also by western blotting or gel particle agglutination tests.

Tests are now available to detect the P24 antigen in serum as well as antibodies to this protein. These tests together with CD4 cell counts are of particular value in monitoring asymptomatic HIV-positive individuals to predict transition from carrier state to AIDS.

HIV testing is unique amongst medical investigations for the constraints and special considerations which apply. These have arisen because of the connotations of lifestyle associated with the onset of this epidemic. Marked and often irrational prejudice has been exhibited towards individuals who have been found to be HIV-positive. There is moreover the consideration that there is no curative therapy for the underlying disease. As a result the considerations of confidentiality and consent have assumed proportions unprecedented in the field of investigative medicine. At the same time the need for epidemiological studies of the spread of the disease seems of ever greater importance, particularly with the involvement of low-risk members of the heterosexual population. Medical and lay opinion is still divided on the ethics, legality and propriety of various testing programmes. It is as well therefore to define the terms used in this debate, as misunderstanding only adds to the general confusion on the issues.

CONSENT TO TESTING

Because of the nature of the disease, confidentiality has to be respected. A variety of approaches to testing can be used:

1. *Attributable* or open testing, where the blood sample is clearly marked with a symbol or number related to the individual.
2. *Unattributable* is the converse: personal data are removed although cohort data (e.g. age, sex, geographic origin) may be preserved.
3. *Compulsory* testing is the obligatory testing of a population whose membership is not voluntary (e.g. a prison).
4. *Mandatory* testing is obligatory testing of all members of a population, but membership of this population is voluntary (e.g. blood or other tissue donation).

Consent may be implied (explicit consent not required) or explicit. The General Medical Council (1988, 1989) requires explicit consent in the UK for HIV testing and regards failure to do this as unethical practice. For epidemiological purposes, an exception can be made when HIV testing is an additional and anonymous investigation on a blood sample which has already been taken for routine purposes, e.g. HIV screening in antenatal care.

COUNSELLING

It is recommended by the World Health Organization and widely accepted that HIV testing should be accompanied by counselling, and more particularly that post-test counselling should be available to those for whom a positive test is recorded. It is fundamental that the initiator of a test must be clear that the appropriate support will be available to the recipient of the news of a positive result. This applies most particularly to mandatory testing as is done before blood, semen or milk donation, or tests required, for instance, for insurance purposes. Otherwise the only contentious issue is the scope and extent of pretest counselling.

In the earlier stages of the AIDS epidemic testing was only carried out for reasons of clinical suspicion; later came the issue of testing those in seemingly risky situations who nevertheless were apparently entirely well. Clearly a significant measure of counselling is required in such instances regardless of whether the test is positive and particularly if high-risk activity continues. The expertise and resources to provide such a service were not immediately available.

More recently the issue of testing low-risk individuals has arisen, often as part of a screening programme. The level of pretest counselling required under such circumstances has caused difficulty. Because the provision of in-depth counselling by a trained counsellor for all recipients of the test is obviously not feasible, the responsibility for primary counselling has to devolve upon the professional staff administering the test. Furthermore the desirability of even attempting in-depth counselling on a universal basis for screening programmes has been questioned; there is no doubt that many individuals would resent probing of their private lives as an impertinent intrusion if its relevance were not fully apparent.

The issue is however further complicated by the potentially deleterious effects of merely having a test even though the result is negative. Many insurance companies require an answer to the question 'Have you ever undergone an HIV (AIDS) test?' and an affirmative may indicate loading of the premium or at worst a rejection of the proposal. More recently the Association of British Insurers (1988) has indicated that the mere taking of a test as part of a recognized screening programme will not of itself cause loading of the premium, provided of course that the test itself is negative. This is without prejudice to other considerations and a negative test in a risky situation does not diminish the risk in the eyes of the insurers.

CONFIDENTIALITY

The effect on insurance and mortgages is but one of the unwelcome consequences of HIV testing. There are a number of other sequelae which may stem from having a positive test or even from being suspected of having a positive test. These range from discrimination and ostracism at work to the devastating disruption of a sexual union. This can spread to other family members as well, with the resulting loss of support at the very time when it may be most needed.

IMPLICATIONS FOR OBSTETRICS AND GYNAECOLOGY

There are several theoretical as well as practical implications.

Impact of pregnancy on HIV

Accurate data on the progress of the disease process in pregnancy are scanty. An initial report suggested that pregnancy might accelerate the course of the disease (Semprini et al 1987). This report was based upon observations of pregnant women whose HIV status had become apparent because AIDS had been diagnosed in an infant produced in an earlier pregnancy. Subsequent studies have not sustained this view although there is some circumstantial evidence that nutritional status is relevant and pregnancy may add to deprivation under adverse circumstances.

If pregnancy is the trigger which activates recognition of a woman's seropositive status, then clearly those responsible must be aware of and prepared for the impact on her social and medical environment and of the need for continuing support and medical care. The total environmental impact of the discovery of HIV seropositivity amply justifies termination of pregnancy if that is what is requested by the individual. There is not, however, a medical need to promote such an intervention.

The impact of HIV on pregnancy

The complex interface between systemic disease and pregnancy covers the entire process from conception through placentation, embryogenesis, fetal development and parturition to lactation and involution. Many of the data relate to pregnancies in individuals with other relevant factors often secondary to lifestyle, such as intravenous drug abuse. There is no evidence of a conceptional problem nor of major defects in embryogenesis. A mild dysmorphic syndrome has been described (but its existence has not been confirmed by other workers and its origin may be multifactorial (Quazi et al 1988)). There is little evidence for a tendency to preterm labour and intrauterine growth retardation. These are in any event features associated with lifestyle phenomena. There is however well documented evidence of transplacental infection. The proportion of babies so affected is not yet known for certain (see above) but is of the order of 1 in 4.

The natural history of paediatric AIDS is outside the scope of this chapter but the relevance is clear. This is a consideration which needs to be taken into account by any seropositive woman when deciding whether to have a termination. Because immunoglobulin G antibodies cross the placenta and are only slowly eliminated from the neonate, the determination of whether a potentially infected infant is actually infected may take a considerable time. Nevertheless the consensus view is that early knowledge of this potential situation is now of benefit in the provision of proper care to a neonate. For all practical purposes a negative test eliminates HIV infection from the differential diagnosis; a positive result declares a potential risk which may only be determined by virus culture, antigen studies or differential antibody changes.

Pregnancy is thus unique with respect to HIV status and testing because two therapeutic decisions hang on the results of such a test — the decision to terminate or continue with the pregnancy and a perceived need to modify the management of any infant born.

Breast-feeding

Anecdotal reports have provided persuasive evidence that under some circumstances (perhaps when there is viraemia) infection may be transmitted via breast milk. Epidemiological studies however seem to indicate that this route of transmission is unlikely to be a major feature in the development of the epidemic. After much debate the UK Department of Health has recommended that where a safe alternative exists it is preferable for a woman who is known to be HIV seropositive not to breast-feed her infant. Similar advice is not now given to untested women from so-called high-risk categories whose definition is insufficiently precise for this purpose. It is particularly important to recognize that this advice is given for the UK only and cannot be construed as applicable to other countries where, for instance, the safety of artificial feeding cannot be assured, and where the benefits of breast-feeding outweigh the risks.

Tissue donation

Obstetrics and gynaecology as a specialty covers a number of areas in which tissue donation occurs. HIV transmission occurs with gamete donation and donor insemination (Stewart et al 1985). Oocyte and embryo donation are now features of some assisted reproduction programmes. In addition, material consisting of secundines or fetal tissues from abortions may be harvested for donation purposes. Such materials include amnion, fetal brain, fetal pancreas and paternal lymphocytes for immunotherapy.

The banking of expressed breast milk for donation other than to a woman's own infant is accepted practice and is an extension of the time-honoured procedure of wet nursing. All forms of tissue donation are now covered by policies and guidelines to eliminate the risk of transmission of HIV infection. These include the counselling of donors and elimination of all those in putative high-risk groups and the mandatory testing of those who agree to be donors.

In the case of semen donation, cryopreservation and repeat testing to allow for the window between the acquisition of infection and the appearance of antibodies in the blood is recommended. In other circumstances storage, delay and repeat testing may not be feasible. Certain groups may undertake unsupervised donations of fresh unscreened semen and this should be regarded as unsafe practice.

SAFE CLINICAL PRACTICE

For reasons discussed above, clinical testing will never suffice to identify all occult carriers of HIV infection. The practice of obstetrics, midwifery and gynaecology exposes the participants to a greater risk of direct contact with blood and blood-stained fluid than almost any other discipline except perhaps orthopaedic surgery. The joint working party of Royal Colleges and Faculties addressed the subject in depth and still adheres to the view that whereas a single tier of universal precautions is appropriate for the care of the neonate, a two-tier policy for safe clinical practice in maternal care remains applicable in low-prevalence areas (Royal College of Nursing 1986). The extra precautions envisaged for the management of HIV-positive women in labour and delivery are those commonly currently employed for prophylaxis against the spread of hepatitis B.

What is less widely appreciated is that coincident with the above is the recommendation that significant changes relating to blood spills should be introduced into ordinary clinical practice. There is now a formal recommendation to all health care workers to avoid all personal contact with spilled blood as well as for an active policy of containment and decontamination of blood spills to minimize the risk of secondary contamination of others not directly involved at the time of fresh blood spillage. In essence these recommendations call for the use of task-related degrees of protection:

1. The wearing of latex and rubber gloves and an apron is the minimum when personal contact with spilled body fluids is to be avoided. In many active situations such as delivery a gown is also required.
2. In addition disposable overshoes or protective footwear should always be available when there is risk of contamination at floor level.
3. Finally for those potentially or actually exposed to splashing at any level additional face protection is essential for eyes, nose and mouth (e.g. spectacles and mask or visor. Moreover ordinary overshoes do not afford protection to personal footwear nor to clothing below the level of an apron, so that boots or overboots are required by active participants for an effective containment policy. It is a corollary that soiled protective gear should be safely divested before leaving the clinical area.

The most important recommendations, however, relate to safe practice in handling sharps. Nearly all seroconversions have followed sharps injuries, which are almost always preventable, particularly those involving syringes and needles. Deep pelvic surgery is always difficult and extra care is necessary in known high-risk situations, which therefore require the involvement of fully trained staff. It is worth mentioning that needlestick injury has occurred through wearing open-toed or fenestrated footwear in a clinical area such as an operating theatre. A routine must be established for first aid in the case of inadvertent injury. This will include liberal washing of eyes or wounds, and in the care of wounds, encouraging free bleeding without scrubbing or trauma. It is worth preserving but not necessarily testing a blood sample from the health care worker.

In the operating theatre the objective must be to approximate to universal high-level precautions. These will include the acceptance of eye protection by all working in close proximity to open major surgery. It will also include the provision of waterproof gowns (at least those which are impermeable in the forearm and bib) for all so engaged. It will moreover involve tight clinical practice in the control and decontamination of soiled linen and working clothes and the chemical decontamination of blood spills in the operating theatre on the floor, table and other equipment. Techniques for the decontamination of endoscopes are under active consideration. There is no doubt that autoclaving is the preferred method of sterilization but as yet few working endoscopes are capable of withstanding such a procedure. The question of double-gloving for surgical procedures is one which the individual surgeon must make.

In the delivery suite second-tier precautions in known or suspected high-risk situations follow the above lines. In the puerperium segregation is not regarded as necessary except that most units would prefer dedicated toilet facilities to be used.

The care of the neonate born to a seropositive mother is a long-term concern of the paediatric unit which raises many issues such as the clash of interest between confidentiality and information given to health care workers on a 'need to know' basis. There is little doubt that several individuals concerned with the care of the baby do need to know. How this information is supplied on a confidential basis has not been fully resolved.

MANAGEMENT

The importance of continuing care and counselling cannot be overestimated, particularly in view of the complicated lifestyle and socioeconomic circumstances of many of these individuals. This must include attention to public health measures such as safer sex.

The treatment of the known complications of AIDS does not really fall within the purview of obstetrics and gynaecology. When pregnancy occurs in a known sufferer from AIDS or ARC, careful clinical monitoring is essential. Serial T cell counts may be predictive of deterioration and non-specific symptoms should be regarded with suspicion. Opportunist infections such as occur with *Pneumocystis carinii* require rigorous therapy which may carry its own risks. Candidiasis is perhaps the infection with which obstetricians may be more familiar.

Prophylactic use of zidovidine is under investigation; other studies are attempting to harness the CD4 antigen receptor protein for targeting of virus-infected cells. Deoxyinosine, a drug which inhibits reverse transcriptase activity, is also under study.

FUTURE OUTLOOK

It is a matter of speculation how rapidly HIV infection will spread into the notionally low-risk population and this will be of immediate relevance to the practice of obstetrics and gynaecology. Debate is current on the best methods of monitoring the situation but clearly information must be obtained if sensible and adequate health care provision is to be made.

The clinical approach to the established disease is not totally nihilistic. Disease progress is related in some way to general health which therefore needs to be maintained and the vigorous treatment of incidental and opportunist infection appears to play an important part. While work an methods of direct treatment of the underlying viral infection continues other measures of support for the deprived immune system are under trial and the use of the agent zidovidine in the management of paediatric HIV infection is under experimental consideration. A balanced and positive approach to the situation is required with specific avoidance of the widespread reactions of denial, hyper-anxiety and recrimination. Health care workers have a duty to respond to the needs of patients with sensitivity and without personal reservation.

KEY POINTS

1. Infectivity of HIV is lower than that of hepatitis virus.
2. Pregnancy per se does not accelerate the course of HIV.
3. HIV may cause dysmorphic syndromes in the fetus and one in four pregnancies will have transplacental infection.
4. There is no evidence for major defects in embryogenesis, preterm labour or intrauterine growth retardation.
5. Transmission via breast milk is not a major source of infection but it is preferable for an HIV positive woman not to breast feed.
6. Donor material (i.e. fetal tissues, milk, oocytes and semen) should not be accepted from an HIV positive person.
7. Precautions against the spread of HIV infection during labour, delivery and at surgery should be those commonly employed against the spread of hepatitis B.
8. HIV infection is increasing amongst women and those attending antenatal clinics.

REFERENCES

Association of British Insurers 1988 ABI fact file: AIDS and insurers. Association of British Insurers, London

Barré-Sinoussi F, Nugeyre M T, Cherman J C 1985 Resistance of AIDS virus at room temperature. Lancet ii: 721–722

Davison C F, Ades A E, Hudson C N, Peckham C S 1989 Antenatal testing for human immunodeficiency virus. Lancet ii: 1442–1445

European collaborative study 1988 Mother-to-child transmission of HIV infection. Lancet ii: 1039–1042

General Medical Council 1987 Duties of doctors infected with human immunodeficiency virus. General Medical Council, London, pp 17–19

General Medical Council 1988 HIV infection and AIDS: ethical considerations. General Medical Council, London

General Medical Council 1989 Letter from President. General Medical Council, London

Heath R B, Grint P C A, Hardiman A E 1988 Anonymous testing of women attending antenatal clinics for evidence of infection with HIV. Lancet i: 1394

Royal College of Nursing 1986 Second report of the Royal College of Nursing AIDS working party. Nursing guidelines on the management of patients in hospital and the community suffering from AIDS. Royal College of Nursing, London

Semprini A E, Vucetich A, Pardi G, Cossu M M 1987 HIV infection and AIDS in newborn babies of mothers positive for HIV antibody. British Medical Journal 294: 610

Stewart G J, Tyler J P P, Cunningham A L et al 1985 Transmission of human T cell lymphotropic virus type III (HTLV III) by artificial insemination by donor. Lancet ii: 581–585

FURTHER READING

Advisory committee on dangerous pathogens 1989 Causative agents of AIDS. Advisory committee on dangerous pathogens, London

Alexander N J, Anderson D J 1987 Immunology of semen. Fertility and Sterility 47: 192–205

British Medical Association 1989 Sterilisation of instruments and control of cross-infection: a BMA code of practice. British Medical Association, London

Centers for Disease Control 1989 Guidelines for prevention of transmission of human immunodeficiency virus and hepatitis B virus to health care and public safety workers. Morbidity and Mortality Weekly Report 38: 1–21

Chin 1988 The global patterns and prevalence of HIV infection in women. In: Hudson C N, Sharp F (eds) AIDS and obstetrics and gynaecology. Royal College of Obstetrics and Gynaecology, London, pp 15–21

Chiodo F, Ricchi E, Costigliola P 1986 Vertical transmission of HTLV-III. Lancet i: 739

Department of Health 1989 HIV infection, breastfeeding and human milk banking. CMO/CNO letter HMSO, London

Department of Health 1989 Guidance for the protection of clinical health care workers against occupational infection with human immunodeficiency viruses and hepatitis viruses. Report of the expert advisory group on AIDS. HMSO, London

Department of Health and Social Security 1986 Acquired immune deficiency syndrome (AIDS) and artificial insemination: guidance for doctors and AI clinics. DHSS publication CMO(86)12. Department of Health and Social Security, London

Department of Health and Social Security 1987 Decontamination of equipment, linen or other surfaces contaminated with hepatitis B or human immunodeficiency virus. DHSS publication HN (87)1. Department of Health and Social Security, London

Department of Health and Social Security 1988 AIDS: HIV infected health care workers. Report of the expert advisory group on AIDS. HMSO, London

Department of Health and Social Security 1988 Decontamination of instruments and appliances used in the vagina. DHSS publication EL(88)MB/210. Department of Health and Social Security, London

Department of Health and Social Security 1989 HIV infection and tissue and organ donation. DHSS publication CMO(87)5. Department of Health and Social Security, London

Hudson C N, Sharp F (eds) Aids and obstetrics and gynaecology. Royal College of Obstetricians and Gynaecologists, London

James K, Hargreave J R 1984 Immunosuppression by seminal plasma and its possible clinical significance. Immunology Today 5: 357–363

Johnstone F D 1988 Termination of pregnancy. In Hudson C N, Sharp F (eds) AIDS and obstetrics and gynaecology. Royal College of Obstetricians and Gynaecologists, London, pp 151–156

Krasinksi K, Borkowsky W, Bebenroth D, Moore T 1988 Failure of voluntary testing for human immunodeficiency virus to identify infected parturient women in a high risk population. New England Journal of Medicine 318: 185

Mortimer P P, Cooke E M, Tedder R S 1988 HIV infection, breastfeeding and human milk banking. Lancet ii: 452–453

Oxtoby M J 1988 HIV and other viruses in human milk: placing the issues in broader perspective. Paediatric Infectious Diseases Journal 7: 825–835

Pedersen C, Nielsen C M, Vestergaard B F et al 1987 Temporal relation of antigenaemia and loss of antibodies to core antigens to development of clinical disease in HIV infection. British Medical Journal 295: 567–569

Quazi Q H, Sheikh T M, Fikrig S, Menikoff H 1988 Lack of evidence for craniofacial dysmorphism in perinatal human immunodeficiency virus infection. Journal of Paediatrics 112: 7–11

Royal College of Obstetricians and Gynaecologists 1990 Revised report. HIV infection in maternity care and gynaecology. RCOG, London

SECTION 7

Pain

58. Physiology and relief of pain

W. G. Brose M. J. Cousins

Pain has plagued mankind for generations. The inconsistent descriptions of individual patients' experiences with pain and the complex interaction of both physical and psychological factors involved in pain perception have delayed the development of effective strategies for treating pain. The last few decades have seen an increase in the understanding of pain and of pain pathways that has promoted development of many more effective treatments for all types of pain.

Pain is a large-scale health problem. Chronic non-cancer pain alone costs approximately 50 billion dollars in the USA every year. This financial burden, in addition to the concern for human suffering, has initiated a change in attitudes of employers, insurance companies and the lay public towards pain.

From a simple point of view, pain is what the patient says hurts. The definition of pain, provided by the International Association for the Study of Pain (1986) is: 'an unpleasant sensory and emotional experience associated with actual or potential tissue damage, or described in terms of such damage'. This definition provides a starting point for a discussion of the intricate association between the sensory mechanisms of pain and the psychological aspects. A review of the current neurological and pharmacological information that describes the wiring diagram for the network of pain transmission, and a discussion of neurochemical mediators affected by psychological factors, will provide insight to effective treatment modalities employed in pain relief.

NEUROLOGICAL MECHANISMS OF PAIN

General considerations

Rather than a simple pathway for pain transmission, very complex interactions of many different peripheral and central nervous system structures, from the skin surface to the cerebral cortex, are now known to be involved in the processing of pain. It is now possible to consider blockade of any of these pathways and/or antagonism of involved neurotransmitters to treat specific pain problems.

Presentation of these various treatment options is best preceded by a brief discussion of certain established parts of this complex pathway for pain transmission. Yaksh (1988) summarized the detailed neurophysiological and neuropharmacological findings from 1913 until 1986.

Peripheral sensory receptors

Early descriptions of peripheral nerves indicated that they

were modality-specific and that each class of nerve fibre was responsible for only one type of sensation (Muller 1844). Recent neurophysiological evidence has established the existence of specific receptors (nociceptors) for signalling noxious stimulation. These nociceptors are characterized by a high threshold to all naturally occurring stimuli and by a progressively augmenting response to repeated or increasingly noxious stimuli (sensitization).

Cutaneous pain sensation

Mechanosensitive nociceptors respond to pressure. These receptors in the trunk have fairly large receptive fields while those in the face have smaller fields. Thermoreceptive nociceptors respond to normal heating and cooling and to noxious thermal stimuli. Mechanothermal nociceptors are activated by high-intensity heat or pressure. They have small receptive fields and are probably responsible for the 'first pain'. Polymodal nociceptors respond to many different noxious stimuli. These are the most common of all and are activated by pressure, temperature and chemical stimuli.

Skeletal muscle pain

Group III and IV nociceptors found in skeletal muscle respond to chemical agents that are released locally during muscle contraction. Metabolic byproducts alone do not trigger these receptors.

Cardiac muscle pain

Cardiac muscle afferents are activated by high-intensity mechanical stimulation, heat and chemical agents. Humoral agents released locally may be responsible for the pain seen with angina. Prostaglandins are released following myocardial hypoxia and together with histamine, bradykinin and serotonin have been shown to stimulate these receptors.

Joint pain

Group III nociceptors activated by deformation or expansion within the joint will relay pain messages. These receptors also appear to be sensitized by certain chemical substances injected into the joint (e.g. urate crystals, endotoxin, prostaglandin).

Visceral pain

These nociceptors have not been well identified. Pain is seen in response to mechanical distension, thermal and chemical stimuli.

Primary afferent transmission

After a noxious stimulus has been detected by a nociceptor

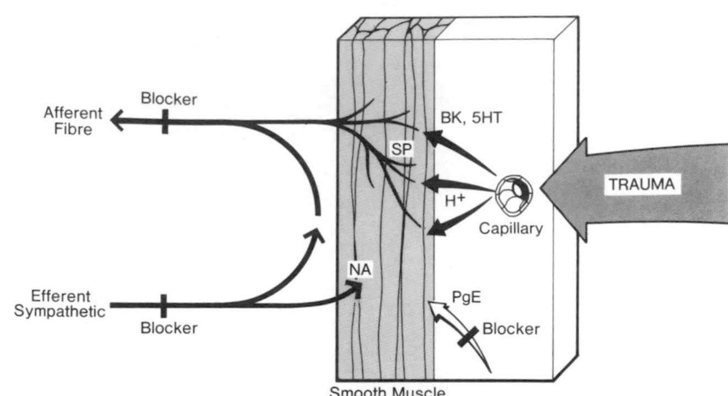

Fig. 58.1 Local tissue factors and peripheral pain receptors. The physical stimuli of trauma, the chemical environment (e.g. H^+), analgesic substances such as serotonin (5HT) and bradykinin (BK) and microcirculatory changes may all modify peripheral receptor activity. Efferent sympathetic activity may increase the sensitivity of receptors by noradrenaline (NA) release. Substance P (SP) may be the peripheral pain transmitter. Points of potential blockade of nociception are shown as 'Blocker'. Other potential sites involve BK, 5HT, NA, SP and prostaglandin E (PgE). From Phillips & Cousins (1988) with permission.

the resultant impulse travels from the point of origin via the primary afferent nerve.

There are vesicles in primary afferent terminals visible on electron microscopy. These probably provide the substrate for various peripherally active agents. Substance P is an undecapeptide found in small-diameter primary afferent neurones. This peptide is transmitted to the periphery and is released from the end of the nerve. Serotonin, histamine, acetylcholine, bradykinin, slow-reacting substance in anaphylaxis and potassium all excite primary noxious afferents. Prostaglandins sensitize the afferent nerves (Fig. 58.1).

Lesions of these peripheral nerves do not necessarily correlate with presence or absence of pain. The gate theory of pain promoted by Melzack & Wall (1965) explains the pain in some diseases whose primary lesion is demyelination of large-fibre afferents. The loss of large-fibre input in these cases leads to an open gate that allows transmission of all noxious stimuli which might otherwise be blocked by large-fibre afferent transmission closing the gate. However, a simple balance of large-fibre and small-fibre activity is far too simplistic a view of pain modulation at the spinal cord level.

Peripheral nerve injuries can also lead to pain. This may be due to increased activity in sympathetic fibres near the damaged area; neuroma formation due to sprouting from damaged axons; collaterals from intact neighbouring fibres, or changes in dorsal root ganglion cells or in central terminals of damaged axons.

Spinal cord terminals of primary afferents

Dorsal and ventral roots

The cell bodies of all primary afferent fibres except the trigeminal ganglion are in the dorsal root ganglia adjacent to the spinal cord. The dorsal root enters the spinal cord and fibres bifurcate into both cephalad and caudad-projecting branches. The smaller fibres ascend and descend for one to two segments where they enter the Lissauer tract. A small number of fibres will cross to the opposite side and some non-myelinated C fibres travel in the ventral root. This explains the incomplete pain relief that is seen following ablation of a unilateral dorsal root entry zone.

Dorsal horn

Impulses terminate in the ipsilateral dorsal horn of the spinal cord. The dorsal horn is organized into distinct lamina into which specific primary afferent fibres terminate (Fig. 58.2). Lamina I is a thin superficial layer of neurons also known as the zone of Waldeyer. The neurons with cell bodies in this lamina receive projections from both skin and muscle. These then project to the thalamus by way of the contralateral spinothalamic tracts, the ipsilateral dorsal white matter and the ipsilateral dorsal grey matter for several segments.

Laminae II and III are grouped together because of physiological and morphological similarity. This region is also known as the substantia gelatinosa. It acts as a modulating centre for small and large fibres which terminate in this region. Afferent input is from noxious stimulation as well as light touch and pressure sensations. The axons of most of these cells are short and only a few of them project to the thalamus through the contralateral anterolateral columns.

Laminae IV and V comprise the nucleus proprius. Many of these cells respond to a wide range of inputs and are called wide dynamic range (WDR) neurons. The WDRs receive input from a large field. While the receptive fields of the individual afferents may be quite small, the corresponding WDR has a larger receptive field, and closely related fields input to a single WDR, accounting for the somatotopic convergence seen in stimulation of different areas. Sympathetic afferents also converge on the WDR associated with the same spinal segment.

Lamina X lies centrally and receives input from fibres associated with noxious stimulation which terminate on cells with small receptive fields. They ascend ipsilaterally and contralaterally in the ventrolateral tract to the reticular formation. The convergence of somatic and visceral nociceptive afferents on the same dorsal horn explains referred pain. The presence of viscero/somatic, muscle/somatic, and viscero/viscero convergence seen in the laminae of the dorsal horn helps to explain some of the peculiar characteristics of non-somatic pain (Fig. 58.3).

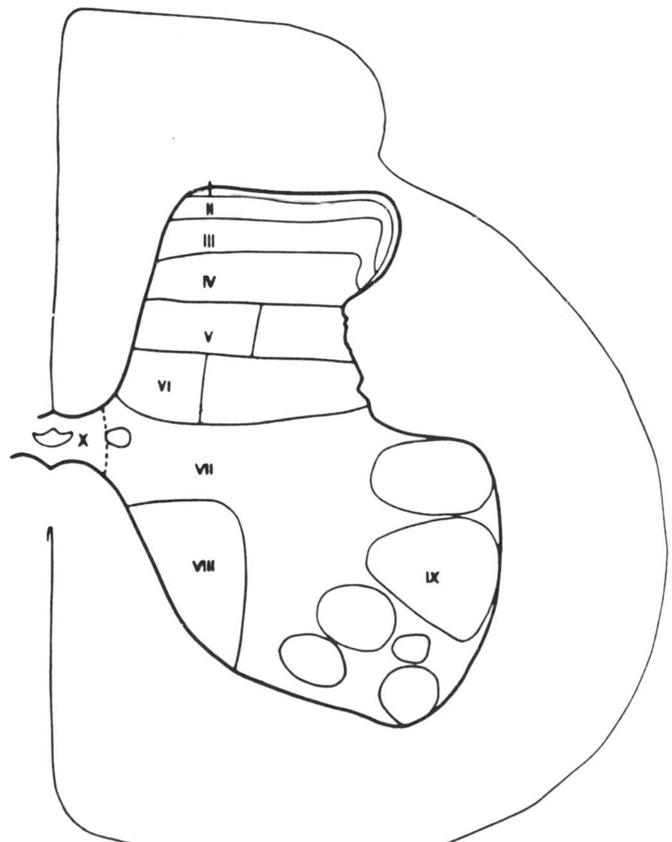

Fig. 58.2 Schematic drawing of the lamination of the ventral cell column of the VIIth lumbar spinal cord segment in the full-grown cat. From Rexed (1952) with permission.

Ascending sensory pathways

The spinothalamic and spinoreticular systems are the most important tracts associated with pain transmission in humans. Axons from laminae I, IV, V, VII and VIII make up the spinothalamic tract and ascend predominantly in the contralateral ventral quadrant of the spinal cord. Crossed fibres predominate, but perhaps 25% ascend on the ipsilateral tract.

Brainstem processing

The brainstem is involved in transmission of all ascending and descending information but nociceptive systems send numerous collaterals to the medullary and pontine reticular formation. Descending connections between the raphe nuclei and the spinal cord may suppress dorsal horn transmission of noxious information.

Thalamic relays

Several nuclear groups of the thalamus are associated with the relay of nociceptive afferent impulses. The posterior nuclear complex receives primary input from the spinothalamic system and the dorsal columns before projecting on to the posterior portion of the somatosensory cortex. The ventrobasilar complex receives input from the dorsal columns and projects to the somatosensory cortex. The intralaminar nuclei receive input from the spinothalamic tract and from the spinal reticular formation.

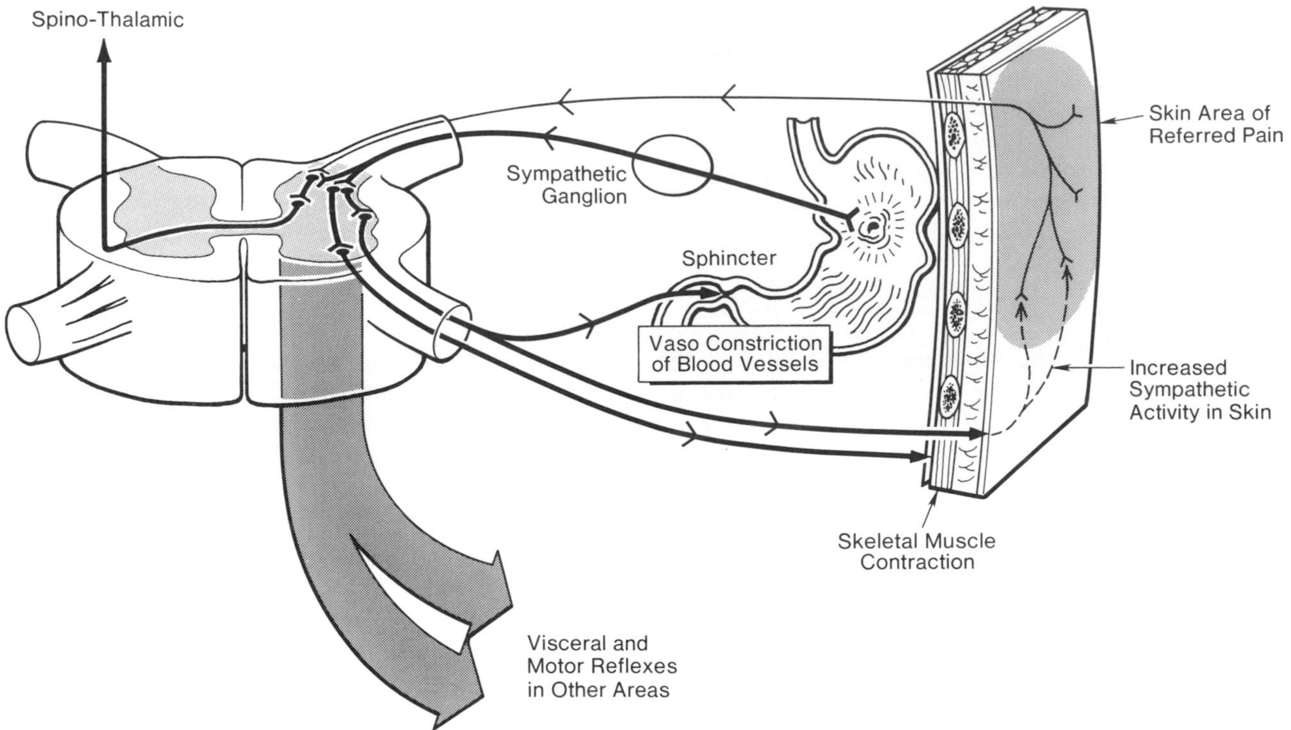

Fig. 58.3 Visceral pain: convergence of visceral and somatic nociceptive afferents. Visceral sympathetic afferents converge on the same dorsal horn, as do somatic nociceptive afferents. Visceral noxious stimuli are then conveyed, together with somatic noxious stimuli, by means of the spinothalamic pathways to the brain. Referred pain is felt in the cutaneous areas corresponding to the dorsal horn neurons upon which visceral afferents converge. This is accompanied by allodynia and hyperalgesia in this skin area. Reflex somatic motor activity results in muscle spasm, which may stimulate parietal peritoneum and initiate somatic noxious input to the dorsal horn. Reflex sympathetic efferent activity may result in spasm of sphincters of viscera over a wide area causing pain remote from the original stimulus. Reflex sympathetic efferent activity may result in visceral ischaemia and further noxious stimulation. Also, visceral nociceptors may be sensitized by noradrenaline release and microcirculatory changes. Increased sympathetic activity may influence cutaneous nociceptors, which may be at least partly responsible for referred pain. Peripheral visceral afferents branch considerably, causing much overlap in the territory of individual dorsal roots. Only a small number of visceral afferent fibres converge on dorsal horn neurons compared with somatic nociceptive fibres. Also, visceral afferents converge on the dorsal horn over a wide number of segments. Thus dull, vague visceral pain is very poorly localized. This is often called deep visceral pain. From Cousins (1988) with permission.

This information is projected diffusely to the cortex, including the frontal, parietal and limbic areas.

Cerebral cortex

S2 appears to be the principal cortical region involved with the reception and perception of noxious information. Berkley & Palmer (1974) demonstrated that bilateral ablation of the posterior region of S2 produces an increase in nociceptive threshold.

Descending modulations

So far, the discussion of pain pathways has been limited to the rostral projection of primary noxious stimuli. However, uncoupling of pain stimulus and response is observed as the absence of pain in some individuals injured in battle or during a sporting event. This shows the need to consider the modulating influences on pain transmission.

Modulation of pain stimuli can occur at many different levels in the pathway. Melzack & Wall (1965) in their proposal of the gate control theory predicted modulation of small-fibre activity by the presence of large-fibre activity in the same region of the dorsal horn.

Hagbarth & Kerr (1954) demonstrated the existence of descending long tract systems to modulate spinal-evoked activity. Virtually every pathway carrying nociceptive information is under modulatory control from supraspinal systems.

NEUROPHARMACOLOGY

Pharmacology of pain

Basic research on the processing of nociceptive information by the central nervous system has lead to an improved understanding of pain and its treatment (Fig. 58.4). By using this simplified picture of the pain pathway we can focus on pharmacological intervention at different points in the pathway and determine a clinical effect on the relief of pain.

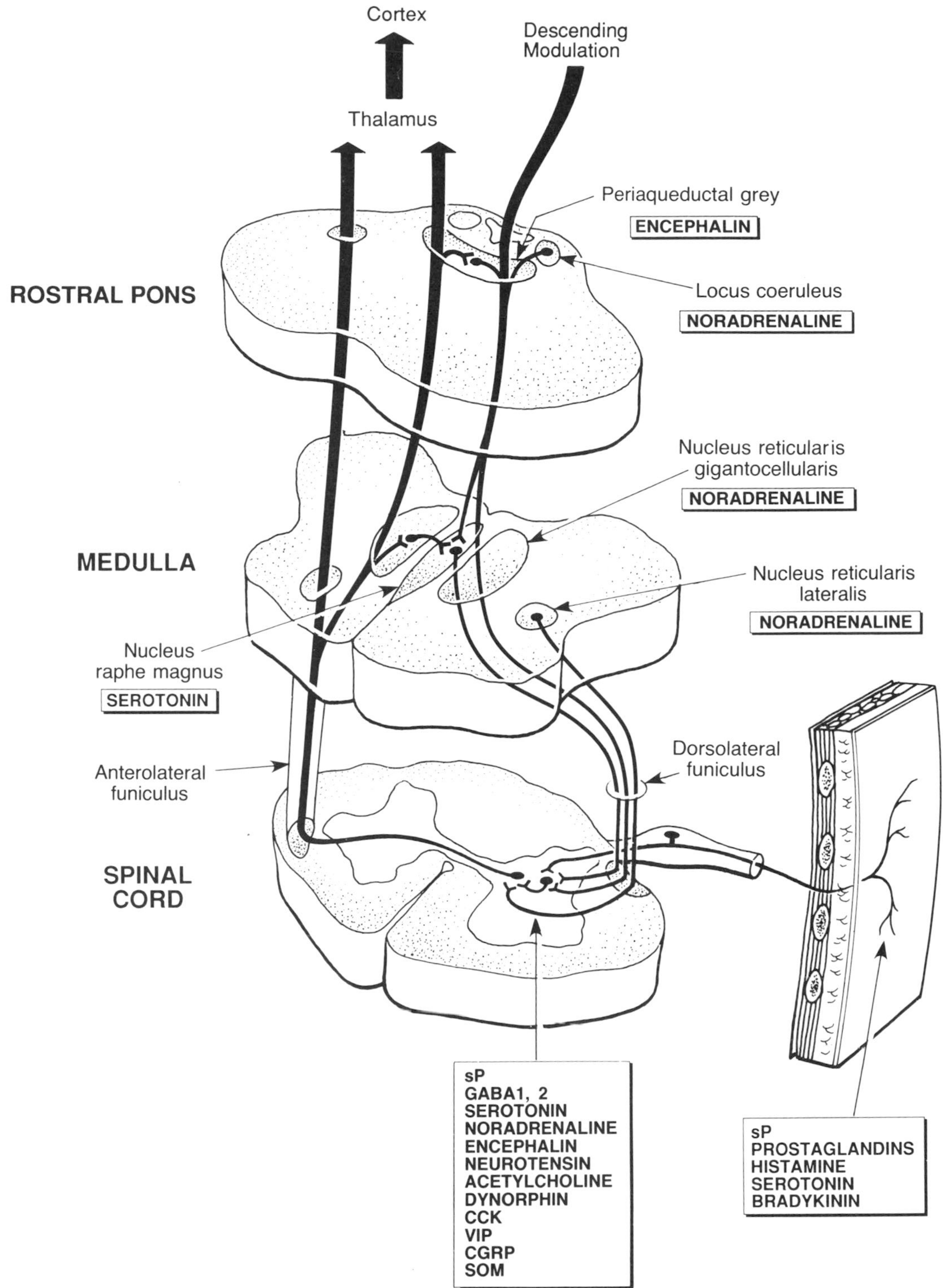

Fig. 58.4 Schematic drawing of nociceptive processing, outlining ascending (left side of drawing) and descending (right side) pathways. Stimulation of nociceptors in the skin surface leads to impulse generation in the primary afferent and levels of various endogenous algesic agents (substance P, prostaglandins, histamine, serotonin, bradykinin) increase near the area of stimulation in the periphery. The noxious impulse is conducted to the dorsal horn of the spinal cord where it is subjected to local factors and descending modulation. Projection neurons take the signal from the dorsal horn and ascend in the anterolateral funiculus to end in the thalamus. En route, collaterals of the projection neurons activate multiple higher centres including the nucleus reticularis gigantocellularis. Neurons from the nucleus reticularis gigantocellularis project to the thalamus and also activate the periaqueductal grey of the midbrain. Encephalinergic neurons from the periaqueductal grey and noradrenergic neurons from the nucleus reticularis gigantocellularis activate descending serotonergic neurons of the nucleus raphe magnus. These fibres join with noradrenergic fibres from the locus coeruleus and nucleus reticularis lateralis to send descending modulatory impulses to the dorsal horn via the dorsolateral funiculus. Multiple endogenous peptides which are involved with processing or modulation of noxious information at the dorsal horn are listed in the figure: substance P (sP); gamma-aminobutyric acid (GABA); serotonin, noradrenaline, encephalin, neurotensin, acetylcholine, dynorphin, cholecystokinin (CCK), vasoactive intestinal peptide (VIP), calcitonin gene-related peptide (CGRP), somatostatin (SOM).

Peripheral desensitization

The local circuitry involved in the detection of a noxious stimuli from the periphery is shown in Figure 58.1. Following trauma to a peripheral site, an inflammatory reaction including the activation of complement and coagulation/fibrinolytic pathways will begin. Local release of histamine, serotonin, prostaglandins and substance P has been observed. Subsequent changes in the local environment such as decreased tissue pH, changes in the microcirculation and increase in efferent sympathetic activity all appear to increase the response of peripheral nociceptors.

Numerous drug therapies have been tried to interrupt these peripheral processes. Blockade of pain by aspirin-like drugs is such a peripheral action, acting through inhibition of cyclo-oxygenase, the enzyme responsible for the synthesis of prostaglandins, prostacyclins, and thromboxanes, all of which may mediate local pain response (Juan 1978). Topical capsaicin depletes substance P from cutaneous nerve endings. The initial effect is a burning pain followed by insensitivity to subsequent painful stimuli.

Blockade of sympathetic fibres can eliminate the pain of causalgia in some patients and the burning pain and hyperalgesia seen with this syndrome can be reproduced with local noradrenaline.

Neural blockade

In 1902 Cushing suggested that nerve block could prevent the pain and shock of amputation. Later (1910) Crile proposed that disruption of the pain pathway might improve outcome from trauma. Since then many investigations have proven the benefit of neural blockade in trauma or surgery.

Neural blockade can occur at any point along the pain pathway. The most common sites are peripheral nerves, somatic plexuses and dorsal roots. These blocks can be performed with relatively short-acting agents such as local anaesthetics for acute pain, or long-acting (permanent) blockade with alcohol or phenol for chronic pain. The disadvantage with permanent techniques is that they are neither specific for pain fibres nor are they reliable for protracted pain problems. The lack of anatomical separation of fibres carrying pain, motor and other sensory information results in varying amounts of sympathetic, somatic, and perhaps motor dysfunction. While these side-effects may be well tolerated in certain acute situations or in chronic cancer pain where the life expectancy is short, the use of these techniques in other chronic conditions is inappropriate.

Opioid analgesia

There are many endogenous opioid chemicals that have analgesic effects. These include the encephalins and beta-endorphin. There are at least four different types of opioid receptors in the brain and spinal cord (Table 58.1). Intrathecal opioids produce dose-dependent, stereospecific, naloxone-reversible analgesia and are important clinical tools to combat pain.

Table 58.1 Pharmacodynamic effects obtained when an opioid agonist interacts with the various types of opioid receptor

Effect	Receptor subtype			
	Mu	Kappa	Sigma	Delta
Pain relief	Yes	Yes, especially at spinal cord level	Yes	Yes
Sedation	Yes	Yes		
Respiratory effects	Depression	Depression but not as much as for mu (may reach plateau)	Stimulation	Depression
Affect	Euphoria		Dysphoria	
Physical dependence	Marked	Less severe than with mu		Yes
Prototype agonist (other drugs with predominantly agonist activity)	Morphine (Pethidine) (Methadone) (Fentanyl) (Heroin) (Codeine) (Propoxyphene) (Buprenorphine)	Ketocyclazocine (Nalbuphine) (Dynorphine) (Butorphanol) (Nalorphine) (Pentazocine)	SKF 10,0 47	Encephalins

From Burrows et al (1987) with permission.

Brain receptors

For centuries opium has been known to possess analgesic properties. Its main site of action is the periaqueductal grey matter of the midbrain and midline medullary nuclei (Fig. 58.4).

Spinal cord receptors

There is a growing appreciation of opioid systems in spinal function. Opioids administered systemically will produce inhibition of nociceptive reflexes in spinal transected animals. Also, administration of opioids to the dorsal horn of the spinal cord will inhibit the discharge of nociceptive neurons. Multiple discrete populations of opioid receptors have been identified.

Other non-opioid systems appear to be functioning at this level to produce analgesic effects. Baclofen (beta-(p-chlorophenyl) gamma-aminobutyric acid; GABA) produces a dose-dependent analgesic action when it is injected intrathecally in cats. This analgesia was not affected by naloxone. An intrathecal preparation of morphine, serotonin and baclofen demonstrated synergistic analgesia (Yaksh 1988). This suggests that these analgesic actions were not via a common pathway (Fig. 58.5).

The substantia gelatinosa receives collaterals of nociceptive information which is subject to extensive modulation at the spinal level. Chemical mediators associated with analgesia at this level include opioids, serotonin, noradrenaline, GABA, neurotensin and cholinergic agents (Table 58.2).

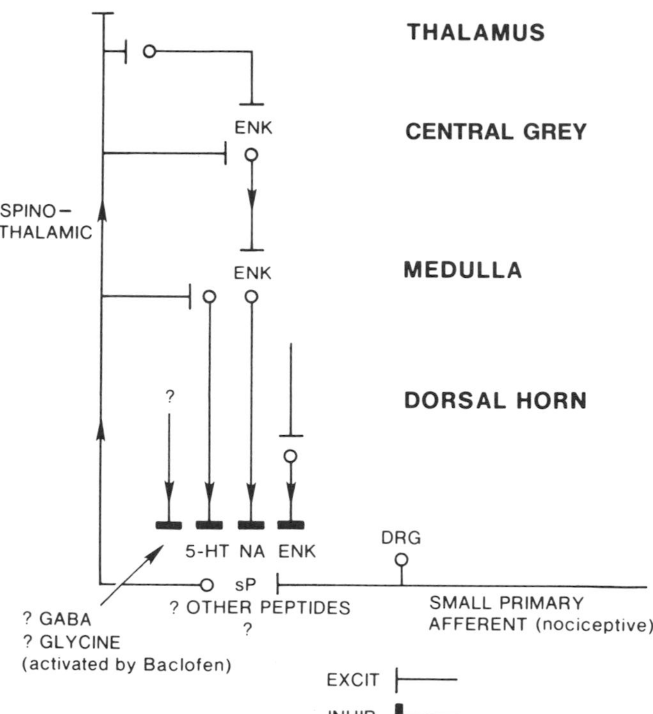

Fig. 58.5 Model of pain transmission. Proposed excitatory (excit) and inhibitory (inhib) pathways and transmitters are shown. DRG = Dorsal root ganglion; sP = substance P; 5-HT = serotonin; NA = noradrenaline; ENK = encephalin; GABA = gamma-aminobutyric acid. Primary afferent nociceptive impulses are conducted by way of DRG to spinothalamic and spinoreticular neurons in the dorsal horn with sP as a transmitter. Collaterals supply medulla and central grey matter. Encephalin activates descending pathways (GABA, 5-HT, NA), which inhibit primary afferent transmission. Within the dorsal horn there are local encephalin (opioid) inhibitory systems. From Cousins et al (1988) with permission.

Electrical stimulation

The prediction that large-fibre activity could block certain noxious information at the level of the dorsal horn was shown to have clinical value when transcutaneous electrical nerve stimulation (TENS) was introduced. The success of TENS in certain pain problems has provided enthusiastic support for development of other treatment modalities based on research theory. Dorsal column stimulation (DCS) excites descending inhibitory pathways with electricity to provide analgesia. DCS has had mixed success

Table 58.2 Spinal neurotransmitters, receptors and ligands

Neurotransmitter systems	Proposed receptor	Endogenous ligand	Exogenous ligand
Opioid	Mu	Beta-endorphin; met/leu-encephalin	Morphine
	Delta	Met/leu-encephalin	DADL
	Kappa	Dynorphin	U50488H
Adrenergic	$Alpha_1$	Noradrenaline	Methoxamine
	$Alpha_2$	Noradrenaline	Clonidine
	Beta	Adrenaline	Isoproterenol
Serotonergic	5-HT	Serotonin	Serotonin
Gabaergic	1	GABA	Baclofen
	2	GABA	Muscimol
Neurotensin		Neurotensin	Neurotensin
Cholinergic	Muscarinic	Acetylcholine	Oxotremorine

From Burrows et al (1987) with permission.

but it does appear to have a place in certain deafferentation pain syndromes.

The success of central morphine microinjection techniques may have prompted Reynolds (1969) to demonstrate similar results in animals using electrical stimulation of the periaqueductal grey matter. Naloxone-reversible analgesia has been shown in humans following implantation of brainstem electrodes. Electrical stimulation seems to have found a place in pain management by exciting intrinsic mechanisms used for the modulation of nociceptive information.

GENERAL ANAESTHESIA

Goals of general anaesthesia

General anaesthesia has developed over the last 150 years to provide good operating conditions while rendering the patient insensitive to the physiological changes associated with surgical trauma. The aims of anaesthesia are hypnosis, amnesia, analgesia, ablation of autonomic responses to surgical stimuli, maintenance of physiological homeostasis, a quiet operating field, and rapid recovery free from any sequelae.

Mechanism of anaesthesia

The precise mechanism of general anaesthesia has not been elucidated. There is a progressive dose-dependent reversible depression of nervous system function. Whatever the mechanism of action, all inhalational and intravenous anaesthetics depress or alter the function of every cell in the body.

Drugs used in general anaesthesia

Modern general anaesthesia employs many different drugs alone or, more usually, in combination.

Benzodiazepines

Benzodiazepines provide anxiolysis, amnesia, sedation and hypnosis. The most commonly used drug in this group is diazepam. However its long duration of action may delay recovery from anaesthesia. Shorter-acting drugs include lorazepam, flumazepam and midazolam. Midazolam is employed both as a preoperative medication and as an induction agent.

Barbiturates

The intravenous barbiturate thiopentone is one of the most widely employed drugs for induction of anaesthesia. It acts quickly and the effects disappear rapidly. Although safe when used properly, thiopentone has a pronounced myocardial depressant effect and can induce histamine release. Methohexitone is three times as potent as thiopentone and is cleared four times faster. However it causes hiccups, myoclonic jerking and lowers the threshold for seizures.

Oxygen

Careful attention is focused on maintaining adequate tissue oxygenation through monitoring the fraction of oxygen in the inspired gases. The pulse oximeter allows the blood oxygen saturation to be monitored.

Nitrous oxide

Nitrous oxide is commonly used to quicken the induction of anaesthesia by adding it to a mixture of oxygen and volatile agent. It provides some amnesia and analgesia while allowing a more rapid increase in the concentration of volatile agent to achieve anaesthesia. The effects of nitrous oxide are rapidly reversible.

Volatile anaesthetics

The history of volatile agents in anaesthesia began in October 1846 when William Morton administered diethyl ether to a patient for resection of a jaw tumour. Since then many agents have been employed. These drugs can be utilized for induction and maintenance of anaesthesia and provide amnesia, analgesia, hypnosis and some degree of muscle relaxation. Halothane, enflurane and isoflurane are used most commonly in the western world but ether is still widely employed elsewhere.

Opioids

Opioids are included in general anaesthesia for their analgesic effects. This reduces the dose of volatile agents and allows the patient to emerge from anaesthesia painfree.

Autonomic agonists and antagonists

Some drugs used in anaesthesia have autonomic effects. Bradycardia can be seen following administration of morphine or fentanyl, tachycardia following volatile agents and some neuromuscular blocking agents. Hypotension is associated with high doses of barbiturates, volatile agents and some muscle relaxants. These unwanted effects are prevented by drugs which act on the autonomic system.

Parasympatholytic drugs like atropine are used to achieve changes in heart rate as well as drying of oral secretions. Parasympathomimetic drugs such as neostigmine reverse the effects of non-depolarizing muscle relaxants. Sympathomimetic drugs including isoproterenol, dopamine and ephedrine are used to increase beta- or alpha-adrenergic activity. Sympatholytic drugs such as propranolol or phentolamine may be used to reduce heart rate and blood pressure in selected patients.

Neuromuscular blocking agents

Neuromuscular blocking drugs were developed to allow good muscle relaxation without providing unnecessarily deep levels of inhalational anaesthesia. These drugs prevent the transmission of nerve impulses across the neuromuscular junction by occupying the receptors on the motor end-plate (Table 58.3). The particular advantage provided by these drugs is to allow lighter levels of general anaesthesia while providing excellent operating conditions. However, care must be taken to assure adequate levels of analgesia and hypnosis as the muscle relaxant will prevent any voluntary movement which might be a signal of awareness.

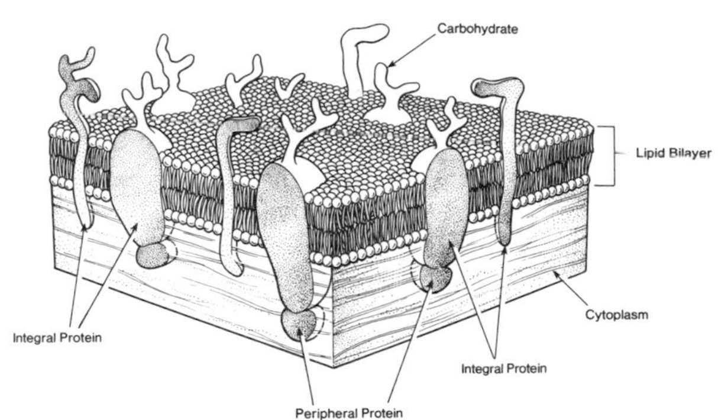

Fig. 58.6 Axonal membrane. The axonal membrane is similar to the plasma membrane of other cells. This diagram is modified from the classic Singer–Nicholson fluid–mosaic model. Carbohydrate molecules attach to proteins on the extracellular surface of the lipid membrane. The lipid bilayer consists of densely packed phospholipids which freely diffuse laterally in the plane of the membrane. Integral proteins on the cytoplasmic surface are associated with enzymatic and receptor functions. From Strichartz (1988) with permission.

REGIONAL ANAESTHESIA

Regional anaesthesia refers to the technique of rendering one part of the body insensitive to surgical stimulus. This discussion of regional anaesthesia will include the factors which determine the desired effect of local anaesthetics as well as the current applications of individual agents.

Mechanism of action

All local anaesthetics reversibly block conduction of nerve impulses along the axonal membrane (Fig. 58.6). Local anaesthetics act by interfering with the function of sodium channels (Hille 1966, 1977). They may bind inside the channel after gaining access to the axoplasm (Skou 1954; Strichartz 1973; Calahan & Almers 1979) or act within the hydrophobic core of the axonal membrane.

Pharmacokinetics

The three major mechanisms which dictate the movement of local anaesthetics within the body are bulk flow, diffusion and vascular transport. Direct injection is used to provide access to the site of action with regional anaesthesia. Bulk flow is determined by tissue resistance of the

Table 58.3 Some features of muscle relaxants

Drug	Dose (mg/kg)	Duration	Histamine release	Cardiac muscarinic receptors	Effect on autonomic ganglia	Elimination
Suxamethonium (succinylcholine)	1	Short	Slight	Stimulation (especially in children)	Stimulation	Plasma hydrolysis kidney <25%
d-Tubocurarine	0.5	Long	Moderate	None	Moderate blockade	Liver>kidney
Gallamine	2	Long	None	Strong blockade	None	Kidney primarily
Metocurine	0.4	Long	Slight	None	Slight blockade	Kidney primarily
Pancuronium	0.1	Long	None	Weak blockade	None	Kidney>liver
Alcuronium	0.25	Long	Slight (very occasionally severe)	None	Slight blockade	Kidney>liver
Vecuronium	0.1	Medium	None	None	None	Liver>kidney
Atracurium	0.3	Medium	Slight	None	None	Hoffman elimination; ester hydrolysis

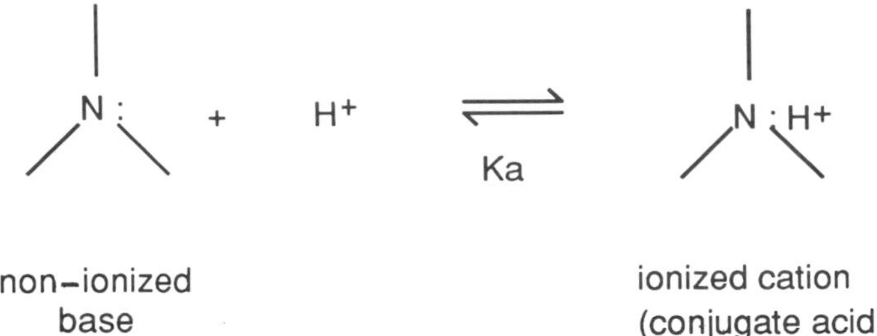

Fig. 58.7 Local anaesthetics are weak bases with pKa > 7.4. They are dispensed in acidic solution as hydrochloride salts where the non-ionized base is in equilibrium with the conjugate acid.

body planes into which it is injected but diffusion depends largely on the characteristics of the drug: the molecular weight of the agent, its lipid solubility, the degree of ionization of the drug (Fig. 58.7) and the amount of protein binding (Table 58.4).

Toxicity

Systemic absorption accounts for most of the toxicity observed with local anaesthetics. The most common toxicity seen in humans involves the central nervous system but, while cardiovascular toxicity is less frequent it is more difficult to treat and often results in some morbidity (Fig. 58.8). Central nervous system toxicity progresses from dizziness and lightheadedness to seizures and finally to coma. Cardiovascular toxicity occurs because of a direct effect on cardiac muscle and vascular smooth muscle. Reduced cardiac output and vasodilation may occur.

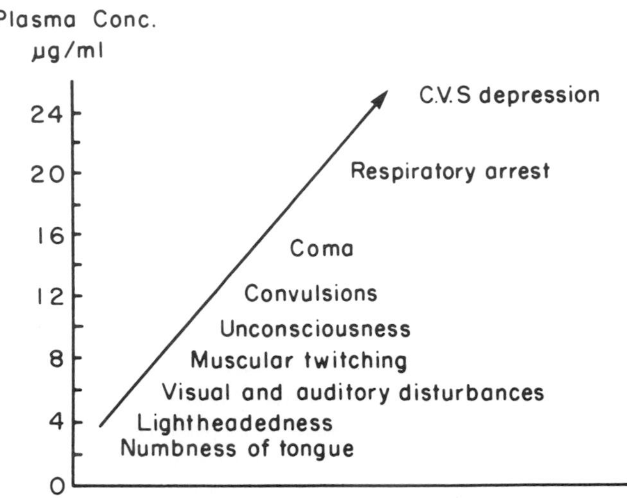

Fig. 58.8 The relationship of signs and symptoms of local anaesthetic toxicity to plasma concentrations of lignocaine. From Covino (1988) with permission.

Bupivacaine may cause ventricular fibrillation which is refractory to resuscitation. Pregnancy, acidosis and hypoxia potentiate this effect.

Local anaesthetics

Cocaine was the first local anaesthetic introduced into clinical use but deaths associated with its high toxicity led to the search for safer alternatives (Fig. 58.9). Procaine is rapidly metabolized and provides no mood elevation but the long latency and short duration of action are disadvantages. 2-Chloroprocaine is rapid-acting with low

Table 58.4 Physiochemical properties of local anaesthetics

Agent	Physiochemical properties					Biological properties		
	Molecular weight (base)	pKa* (25°C)	Partition coefficient	Aqueous solubility*	Per cent protein binding	Equieffective anaesthetic concentration†	Approximate anaesthetic duration (min)‡	Site of metabolism
Esters								
Procaine	236	9.05	0.02	?	5.8	2	50	Plasma
Chloroprocaine	271	8.97	0.14	?	?	2	45	Plasma
Tetracaine	264	8.46	4.1	1.4	75.6	0.25	175	Plasma
Amides								
Prilocaine	220	7.9	0.9	?	55	1	100	Liver‡
Mepivacaine	246	7.76	0.8	15	77.5	1	100	Liver
Lidocaine	234	7.91	2.9	24	64.3	1	100	Liver
Bupivacaine	288	8.16	27.5	0.83	95.6	0.25	175	Liver
Etidocaine	276	7.7	141	?	94	0.25	200	Liver

* Aqueous solubility: mg HCl salt/ml at pH 7.37 and 37°C.
† Data derived from rat sciatic nerve-blocking procedure.
‡ Peripheral metabolic sites are also active.
Adapted from Cousins & Bridenbaugh (1988) with permission.

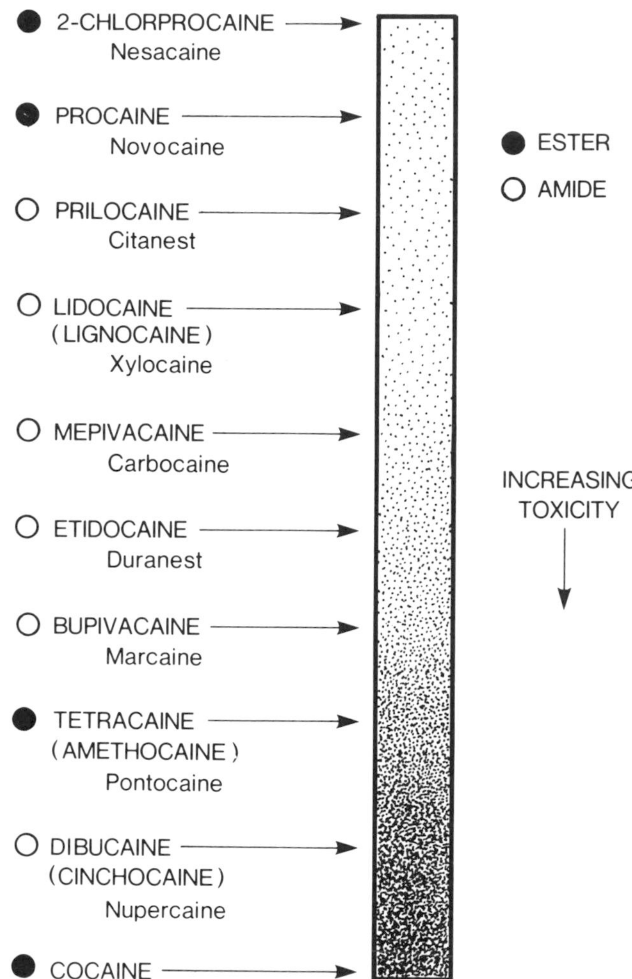

Fig. 58.9 Spectrum of local anaesthetic agents arranged in approximate order of increasing toxicity. It should be noted that comparisons of all agents at equivalent dosages under the same conditions have not yet been made in humans. From Covino (1988) with permission.

systemic toxicity and is used widely in epidural analgesia.

The remaining local anaesthetics are amides which are more stable. Prilocaine is similar to lignocaine in terms of anaesthetic profile and is the least toxic of all amide local anaesthetics. Bupivacaine produces significant sensory blockade without dominant motor block (Fig. 58.10), a characteristic which has led to its wide use in labour. However it is four times as toxic as lignocaine.

ACUTE PAIN MANAGEMENT

General

The importance of acute pain in signalling potential damage to the organism cannot be overlooked but once these warning signs have been heeded and treatment initiated, acute pain no longer serves a useful purpose. The most common forms of analgesia used to treat such acute pain are analgesic drugs and neural blockade.

Analgesic drugs

Non-steroidal anti-inflammatory drugs (NSAIDs)

These act by inhibiting the synthesis of prostaglandins by inactivation of the enzyme cyclo-oxygenase which catalyses the formation of cyclic endoperoxides from arachidonic acid. Prostaglandins are formed in damaged tissue and appear to be involved in sensitizing the peripheral nociceptors to painful stimuli.

The indications for NSAIDs range from the treatment of aches and pains, and dysmenorrhoea to long-term therapy for arthritis and degenerative joint diseases. Indeed they may be more effective than opioids in bone pain and are valuable in cancer patients with bone metastases. In contrast to the opioid drugs there has not been a clear demonstration of a relationship between blood levels of NSAIDs and pain relief.

Most may be classified into one of two groups based on their elimination half-lives (Table 58.5). The drugs in group 2 have longer half-lives ranging from 6 to 60 h. Although these agents are excreted by the kidneys, dose adjustment is not necessary for patients with renal failure.

Side-effects of NSAIDs include gastric irritation, salt and fluid retention, platelet inhibition and tinnitus. Paracetamol does not cause gastric side-effects but has potential for liver damage with excessive doses.

Antidepressants

Many of the antidepressant drugs block the uptake of noradrenaline and scrotonin in the central nervous system (Table 58.6). Pain relief usually occurs in 2–7 days, as compared with the accepted time for antidepressant effect of 3–4 weeks. Side-effects from tricyclic antidepressants include anticholinergic and adrenergic effects. Dry mouth is the most common, and can be relieved by increased fluid intake and salivary stimulants such as sugarless candy. Blurring of vision is also common and usually interferes with reading. Constipation has also been described.

Opioids

Opioids are extremely effective agents in treating acute pain. Many misconceptions surround the use of opioid drugs. In particular, the risk of addiction is greatly overstated. It is important to realize that there may be as much as a fourfold variability between patients in the minimum effective dose of opioids needed to relieve pain. It is

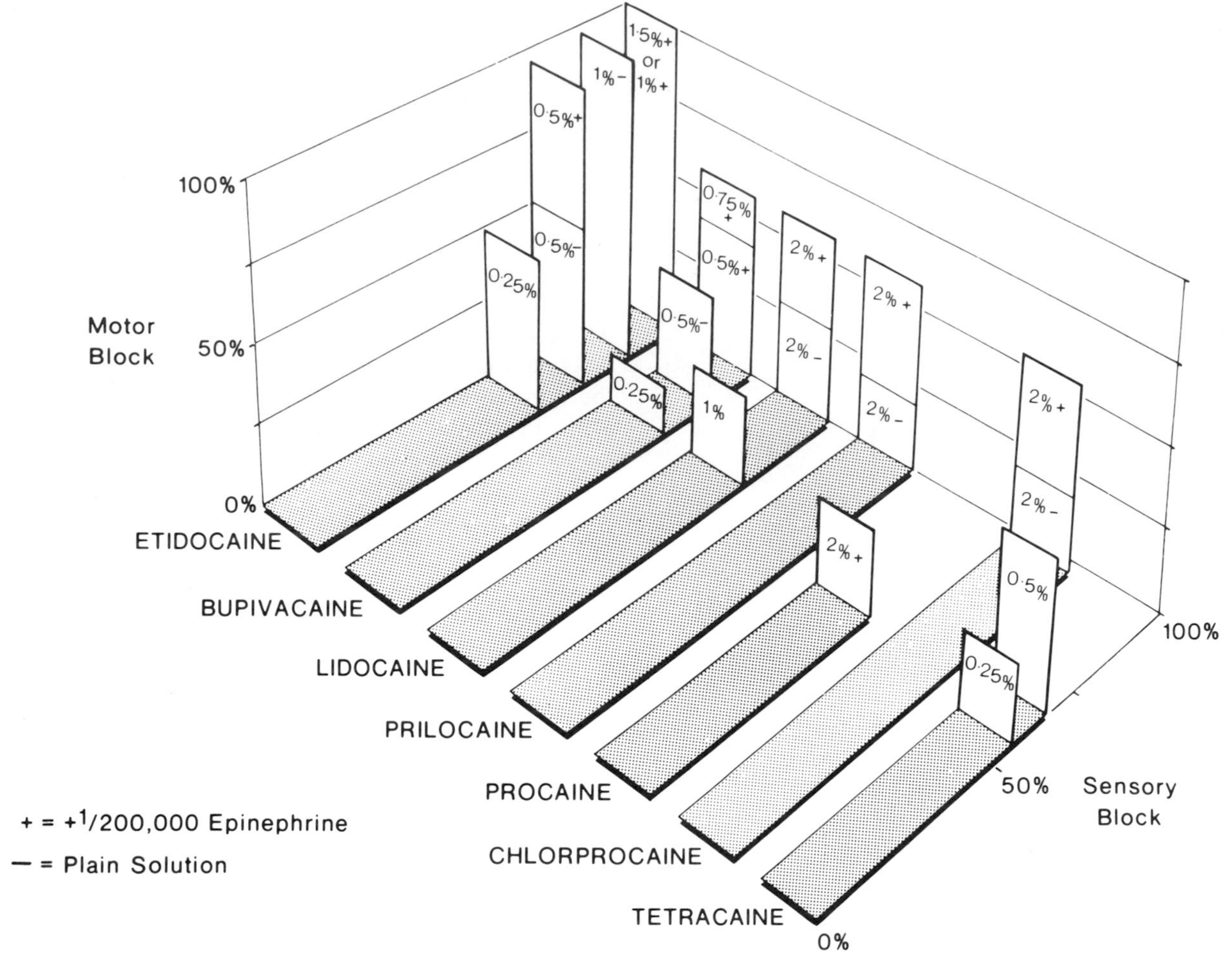

Fig. 58.10 Comparison of relative motor blockade and sensory blockade induced by different agents in epidural block. This illustration is based on subjective clinical data and only approximate comparisons can be drawn. From Covino (1988) with permission.

Table 58.5 Terminal half-life, recommended dose, influence of food on absorption and incidence of gastric erosion from NSAIDs

Drug	Terminal half-life (h)	Oral dose and frequency (mg/h)	Effect of food on absorption	Incidence of gastric erosion
Aspirin	0.2–0.3	600–900/4	a	+++
Salicylate	2–3	600/4	a	++
Difusinal	8–12	500/12	a	+
Diclofenac	1.5–2	25–50/8	a	+
Ibuprofen	2–3	200–400/8	a	+
Naproxen	12–15	250–375/12	c	+
Fenoprofen	2–3	400–600/6	b	+
Indomethacin	6–8	50–75/8	a	++
Sulindac	6–8	100–200/12	b	+
Piroxicam	30–60	20–30/24	a	+
Flufenamic acid	8–10	500/6	a	–

a = Decrease in rate of absorption, no change in oral bioavailability; b = decrease in rate of absorption and oral bioavailability; c = no change in rate of absorption and oral bioavailability.
+ = Low incidence of gastritis; ++ = intermediate gastritis; +++ = high incidence of gastritis.
Adapted from Burrows et al (1987), with permission.

Table 58.6 Terminal half-life, recommended daily doses and other properties of antidepressant drugs

Drug	Amine group	Terminal half-life (h)	Inhibitor concentration* NA	Inhibitor concentration* 5-HT	Recommended daily dose (mg)
Amitriptyline	3	20–30	4.6	4.4	50–150
Nortriptyline	2	18–36	0.9	17	50–150
Protriptyline	2	50–90	—	—	10–50
Clomipramine	3	20–30	4.6	0.5	50–75
Imipramine	3	20–30	4.6	0.5	50–75
Desipramine	2	12–24	0.2	35	75–150
Doxepin	3	10–25	6.5	20	75–150
Dothiapen	3	20–30	—	—	50–100
Mianserin	3	10–20	20	130	20–50
Nomifensine	1.3	2–4	2	120	75–150
Zimelidine	3	5–10	630	14	200–300

* Inhibitor concentration (IC_{50}) represents the antidepressant concentration ($\times 10^{-8}$ M) required to inhibit the uptake of either noradrenaline (NA) or serotonin (5-HT) by 50% using rat midbrain synaptosomes.
1 = Primary amine group; 2 = secondary amine group; 3 = tertiary amine group.
Adapted from Burrows et al (1987) with permission.

impossible to predict how much will be required for any patient. Therefore, the dose for each individual must be titrated to the desired effect.

The pure opioid agonists all give pain relief, sedation, euphoria and respiratory depression (Table 58.7). The partial agonists were developed to provide pain relief without significant respiratory depression and with less tendency towards physical dependence. However, the clinical results with partial agonists have been unimpressive in terms of analgesia or sparing of respiratory effects. The correlation between analgesia and blood concentration of opioids is an essential key to the planning of opioid dosing.

In addition to an individualized plan of effective analgesic therapy, the use of opioids involves the management of side-effects. The major side-effects which limit the effectiveness of opioid therapy are nausea, vomiting, sedation, respiratory depression and constipation. Rather than restrict the dose of opioids, other medications should be given to treat these side-effects. Nausea and vomiting are frequently responsive to drugs such as metoclopramide, phenothiazines or buterophenones. Respiratory depression is immediately reversible with naloxone but the action of naloxone is short-lived and repeated doses may be required.

Delivery systems

The association between stable blood levels of opioids and continuous analgesia must be remembered when planning systemic opioid therapy. The effective dose of opioid medication is the minimum dose which provides acceptable pain relief with a low incidence of side-effects.

Oral. Following oral administration, a significant percentage of the dose is metabolized in the liver to inactive products before the opioids reach the systemic circulation (Mather & Gourlay 1984). This is referred to as the hepatic first-pass effect. This, and poor oral bioavailability seen with certain opioids, leads to the incorrect perception that oral administration of opioids is ineffective.

Oral bioavailability ranges from zero for heroin to 80% for methadone. Morphine oral bioavailability ranges from 10 to 40%, leading to very wide fluctuations in oral dosing requirements between different patients. Satisfactory analgesia can be obtained by oral administration of opioids if the dose is titrated to the needs of the individual patient.

Rectal. This route has been advocated for patients who cannot swallow, or who have a high incidence of nausea or vomiting following oral administration. Pain relief for 6–8 h follows 40 g rectal meperidine, but there is a significant latency of 2–3 h following administration.

Intramuscular. This is the most commonly used route for managing postoperative pain with morphine or meperidine. The typical prescription would read: 'Morphine 10 mg intramuscularly every 3–4 h as needed for pain'. This approach provides inadequate analgesia. The patient may not request medication despite experiencing severe pain. The nurse may not administer the medication. The dose may not be adequate for the patient's needs. Even withstanding all of these potential problems, the variable blood levels seen following intramuscular injection usually result in periods of pain alternating with periods of

Table 58.7 Dose, pharmacokinetic parameters, minimum effective concentration (MEC) and duration of pain relief for various opioid drugs

Opioid	Dose (mg)		Pharmacokinetic parameters					
	i.m./i.v.	Oral	Terminal half-life (h)	Clearance (l/min)	Bioavailability (%)	MEC ng/ml)	Duration of pain relief (h)	Comments
Heroin	5	15	0.05	2–22	0		2–3	Very soluble, rapidly converted to 6-monoacetyl morphine and morphine in vivo. Zero oral bioavailability
Morphine	10	40	2–4	0.85–1.1	10–40	10–40	3–4	Standard opiate to which new opioids are compared. New sustained-release formulation available in some countries — of considerable benefit in chronic cancer pain
Codeine	30	60	2–3	0.6–0.8	50		3–4	Weak opiate, frequently combined with aspirin. Useful for pain with visceral and integumental components
Meperidine	100	300	3–5	0.6–0.8	30–60	200–800	2–4	Not as effective in relieving anxiety as morphine. Suppositories (200–400 mg) have slow onset (2–3 h) but can last for 6–8 h
Methadone	10	10–15	10–80	0.1–0.3	70–95	20–80	10–60	Duration of pain relief ranges from 10 to 60 h both postoperatively and for cancer pain. Variable half-life. Requires initial care to establish dose for each patient to avoid accumulation. Otherwise of great value
Dextromoramide	7.5	10					2	Methadone-like chemical structure. Short-acting. Useful in covering exacerbation pain. Supposed good oral bioavailability (oral compared to parenteral doses)
Oxycodone	10	30					4–6	Suppository (30 mg) can provide pain relief for 8–10 h.
Hydromorphone	2	4–6	2–3	0.4	50–60	4	4–5	More potent but shorter-acting than morphine
Fentanyl	0.1	NA	3–6	0.7–0.9	NA	0.6–2	0.5–1	Potent opioid. Usually administered by i.v. injection. Short duration of pain relief. Therefore repeated doses on the basis of pain-relieving effects may cause accumulation and respiratory depression. Transdermal patch under evaluation
Alfentanil	0.5	NA	1–3	0.2–0.6	NA	250	0.1–0.3	Rapid and short-acting opioid with small initial volume of distribution. Pharmacokinetic characteristics make this drug suitable primarily for continuous i.v. infusion
Sufentanil	0.02	NA	2–5	0.5–1	NA	?	0.5–1	More potent drug, similar to fentanyl. Small doses utilized make the determination of MEC from blood extremely difficult. Only available as i.v. form
Propoxyphene	65	130	8–24	0.9–1.2	40		4–6	Weak opioid. Unacceptable incidence of side-effects
Buprenorphine	0.3	0.8	2–3	0.9–1.3	30		6–8	Available as a sublingual tablet in many countries — appears useful in treatment of cancer pain
Nalbuphine	10	40	4–6	0.9–1.5	20		3–6	Oral form unavailable in many countries. Value in treatment of chronic pain not established

NA = Data not available
Adapted from Burrows et al (1987) with permission.

toxicity (Austin et al 1980). Intramuscular infusion and intramuscular patient-controlled analgesia (PCA) produce analgesia similar to intravenous administration, but with higher doses.

Subcutaneous. Subcutaneous administration of opioids has been used for decades to provide analgesia. More recently, continuous infusion of subcutaneous morphine has been demonstrated to provide equivalent analgesia and blood levels to intravenous infusion.

Intravenous. Intermittent intravenous injection and continuous infusion provide rapid and effective analgesia. A loading dose followed by a continuous infusion is the simplest method. Providing the loading dose as an infusion over 10–15 min followed by the maintenance rate allows good analgesia to be established rapidly with minimum toxicity. Subsequently, the maintenance rate should be titrated to patient comfort.

Patient-controlled analgesia. The wide interpatient variability in analgesic requirements necessitates individual titration of opioid dose to achieve adequate analgesia. While the physician can do this by careful evaluation of the patient, PCA allows the patient to decide when a dose should be administered and how often. The most commonly used method of PCA is a bolus demand form in which the physician prescribes a bolus dose range that can be adjusted if inadequate analgesia or toxicity develops from a single demand. In addition, the minimum time between doses is determined by the physician, to avoid potential toxicity from repeated demands before the peak effect of each bolus has been experienced. Higher patient satisfaction and lower pain scores are reported when this therapy is compared with other forms of parenteral opioid analgesia.

Spinal. The term 'spinal opioids' is used to describe intrathecal, epidural and intracerebroventricular administration of opioids. The remainder of this section will relate to epidural opioids except where specifically stated.

Movement of the drug into the cerebrospinal fluid by diffusion across the dura mater, transfer across the arachnoid granulations and vascular uptake all regulate the

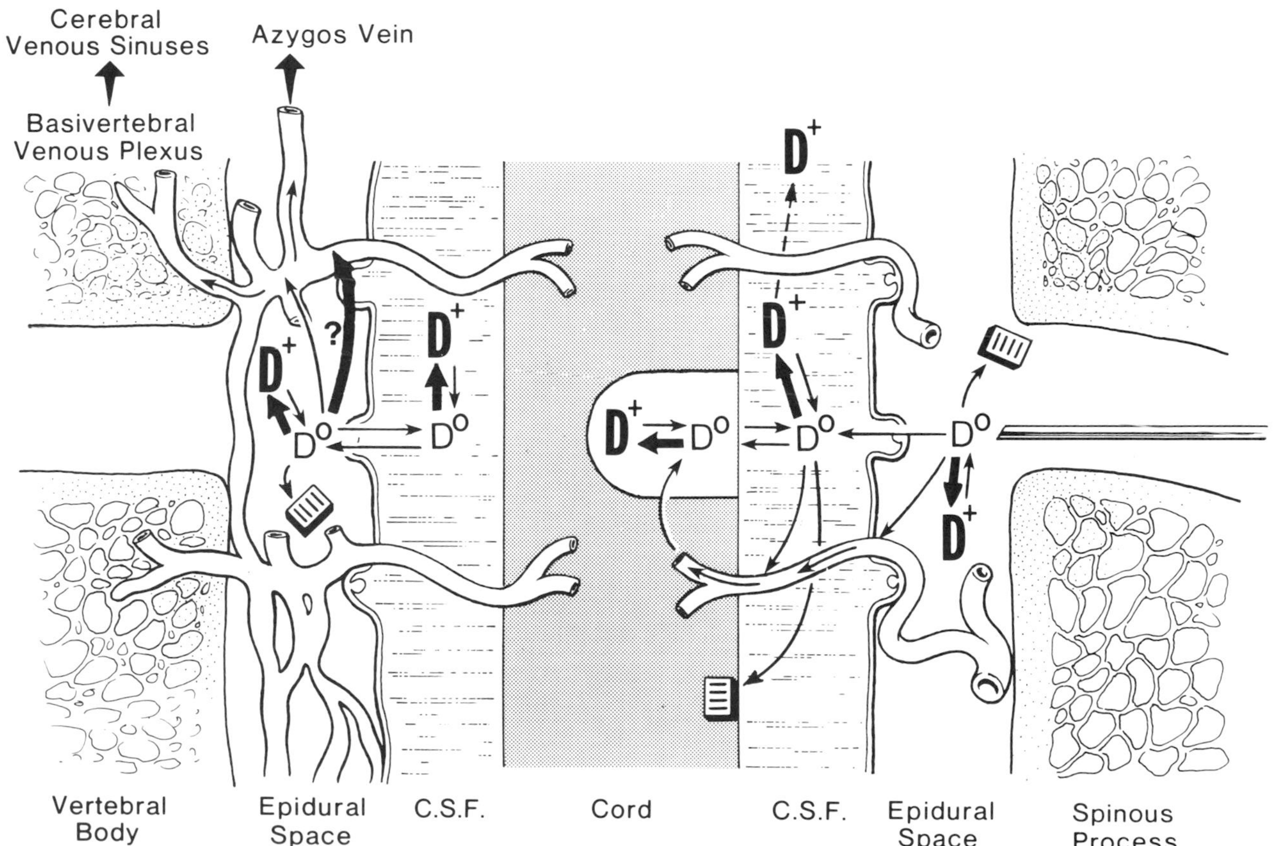

Fig. 58.11 Pharmacokinetic model of epidural injection of a hydrophilic opioid such as morphine. D^0 = Unionized, lipophilic drug; D^+ = ionized, hydrophilic drug. An epidural needle is shown delivering drug to the epidural space. The role of absorption by way of the radicular arteries remains speculative. The shaded area represents non-specific binding sites. CSF = Cerebrospinal fluid. From Cousins (1988) with permission.

Table 58.8 Comparison of actions and efficacy of spinally administered opioids and local anaesthetics

	Opioids	Local anaesthetics
Actions		
Site of action	Substantia gelatinosa of dorsal horn of spinal cord*	Nerve roots (long tracts in spinal cord)
Types of blockade	Presynaptic and postsynaptic inhibition of neuron cell excitation	Blockade of nerve impulse conduction in axonal membrane
Modalities blocked	Selective block of pain conduction	Blockade of sympathetic and pain fibres, often also loss of sensation and motor function
Type of pain/efficacy		
Surgical pain	Partial relief	Complete relief possible
Labour pain	Partial relief	Complete relief
Postoperative pain† Early first 24 h	Partial to complete relief (high dose)	Complete relief
After first 24 h	Complete relief (low dose)	Complete relief
Chronic pain	Complete relief	Impractical (usually)

* And/or other sites where opioid receptors are present.
† Pain after major surgery requires higher doses than after minor surgery.
Adapted from Cousin & Bridenbaugh (1988) with permission.

distribution of epidural morphine (Fig. 58.11). Because diffusion takes place slowly the onset of analgesia is delayed and respiratory depression occurs late.

While some of the physical principles governing the interaction of opioids at the spinal level with their receptors are similar to those seen with spinal local anaesthetics, the drug effects obtained are quite different (Table 58.8). The analgesia obtained from spinal administration of opioids without motor weakness is a major advantage.

The long duration of action seen following the administration of morphine epidurally has led to the increased use of this drug (Table 58.9). The sedation that was seen early in the use of spinal morphine appears to be a dose-related phenomenon. In fact most clinical observations suggest that appropriate doses of spinal morphine result in less sedation than parenteral opioids. Nausea, vomiting, pruritus and urinary retention may also occur. The incidence of severe delayed respiratory depression following epidural morphine is approximately 1/1000 patients. This cannot be predicted reliably.

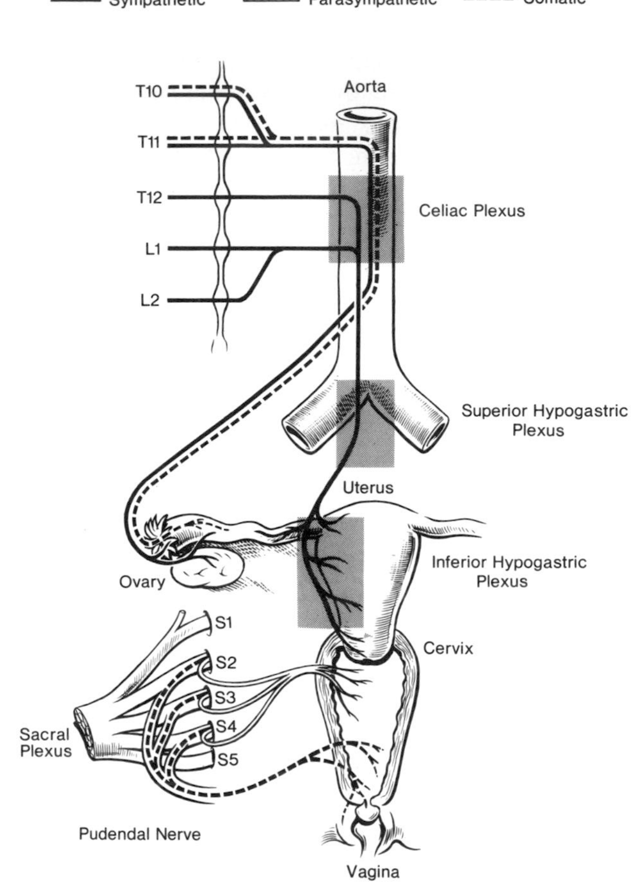

Fig. 58.12 Pain pathways in gynaecological pain. Somatic afferents from the lower vagina are also shown. From Wilson & Cousins (1981) with permission.

Table 58.9 Epidural opioids: latency and duration of postoperative analgesia

Drug	Dose (mg)	Detectable onset (min)	Complete pain relief (min)	Duration (h)
Meperidine	30–100	5–10	12–30	6
Morphine	5–10	23	60	20
Methadone	5	13	17	7
Hydromorphone	1	13	23	11
Fentanyl	0.1	5	20	3
Diamorphine	5	15	30	8

Adapted from Cousins & Bridenbaugh (1988) with permission.

Neural blockade

This section will focus on techniques of neural blockade that can be employed for gynaecological pain.

Choice of local anaesthetic

The differential somatic blockade and the prolonged effect of low concentrations of bupivacaine make it the most logical choice of agent for acute and chronic pain.

Anatomy of neural blockade

Knowledge of the neuroanatomy of the pelvic organs is essential to employ local anaesthetic or permanent neural blockade appropriately (Figs 58.12 and 58.13). The most common error made in many texts is the innervation of the cervix. There is no doubt that pain relief is obtained by blockade of the sympathetic fibres travelling via lumbar ganglia to spinal cord segments T10–L2 rather than somatic nerves S2–4. Successful peripheral blockade of these areas requires precise placement of the local anaesthetic.

Somatic blockade. The lower abdominal wall is innervated by somatic nerve fibres in 10th to 12th thoracic nerves and the ilioinguinal, iliohypogastric and genitofemoral nerves (Fig. 58.14). Pain from this region can be diagnosed and possibly treated by local anaesthetic blockade of the thoracic nerves just below the border of the costal margin, or the ilioinguinal, genitofemoral and iliohypogastric nerves around the anterior superior iliac spine (Fig. 58.14).

Sympathetic blockade. The innervation of the major intra-abdominal organs, including the gonads, is via the

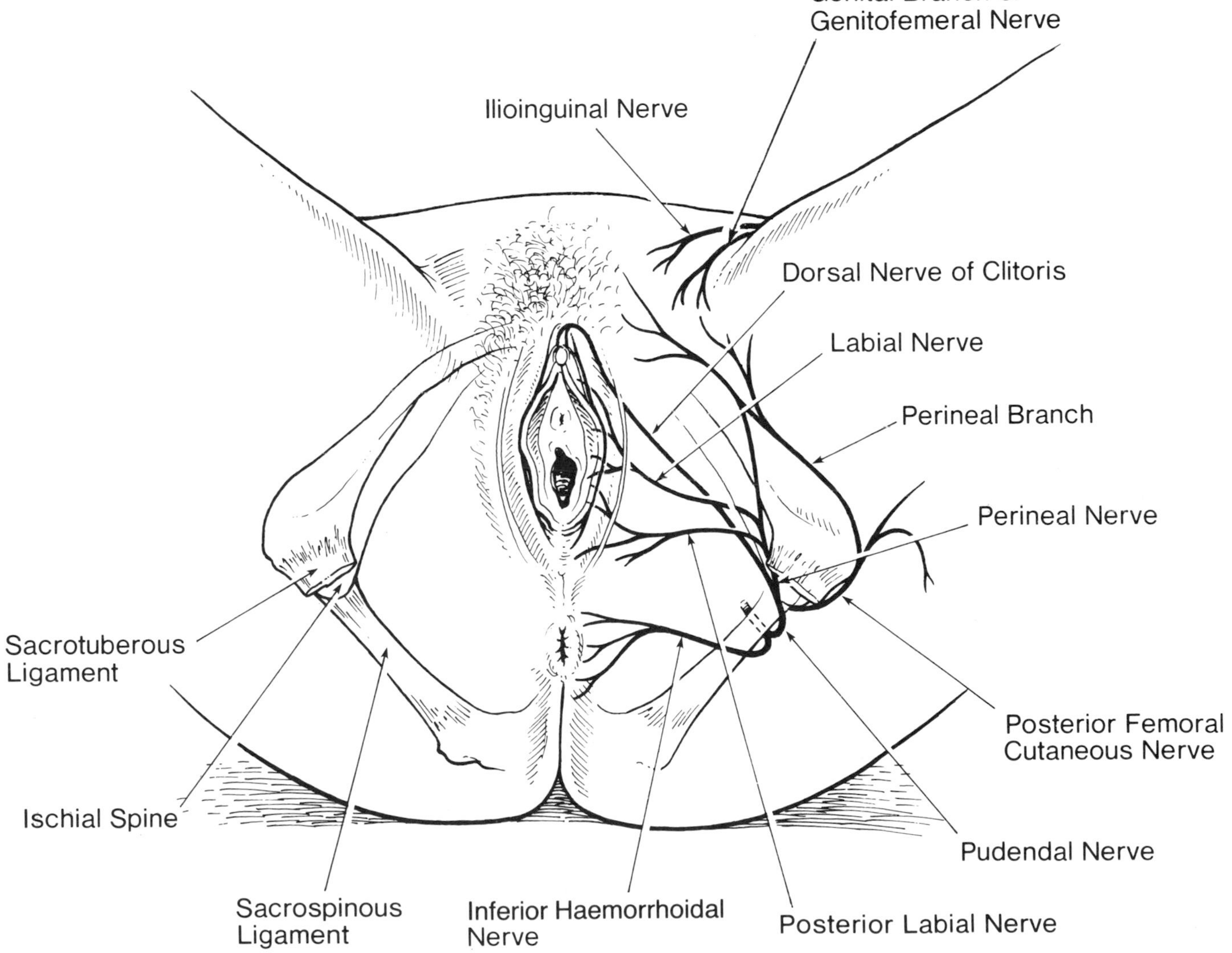

Fig. 58.13 Cutaneous innervation of the perineal region. Modified from Brownbridge & Cohen (1988) with permission.

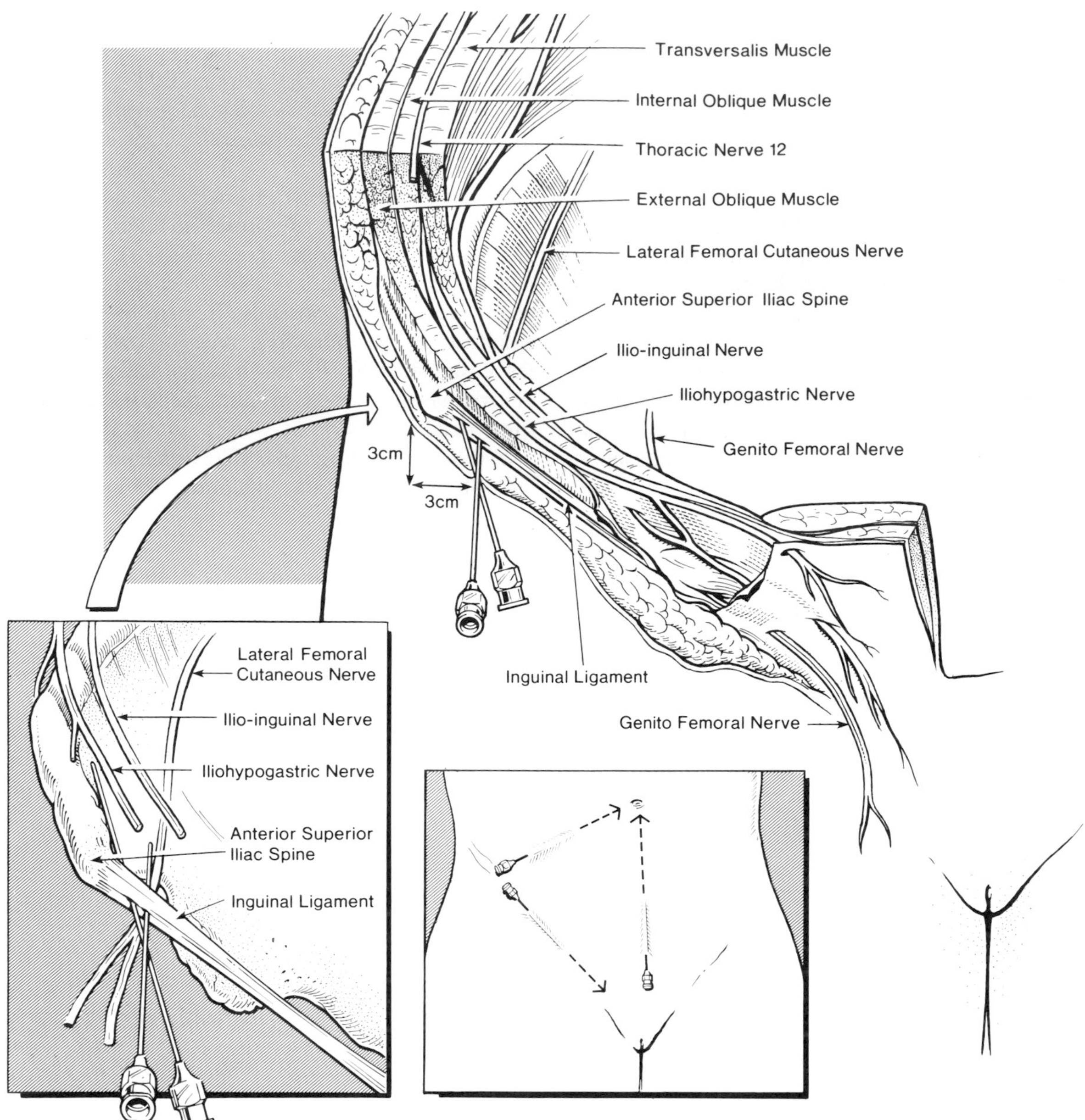

Fig. 58.14 Cutaneous innervation of the lower abdomen. The iliac crest block shown allows the simultaneous blockade of the ilioinguinal, iliohypogastric and lateral femoral cutaneous nerves. **Main picture**: the point of needle is inserted 3 cm caudad and 3 cm medial to the anterior superior iliac spine. The initial direction of the needle is superolateral to reach the inner aspect of the iliac bone. Then it is redirected approximately perpendicular to the long axis of the body. Note the relation of the nerves to the muscles of the anterior abdominal wall. An alternative approach is to insert the needle along a line from the anterior superior iliac spine to the umbilicus. **Inset left**: Bone and ligamentous landmarks in relation to the nerves. **Inset right**: Superficial infiltration for right lower quadrant anaesthesia. Modified from Thompson & Moore (1988) with permission.

sympathetic postganglionic fibres from the coeliac plexus and the inferior hypogastric plexus. Effective blockade of the coeliac fibres can be obtained by administration of local anaesthetic directly adjacent to the plexus in the upper abdomen. This will be followed by many hours of analgesia to the abdominal viscera.

Central neural blockade. Epidural, caudal and spinal administration of local anaesthetic can provide central blockade of the nociceptive fibres of both the body wall and the viscera if the level of blockade includes lower thoracic, lumbar and sacral dermatomes. Continuous techniques with indwelling catheters either in the caudal or lumbar epidural space are widely used in the treatment of postoperative pain.

Transcutaneous nerve stimulation. TENS is a low-intensity stimulation of skin and muscle afferents in a specific segmental distribution. It has value in certain painful conditions and can decrease opioid requirements following surgery.

Acupuncture. Acupuncture analgesia uses stimulation of designated body sites originally by manual rotation of needles to produce a sensation known as *teh chi*. Now low-frequency current (less than 5 Hz) is used to stimulate the needles. This also produces powerful muscle contractions. Acupuncture produces a high-intensity stimulation which is believed to induce a chemical modulation of pain, explaining why the relief is not confined to a local segmental distribution.

Cryoanalgesia. This term refers to the destruction of peripheral nerves by extreme cold to achieve analgesia. This technique was developed to provide destructive blockade of peripheral nerves that had responded favourably to somatic blockade. The alternative destructive techniques, including cutting, crushing and burning, are all associated with development of neuralgia. There is complete functional loss after a cryolesion, but recovery usually occurs in a period of weeks. The clinical limitation of cryoanalgesia is the short duration of analgesia.

Psychotherapy. The effects of anxiety and lack of sleep on pain control are well documented. Open communication between physician and patient will help to dispel any misconceptions about pain and its effective treatment. Methods of self-control using relaxation training (with or without biofeedback) are very helpful for many patients. Learned coping skills can reduce the need for potent analgesic drugs.

CHRONIC NON-CANCER PAIN MANAGEMENT

Classification of chronic pain syndromes

There are many chronic pain syndromes (International Association for the Study of Pain 1986). All pain has both physical and psychological components. As pain becomes more long-standing, psychological sequelae become even more pronounced. A vicious cycle develops of anxiety, sleep disturbance and irritability or anger. In order to treat chronic pain, all aspects of this vicious cycle need to be assessed. To do this more effectively, multidisciplinary pain management units have been developed.

Categories of pain

There are at least three broad categories of chronic pain: nociceptive, neuropathic and psychogenic.

Nociceptive pain results from the stimulation of a nociceptor by a noxious stimulus. This is the type of pain that follow acute injury. Nociceptive pain is often responsive to NSAIDs or opioids.

Neuropathic pain results from a lesion anywhere along the afferent pathway for pain transmission. This could be in the primary afferent neuron, the spinal cord or a higher brain centre. Spinal cord damage or a brachial plexus avulsion are classical examples of this type of pain. The deafferentation syndrome that may develop after this type of neurological lesion usually involves an element of neuropathic pain. This rarely responds to opioid medications and only responds partially to a combination of tricyclic antidepressants and a phenothiazine such as fluphenazine. It may respond to electrical stimulation provided by a dorsal column stimulator.

Psychogenic pain is said to be present when there is clear evidence for a major role of psychological or psychiatric factors in the pain. This diagnosis cannot be made by exclusion of detectable physical damage but requires complete medical and psychiatric evaluation. Contributions from physical factors to the patient's pain problem do not preclude the diagnosis of psychogenic pain.

Multidisciplinary pain treatment

The first goal of a multidisciplinary pain centre is to determine the nature of a patient's pain complaints along the lines described above. An accurate diagnosis permits the selection of appropriate therapy. Cross-specialty collaboration and communication are essential for dealing with these complex problems. Such units form a focus for continued education, training and research.

CANCER PAIN MANAGEMENT

Scope of cancer pain

Cancer pain is a major world health problem (World Health Organization 1986). Severe cancer pain is unrelieved in 30–50% of patients in the developed world and in up to 90% of patients in the developing world. The World Health Organization is collaborating with the International Association for the Study of Pain to establish educational and treatment programmes throughout the world by the year 2000.

Aetiology

Effective treatment of cancer pain depends to a great degree upon good management of the cancer itself. A short course of radiotherapy to localized bone metastases can completely relieve pain. Even when treatment of the cancer is no longer possible it is important to define all of the pain sites and to determine the aetiology of pain at each site. Over 30% of patients with cancer have pain in more than one site.

In considering cancer pain it is useful to recognize some of the common pain syndromes related to cancer (Table 58.10). They may be due to the tumour or to the therapy

Table 58.10 Pain syndromes in patients with cancer: pain directly caused by cancer (primary or metastatic)

Mechanism	Common sites and characteristics of pain
Infiltration of bone by tumour	Dull, constant aching ± muscle spasm
Base of skull (jugular foramen, clivus, sphenoid sinus)	Early-onset pain in occiput, vertex, frontal areas respectively
Vertebral body (subluxation atlas, metastases C7–T1, L1, sacral)	Early-onset pain in neck and skull, neck and shoulders, mid-back, lower back and coccyx, respectively ± neurological deficit
Metastatic fracture close to nerves	Acute-onset pain + muscle spasm
Infiltration or compression of nerve tissue by tumour	
Peripheral nerve (± peripheral and perivascular lymphangitis)	Burning constant pain in area of peripheral sensory loss ± dysaesthesia and hyperalgesia ± signs of sympathetic overactivity
Plexus Lumbar	Radicular pain to anterior thigh and groin (L1–L3) or to leg and foot (L4–S2)
Sacral	Dull aching midline perianal pain + sacral sensory loss and faecal and urinary incontinence
Brachial	Radicular pain in shoulder and arm ± Horner's syndrome (superior pulmonary sulcus or Pancoast syndrome)
Meningeal carcinomatosis	Constant headache ± neck stiffness or low back and buttock pain
Epidural spinal cord compression (± vertebral body infiltration)	Severe neck and back pain locally over involved vertebra, or radicular pain
Obstruction of hollow viscus	Poorly localized, dull, sickening pain, typical visceral pain
Occlusion of arteries and veins by tumour	Ischaemic pain like rest pain (skin) or claudication (muscle) or pain ± venous engorgement
Stretching of periosteum or fascia, in tissues with tight investment by tumefaction	Severe localized pain (e.g. periosteum) or typical visceral pain (e.g. ovary)
Inflammation owing to necrosis and infection of tumour (± superficial ulceration)	Severe localized pain (e.g. perineum), visceral pain (e.g. cervix)
Soft-tissue infiltration	Localized pain; unsightly and foul-smelling if ulcerated
Raised intracranial pressure	Severe constant headache, behavioural changes, confusion, etc.

From Cousins & Bridenbaugh (1988) with permission.

Table 58.11 Pain syndromes in patients with cancer: pain associated with cancer therapy

Mechanism	Common sites and characteristics of pain
Following surgery	
Acute postoperative pain	Wound or referred pain; back or other sites (owing to posture during surgery)
Nerve trauma	Neuralgic pain in area of peripheral nerve or spinal nerve
Entrapment of nerves in scar tissue	Superficial wound scar; hypersensitivity of area supplied by scarred nerves (e.g. perineum)
Amputation of limb or other area (breast)	Localized stump pain (neuroma) or phantom pain referred to absent region
Following radiotherapy	
Acute lesions or inflammation of nerves or plexuses	Pain associated with motor and sensory loss
Radiation fibrosis of nerves or plexuses	E.g. brachial plexus, lumbar plexus; diffuse limb pain, 6 months to many years after radiation ± lymphoedema and local skin changes ± sensory loss ± motor loss (difficult to distinguish from tumour recurrence)
Myelopathy of spinal cord	Brown-Séquard syndrome (ipsilateral sensory and contralateral motor loss) with pain at level of spinal cord damage or referred pain
Peripheral nerve tumours owing to radiation	Painful enlarging mass in area of radiation along line of peripheral nerve or plexus
Following chemotherapy	
Vinca alkaloids (vincristine/vinblastine)-induced peripheral neuropathy	Burning pain in hands and feet associated with symmetrical polyneuropathy
Steroid pseudorheumatism owing to slow as well as rapid withdrawal of steroid treatment	Diffuse joint and muscle pain with associated tenderness to palpation but no inflammatory signs. Pain resolves when steroid reinstituted
Aseptic necrosis of bone (femoral or humoral head) with chronic steroid therapy	Pain in knee, leg, shoulder with limitation of movement; bone scan changes delayed after pain onset
Postherpetic neuralgia, following herpes zoster infection in area of tumour or area of radiotherapy with onset during chemotherapy	Continuous burning pain in area of sensory loss, painful dysaesthesia, intermittent shock-line pain

From Cousins & Bridenbaugh (1988) with permission.

(Table 58.11). In many cases the pain is unrelated to the malignancy (Table 58.12).

Analgesic ladder

The World Health Organization guidelines for treatment of cancer pain are formulated around the concept of an analgesic ladder (Table 58.13). Opioids are just as effective given orally as parenterally if proper dosing regimens are used. Because almost all patients receiving morphine become constipated, a laxative such as docusate with casanthranol should be prescribed when the morphine is started. The analgesic ladder was successful in treating over 80% of patients, without the need for other measures. In developed countries, the challenge lies in education and the implementation of the simple principles behind this technique.

Table 58.12 Pain syndromes in patients with cancer: pain unrelated to cancer or cancer therapy

Mechanism	Common sites and characteristics of pain
Neuropathy (e.g. diabetic)	Burning pain in hands, feet
Degenerative disc	Back pain ± radicular pain
Rheumatoid arthritis	Joint pain on movement
Diffuse osteoporosis	Back pain, limb pain (may be like causalgia)
Posture abnormalities after surgery	Back pain and muscle spasm ± radicular pain
Myofascial syndromes owing to anxiety	Local pain in muscle with muscle spasm ± referred pain; trigger areas in muscle
Headache	Typical migraine or tension type

From Cousins & Bridenbaugh (1988) with permission.

Table 58.13 Analgesic ladder in cancer pain

Step	Medication
Step 1	Paracetemol, aspirin or other NSAIDs ± adjuvants* (coanalgesics)
Step 2	Codeine, dextropropoxyphene (or ? oxycodone) ± NSAID ± adjuvants*
Step 3	Morphine, methadone ± NSAIDs ± adjuvants*

NSAIDs = non-steroidal anti-inflammatory drugs.
* Psychotropics (anxiolytics, antidepressants), anticonvulsants, steroids, etc.

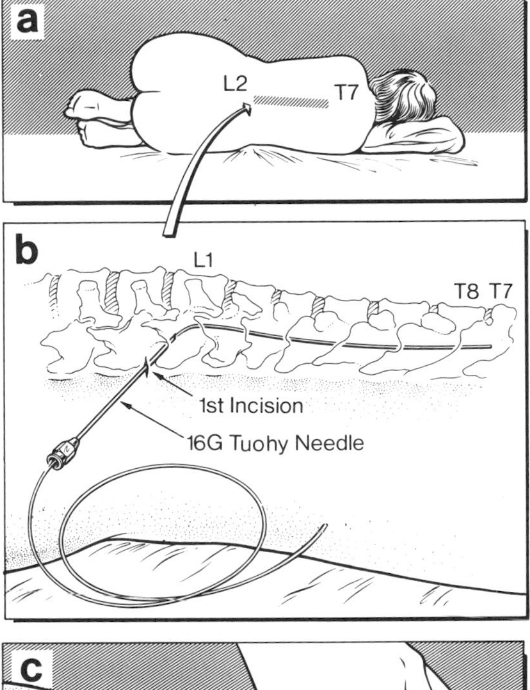

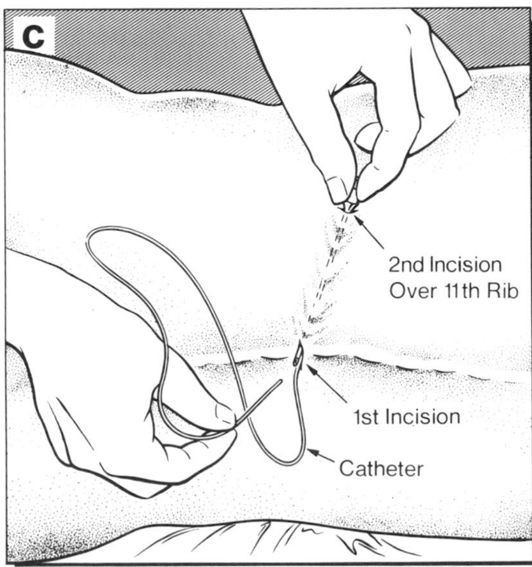

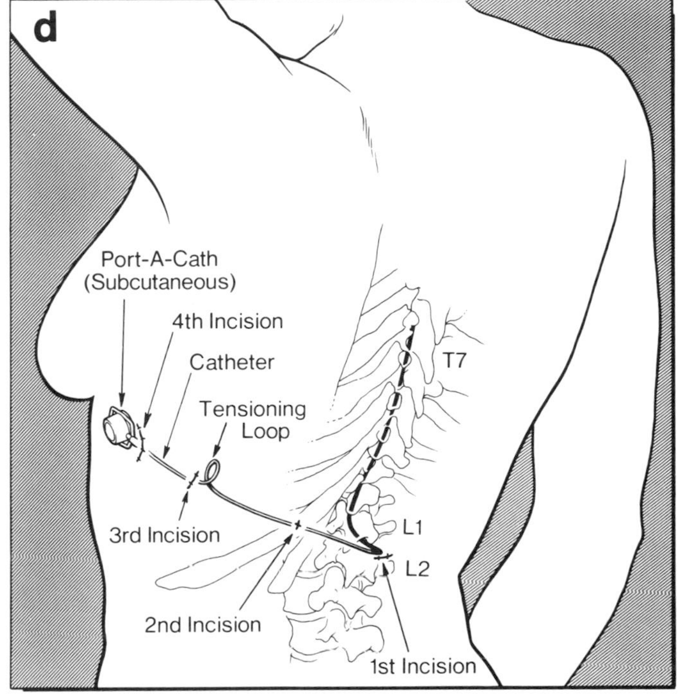

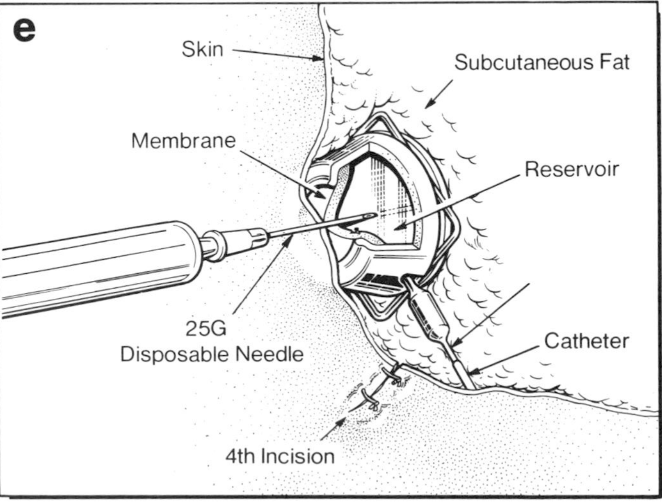

Fig. 58.15 Implantation of epidural portal system. (**a**) Position patient before implantation. (**b**) Insertion of 16-gauge epidural catheter through a Tuohy needle. (**c**) Tunnelling technique used to relocate the end of the epidural catheter on the anterior chest wall. (**d**) Portal attached to the inserted epidural catheter. (**e**) Injection technique and exposed view of the epidural portal. From Cousins et al (1988) with permission.

Neural blockade in cancer pain

Patients who exhaust the analgesic ladder or who develop toxicity may benefit from neurolytic blockade. The usual approach is to begin with the least invasive techniques. The use of spinal opioids or of continuous subcutaneous opioid infusions continues to decrease the need for neurodestructive techniques.

The spinal administration of opioids is appropriate for pain in virtually any region of the body. Epidural cannulae implanted with skin-tunnelling techniques may be left in place for long periods of time (Fig. 58.15). The shortcomings of this therapy include formation of a fibrous sheath around the catheter, development of hyperaesthesiae in a minority of patients who receive high doses of spinal morphine, eventual loss of efficacy due to opioid tolerance, and resistance of certain neuropathic pains.

Neurolytic blocks are most appropriate for pain which is unilateral and relatively localized. They are most successful for pain in a localized region of the thorax (subarachnoid alcohol block), and for pain in the upper abdominal region (splanchnic and coeliac plexus block). Pain in the sacral dermatomes in patients who have reached the stage of requiring permanent bladder catheterization can be successfully treated with subarachnoid and sacral root blocks. More diffuse pain states have also been treated with chemical hypophysectomy (alcohol pituitary ablation).

KEY POINTS

1. Local release of substances such as serotonin and bradykinin, efferent sympathetic activity and microcirculatory changes may all modify peripheral pain receptor activity.
2. Nerve fibres from the dorsal root ganglion ascend and descend one to two segments and some cross to the opposite side, explaining the incomplete pain relief that is seen following ablation of a unilateral dorsal root entry zone.
3. Response to pain can be modulated at many different levels.
4. Visceral and somatic afferents converge in the dorsal horn with the result that pain from an organ is referred to the area of skin innervated by fibres going to the same dorsal horn. Reflex sympathetic activity may cause smooth muscle spasm over a wide area, causing pain remote from the original site. Visceral afferents go to the dorsal horn in several segments, so visceral pain is poorly localized.
5. Systemic absorption accounts for most of the toxicity observed with local anaesthetics: central nervous system toxicity is manifest by dizziness, lightheadedness, and finally coma; cardiovascular toxicity caused by a direct effect on cardiac muscle and vascular smooth muscle results in reduced cardiac output and vasodilation. Bupivacaine may cause ventricular fibrillation which is refractory to resuscitation.
6. Non-steroidal anti-inflammatory drugs are more effective than opioids in bone pain.
7. The risk of addiction to opioids when used for pain is very low.
8. Satisfactory analgesia can be obtained by oral administration of opioids if the dose is titrated to the needs of the individual patient.
9. Patient-controlled analgesia gives higher patient satisfaction and lower pain scores than other form of parenteral opioid analgesia.
10. Because diffusion of epidural opiates takes place slowly, the onset of analgesia is delayed and respiratory depression occurs late.
11. Naloxone may need to be given in repeated doses when the systemic levels of opiates are high after oral or parenteral administration, or when respiratory depression follows epidural administration, because the plasma concentration of opioids may remain dangerously elevated long after the effect of a single dose of naloxone has worn off.
12. Cancer patients taking morphine for pain will almost always require a laxative. This should be prescribed when the morphine is started.

REFERENCES

Austin K L, Stapleton J V, Mather L E 1980 Multiple intramuscular injections: a major source of variability in analgesic response to pethidine. Pain 8: 47–62

Berkley K J, Palmer R 1974 Somatosensory cortical involvement in response to noxious stimulation in the cat. Experimental Brain Research 20: 363–374

Brownbridge P, Cohen S E 1988 Neural blockade for obstetrics and gynaecological surgery. In: Cousins M J, Bridenbaugh P O (eds) Neural blockade in clinical anesthesia and management of pain, 2nd edn. J B Lippincott, Philadelphia

Burrows G D, Elton D, Stanley G V (eds) 1987 Handbook of Chronic pain management. Elsevier Science, Amsterdam

Calahan M D, Almers W 1979 Interactions between quaternary lidocaine, the sodium channel gates and tetrodotoxin. Biophysiology Journal 27: 39–56

Cousins M J 1988 Introduction to acute and chronic pain: implications for neural blockade. In: Cousins M J, Bridenbaugh P O (eds) Neural blockade in clinical anesthesia and management of pain, 2nd edn. J B Lippincott, Philadelphia

Cousins M J, Cherry D A, Gourley G K 1988 Acute and chronic pain: use of spinal opioids. In: Cousins M J, Bridenbaugh P O (eds) Neural blockade in clinical anesthesia and management of pain, 2nd edn. J B Lippincott, Philadelphia

Cousins M J, Bridenbaugh P O (eds) 1988 Neural blockade in clinical anesthesia and management of pain, 2nd edn. J B Lippincott, Philadelphia

Covino B J 1988 Clinical pharmacology of local anaesthetic agents. In: Cousins M J, Bridenbaugh P O (eds) Neural blockade in clinical anesthesia and management of pain, 2nd edn. J B Lippincott, Philadelphia

Crile G W 1910 Phylogenetic association in relation to certain medical problems. Boston Medical and Surgical Journal 163: 893

Cushing H 1902 On the avoidance of shock in major amputations by cocainization of large nerve-trunks preliminary to their division. Annals of Surgery 36: 321

Hagbarth K E, Kerr D L B 1954 Central influences on spinal afferent conduction. Journal of Neurophysiology 17: 295–307

Hille B 1966 The common mode of action of three agents that decrease the transient change in sodium permeability in nerves. Nature 210: 1220–1222

Hille B 1977 The pH dependent rate of action of local anaesthetics on the node of Ranvier. Journal of General Physiology 69: 475–496

International Association for the Study of Pain, subcommittee on taxonomy 1986 Classification of chronic pain; description of pain terms. Pain 3 (suppl): S1–S225

Juan H 1978 Prostaglandins as modulators of pain. Journal of General Pharmacology 9: 403

Mather L E, Gourlay G K 1984 The biotransformation of opioids. In: Nimmo W S, Smith G (eds) Opioid agonist/antagonist drugs in clinical practice. Excerpta Medica, Amsterdam, pp 31–47

Melzack R, Wall P D 1965 Pain mechanisms: new theory. Science 150: 971–975

Muller J 1844 Von den Ergentumlichkeiten der einzelnen Nerve. In: Kobling L (ed) Handbuch der Physiologie des Menschen. Holscher, Coblenz, pp 667–682

Phillips G D, Cousins M J 1988 Neurologic mechanisms of pain and the relationship of pain, anxiety and sleep. In: Cousins M J, Bridenbaugh P O (eds) Neural blockade in clinical anesthesia and management of pain, 2nd edn. J B Lippincott, Philadelphia

Rexed B 1952 Cytoarchitectonic organisation of spinal cord in cat. Journal of Comparative Neurology 96: 415

Reynolds D V 1969 Surgery in the rat during electrical analgesia induced by focal brain stimulation. Science 164: 444–445

Skou J C 1954 Local anaesthetics: VI. Relation between blocking potency and penetration of a monomolecular layer of lipoids from nerves. Acta Pharmacologica Toxicologica 10: 325–337

Strichartz G R 1973 The inhibition of sodium currents in myelinated nerve by quaternary derivatives of lidocaine. Journal of General Physiology 62: 37–57

Strichartz G R 1988 Neural physiology and local anaesthetic actions. In: Cousins M J, Bridenbaugh P O (eds) Neural blockade in clinical anesthesia and management of pain, 2nd edn. J B Lippincott, Philadelphia

Thompson G E, Moore D C 1988 Coeliac plexus, intercostal and minor peripheral blockade. In: Cousins M J, Bridenbaugh P O (eds) Neural blockade in clinical anesthesia and management of pain, 2nd edn. J B Lippincott, Philadelphia

Wilson P, Cousins M J 1981 Gynaecological pain. In: Coppleson M (ed) Gynecologic oncology. Churchill Livingstone, Edinburgh

World Health Organization 1986 Cancer pain relief. Australian Government Publishing Service, Canberra

Yaksh T L 1988 Neurologic mechanisms of pain: In: Cousins M J, Bridenbaugh P O (eds) Neural blockade in clinical anesthesia and management of pain, 2nd edn. J B Lippincott, Philadelphia, pp 791–845

59. Acute pelvic pain

J. M. Frappell S. L. Stanton

INTRODUCTION

Pain is a symptom which the patient brings to the doctor and is not a diagnosis in itself. Acute pelvic pain is one of the commonest problems in everyday gynaecology, and yet is one which can present a difficult diagnostic conundrum. Women with acute pelvic pain are usually seen as emergency admissions, often by relatively inexperienced doctors, and do not arrive conveniently labelled as 'gynaecological' or 'surgical' problems (Paterson-Brown et al 1988). The cornerstones of management remain a thorough history and detailed physical examination coupled with an open mind. In addition, the use of the laparoscope where the diagnosis is in doubt has revolutionized the management of these cases.

Pain may be produced by a variety of processes both physiological and pathological and of course may be arising from organs other than those of the female genital tract. Pelvic pain frequently has a psychological background, although this is more commonly found in women who present with chronic pain to the outpatient clinic (Gomez & Dalby 1977). An acute episode which presents as an emergency is more likely to have a clearly identifiable cause with a specific line of management which often involves surgery.

INNERVATION

Pelvic pain may be somatic or visceral. Somatic pain comes from the vulva, perineum and lower vagina (transmitted via the pudendal nerve S2–4) or from the peritoneum covering the abdominal wall which is supplied by the same nerve roots as supply the overlying skin (dermatomes). Visceral pain originates from the abdominal and pelvic organs and is transmitted via the autonomic nervous system (T10–L1). Visceral and somatic pain perceptions are different. The viscera are insensitive to thermal and tactile sensations, and are poorly localized in the cerebral cortex. Stimuli that produce pain include the following:

1. Distension and contraction of a hollow organ.
2. Rapid stretching of the capsule of a solid organ.
3. Chemical irritation of the parietal peritoneum.
4. Tissue ischaemia.
5. Neuritis secondary to inflammatory, neoplastic or fibrotic processes in adjacent organs.

CLASSIFICATION

Classification of pain by pathology is of little practical use other than to remind the clinician of the large variety of conditions that may present in this way (Tables 59.1 and 59.2). A more helpful approach is to define the urgency of the problem, as this will influence the patient's early management. Acute pelvic pain can be divided into two main problem categories:

1. *Urgent*: Here the woman is ill and may need to be resuscitated quickly with intravenous fluids (including blood) for hypovolaemic or septic shock or dehydration. These patients will often require urgent surgery both to confirm the diagnosis (e.g. ruptured ectopic pregnancy, advanced peritonitis) and to perform the appropriate treatment.

Table 59.1 Gynaecological causes of pain

Pregnancy-related	Abortion, ectopic pregnancy, fibroid degeneration, round ligament stretch
Physiological	Menstruation, ovulation
Ovarian	Cyst accident (torsion, rupture, haemorrhage), polycystic ovarian syndrome
Infection	Pelvic inflammatory disease, tubo-ovarian abscess, septic abortion
Endometriosis	
Neoplasia	Benign Fibroids Ovarian cyst Malignant disease of genital tract

Table 59.2 Non-gynaecological causes of pain

Urinary tract	Infection, calculus, retention, urethral syndrome, malignancy
Gastrointestinal	Appendicitis, gastroenteritis, constipation, diverticulitis, strangulated hernia, inflammatory bowel disease, malignancy, volvulus, mesenteric infarction, irritable bowel syndrome

2. *Subacute*: These are women with pain of acute onset but who are not desperately ill and in whom the diagnosis may be uncertain. They do not therefore require emergency surgery immediately, but can be safely observed on the ward over the next 12–24 hours whilst appropriate investigations are carried out. The passage of time alone may be all that is required for continued observation and further examination to make the diagnosis apparent.

HISTORY

A well taken history is the single most important part of making a diagnosis, and the time-honoured aphorism 'Listen to the patient and she will tell you the diagnosis' is nowhere more true than in acute pelvic pain. Whilst taking the history one has a golden opportunity to observe the patient's general condition and demeanour which can give valuable clues as to the cause of the pain, how ill she is, and whether or not urgent surgery is likely to be necessary. A good place to start the history is to go back to the time when the patient last felt well before the onset of any pain. She should then be allowed to tell her story in her own words and in a chronological order, rather like Humpty Dumpty's advice to Alice in *Through the Looking Glass*: Start at the beginning, go through to the end, and then stop'. Interruptions should be kept to a minimum and points of uncertainty clarified when the patient has finished her story.

The following points should all be covered, although obviously they will not necessarily be in the same order, nor weighted with the same emphasis. The age of a patient, particularly whether or not she is in her reproductive years, will obviously influence one's thoughts as to the likely diagnosis.

Mode of onset and nature of pain

Pain of very sudden onset, prior to which the patient felt perfectly well, tends to suggest an underlying mechanical problem such as torsion or rupture of an ovarian cyst, whereas pain caused by infection, e.g. appendicitis or pelvic inflammatory disease (PID) tends to be slower to arrive, duller in natural and more poorly localized. In such cases it is only when the parietal peritoneum adjacent to inflamed organs becomes inflamed itself that the pain becomes sharper and more clearly localized, as in the classical description of acute appendicitis where the initial 'visceral' pain is poorly localized in the periumbilical region to be replaced after 12 hours or so by 'somatic' pain localized in the right iliac fossa.

Colicky pain suggests muscle contraction in a hollow organ, such as a uterus expelling a pregnancy, a ureter expelling a calculus and intestine trying to overcome obstruction. By contrast, dull aching or throbbing pain is indicative of inflammation.

Timing

As well as the duration of the pain, it is important to know if the pain is constant or intermittent, and whether the current episode is a more severe exacerbation of a similar pain which has been grumbling on for some weeks or months or is an entirely new event prior to which the patient was fit and well. Constant pain suggests either an ischaemic event or an inflammatory aetiology.

Timing also encompasses the relationship of the pain to other events. In gynaecological cases one thinks particularly of the menstrual cycle and vaginal bleeding, as complications of early pregnancy are one of the commonest causes of acute pain in young women. Whether the pain occurred before or after the onset of vaginal bleeding may help to differentiate between threatened abortion and tubal pregnancy. In acute appendicitis there is a typical temporal relationship between the onset of pain and other more generalized symptoms such as anorexia, nausea, vomiting and bowel upset, although these symptoms may also be features of other inflammatory pathology.

Location and radiation

Although visceral pain is often poorly localized, unilateral pain may point to a localized problem in a particular organ, e.g. ureteric colic, appendicitis, diverticulitis, torsion of an ovarian cyst or tubal pregnancy. In cases where there is a more generalized inflammation of peritoneal surfaces, e.g. from pus in acute salpingitis or from blood in a ruptured ovarian cyst or tubal pregnancy, then the pain is felt more diffusely across the entire lower abdomen and pelvis.

Radiation of pain to the thighs suggests ovarian or ureteric origin. Blood in the pouch of Douglas may cause a sharp pain in the rectum and an urge to defecate, whilst similar irritation of the peritoneal surface of the bladder will produce pain related to micturition without any dysuria. Radiation of pain to the shoulder tips is produced by irritation of the undersurfaces of the diaphragm, usually by blood or from the contents of a perforated viscus. The pain is usually made worse when the patient takes a deep breath or lies flat. In a bleeding tubal pregnancy shoulder tip pain appears only after there has been considerable blood loss when the patient may well be shocked. A similar picture may present in the relatively rare condition of spontaneous rupture of a splenic cyst.

Exacerbating and relieving factors

Pain relieved by lying still and exacerbated by movement points strongly to peritoneal irritation by blood or pus. A history of deep dyspareunia may indicate peritoneal inflammation, but if the pain so caused is well localized to a particular part of the pelvis then it is more likely to be due to a more localized lesion, such as an ovarian cyst, endometriosis, an unruptured tubal pregnancy or a pyosalpinx.

Gynaecological history

The date of the last menstrual period and the usual cycle length are of paramount importance. Pain in the middle of a regular cycle may be due to ovulation (Mittelschmerz = middlepain). One must always ask quite specifically about the nature of vaginal bleeding or discharge, as many women will assume that any bleeding, be it even very light or short-lived, was a period. Although the bleeding associated with ectopic pregnancy caused by shedding of the decidua is usually brownish and quite light in amount, it is sometimes heavy enough to mimic a spontaneous abortion. The passage of a decidual cast which the patient may bring to the hospital with her is highly suggestive of tubal pregnancy, whilst the passage of products of conception confirms a spontaneous abortion. Normal periods themselves can of course be painful, and particularly so in cases of retrograde menstruation when there may be symptoms and signs of peritoneal irritation.

The likelihood of the patient being pregnant obviously depends upon whether she has been sexually active and upon the use of contraception. This may be a difficult area in which to arrive at the truth, particularly in young girls who may wish to conceal knowledge of sexual activity from their parents or in a married woman who has had extramarital relationships whilst her husband has had a vasectomy. Erratic use or impaired absorption of oral contraception may result in pregnancy, whilst an intrauterine contraceptive device can predispose to acute salpingitis and tubal pregnancy. Previous sterilization by tubal occlusion does not rule out the possibility of a pregnancy, which if present is more likely to be lodged in the tube. Of course a normal intrauterine pregnancy can also cause dull cramping pelvic pain which may mimic ectopic pregnancy, whilst a retroverted gravid uterus incarcerated in the pelvis during the first trimester may precipitate acute urinary retention. A women with a previous tubal pregnancy has approximately 10 times the risk of a recurrence in a subsequent pregnancy, i.e. a risk of approximately 1 in 30 against the usual background rate of 1 in 300 pregnancies. A history of infertility and tubal surgery again increases the risk of tubal pregnancy, whilst ovulation induction using injectable gonadotrophins may cause the ovarian hyperstimulation syndrome where pain is due to rapidly enlarging multicystic ovaries and, in extreme cases, the development of ascites.

Vaginal discharge is frequently a confusing symptom, as a brownish loss may be due to old blood, whilst in cases of acute PID there is often no discharge at all. The presence of an offensive, purulent discharge tends to suggest the acute recrudescence of chronic PID. In women over the age of 40, one should remember that discharge may be associated with malignant disease of the uterine body or cervix, and that these may present with acute pelvic pain, although more typically it will have been a chronic problem.

Urinary symptoms

Lower urinary tract infection is common in women, and often results in pelvic pain with associated urgency, frequency and dysuria. With a more severe ascending infection, pain may be felt in the ipsilateral loin and iliac fossa and may be accompanied by rigors and high fever. Remember that in the elderly, infection may cause pain but very little else. Haematuria suggests calculi, neoplasia or a severe cystitis. Acute pelvic pain may be the presentation of acute urinary retention, precipitated by pregnancy, surgery, infection, drugs, neuropathy or rarely neoplasia.

Gastrointestinal symptoms

Anorexia, nausea and vomiting may be the harbingers of intestinal pathology, but they are very non-specific complaints and may be precipitated by many illnesses, or follow a very painful event such as the rupture of an ovarian cyst. Change of bowel habit is equally non-specific, although the onset of pain and diarrhoea together suggests an enteritis (of which infection with *Campylobacter* is now the commonest cause) or inflammatory bowel disease. Diarrhoea or constipation may be features of colonic diverticulitis, which is common amongst elderly patients, but absolute constipation points to a low large bowel obstruction which can be caused by extrinsic pressure from malignant or inflammatory conditions of the pelvic organs. Rectal carcinoma may present with pelvic pain as a leading feature, and is often associated with the passage of blood and mucus per rectum.

CLINICAL EXAMINATION

Examination starts from the moment the patient is first seen, whether it be when she comes through the door of the consulting room or when she is seen in bed on the ward following urgent admission to hospital. The first observation to make is whether or not she looks ill. Although this may not be an easy assessment for an inexperienced doctor to make, with increasing experience one learns to assimilate almost imperceptibly information about the patient from her general appearance and demeanour. Pain caused by peritoneal irritation from blood or pus is exacerbated by movement and so the patient lies still. In contrast severe pain which causes her to writhe around in agony is usually caused by spasm within a muscular organ such as ureteric colic. If the patient is suffering from shock caused by hypovolaemia or septicaemia, she will look pale and listless with the cold clammy extremities associated with peripheral vasoconstriction. Observation of a patient on the ward when she is unaware that she is being watched following admission for acute pain can be very informative. Pain may completely disappear when she is alone or talking to friends. Episodes of severe pain which are not accompanied by a significant rise in the pulse rate may be of psychogenic origin. Conversely a pulse rate of greater than 100 beats/min in association with a systolic blood pressure of 100 mmHg or less means that the patient is shocked and resuscitation with intravenous fluids should be carried out immediately prior to a definitive diagnosis being made. The presence of pyrexia points to an infectious cause, although the temperature can be normal in some cases of PID. The presence of blood in the peritoneal cavity can raise the temperature by a few tenths of a degree, and this may be a presenting feature in a leaking ectopic pregnancy.

A general physical examination should be carried out prior to abdominal examination to look for signs of anaemia, as well as signs of disseminated malignant disease such as enlarged supraclavicular or inguinal lymph nodes, pleural effusion and ankle oedema. The latter may be due to obstruction of venous return by a pelvic mass or lymphatic obstruction secondary to malignant infiltration. Inspection of the tongue may show signs of dehydration in patients who have been vomiting whilst a foul-smelling breath (foetor oris) may be associated with intestinal stasis either from a mechanical obstruction or secondary to a paralytic ileus.

Inspection of the abdomen may reveal distension due to ascites or a large mass, or to distended bowel. This latter may be associated with an ileus caused by intra-peritoneal blood or pus, or due to bowel obstruction when peristaltic movement may be visible (in association with a history of colicky pain and vomiting). The presence of surgical scars makes a diagnosis of small bowel obstruction more likely in the abdomen, although in the patient who has undergone repeated operations one may be dealing with a rare case of Münchhausen's syndrome.

Abdominal palpation should always start as far from the site of maximum pain as possible, gradually working towards it. Tenderness, guarding and rigidity are noted at the same time, as is rebound tenderness. This sign should be elicited unobtrusively during the course of palpation, and preferably should be volunteered by the patient without prompting. Rebound tenderness elicited by extravagant withdrawal of the examining hand whilst asking the patient if it hurts is unlikely to be of great significance! Classically the sight of maximum tenderness in acute appendicitis is over McBurney's point which is at the junction of the lateral and middle thirds of the line between the umbilicus and the anterior superior iliac spine. An inflamed retrocaecal appendix (the anatomical site in 15% of the population) may however cause tenderness in the right loin. The ovarian point is said to be at the junction of middle and medial thirds of the same line, and pressure over this point produces pain identical to that of the pelvic pain syndrome (Beard et al 1986). Although a patient with this syndrome usually presents to outpatients with a chronic history of recurrent pain, she may in some instances present with severe acute lower abdominal pain. Similarly, in cases of the irritable bowel syndrome there may be tenderness in left and right iliac fossae over a palpable sigmoid colon and distended caecum respectively.

The hernial orifices must always be examined as small bowel strangulation, particularly in a femoral hernia, is a common cause of acute pain in elderly women. Any masses should be defined in terms of site and size, regularity of outline, consistency, mobility and tenderness. In the presence of a mass a search for ascites must be made by percussing for shifting dullness or a fluid thrill, although these signs will be absent unless there are several litres of intraperitoneal free fluid. Percussion can also be very helpful in outlining soft-walled swellings such as a benign ovarian cyst or a full bladder. Palpation for enlargement of liver, spleen and kidneys and auscultation of bowel sounds should form part of all abdominal examinations.

Vulval inspection may reveal an obvious malignancy or an infectious lesion such as a Bartholin's abscess or herpes genitalis. Speculum examinations will reveal the presence of blood or pus and give an opportunity to inspect the cervix (to exclude malignancy) as well as to take a cervical smear and microbiological swabs from the endocervix and vaginal fornices. One may also see the threads from an intrauterine contraceptive device or note products of conception in cases of spontaneous abortion.

Bimanual examination is best performed with the patient in the dorsal position, although she should also be examined in the left lateral position if genital prolapse is suspected; rectal examination is essential if gynaecological malignancy or bowel pathology is suspected. One often gains far more information about a pelvic mass (be it inflammatory or neoplastic) from bimanual rectal than vaginal examination. Cervical position and mobility should be assessed initially. A very anterior cervix associated with retroversion of the uterus may cause urinary retention particularly in the first trimester of pregnancy. If the patient does have urinary retention and cannot void spontaneously, she should be catheterized prior to further bimanual palpation. If movement of the cervix produces pain this suggests parametrial inflammation by blood or infection, although lack of pain does not definitely rule out a tubal pregnancy. Fixed retroversion of the uterus suggests fibrosis resulting from chronic infection, endometriosis or advanced malignancy.

The size and consistency of the uterus are next elicited, looking for signs of pregnancy, e.g. Hegar's sign, or enlargement due to fibroids which may be very difficult to differentiate from large ovarian cysts which commonly occupy the midline. Uterine enlargement due to endometrial malignancy is most uncommon unless very advanced, as most women tend to present early due to abnormal bleeding. Tenderness over the uterus and adnexa suggests pelvic infection which is most commonly bilateral. A tubo-ovarian abscess may however be unilateral, particularly in association with an intrauterine contraceptive device. This is unlikely to cause confusion with a case of tubal pregnancy as it is most unusual to elicit an easily palpable mass in such cases.

INVESTIGATIONS

Blood tests

These are not particularly helpful in the differential diagnosis of pain.

Haemoglobin

In acute blood loss, the haemoglobin concentration remains normal until time for haemodilution has elapsed, usually 12–24 h. Therefore serial readings may be necessary for comparison; a rapidly falling level will confirm the diagnosis. In the case of a chronic leaking tubal pregnancy, the patient may have a low haemoglobin resulting from the steady loss of a considerable volume of blood into the peritoneal cavity with surprisingly few physical signs.

The white cell count

This is of little value as it is often normal in cases of acute sepsis such as appendicitis, salpingitis or urinary infection. On the other hand it may be significantly raised to 15×10^6/l or more in normal pregnancy. In cases where chronic sepsis is suspected, e.g. tuberculosis, a differential count may be helpful.

Erythrocyte sedimentation rate

This is unlikely to be significantly elevated in cases of gynaecological pain, but may be elevated in normal pregnancy.

Pregnancy tests

These can be rapidly carried out on the ward using commercially prepared kits which use a monoclonal antibody to test for the beta subunit of human chorionic gonadotrophin. A positive test is diagnostic of a continuing pregnancy which may be intra- or extrauterine. A negative pregnancy test does not exclude a tubal pregnancy.

Bacteriological tests

Swabs

High vaginal swabs are useful for diagnosis of localized vaginitis, e.g. *Candida* or *Trichomonas*, but do not give a reliable picture of organisms infecting the upper reaches of the genital tract. In cases of suspected PID therefore, swabs should be taken from the endocervical canal. For detection of *Chlamydia*, the swabs should be sent in special culture medium or preferably a smear should be made on a special slide which is fixed and *Chlamydia* detected by microimmunoflourescence techniques. In cases of suspected gonococcal infection, swabs should also be taken from urethra and rectum and transported in Stuart's medium, or inoculated directly on to an agar culture plate.

Pus

This is the best material for culturing organisms and should be sent directly in a sterile pot if obtainable on speculum examination of the cervix, or from the peritoneal cavity at the time of a laparoscopy or laparotomy.

Urine microscopy and culture

Urinary tract infection is very common in women, and

testing of a midstream specimen should be performed in all cases. Nephur-test diagnostic strips (Boehringer-Mannheim) will detect the presence of blood, white cells and protein. Positive specimens should then be sent for microscopy and culture. Specimens which contain $> 10^5$ bacteria per millilitre indicate infection of 80% of cases. If two successive specimens show $> 10^5$ organisms per millilitre, this is diagnostic of infection in 95% of cases. In the remainder, the growth is due to contamination of the specimen at the time of collection or to delay in culturing which may give a few contaminant bacteria time to multiply. If it is impossible to obtain a clean-catch specimen, then suprapubic aspiration or a urethral catheter specimen is indicated.

Examination for pus cells in the urine is of little value in the diagnosis of urinary tract infection as their presence may be due to contamination or other disorders of the urinary tract such as glomerulonephritis or urolithiasis. The finding of excess white cells in the absence of bacteria however means that tuberculous infection of the urinary tract should be excluded.

Red cells seen on microscopy in the absence of infection may be a sign of a ureteric or bladder calculus, or of malignancy anywhere in the urinary tract. On the very rare occasion when an acute porphyria is suspected, testing for porphobilinogen should be carried out.

Stool culture

This should be performed where an enteritis is the suspected cause of the pain.

Cytology

Where malignant disease is a possible diagnosis, cytological examination of fluid obtained from ruptured ovarian cysts, ascites or urine should be carried out to look for malignant cells.

Diagnostic imaging

X-rays

Plain abdominal X-rays. Although these are not usually very helpful in the diagnosis of gynaecological pain, they can play an important role in evaluating the acute abdomen. An erect film is the most helpful, and may reveal the dilated bowel with fluid levels seen in intestinal obstruction, free gas under the diaphragm from a perforated viscus, faecal impaction, ureteric calculi, foreign bodies, or swabs and instruments left inside at previous surgery. It may also reveal an intrauterine contraceptive device, although this is better demonstrated by ultrasound which can accurately define its position in the pelvis. Occasionally the solid components of a dermoid cyst may show up, giving an instant diagnosis.

Intravenous urography. This is required for cases where urolithiasis or urothelial malignancy is suspected.

Ultrasound scanning

This is a technique ideally suited for investigation of the pelvis, as it is informative, non-invasive and well tolerated by patients. It can reveal the presence of pelvic masses, and will help to differentiate between ovarian cysts and uterine fibroids. It will exclude intrauterine pregnancy but cannot definitely exclude an ectopic pregnancy. It is also the best method of looking for 'lost coils' and will show whether an intrauterine contraceptive device is inside or outside the uterine cavity.

Computerized tomography and magnetic resonance imaging

These sophisticated scanning techniques have little place in managing cages of acute pelvic pain in the emergency setting. However they can be particularly helpful in the assessment of malignant disease which may present with pain.

Laparoscopy

This is a safe and simple procedure, but it should not become a substitute for proper clinical assessment of the problem, and it should not be performed in cases where a patient clearly requires a laparotomy, e.g. when shocked from acute intraperitoneal blood loss or in the presence of a large mass. It is however the best way to exclude ectopic pregnancy, a situation which has been most eloquently summarized by McFadyen (1981) thus: 'Pregnancy in the fallopian tube is a "black cat on a dark night". It may make its presence felt in subtle ways and leap at you or it may sneak past unobserved. Although it is difficult to distinguish from cats of other colours in the darkness, illumination clearly identifies it'.

Laparoscopy is also an invaluable aid in the diagnosis of PID as the clinical signs and symptoms are very variable and only about 50% of women will be correctly diagnosed on clinical grounds alone (Jacobson 1980). In cases of doubt there is no harm in instituting antibiotic therapy on an expectant basis as this can be discontinued following laparoscopy if the suspected diagnosis of PID turns out to be incorrect. Laparoscopy can also reveal ovarian cyst accidents, such as torsion, rupture or haemorrhage, and acute appendicitis unless the appendix is retrocaecal. At the time of laparoscopy specimens of pus may be obtained for culture, or fluid from ovarian cysts sent for cytological assessment.

CONCLUSION

Acute pelvic pain is a common problem in gynaecology

which is often delegated to relatively inexperienced junior staff. Sound clinical skills of history-taking and examination together with an open mind and the intelligent use of ultrasound scanning and the laparoscope all contribute towards the successful management of these cases.

KEY POINTS

1. Acute pelvic pain is a common symptom in a wide range of gynaecological and non-gynaecological conditions.
2. A thorough history and examination are essential in the assessment of the patient.
3. Initial assessment categorizes the problem as urgent or subacute.
4. Urgent cases are likely to need rapid resuscitation prior to immediate surgery.
5. In sub-acute cases the most helpful investigations are ultrasound scanning and laparoscopy.
6. Laparoscopy should not be performed in cases where laparotomy is clearly required, i.e. in the presence of hypovolaemic shock or a large mass.
7. PID is reliably diagnosed on clinical grounds alone in only 50% of cases.

REFERENCES

Beard R W, Reginald P W, Pearce S 1986 Pelvic pain in women. British Medical Journal 293: 1160–1162

Gomez J, Dally P 1977 Psychologically mediated abdominal pain in surgical and medical outpatient clinics. British Medical Journal 1: 1451–1453

Jacobson L 1980 Differential diagnosis of acute pelvic inflammatory disease. American Journal of Obstetrics and Gynecology 138: 1006–1011

McFadyen I R 1981 Gynaecological pain in the lower abdomen. Clinics in Obstetrics and Gynaecology 8: 35

Paterson-Brown S, Eckersley J R T, Dudley H A F 1988 The gynaecological profile of acute general surgery. Journal of the Royal College of Surgeons of Edinburgh 33: 13–15

60. Chronic pelvic pain

R. W. Beard P. W. Reginald

INTRODUCTION

Women learn from an early age that many aspects of their gynaecological function, unlike other functional systems of the body, are painful. Commonly the association between gynaecological function and pain is conditioned by what women are told as children by their mothers and older friends. Some pain with menstruation is usual, ovulation is often uncomfortable and it is generally accepted that labour is always painful. What varies from one woman to another is the way in which this physiological pain is perceived when it occurs. The perception of gynaecological pain is determined by many factors ranging from an individual response dependent on personality to specific factors such as expectations, attributions and attitudes to menstruation, femininity and sexual attitudes. This expectation of pain, at least at menstruation, may account for the marked discrepancy between women's reports of menstrual symptomatology on retrospective surveys and those obtained for daily, prospective symptom ratings. Prospective studies consistently yield lower measures of pain and distress than similar studies done retrospectively (Golub 1976; Bosanko 1982). Hence it seems likely that women have a mental 'set' or schema to expect some pain and distress at menstruation. The implications that this has for the process whereby women decide that a given level of distress is abnormal and warrants medical consultation have been largely ignored. Nevertheless, it is obviously important to recognize the close interaction between psychological and somatic factors in the perception of pain.

It should also be recognized that the severity of pain as perceived by any individual is influenced by psychological processes. The literature suggests that pathology is more likely to be attended to and labelled as painful if the patient is anxious, depressed or has been exposed to friends and relatives who experience pain or believe that they have minimal control over pain and illness. Factors such as these may go some way towards explaining how patients may have equivalent degrees of pathology yet report very different levels of pain.

Pelvic pain remains the single most common indication for referral to a gynaecology clinic (Morris & O'Neill 1958) and for diagnostic laparoscopy (Chamberlain & Brown 1978). However it is difficult to be certain what is the true incidence of lower abdominal pain requiring medical or surgical treatment. Women with pelvic pain alone are usually referred to a gynaecologist whereas those with, for example, associated urinary symptoms go to a urologist. Table 60.1 shows the findings at laparoscopy summarized from five studies of women with chronic pelvic pain. A total of 553 women were investigated and the commonest abnormality found was adhesions after pelvic inflammatory disease or surgery (20%), followed by endometriosis (12%) and other conditions (3%). The most striking finding was an apparently normal pelvis in 65% of all the women studied. Figure 60.1 shows similar findings on a small group of women, some with acute and others with chronic pelvic pain, studied by Stacey et al (1989). Of particular interest in this study is the fact that, even amongst women with acute pain, 44% had a normal pelvis on laparoscopy. These negative findings are so striking that one has to question the validity of any diagnosis of pelvic pain based on laparoscopy alone, with the exception of obvious conditions like ectopic pregnancy.

Table 60.1 Laparoscopic findings in women with chronic pelvic pain

Author	Number of cases	Normal pelvis	Adhesions (PID)	Endometriosis	Others
Liston et al (1972)	134	102	21	6	5
Pent (1972)	38	18	13	7	—
Lundberg et al (1973)	95	37	32	13	13
Levitan et al (1985)	186	168	14	4	—
Rapkin (1986)	100	36	26	37	1
Total	553	361 (65%)	106 (20%)	67 (12%)	19 (3%)

PID = Pelvic inflammatory disease.

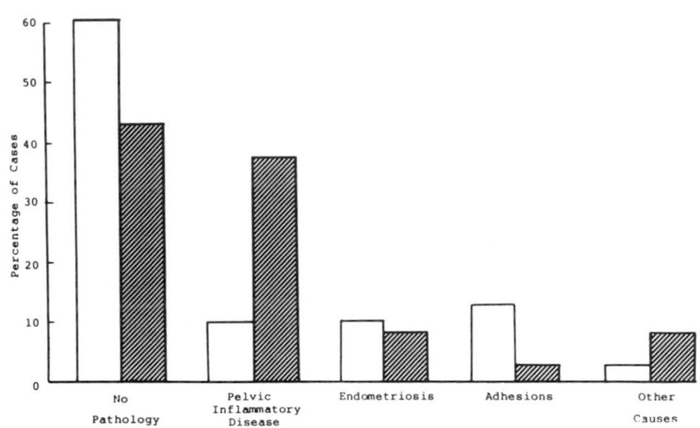

Fig. 60.1 Distribution of cases of acute (hatched boxes, n = 37) and chronic (open boxes, n = 39) pelvic pain according to diagnosis at laparoscopy. Adapted from Stacey et al (1989).

SENSORY AND MOTOR NERVE SUPPLY TO THE PELVIS

Pelvic organs have both a sympathetic and a parasympathetic nerve supply. The pain impulses from the uterus, medial part of the fallopian tubes and upper part of the vagina travel through the visceral efferents to Frankenhauser's paracervical plexus of nerves. From this plexus, the impulses travel to the inferior, middle and superior hypogastric plexus and enter the lumbar and lower thoracic sympathetic chain passing to the spinal cord through the posterior nerve root at the level of T10 to L1 and travelling to the neurones in the posterior lateral tract of Lissauer and the dorsal horn. The impulses are subjected to various modulating influences here and some pass through the spinothalamic tract to reach the sensory cortex. Sympathetic nerves from the ovary, lateral part of the fallopian tubes and from the peritoneum of the broad ligament travel along the ovarian vessels to enter the aortic plexus. The parasympathetic fibres travel along the pudendal nerves and enter the spinal cord at S2–4. The combination of sympathetic and parasympathetic innervation of pelvic organs is accompanied by different reflex arcs from the thoracolumbar and sacral visceral afferent fibres conveying to the spinal cord pressure as well as pain impulses. Pain originating from any one of these pelvic organs is also experienced by the skin areas supplied by the somatic afferent fibres of the same spinal segment. This is termed 'referred pain'. Accordingly, the pain arising from the ovaries is referred to the area of the abdominal wall just below and lateral to the umbilicus (the ovarian point); pain from the uterus and cervix goes to the lower abdominal wall supplied by the 12th thoracic nerve, and pain from the bladder and vagina to the skin area over the pubic bone and groin. In addition, because of their dual innervation, pain from the uterus and cervix can be referred to the skin area over the dorsum of the sacrum (S2–S4).

CAUSES OF PELVIC PAIN

Adhesions

Adhesions are found in about 20% of women investigated by laparoscopy for chronic pelvic pain (Table 60.1). Controversy still exists as to whether adhesions can be the cause of such pain (Alexander-Williams 1987). A retrospective study by Rapkin (1986) concluded that adhesions were rarely a cause of pain. Women being investigated by laparoscopy for chronic pelvic pain were compared with a group being investigated for primary infertility. The author reported that more women in the fertile group had adhesions (38 compared with 26%) and only 12% of them complained of pain even though the nature and distribution of the adhesions were similar in both groups. A study by Kresh et al (1984) came to an opposite conclusion, but neither study took into account that the majority of pelvic pain women had had previous surgery for the pain which predated the appearance of adhesions. It seems likely that it is the site of the adhesions which determines whether or not pain is caused. For example, adhesion of bowel to the back of the broad ligament rarely causes pain whereas adhesion of an ovary in the same position, whether from inflammation or endometriosis, does cause pain.

Trapped or residual ovary syndrome

This occurs in women who have had a hysterectomy with conservation of one or both ovaries, although occasionally it is seen after pelvic inflammatory disease. It is characterized symptomatically by pelvic pain, deep dyspareunia and a fixed tender ovary felt at the angle of the vault of the vagina. It is a relatively rare cause of chronic pelvic pain and occurs in only 1–3% of all cases of hysterectomy with conservation of the ovaries (Renaer 1981). Christ & Lotze (1975) reported that among women with a trapped ovary, 77% complained of chronic pelvic pain, 67% of dyspareunia and an asymptomatic pelvic mass was found in 14%.

At laparoscopy most women with a trapped residual ovary have extensive pelvic adhesions involving the ovaries which appear to be enlarged and cystic. The pain is likely to be due to the tension within a developing follicle in an ovary covered with adhesions. Pathological examination of a trapped ovary commonly reveals multiple cystic follicles and periovarian adhesions.

Pelvic pain may be relieved by ovarian suppression but the most effective treatment of the condition is removal of these ovaries. Frequently the adhesions are extremely dense and tough and in order to avoid damage to surrounding structures such as the ureter it is advisable to employ blunt rather than sharp dissection to free the ovary.

Ovarian remnant syndrome

Ovarian remnant syndrome is defined as the persistence of functioning ovarian tissue following an apparently complete bilateral oophorectomy. This occurs most commonly following surgery for extensive endometriosis, pelvic inflammatory disease or inflammatory bowel disease and is probably more common than has previously been thought. Pettit & Lee (1988) reported 31 cases seen within a period of 5 years. The patient complains of a constant dull ache in the pelvis or intermittent sharp pain that is exaggerated during intercourse or pelvic examination. Clinical diagnosis of this condition is difficult because the remaining ovary is usually small and located on the pelvic side-wall. Laparoscopic examination reveals adhesions through which the ovary may not be visible, thereby preventing accurate assessment but ultrasound or computerized tomography scan is often helpful. The finding of follicle-stimulating hormone levels in the premenopausal range, in the absence of exogenous administration of hormones, is a useful confirmatory test.

Ovarian suppression using oral contraceptives or medroxyprogesterone acetate (Provera) should be tried first more for diagnostic than therapeutic purposes. However, surgical removal of the ovarian remnant is usually necessary although it may involve prolonged dissection by an experienced surgeon to avoid ureteric injury.

Endometriosis

Endometriosis is a poorly understood disease with a variable clinical presentation. The condition is typified by the abnormal implantation of endometrium outside the uterine cavity in local and distant sites from the pelvis (see Ch. 30).

Dysmenorrhoea, dyspareunia, pelvic pain and infertility are the characteristic symptoms of endometriosis. However, a recent study (O'Connor 1987) has shown that only 39 (5%) of 717 patients with endometriosis had all the above symptoms and 155 (22%) had no symptoms at all. Generally, asymptomatic endometriosis is detected during investigation for infertility or some other condition requiring laparoscopy or laparotomy.

The condition may occur at any time after puberty and is often progressive until near the menopause, suggesting that it is modulated by oestrogen, though there is still no certain knowledge of the pathogenesis of the condition. Cyclical bleeding leads to intense fibrosis around the endometrial deposits and is thought to be one of the reasons why women with the condition frequently suffer severe dysmenorrhoea.

An alternative explanation is based on the observation (Schmidt 1985) that women with endometriosis not only have more peritoneal fluid in the pouch of Douglas than normal control women, but that this fluid contains significantly more prostaglandins, in particular prostaglandin E_2 and $F_{2\alpha}$. It is possible that these compounds, which are vasoactive, cause vascular stasis leading to the release of pain-producing substances. This explanation is supported by the knowledge that prostaglandin inhibitors provide effective pain relief in women with dysmenorrhoea associated with endometriosis.

Although congestive dysmenorrhoea is the commonest symptom among women with endometriosis, many women report that the nature of their period pain changed from premenstrual pain to pain commencing after the onset of menstrual bleeding. Any woman presenting in the reproductive years with unexplained lower abdominal pain, the site of which is constant, and which is exacerbated by menstruation should be suspected of having endometriosis.

Treatment of endometriosis

Treatment for the relief of pelvic pain due to endometriosis has to be individualized, as it is dependent on such factors as the age of the patient, desire for conservation of fertility, severity of pain including disturbance to daily life and the site of the deposits. In general the following guidelines can be used in planning the treatment of women with endometriosis. In the presence of symptoms medical treatment should always be tried before resorting to surgery. The only exception to this rule is when the endometriotic deposit is isolated, as with chocolate cysts of the ovary, adenomyosis and isolated symptomatic deposits.

Analgesics and ovarian suppression. Analgesics and anti-prostaglandin agents are used for treating young women with dysmenorrhoea who still wish to become pregnant. For this purpose mefenamic acid (Ponstan) is an extremely effective and safe anti-prostaglandin.

A variety of ovarian suppression regimens are available and are discussed at length in Chapter 30.

Surgery. Surgical removal is a most successful procedure for isolated endometrial deposits which are causing pain, and can sometimes be done without the need to resort to a laparotomy. Presacral neurectomy has been advocated in the treatment of endometriosis and pelvic pain (Polan & de Cherney 1980) but this is not widely practised in this country.

Adenomyosis is more difficult to treat because it responds poorly to medical treatment and is difficult to remove by local excision. Hysterectomy may be indicated but it is often necessary to adopt a more conservative approach because of the wish of these women — who are commonly aged less than 40 years — to avoid such a drastic solution.

Neural causes

Entrapment of the iliohypogastric nerve

This may follow a Pfannenstiel incision leading to intermittent sharp pain induced by physical activity. The pain is said to be usually felt at the incision site, radiating into the labia and upper inner aspect of the thigh. It is suggested that nerve entrapment occurs as a result of nerve damage by incision or suture leading to the formation of a neuroma, or entrapment of the nerve by scar tissue. Ilioinguinal nerve entrapment is also reported and may occur between internal oblique and transverse abdominis muscle, leading to lower abdominal pain. Hahn (personal communication 1989) reports that in a study of 46 patients with ilioinguinal nerve entrapment, 88% had hyperaesthesia in the inguinal region, 52% had dysaesthesia and 75% had tenderness which could be elicited at the assumed site of nerve entrapment just medial to and below the anterior superior iliac spine. Injection of local anaesthetic (0.5% bupivacaine) to block the ilioinguinal and iliohypogastric nerves is an important diagnostic tool in the assessment of patients complaining of pain after Pfannenstiel incision. Relief of pain is said to be diagnostic of nerve entrapment.

Repeated nerve blocks should be tried first and surgical resection of the nerve is only justified when recurrent nerve blocks have failed to produce permanent relief of symptoms.

Trigger points

Trigger points are areas of hypersensitivity on the abdominal skin and in the abdominal wall. They are located in single unilateral dermatomes, most often in the abdominal wall which, on compression or stretching, reproduce the same painful sensations complained of by the patient. There have also been described trigger points in the paracervix and sacrum suggesting they could be a primary source of pelvic pain. On the abdominal wall they may be identified by inserting a 22-gauge needle into the fat pad above the fascia. Movement of the tip of the needle reproduces the pain sensations complained of and injection of a local anaesthetic into the point temporarily blocks the sensation of pain. Slocumb (1984) studied 131 patients with pelvic pain of whom 89% had painful trigger points on the abdominal wall, 71% in the vagina and 25% on the sacrum. He treated these women by injecting bupivacaine (0.25%) into the located site of the trigger point. The results were available on 122 patients, of whom 89% reported complete or partial relief of pain 3–36 months after treatment. This suggests that the women in Slocumb's study form a complex group, perhaps with various underlying causes for their pain. No information was given as to whether these women had had a laparoscopy to rule out the presence of pelvic pathology, although 14 subsequently had pelvic surgery, including adhesiolysis, and a variety of medical treatments — anti-prostaglandins, anti-depressants, medroxyprogesterone acetate and ovarian suppression using oral contraceptives. These results are difficult to interpret because there was no standardized approach to investigation and diagnosis. It is clear that the group of women studied had a variety of causes for their pain, including recognizable pelvic pathology. The validity of Slocumb's assertion that injection of a local anaesthetic into a trigger point cures the pain must remain speculative.

Chronic pelvic inflammatory disease

Chronic pelvic inflammatory disease is a consequence of acute pelvic infection leading to permanent damage to tissues such as the parametrium, tubes and ovaries. Peritoneal adhesions may lead to hydrosalpinges, tubo-ovarian masses, fixity and distortion of the pelvic organs, and the 'trapped ovary' already referred to. The diagnosis of chronic pelvic inflammatory disease implies an active but subclinical infective process. There is little evidence that this is so, and it is more likely that if the condition is progressive, it is due to recurrent infections.

Some women with chronic pelvic pain give a history of pain which started with an acute attack of salpingitis. Such a history is commonly the product of a diagnosis made at the time without adequate investigation. Many investigators (Murphy & Fliegner 1981; Brihmer et al 1987) have confirmed the laparoscopic findings of Stacey et al (1989) shown in Figure 60.1 which reveal that even in cases of acute pelvic pain many women have no evidence on laparoscopy of pelvic inflammatory disease. Equally women with laparoscopic evidence of chronic pelvic inflammatory disease do not necessarily give a history of acute pelvic inflammatory disease as infection with *Chlamydia*, a major cause of salpingitis, is often asymptomatic. These observations reveal how unwise it is to make a diagnosis in young women with lower abdominal pain of such a potentially serious condition without the use of a laparoscope.

Pain due to acute pelvic inflammatory disease often resolves completely after appropriate treatment, with disappearance of pelvic sepsis leaving no residual adhesion or tubal occlusion. However, some women continue to complain of pelvic pain that may be associated with tubo-ovarian adhesions. Cultures from the cervix or from pelvic organs are usually negative unless there is an acute re-infection. The actual cause of chronic pelvic pain in such cases is not clear. It could be due to recurrence of acute infection when the patient presents with signs and symptoms of acute salpingitis. Some women with chronic pelvic inflammatory disease complain of constant unilateral or bilateral pelvic pain and dyspareunia. Pelvic examination reveals generalized pelvic tenderness and thickening of adnexal tissue with or without the presence of tubo-ovarian mass. A standard investigation approach which includes laparoscopy, pelvic ultrasound and pelvic venography excludes conditions such as ovarian entrapment and pelvic congestion.

Antibiotic treatment is usually effective in women with acute pelvic inflammatory disease and symptomatic relief with analgesics provides temporary help. Long-term antibiotic treatment of chronic pelvic infection is of limited value and more often an extensive dissection of adherent pelvic structures combined with a total hysterectomy and bilateral oophorectomy is necessary in those women with persistent disabling pelvic pain.

Irritable bowel syndrome

This is an example of a non-gynaecological psychosomatic condition which is often confused with gynaecological causes of lower abdominal pain and, equally, is frequently mistakenly diagnosed when no gynaecological cause has been found.

The condition occurs more commonly in women with a frequency ranging from 56 to 90% (Thompson & Heaton 1980; Harvey et al 1987). Sufferers tend to be polysymptomatic, the predominant symptoms being colicky abdominal pain and frequent loose motions alternating with bouts of constipation. Urgency and frequency of micturition, backache and dyspareunia are common as are psychological correlates such as lassitude, fear of serious disease and palpitations. It has been suggested that individuals with irritable bowel syndrome tend to be over-anxious, highly sensitive people who complain more about minor ailments (Heaton 1983).

The condition with which irritable bowel syndrome is most likely to be confused is pelvic congestion. The tendency to be polysymptomatic is common to both groups, but the similarity ceases there. Bowel symptoms predominate in irritable bowel syndrome which is why the condition generally leads to referral to the gastroenterologists, whereas the absence of such symptoms is striking in women with pelvic congestion. There is good evidence of abnormal sensitivity of the large bowel to distension with irritable bowel syndrome which responds to treatment with anti-cholinergic drugs.

Treatment

The treatment of irritable bowel syndrome reveals the dichotomy that exists between those who regard the condition as predominantly somatic in origin and those who consider psychological factors as being of paramount importance. A controlled trial of psychotherapy for irritable bowel syndrome which took the form of 10 1-hour sessions was reported by Svedlund et al (1983). In total, 101 men and women with irritable bowel syndrome on conventional treatment with bulk-forming agents and anti-cholinergic drugs were randomly allocated to psychotherapy and a control group. Fifteen months after completion of treatment the psychotherapy group showed a significant improvement over the control group in terms of bowel function and abdominal pain. It is of interest that the initial early improvement observed in the control group tended to regress.

Similar results were reported by Harvey et al (1987) from their study of the short- and long-term results of treatment with reassurance, a bulking agent and an anti-spasmodic drug in 104 individuals. At 5–7 years after treatment started, 23% of these individuals had no symptoms, 45% had occasional minor symptoms, while the remainder were not significantly improved. The authors comment:

> Patients often find that tension worsens their IBS. There is a high prevalence of anxiety or depression among such patients and many doctors believe that the symptoms of IBS in most patients are simply a reflection of their personality disorder. Their good initial and long-term response to physical treatment suggests that most do not have any causative personality disorder but that as their condition is explained and treated their anxiety or depression improves.

The success of different approaches to treating irritable bowel syndrome should not be regarded as conflicting and does suggest that the careful integration of physical and psychological approaches may lead to the most beneficial interventions.

PELVIC CONGESTION

There is obviously a need to find an explanation for the 65% of women who complain of chronic pelvic pain for which no cause can be found. Over the last 150 years gynaecologists have recognized what a disabling symptom this can be and, for a condition for which no cause has been found it is surprising how consistent the description of pelvic vascular stasis or congestion has been. Gooch (1831) referred to 'a morbid state of the pelvic blood vessels' as evidenced by their appearance of fullness. Lawson Tait (1883) advocated bilateral oophorectomy as the best treatment for the condition which he considered was due to ovarian hyperaemia. Taylor in a series of classic publications (1949a–c) coined the term 'the pelvic congestion syndrome'. Histological studies have described the presence of pelvic varicosities in these women whilst venographic studies have demonstrated the presence of dilated pelvic veins with associated congestion. Further evidence for chronic pelvic congestion comes from the careful histological study of Stearns & Sneeden (1966) who described hysterectomy specimens from women with a long history of pelvic pain for which no cause could be found as follows:

> The typical uterus weighed 135–150 g or more with a cavity length of 8.5–10.0 cm (normal 6–8 cm). Sections of the cervix revealed sub-epithelial pale staining bands of oedematous fibrous connective tissue containing dilated lymphatics and blood-filled vascular spaces. There was also oedema, lymphangiectasia and telangiectasia in the subserosal layer.

Causes

Anatomical considerations

The network of veins draining the pelvis have certain characteristics that make them unique in the body. They are thin-walled and unsupported with relatively weak attachments between the adventitia and the supporting connective tissue; they are also notable for their lack of valves. These characteristics enable them to accommodate the sudden changes in blood flow that occur during orgasm, and the progressive increase in volume as the uterus grows during pregnancy. Hodgkinson (1953) estimated that the capacity of pelvic veins increased 60-fold by late pregnancy. These features make them vulnerable in the non-pregnant state to chronic dilatation and stasis with resultant vascular congestion. Factors which further contribute to this tendency to dilatation are weakening of the fascial supports during parturition, and the vasodilating effects of cyclically fluctuating hormones draining the ovaries to which they are exposed in high concentration as vessels draining the ovaries.

The cause of pain due to pelvic congestion remains speculative. The likely possibility is an increased dilatation of the pelvic veins with a concomitant reduction in flow leading to venous congestion and stasis, which may on occasions be so marked as to lead to release of pain-producing substances. Studies by our group have shown that the intravenous administration of the selective venoconstrictor, dihydroergotamine, is followed by a 30% reduction in the diameter of dilated pelvic veins (Reginald et al 1987). This effect is accompanied by a visible increase in pelvic blood flow with the more rapid disappearance of dye and a reduction in pain. The delayed pain response to intravenous dihydroergotamine of 3–4 hours, despite an immediate venoconstricting effect, with the improvement coinciding with the clearance of pain-producing substances from the pelvic tissues, supports the likelihood that congestion is the cause of the pain.

The possibility that distension of the pelvic veins is also a cause of pelvic pain cannot be dismissed. One of the most consistent symptoms in women with pelvic congestion is an increase in pain on standing or bending forwards, while lying down commonly alleviates the pain. Compression of the ovarian vein by the abdomen at the ovarian point as it crosses the transverse process of the second and third lumbar vertebrae results immediately in referred pain at the site of the ovary on that side. The interpretation of these results is complicated by the known vascular changes accompanying a decrease in pelvic blood flow that occurs on standing (Beard et al 1986).

Hormonal factors

It seems likely that pelvic congestion is a product of ovarian dysfunction. The condition only occurs in women of reproductive age and suppression of ovarian function leads to a significant reduction in pain, and oophorectomy to the disappearance of this pain (see section on treatment, below). The high prevalence of cystic ovaries and of an enlarged uterus with thickened ovaries further supports this view. If an ovarian hormone such as oestradiol is directly or indirectly responsible for the venous dilatation it is likely that the reason why these changes are mainly confined to the pelvic veins is because of the much higher concentration of ovarian hormones in the ovarian vein effluent than in peripheral blood. The exact nature of the ovarian dysfunction and why it leads to pelvic congestion in some women and not in others still needs to be determined.

Stearns & Sneeden (1966) considered that a hormonal factor was the most likely cause of pelvic congestion. McCausland et al (1963) reported a 30% increase in venous distensibility a week prior to menstruation and implicated progesterone as the cause, although the possibility that oestrogen played a part was not ruled out. Barwin & McCalden (1972) demonstrated during in vitro experiments that the contractions produced by field stimulation on the smooth muscle in the veins of humans could be blocked by 17-β oestradiol and progesterone. McCausland and coworkers (1961) showed the effect of pregnancy on venous distensibility and thought this was mediated through oestrogen and progesterone on the smooth muscle of the vessel wall. They concluded that increased distensibility contributes to the production of dilated veins in pregnancy.

Psychological factors

The failure in the past to identify a clear organic cause for pain has led to the search for psychological disturbance in women with this condition. Some studies (Benson et al 1959; Magni et al 1984) reported mood disturbance or high levels of psychopathology. However, global measures of psychological disturbance do not seem to play a causal role in chronic pelvic pain, whereas specific differences in attitudes to illness, sexual problems and exposure to death and illness do. Women with previously unexplained pelvic pain report a greater number of deaths and illnesses among family members and close friends. It is likely that this greater exposure to illness acts in some patients to cause a greater attention to health and illness and a closer monitoring of their physical state. They are likely to be paying greater attention to physiological changes in their bodies, leading them to label relatively minor sensations as 'painful'. It seems reasonable to suggest that their preoccupation with physiological changes also leads to them attending to and labelling sensations resulting from pelvic congestion as painful.

A diagrammatic representation of the possible interaction between the different psychological influences discussed above and the somatic changes identified by the venographic studies is provided in Figure 60.2. In this model, women who develop pain associated with pelvic congestion have a predisposition to respond to stress by changes in pelvic blood flow that are either greater in magnitude or take longer to return to baseline levels than normal. The experience of pain then leads to 'pain behaviours', particularly if these are reinforced by concerned family members. Feedback loops may arise at several of these levels of pain experience. Being in pain, for example, is likely to direct further attention to the pelvis and strengthen the central schema or expectation of pain.

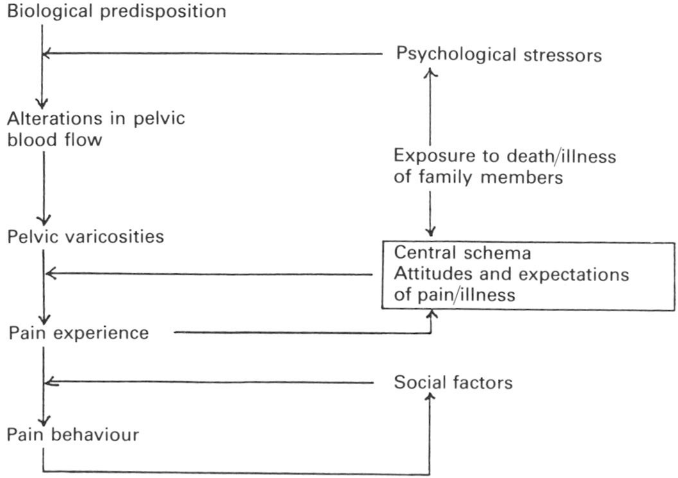

Fig. 60.2 Possible mode of interaction between psychological and somatic factors in pelvic pain associated with pelvic congestion. From Beard & Pearce (1989).

Such a model is clearly speculative and should give rise to experimental investigations to test some of the hypothetical links. However, it does suggest a number of potential levels of intervention. Treatment could be directed at the somatic level or at the alteration of the central schema or manipulation of expectations influencing pain perception. Alternatively, it could be directed towards altering pain behaviours and the responses to pain and attitudes of family members.

Clinical presentation

Women with pain due to pelvic congestion are always in the reproductive age group with a mean age of 32 years, and can be nulliparous or parous. The duration of the pain varies from 6 months to 20 years. Typically the pain is dull and aching similar to dysmenorrhoea and is interspersed with acute episodes. It is situated, more commonly, in one or other iliac fossa but occurs occasionally on the contralateral side. These women commonly have a number of other complaints such as vaginal discharge, backache, headache and urinary symptoms although bowel symptoms are uncommon. They may have a history of being treated on a number of occasions for pelvic inflammatory disease (46%) and have often had some form of lower abdominal surgery such as the removal of simple cysts of the ovary or appendectomy (48%). Menstrual cycle defects are common (54%) and congestive dysmenorrhoea is often present (66%). The frequency of regular sexual intercourse is diminished (46%) and apareunia is common. The most usual reason given for this change in sexual activity is deep dyspareunia (71%) and postcoital ache (65%), which is one of the most consistent findings in women with pelvic congestion. There is often a history of serious illness in family members and close friends, and many report major losses in childhood in this group, such as the separation from parents as a result of divorce. A detailed comparison of psychological differences between women with pelvic congestion and those with clear pathology is presented by Pearce (1988).

Physical signs

On examination the abdomen feels soft and, unless the woman is having an acute attack of pain, it is unusual to elicit tenderness on pressure in either iliac fossae. However, deep pressure over the ovarian point (the junction of the upper and middle third of a line drawn from the umbilicus to the anterior–superior iliac spine) commonly elicits pain in the iliac fossa (77%). Vaginal examination may reveal a visibly congested vagina with a blue or violet colour and an eroded cervix. If the woman is experiencing moderate or severe pain, the whole pelvis will be tender, but typically in a quiescent phase it is only the ovaries and sometimes the uterus which on gentle compression are tender.

Although a provisional diagnosis can be made from a good history and clinical examination, a definitive diagnosis can only be made by further investigation. A full blood count is nearly always normal and investigations such as urine culture, intravenous pyelography and barium enema are only useful when urinary or bowel disturbance is complained of. The following investigations should be done routinely.

Investigations

Laparoscopy

Laparoscopy is usually done to exclude pelvic endometriosis and pelvic inflammatory disease as relatively infrequent causes of chronic pelvic pain. When pelvic congestion is present the whole pelvis may appear hyperaemic, leading to a mistaken diagnosis of acute pelvic inflammatory disease. Large dilated pelvic veins on the back of the broad ligament and/or infundibulopelvic ligament may be seen at the start of the laparoscopy; these then disappear. Careful inspection will often reveal bulky mobile ovaries with multiple subcortical follicular cysts. An excess of straw-coloured fluid is often seen in the pouch of Douglas.

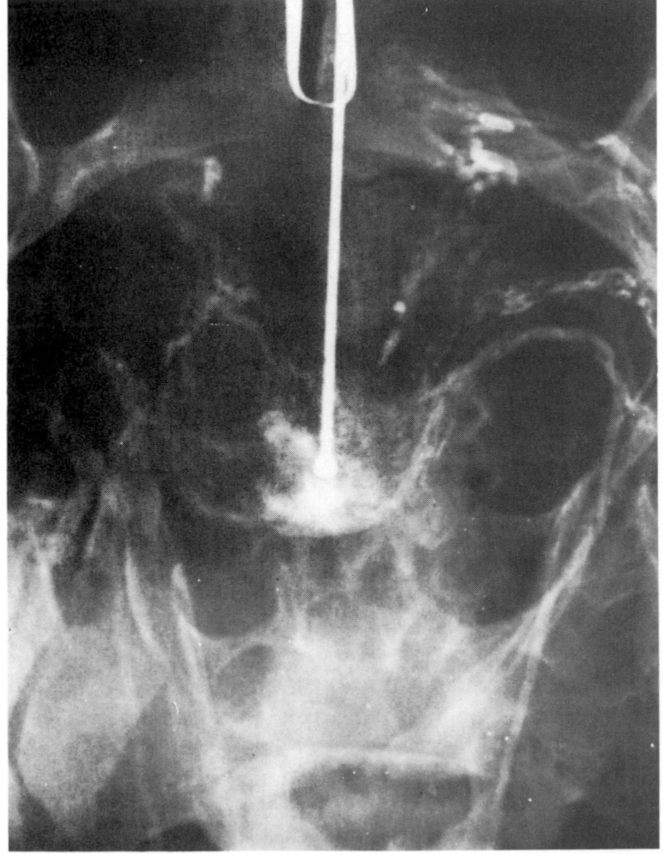

Fig. 60.3 Normal venogram: end of injection.

Pelvic venography

Pelvic venography is a technique developed by Topolanski-Sierra (1958) for displaying the pelvic veins and observing the rate of venous blood flow. The patient is premedicated with intravenous benzodiazepam. A radiopaque dye, which has previously been warmed, is injected over 1–2 min into the myometrium. The passage of the dye through the uterine, vesical and ovarian veins and into the common iliac veins is observed on a fluoroscopic screen. In a normal woman all the dye disappears by 20 s after the injection, and when it is visible the diameter of the ovarian vein is less than 4 mm (Fig. 60.3). Women with pelvic pain syndrome have evidence of dilated veins, particularly the

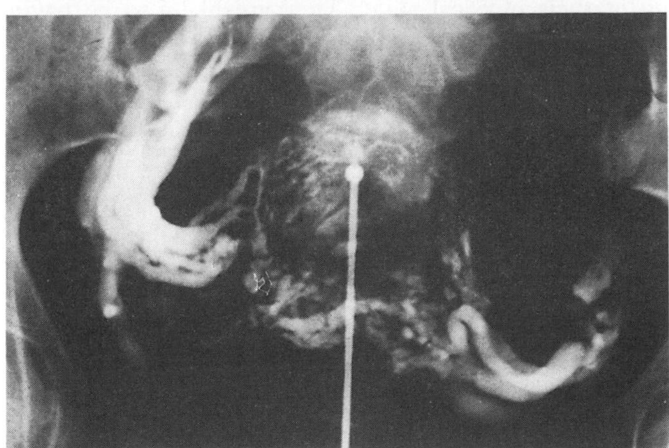

Fig. 60.4 Abnormal venogram: end of injection.

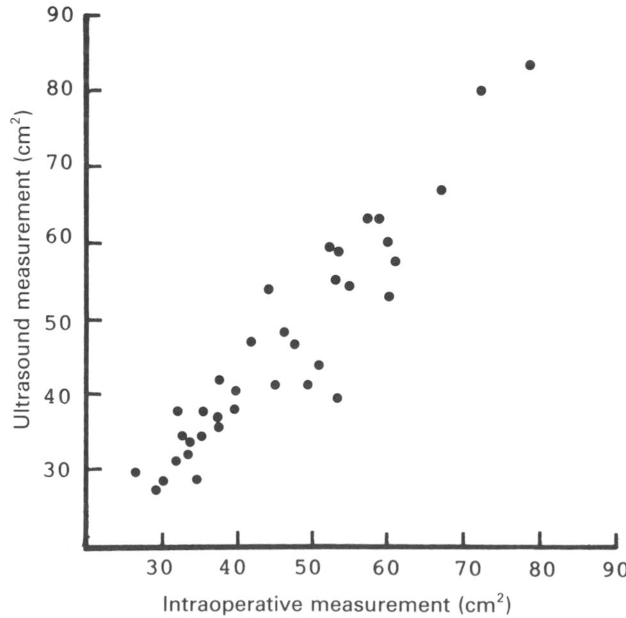

Fig. 60.5 Comparison of ultrasound and intraoperative caliper measurements of uterine cross-sectional area. $n = 38$; $r = 0.94$. From Saxton et al (1990).

Table 60.2 Measurement of uterine cross-sectional area (length × breadth) and thickness of endometrium on days 10–14 of the cycle in women with regular cycles (Adams et al 1990). The prevalence of cystic ovaries in women with pelvic congestion is compared with that in normal women (Polson et al 1988)

	Cross-sectional area of uterus in cm^2 (s.d.)	Endometrial thickness in mm (s.d.)	Presence of cystic ovaries
Pelvic congestion	39.1 (6.1)	11.5 (3.1)	56%
Normal	28.3 (6.2)	7.5 (1.8)	23%

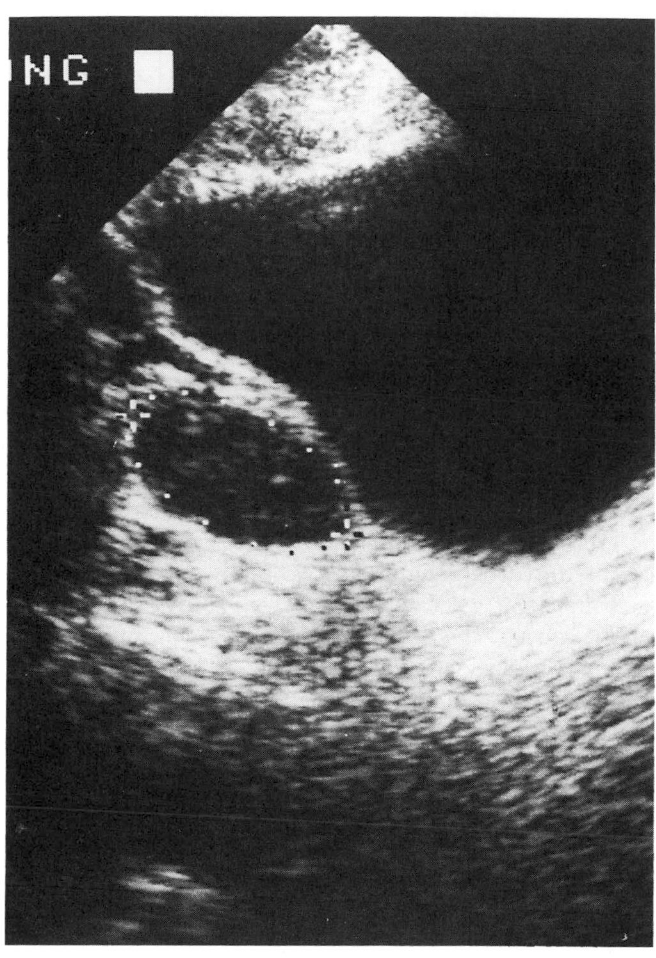

a

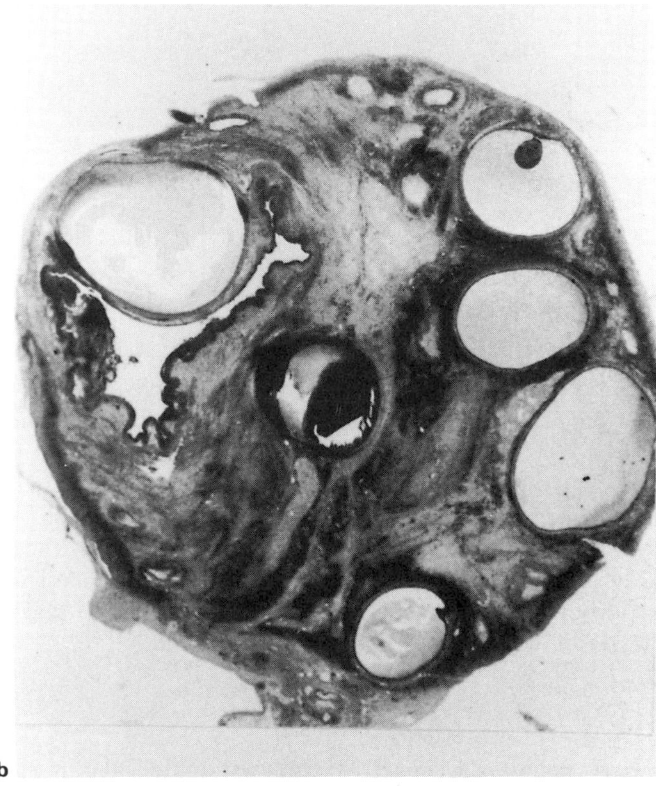

b

Fig. 60.6 (**a**) Ultrasound scan showing a cystic ovary. From Saxton et al (1990). (**b**) Photomicrograph of the same ovary. From Saxton et al (1990).

ovarian vein (range 4–15 mm), delayed disappearance and pooling of dye (Fig. 60.4). A venographic study of women complaining of pelvic pain (Beard et al 1984) showed that pelvic congestion, defined as dilated pelvic veins and vascular stasis with delayed disappearance of dye, was a common finding in the women with no apparent cause for their pelvic pain. Using a scoring system for grading the abnormality of the venogram it was found that with venography a diagnostic sensitivity of 91% and specificity of 89% could be achieved.

Ultrasonography

Abdominal ultrasound scanning is used to display and measure the pelvic organs. The size of the uterus can be measured with considerable accuracy, as shown in Figure 60.5 (Saxton et al 1989). Recent studies, summarized in Table 60.2, have shown that women with pelvic congestion have an enlarged uterus, thicker endometrium and that 56% have cystic ovaries (Fig. 60.6). It is also possible to show dilated veins in the broad ligament (Fig. 60.7) and by use of a vaginal ultrasound probe, dilated veins in the cervix. Ultrasound scanning and pelvic venography are complementary diagnostic techniques to each other, providing information on the structure of pelvic organs and the function of the pelvic venous circulation.

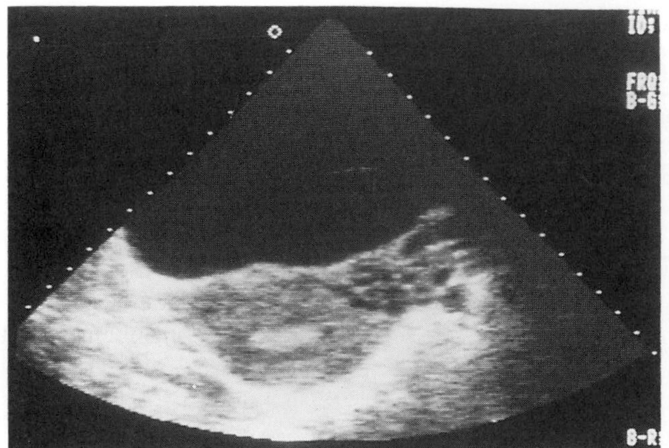

Fig. 60.7 Ultrasound scan showing transverse section of the uterus with the uterine cavity and dilated veins to the left of the uterus.

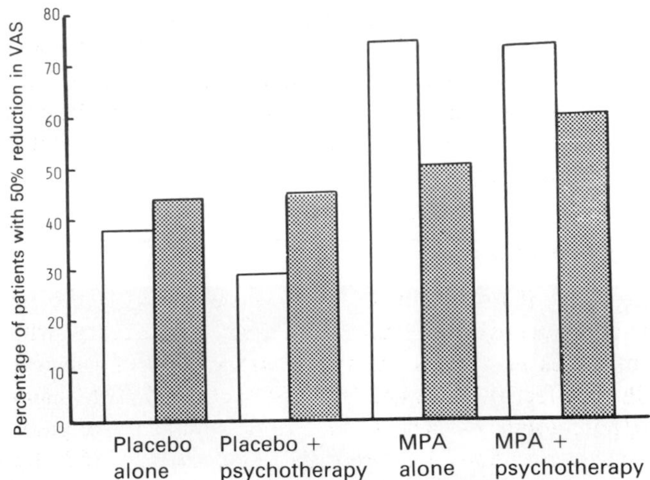

Fig. 60.8 Percentage of patients with 50% reduction in visual analogue scale (VAS) pain-rating at the end of treatment with medroxyprogesterone acetate (MPA) (4 months; open boxes) and 6 months after completion of treatment (10 months; hatched boxes).

Treatment

Women with pelvic congestion are in the reproductive period of life so medical treatment is preferable to surgery. The temptation to recommend surgical treatment of some form is considerable because of the lack of confidence in medical treatment as a means of achieving a permanent cure for pain and the strong desire most women who suffer from the condition have to obtain a final solution without delay. It should be understood when reading the following section that the characterization and management of pelvic congestion are still in a developmental phase.

Medical treatment

Suppression of ovarian activity is based on the concept that pelvic congestion is the result of oestrogen activity. Luciano et al (1986) reported that the progestogen medroxyprogesterone acetate in a dose of 50 mg/day reduces secretion of oestrogen to a blood concentration equal to that found in the early part of the follicular phase of the cycle. The advantage of avoiding total suppression of oestrogen secretion is that unpleasant side-effects do not complicate the treatment.

A pilot study of 21 women with proven pelvic congestion treated with oral medroxyprogesterone acetate 30 mg/day for 6 months was undertaken (Reginald et al 1989). By the end of treatment three-quarters of the women showed a significant reduction in pain as rated by the visual analogue scale. Venography done at this time showed a diminution in the diameter of the pelvic veins with a striking reduction in congestion. In the light of this pilot study a double-blind randomized controlled trial of treatment with medroxyprogesterone acetate and/or psychotherapy was done (Farquhar et al 1989). Figure 60.8 shows a statistically significant benefit in terms of a reduction in pain after 4 months' treatment with medroxyprogesterone acetate alone. Six months after stopping treatment the beneficial effects of treatment with medroxyprogesterone acetate alone were still present but were no longer greater than in the placebo group. However, the group treated by medroxyprogesterone acetate plus psychotherapy showed the greatest benefit at this time.

Oral dihydroergotamine is useful in the treatment of postcoital ache due to pelvic congestion. Unfortunately the manufacturers (Sandoz) have now withdrawn this drug and further studies of drugs with a similar selective venoconstrictor activity in the treatment of both deep dyspareunia and postcoital ache are needed.

Psychological interventions

Psychological interventions have largely been investigated for their value in the management of women with unexplained pelvic pain, but given the involvement of psychological processes in the perception of all kinds of pain, there is no a priori reason why they should be any more beneficial for women with unexplained pelvic pain than, for example, women with endometriosis. Strategies which help women to be distracted from the painful stimulation and to cope despite the pain may be helpful for all forms of pelvic as well as other chronic pain conditions. Where pathology is identified, other treatment approaches may also be indicated and it is likely that advances in pain management will involve a closer integration of pharmacological, surgical and psychological methods of pain control. To date, however, psychological approaches have been almost exclusively used for unexplained pelvic pain whilst medical and surgical approaches are used for conditions with visible pathology.

Relaxation training has been recommended in the treatment of women with pelvic pain (Beard et al 1977). This form of treatment has the inevitable drawback of requiring a considerable amount of time from a therapist. However, many of the patients are emotionally disturbed and it is likely that any improvement in pain is likely to be more long-lasting if treatment includes some form of counselling or psychotherapy.

Surgical treatment

Logically, if ovarian dysfunction is the cause of the pain of pelvic congestion, then any form of surgery which diminishes or ablates the functional activity of the ovary will be effective. Lawson Tait (1883) claimed that bilateral oophorectomy was always successful in curing the pain of pelvic congestion. Dudley (1888) and Railo (1968) have reported that division of the ovarian veins is a successful method of treatment while Rundquist et al (1984) reported that in 15 women who had had a ligation of the left ovarian vein and who were followed up for 5–6 years, 8 had no pain while 3 showed marked improvement. Our preliminary results do not support those findings.

The statement by Taylor (1959) that 'premature resort to surgery is the characteristic error in the treatment of women with pelvic pain' is even more apposite today now that effective medical treatment is available. Nevertheless it is our experience that there is a minority of women for whom surgery is eventually the only solution. These are usually women aged 28–35 years who have completed their family and who have failed to respond to all forms of medical treatment. Initial follow-up for a year after hysterectomy and bilateral salpingo-oophorectomy followed by hormone replacement therapy has shown a complete resolution of pain with a return to a normal social and sexual life. These preliminary results are encouraging but should not be regarded as an indication for primary treatment of pelvic congestion by hysterectomy and bilateral oophorectomy. In our large experience of managing more than 1000 women who have come to the clinic complaining of pelvic pain, only 35 have eventually required this operation. The remaining women have been managed successfully by a variety of medical and psychological interventions.

KEY POINTS

1. Sensory innervation of the pelvis is via both sympathetic and parasympathetic nerves.
2. The sympathetic innervation of the uterus, medial part of the fallopian tube and upper part of the vagina travels via paracervical and hypogastric plexus to enter the spinal cord through the posterior nerve roots at the level of T10–L1.
3. The sympathetic innervation of the lateral part of the fallopian tube, ovary and broad ligament travels along the ovarian vessels to the aortic plexus.
4. Parasympathetic fibres travel along the pudendal nerve and enter the spinal cord at S2–S4.
5. 44% of patients undergoing laparoscopy for acute pelvic pain will have a normal pelvis.
6. Of patients laparascoped for chronic pelvic pain, 65% will have a normal pelvis, 20% adhesions and 12% endometriosis.
7. Trapped or residual ovary syndrome occurs in 1–3% of cases after hysterectomy.
8. 22% of patients with endometriosis will be asymptomatic, but only 5% will have all of the classic symptoms of endometriosis (dysmenorrhoea, dyspareunia, pelvic pain and infertility).
9. Chronic pelvic pain can be caused by entrapment of the iliohypogastric nerve in a pfannenstiel incision.
10. The commonest infective organism in pelvic inflammatory disease is Chlamydia.
11. Pelvic congestion occurs in women of reproductive years.
12. Pelvic congestion may occur in nulliparous women.
13. Pelvic congestion can be diagnosed by venography, laparoscopy or vaginal ultrasound.
14. Pelvic congestion can be treated medically by medroxyprogesterone acetate 50 mg/day for 6 months.
15. Pelvic congestion can be treated surgically by total abdominal hysterectomy and bilateral salpingo-oophorectomy followed by hormone replacement therapy.

REFERENCES

Adams J, Reginald P W, Franks S, Wadsworth J, Beard R W 1990 Uterine size and endometrial thickness and the significance of cystic ovaries in women with pelvic pain due to congestion. British Journal of Obstetrics and Gynaecology 97: 583–587

Alexander-Williams J 1987 Do adhesions cause pain? British Medical Journal 294: 659–660

Barwin B N, McCalden T A 1972 The inhibitory action of estradiol-17 β and progesterone on human venous smooth muscle. Journal of Physiology 227: 41P

Beard R W, Pearce S 1989 Gynaecological pain. In: Wall P D, Melzack R (eds) Textbook of pain, 2nd edn. Churchill Livingstone, Edinburgh, pp 466–481

Beard R W, Belsey E N, Lieberman M B, Wilkinson J C M 1977 Pelvic pain in women. American Journal of Obstetrics and Gynecology 128: 566–570

Beard R W, Highman J W, Pearce S, Reginald P W 1984 Diagnosis of pelvic varicosities in women with chronic pelvic pain. Lancet ii: 946–949

Beard R W, Randall N J, Reginald P W, Sutherland I A, Wertheim D F B 1986 Postural changes in pelvic blood flow in women. Journal of Physiology 374: 9p

Beard R W, Reginald P W, Wadsworth J 1988 Clinical features of women with chronic lower abdominal pain and pelvic congestion. British Journal of Obstetrics and Gynaecology 95: 153–161

Benson R, Hanson K, Matarazzo J 1959 Atypical pelvic pain in women: gynecologic psychiatric considerations. American Journal of Obstetrics and Gynecology 77: 806–823

Bosanko C 1982 An investigation of factors influencing menstrual cycle complaints with particular reference to the attitude of women and their partners towards menstruation. Dissertation for M Clin Psychol, University of Liverpool

Brihmer C, Kallings I, Nord C E, Brundin J 1987 Salpingitis; aspects of diagnosis and etiology: a 4 year study from a Swedish capital hospital. European Journal of Obstetrics, Gynecology and Reproductive Biology 24: 211–220

Chamberlain G, Brown J C (eds) 1978 Gynaecological laparoscopy. Report of the working party on gynaecological laparoscopy. Royal College of Obstetricians and Gynaecologists, London

Christ J L, Lotze E C 1975 The residual ovary syndrome. Obstetrics and Gynecology 46: 555–566

Dudley A 1888 Varicocoele in the female. What is its influence on the ovary? New York Medical Journal 48: 174–177

Farquhar C M, Rogers V, Franks S, Pearce S, Wadsworth J, Beard R W 1989 A randomised controlled trial of medroxyprogesterone acetate and psychotherapy for the treatment of pelvic congestion. British Journal of Obstetrics and Gynaecology 96: 1153–1162

Golub S 1976 The effect of premenstrual anxiety and depression on cognitive function. Journal of Personality and Social Psychology 34: 99–104

Gooch R 1831 On some of the most important diseases peculiar to women. Republished by the Sydenham Society, London 1859, pp 299–331

Harvey R F, Mauad E C, Brown A M 1987 Prognosis in the irritable bowel syndrome: a 5-year prospective study. Lancet i: 963–965

Heaton K W 1983 Irritable bowel syndrome: still in search of its identity. British Medical Journal 287: 852–853

Hodgkinson C P 1953 Physiology of the ovarian veins during pregnancy. Obstetrics and Gynecology 1: 26–37

Kresh A J, Seifer D B, Sachs L B, Barrese I 1984 Laparoscopy in 100 woman with chronic pelvic pain. Obstetrics and Gynecology 64: 672–674

Levitan Z, Eibschitz I, de Uries K, Hakim M, Sharf M 1985 The value of laparoscopy in women with chronic pelvic pain and a 'normal pelvis'. International Journal of Gynaecology and Obstetrics 23: 71–74

Liston W A, Bradford W P, Downie J, Kerr M G 1972 Laparoscopy in a general gynaecological unit. American Journal of Obstetrics and Gynecology 113: 672–677

Luciano A A, Turksey R N, Dlugi A M, Carleo J L 1986 Endocrine consequences of oral medroxyprogesterone acetate (MPA) in the treatment of endometriosis. Proceedings of the 68th Annual Meeting of the Endocrine Society, Anaheim, California. Abstract 694 p 204

Lundberg W I, Wall J E, Mathers J E 1973 Laparoscopy in the evaluation of pelvic pain. Obstetrics and Gynecology 42: 872–876

Magni G, Salni A, Leo D, Ceola A 1984 Chronic pelvic pain and depression. Psychopathology 17: 132–136

McCausland A M, Hyman G, Winsor T, Trotter A D Jr 1961 Venous distensibility during pregnancy. American Journal of Obstetrics and Gynecology 81: 472–478

McCausland A M, Holmes F, Trotter A D Jr 1963 Venous distensibility during menstrual cycle. American Journal of Obstetrics and Gynecology 68: 640–643

Morris N, O'Neill D 1958 Outpatient gynaecology. British Medical Journal 2: 1038

Murphy A, Fliegner J 1981 Diagnostic laparoscopy. Role in the management of acute pelvic pain. Medical Journal of Australia 1: 571–573

O'Connor D T 1987 Endometriosis. Churchill Livingstone, Edinburgh

Pearce S 1988 The concept of psychogenic pain. Current Psychological Research and Reviews 6: 219–228

Pent D 1972 Laparoscopy: its role in private practice. American Journal of Obstetrics and Gynecology 113: 459–468

Pettit P D, Lee R A 1988 Ovarian remnant syndrome: diagnostic dilemma and surgical challenge. Obstetrics and Gynecology 71: 580–583

Polan M, de Cherney A 1980 Presacral neurectomy for pelvic pain infertility. Fertility and Sterility 321: 557–560

Polson D W, Adams J, Wadsworth J, Franks S 1988 Polycystic ovaries — a common finding in normal women. Lancet i: 870–872

Railo J E 1968 The pain syndrome in ovarian varicocoele. Acta Chirurgica Scandinavica 134: 157–159

Rapkin A J 1986 Adhesions and pelvic pain: a retrospective study. Obstetrics and Gynecology 68: 13–15

Reginald P W, Beard R W, Kooner J S et al 1987 Intravenous dihydroergotamine to relieve pelvic congestion with pain in young women. Lancet ii: 351–353

Reginald P W, Pearce S, Beard R W 1989 Pelvic pain due to pelvic congestion. In: Studd J (ed) Progess in obstetrics and gynaecology. Churchill Livingstone, Edinburgh, pp 275–292

Renaer M 1981 Chronic pelvic pain in women. Springer-Verlag, Berlin, p 100

Rundquist E, Sandholm L E, Larsson G 1984 Treatment of pelvic varicosities causing lower abdominal pain with extra peritoneal resection of the left ovarian vein. Annales Chirurgiae et Gynaecologiae 73: 339–341

Saxton D W, Farquhar C M, Rae T, Beard R W, Anderson M C, Wadsworth J 1989 Accuracy of ultrasound measurements of female pelvic organs. British Journal of Obstetrics and Gynaecology 97: 695–699

Schmidt C 1985 Endometriosis: a reappraisal of pathogenesis and treatment. Fertility and Sterility 44: 157–173

Slocumb J C 1984 Neurological factors in chronic pelvic pain: trigger points and the abdominal pelvic pain syndrome. American Journal of Obstetrics and Gynecology 149: 536–543

Stacey C M, Munday P E, Beard R W 1989 Pelvic inflammatory disease: diagnosis and microbiology. Presented at the Silver Jubilee Congress of Obstetrics and Gynaecology, London

Stearns H C, Sneeden U D 1966 Observations on the clinical and pathological aspects of the pelvic congestion syndrome. American Journal of Obstetrics and Gynecology 94: 718–732

Svedlund J, Ottosson J O, Sjodin I, Doteval G 1983 Controlled study of psychotherapy in irritable bowel syndrome. Lancet ii: 589–592

Tait 1883 The pathology and treatment of the diseases of the ovaries. William Wood, New York

Taylor H C 1949a Vascular congestion and hyperemia I: psychologic basis and history of the concept. American Journal of Obstetrics and Gynecology 57: 211–230

Taylor H C 1949b Vascular congestion and hyperemia II: the clinical aspects of the congestion — fibrosis syndrome. American Journal of Obstetrics and Gynecology 57: 637–653

Taylor H C 1949c Vascular congestion and hyperemia III: etiology and therapy. American Journal of Obstetrics and Gynecology 57: 654–668

Taylor H C 1959 The pelvic pain syndrome. Journal of Obstetrics and Gynaecology of the British Empire 66: 733–761

Topolanski-Sierra R 1958 Pelvic phlebography. American Journal of Obstetrics and Gynecology 76: 44–52

SECTION 8

Legal and General

61. The gynaecologist as defendant and expert witness

R. V. Clements M. Puxon

THE LEGAL FRAMEWORK

Gynaecologists, like any other practitioners, may find themselves in legal conflict with their patients when anything goes wrong with treatment. While there are particular risk areas in gynaecology (see Ch. 62), practitioners in this field face the same traps and snares as do all medical workers, indeed all who offer their professional services to the public.

Two types of action may arise: breach of contract and negligence, which is a breach of duty.

Breach of contract

Whenever a practitioner agrees to advise or treat a patient, it is an implied term of that agreement that he will 'bring a fair, reasonable and competent degree of skill' to the care of that patient (Tindal 1838).

> An attorney does not undertake that at all events you shall gain your case, neither does a surgeon undertake that he will perform a cure; nor does he undertake to use the highest possible degree of skill (Tindal 1838).

But if the surgeon fails to comply with the standards of that profession he will be in breach of the contract and liable for the return of any fees that may have been paid and damages for any resultant loss or suffering to the patient. The surgeon will also be liable to compensate the patient for any loss (such as loss of earnings) or expenses incurred, including the cost of further treatment.

Negligence

In practice most actions against doctors are brought in negligence, which is a tort — a wrongful act at common law, for which the law provides a remedy. The test of fault, however, is the same whether the alleged breach is of the contract or of the duty all professional people have to their clients.

It is not always appreciated that the doctor is in the same position before the law as any other professional person who offers skills, whether lawyer, accountant, surveyor or architect. The level of skill required is that which other members of that particular profession regarded as fair and reasonable at the time of the alleged act of negligence. Thus the standard imposed is that of one's peers — not of the public, nor of the judge, although it will be the judge's decision, after hearing all the evidence, to decide what was in fact the accepted standard of care at the time.

This has been the position for at least 30 years, and it was finally given the accolade of the House of Lords in the case of *Whitehouse* v. *Jordan* (1980) when Lord Edmund Davis said this:

> Doctors and surgeons fall into no special category and . . . I would have it accepted that the true doctrine was enunciated by *McNair J in Bolam* v. *Friern Hospital Management Committee (1957)* in the following words: '. . . where you get a situation which involves the use of some special skill or competence, then the test as to whether there has been negligence or not is not the test of the man on the top of a Clapham omnibus (a well known figure in law) because he has not got this special skill. The test in the standard of the ordinary skilled man exercising and professing to have that special skill'.
>
> If a surgeon fails to measure up to that standard in *any* respect ('clinical judgment' or otherwise), he has been negligent and should be so adjudged.

Such, then, is the test for *all* professional people and short of legislation, that ruling of the House of Lords will remain the touchstone of medical liability at every level, from the most eminent down to the newly qualified. It must be emphasized that in deciding whether a doctor has been negligent, the law is not concerned with general ethics but only with the interest of the patient within the bounds already defined.

That does not necessarily mean that the same standards will apply to the consultant gynaecologist as to the junior house officer, but if a service is offered, then the practitioner who carries out that service will be judged by the standards expected by the profession for that particular service; if there is no one adequately trained to do the job properly, it will not be a defence to the health authority or even the doctor concerned if something goes wrong because of the doctor's inexperience. The provision of adequate skilled staff is a problem for Parliament rather than for the law (*Wilsher* v. *Essex Area Health Authority* 1987): if no one properly trained is available, the operation should not be carried out.

Burden of proof and causation

To succeed with an action, the plaintiff must prove on the balance of probabilities that the defendant was negligent. The defendant does not have to prove that he was *not* negligent.

Even if negligence is proved, there can be no finding of liability against the doctor unless the plaintiff can also prove, again on the balance of probabilities, that the injuries and loss complained of were directly caused by that particular negligence. The plaintiff in a medical negligence claim thus has a difficult task. It is right that this should be so, but it is also right that when there is negligence, the patient should be properly compensated.

Expert witness

In deciding whether the defendant has been negligent the judge will have to hear expert evidence called by both the plaintiff and the defendant. If the experts on both sides differ in their views of what was the proper course of action for the defendant to take in the particular circumstances, as frequently happens when a case comes to court, this will usually indicate that there is a competent body of medical opinion holding the contrary view to that put forward by the plaintiff in her allegation that the defendant fell below the appropriate standards. It may be that the experts on the two sides will come together during the process of questioning and cross-examination during the trial; if not the judge can accept or reject the medical evidence on one side or the other, assessing the credibility of the witnesses. But the judge must not choose between the two views put forward simply because he prefers the opinion of one expert to the other: see the House of Lords' ruling in *Maynard* v. *West Midlands Regional Health Authority* (1985).

Would it not be better if the experts on both sides could come together without a time-consuming and expensive hearing in court, thrash out their differences and resolve the issues as to whether the management of the case could or could not be supported by a responsible body of the profession, and whether the resulting injuries were in fact caused by the failure of the surgeon? Under recent Rules of Court (referred to below 1) it is hoped that experts will in many cases meet before the hearing; if it then appears to both sides that there is substantial support for the treatment given by the defendant, the plaintiff will almost certainly be advised not to pursue her claim, or perhaps to settle for a modest sum where there is an element of doubt as to her chances of discharging the burden of proof.

It is certainly very important, both from the public's point of view and that of the medical profession, that experts of high calibre should be readily available to give their independent disinterested opinions on these cases. Good opinions, given at an early stage, will often avert litigation or produce a reasonable settlement without a court hearing.

Consent

An increasingly important risk area for all doctors is the question of consent. No one may lay hands on another against their will without running the risk of criminal prosecution for assault and, if injury results, a civil action for damages for trespass or negligence. In the case of a doctor, consent to any physical interference will readily be implied: a woman must be assumed to consent to a normal physical examination if she consults a gynaecologist, in the absence of clear evidence of her refusal or restriction of such examination. The problems arise when the gynaecologist's intervention results in unfortunate side-effects or permanent interference with functions, whether or not any part of the body is removed. For example, if a gynaecologist agrees with the patient to perform a hysterectomy and removes the ovaries without her specific consent, that will be a trespass and an act of negligence. The only available defence will be that it was necessary for the life of the patient to proceed at once to remove the ovaries because of some perceived pathology in them.

What is meant by consent? The term 'informed consent' is often used, but there is no such concept in English law. The consent must be *real*: that is to say, the patient must have been given sufficient information for her to understand the nature of the operation, its likely effects, and any complications which may arise and which the surgeon in the exercise of his duty to the patient considers she should be made aware of — only then can she reach a proper decision. But the surgeon need not warn the patient of remote risks, any more than an anaesthetist need warn the patient that a certain small number of those anaesthetized never recover consciousness or suffer cardiac arrest. Only where there is a recognized risk, rather than a rare complication, is the surgeon under an obligation to warn the patient of that risk. He is not under a duty to warn the patient of the possible results of hypothetical negligent surgery.

The duty to inform the patient before she consents to any physical intrusion is judged by the same criteria as apply to all other aspects of treatment. Lord Diplock said in the House of Lords in 1985:

> The doctor's relationship with his patient which gives rise to the normal duty of care to exercise his skill and judgement to improve the patient's health . . . is . . . a single comprehensive duty covering all the ways in which a doctor is called upon to exercise his skill and judgement . . . *including warning of something going wrong however skilfully the treatment advised is carried out* (*Sideway* v. *Bethlem Royal Hospital Governors* 1985).

In advising an operation, therefore, the doctor must do so in the way in which a competent gynaecologist exercising reasonable skill and care in similar circumstances would have done. In doing this he will take into account the personality of the patient and the importance of the operation to her future well-being. It may be good practice not to warn a very nervous patient of any possible complications if she requires immediate surgery for, say, a malignant condition. The doctor must decide how much to say to her taking into account his assessment of her personality, the questions she asks and his view of how much she understands. If the patient asks a direct question, she must be given a truthful answer.

To take the example of hysterectomy, while the surgeon will tell the patient that it is proposed to remove her uterus and perhaps her ovaries and describe what that will mean for her future well-being (sterility, premature menopause), she will not be warned of the possibility of damage to the ureters, vesicovaginal fistula, fatal haemorrhage, or anaesthetic death. Where the surgeon feels that there is information which should be imparted to the patient, but her condition and the urgency of the matter make it advisable and in her interest not to go into much detail, it is wise to tell her husband or a close relative of any possible complications. The important thing is not to mislead the patient in any way without some very cogent reason, and then only after careful consideration and discussion with colleagues and perhaps relatives. Where the surgeon feels in a dilemma, in the end he must resolve it alone, but should always make a contemporaneous note recording the reasons for his decision. This will be strong support for his evidence for rebutting any later charge of assault or negligence.

The consent form

The signing of a consent form is some evidence that the patient has been given an opportunity to decide whether or not to undergo the operation after full information, but it is not as important as the evidence of the surgeon as to what he said to the patient and whether or not she understood. The 'catch-all' clause giving the surgeon permission to do anything necessary does not give roving authority to remove whatever he fancies may be for the good of the patient. The surgeon cannot, for example, construe a consent to termination of pregnancy as a licence to sterilize the patient. Explanation of the law on consent is provided in a new DHS publication (A Guide to Consent for Examination or Treatment: NHS Management Executive 1990) which includes model consent forms.

The surgeon needs no consent for any emergency procedure. But as one of the aims of good medical practice is to avoid misunderstandings later, it is wise to discuss any emergency with relatives if this is practicable, as part of the general policy of open communication which is so important in the avoidance of litigation.

Consent of third parties

Only the individual concerned can, strictly, give consent for any interference with her body. It is the practice to obtain the consent of a parent for operation on a minor (i.e. under 18), but since the Family Law Reform Act of 1969 a minor who has attained the age of 16 years can give effective consent to any surgical, medical or dental treatment without parental consent. If such consent is refused for an operation on a girl under 16 years, and that operation is regarded as essential for the well-being of the girl, the only course is for her to be made a ward of court, and the court's consent obtained. Sometimes a local authority will take this step or a parent or medical practitioner may do so. Where the minor is a ward of court, even if she is over 16 years, the court's consent must be obtained to any intervention. This is something of an anomaly.

In this country (although not in some states of America) the courts cannot order a surgeon to operate.

Consent for the mentally handicapped

A further problem as to consent arises in those cases where an adult is incapable of giving consent by reason of mental disability. In the case of *F* v. *West Berkshire Health Authority* (1985) the House of Lords ruled that no court has jurisdiction to give or withhold consent to such an operation in such an adult (unlike the position with a minor) but that the court can make a declaration that the proposed operation is lawful 'in the circumstances in the best interests of the woman'. They went on to say that although such a declaration is not necessary to establish the lawfulness of the operation, 'in practice the court's jurisdiction should be invoked whenever such an operation is to be performed'. In view of this ruling, any gynaecologist who believes such a patient requires sterilization, having come to that decision applying the standards laid down in the Bolam test (*Bolam* v. *Friern Barnet* 1957), should ensure that an application is made to the court for approval of the lawfulness of the operation. Lord Brandon said:

> The applicant should normally be those responsible for the care of the patient or those intending to carry out the proposed operation or other treatment if it is declared to be lawful — *i.e. the health authority or the surgeon* (*F* v. *West Berkshire Health Authority* 1985).

But their Lordships stressed that the doctor would have a common law duty to operate in such circumstances if it was in the best interests of the patient. If, therefore, for some reason no application to the court were made, it would seem that a surgeon could not be held guilty of trespass or negligence if he went on to operate, always keeping within the Bolam principle.

Husband's consent

The consent of a husband is never required for surgery on his wife, not even for sterilization. Nor can he prevent her from having an abortion within the law. But if the woman is unable to give real consent because of her condition, it is a wise precaution to discuss the case fully with the husband, always provided that she waives the duty of confidentiality. But if he does not give his consent, the surgeon must decide independently whether or not to operate, and it will be the surgeon's duty to do so if he believes it necessary.

Abortion

A gynaecologist who undertakes to terminate a pregnancy or to sterilize a patient will be liable in damages if the child is nevertheless born alive, or if the woman becomes pregnant as a result of negligence. But there is no right of action in English law for permitting a 'wrongful life'.

In a case in 1982 (*McKay* v. *Essex Health Authority* 1982) the Court of Appeal decided that a gynaecologist who failed to diagnose rubella in the mother, and thus failed to terminate her pregnancy as she would have wished if she had been told of the risks, was not liable to the child for the handicaps he suffered.

A negligent failed abortion can give rise to a claim for damages. In 1979 an unmarried woman was awarded damages for pain and suffering, loss of earnings and reduced chance of marriage because she went to term after an attempted aspiration abortion at the 7th week (*Sciuriaga* v. *Powell* 1980). She did not claim the expense of bringing up the child as she had an affiliation order. The judge held that the gynaecologist had been negligent and rejected the defence that she should have mitigated her damages by having a mid-term abortion when it was discovered that she was still pregnant, saying that it was reasonable for her to refuse termination after she had felt fetal movement. The defence that has been raised in such cases, that it is contrary to public policy to allow a mother to claim damages for the birth of a child who is a source of joy and satisfaction to her, has been rejected by the courts.

Sterilization

Failed sterilization claims have become frequent and most of them settle before coming to court. Lack of advice as to the risk of failure of the operation has caused particular problems. The question as to whether the standard of information before consent is obtained for the operation should be different where it has been performed on contraceptive rather than therapeutic grounds was considered in a case brought in 1987 by a woman who became pregnant after a sterilization (properly performed), alleging that she had not been warned of the risks of failure (*Gold* v. *Haringey Health Authority* 1987). She claimed that if she had been so warned and had been properly advised as to the alternatives she and her husband would have elected for him to have a vasectomy. The Court of Appeal held that the standard of care required of a doctor was the same whatever the context in which the advice was given, and although the experts agreed that at the date of the hearing (1987) they personally would have advised as to the risks of failure, at the date of the operation (1979) there was a responsible body of doctors who would not have done so. The plaintiff therefore failed. If the failure to give such advice had occurred more recently she would probably have succeeded — depending entirely on the medical evidence.

The costs of medical litigation

While all practitioners are covered either by insurance through their medical defence organizations or by NHS indemnity, it is not only the legal costs of fighting a case that have to be considered. The harassment, the waste of time and the emotional strain of threatened and actual litigation are things that every professional person would wish to avoid, and it bears particularly hard upon a surgeon. The doctor–patient relationship is a precious one, but the price that is paid for it includes the risk of conflict arising. The best way to avoid litigation is to ensure that no medical accidents occur, but this is a counsel of perfection. The next best thing is to ensure that the patient understands before any operation what is entailed, and, if something goes wrong, that she is properly treated and given all the information necessary for her to understand what has gone wrong and what is being done to put it right.

Many claims for medical negligence arise because the patient has been kept in the dark; lack of knowledge and understanding breeds suspicion, and even when there has been no error on the part of the doctor, the patient and her friends and relations can come to believe that there is something wrong because information has been kept away from her. Good communication between doctor and patient in this case, as in many others, will avoid trouble. Defensive medicine is not the answer: cooperation with the patient throughout, when this is practicable, combined with the courage to take decisions in the interest of the patient, will always be respected by the Courts and hopefully the claim will not get as far as that.

THE GYNAECOLOGIST AS DEFENDANT

A doctor's first duty is always to the patient: the doctor's duty to his peers comes second. After a medical accident a doctor is naturally concerned about his own responsibility, criticism by peers, the possibility of litigation, the fear of appearing in court and ultimately a finding of negligence. But the clinician's first concern should be for the consequences of the accident for the patient. One's duty is to establish what went wrong, find out why, explain to the patient, seek to rectify the damage and see that she is properly advised about her legal rights. Only after these duties have been discharged should peer loyalty arise.

The practitioner's duty of care does not cease, and indeed may increase, when a suspicion of an accident arises. The doctor should appreciate the injured patient's difficulties in understanding her legal position and in pursuing any claim she may have.

Any professional person — solicitor, doctor or other — has a duty to inform the client when injury may be the result of negligence, so that he or she may take independent advice. The Master of the Rolls made this clear in his address to the Medico-Legal Society in 1985. After referring to the lawyer's duty to his client, he continued:

> But what about doctors? Should not the same rule apply? Indeed, I think there is a much stronger case for such a rule in the case of doctors. The relationship between doctor and patient is so much closer than between lawyer and client. The patient is therefore so much more trusting. . . . Is not a policy of keeping silent when you think you may have been negligent an abuse of that trust? . . . If a doctor thinks that he may have been negligent and damage has undoubtedly resulted . . . should it not be part of the doctor's professional duty to give full and frank disclosure to the patient of what he did and why he did it and *to suggest to the patient that he takes independent medical and legal advice.*

(But see page 809 as to the difficulties which may arise with crown indemnity.)

Avoidance of litigation

Many doctors feel that the Courts set unreasonable standards for them and that this forces them into a practice of defensive medicine, that is treatment which is for the protection of the doctor and not for the good of the patient. The standards of proof however are the same for all who practise a skill, as we will see, and the potential defendant should bear in mind that the standards set by the Courts are those of the experts called to give independent evidence. There is no danger that a doctor will be found negligent if the care given is to a standard acceptable to the doctor's peers.

The Courts do not impose defensive medicine — indeed, judges are well aware of the danger of so doing, and are anxious not to interfere with doctors' discretion.

The first necessity in avoiding litigation is to maintain a reasonable standard of care. The doctor must not undertake intervention when the requisite facilities and expertise are not available. It is no defence to a charge of negligence that suitably skilled back-up was not available (*Wilsher* v. *Essex Area Health Authority* 1987).

The second requirement is meticulous contemporary notekeeping, including a full history, the advice given in relation to surgery, a precise account of surgical technique or other treatment, and full details of postoperative management. The discharge letter (or summary), in particular, requires meticulous care and accuracy, remembering that at some later stage it may be subjected to a critical, even adversarial, examination.

The third essential is good communication. The patient must be kept informed at all times. Part of the duty of care is to ensure that the patient understands as far as possible the options available for treatment. It is sometimes necessary to canvass with the patient the possibility of poor outcome, particularly if the procedure is elective. When things go wrong, a full and frank disclosure to the patient is desirable (but see page 797). This is not necessarily the same as an admission of liability. However where there is no other satisfactory explanation (e.g. a retained swab) even an admission of fault may well be appropriate.

In matters relating to consent it is essential that the explanatory material given to the patient is fully reported in the notes and that the patient's questions are properly answered. The limited value of the consent form is dealt with on page 793.

As soon as possible after an accident has occurred, all the staff concerned should be asked to produce a report while the incident is still fresh in their minds. It is particularly important that nurses and junior doctors are asked to write a contemporary account since by the time an action arises, they may have left the employment of the health authority and, in any event, may have forgotten the details of their involvement.

Doctors who are concerned with techniques at the horizon of medical research, such as organ transplants, artificial conception techniques and embryo research would do well to stick closely to such ethical guidelines as have been laid down, or to seek advice from the appropriate ethical committee (and see page 801).

What to do when a complaint is made

Whatever the nature of the complaint, if the doctor–patient relationship is continuing, the first step should be to see the patient and give a full explanation. Where the complaint is of an administrative nature, the appropriate hospital manager should be immediately involved. In any event, the doctor should consult the appropriate medical defence organization immediately, as he may need expert advice on how to handle the situation.

Letter before action

Where the complaint relates to clinical management and there is a possibility of litigation, there will usually be a letter from the patient's legal advisers (the letter before action). Such a letter requires prompt response if unnecessary delays and accompanying legal charges are to be avoided. The doctor should not correspond with the patient's solicitors, save only to acknowledge the letter. Defensible actions may be prejudiced as a result of inappropriate correspondence. The doctor should immediately pass on the letter of complaint to the appropriate manager who will consult with the legal advisers of the health authority. The 'letter before action' will usually require disclosure of the clinical records. Most such letters nowadays state that the plaintiff's solicitors will not agree to restriction of disclosure of notes to a medical adviser but the plaintiff's solicitors can obtain a court order for full disclosure if this is refused and certain conditions are fulfilled (*Lask* v. *Gloucester Health Authority* 1985). There is no legal basis for restriction of disclosure; it is essential that the lawyers see the records in order to advise on liability.

Documents to be disclosed

Correspondence and other communications between the solicitors and client are privileged from production to the plaintiff even though no litigation was contemplated or pending at the time they were written, provided that they are of a confidential nature and the solicitor was acting in a professional capacity, giving legal advice or getting it on behalf of the client (e.g. from counsel).

The general principle is that communications between a solicitor and a third party, whether directly or through an agent, which are written after litigation is contemplated or commenced for the purpose of giving or obtaining advice or evidence in regard to that litigation, are privileged. This privilege includes documents which are obtained by a solicitor with a view to enabling him to prosecute or defend an action, or to give advice with reference to existing or contemplated litigation.

However, reports of accidents and similar documents which are made before litigation is commenced to put the managers or solicitors fully in the picture can cause difficulty. This is because the reports have a dual purpose, that of producing as clear an account of the incident as soon as possible so that the facts may be ascertained and any necessary action taken, as well as that of providing a basis on which solicitors may be instructed if necessary and proceedings defended (or settled) if they are instituted. In general, such documents are not privileged.

For example, in the case of *Lask* v. *Gloucester Health Authority* (1985), the Court of Appeal held that a confidential accident report (which HM(55)66 requires to be completed by health authorities both for the use of solicitors in case litigation arises in respect of the accident, and also to enable action to be taken to avoid repetition of the accident) was not privileged since the *dominant* purpose of its preparation had not been for submission to solicitors in anticipation of litigation.

Medical notes are never protected from disclosure. Such non-privileged documents, including the nursing Kardex, notes or extracts from the relevant nursing books, consent forms, X-rays, pathology reports and other laboratory investigations, should be included in the case notes which are disclosed. A consultant in charge of the case is well advised to examine these records in detail and to make sure that all the appropriate documents are copied, before releasing them to the legal advisers of the health authority. At this point, the consultant in charge of the case should prepare an immediate assessment for the assistance of the health authority and their respective solicitors.

The role of medical defence organizations

The role of the defence organizations has been radically altered by the introduction of NHS indemnity (see below) and the responsibility for the conduct of cases within NHS provider units now becomes the sole responsibility of those units. They may choose to employ the defence organizations; in any event doctors in private practice and general practitioners will still need to rely upon the defence organizations to conduct their defence. Defence unions have advised their members on disclosure in the circumstances of a medical accident as follows.

> . . . when something has gone wrong in practice, explain the facts to the patient, parent or relative and strive to rectify the problem sympathetically. Junior staff should enlist and receive the help of senior colleagues.
>
> The Council and Secretariat of the Society advocate a full and proper communication with patients. In circumstances where complications and errors arise it is proper that objective, factual information, with appropriate clinical reassurance, is provided. Adequate explanations, ideally from the responsible consultant or principal, assist in reducing fear and uncertainty which may give rise to complaints and claims. The Society does not encourage members to withhold objective, factual information or expressions of sympathy (Medical Protection Society 1987).

A full explanation of the circumstances of an accident is not the same as an admission of liability. However, when liability is undeniable, it is clearly right, and indeed in their own interests, that the medical defence organizations or the health authority should settle the case as soon as possible.

The defence lawyers will eventually need to rely upon the defendant doctor to give evidence; the doctor must make it clear at an early stage what his evidence will be.

The defendant doctor does well to understand the position of the defence organizations. The lawyers they instruct are acting for the organization corporately, not for the individual doctor concerned, and they will act on the instructions not of the doctor but of the organizations, who will in turn act on their perception of the interests of their members as a whole. If there is a conflict between these interests, the doctor may be well advised to take independent advice.

Meeting legal advisers

It is essential at an early stage in the proceedings that the defendant doctor should give a full explanation of his part in the case, the reasons for acting as he did and an assessment of his own and others' responsibilities. The doctor should try to ensure that the expert chosen to help the defence is the right one who has appropriate recent experience in circumstances similar to those of the defendant doctor. If he works in a busy district hospital, it may be little help to have a retired academic give expert evidence.

It is essential that the defendant doctor should understand the expert evidence which is to be given on his behalf. He should read the expert's report and make sure he agrees with it or comment accordingly. The defendant should read all of the authorities upon which the expert seeks to rely.

When the case is to be defended, the doctor must ensure that he attends a conference with counsel at which the experts are also present so that it is certain that due weight is given to the doctor's own evidence and it corresponds with the experts' view.

Appearing in court

Before appearing in court the defendant doctor will have the opportunity to read the expert evidence from the plaintiff. This will indicate where the main thrust of cross-examination will lie. The doctor should become familiar with the authorities upon which the plaintiff's experts rely and make sure that his own experts fully understand the case.

Although a witness of fact, the defendant doctor is inevitably an expert in his own field; nevertheless he should be encouraged to concentrate on the facts.

In giving evidence the defendant doctor must be modest, succinct and intelligible.

THE GYNAECOLOGIST AS EXPERT WITNESS

Definition

The salient feature of an 'expert' witness is that he is unconnected with the case in question and can give an independent opinion of the standards of care provided by the defendant. He must have specialized knowledge and experience in the particular field relevant to the facts under investigation: in a gynaecological case, for example, an expert may be called who is a general practitioner, or perhaps a scientist working within a much narrower area such as immunology or genetics. Thus several experts may be called in any one case to deal with different aspects of management.

It is desirable that the expert should have current practical contact with his specialty, although often an eminent practitioner who has retired may have the additional assets of time and opportunity to apply a lifetime's experience to an area with which he is familiar. The expert should not be tempted to stray outside his own particular field of expertise.

The role of the expert

When the expert is first asked for an opinion, he should approach the analysis of the case in an objective fashion, forming an opinion without fear or favour. He must give a clear indication of an assessment of the standards of care, but once that opinion has been formed he cannot be disinterested although should at all times remain balanced. In an adversarial system, the expert who gives evidence on behalf of either plaintiff or defendant becomes part of the team assembled to conduct the litigation and will have a responsibility to assemble evidence and advise the lawyers on the best way of presenting it. He will be expected not only to justify his own opinion but also to deal with contrary arguments advanced by the other side.

When giving evidence in court the expert will be subjected to cross-examination in which his views will be challenged and contrary views advanced; he must be able to marshal the evidence in such a way that the independent opinions advanced can be justified. The expert should be able to support these views from textbooks, the literature and acceptable statistics.

The medical report

It is an essential prerequisite for a plaintiff's expert to interview the plaintiff whilst in possession of all the medical records, so as to compare her version of events with the written record. Similarly, it is unrealistic to expect a defence expert to fulfil his role without the opportunity of discussing management with the doctors concerned.

The first and largest part of the report is a careful analysis of all the hospital notes. If the notes are incomplete, the expert must advise the solicitors to enquire for the missing documents, and should not take no for an answer. The expert should then reconstruct in a report the events in a way which an intelligent educated layman will understand. Although it is not essential to include all the details of the events of the case in the report, it is often helpful to the Court to do so in a detailed and explicit form.

In the second part, the expert should go on to explain the technical matters involved. For instance, where a urinary fistula has developed as a result of gynaecological surgery, it is essential to explain in the report how such injuries may be caused, the anatomical arrangements (if necessary with diagrams) and their possible sequelae for the plaintiff. Such explanatory material may well be separated from the main narrative into appendices.

The third part of the report should relate the case in point to this technical explanation. It should give a critical appraisal of the standards of care. Finally, the expert should give an unequivocal assessment of the standards of care and, if he believes these to be defective, should list the areas in which care fell short of the reasonable standard to be expected. In this discussion the expert should if possible avoid the use of the term 'negligence' since this is a question of law and may be misunderstood by doctors; in any event, it is for the Court to decide after hearing evidence what is acceptable to the profession and hence whether the care was negligent.

In forming this opinion the expert will refer to standard textbooks, for they define what is an acceptable standard. It is sometimes useful to refer to learned scientific papers, but they often reflect matters that are still under debate and on which there may well be more than one opinion. Such articles can be particularly useful to rebut the view that a particular practice is not acceptable, or conversely to establish that there is a responsible body of medical opinion of a contrary view. It is important that such references should antedate the accident.

Disclosure of reports

The initial report is prepared for the use of counsel in drafting or rebutting the statement of claim. It will often need to deal with contrary arguments and discuss controversial areas. After the pleadings are closed there will at some stage before the trial be an exchange of experts' reports in accordance with recent changes in the Rules of Court (order 38, rule 37). In all personal injury cases the Court may order disclosure of experts' written reports to the other party or parties:

> When in any cause or matter an application is made in respect of oral expert evidence, then, unless the Court considers that there are special reasons for not doing so, it shall direct that the substance of the evidence be disclosed in the form of a written report or reports to such other parties and within such period as the Court may specify.

There may already have been voluntary exchange or exchange within the provisions for automatic disclosure under order 25, rule 8. But in any event parties are now bound to disclose their evidence in medical negligence cases well before the trial, and may not rely on any evidence that has not been disclosed to the other side.

The initial report may not be suitable for disclosure, and both expert and counsel should be aware that it is not intended for such a purpose. Should the matter reach the Courts, a separate report, often shorter and perhaps modified in the light of disclosure of further facts or documents, would be appropriate for exchange. Counsel may wish to draft this final report independently but the doctor must ensure that it represents his own views.

The Court also has the power to order a 'without prejudice' meeting between the experts (order 38, rule 38):

> In any cause or matter the Court may, if it thinks fit, direct that there be a meeting 'without prejudice' of such experts within such periods before or after the disclosure of their reports as the Court may specify, for the purpose of identifying those parts of their evidence which are in issue. Where such a meeting takes place the experts may prepare a joint statement indicating those parts of their evidence on which they are, and those on which they are not, in agreement.

The effect of these changes in the rules should be to resolve many cases before trial, or at best to narrow the issues.

Conference

The earlier the expert is involved in a meeting with solicitors and counsel, the better. If possible this should take place before any report is written: this will ensure that the expert's mind is directed to the legal issues, what has to be proved, and where the other side will direct its attack. This will mean that counsel has a report on which to draft the pleadings with confidence, and there should then be no need to amend them later. Time spent in conference is thus well worth the time and expense, as it saves both in the long run. Neither the plaintiff nor the defence can mount their cases properly without early and full consultation between the lawyers, the expert (or experts — there may be more than one), and the client, either patient or doctor.

The pleadings

Pleadings are the formal statements of each party's case. Their importance is that they set out the case on each side, define the allegations and limit the area of dispute, for no evidence can be given that does not relate to allegations in the pleadings. The plaintiff's statement of claim sets out the main events relating to the complaint, then lists the 'particulars of negligence' alleged and gives an account of the damages suffered. The defendant doctor and any other defendant (often the health authority) will then prepare their defence.

The next stage in pleading will probably be a request for 'further and better particulars' of the statement of claim or the defence. Those particulars will almost certainly need to be drafted with the expert's help; in any event they should not be served without his approval as the advocates will be bound by these particulars in the conduct of the case.

Evidence in court

To the uninitiated, the giving of expert evidence is often a daunting experience. But there are some simple rules which help. It should be remembered that most judges today, especially in the High Court, have a basic scientific knowledge which enables them to understand even the most difficult medical problem; the judge will probably have read the medical reports and done the necessary 'homework'; above all, he will have empathy with the experts and some common professional understanding.

On a more practical level, the expert must understand that the judge will take down in longhand all the germane points of the evidence, often word for word. It must therefore be given to the judge in a way which he can comprehend and note. The expert should face the judge when giving evidence and do it in a modest although firm manner and at a speed commensurate with the judge's requirement to take notes.

In cross-examination the expert's views will be attacked with varying degrees of effectiveness. Sometimes it will be necessary to concede a point in cross-examination. To do so gracefully will enhance the expert's authority and credibility. The expert should take time to answer questions if necessary. He should bear in mind the 'bottom line' beyond which he is not prepared to retreat. If the expert's opinion has been stated clearly in the report and he has thought out the implications fully, there should be no difficulty in withstanding cross-examination.

It is important that the expert should hear the evidence given by the expert on the other side and he should be readily available to counsel during cross-examination; without expert advice, counsel may be unable to cross-examine effectively.

FUTURE TRENDS

Rising expectations, increasing public awareness of scientific and specifically of medical progress, avid interest in the more lurid aspects of professional conduct of all kinds — greatly encouraged by the media — are all likely to increase medical litigation. Escalating damages in all accident claims, not only those for medical mishap, are inevitable as the costs and potential of caring increase. These are widely publicised, naturally making patients more aware of the significance of any unfortunate sequelae of treatment. Whilst it is to be hoped that these developments will be offset, to some degree at least, by greater understanding by doctors of their patients' desire to have and their capacity to receive full information about their condition, any proposed treatment, and any accidents which occur, we have to face the inevitability that claims will increase in both number and value. In this chapter we have tried to show how these can best be dealt with, to abort those based on ignorance or misunderstanding and to handle the serious ones in such a way as to minimize the injury to both the plaintiff and defendant.

In gynaecology there are several areas which threaten to become fertile fields for the disaffected patient; there are also some hopeful signs of change, some of which are controversial but should be examined with a view to progress.

'No fault' compensation

Perhaps the most superficially attractive reform of accident litigation, this concept seems to raise more doubts than it solves (see Ch. 62).

No system yet devised would protect the doctor entirely from the miseries of legal claims; what might be the greatest benefit is a reduction of the gap between doctor and patient once a claim arises, since the patient would need the doctor's help in quantifying the claim and the doctor would not have such a direct interest in the payment of damages.

One cause for concern in the 'no fault' concept is that the element of audit is removed. Otherwise, it does not appear to have any particular relevance to gynaecology.

National Health Service (NHS) indemnity

Since 1 January 1990 new regulations have governed the

handling of claims for alleged medical negligence against medical and dental personnel employed in the hospital and community health services. Health authorities thereafter (subject to some complex transitional provisions) assumed all responsibility for new and existing claims against their doctors, who are no longer required as a condition of their employment to subscribe to a professional defence organization.

The circular establishing the new arrangements (HC(89)34) sets out the mechanism for dealing with claims lodged after the 1st January 1990. After that date the responsibility for defending and indemnifying claims rests entirely with the health authority. Doctors do not require separate representation by solicitors instructed by defence bodies. This means there will be no longer up to three legal firms dealing with a single case and no need for negotiation on apportionment of liability. Overall defence costs are thereby reduced.

A further Department of Health circular of September 1990 advised that, even where more than one health authority was sued, only one firm of solicitors should act for all defendants, further reducing disputes over apportionment. Health authorities are instructed not to enter into commercial insurance arrangements without approval (which must come from the treasury); trusts can seek insurance cover in the commercial market but not for medical negligence. Individual units and trusts will have to suffer the financial consequences of lost cases. Loans will be available from regional health authorities (for directly managed units) and from the Department of Health (for trusts). The costs of medical negligence should be reflected in the charges a unit or trust makes for its services. Loans of £100 000 or less must be repaid within 1 year, rising to 10 years for those of more than £900 000. Payments into court are only covered by the loan scheme once a claim is finalized. Health authorities and trusts may therefore be unable to afford large payments into court to protect their position on costs.

Nevertheless, health authorities seem likely to benefit from an end to the involvement of the defence bodies since they will gain control of cases and be able to conduct their own risk management programmes.

The procedure for cases current before the beginning of 1990 is more complex. In December 1989 a Department of Health circular strongly advised health authorities to continue employing defence bodies to deal with claims notified before 1 January 1990; this would ensure that the defence bodies reinsurance cover remained valid.

Work done outside the NHS contract, including Category 2 work, Samaritan acts and disciplinary proceedings, is not covered by this indemnity; individual doctors therefore need to have continued cover from their medical defence organizations, and a scale of revised premiums has been set out to take account of the NHS cover and the amount of 'risk' practice undertaken by individual doctors outside that cover. Premiums for those with no substantial commitment outside their NHS contracts will be low. For private practice indemnity, the premiums are linked to income.

Some concern has been expressed by doctors about the new arrangements. They fear that their interests will not be properly addressed or understood by the health authorities, and they are anxious about the loss of advice previously given by the medical defence organizations. In some cases the authority will choose to use the services of a medical defence organization as agent, but this is not obligatory and may not remedy the lack of independent advice. The circular does address these fears to some extent, in that it requires health authorities to take into consideration four matters:

1. The views of the practitioner(s) concerned.
2. The potentially damaging effects on the professional reputation(s) of the practitioner(s) concerned.
3. Any point of principle or of wider application raised by the case.
4. The costs involved.

It is likely that any matter which affects the doctor's reputation will reflect upon the authority, so that their interests will usually coincide. But if a doctor wishes to be separately represented in a case he is entitled to make separate arrangements, at the risk of paying his own costs. To quote the circular:

> The Health Authority may welcome a practitioner being separately advised without cost to the Health Authority. However, if a practitioner claims that his interests in any case are distinct from those of the Health Authority and wishes to be separately represented in the proceedings, he will need the agreement of the Plaintiff, the Health Authority and the Court. If liability is established, he would have to pay not only his own legal expenses, but also further costs incurred as a result of his being separately represented.

Procedural reform

One of the greatest defects of negligence litigation at present is delay. As a judge said despairingly in a recent case where the plaintiff sought to amend pleadings at the trial, 7 years after issue of the writ and 9 years since the operation: 'I never seem to try a case that is less than 9 years old!' This is scandalous: memories fade, documents are lost, registrars are in the Antipodes — worse than these practical defects, the years may have caused deprivation of rightful damages much needed by the plaintiff, and will almost certainly have built up resentment and even bitterness on both sides.

The new Rules of Court (p. 798), if properly used, could narrow issues and avoid the delays which result from neither side understanding what the case is about; as Mustill (1987) said in the Court of Appeal:

> The parties realised, soon after the case began, that they

> had misunderstood what the case was about. As was stated before us, it was fought 'in the dark'. It lasted four weeks instead of the allotted five days which not only imposed great pressure of time on all concerned, but meant that the scheduling of the expert witness was put quite out of joint . . . Nearly 150 pages of medical literature were put in, without prior exchange, or any opportunity for proper scrutiny.
>
> All this could have been avoided if there had been adequate clarification of the issues before the trial . . . I believe that practitioners do their clients and the interests of justice no service by continuing to pursue this policy of concealment . . . To me it seems wrong that in this area of the law, more than in any other, this kind of forensic blind-man's buff should continue to be the norm.

This should not happen again, but unhappily delays can occur from many different causes; some of these lie in the control of doctors and their legal advisers, but probably more are the responsibility of plaintiffs' lawyers. All the surgeon can do, whether as defendant or expert, is to cooperate fully and promptly with the lawyers, and if appropriate bring such pressure to bear as is possible to hasten matters.

Any action taken to expedite will have the full support of the judges, who will in future be increasingly vigilant to ensure that both sides not only get justice, but get it quickly.

New areas of risk in gynaecology

Although no case has yet come before the Courts of surgery for the convenience of the surgeon 'lacking in conscience or care' (Jeffcoate 1957), there may well be claims in the future for unnecessary pelvic surgery, undertaken to deal with a difficult patient in place of troublesome attempts at an accurate diagnosis.

Those who break barriers will always attract criticism, and this easily crystallizes into litigation. The whole area of artificial conception is a potential minefield: at present no specific law exists (save for a minimal piece of reactive legislation in a feeble attempt to control surrogacy) (Surrogacy Arrangements Act 1985) but that does not mean that practitioners are immune from the civil law.

Communication is the watchword, as always, but in these new fields, where surgery is neither life-saving nor truly necessary, and often fails, communication becomes vital to a happy outcome on all sides.

Assisted reproduction

From October 1991 most forms of assisted reproduction were brought under the control of the Human Fertilisation and Embryology Authority (HFEA). This was set up by the Human Fertilisation and Embryology Act, 1990 which defined the legal limits and conditions which were in future to govern all medical services for the purpose of 'assisting women to carry children' ('treatment services') and the storage of and research upon gametes and embryos.

(The Act does *not* control surrogacy, save to spell out that surrogacy contracts are unenforceable. It does amend the Abortion Act and the Infant Life Preservation Act to legalize termination of pregnancy up to term where there is a serious threat to the life or health of the mother, or 'substantial risk' of a seriously handicapped child.)

Under the Act no creation, storage, or implantation of embryos, or research thereon, is legal unless licensed by HFEA, which has the power to grant, vary or revoke licences (subject to appeal to the High Court or the Court of Session), to inspect the premises and activities of licensees, and to advise them. The HFEA must also publish a Code of Practice for the guidance of licensees, setting out the manner in which treatment services should be carried out. It is important to distinguish between the edicts of the Act and those of the Code of Practice: the former are mandatory, the latter persuasive; a breach of the former is a criminal offence, which will result in the loss of the licence and possible prosecution, whereas a breach of the Code is *not* a criminal offence, although it may result in the loss or suspension of the licence.

Licences for treatment services — which include in vitro fertilization, other embryo implantations, artificial insemination and egg donation — are granted to the 'responsible person' in charge of the unit (both being specified in the licence) and continue in force until suspended or revoked. Licenses for research are granted for each specific project, and the Authority requires that the protocol should be approved by the appropriate ethics committee. Thus any unit conducting research requires an ethics committee, whereas a unit providing treatment services only is not required by the Code to have one (as it was under the ILA), although most will wish to do so for their own protection and for guidance through a complicated Act and the Code of Conduct, which will undoubtedly be revised frequently.

Any gynaecologist undertaking treatment services as defined in the Act will be well advised to familiarize himself, directly or through his ethics committee, with the provisions of the Act and the current Code. Since undertaking such treatment without a licence, or in breach of its terms, is liable on conviction to a fine or a term of imprisonment for up to 2 years, the rules governing these licences are of vital interest to all practitioners carrying out any sort of assisted reproduction.

The removal of ova for research, or for egg donation, and oophorectomy to facilitate hormone replacement therapy will require meticulous adherence to professional standards in the giving of advice. In all these cases, and others involving any element of experiment, full discussion with colleagues as well as the patient and detailed note-keeping, together with reasoned correspondence with the general practitioner and perhaps other workers in the same field, will minimize the risks of litigation or even complaint.

KEY POINTS

1. The surgeon does not necessarily undertake to perform a cure but must comply with the standards of care at the time. He will be judged as the ordinary skilled man exercising and professing to have that special skill.
2. Consent for an operation is real and means that the patient must be given sufficient information for her to understand the operation, its likely effects and recognized complications.
3. A minor can be made a ward of court if parents refuse permission for surgery.
4. For a mentally handicapped person, a court can declare the operation lawful if it is in the best interests of the patient.
5. A failed termination or sterilization can be the basis for a claim for negligence, especially when advice about risks of failure has not been given.
6. A doctor's first duty is to the patient and then to his peers.
7. Litigation is avoided by maintaining a reasonable standard of care, keeping meticulous and contemporary notes and good communication with the patient and relatives.

REFERENCES

Bolam v. Friern Barnet 1957 2 All England Law Reports pp 118, 121
F v. West Berkshire Health Authority 1985 (Mental Health Act Commission intervening) 2 All England Law Reports 2: 545
Family Law Reform Act (1969) Act of Parliament
Gold v. Haringey Health Authority 1987 2 All England Law Reports p 888
Jeffcoate T N A 1957 Principles of gynaecology, 1st edn. Butterworths, London
Lask v. Gloucester Health Authority 1985 The Times 13 December
Maynard v. West Midlands Regional Health Authority 1985 1 All England Law Reports p 635
McKay v. Essex Health Authority 1982 2 All England Law Reports p 771
Medical Protection Society 1987 Annual report. Medical Protection Society
Medico-Legal Journal 1985 53: 57
Mustill L J 1987 Medical Protection Society Annual Report p 461
Sciuriaga v. Powell 1980 Unreported; considered in Emeh v. Kensington and Chelsea and Westminster AHA 1984 3 All England Law Reports p 1044
Sideway v. Bethlem Royal Hospital Governors 1985 1 All England Law Reports p 643
Surrogacy Arrangements Act (1985) Act of Parliament
Tindal Chief Justice In: Lanphier v. Phipos 1838 Carrington and Paynes Reports, pp 475, 479
Whitehouse v. Jordan 1980 1 All England Law Reports p 650
Wilsher v. Essex Area Health Authority 1987 2 Weekly Law Reports p 466

62. Medicolegal aspects

E. M. Symonds

Indemnity cover for doctors in the UK has been provided by the medical defence organizations for more than 100 years. These organizations are not insurance companies and originally arose, as stated in the original memorandum of the Medical Defence Union, out of the need:

1. To support and protect the character and interests of medical practitioners practising in the UK.
2. To promote honourable practice and to suppress or prosecute unauthorized practitioners.
3. To advise and defend or assist in defending members of the Union in cases where proceedings involving questions of professional principle or otherwise are brought against them.

Clifford Hawkins (1985), in his history of the medical defence organizations, refers to the original trigger for the formation of these societies as the case of Dr David Bradley who in 1884 was found guilty of attempted criminal assault against a woman patient who alleged that Dr Bradley had raped her. A letter from Lawson Tait to the *British Medical Journal* drew attention to the unsatisfactory nature of this judgement. The case was re-examined and the Home Secretary eventually granted a free pardon. It was the lack of proper expert evidence that had resulted in the initial conviction. It was apparent that some proper organization was necessary to defend the interests of doctors and dentists in resisting this type of claim.

THE MEDICAL DEFENCE ORGANIZATIONS

The Medical Defence Union

This was the first of the defence organizations, and it was founded in 1887 with Lawson Tait as the first President. He was a man of great presence and a distinguished surgeon and gynaecologist.

In 1893 he resigned as President because of his difficult personality and because of internal difficulties, and the Medical Defence Union moved its office from Birmingham to London.

The Medical Protection Society

The new constitution of the Medical Defence Union introduced by Lawson Tait led to internal dissent on the Council, as it proposed to concentrate too much power in too few hands running the organization. Dr Hugh Woods led a dissenting group and in conjunction with a group of dissatisfied members, he formed the London and Counties Medical Protection Society Ltd (1892). The title was subsequently changed after the Second World War to the Medical Protection Society.

The Medical and Dental Defence Union of Scotland

The Medical and Dental Defence Union of Scotland was formed in 1902 specifically to serve graduates from Scottish schools and doctors working in Scottish hospitals.

Despite the establishment of three different organizations, the essential purpose of the societies has remained constant to the original functions discribed by the constitution of the Medical Defence Union.

THE MEDICAL DEFENCE ORGANIZATIONS AND INSURANCE COMPANIES

In 1974, the Insurance Companies Act defined a system of requirements and powers for the Secretary of State to regulate the affairs of insurance companies. In many countries doctors are covered by insurance companies and whereas the medical defence organizations are mutual, non-profit-making defence associations which provide effectively unlimited cover for any person in membership at the time of a specific event whenever the claim is initiated, insurance companies can load premiums, refuse membership because of multiple claims, settle claims out of court if there is a pecuniary advantage, and require additional insurance to cover retired members and their estates.

This was far removed from the generous cover and support given by the defence organizations. However, a close scrutiny of events over the last 5 years shows that the medical defence organizations are, indeed, being forced into pathways that are rapidly becoming indistinguishable from the activities of ordinary insurance companies.

THE MEDICOLEGAL FRAMEWORK IN THE UK

Under English law, professional negligence and liability are covered under the laws of civil tort. Until recently, actions against a doctor for negligence could also be based on breach of contract but the judiciary have in recent years largely removed this option. Thus, in English law all legal issues for the recovery of damages in medical practice fall within the law of negligence. What exactly constitutes negligence is difficult to define. The most widely accepted definition, and the one most commonly applied in the courts, arises from the direction given by Mr Justice McNair in 1957 in the case of *Bolam v. Friern Hospital Management Committee* and this reads as follows:

> In the ordinary case which does not involve any special skill, negligence in law means this: some failure to do some act which a reasonable man in the circumstances would do, or doing some act which a reasonable man in the circumstances would not do: and if that failure or doing of that act results in injury, then there is a cause of action.
>
> How do you test whether this act or failure is negligent?
>
> In an ordinary case it is generally said that you judge that by the action of the man in the street. He is the ordinary man. In one case it has been said that you judge it by the conduct of the man on the top of a Clapham omnibus. He is the ordinary man. But where you get a situation which involves the use of some special skill or competence, then the test whether there has been negligence or not is not the test of the man on the top of a Clapham omnibus, because he has not got this special skill. The test is the standard of the ordinary skilled man exercising and professing to have that special skill.
>
> A man need not possess the highest expert skill to be at risk of being found negligent. It is well established law that it is sufficient if he exercises the ordinary skill of an ordinary competent man exercising that particular art.

As Butcher (1990) has pointed out, this judgement failed to take account of the status of the doctor involved. The matter was eventually addressed by the Court of Appeal in the case of *Wilsher v. Essex Health Authority* when it was decided that:

> it must be recognised that different facts make different demands. If it is borne in mind that the structure of hospital medicine envisages that the lower ranks will be occupied by those of whom it would be wrong to expect too much, the risk of abuse by litigious patients can be mitigated.

Nevertheless, the level of skill to be expected of a doctor in training as a specialist is still a grey area and the desire for courts to compensate plaintiffs has led to unrealistic expectations of clinical skills.

There are also serious difficulties in deciding where complications of particular procedures are acceptable and where the complications are considered to arise from unsatisfactory skills.

The procedure of a claim

Anyone may commence proceedings against any other person and there is no real way by which this process can be screened. The initial claim made by the plaintiff leads to the issuing of a writ of summons from the court and this must contain a summary of the nature of the claim. It does not have to be precise. The action is usually initiated at the solicitor's request for the production of case notes as an indication of threatened legal action.

The service of a claim has to be personal, but in the past the service has generally been accepted by the doctor's defence organization. It is not clear who will accept service in the future as this has not been stated by the Department of Health, but one assumes it will be accepted by the health authorities' and Trust Hospitals' solicitors. After the service of a statement of claim, the defendant has to serve a defence. Under the Scottish system, considerable detail must be supplied and both sides are then entitled to ask for further and better particulars of the statement of claim.

Before the case comes to court, there is a process of discovery of documents which have not already been revealed, the exchange of expert reports and sometimes a meeting of experts to define the areas of agreement and disagreement. The action is then set down for trial and a date is fixed.

Legal aid

The availability of legal aid is determined by the disposable income of the applicant. The opinion of one expert adviser is then sought as well as counsel's opinion on the likelihood of the claim being successful. If this opinion is favourable, then the certificate is extended to summons for directness and if the advisers still advise that the claim should succeed, then the certificate is extended to trial.

The statute of limitations

In the case of obstetricians, the course of legislation in this field has been entirely adverse.

Claims alleging brain damage can be commenced up to 21 years after birth and longer if there is mental incapacity.

This effectively makes defence of any case impossible because the case notes will often not be available or will be indecipherable and the medical and midwifery staff involved will almost certainly have no recollection of the nature of the events involved in the management of the case.

Actions for negligence causing injury have to be commenced within 3 years of the event, but this period can be extended if it can be shown that there was no knowledge within the 3-year period that the injury was significant or if the plaintiff is under the age of 18 years.

MEDICAL LITIGATION IN THE USA

The system of litigation in the USA is adversarial and cases are heard in front of a judge and jury. In the UK, cases are heard in front of a judge but no jury and since 1988 this also applies in Eire.

The decision made by both judge and jury is, therefore, highly dependent on the presentation of the case and the experts on either side. It has to be said that this principle also applies in the UK, although not to the same degree.

Contingency fees are a feature of the American system: this means that the lawyers take up to 40% of the award if the case is won by the plaintiff, but do not charge if the case is lost.

Although it is generally believed that this process entirely favours the plaintiff, this is probably not true. Unless the courts are strongly biased against the medical profession, there is a real risk that the lawyers may lose heavily if a frivolous claim is taken to court. Experienced lawyers, therefore, tend to avoid situations where they are unlikely to have a successful case. Moves towards a similar process in the UK have so far largely been resisted, but it is uncertain in the British courts whether such changes would favour the plaintiff or the defendant.

The cost of settlements in the USA has been substantially enhanced by the fact that these matters are determined by the juries and that there appears to be no limit to the sums awarded for pain, suffering and loss of amenity. This has so far been restricted in the UK because the awards are determined by judges within proscribed agreements. Many of the American states now have a cap on damages in order to limit professional liability. In two states, West Virginia and Florida, a system of no-fault compensation has been introduced for claims concerning birth-related injuries as a result of the virtual breakdown of the obstetric services.

It seems likely that at some stage, the whole structure of civil tort and professional indemnity will have to be changed towards a genuine insurance system with costs being met by a consortium of insurers involving the state legislature, doctors and hospital insurers.

The cost of litigation simply diverts revenue away from patients suffering disabilities related to their illnesses and greatly increases the cost of overall medical care.

NO-FAULT COMPENSATION

New Zealand

The first system of no-fault compensation was introduced in New Zealand in 1974 (Blain 1983). It has much broader connotations than medical malpractice and was specifically designed to avoid the inefficiencies of the common law system which, in subjects which always carry an element of uncertainty on causality, carries some of the features of a lottery. Does the woman who bears a child with cerebral palsy need any less support if the condition is congenital than if the child's injury is apparently birth-related? In the case of *Whitehouse* v. *Jordan*, Lord Justice Lawton stated in 1981: 'The victim of medical mishaps of the present kind should be cared for by the community, not by the hazards of litigation'.

The New Zealand system has taken account of these problems and has now been functioning for 16 years. The scheme is administered by the Accident Compensation Corporation Scheme and part of the funds are provided from general taxation and part from employers' contributions and a levy on the self-employed.

Payments are based on loss of earnings, reasonable medical expenses and other out-of-pocket expenses. There is no contribution for pain and suffering. If the Commission rejects the claim, the plaintiff may bring action in court for negligence, but if compensation is accepted, the right to go to court is lost.

The Swedish patient insurance scheme

Sweden introduced a patient insurance scheme in 1975 (Oldertz 1984). Decisions are made on objective facts and on the nature of the injury and the disabilities resulting from it. The circumstances leading to the injury are considered to be of little importance, although disciplinary actions can he invoked by other mechanisms where this is considered to be appropriate. Decisions are made by a consortium of Swedish insurers and if the patient wishes to appeal against the level of compensation, he or she can apply to a consulting claims panel.

The main concern with patient insurance systems is the

relatively low level of compensation and the cost generally to the community. However, overall, with the removal of legal costs, there seems little doubt that this is a much more efficient method of compensation and ensures that medical practice and new developments are not distorted by the legal process.

TYPES OF GYNAECOLOGICAL CASES IN LITIGATION

General surgical problems

Litigation arises from the general problems that beset all surgical procedures. There is no defence to leaving swabs, packs or instruments in the abdominal cavity or in the vagina and these matters almost invariably attract an out-of-court settlement. Fortunately, gynaecological procedures are rarely subject to the problem of performing the wrong operation. However, occasionally a patient is sterilized when her name is put on the operating list for diagnostic laparoscopy one ahead or one behind a patient put on the operating list for sterilization.

These are all matters that can be avoided by good practice and the responsibility lies with the theatre staff and the surgeon to ensure that swab and instrument counts are correct at the end of the operation and that the lists are correct with the patient receiving the correct operation. One common source of litigation results from the retention of swabs after repair of an episiotomy. In this situation, swab counts are often forgotten and the obstetrician usually relies on directly checking the vaginal cavity at the end of the procedure.

Complications of sterilization

Failed sterilization

Most claims in relation to sterilization relate to failure of the procedure. Until the 1980s, it was uncommon to advise patients of the risk of failure of sterilization. Indeed, even today the only reasons for telling the patient of this possibility are medicolegal and to make the patient aware of the possibility of failure so that early termination of pregnancy can be sought should this happen. In the Particulars of Negligence, it is often alleged that had the patient been informed of the risk of failure, she would not have been sterilized or would have persuaded her partner to have a vasectomy or would have continued to use contraception. In practice, since gynaecologists began to advise patients of the risk of failure, there is no evidence that women in any way change their intention to be sterilized.

In the recent case of *Gold* v. *Haringey Health Authority* (1987) these issues were thoroughly rehearsed and it was agreed after resort to the Court of Appeal that a significant body of gynaecologists did not warn of the risk of failure in 1979 (Brahams 1987). In his original judgement, Mr Justice Schiemann held that there was a duty to counsel the patient about alternative methods of family planning, including vasectomy. As a result of these cases, it is generally agreed that a statement should be included in the consent form to the effect that 'there is a possibility that I may not become or remain sterile'. In fact, it is difficult to sustain an argument that signing a form that acknowledges that the failure to render a patient sterile in the first instance has any value in protecting the surgeon from accusations of negligence.

Claims have also been made in relation to the failure to warn the patient of the risk of ectopic pregnancy.

The other source of claims rests with the accusation that the procedure was faulty. It is now generally recognized and acknowledged by the Courts that all tubal occlusive techniques may fail because of recanalization of the tube, but this rarely occurs less than 1 year after the procedure has been performed. Early failure usually indicates that the technique was faulty. In the case of clip sterilization, this means that either one or both clips were applied to the wrong structure or that the clip fell off or extruded the tube.

Different forms of sterilization tend to have different failure rates, but provided the technique is generally acceptable to practising consultants, its use can be defended. In the case of *Gold* v. *Haringey Health Authority*, it was alleged that placement of clips across the proximal part of the ampulla instead of the isthmus was negligent, even though there was evidence that the clip completely enclosed the tube. This allegation was not successful. It is particularly helpful to the Courts if the tubes are photographed in cases of failed sterilization if a second procedure is undertaken.

Implantation before sterilization

In some cases, actions have been brought for failure of sterilizations performed in the second half of the menstrual cycle where implantation has already occurred, even though the period has not been missed. Such allegations can usually be defended provided that the period is not actually overdue. In this case, modern pregnancy tests can detect the presence of human chorionic gonadotrophin within 7 days of the last menstrual period and if serum human chorionic gonadotrophin measurements are available, this may indicate a pregnancy before the last period is missed. An alternative scenario is to perform a diagnostic curettage in all patients sterilized in the second half of the menstrual cycle, but this theoretically raises the risk of performing an illegal termination of pregnancy.

Hazards of laparoscopy

The risks of laparoscopy are well established and have been known since the Royal College of Obstetricians and

Gynaecologists report on laparoscopy in 1978 (Chamberlain & Carron-Brown 1978). In general terms, problems such as bowel perforation, damage to vessels and difficulties with insufflation can be defended provided that the surgeon is known to have adequate experience or to be properly supervised if inexperienced. Claims commonly arise from the failure to recognize damage to the gut with consequent delayed recognition of the development of peritonitis. The use of unipolar diathermy within the peritoneal cavity also leads to delayed perforation of bowel and claims of negligence. With the extensive use of clips or other occlusive devices instead of diathermy, these claims are now becoming very rare.

Termination of pregnancy

In view of the number of terminations that are performed, it is not surprising that the defence organizations have received a large number of claims involving termination of pregnancy. Claims may arise from interpretation of the 1967 Abortion Act or from complications in performing the abortion. In fact, the vast majority of claims are related to the abortion procedure. These difficulties were reviewed by Symonds (1985) in the Royal College of Obstetricians and Gynaecologists' working party on litigation.

'Failed termination'

Continuation of a pregnancy after attempted termination is a common source of litigation. The problem usually arises in early terminations where the gestation sac is missed by the suction curette, but sometimes occurs with later pregnancies. It is usually possible to recognize products of conception in the suction curette or in the suction flask, but sometimes these can be obscured by blood and decidual material. A common defence offered in these cases is that the uterus was bicornuate and that a fetus was removed from one horn, but left intact on the other side. This defence is unlikely to succeed unless there is proven evidence that the woman does have a double uterus. It is often alleged by solicitors for plaintiffs that the products of conception should have been submitted for histological confirmation, but this is not standard procedure in the UK and most laboratories would not welcome such a policy.

The only way that the consequences of mishaps of this type can be avoided is to ensure that all women have a follow-up 6-week visit to the consultant clinic or to the general practitioner so that there will be a chance to recognize an on-going pregnancy.

Incomplete evacuations

Incomplete evacuations are common and sometimes lead to claims, particularly where they cause severe secondary complications from haemorrhage or infection. However, provided the proper steps are taken to complete the evacuation of the uterus, these claims can generally be resisted as the retention of placental tissue or fetal parts is not evidence of negligent management.

Damage to viscera

Perforation of the uterus often occurs during evacuation of the uterus, either during the performance of a therapeutic termination or following a spontaneous abortion. Injuries to the uterus may affect the cervix or the body of the uterus. Excessive dilatation of the cervix may result in damage to the cervix and may be difficult to defend, but the commonest injuries result from perforation of the uterine fundus by the dilators or polyp forceps or by the curette. It is possible to defend claims based on these accidents provided that the problem is recognized and that the appropriate action in taken.

However, extensive damage to the uterus and to bowel as a result of these procedures may be difficult to defend if it is considered that the surgeon's performance was substandard.

Oral contraception

Claims related to oral contraception are not particularly common and this is perhaps surprising in view of their widespread usage. However, patients should be advised of the diminished efficacy of the pill if they are taking anticonvulsants, some antibiotics and tranquillizers and anti-inflammatory compounds. Furthermore, with the modern low-dose pills, missing a pill may result in ovulation and pregnancy.

Good advice can identify these problems and ensure that the doctor is not blamed if failure occurs. It is, perhaps, a reflection on the fact that information about the pill has been widely disseminated that there is a relatively low rate of claims in this field.

Intrauterine devices

Contraception with intrauterine devices enjoyed a time of popularity which is now in decline. Product liability is slowly removing intrauterine devices from the market, despite the fact that for those women who they suit, they are a particularly useful form of contraception. Claims commonly arise from perforation of the uterus either at the time of insertion or at a later date. If the loop strings cannot be seen in the vagina then it is essential to ascertain the whereabouts of the device and to make a decision about its removal. Some claims have arisen concerning long-term problems with pelvic infections and subfertility.

It is important that care is taken to keep the patient properly informed of potential complications. Correct procedure in inserting a device is also important if a defence is to be sustained against allegations arising from uterine perforation.

Complications arising from hysterectomy

Damage to adjacent viscera

The proximity of bladder and bowel to the uterus means that damage to the bladder, ureters and bowel is a recognized hazard of either vaginal or abdominal hysterectomy.

Urinary fistulae are commonly the basis for medicolegal claims. Despite the fact that vesicovaginal and ureterovaginal fistulae are a recognized complication, can it be assumed that they can always be defended? If one ureter is damaged during a difficult hysterectomy where there is extensive pelvic disease, then it should be possible to defend this action as being the sort of complication that any competent gynaecological surgeon can have and almost invariably has met in a professional lifetime. However, if both ureters are ligated during the performance of a routine hysterectomy, it is unlikely that any expert would want to defend such a case in court. The same considerations apply to damage of the bladder or bowel.

Procedures undertaken for urinary incontinence may also result in bladder damage. This may be an acceptable complication depending on the nature of the disease and the skill of the surgeon.

Cervical cytology and carcinoma of the cervix

Various claims have arisen in recent years where either abnormal cervical smears have been filed without any decision or action being taken until an invasive carcinoma has developed, or where the interpretation of the smear has itself been faulty.

The latter event is relatively uncommon, whereas the failure to act on abnormal cytology occurs relatively frequently, usually as a result of reports being filed in casenotes without receiving proper attention. It is, therefore, essential that a good chain of command is established to make certain that all abnormal smear tests are drawn to the attention of the general practitioner or gynaecologist so appropriate action can be taken.

These items form the common basis of claims in gynaecology. There are many other less common sources of litigation which have not been listed.

VALUATION OF A CLAIM — THE QUANTUM

Trials are commonly held to decide on both liability and quantum, but sometimes these events may be split. In forming a judgement about quantum, the judge may take account of the following factors:

1. Pain, suffering and loss of amenity: these factors are difficult to quantify and in the USA this has resulted in unrealistic damages being set by juries. However, damages in British courts tend to be agreed at reasonably fixed levels.
2. Medical and nursing care costs, including those incurred by the relatives in looking after the plaintiff.
3. Future costs of accommodation.
4. Loss of earnings because of incapacity.

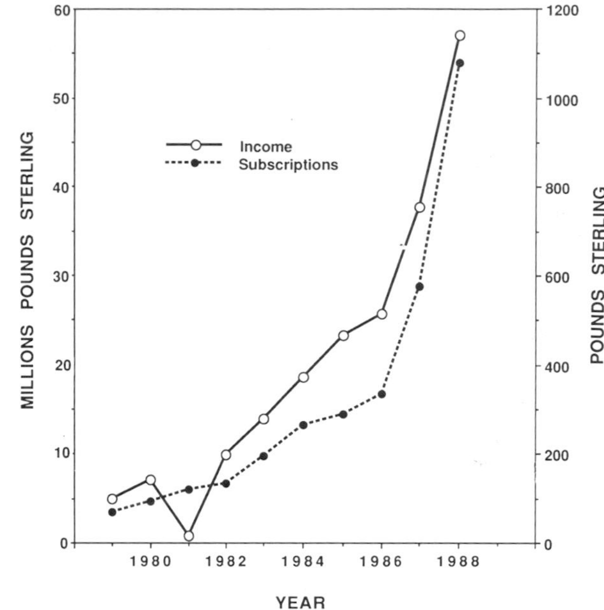

Fig. 62.1 The cost of members' subscriptions and subscription income 1979–1988, derived from Medical Defence Union annual reports.

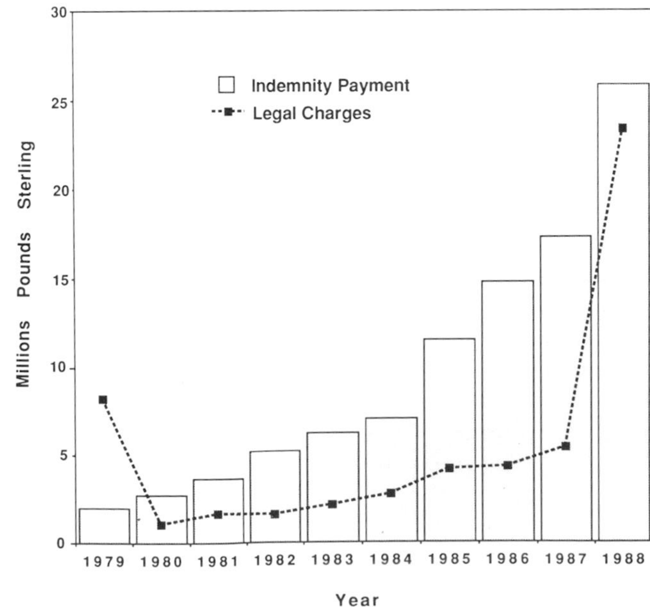

Fig. 62.2 Indemnity payments and legal charges and disbursements 1979–1988, derived from Medical Defence Union annual reports.

The cost of settlements for long-term disabilities is therefore very high, depending on the extent of the disability and life expectancy. This particularly applies to birth-related injuries.

CROWN INDEMNITY

The decade of the 1980s witnessed a massive escalation in malpractice litigation. This is reflected in the subscriptions paid and the income of the Medical Defence Union over the last decade (Fig. 62.1). By 1989, it was becoming apparent that the costs could not be contained within the salary structure of full-time consultants and staff in training. This problem was brought to crisis point by the proposal to introduce differential rates for high-risk specialties. Effectively, this meant that doctors working in high-risk disciplines such as obstetrics, orthopaedics, anaesthesia and neurosurgery would be unable to pay the subscription rates and that these disciplines would become untenable within a relatively short time-span. The Government, therefore, introduced crown indemnity. Liability for patients treated within the National Health Service will be met by the Department of Health.

Examination of the costs for settlements and for legal services and disbursements shows the problem that health authorities have assumed by taking over these responsibilities (Fig. 62.2). This takes no account of the time and effort that will need to be made for defendants and expert witnesses under the civil tort system in the future. In other words, crown indemnity provides a short-term solution for the malpractice crisis, but it will eventually distort patient services and medical recruitment in specific high-risk disciplines. In obstetrics, it must be remembered that the processes of litigation apply to anyone attending upon the labour of any mother.

KEY POINTS

1. Negligence is judged by the standard of the ordinary skilled doctor exercising that special skill and should take into account the level of training of the doctor.
2. For brain damage at birth, the statute of limitations extends up to 21 years after delivery. Other actions for negligence have to be commenced within 3 years of the event causing injury.
3. Surgical litigation can be minimized by good theatre practice.
4. It is the obstetrician's responsibility to check the vagina after repair of episiotomy, to ensure no swabs are left behind.
5. It is important to counsel every patient undergoing sterilization about the risks of failure and ectopic pregnancy.
6. A follow-up visit after termination of pregnancy will enable an ongoing pregnancy to be detected.
7. It is important to inform the patient about likely complications, risks and success rates of any procedure.
8. With an abnormal cervical smear it is prudent to ensure that the general practitioner is also informed of the results.

REFERENCES

Blain A P 1983 Accident compensation in New Zealand, 2nd edn. Butterworth, Wellington, New Zealand

Bolam v. *Friern Hospital Management Committee*. All England Law Report 1957, pp 118, 121

Brahams D 1987 Pregnancy following sterilisation: two cases fail. Lancet i: 638

Butcher C 1990 In: Chamberlain G, Orr C (eds) How to avoid problems in obstetrics and gynaecology. Members of the Joint Medicolegal Committee of the Royal College of Obstetricians and Gynaecologists and the Medical Defence Organisations. Royal College of Obstetricians and Gynaecologists, London

Chamberlain G, Carron-Brown J 1978 In: Gynaecological laparoscopy. Royal College of Obstetricians and Gynaecologist, London

Chamberlain G, Orr C 1990 How to avoid medico-legal problems in obstetrics and gynaecology. Royal College of Obstetricians and Gynaecologists, London

Hawkins C 1985 In: Mishap or malpractice. Blackwell Scientific Publications, Oxford, pp 1–2

Lawton Lord Justice In *Whitehouse v. Jordan*. All England Law Reports 1 1981: 267

Oldertz C 1984 The Swedish patient insurance system — 8 years of experience. Medico-legal Journal 52: 43–59

Symonds E M 1985 Medico-legal aspects of therapeutic abortion. In: Chamberlain G W P, Orr C J B, Sharp F (eds) Litigation and obstetrics and gynaecology, Proceedings of the 14th study group of the RCOG. Royal College of Obstetricians and Gynaecologists, London, pp 123–129

Wilsher v. *Essex Health Authority*. Weekly Law Reports 1987, p 466

63. Forensic gynaecology

R. E. Roberts F. Lewington

RAPE

Nature of assault

Sexual assaults on older girls and adult women may involve rape (vaginal penetration), buggery (anal penetration), oral assault (involving both masturbation and ejaculation) and attempts at these assaults, as well as a range of other indecent acts on various parts of the body. All may be accompanied by actual physical injury or threat of the same. However, it is extremely rare for such victims to be severely wounded, although some may bear defence wounds on the hands or knifetip wounds, particularly on the neck. It is not unusual for victims to have no injuries whatsoever through fear or intimidation. Where the attacker fails in his aims, women may be subjected to a variety of indecent and physical assaults and may be made to perform indecent acts themselves. It is important to remember that the outcome is known when the person presents to the hospital or doctor, but at the time of the attack, extreme fear of death or serious mutilation may well have precluded rational behaviour.

The true frequency of these assaults will never be known since many women will not even seek help from a friend or relative or consult their general practitioner. The data for the charts (Figs 63.1–63.4) are taken from actual referrals to St Mary's Centre, Manchester, a special hospital-based centre which offers a confidential service on a self-referral basis to adults who have been sexually assaulted. The Centre also provides examination facilities for persons reporting to the police and for self-referrals who later wish the police to be informed. These four figures show the source of referral to the Centre, the age of the complainants, the location of the assaults and the frequency of rape and other offences.

Immediate assessment

Management

Women who are injured are likely to report to the police

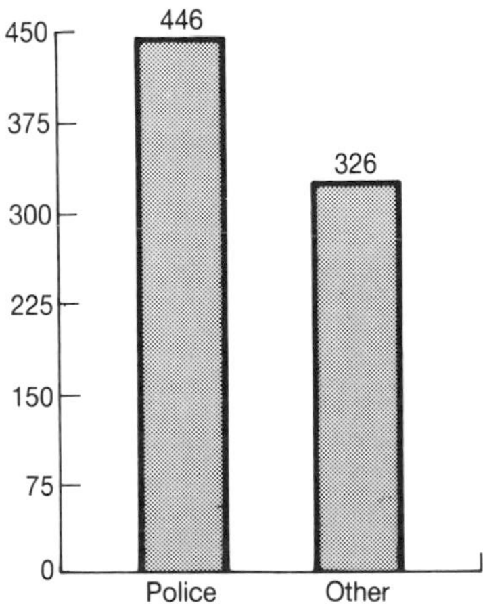

Fig. 63.1 Sources of referral to St Mary's Centre, Manchester. Cases reported to Greater Manchester police are investigated at the Centre. The same service is offered to those reporting directly to the Centre and those who are referred by other agencies such as doctors or social workers.

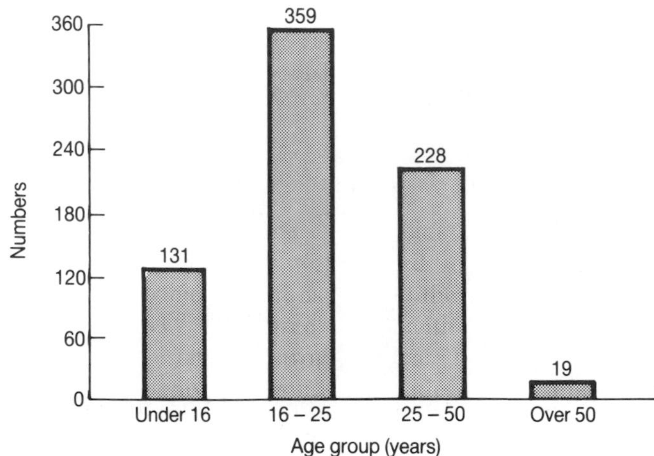

Fig. 63.2 The ages of patients examined at St Mary's Centre, Manchester.

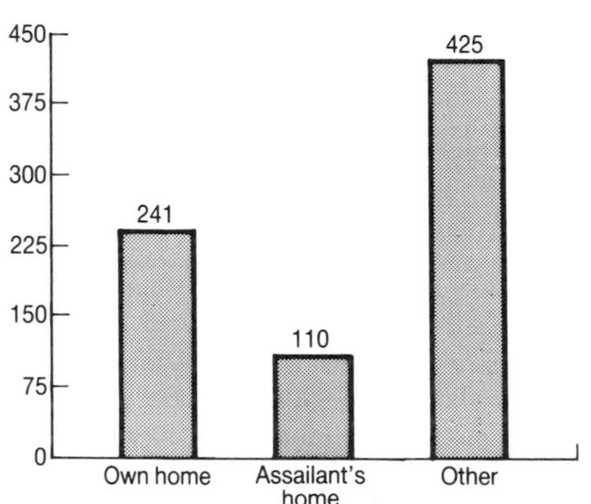

Fig. 63.3 The location of assaults on patients examined at St Mary's Centre, Manchester.

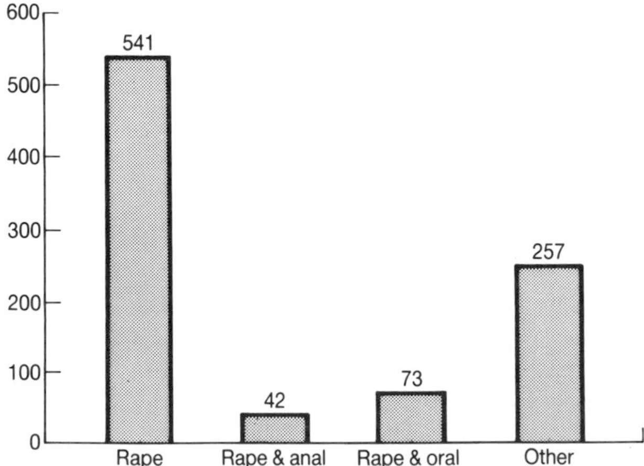

Fig. 63.4 The frequency of rape and other offences among patients examined at St Mary's Centre, Manchester.

or to a Casualty Department shortly after the assault. Others may do so, or only after a few days tell their family doctor, or come to Casualty or a Sexually Transmitted Disease clinic. Patients seeking help from the medical profession should be asked if they wish the police to be informed; if so this should be done without delay.

Reporting to the police

Reasons why women do report

1. For justice
   a. to have the offender punished.
   b. to prevent him attacking others.
2. Degrading acts such as buggery or oral sex may have occurred.
3. Cry for help.
4. Fear of pregnancy or infection.
5. (Rarely) malicious or political.

Reasons why women do not report

1. Afraid of not being believed.
2. The offender is personally known to them.
3. Afraid of reactions of others — family or friends.
4. Fear of court.
5. Wish to forget.

Police forces should have a team of trained forensic physicians (of both sexes) to carry out the forensic medical examination. The woman should have the choice of gender of the examiner. She will usually be examined in a special examination suite or in the doctor's surgery. Alternatively the forensic physician will attend the hospital and take all forensic specimens in the Casualty Department, ward or theatre as appropriate.

Whilst awaiting the arrival of the forensic physician the hospital staff should avoid removing clothing or cleaning away evidence but must remember that the patient may be injured and need medical care.

In many parts of the world there will be no forensic examiner and untrained staff will have to carry out the investigation. A brief outline of the procedures to be followed is given here but staff should have reference to more detailed information (McLay 1990).

Special consent — forensic medical examination

The reasons for the medical examination should be explained and consent obtained for it.

If the assault has been reported to the police it is important that the woman understands the role of the doctor. Confidentiality is implied in most medical situations. If the doctor is carrying out the examination at the request of the police, the complainant must be told at the outset that the medical findings will be reported to them and written consent must be obtained for this.

Partial and delayed reporting to police

If the woman wants to be examined but has not decided whether to report, confidentiality must be respected even if the doctor becomes aware that a serious offence has been committed. Often a woman will allow limited information such as time, site and nature of the attack to be reported but will not at that stage feel able to be interviewed by a police officer. Such wishes must be respected. In these cases a full and careful examination should be made so that evidence is preserved should the offence be reported later.

When the woman has regained some control of her life after sympathetic and skilled care at the crisis point, she may well decide of her own free will to report to the police.

Later presentations

It is worth carrying out a full forensic examination, including the gathering of specimens, if up to a week has elapsed after the assault, but the chances of obtaining forensic evidence are much diminished after 48 hours. There may be evidence of previous injuries, such as bruises, scars or bite marks.

A woman presenting to a gynaecologist with vague symptoms may have been the subject of rape or previous abuse in childhood. Sometimes she may wish to report the matter to the police even after many years. Many women are repeatedly assaulted by their partners. They often feel that serious harm has been done and seek medical investigation.

Notes on the medical examination

The doctor should record carefully everything that has been observed and remember that rape is not a medical diagnosis. Careful recording of observations is what is required and not a value judgement based on incomplete knowledge of the facts.

It is most important that notes are clear, legible, full and contemporaneous. They are the doctor's evidence and the basis on which a statement will be written if required. The notes remain the doctor's personal property but may be called for in court for inspection by the judge and counsel and may be shown to the jury. Specific questions may be asked regarding particular entries.

The medical examination should be of the whole body. It is important to remember that a woman who has been sexually assaulted may not be injured physically. In the vulval area in a sexually active woman there is unlikely to be any sign of trauma unless excessive force was used or objects inserted.

Record

The following details should be recorded:

1. Day, date, time and place of the examination and persons present.
2. Written consent to the examination, permission for photographs of relevant injuries to be taken and for findings to be reported to the police.
3. History of the attack
   a. Physical assault.
   b. Removal of or damage to clothing.
   c. Sexual assault.
   d. Drugs/alcohol involved.
   e. Actions afterwards (washing, bathing, urination, defecation, drinks, medication).
   f. Previous sexual intercourse (if within 2 weeks).
   g. Alcohol or drugs taken immediately prior to the assault.
4. General history
   a. Previous health.
   b. Operation.
   c. Medications.
   d. Gynaecological history.
   e. Obstetric history.
5. State of clothing
   a. Torn or damaged.
   b. Obvious materials adhering (e.g. dust, soil).
   c. Obvious stains (position, colour, wet, dry).

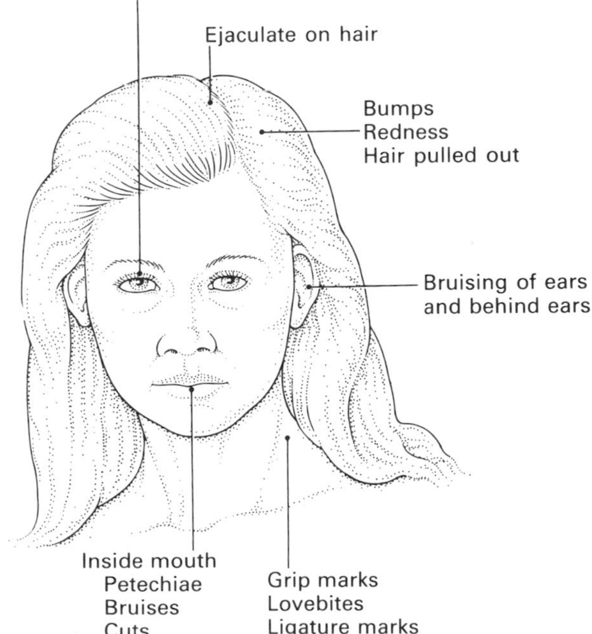

Fig. 63.5 The signs of injury to the head which are likely to be found following sexual assaults.

6. Ask how she feels — record what she says.
7. Examine the whole body and inside the mouth. Measure and chart the injuries. Measure to fixed body points. Photograph if possible.

The various important possible signs of injury to the head, the front of the body, the vulva and anus are indicated in Figures 63.5–63.7.

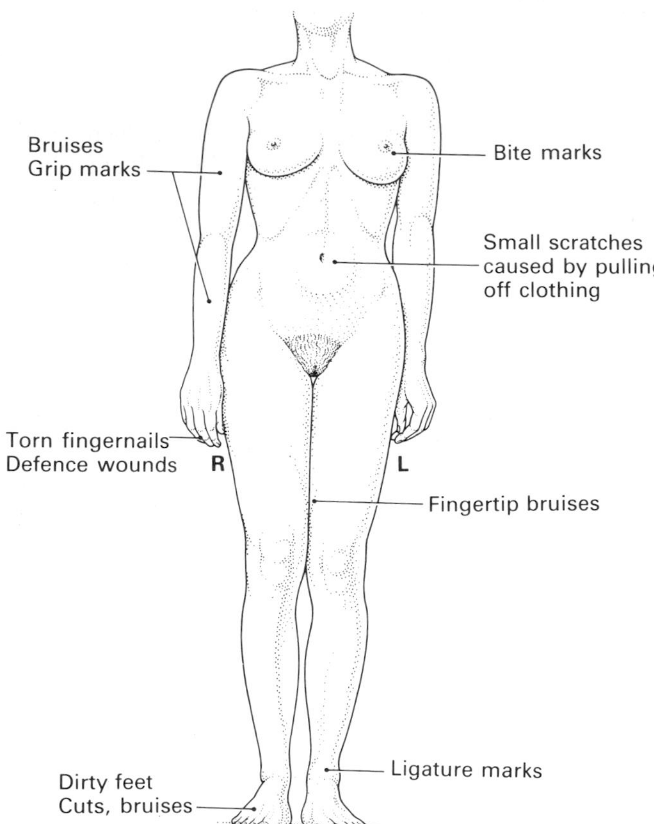

Fig. 63.6 The signs of injury to the body which are likely to be found following sexual assaults.

Forensic samples

The doctor must record exactly how samples were obtained, their labelling, sample number and sealing and to whom they were handed. Also the times when vaginal swabs, preserved blood and urine samples were taken should be recorded.

The forensic samples fall into two categories: evidential samples and control samples (hair, blood and saliva) for comparison purposes. The usefulness of evidential samples will depend not only on the nature of the indecent acts but also on the time since the assault and the woman's actions subsequently.

Time limits for the survival and detection of spermatozoa and seminal fluid from the vagina, anus and mouth and on unwashed clothing and bedding are given in Table 63.1.

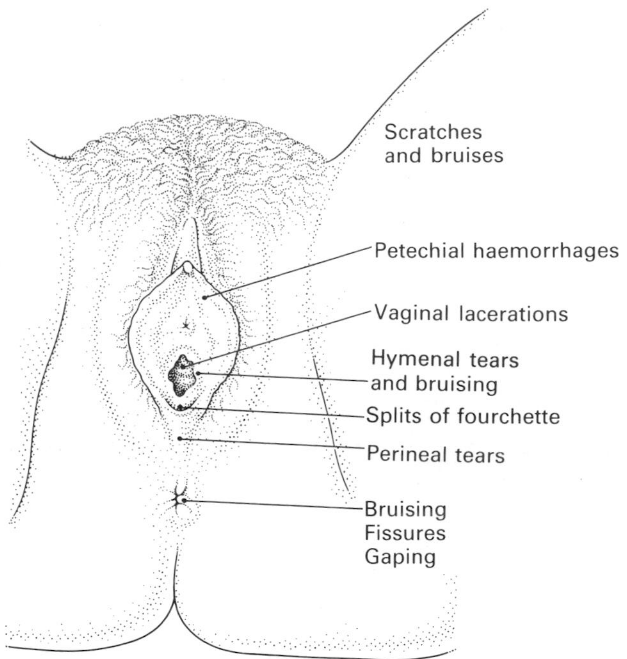

Fig. 63.7 The signs of injury to the vulval area and anus which are likely to be found following sexual assaults.

Taking the specimens

Clothing. Complainants should stand on a sheet of paper when undressing so that any debris which falls can be collected. The paper should be folded and retained as a sample. Place each item of clothing in a separate bag as it is removed. Secure obvious tufts of fibres in place with clear adhesive tape.

Skin swabs. Skin should be swabbed with a slightly moistened swab (water not saline):

1. for blood, if and where seen.
2. for semen, from areas where assailant ejaculated or wiped his penis.
3. for saliva, from areas licked, bitten or spat upon.

A control swab should be taken from an unstained area of skin.

Mouth swab and saliva sample. Swabs from inside the mouth and around the teeth and gums should be taken if oral assault is alleged within the past 24 hours. A liquid saliva sample (10 ml) should also be taken.

Fingernail samples. Cuttings should be taken if blood, fibres or other debris is seen.

External vaginal and anal swabs. These should be taken from around the introitus and anal margin. The vulval and anal areas should then be washed and dried.

Low vaginal swab. This should be taken by separating the labia.

Vaginal examination. A warmed, moistened (but not lubricated) small disposable speculum should be inserted

Table 63.1 Time limits for the detection of spermatozoa and seminal fluid

	Spermatozoa	Reference	Seminal fluid	Reference
Vagina	6 days	Davies & Wilson (1974)	12–18 h	Davies & Wilson (1974)
Anus	3 days	Willott & Allard (1982)	3 h	MPFSL* unpublished
Mouth	12–14 h	Willott & Crosse (1986)	—	
Clothing/bedding	Until washed		Until washed	

* Metropolitan Police Forensic Science Laboratory.

and the walls inspected for injury. Take one or more high vaginal swabs from above the speculum. If a pool of fluid is present, use a pipette to obtain a larger sample. Take an endocervical swab.

Internal anal swab. If buggery is alleged, take internal anal swabs using a small disposable proctoscope. It is usually not possible to insert a proctoscope without a lubricant. Record the use of the lubricant. Take swabs from above the proctoscope to ensure that they are not contaminated. Vaginal swabs must be taken in all suspected buggery cases to establish whether semen found on anal swabs could have drained from the vagina.

Hair samples. Comb the pubic hairs for debris and loose hairs which could have come from the assailant. Cut about 10 pubic hairs close to the skin as a control sample. Similarly take head hair combings and at least 10 pulled hairs from different parts of the head.

Blood samples. Two blood samples are required, one with preservative (sodium fluoride) and anticoagulant (potassium oxalate) for alcohol assay and one with ethylenediaminetetraacetic acid for grouping and DNA profiling.

Urine samples. If drugs are thought to have been involved in the assault, a preserved urine sample should be taken.

Dirt and debris. Swab any areas of dirt or debris.

Control. A control unused swab should be included with the specimens.

Labelling and sealing specimens

Label each specimen with the following:

1. Name of the patient.
2. Date taken.
3. Person taking sample.
4. Type of sample.
5. Sample number.

The accepted way to number samples incorporates the doctor's initials followed by the number of the specimen, e.g. ABC/1 saliva sample; ABC/2 mouth swab.

It is most important to be able to confirm in court that specimens were transferred intact between the doctor and the forensic scientist. Police forces issue individual sealing instructions, all of which are basically as follows. After labelling, the container or bag is fastened with clear adhesive tape. Freezer tape should be used for blood, urine and saliva bottles, swabs and any other items to be refrigerated or frozen. The tape must be wound completely around the neck of bottles and swab caps. When sealing bags the top should be turned over at least 2.5 cm, turned over again and fastened with a strip of adhesive tape sufficiently long for the free ends to be fastened to the reverse of the bag. Many police forces are introducing specially manufactured tamperproof bags which incorporate a court label in the self-adhesive flap of the bag.

If a woman police officer is present during the examination she will often label and seal specimens as they are taken by the doctor.

Storage of items

Forensic specimens can be stored for months or years in a freezer and used as evidence later if properly packaged and identified.

The following can be *frozen*:

1. Swabs.
2. Saliva samples.
3. Preserved blood for solvent analysis.

The following should be *refrigerated*:

1. Preserved blood for drugs/alcohol assay.
2. Blood for grouping and DNA profiling (short-term; for long-term storage freeze the specimen).
3. Urine samples.
4. Fingernail cuttings.

The following should be kept at *room temperature*:

1. Clothing.
2. Hair samples.

Sexually transmitted diseases

After the forensic specimens have been taken, swabs

should be taken for sexually transmitted diseases, not because one would expect to find evidence of disease which had been transmitted in a recent rape, but for the medical care of the woman. A high vaginal swab for *Trichomonas*, endocervical swabs for gonococci and *Chlamydia*, and urethral, anal and oral swabs can easily be taken and placed in the appropriate transport media.

Follow-up is essential and a thorough sexually transmitted disease screen should be done about 7 days later. The question of human immunodeficiency virus infection should be thoroughly considered and discussed at that stage.

Pregnancy

The question of pregnancy must be discussed and appropriate measures taken. Postcoital contraception should be offered if within 72 hours of the attack or the insertion of a coil should be considered.

Reassurance

Finally, some time should be spent discussing the medical findings and problems.

In ideal circumstances a trained rape counsellor will take over the support of the complainant and trained sympathetic police officers will continue the investigation.

Long-term psychological counselling

To be subjected to sexual assault can be one of life's most traumatic experiences. It forces women to question themselves and their world because it destroys their sense of trust and their sense of control over their lives. The guilt and shame at having been raped are already apparent when women are seen shortly after the offence.

Women often feel guilty about not having struggled or resisted and it is all too easy for family, friends and professionals such as doctors and police officers to give the impression that not enough was done to avoid being raped.

The degree of psychological trauma is not proportional to the physical injuries sustained and may even be greater in those who are given the impression that they should have done more to prevent the assault than in those who have injuries.

It is important to reassure the woman that the responsibility lies with the offender, whatever the circumstances.

In the few weeks following, severe emotional reactions are common and may necessitate medical help. Many women seek some form of help during the early weeks but may not be able to talk about the real problem. In a hospital clinic they may tell a sympathetic nurse what has really happened but be unable to tell the doctor. Patients in trouble will offer the doctor a physical complaint such as menorrhagia when the real trouble is too painful to discuss.

Rape trauma

Rape trauma was described by Burgess & Holstrom (1974). It is a post-traumatic stress disorder. The essential feature is the development of characteristic symptoms following a psychologically distressing event outside the range of normal experience which at the time has been accompanied by feelings of intense fear, terror and helplessness.

Symptoms include:

1. Re-experiencing the traumatic event.
2. Avoidance of stimuli associated with the event.
3. Numbing of general responsiveness.
4. Increased arousal.

A prevailing myth about women who have been raped is that they are hysterical and tearful. Many are in a state of shock and disbelief but may appear to be acting normally, even unconcernedly and may describe what has occurred in an almost matter-of-fact way. A woman who is used to dealing with strangers, for example a business executive, may present her story in a detached way as though she were dealing with customers.

Women who initially present in a state of shock and appear to be in control will often break down a few days later and become very distressed.

Sometimes the detailed medical examination does not cause distress when conducted immediately after an assault but if it is carried out a few days later the intimate part of the examination often appears to cause distress and the sensation of the genitalia being touched for the first time after the assault brings back the feelings experienced at the time.

Emotional reactions commonly include shame, guilt and self-blame. Some women become very angry and wish for revenge. Perceived lack of concern as well as insensitive remarks will cause disproportionate upset in the traumatized woman. Thoughts continually return to the circumstances of the rape and the event is relived many times.

Sleep pattern disturbances are common. Difficulty in getting to sleep, waking in the night and nightmares may occur. Eating disorders may also be experienced but are less common.

Physical symptoms specific to the areas which have been injured may be present but psychosomatic symptoms related to these may occur later.

Complaints of vaginal soreness, discharge and menstrual irregularities will commonly lead to the woman seeking help.

The long-term effect

Women may appear to have recovered from the attack and be functioning well only to be set back by situations of stress.

The woman who has been raped will never be quite the

same again. She may recover, become a survivor and even be stronger and more able to cope with adversity afterwards, or may be permanently psychologically scarred or disabled by the experience.

A number of factors will influence the outcome:

1. Previous personality including previous experience of child abuse or rape.
2. The family circumstances and people available for support. Unsupported single women living alone in a large city will find coping much more difficult than those with supportive family and friends.
3. The way the problem is handled by police officers, medical practitioners, hospital staff and the courts.
4 Those who receive psychological help such as counselling, ideally from trained rape counsellors but also from lay counsellors such as those in victim support schemes or from ministers of religion, are generally thought to recover better than those who do not receive such help. Nurses in gynaecological clinics and casualty departments can be of great help.

Physical symptoms may present years after the rape. Sexual dysfunction is common; fears and phobias may develop. Women become afraid of going out, sleeping alone, going in lifts and may be unable to stay in their own home if that is where the rape occurred. Many women will move to a different town after the rape.

The partners and family of the woman who has been raped also suffer considerable stress. Parents and husbands may, after initially being supportive, start to blame the woman and when the rape trauma symptoms persist, become impatient with the continuing disruption of their lives.

Counselling

Where a rape is reported immediately, crisis intervention is indicated. Comfort and support with a caring attitude being shown are more important at this stage than specific counselling skills. It is important not to appear to be judging or critical.

Those who have been raped in the past may develop psychiatric conditions such as depression, suicidal behaviour, drinking or drug abuse and will need appropriate professional help for these problems.

The woman who has not reported the rape to anyone may present with severe psychological problems and with complex physical and particularly gynaecological disorders.

We do not know how many people have been raped in the past and have not sought help about it and yet have 'survived' and lived effective and reasonably happy lives. Certainly many sexual offences are unreported.

False complaints of rape

Any complaint of rape is a cry for help and the woman making the complaint is in great trouble.

It is almost impossible for a doctor to be able to tell whether a person is lying or not unless the story is so fanciful as to be incapable of being true or the details of the alleged rape repeatedly change.

The doctor must be careful not to jump to the conclusion that because the circumstances described are outside his or her experience they must be imagined.

Many complaints of rape are based on fact, but the details have been altered perhaps to offer what is perceived as a more acceptable story. Sometimes self-inflicted injuries such as superficial injuries to the face, breasts and arms will be added on in someone who feels dirty and abused or who feels that she will not be believed unless injured.

Sometimes a stranger may be alleged to have raped when the offender is known but the woman does not want him to go to prison.

A common presentation is for the woman to complain of rape when the real reason for feeling degraded is that buggery or oral sex has occurred.

Many women, even sexually experienced ones, find it impossible to talk about these offences and only during the medical examination when signs of trauma to the anus are found may the real truth emerge.

Some young women may falsely say that they have been raped because their parents are angry at their late arrival home and may already have rung the police. Sympathetic support and understanding from a specially trained police officer and doctor will usually evaluate these cases relatively easily and speedily and advice and the prescription of the morning-after pill will help to resolve the situation.

CHILD SEXUAL ABUSE

Professionals have become increasingly aware of child sexual abuse in recent years. It is not known if the incidence is rising, but more cases are being reported. Children are now much more likely to be believed when they tell someone about abuse. Spontaneous statements by children are likely to be true and must be treated very seriously indeed.

Child sexual abuse is any use of children for the sexual gratification of adults.

It includes:

1. Exposure, e.g. pornographic photography, exposing children to indecent acts by others in real life or on video.
2. Contact, e.g. indecent fondling of the child, masturbation of adult by child, intercrural intercourse.
3. Penetration, oral, vaginal and anal.
4. Penetration with force.

Full sexual intercourse is unusual before the age of 8 or 9, though buggery may occur in younger children. The commonest offences are those of contact, such as indecent fondling progressing to penile contact without penetration.

It is unusual for there to be general physical injuries because the child can be abused by a process of seduction and/or intimidation without the need to use force.

Presentation

The matter may present in a number of ways:

1. A direct or indirect statement from the child.
2. Accidental revelation, e.g. when the child is overheard discussing abusive acts.
3. Perceived abuse, where teachers, social workers or others interpret the child's behaviour as indicating abuse.
4. Physical symptoms, e.g. vulval or anal soreness or discharge.
5. Other maltreatment, where the child is physically abused or fails to thrive.
6. Allegations by others, especially in custody disputes.

Where there is a clear statement by the child, the investigation is relatively straightforward. In the other categories the very greatest caution must be exercised and a careful multidisciplinary assessment is essential before a conclusion can be reached. Often it will be impossible to be certain and this must be accepted. The assessment and diagnosis will never be 100% correct and errors will be made, both in over-diagnosis and under-diagnosis.

Great emphasis has been laid recently on the amount of undiscovered abuse but the damaging effect on children and their families of over-diagnosis has not always been appreciated.

Most child sexual abuse takes place within the family or is perpetrated by persons — usually men — who are known to the child. Stranger abuse and rape are much less common.

Where a child has recently been raped the forensic investigation will be carried out as for the adult woman. In some cases an examination under anaesthetic will be necessary. The careful gathering of forensic evidence and the recording of injuries are vital.

It may be helpful for joint examinations to be carried out by a forensic examiner and a paediatrician or gynaecologist. This is particularly important where neither doctor has a wealth of experience in child abuse investigations.

Most child sexual abuse does not present as an emergency. It has usually been going on for some time and is escalating in its intrusiveness.

It is important to assure the child that no blame attaches to her, either for allowing or taking part in the abuse, or for not reporting at the outset. It is very difficult for a child, for example in a family where the new stepfather pays her special attention and gives treats, to complain if when bathing her or putting her to bed he touches her genitals 'accidentally'. Only when it becomes outside the range of normal behaviour (and this can be difficult for a child to know) will she tell someone. The child may retract the story when she discovers how seriously the matter is viewed and realizes what the consequences of her disclosure may be. The child and her family must be treated with care and consideration, whatever has happened. Remember that if an allegation of child sexual abuse is made the consequences for the family may be catastrophic and the mother may see her whole world collapsing about her.

Factors which may *indicate child sexual abuse*

1. Change in behaviour
   a. Clinging.
   b. Irritable.
   c. Quiet.
2. Regression, e.g. wetting and soiling.
3. Sleep disturbance and nightmares.
4. Poor school performance.
5. Sexualized behaviour.
6. Running away from home.
7. Self-mutilation.
8. Overdoses.
9. Drug abuse.
10. Promiscuity.

It is important to remember that there are many other causes of such problems.

Medical problems which may *indicate child sexual abuse*

1. Recurrent vulval soreness or discharge.
2. Urinary symptoms without infection.
3. Vague complaints, such as abdominal pain.
4. Infections
   a. Gonorrhoea.
   b. *Trichomonas*.
   c. *Chlamydia*.
   d. Condylomata acuminata.
5. Signs of injury to genitalia or anus.
6. Pregnancy.

A teenage girl may present with vague gynaecological problems or may ask to go on the pill. Sexual abuse should be suspected if the girl seems evasive or unhappy and is not able to talk about her problem or say who her sexual partner is. Some complaints of rape are masked presentations of child sexual abuse. Injuries to the genitalia may be claimed to be accidental when they are due to abuse.

Medical examination

The medical examination is only one part of the investigation of child sexual abuse. In all cases a careful multidisciplinary approach is essential with information from a number of professionals being pooled. The findings can only be evaluated in the context of a full assessment including careful inquiry about family habits and social patterns. It is rarely possible to make a diagnosis on the medical findings alone. Only the presence of semen or pregnancy can prove with certainty that abuse has occurred. If paternity is the issue, e.g. in a suspected incestuous relationship, the police may well ask for release of the fetus for DNA profiling studies if there is a termination.

The child may be referred for medical examination because she has said that abuse has occurred, or because there is medical concern.

It is important that any medical examination does not constitute an abuse of the child. If no penetration has occurred the child may perceive the medical examination as being worse than the alleged abuse. In many cases a careful and thorough inspection, without any touching, may be all that is indicated.

The number of examinations should be kept to a minimum. Where there is no forensic urgency the examination should be arranged for a convenient time within the next few days but the anxieties of the parents and child and the need for the police to have as much information as possible before they interview the alleged perpetrator indicate that it should be carried out as expeditiously as possible.

The examination should be conducted in quiet, private surroundings and not behind curtains in a busy casualty department.

The child should be treated with consideration and respect. She should be told what is to happen and invited to help. A full general examination should be carried out, both to let the child settle down and to find any general injuries or abnormalities. Height and weight, the state of nutrition and general paediatric information should be recorded.

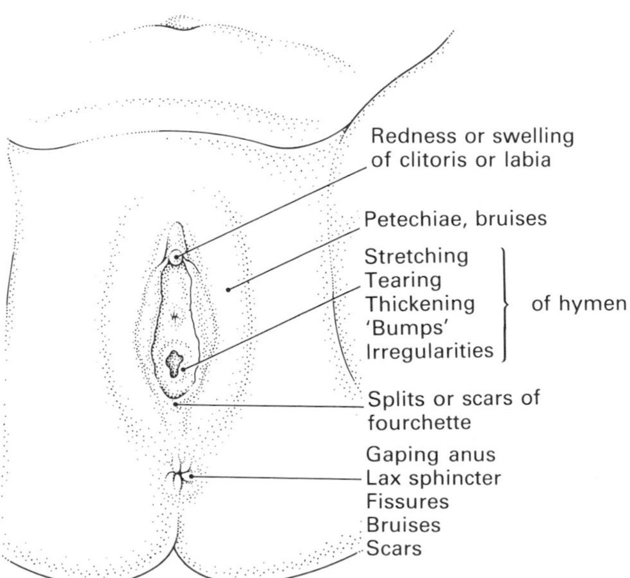

Fig. 63.8 The signs of injury to the vulval area and anus which are likely to be found following child sexual abuse.

The behaviour of the child should be noted and the apparent relationship with the parent observed and recorded.

The preschool child is usually most easily examined on the mother's knee, though some will happily lie on the examination couch. Older children may wish to be examined without the parent present, but the parent or carer must stay nearby.

The medical examination of the genitalia and anus should try to answer the following questions:

1. Is the finding normal or abnormal?
2. If abnormal, is there some innocent explanation or is it due to abuse?
3. If due to abuse:
   a. What caused it?
   b. How was it caused?
   c. How often has it occurred?

It may not be possible to answer these questions, but they must be considered.

Possible causes for abnormal findings

1. Congenital deformity.
2. Medical condition/infection.
3. Medical treatment.
4. Family remedies.
5. Poor hygiene.
6. Cleansing, e.g. bubble baths, disinfectants.
7. Accidental injury.
8. Self-inflicted injury.
9. Abuse/assault.

Medical findings which may indicate abuse

In many children who have been sexually abused there will be no medical findings. The absence of signs of recent or healed injuries does not negate the allegation or suspicion. Possible findings in the vulval and anal areas are shown in Figure 63.8.

General injuries

There may be signs of previous non-accidental injury or neglect. Bruises, particularly grip marks on the lower face, the arms or legs or over the pelvis may be seen. Inside the mouth the frenulum may be torn, bruising may be seen inside the cheeks where the face has been gripped, or there may be patchy petechial haemorrhages on the roof of the mouth caused by forceful insertion of the penis. Love bites caused by sucking and tongue pressure are unusual in children.

The vulval area

Rubbing and fondling of the genitalia may cause patchy or

general redness and occasionally the skin over the clitoris may be reddened and swollen.

Pushing the penis against the genital area may cause stretching and slight tearing of the hymenal orifice. Small splits of the fourchette may be seen or may heal leaving fine scars but scarring is not invariable. Friability of the fourchette may occur with non-specific vulvitis as well as with abuse.

The introitus may become stretched and widened by repeated rubbing without there being any tears in the hymen. Care must be taken to distinguish a prominent vestibule from the hymenal opening.

Labial adhesion may sometimes be caused by rubbing which has been sufficient to produce superficial trauma, causing the edges to stick together as they heal but adhesions are usually associated with low oestrogen status and are almost certainly innocent.

Hymen

It is essential to spend some time looking at the hymen before coming to a definite conclusion about it. As the child settles down, the orifice will open up and sometimes will appear to vary in size. The edge of the hymen can often be thoroughly inspected by gently pulling the labia forwards and down, but in some cases it is necessary to insert a small glass probe and display the edge of the hymen over the glass. Occasionally, tears in the hymen not seen previously will become apparent. The edge of the hymen should be carefully inspected with a magnifying light. Occasionally, whitish scars will be seen, particularly in the posterior half, or increased vascularity and distorted blood vessels may be present where there has been previous damage. Clean tears of the hymen caused by one episode of interference may heal leaving no trace. The presence of bumps on the edge of the hymen is thought to be an indicator of previous damage and may be caused by the healing of slight tears.

The area surrounding the urethra may show bruising or petechial haemorrhages when pressure has been exerted there, but it is unusual to get tears of the hymen in the anterior part because the urethra supports and buttresses it. Errors have occurred in mistaking a normal crescentic hymen for tears.

The size of the introitus is of less significance than the condition of the hymen though it is helpful to make some estimate of its size in both the anterior–posterior and side-to-side planes. A diagram should be made of the shape and character of the hymen and should record whether any measurement has been made visually, by using a measure or by inserting glass rods.

In young children no attempt should be made to insert a finger into the vagina.

At the time of the examination, swabs should be taken for sexually transmitted diseases. This can be done gently using a swab moistened in saline or tap water or it is quite possible to allow the child to take the swab herself thereby reducing the degree of stress and trauma.

Examination of the anus

In all cases of possible child sexual abuse, the anus should be inspected. The presence of fissures, scars, skin tags and engorged veins should be noted. The anus may dilate as the buttocks are separated and the degree of dilatation should be recorded. With firm pressure on the buttocks many children will show some degree of opening of the external sphincter and in some the internal sphincter will also open, particularly if faeces are present in the rectum. The significance of anal dilatation is at present unproven. It has been claimed as a significant diagnostic pointer to anal abuse but it is increasingly being reported that anal dilatation occurs commonly in normal children, particularly in very small children. In more than 50% of cases where anal abuse has occurred there will be no medical signs.

Differential diagnosis

Many children are referred to paediatricians and gynaecologists because of vulval soreness or discharge. Some of them have been sexually abused but many have not. During the examination the child can be asked what made her sore and will sometimes make a spontaneous disclosure of abuse. If this occurs the questions, as well as the answers, should be recorded. Care must be taken to avoid leading questions which suggest the answer.

Accidental injuries caused by falling astride bicycle crossbars and the like are common. Usually there is bruising of the outer vulval area and sometimes splits are seen between the labia minora and majora. The hymen is not damaged in this type of accident but occasionally may be torn if there is a shearing force such as that caused by being run over by a car wheel or if there is a fall on to a sharp object. The findings should be entirely consistent with the history given. The ordinary principles of medicine should apply to this subject as to any other and investigations should be completed before a diagnosis is made.

Reassurance

After the examination, with the child dressed, the doctor should spend some time talking to both the child and the carers about the examination and findings. Children who have been sexually abused feel guilty and blame themselves for what has happened and it is important for the doctor, as well as for other investigators, to reassure the child that it is not her fault.

Children often feel that they have been seriously physically damaged and will not be able to grow up normally and have babies. A few minutes spent reassuring the child that whatever has happened she is absolutely normal and is the same as everyone else can be of enormous benefit in starting the process of recovery and minimizing the damaging effects of the abuse.

Counselling

At present, services for sexually abused children are patchy and variable. Local authority and voluntary sector social workers are becoming more aware of the problem and training is improving. Long-term counselling for families, including the perpetrator, and for the child may be needed. In some areas treatment programmes under the jurisdiction of the court may be available, such as those of Giaretto et al (1978) in California. Incest survivor groups can often be helpful, provided that their members have come to terms with their own problems.

In many places there will be little, if any, satisfactory long-term help and the damaging effect of child sexual abuse with its consequences of poor self-image and a failure of the abused person to reach her potential in life will be apparent for many years and will leave scars not only on the victim, but on her family and friends.

How the problem is handled in the first 48 hours after the matter comes to light and in particular the therapeutic effect of skilled and sympathetic medical intervention can do a great deal to minimize these effects and to ensure that the child does not become a permanent loser in life.

INVESTIGATIONS

Laboratory examinations and interpretation of results

The laboratory examination (Keating 1988a, 1988b) is based on Locard's exchange principle 'that every contact leaves a trace' (Locard 1928). The evidential trace materials are of two types: loose debris and stains.

The examination seeks to investigate possible links between the suspect, the victim, the scene of the assault (e.g. child's bed) and items used in the assault (e.g. a bottle neck or broom handle which may have been forced into the vagina or anus).

The materials examined will include those gathered by police investigators in addition to samples taken by doctors examining both victims and suspects.

The amount of evidence detected will depend on the nature of the assault, the time-interval since it happened and subsequent handling of evidential materials, e.g. seminal stains on underwear may have been removed by washing.

The scientific examination may also concern the analysis of preserved blood and urine samples for alcohol, drugs and solvents.

In sexual assaults the evidentially most useful materials are:

1. Semen, blood, saliva, vaginal fluid, lubricants, faeces and urine detected as stains on swabs, clothing, bedding, carpets, etc.
2. Textile fibres, hairs and vegetation detected as loose debris in body samples and on clothing and bedding.
3. Drugs, alcohol, and solvents detected in blood and urine samples.

The examination will involve locating the materials, e.g. invisible semen and saliva stains, their identification and comparison with known control samples to establish their origin, e.g. comparison of a DNA profile from a seminal stain with that obtained from a blood sample from a possible suspect, or pubic hairs removed from a child's mouth with those in a pubic hair sample from the suspected perpetrator.

The trace materials are not usually in a good condition, stains are often small and mixtures frequently occur. A blood-stained vaginal swab could be examined for semen and saliva or an external anal swab for lubricants and semen.

The presence of semen provides the most conclusive evidence of sexual intercourse (but not assault) and the laboratory examination will concentrate on the detection and grouping of any seminal stains on swabs, clothing, bedding etc. Stains may be identified by the presence of spermatozoa or biochemical constituents of the seminal fluid (including acid phosphatase, choline and prostaglandins). Spermatozoa usually persist for much longer (up to 6 days in the vagina) than the chemical constituents (Davies & Wilson 1974), but may be absent (e.g. naturally or after a vasectomy). The longest time-interval for the detection of spermatozoa on anal and rectal swabs is 46 and 65 h respectively (Willott & Allard 1982) and from the mouth 21 h (Davies 1986). It is possible to detect spermatozoa and seminal fluid in stains on unwashed clothing and bedding for many months after the assault.

In an allegation of buggery, anal swabs from a victim should be examined in conjunction with vaginal swabs. The finding of semen on anal swabs is indicative of buggery only when there is no semen on the vaginal swabs.

Many stains contain relatively large quantities of vaginal material and few spermatozoa. Treatment of stains with a proteinase (to digest epithelial cells) greatly improves the chances of detecting the relatively few spermatozoa present (Chapman et al 1989).

Assay of acid phosphatase activity using *p*-nitrophenyl phosphate as substrate is used to provide more certainty of the presence of seminal fluid on vaginal swabs in the absence of spermatozoa, and for estimation of the time-interval between intercourse and the taking of the swabs in cases where the time of assault is doubtful (Allard & Davies 1978; Davies 1978).

In order to interpret laboratory findings scientists will need to know the exact time when the doctor took the vaginal swabs and preserved blood and urine samples. The laboratory will also require information from the medical examination of the complainant regarding:

1. Previous sexual intercourse (if within 2 weeks of the assault).
2. Contraception on that occasion.
3. Source of any bleeding.
4. Infectious diseases.
5. Current medication.

The advent of DNA profiling and its adaptation for criminal investigations (Gill et al 1985) has made it possible to link seminal stains to a suspect with a high degree of probability.

DNA profiling, also known as genetic fingerprinting or DNA fingerprinting, was originally described by Professor Alec Jefferys at Leicester University (Jefferys et al 1985). He discovered that there are hypervariable regions in the DNA structure where the base sequence differs markedly between individuals. Within these hypervariable regions there are short sequences of DNA which are repeated many times. The length of each repeated sequence, the number of repeats and their exact location within the molecule are exactly characteristic of the individual. These sequences can be visualized by the laboratory process using a radioactive DNA probe to reveal a unique multiple-band pattern on an X-ray film — the DNA profile (Gill et al 1985). This involves comparison of DNA profiles from the seminal stains with those of blood samples from suspects. DNA profiling is particularly successful for the elimination of possible suspects.

DNA profiling is not suitable for grouping seminal stains where there are few or no spermatozoa. Such stains may be grouped using the ABO, Lewis/secretor, phosphoglucomutase, glyoxylase and peptidase A systems, of which the ABO system is the most useful and successful.

DNA profiling is routinely used for seminal stains with a sufficient concentration of spermatozoa. In addition this technique can be used to identify the source of other body fluid stains such as blood, vaginal fluid, saliva, urine and nasal mucus, provided they contain sufficient cellular material.

In the forensic situation many of the samples to be analysed yield insufficient DNA for analysis with the standard multilocus probes; also the DNA may be partially broken down due to age or storage conditions. A new generation of DNA probes known as single-locus probes have been developed and are now routinely used in forensic examinations. These probes examine the DNA at a single locus and produce a profile of only two bands in any individual. These probes are particularly useful for the examination of stains containing mixtures of body fluids from more than one person, e.g. a mixture of semen and vaginal fluid on a sheet, a vaginal swab stained with semen from two or more assailants. Two or more single-locus probes can be used sequentially on a single stain to produce for example a six-band pattern using three probes.

DNA profiling using both single-locus and multilocus probes is particularly useful in situations of disputed paternity. Successful results can be obtained from fetal material, e.g. obtained by the termination of a pregnant teenage girl.

Future trends

Three important areas of research at present are:

1. The need to reduce the length of time required to produce a result (at present in excess of 2 weeks).
2. The need to accumulate further statistics regarding band frequency in specific ethnic groups.
3. Reduction in sample size is needed, including the replication of small amounts of DNA (polymerase chain reaction) to give sufficient material to yield a DNA profile. A significant consideration in this work is the need to eliminate replication of possible contaminants.

COURT PROCEEDINGS

Preparation of the patient for court

It has been said that a woman is raped three times: firstly by her assailant, secondly by the medical examination and thirdly in the court.

Doctors are increasingly aware of the problems of raped women and likely to offer a more understanding and sympathetic approach than has sometimes been the case in the past.

The ordeal of giving evidence in court, however, is still considerable, though improved arrangements are often made now to allow witnesses to sit in a private waiting area and to be kept informed at all times what is happening.

The period of waiting for the court hearing, which may be many months, can be very stressful and when the episode has to be relived in the court and the woman's account is perhaps vigorously cross-examined, all the symptoms experienced at the time of the offence may return.

Law enforcement officers are likely now to ensure that the woman is aware of what is likely to happen. A police officer or rape counsellor may take the woman to see the court before the hearing and familiarize her with the procedure.

The woman often feels that she is on trial as well as the defendant and that if he is found not guilty this implies that she is guilty. It is helpful to explain that a criminal trial requires a burden of proof beyond that where it is the word of one person against another so that the judge may advise the jury that it is unsafe to convict in such circumstances. This does not mean that she has not been believed.

It is most important for her to be strongly assured that if she tells the truth she has nothing to fear. She can retain her self-respect whether the whole truth comes out in the court or not, and whether the defendant is found guilty or not.

When a court case is concluded, whether successfully or not, the woman may suffer an acute episode of stress and even if under the care of a counsellor, may take an overdose of drugs or need more help.

If the man is convicted, she may feel guilt that she has caused him to go to prison. If he is acquitted she may feel that reporting the crime was a waste of time; she may also be afraid of retaliation or revenge from the defendant or his family or friends.

In the case of child witnesses, special arrangements are now made to reduce the stress, but the court case is described by survivors as being the most traumatic event following the disclosure.

Children may now give evidence by live video link or be screened from the alleged perpetrator and in some countries prerecorded video evidence is accepted. There are legal difficulties in permitting this as an accused man has the right to see and hear his accuser and the jury should see as well as hear the witness give evidence.

At present the legal system appears to safeguard the rights of the defendant but pays insufficient regard to the needs and rights of the aggrieved person.

Redressing the balance without removing the inalienable right of the citizen in common law jurisdiction to be regarded innocent until proved guilty is fraught with difficulty.

Presentation of the doctor's evidence (see Ch. 62)

Doctors are often afraid of court and may try to avoid being involved in matters which may require them to give evidence in court. The subjects of rape and child sexual abuse are distasteful and upsetting but the people who suffer such violations deserve skilled and professional help. The doctor should not 'pass by on the other side' but should use the skills of medicine and surgery to help.

It is important to remain objective and impartial whilst offering care and help. It is not possible to remain unaffected by what is seen and heard but it is important not to become emotionally involved and appear to be biased in favour of the complainant when giving evidence.

The doctor should not try to be a detective or social worker but should approach these problems as any other medical problem, using medical skill and training. In all cases the patient should be treated with courtesy and consideration.

Documentation and reports

Full, clear and legible notes should be made at the time of the examination. Those facts which it is important to record in rape examinations have already been listed above. Recording the following data is essential preparation for the court hearing:

1. Name, age and date of birth of the complainant.
2. Day, date and place of the examination.
3. Time of start and finish of the examination and when notes were completed.
4. Who requested the examination.
5. Purpose of the examination/nature of the assault.
6. Who gave consent to the examination.
7. Who was present during the examination.
8. Details of any findings.
9. If forensic samples were taken, from
   — where they were obtained, their
   — labelling and sealing and to whom they
   — were handed.

In cases of child abuse the following are essential:

1. The position in which the child was examined.
2. What instruments were used.
3. What the child said during the examination. Record the questions, which should be non-leading, i.e. not suggesting the answer, as well as the answers.

A differential diagnosis should be considered and if possible a diagnosis reached. It is important to remember, however, that neither rape nor child sexual abuse is the subject of a medical diagnosis but that an opinion should be offered as to whether the findings observed are consistent with the history given, or whether there is another more likely explanation.

The doctor may be called as a professional witness to describe what was found at the time of the examination. Usually, having described the findings, the doctor will be asked to give an opinion as to what may have caused the findings and then becomes an expert witness.

After the examination-in-chief, which in a criminal trial is usually conducted by counsel for the prosecution, the doctor will be cross-examined by the opposing side. Counsel for the defence is allowed to ask leading questions and can suggest answers to the witness. The doctor should be careful to agree only with that part of the answer which is accurate and not to be led into making statements with which he or she is unhappy.

It is important, in giving evidence, to keep one's answers simple and as brief as possible. The longer one speaks, the more likely one is to make an error which will be picked up by the opposing counsel.

Before giving evidence in court, it is important to read carefully through the notes and refresh one's memory about the case. If there are any points where medical expertise is required, then the appropriate textbooks or journals should be consulted.

Always remember that the doctor's task is to assist the court from the basis of his or her special knowledge. If the doctor makes a careful, thorough and unbiased examination at the time, provides thorough and comprehensive notes, prepares the night before the case and, as Bernard Knight (1987) said: 'dresses up, stands up, speaks up and shuts up', there will be nothing to fear.

> Truth or the nearest reasonable approach to it that is possible from what is observed is the sole aim.
>
> The doctor who properly says he does not know or feels inadequately qualified to advise acquires more respect than one who 'ventures an opinion' (Simpson 1986).

KEY POINTS

1. The frequency of assault on women is unknown.
2. Chances of forensic evidence are diminished after 48 hours.
3. Careful recording of observation and labelling of samples and specimens are mandatory.
4. It is important to treat the physical and psychological effects of trauma.
5. Most child abuse takes place within the family or by someone known to the child and usually does not present as an emergency but rather as a chronic situation which has become worse.
6. In more than 50% of cases where anal abuse has occurred, there will be no medical signs.
7. DNA profiling (genetic fingerprinting) provides great accuracy in detecting source of body fluids, e.g. semen, vaginal fluid, saliva and blood.
8. Single locus DNA probes are particularly useful when disputed paternity exists.
9. Many women and children will not admit to an assault because of shame and a fear of not being believed.

REFERENCES

Allard J, Davies A 1978 Further information on the use of *p*-nitrophenyl phosphate on vaginal swabs examined in cases of sexual assault. Medicine, Science and the Law 19: 170–172

Burgess A W, Holstrom L L 1974 Rape trauma syndrome. American Journal of Psychiatry 131: 980–986

Chapman R L, Brown N M, Keating S M 1989 The isolation of spermatozoa from sexual assault swabs using proteinase K. Journal of the Forensic Science Society 29: 207–212

Davies A 1978 A preliminary investigation using *p*-nitrophenyl phosphate on vaginal swabs examined in cases of sexual assault. Medicine, Science and the Law 18: 174–178

Davies A 1986 The sexual abuse of children: cases submitted to a police laboratory and the scientific evidence. Medicine, Science and the Law 26: 103–106

Davies A, Wilson E 1974 The persistence of seminal constituents in the human vagina. Forensic Science 3: 45–55

Giaretto H, Giaretto A, Sgroi S M 1978 In: Sexual assault of children and adolescents. Lexington Books, Lexington, Massachusetts, pp 231–240

Gill P, Jeffreys A J, Werrett D J 1985 Forensic applications of DNA fingerprints. Nature 318: 577–579

Jeffreys A J, Wilson V, Thein S L 1985 Individual-specific fingerprints of human DNA. Nature 314: 67–73

Keating S M 1988a The laboratory approach to sexual assault cases. Part I. Sources of information and acts of intercourse. Journal of the Forensic Science Society 28: 35–47

Keating S M 1988b The laboratory approach to sexual assault cases. Part II. Demonstration of the possible offender. Journal of the Forensic Science Society 28: 99–110

Knight B 1987 Legal aspects of medical practice, 4th edn. Churchill Livingstone, Edinburgh

Locard E 1928 Dust and its analysis. Police Journal 1: 177–192

McLay W D S (ed) 1990 Clinical forensic medicine. Association of Police Surgeons

Simpson K 1986 Textbook of forensic medicine, 9th edn. Edward Arnold, London

Willott G M, Allard J E 1982 Spermatozoa — their persistence after sexual intercourse. Forensic Science International 19: 135–154

Willott G M, Crosse M M 1986 The detection of spermatozoa in the mouth. Journal of the Forensic Science Society 26: 125–128

FURTHER READING

Jones D P H, McQuiston M G 1988 Interviewing the sexually abused child. Royal College of Psychiatrists, Gaskell, London

Krugman R D 1986 Recognition of sexual abuse in children. Paediatrics in Review 8: 25–30

Meadow R (ed) 1989 ABC of child abuse. British Medical Journal

Steiner H, Taylor M 1988 Description and recording of physical signs in suspected child sexual abuse. British Journal of Hospital Medicine 40: 346–351

Underhill R, Dewhurst C J 1978 The doctor cannot always tell. Medical examination of the 'intact' hymen. Lancet 375

64. Medical ethics

M. C. Macnaughton

BACKGROUND ETHICAL PRINCIPLES

In western culture there are three ethical principles. These are:

1. *Respect for persons*. There are two parts to this principle:
   a. Autonomy: this requires that competent people be governed by their own wishes and preferences and that competence be presumed in the case of adult persons and in adolescents who show on a case-to-case basis that they possess adequate understanding and a capacity to bear the consequences of autonomous decision-making.
   b. Protection of the vulnerable: this requires that guardianship be exercised over children, adolescents and impaired adults who are incapable of autonomy.
2. *Beneficence*. This principle goes beyond the negative medical ethic 'do no harm' by imposing a positive duty to seek good, if necessary by initiating action that will advance the welfare of individuals and communities.
3. *Justice*. This principle is directed to the achievement of fairness in dealings among peoples, for instance by seeking to ensure that the intended beneficiaries of a development will bear its risks and pay its costs appropriately and that one group of people will not be sacrificed to the benefit of another.

Traditional western ethics has tended to concentrate on ethical relationships between individuals. Other religious and political cultures have given primacy to the collectivity of the group or state as the focal point of ethical concern and have considered the individual only in so far as the individual owes duties to the state and enjoys rights to protection through membership of the group or nation. Ethical principles can therefore be applied at several different levels. There are at least four levels of ethics:

1. *Microethics*. This is concerned with interaction between individuals and provides the level at which most western ethical discussion is conducted. Microethics addresses the duty an individual owes to each other individual and the expectations that each individual may properly have of each other individual.
2. *Mesoethics*. This occupies the middle ground between microethics and macroethics. Mesoethics is usually considered as administrative, management or bureaucratic ethics that deals mainly with resource allocation. Mesoethics is being developed particularly with respect to health resource allocation, as between the public and private sectors.
3. *Macroethics*. This is concerned with the discharge of governmental or other collective responsibilities. Macroethics might deal with the ethics of allocation of a national budget between sections such as health and defence.
4. *Megaethics*. Megaethics is concerned with the survival of the human species but has application to population policy, for example human habitation that causes deforestation, loss of rainforests and agricultural practices to support population growth that result in the spread of deserts. In the case of infertility, megaethical issues may be involved when natural varieties are endangered through genetically linked infertility and also when the dysgenic are assisted through artificial means to reproduce their kind. Megaethics, therefore, raises more pervasive and enduring issues affecting human stock and racial varieties than are addressed by macroethics.

With regard to some of the new techniques which have become available in our pluralistic society it is not to be expected that any one set of principles can be enunciated which will be completely acceptable by everyone. The law itself binding on everyone in society whatever their beliefs is the embodiment of a common moral position. Within legislation, however, there is room for different and perhaps more stringent moral rules. What is legally permissive may be thought of as the minimum requirement for a tolerable society. Individuals or communities may voluntarily adopt more exacting standards. The question is ultimately in what sort of society can we live with a clear conscience?

ETHICS AND ARTIFICIAL REPRODUCTION

Artificial reproduction is defined as where some third party has to intervene in the process of reproduction.

Donor insemination

Donor insemination (DI) is where seminal fluid of a third person is used to inseminate the wife of a man who is infertile. The resultant child is not the genetic child of the husband of the woman, although it may be the social child. A child born by this technique was until recently in England and Wales illegitimate but recently a law has been passed implementing one of the recommendations of the Warnock Report (1984). This was that, provided the husband agrees to his wife being inseminated in this way with material from a donor, a child born of DI is legitimate in law.

However, while this removes a legal problem it does not necessarily remove an ethical problem. Many of the children born as a result of DI are not told of their origin. It is particularly essential that the child should know of its origins if the reason for the artificial insemination was a genetic one. The result of this problem is that the secrecy involved in DI obliges the practitioner, the husband, the wife and the donor to conspire together to deceive the child and society as to the child's true parentage and genetic identity.

The question of the donor also gives rise to ethical considerations. At present there is a regrettable ignorance and uncertainty about his motives, about the effect of his action upon himself both in the short and long term and about his suitability for the role of father of a child to which he will forever remain unrelated.

There have been difficulties also about the production of semen for DI but the giving of semen for examination or for assisted insemination of a wife would now be considered to be done for a proper end and therefore licit in Anglican moral theology. Formal Roman Catholic discipline would still appear to forbid it although some Roman Catholic moral theologians are now quoted who would permit it (Mahoney 1984). The basic moral requirement is that a man should take full responsibility for his offspring. To moralists, for whom this requirement is paramount, it is not enough that the donor will know that someone will be responsible for his child. The responsibility is exclusively his because of the moral relationship which derives from paternity. To beget a child without the possibility of a continuing father–child relationship is to withdraw biological from personal potential. In a defined sense, therefore, the donor's action made possible by human science is anti-human. It isolates biological potential from human potential. The DI donor in this respect is a social isolate without continuing responsibility.

The question as to whether donors should be paid has clear moral implications. Implications as to motive and even clearer scientific implications are highly relevant to medical practice. The problem with paid donors is that the donor may be tempted to withhold some information about himself that would, if known, make him unacceptable as a donor. The Warnock Committee (1984) recommended that there should be a gradual move towards a system where semen donors should be given only their expenses.

DI is now considered by society to be an acceptable form of treatment where the husband is infertile. This social acceptance has occurred only in about the last 30 years: in 1960 the Feversham Committee set up by the Government to consider DI considered that the majority within both society and the medical profession was opposed to the practice of DI. It concluded that DI was an undesirable practice, strongly to be discouraged!

In vitro fertilization

A full decade has passed since the birth of Louise Brown — the first child to be born as a result of in vitro fertilization (IVF). Initially this type of therapy was used for women with damaged or diseased fallopian tubes but more recently it has been utilized in the treatment of oligospermia and unexplained infertility.

Many people regard IVF as an exciting possibility for helping the childless but there are those who are deeply worried by its development (Torrance 1984). These people either feel that IVF is fundamentally wrong or are worried about its consequences. Those who feel that it is fundamentally wrong consider that this practice represents a deviation from normal intercourse and that the unitive and procreative aspects of intercourse should not be separated. Those who hold this view believe that it is an absolute moral principle which must be upheld without exception.

The arguments based on consideration of the consequences are slightly different. These reservations start when IVF results in more embryos being brought into existence than will be transferred to the mother's uterus. It is argued that it is not acceptable deliberately to produce embryos which have a potential for human life when that potential will never be realized. A mesoethical problem that arises is the argument which asks whether the country can afford such special treatment which benefits only a few when the money might be better spent elsewhere with beneficial effects for more people. However, it does seem that the use of IVF has been generally accepted in the UK, although most of the funds now come from the private sector.

When the use of donor material for IVF is considered then other ethical issues arise. DI has been used in cases of IVF where the husband is infertile and the wife requires IVF. There is little difference between this technique and DI as described above. It is now possible for a woman to donate an egg to another woman and this does not seem to be very different from semen donation. Embryo donation is also possible now and this gives rise to ethical problems since the woman who carries the child may have made no contribution to its genetic make-up: concern has been expressed about this (see below).

Freezing and storing of embryos

It is now common practice to freeze and store embryos. There are some who object to this practice, arguing that it is tampering with the creation of human beings and is unethical. A particular difficulty arises when one or both of the parents of the embryo die. The Government White Paper has suggested that when embryos are to be stored the couple who have provided the gametes should state what should happen to the embryo if such an event should occur.

Embryo research

Perhaps the most contentious issue in IVF is the question of human embryos and research. It was the development of IVF that, for the first time, gave rise to the possibility that human embryos might be brought into existence which would have no chance of implanting because they were not transferred to a uterus and therefore had no chance of being born as human beings. What then are the moral rights of the embryo? There are some people who hold that if an embryo is human and alive it follows that it should not be deprived of a chance of development and, therefore, that it should not be used for research. These people would give moral approval for IVF only if each embryo produced were to be transferred to the uterus. Others argue that while one does not deny that human embryos are alive, one can also say that eggs and sperm are alive and embryos are just another stage further on in development. Furthermore, embryos are not yet human persons and if it could be decided when an embryo became a person it might be easier to decide when research could be undertaken. Some state that when life or personhood begins is simple — that is, at the moment of fertilization — and that the embryo has moral rights from that time. These questions are, however, very complex amalgams of factual and moral judgement.

The answer to the question about the status that ought to be accorded to the human embryo must necessarily be in terms of ethical and moral principles and not facts. Perhaps the most reasonable attitude is that taken by Dunstan & Sellar (1988) who record the traditional attempt to grade the protection accorded to the nascent human being according to the stages of its development. This tradition is challenged today by those who claim absolute protection from the moment of conception. But a choice has to be made. Uterine life must be protected at some point. If that point is put too early, forbidding observation and experimental use of pre-implantation embryos in the early stages of cell division, much useful research of potential human benefit will be inhibited and that includes the improvement of the chances of successful pregnancy for lack of which many extra embryos are sacrificed at present. It is most important that embryo research should continue in the manner recommended by the Warnock Report (1984), that is up to 14 days after fertilization, and under the supervision of a statutory licensing authority which would prohibit certain types of research such as cloning, gestation of human embryos in other species and trans-species fertilization. The term 'pre-embryo' is now used to refer to an embryo before the stage when differentiation has occurred, that is before 14 days when the primitive streak first appears.

Surrogacy

A surrogate mother is a woman who carries a fetus and bears a child on behalf of another person or persons, having agreed to surrender the child to this person or persons at birth or shortly thereafter. There is little doubt that surrogacy by sexual intercourse has always been practised in some small measure to alleviate childlessness. What has changed is that developments in artificial insemination and in IVF now make it possible for surrogacy to proceed without intercourse and the fact that actual fertilization can be carried out outside the human body. This means that a husband and wife, where the wife has no uterus as the result of an operation, could produce semen and eggs which could be used to form embryos which would then be inserted into the uterus of another woman who would carry the child during her pregnancy and when the baby was delivered hand it over to the genetic parents who had provided the gametes. The carrying mother would then not have made any contribution to the genetic make-up of the child. As the Warnock Committee stated (1984), it is not difficult to envisage circumstances where serious arguments could develop as to whether the genetic mother or the carrying mother ought to be regarded as the true mother of the child. The resolution of this issue could be of great importance in questions of inheritance or citizenship.

Surrogacy can be performed for a number of reasons but surrogacy for convenience where the woman is physically capable of bearing a child is ethically unacceptable. Even in compelling medical circumstances, the danger of exploitation of one human being by another appears to most people to outweigh the potential benefits in most cases. This becomes positively exploitative when financial interests are involved. As a result of some cases of commercial surrogacy agencies being set up in the UK the British Government in 1985 enacted the Surrogacy Arrangements Act, the only surrogacy act in the world at present. Basically the act states that no person shall on a commercial basis do any of the following in the UK:

1. Initiate or take part in any negotiation with a view to the making of a surrogacy arrangement.
2. Offer to agree to negotiate the making of a surrogacy arrangement.
3. Compile any information with a view to its use in making or negotiating the making of surrogacy arrangements.

Anyone guilty of contravening this act is guilty of an offence.

The present position is that the Government does not intend to legislate further and therefore surrogacy, in a very minor way, will probably continue. A working party of the British Medical Association (1989) has issued guidelines to doctors as to how they should act when approached by a couple wishing to make a surrogate arrangement.

THERAPEUTIC ABORTION

The ethics of therapeutic abortion have been debated for many years and the debate continues. In almost every session of British Parliament an attempt has been made to change the 1967 Abortion Act. Strong pressure groups desire to have abortion made illegal again and others have wished to change the Act so that the age of viability is 24 weeks. This latter desire is certainly a reasonable one since modern neonatal care has made it possible for babies born at an earlier period of gestation to survive without handicap. In 1985 a report on fetal viability and clinical practice was produced by a representative committee of the Royal College of Obstetricians and Gynaecologists, the British Paediatric Association, the Royal College of General Practitioners, the Royal College of Midwives, the British Medical Association and the Department of Health and Social Security. This Committee recommended that the gestational age after which a fetus is considered as viable should be changed from the present limit of 28 weeks (196 days) to 24 weeks' (168 days') gestation. As a result of the Human Fertilisation and Embryology Act 1990, the Abortion Act of 1987 was amended to reduce to 24 weeks the upper limit for the termination of pregnancy. However, there are three exemptions to the new limit: if the termination is necessary to prevent grave permanent injury to the physical or mental health of the woman; if there would be a risk to the life of the pregnant woman greater than if the pregnancy were terminated; if there is a substantial risk that the child would suffer such physical or mental abnormalities as to be seriously handicapped.

Carol Gilligan, who has studied the ethical thinking of women facing the dilemma of an unwanted pregnancy, feels that women do not approach this problem as a case of conflicting rights or principles but rather in terms of the meaning and demands of the concept of responsibility (Gilligan 1982). Many women see the ethical problems as being the tension between acting selfishly and acting responsibly. Respecting a fetus's right to be nurtured and developed involves a complex pattern of activities which form a prominent, demanding and in some cases permanent part of a woman's life (Bolton 1979). To continue a pregnancy a woman must assess the resources available to her in terms of a complex and broad range of responsibilities which would fall on her shoulders if she chooses this course. These responsibilities, such as making sure her lifestyle during pregnancy does not harm the developing fetus, are not necessarily logically entailed by the woman's decision to continue the pregnancy. However, because of the nature of society and the role-related responsibilities of women and mothers, careful consideration of these responsibilities is ethically demanded of the pregnant woman. If the doctor has accepted the responsibilities of assisting a woman in the important task of controlling her fertility an unintended pregnancy confronts both the woman and doctor with serious questions of responsibility. This issue is most clear-cut where a pregnancy follows a gynaecologist's performance of sterilization. In such a case the gynaecologist may have a prima facie obligation to provide an abortion if the woman involved is unable to assume the responsibility of nurturing the fetus and bearing a child.

There are those who object to abortion in all circumstances for religious or other reasons but in a pluralistic society this view should not be the basis for legislation. These groups will not wish to take part in abortion practice at all but that does not mean that their view should prevail over all others. Taken in the world context where 100 000 women die each year of illegal abortion, mainly in countries where abortion is illegal, it could be argued that it is unethical not to allow therapeutic abortion which would result in the saving of very many lives of these women and mothers.

Since abortion involves terminating pregnancy and thereby ending the life of a developing fetus it is always an ethical judgement involving the choice of an action that is felt to be 'less wrong' than another. A fundamental ethical consideration in any analysis of the ethics of abortion involves prevention of the problem that places women and their physicians in this 'no-win' situation: accidental or unintended pregnancy. Women, doctors, politicians and many others in society must consider this important moral situation. From the doctor's point of view a complex set of ethical duties, obligations and responsibilities is owed to the woman considering termination of pregnancy. There are situations in which termination of pregnancy can be a physician's ethical duty.

STERILIZATION

Most governments and individuals throughout the world recognize family planning as a basic human right. Individuals must be free to choose sterilization as long as there is no legal prohibition or personal objection and doctors and others must provide suitable counselling to those wishing this procedure. At all times it must be entirely voluntary. Public policy in the area of contraceptive sterilization addresses the most important human rights — the right of procreation and the rights of individuals versus the needs of society, involving strong and deeply felt religious and ethical convictions.

Where sterilization is not illegal there is no particular ethical problem involved. A major ethical difficulty arises, however, in the case of the mentally handicapped. In this case the individual's ability to provide informed consent for sterilization is questionable or absent. If a patient is or is considered to be mentally incapacitated serious consideration must be given to a variety of issues before a sterilization procedure is performed. The initial premise should be that non-voluntary sterilization is generally not ethically acceptable in our society because of the violation of privacy, bodily integrity and reproductive rights that it represents. In some unusual situations, however, sterilization may be considered a reasonable part of the overall health care of a person who is mentally incapacitated or incompetent. Consideration must also be given to alternative methods of management before surgical sterilization is performed.

Of course, individuals who are mentally handicapped are not necessarily incapable of providing informed consent for sterilization. It is often difficult to determine their capacity, however. One must ensure that decisions to request sterilization are not coerced and that other professionals involved in the care of the patient are always consulted. At all times the best interests of the patient should be the primary consideration. It should be ascertained that the mental condition is permanent; that there is a reasonable likelihood that she is fertile and may have sexual intercourse, and that even if no health risks are incurred by pregnancy the burdens of child-bearing, parenting etc. are considered as well as the risk to the resulting child. In the UK at the present time it would be unwise for a doctor to sterilize a mentally handicapped person without having the permission of the court.

CONTRACEPTION AND THE YOUNG

This is a difficult problem and from an ethical point of view involves the autonomy of the individual. The crux of the matter is the question of consent and whether the person involved is competent to give consent. If a doctor considers that a young person shows that she possesses adequate understanding and a capacity to bear the consequences of her decision-making then it is ethically justifiable to give contraceptive advice. In this case the ethical and legal aspects are confused. If a young girl asks for contraceptive advice because she is intending to engage in sexual intercourse then it could be considered unethical to refuse to help unless the doctor had some moral or religious objection. However, in this case there are legal aspects to be considered and it is not easy to separate the ethical and legal problems. It is possible that a doctor in the UK who gives contraceptive advice to a girl under 16 may be aiding and abetting the offence of unlawful sexual intercourse. It would be advisable for the doctor in this case to endeavour to persuade the girl to involve her parents or guardian at an early stage in the consultation. If the girl refuses, the doctor should prescribe contraception and respect her confidentiality if this is considered to be in her best interests. This view was challenged in the High Court by a mother who sought declarations that this advice which had been given in a health department circular was unlawful. In this case the court decided that it was lawful for the doctor to give advice if he considered that a girl under 16 asking for contraception showed that she possessed adequate understanding and a capacity to bear the consequences of a decision. This is the first ethical principle of respect for persons (autonomy of the person) which was upheld by this judgement and this is the position at the present time (1990).

ACQUIRED IMMUNE DEFICIENCY SYNDROME (AIDS)

In gynaecological practice doctors may become involved in managing patients with AIDS. The performance of pelvic examinations where the vaginal secretions may contain the virus; infertility where the woman or her partner may be human immunodeficiency virus (HIV)-positive; gynaecological surgery where the patient operated upon may be HIV-positive — all have consequences for gynaecological practice. A further facet of gynaecological practices is in family planning. Useful guidelines regarding the prevention of the spread of infection are given in the Report of the Royal College of Obstetricians and Gynaecologists subcommittee (1987) on problems associated with AIDS in relation to obstetrics and gynaecology and in the case of family planning by the Family Planning Association and the National Association of Family Planning Doctors (1987). The Royal College of Obstetricians and Gynaecologists' document explores the implications of HIV for gynaecological practice and draws attention to the importance of family planning and well-woman services in the extension of its traditional role of preventive health care to include the prevention of the spread of HIV infection.

The ethical aspects of AIDS revolve round the question of informed consent and the General Medical Council of the UK has indicated this in a letter to all UK doctors (1988). Doctors are expected in all normal circumstances to be sure that their patients consent to the carrying out of investigative procedures involving the removal of samples or invasive techniques, whether these investigations are performed for the purpose of routine screening or for the more specific purpose of differential diagnosis. The General Medical Council believes that this principle should apply generally but that it is particularly important in the case of testing for HIV infection because of the serious social and financial consequences which may ensue for the patient from the mere fact of having been tested for the condition. These problems would be better resolved by developing a spirit of social tolerance than by medical action but they do present the doctor with a particular ethical dilemma in connection with the diagnosis of HIV infection or AIDS. They provide a strong argument for each patient to be given the opportunity to consider in advance the implications of submitting to such a test and deciding whether to accept or decline it. Where blood samples are taken for screening purposes, as in antenatal clinics, there will usually be no reason to suspect HIV infection but even so the test should be carried out only where the patient has given explicit consent. Only in the most exceptional circumstances where a test is imperative in order to secure the safety of persons other than the patient and where it is not possible for the prior consent of the patient to be obtained can testing without explicit consent be justified. It is also important that confidentiality be maintained and here there may be a conflict between micro- and macro-ethics where a patient refuses to be tested and the doctor has to consider the effect of this refusal on others and society. These matters can usually be resolved by proper counselling and discussion but they can present difficult ethical problems.

Contraception

HIV infection and contraception are inextricably linked in several ways. One key issue is how contraceptive use modifies the sexual transmission of HIV; the other concerns the role contraceptives play in preventing pregnancy. Unfortunately the contraceptive methods that reduce sexual transmission of HIV infection are not necessarily the most effective in preventing pregnancy and those methods most effective in preventing pregnancy may not be the safest for women with HIV. Efficacy in preventing pregnancy takes on a particular importance for many HIV infected women because of perinatal transmission of HIV. These are dilemmas which face people making choices or giving advice about which contraceptive method to use in the context of HIV. The dilemma is exacerbated by a frustrating lack of data on the issue and it will be difficult to generate the information. Epidemiological studies which would provide the much-needed information face insurmountable logistical and ethical problems which have been mentioned in connection with screening.

THE ROLE OF GOVERNMENT AND OTHER BODIES IN MEDICAL ETHICS

Ethical matters in connection with medical practice concern society in general and no more so than in connection with artificial reproduction, abortion, sterilization and surrogacy etc. It is appropriate, therefore, that legislation should be enacted in relation to these matters. The legislation so far enacted is in connection with abortion and surrogacy. The Human Fertilisation and Embryology Act 1990, now in force, governs the provisions of artificial reproduction following the recommendations of the Warnock Report (1984). A free vote was allowed in the context of embryo research.

The Royal College of Obstetricians and Gynaecologists has an ethical committee which produces guidelines as to what is considered good ethical practice in the specialty. In both these regards it is essential that there is substantial lay representation in the bodies which are established. In 1985 the Royal College of Obstetricians and Gynaecologists and the Medical Research Council set up the Voluntary Licensing Authority which consists of four fellows of the Royal College Obstetricians and Gynaecologists, four members of the Medical Research Council and six lay members plus a lay chairman. This body has concerned itself with good practice in centres where artificial reproduction is performed and has been successful in reassuring the public about these practices. This was replaced first by an Interim Licensing Authority then, from August 1991, by the Human Fertilisation and Embryo Authority. This is a statutory body with legal powers to control practices in this area.

KEY POINTS

1. Donor insemination raises moral and ethical questions about the identity of the donor and the right of the child to know this.
2. It is important to be aware of local legislation on issues such as sterilization and contraception for minors.
3. A patient's confidence and consent have to be respected when taking HIV tests.

REFERENCES AND FURTHER READING

Bolton M B 1979 Responsible women and abortion decisions. In: O'Neill O, Ruddick W (eds) Having children. Oxford University Press, New York

British Medical Association 1989 Report of a British Medical Association working party on surrogacy. British Medical Association, London

Dunstan G R, Sellar M J 1988 The status of the human embryo. King Edward's Hospital Fund for London

Ethical considerations of the new reproductive technologies 1988. Fertility and Sterility 49 (suppl 1)

Family Planning Association 1987 AIDS (Acquired immune deficiency syndrome). Provisional guidelines from the Family Planning Association and the National Association of Family Planning Doctors 1987. British Journal of Family Planning 13: 11–15

Feversham (Chairman) Home Office and Scottish Home Department Departmental committee on human artificial insemination report 1960 HMSO, London

General Medical Council letter 1988 HIV infection and AIDS: the ethical considerations. General Medical Council, London

Gilligan C 1982 In a different voice: psychological theory and women's development. Cambridge, M A, Harvard University Press

Human fertilization and embryology: a framework for legislation 1987. HMSO, London

Mahoney J 1984 Bioethics and belief. Sheed and Ward, London

National Commission for the Protection of Human Subjects of Biomedical and Behavioral Research 1979 Ethical principles and guidelines for the protection of human subjects of research. US Government Printing Office, Washington

Report on fetal viability and clinical practice 1985 Royal College of Obstetricians and Gynaecologists, London

Report of the Royal College of Obstetricians and Gynaecologists on problems associated with AIDS in relation to obstetrics and gynaecology 1987 Royal College of Obstetricians and Gynaecologists, London

Royal College of Obstetricians and Gynaecologists 1990 Revised report. HIV infection in maternity care and gynaecology. RCOG, London

Scottish Maternal and Perinatal Report 1989 SHHD, Edinburgh

Statement of Policy 1988 Ethical considerations in sterilization. American College of Obstetricians and Gynecologists, Washington, USA

Torrance T F 1984 Test-tube babies — morals, science and the law. Scottish Academic Press, Edinburgh

Warnock M (Chairman) Report of the committee of inquiry into human fertilization and embryology 1984 HMSO, London

65. Lower intestinal tract disease

M. M. Henry

Functional disorders of the anorectum are frequently the consequence of the same aetiopathological mechanisms as those giving rise to disturbance of function within the genitourinary tract and therefore a brief account can be justified in a text largely concerned with gynaecological disease. Patients frequently have symptoms referable to both systems, suggesting that a combined approach to management should be offered such patients wherever possible. In practice, as a consequence of ever-increasing degrees of specialization, this is rarely achieved.

Table 65.1 Factors responsible for normal anorectal continence

Anal sphincters	Internal sphincter Innervated hypogastric and sacral parasympathetic nerves
	External sphincter Innervated pudendal nerves
Pelvic floor	Anorectal angle (flap-valve) Innervated from above by direct branches of the sacral plexus
Sensory factors	Receptors in the pelvic floor Rectosphincteric inhibitory reflex (sampling)
Miscellaneous factors	Valves of Houston Anal cushions Vectors acting in the cephalad direction

PELVIC FLOOR AND ANORECTAL CONTINENCE (Table 65.1)

It is generally believed by proctologists that the pelvic floor plays a key role in the maintenance of anorectal continence in the normal state. If a pressure probe is inserted into the rectum and withdrawn caudally through the anal canal at centimetre intervals a step-wise increase in pressure is recorded over an area approximately corresponding to the internal anal sphincter (IAS) (Fig. 65.1). Resting anal pressure has been shown to be largely a function of IAS contraction with a smaller contribution made by the external anal sphincter (EAS) (Bennett & Duthie 1964). If the subject is requested to contract the EAS maximally, the intra-anal pressure increases by a factor of 100%.

The role of the IAS and EAS in anorectal control continues to be disputable. Surgical division of the IAS [manual dilatation of the anus (MDA), sphincterotomy] rarely gives rise to any significant functional deficit. Inter-

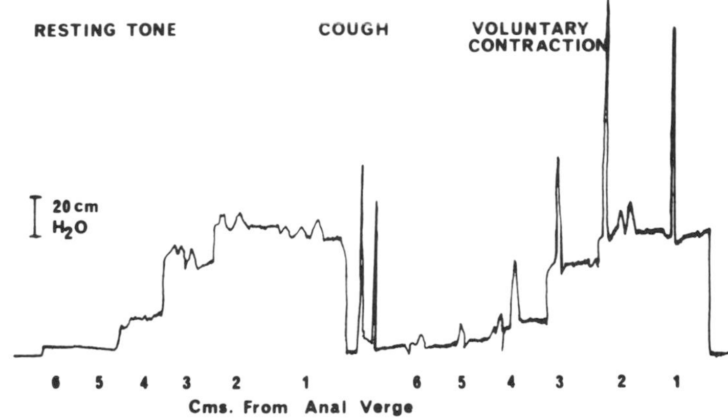

Fig. 65.1 A normal anal pressure profile. In the first section of the tracing the pressure probe has been inserted into the rectum and is withdrawn at centimetre intervals with the patient in the resting state and lying in the left lateral position. The internal sphincter is responsible for a zone of high pressure (maximum 60 cm water) over the distal 4 cm. The pressure profile is repeated but on this occasion the patient is requested to contract the external anal sphincter. Intra-anal pressures are thereby increased during contraction by at least a factor of two times.

nal sphincter loss in most patients leads usually to only a minor degree of incontinence, mostly restricted to loss of control to flatus and to liquid stool. On the other hand, some patients who develop severe faecal incontinence may be found on physiological testing to have idiopathic IAS deficiency as the primary abnormality with relative sparing of the EAS and pelvic floor muscles. Similarly, the true function of the EAS as a separate entity remains uncertain since division of the muscle ring again, in most patients, does not give rise to significant anorectal incontinence other than urgency and soiling in the presence of diarrhoea. However, some patients with neuropathic damage of the EAS (see below) where the pelvic floor is relatively spared may experience severe functional disturbance.

The puborectalis, on account of its intimate relationship to the lower rectum and upper anal canal, is the most relevant of the levator muscles. In company with the remainder of the muscles which comprise the pelvic floor and the EAS this muscle displays the unusual property (for skeletal muscle) of continuous resting electrical tone. This is maintained without unconscious effort, during sleep (Floyd & Walls 1953), and has been demonstrated to be the consequence of a spinal reflex (Parks et al 1962). Hence disruption of any limb of the reflex (e.g. tabes dorsalis, which destroys the afferent limb) will result in complete cessation of resting tone and anorectal incontinence.

Contraction of the puborectalis muscle in turn generates an angle between the lower rectum and upper anal canal — the anorectal angle (Fig. 65.2). Dispute again rests on the true importance of this anatomical entity. Parks (1975)

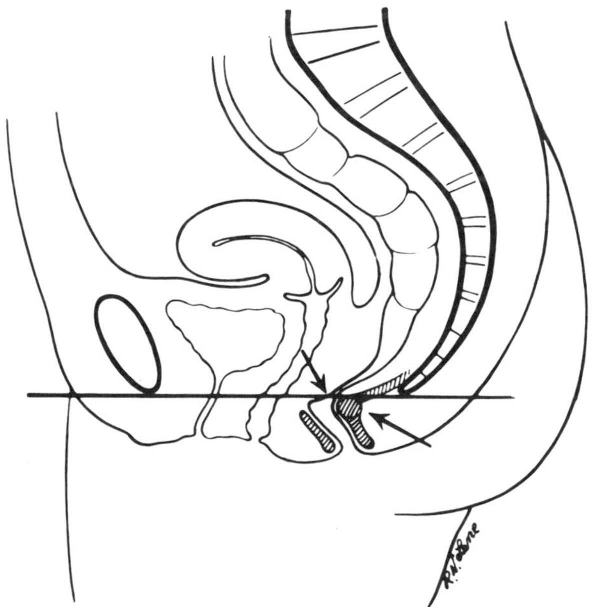

Fig. 65.2 The normal anorectal angle created by the forward pull of the puborectalis muscle (lower arrow). Abdominal pressure is conducted onto the anterior rectal wall (upper arrow) helping to prevent leakage of rectal contents when intra-abdominal pressure is raised (e.g. by coughing, lifting, etc).

believed that the angle is of prime importance to the maintenance of normal control because it permitted a flap-valve mechanism to operate. He believed that intra-abdominal pressure was conducted through the anterior rectal wall such that any increase (e.g. from coughing or sneezing) caused it to close over the top of the anal canal, and so effectively excluded the anus from intrarectal contents. However, Bartolo (1986) failed to demonstrate by cineradiographic techniques any increase in the angle in a group of normal controls in whom intra-abdominal pressures were increased by performing the Valsalva manoeuvre. It could be argued that this manoeuvre does not exactly reproduce the physiological conditions (e.g. coughing) under which the normal continence mechanisms are threatened. There is no question, however, that during a cough impulse there is a considerable recordable reflex increase in the pelvic floor muscle electrical activity (presumably to cause an increase in angulation) and on sigmoidoscopy the anterior rectal wall can be clearly seen moving downwards as it is forced on to the upper limit of the anal canal.

The sensation of a full rectum, alerting the individual to the possibility of an impending need to defecate, is also an important element of continence. Sensory receptors have never been clearly identified within the wall or mucosa of the rectum itself and sensation seems to be preserved in patients undergoing rectal excision and coloanal anastomosis (Lane & Parks 1977). These lines of evidence suggest that the requisite receptors probably reside in the pelvic floor muscles which cradle and lie in intimate contact with the rectum. Evidence in favour is the demonstration of stretch receptors (Winkler 1958) and muscle spindles (Walls 1959) in these muscles.

An important contributing factor to sensation facilitates a locally mediated visceral reflex, referred to as the recto-sphincteric inhibitory reflex. The reflex, first described by Gowers (1877), refers to inhibition of the internal anal sphincter as a consequence of rectal distension (e.g. by flatus or by faeces). The reflex can be shown to be independent of extrinsic neural sources and is abolished by rectal myotomy (Lubowski et al 1987), confirming that it is mediated via the intramural neural pathways (Meissner's and Auerbach's plexuses). Under normal conditions the function of the reflex acts by permitting a small sample of rectal contents to enter the proximal anal canal in response to the IAS relaxation. At the dentate line they make direct contact with the profuse sensory receptors which are concentrated at this level and permit discrimination at cortical level between faeces or flatus. If faeces are perceived to be present there is vigorous contraction of the EAS and anal contents are propelled back to the rectum until it is propitious for defecation to proceed. Sampling occurs on a regular and frequent basis during the daytime in the normal individual.

There are certainly other factors which may play an uncertain role and possibly others which have yet to be revealed. Those that are recognized include vectors which oppose the prograde flow of colonic contents; valves of Houston which similarly oppose prograde flow, and anal canal cushions (haemorrhoids) which may contribute to continence by surface tension effects.

DEFECATION

Once the circumstances are propitious for defecation, certain complex physiological mechanisms are instituted which, like those responsible for continence, are incompletely understood. There is no dispute that, under normal and ideal circumstances, defecation is preceded by a reflex inhibition of electrical activity within the pelvic floor and EAS. This in turn facilitates defecation by causing increased obliquity of the anorectal angle. The passage of the faecal bolus is further assisted by reflex relaxation of the IAS (in response to rectal distension). The actual vector forces responsible for evacuation probably arise from intra-abdominal pressure rather than from peristaltic activity within the rectum itself. At the completion of the defecatory effort there is a rapid burst of electrical activity in the EAS and pelvic floor to restore the anorectal angle; this has been identified as the closing reflex by Porter (1962). At the same time tone is regained within the IAS.

The central mechanisms in the nervous system controlling defecation are ill understood. Urge incontinence is a feature of inflammatory conditions of the rectum and of spinal and cerebral disorders alike. Recent evidence suggests that there is a fast-conducting, direct pyramidal pathway to the sacral anterior horn cells supplying the pelvic floor and EAS; this suggests that the cortex plays an important role in the normal control of these muscles.

INVESTIGATION OF PELVIC FLOOR DISORDERS

The last decade has seen a marked development in techniques designed to provide an objective assessment of pelvic floor function as a direct consequence of an accelerating interest in the treatment of functional disorders of these muscles.

Manometry

This is the most endurable method since it is simple, cheap, and a relatively non-invasive means of assessing IAS (resting pressure) and EAS function (squeeze pressure). Pressures can be recorded simply, either by using water-filled balloons or by a water perfusion system. The latter is vulnerable because intrusion of faecal contents may readily introduce artefact. For more accurate measurement more expensive and complex systems are available (e.g. microtransducer catheter). These are generally only requisite needs in units where research rather than service commitments predominate. The recording system should then be connected via a suitable transducer to a device capable of producing a clear and preferably permanent tracing.

Manometry, is currently the only practical method for assessing IAS function and also the only means of testing the integrity of the rectosphincteric inhibitory reflex. Assessment of EAS manometrically is less satisfactory since it requires the subjectivity of the patient's ability to comprehend and co-operate during maximal voluntary contraction.

Electromyography (EMG)

A more accurate approach to the assessment of EAS and pelvic floor function is gained by conventional and more especially by single-fibre EMG (SF EMG). The former employs relatively broad-diameter needles recording from a wide surface area and as such is only useful in identifying skeletal muscle. This may be important after muscle has been divided (e.g. following third-degree perineal tear) to provide the surgeon with anatomical detail of the position of the retracted EAS prior to repair. In children EMG exploration may be helpful in identifying the pelvic floor in rectal atresia prior to pull-through surgery.

To determine if the skeletal muscle under investigation has undergone denervation (see below) the more sophisticated technique of SF EMG has to be employed. With concentric needle electrodes individual muscle fibre action potentials cannot be recognized reliably within the motor unit action potential. Single-muscle fibre action potentials

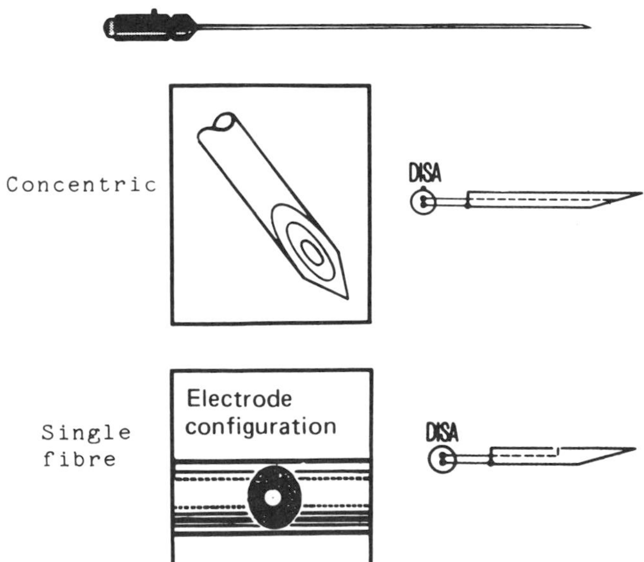

Fig. 65.3 Electrodes employed for electromyography. Upper electrode is of conventional concentric type with its recording surface at the tip. The lower electrode is of single-fibre type with its recording surface situated on the surface of its shank near the tip.

can be recorded extracellularly by using an electrode whose recording surface consists of a central wire which opens at the mid-shaft of the electrode in a small circular leading-off surface of 25 mm diameter (Fig. 65.3). In normal muscle the recordings of motor units are made in which one of two single-muscle fibre action potentials are obtained within the uptake area of the electrode. In muscle which has been denervated and subsequently re-innervated the number of components will be increased. An average of the positive components is taken from 20 different sites in the muscle and the figure is referred to as the fibre density for that muscle. The fibre density for normal EAS is 1.5 ± 0.16 (Neill & Swash 1980).

Nerve stimulation studies

Having established that denervation has occurred within the pelvic floor muscles it may be relevant to determine whether the anatomical site of the neurological damage is central (cauda equina) or peripheral (pudendal nerves).

The central component is studied by means of transcutaneous lumbar spinal stimulation (Merton et al 1982). A single impulse of 800–1500 V decaying with a time constant of 50 μs is delivered through an electrode placed over the spinous process of L1 and repeated at L4. The evoked contraction associated with the pelvic floor response can be detected either by surface or needle electrode. Pathology affecting the cauda equina will give rise to a more pronounced delay at L1 than L4. If the neuronal damage results from peripheral disease the delay at L1 and L4 will be increased to similar degree (Snooks et al 1985a).

The peripheral component (i.e. pudendal nerves) is tested by means of a disposable glove stimulating electrode, which comprises a glove consisting of two stimulating electrodes at the tip and two recording electrodes at the base of the glove. The glove is inserted into the rectum and with the patient in the left lateral position the tip of the glove is brought into contact with the pudendal nerve at the level of the ischial spine. The nerve is then stimulated electrically with a square-wave stimulus of 0.1 ms duration and 50 V amplitude and the evoked response in the EAS is detected electrically by the surface recording electrodes situated at the base of the glove. The procedure is then repeated for the opposite side and the latency of the EAS muscle response is measured on the paper print-out of the EMG apparatus from the onset of the stimulus to the onset of the response. The normal value of the pudendal response is 2.1 ± 0.2 ms and for the perineal response is 2.4. ± 0.2 ms.

Evacuation proctography

The dynamics of the pelvic floor can be studied visually by employing cine-radiographic techniques using video films on which have been superimposed simultaneous EMG and anal pressure recordings (Womack et al 1985). As discussed below, these techniques may be of specific value in the investigation of the constipated patient to identify the subgroup with pelvic floor outlet obstruction.

PATHOPHYSIOLOGY OF FUNCTIONAL ANORECTAL DISEASE

Porter (1962), by employing conventional EMG techniques, made the observation that many patients with rectal prolapse and faecal incontinence could be shown to have abnormal electrical activity of the pelvic floor. The explanation for these changes was clarified by histochemical studies of pelvic floor muscle biopsies in which features consistent with denervation were demonstrable (Parks et al 1977). That these muscles have been denervated in patients with rectal prolapse and faecal incontinence was later confirmed by electrophysiological studies (Neill & Swash 1980). Application of nerve stimulation studies showed that the site of neuronal damage was peripheral (pudendal) in most patients (Snooks et al 1985a). Denervation has since also been demonstrated to be an important feature in patients with constipation (Snooks et al 1985b); solitary rectal ulcer syndrome (Snooks et al 1985c); urinary incontinence (Snooks & Swash 1984) and the descending perineum syndrome (Henry et al 1982).

The source of the denervation is almost certainly multifactorial and is still a subject for speculation. There seems to be no doubt that many patients develop pelvic floor failure as a consequence of traumatic childbirth (Snooks et al 1984). The innervation to the pelvic floor may be damaged by vaginal delivery, but not by Caesarean section; the damage is most prominent in multiparae and correlated most strongly with a prolonged second stage of labour and with forceps delivery. Pudendal nerve injury may also be the consequence of a peripheral neuropathy such as diabetes mellitus (Rogers et al 1988) or direct injury from surgery or road traffic accident (e.g. fracture of the pelvis). Lower motor neuron lesions may result from disease affecting the cauda equina (e.g. tumour or trauma), but these are generally considered to be rare. As discussed below, in the descending perineum syndrome, pelvic floor descent is thought to cause a direct stretch injury to the pudendal nerves of sufficient degree to induce anorectal and/or urinary incontinence. Pathophysiology will be discussed in further detail below.

DISORDERS OF THE PELVIC FLOOR

Faecal incontinence

The consequences for the individual affected by anorectal incontinence are often serious since such people may find themselves in a state of social and professional isolation.

The estimated community prevalence is 4.9/1000 in men and 13.3/1000 in women over the age of 65 years (Mandelstam 1985). At St Mark's Hospital, London, of those who present for treatment, the disorder appears to be most common in middle age and is eight times more common in women.

Minor faecal incontinence is defined as the inadvertent passage of flatus or soiling in the presence of diarrhoea. This clinical state is frequently associated with poor internal sphincter function which in turn may be the consequence of previous anal surgery (e.g. anal stretch, sphincterotomy, haemorrhoidectomy or fistula surgery). Soiling may also accompany minor anal disorders such as anal condylomata, second- and third-degree haemorrhoids and prolapsing fibrous anal polyps. Partial denervation of the pelvic floor and EAS may similarly give rise to a less severe form of incontinence in which the deficit is only revealed by the challenge of liquid stool. Constipation and faecal impaction are often associated with spurious diarrhoea and soiling, partly because of the reflex internal sphincter relaxation which develops in response to rectal distension (by faeces).

Clearly these patients are not usually greatly restricted or stressed and the management is largely conservative. Local anal pathology should be looked for on clinical examination and treated accordingly. Where impaction is encountered, normal function can be frequently readily recovered by the use of aperients and rectal washouts. If the IAS alone is deficient, surgery is unlikely to benefit the patient and management is usually a combination of codeine phosphate (to constipate) and an irritant suppository (to induce complete rectal evacuation).

Patients with major faecal incontinence are greatly disabled and stressed by frequent unheralded passage per anum of stools of normal consistency. Incontinence pads require frequent changing and only deal with the soiling to a limited degree, particularly if there is associated urinary incontinence as well.

As discussed above, the majority of patients will be women in middle age with a history of obstetric trauma which precedes the onset of incontinence by a period varying from several days to several decades. After the sixth decade, muscle denervates as a normal physiological response to ageing and this contributes further to loss of pelvic floor function and helps to explain why some patients fail to develop problems until later life. Sometimes there is a history of straining with perineal descent (see below) and, particularly in the elderly, a history of rectal prolapse should be enquired into. Previous trauma responsible for division of the anal sphincter ring (e.g. fracture of the bony pelvis, third-degree perineal tear, anal fistula surgery, sexual assault) may be relevant and if there is a short history of incontinence in association with a history of perineal pain and/or disseminated neurological symptoms, a neurological cause should be considered.

Examination of patients with anorectal incontinence is customarily conducted with the patient in the left lateral position having first examined the abdomen. On inspection, soiling of the perianal skin with faecal matter may be apparent and when the patient is requested to strain there may be perineal descent accompanied by genital and/or rectal prolapse. The anal canal itself may gape (if there is IAS deficiency) and on digital examination of the anus both resting tone (IAS) and squeeze tone (EAS) may be deficient. The angle and posterior 'bar' created by the forward pull of the puborectalis muscle may be found to be significantly reduced or absent. The anal reflex will be absent to clinical testing and there may be diminished sensation in the perianal skin.

Before embarking on treatment, these patients should be investigated according to the approximate protocol described above. If a neurological or central cause is suspected, lumbar myelography should be included. All patients with rectal symptoms should undergo sigmoidoscopy and, where relevant, a barium enema to exclude malignancy. If there are urological symptoms, urodynamics including videocystourethrography should be considered.

Treatment

By virtue of the degree of their disability these patients require energetic and usually surgical treatment. Where there is complete rectal prolapse, rectopexy is indicated (see below). The majority of patients with prolapse regain near-normal anorectal continence if the prolapse is successfully controlled. In the small subgroup who remain incontinent, pelvic floor surgery can be considered as a secondary procedure.

Anal sphincter repair can be responsible for near-total recovery of function in 80% of patients, provided that there is no coincidental denervation of the muscle (Laurberg et al 1988). Before surgery patients should be investigated physiologically to determine if there is denervation and the position of the retracted ends of EAS. The operation is usually performed with the patient in the lithotomy position and some surgeons prefer to carry out a defunctioning colostomy to permit the repair to heal in a relatively uncontaminated environment. The fibrous scar filling the space between the retracted muscle is excised and the mucosa approximated with an absorbable suture. The muscle is then repaired by an overlapping technique using non-absorbable suture material (Fig. 65.4). The wound is left to heal by secondary intention.

In the presence of established denervation of the pelvic floor the preferred procedure in the UK is the operation devised by the late Sir Alan Parks (post anal repair). The procedure can restore continence in between 60 and 80% of patients, for reasons which are obscure. Parks (1975) originally believed that the anorectal angle could be restored but there is very little evidence to support this. It

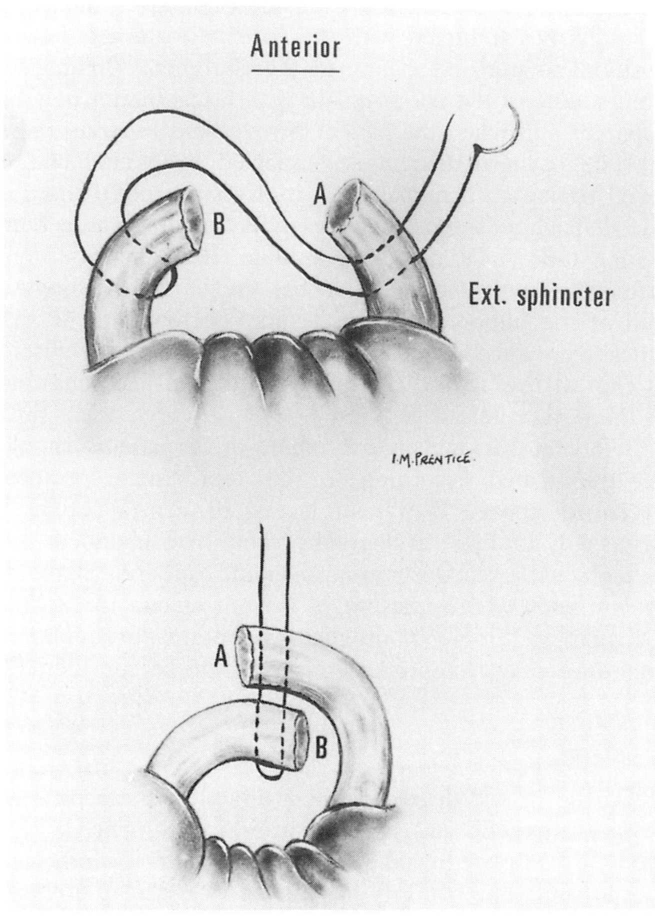

Fig. 65.4 External anal sphincter repair. The muscle ends are overlapped and sutured with a non-absorbable material.

seems more likely that improved function is the consequence of increasing the length of the anal canal and of improving the mechanical advantage of the muscle fibres (Womack et al 1988).

A V-shaped incision is created just behind the anus and the space between the IAS and EAS dissected until Waldeyer's fascia is reached. The fascia has to be divided to obtain access to the pelvis. The levator muscles and EAS are then plicated sequentially using non-absorbable suture material. The skin is partially closed, leaving a portion of the wound to heal by secondary intention (Henry & Porter 1988).

Should repair procedures fail to induce a satisfactory symptomatic improvement, a colostomy is frequently a perfectly acceptable alternative and should not be excluded from consideration.

Rectal prolapse

Although this condition is seen at any age, it is most common at the extremes of life. In children, the disorder may be associated with mucoviscidosis; if not, it is usually a transient phenomenon requiring little treatment. There is no doubt that in adults the majority are associated with pelvic floor denervation (Neill et al 1981). The weak pelvic floor favours prolapse of the anterior rectal wall which in turn initiates a rectorectal intussusception. In some patients the aetiology remains obscure, although malnutrition and chronic constipation are important aetiological factors.

The prolapse may develop only during defecation or alternatively may be permanently down, requiring frequent manual replacement. Sometimes patients are unaware of the prolapse and present with faecal incontinence occurring as a consequence of pelvic floor denervation and IAS damage caused by the trauma of the prolapsing four layers of oedematous bowel wall. Rarely, the prolapsing segment may undergo strangulation and subsequent rupture.

Treatment

Most patients with this condition require surgical treatment since persistent prolapse probably gives rise to cumulative anal sphincter damage. The preferred procedure in the UK is rectopexy, an operation whereby the rectum is tethered to the sacrum by employing an inert implant (polyvinyl alcohol sponge or mersilene; Wells 1959). The mortality of this procedure is of the order of 2% — remarkably low, considering the age group. The relapse rate in differing series ranges from 3 to 12%. For the anaesthetic risk, the perineal procedure devised by Delorme (1900) is favoured by some surgeons. The redundant mucosa is excised and the underlying muscle plicated via a peranal approach.

Descending perineum syndrome, perineal pain syndrome and solitary rectal ulcer syndrome

These conditions are discussed under a single heading since they are closely allied to each other and may be different manifestations of the same entity. The plane of the perineum normally lies above that of the bony outlet of the pelvis both in the resting state and during straining. In patients with the descending perineum syndrome, however, the perineum balloons downwards well below the bony pelvis, particularly during straining (Henry et al 1982). The pelvic floor muscles are usually denervated and it is far from clear whether this is a primary or secondary event. It can be demonstrated that pelvic floor descent produces a stretching force on the pudendal nerve to the order of 20–30%. This leads to an increased length of pudendal nerve and produces severe neuropraxia. Hence many patients with this condition may later develop faecal incontinence when the denervation has become well established. In the early stages, there is often prolapse of the anterior rectal mucosa into the lumen of the anal canal. This has the effect of obstructing the passage of the faecal bolus during defecation, so causing the patient to strain excessively to achieve evacuation. At the completion of the defecatory act the redundant mucosa may remain within the anal canal where it is perceived as retained faecal matter. The patient then strains fruitlessly in an attempt to void what is in essence part of the rectal wall. Sometimes patients describe the need to insert a finger into the rectum to push back the redundant mucosa prior to defecation.

Because the pudendal nerve is a mixed nerve, sensory symptoms sometimes predominate. Usually this takes the form of continuous perineal pain (the perineal pain syndrome) provoked by prolonged standing and relieved by lying flat. The pain is unremitting, not related to defecation and is usually refractory to treatment.

Perineal descent is also associated with a condition in which there is a shallow solitary discrete ulcer within the mid-rectum (solitary rectal ulcer syndrome). The ulcer is usually sited anteriorly or anterolaterally at a level varying from 4 to 10 cm from the anal verge. These patients similarly strain excessively at defecation and it is considered that the ulcer is traumatic in origin: it is caused by direct contact between the prolapsing anterior rectal wall and the contracting puborectalis. Patients with this syndrome, in addition to straining and constipation, also complain of perineal pain. The ulcer itself gives rise to bleeding which can be substantial, and a mucous discharge which is sufficient to cause them to wear incontinence pads throughout the day.

Treatment

The treatment of these three disorders is frequently disappointing, particularly where pain is a principal symptom. In the early stages of the disorder some improvement may be obtained by treating the anterior rectal mucosal prolapse (by banding or by injection sclerotherapy) and by improving bowel function to avoid straining. The bleeding and mucous discharge associated with a solitary rectal ulcer can be cured by rectopexy, which prevents prolapse of the anterior rectal wall.

The irritable bowel syndrome

The diagnosis of the irritable bowel syndrome (IBS) is only made after other pathology has been excluded. The condition is a spectrum of symptoms, any combination of which can present. There is no objective test to enable the clinician reliably to diagnose IBS and there is no recognized underlying aetiopathology. There appears to be strong evidence to support the concept that there is a disorder of motility but whether this is primary or secondary is unresolved (Rogers et al 1989). Episodes of pain correlate with periods of elevated intraluminal pressure in the colon (and possibly small bowel).

The range of symptoms associated with IBS is listed in Table 65.2. The site of the abdominal pain can vary from patient to patient and within individual patients. There is usually a clear relationship between symptoms and periods of stress and/or anxiety. Alteration in bowel habit is almost always present; usually there are periods of constipation alternating with periods of diarrhoea.

Table 65.2 Symptoms associated with irritable bowel syndrome

Severe colicky abdominal pain
Abdominal distension
Constipation
Diarrhoea
Mucus per rectum
Anxiety/depression
Relationship to stress

Treatment

Treatment should always be medical since surgery plays no role in management, except rarely as part of the investigative process (i.e. laparotomy). Some relief may be obtained by a combination of increasing dietary bulk and by the use of antispasmodics (e.g. mebeverine) but probably the most important role for the clinician is one of reassurance and support.

Constipation

A patient is defined as suffering from constipation if she or he complains of either infrequent defecation (less than two bowel actions per week) or difficult defecation (straining and difficulty in evacuating the rectum). Under normal conditions, the first priority must be the exclusion of an

Table 65.3 Classification of constipation in adults

No structural abnormality of anus, rectum or colon and no associated physical disorder
Faulty diet
Pregnancy
Old age
Idiopathic slow-transit constipation
Irritable bowel syndrome
Structural disease of anus, rectum or colon
Anal pain/stenosis
Colonic stricture
Aganglionosis
Megarectum/megacolon
Secondary to abnormality outside colon
Endocrine/metabolic
Hypothyroidism
Hypercalcaemia
Porphyria
Neurological
Sacral outflow/spinal cord disorders
Cerebral disorders
Systemic sclerosis and other connective tissue disorders
Psychological
Drug side-effect

From Lennard Jones (1985).

obstructing lesion such as carcinoma, hence sigmoidoscopy and barium enema should be regarded as mandatory. A classification of the important causes of constipation is provided in Table 65.3.

Where no obvious underlying cause can be identified (idiopathic constipation) the standard investigative approach is to investigate colonic transit and pelvic floor function in an attempt to distinguish between those patients with slow-transit constipation and those with pelvic floor dysfunction. It is often not possible to demarcate the two abnormalities since some patients can be shown to have a combination of the two.

Slow-transit constipation

This can be defined by the simple radiological technique described by Hinton & colleagues (1969). A capsule containing 20 radio-opaque solid markers is ingested and on the 5th day a plain abdominal X-ray is performed. Under normal circumstances a minimum of 80% of the markers should have been voided; if more than 20% remain the patient can be assumed to have delayed colonic transit.

This condition is prevalent in women at the time of the menarche and can be associated with severe degrees of constipation with bowel function proving refractory to large doses of laxatives. The colon is of normal diameter, in distinction to primary megacolon, a functional disorder which affects men and women in equal numbers. For the moment the aetiology of this difficult clinical problem remains entirely obscure. Since women are predominantly affected a hormonal basis has been suspected but not proven.

Pelvic floor dysfunction

Recently it has become clearly established that some patients have normal transit but are quite unable to empty a full rectum. This occurs in some patients because of increased electrical activity within the pelvic floor musculature during attempted defecation (paradoxical contraction). The cause for this abnormality has not been explained. In some patients this may be a behavioural abnormality which is the result of an abnormal pattern of defecation perhaps instituted from early childhood. In other patients the disorder is due to spasticity of the muscle from upper motor neuron lesions; this is frequently observed in patients with multiple sclerosis, for example. Patients with denervated pelvic floor musculature secondary to lower motor neuron lesions (e.g. obstetric trauma to the pudendal nerves) may similarly experience difficulty with evacuation, presumably because an intact pelvic floor is necessary to assist with rectal evacuation.

Patients with this condition experience enormous difficulties with evacuation and frequently have to insert a digit into the anal canal to force the unyielding puborectalis muscle backwards and thereby assist the free passage of faeces.

The investigation which has become of key value in identifying this group is evacuation proctography (Mahieu et al 1984). A barium paste is introduced into the rectum and cine-radiography is performed while the patient attempts defecation. The films are studied for paradoxical puborectalis contraction and intrarectal intussusception. In the latter case, obstructed defecation is the consequence of prolapsing rectum which may not be overt and thereby diagnosable by other methods.

Treatment of constipation

Under normal circumstances, dietary adjustments and/or simple laxatives are adequate means of restoring normal bowel function in the majority of patients where there is no underlying obstructive cause (e.g. carcinoma). In the severe forms of idiopathic constipation associated with slow transit, surgery may be required. It is now generally accepted that partial resection (i.e. sigmoid colectomy) leads to an early recurrence of symptoms and this procedure has now been abandoned. The treatment of choice for well documented slow-transit constipation is total colectomy with ileorectal anastomosis. This operation restores normal bowel function, frequently at the expense of causing moderately severe diarrhoea. The abdominal pain these patients describe preoperatively often persists in the postoperative period, suggesting that the disorder is part of a generalized abnormality of intestinal motility.

Patients with pelvic floor dysfunction are a particular problem in management. Wherever possible conservative measures to induce liquid stool (by laxatives) and to encourage rectal emptying by the use of irritant suppositories (e.g. glycerine) should be employed as forcefully as possible. Biofeedback techniques to encourage the patient to relax the puborectalis during attempted defecation are time-consuming but can prove helpful. Surgical measures to divide the 'tense' puborectalis muscle have not generally proved of value.

KEY POINTS

1. Continence depends on the internal anal sphincter and external anal sphincter and puborectalis. In addition, sensory factors, valves of Houston and anal canal cushions may also play a role.
2. Defecation occurs with relaxation of the pelvic floor, increased obliquity of the anorectal angle and increase in intra-abdominal pressure.
3. Manometry is the most practical method of assessing internal anal sphincter function.
4. The external anal sphincter can be accurately assessed using electromyography.

5. Denervation secondary to traumatic delivery is an important feature in the causation of constipation, solitary rectal ulcer syndrome and descending perineum syndrome.
6. Faecal incontinence is eight times more common in the female than in the male in the middle years and three times more common in the female than in the male when over 65 years.
7. Faecal incontinence is associated with obstetric trauma, physiological denervation associated with ageing, past trauma to the anal sphincter ring including sexual assault, or neuropathy. Surgical repair will cure 60–80% of patients.
8. Rectal prolapse is associated with mucoviscidosis (children), pelvic floor denervation and constipation. Rectopexy will cure 95% of patients.
9. Irritable bowel syndrome is a common cause of abdominal pain in a gynaecological clinic. The condition is often related to stress or anxiety and reassurance and supportive measures, increasing dietary bulk and antispasmodics are the mainstay of treatment.
10. Recent onset constipation may be due to an obstructive lesion such as a carcinoma of the large bowel. Sigmoidoscopy and a barium enema are mandatory investigations.

REFERENCES

Bartolo D C C 1986 Flap-valve theory of anorectal continence. British Journal of Surgery 73: 1012–1014

Bennett R C, Duthie H L 1964 The functional importance of the internal sphincter. British Journal of Surgery 51: 355–357

Delorme R 1900 Sur le traitement des prolapsus du rectum totaux pour l'excision de la muquese rectable au rectocolique. Bulletin des Membres de la Société Chirurgical de Paris 26: 498–499

Floyd W F, Walls E W 1953 Electromyography of the sphincter ani externus in man. Journal of Physiology 122: 599–609

Gowers W R 1877 The automatic action of the sphincter ani. Proceedings of the Royal Society of Medicine 26: 77–84

Henry M M, Porter N H 1988 A colour atlas of faecal incontinence and rectal prolapse. Wolfe Publications, London

Henry M M, Parks A G, Swash M 1982 The pelvic floor muscle in the descending perineum syndrome. British Journal of Surgery 62: 470–472

Hinton J M, Lennard Jones J E, Young A C 1969 A new method for studying gut transit times using radio-opaque markers. Gut 10: 842–847

Lane R H S, Parks A G 1977 Function of the anal sphincters following colo-anal anastomosis. British Journal Surgery 64: 596–599

Laurberg S, Swash M, Henry M M 1988 Delayed external sphincter repair for obstetric tear. British Journal of Surgery 75: 786–788

Lennard Jones J E 1985 Constipation: pathophysiology, clinical features and treatment. In: Henry M M, and Swash M (eds) Coloproctology and the pelvic floor. Butterworths, London, p 367

Lubowski D Z, Nicholls R J, Swash M, Jordan M J 1987 Neural control of internal anal sphincter function. British Journal of Surgery 74: 668–670

Mandelstam D A 1989 Social and economic factors. In: Henry M M Swash M (eds) Coloproctology and pelvic floor. Butterworths, London, pp 217–222

Merton P A, Hill D K, Morton H B, Marsden C D 1982 Scope of a technique for electrical stimulation of human brain, spinal cord and muscle. Lancet ii: 597–600

Neill M E, Swash M 1980 Increased motor unit fibre density in the external sphincter in anorectal incontinence: a single fibre EMG study. Journal of Neurology and Neurosurgery and Psychiatry 43: 343–347

Neill M E, Parks A G, Swash M 1981 Physiological studies of the anal sphincter musculature in faecal incontinence and rectal prolapse. British Journal of Surgery 68: 531–536

Parks A G 1975 Anorectal incontinence. Proceedings of the Royal Society of Medicine 68: 681–690

Parks A G, Porter N H, Melzack J 1962 Experimental study of the reflex mechanism controlling the muscles of the pelvic floor. Diseases of the Colon and Rectum 5: 407–414

Parks A G, Swash M, Urich H 1977 Sphincter denervation in anorectal incontinence and rectal prolapse. Gut 18: 656–665

Porter N H 1962 Physiological study of the pelvic floor in rectal prolapse. Annals of the Royal College of Surgeons of England 31: 379–404

Rogers J, Levy D M, Henry M M, Misiewicz J J 1988 Pelvic floor neuropathy: a comparative study of diabetes mellitus and idiopathic faecal incontinence, Gut 29: 756–761

Rogers J, Henry M M, Misiewicz J J 1989 Increased segmental activity and intraluminal pressures in the sigmoid colon of patients with irritable bowel syndrome. Gut 30: 634–641

Snooks S J, Swash M 1984 Abnormalities of the innervation of the urethral striated sphincter muscle in incontinence. British Journal of Urology 56: 401–405

Snooks S J, Swash M, Henry M M, Setchell M E 1984 Injury to innervation of pelvic floor sphincter musculature in childbirth. Lancet ii: 546–550

Snooks S J, Swash M, Henry M M 1985a Abnormalities in central and peripheral nerve conduction in patients with anorectal incontinence. Journal of the Royal Society of Medicine 78: 294–300

Snooks S J, Barnes P R H, Swash M, Henry M M 1985b Damage to the innervation of the pelvic floor musculature in chronic constipation. Gastroenterology 89: 977–981

Snooks S J, Nicholls R J, Henry M M, Swash M 1985c Electrophysiological and manometric assessment of the pelvic floor in solitary rectal ulcer syndrome. British Journal of Surgery 72: 131–133

Walls E W 1959 Recent observations of the anatomy of the anal canal. Proceedings of the Royal Society of Medicine 52 (suppl): 85–87

Wells C H 1959 New operation for rectal prolapse. Proceedings of the Royal Society of Medicine 52: 602–603

Winkler G 1958 Remarques sur la morphologie et l'innervation du muscle releveur de l'anus. Archives d'Anatomie et Histologie et Embryologie, Strasbourg 41: 77–95

Womack N R, Williams N S, Holmfield J H M, Morrison J F B, Simpkins K C 1985 New method for the dynamic assessment of anorectal function in constipation. British Journal of Surgery 72: 994–997

Womack N R, Morrison J F B, Williams N S 1988 Prospective study of the effects of postanal repair in neurogenic faecal incontinence. British Journal of Surgery 75: 48–52

FURTHER READING

Henry M M, Swash M (eds) 1992 Coloproctology and pelvic floor, 2nd edn. Butterworth–Heinemann, Oxford

66. Psychosexual disorders

A. Parsons

INTRODUCTION

The conditions which we describe as psychosexual disorders show a number of fundamental differences from other conditions described in this book. Firstly, a psychosexual disorder is not a disorder in the same sense as cancer of the endometrium. Although it may have an underlying organic basis, its presentation and prognosis are usually highly dependent on the expectations of both the individual and the society in which she lives. Recognition of a sexual difficulty may depend heavily on the sensitivity of the professionals concerned, but each individual or couple has to define for themselves what should be perceived as a problem.

Secondly, sexual difficulties are, par excellence, a psychosomatic problem (Bancroft 1989). Whilst an enjoyable sexual experience will normally require intact pelvic organs with functioning vascular and neurological mechanisms, the pelvic changes of sexual arousal are inextricably linked with the cognitive processes which determine their sexual meaning for the individual.

Thirdly, disorders may be situational; that is to say, they may occur within the context of one relationship, but not another. Alternatively, they may occur in two different relationships, but be interpreted as a problem in one and not the other.

Clearly then, the recognition of a problem as a psychosexual disorder will be influenced by the expectations of society and of the individual or couples concerned, as well as by those of their professional advisers.

This chapter will address what are commonly referred to as sexual dysfunctions. These are those cases where the sexual response does not appear to be working to the satisfaction of the individuals concerned. Sexual 'deviations' or 'variations' are forms of sexual behaviour or methods of sexual arousal which fall beyond the bounds of what most people consider to be normal and are to some degree culturally determined. These need to be dealt with by people with the expertise to understand the mechanisms underlying abnormal sexual behaviour. They will not be considered further in this chapter.

PATHOPHYSIOLOGY AND CLASSIFICATION

Whilst it is important to realize that no two people or couples will ever present with exactly the same difficulties, a classification is possible based on an understanding of the physiology and anatomy of sexual response. Most of the present conventional wisdom about human sexual response is based on the research findings of Masters & Johnson (1966). It is important to remember that their observations were largely based on 2500 cycles of sexual response in approximately 600 men and women. These subjects were volunteers who were willing to have their sexual response studied under laboratory conditions. Our assumption is that the nature of sexual response for the rest of the population is the same as it was for this group of highly responsive individuals.

Masters & Johnson's classification divides human sexual response into four phases: excitement, plateau, orgasm and resolution. Each phase represents an incremental increase in sexual excitement and each is a necessary precursor for the following phase.

Excitement phase

The excitement or arousal phase is the initial response to sexual stimulation, either physical or psychic. In both men and women this has genital and systemic components. A reflex vasodilation of blood vessels in the genitalia is mediated through two centres in the spinal cord (one at the level of segments T11–L2, the other at S2–S4). In the male, this vasodilation fills the corpora cavernosa of the penis to produce an erection, while in the female, increased vaginal wall blood flow produces a transudate which appears like beads of perspiration on the walls of the vagina and which is the main source of vaginal lubrication. This lubrication is also associated with the ballooning out of the inner two-thirds of the vagina and with varying degrees of engorgement of the vulva. The systemic component of the excitement phase includes changes in pulse and respiratory rates and blood pressure, as well as general vasocongestion, especially over the upper torso and neck. During this phase, arousal increases, but remains vulnerable to interruption. Fatigue, worry or alcohol may all affect the arousal phase, while distracting thoughts or the sounds of other people in the house may easily cause a reversal of the excitement changes.

Plateau phase

The plateau phase is included by some authorities (e.g. Kaplan 1974) as part of arousal. It represents a consolidation of the changes which occur during the excitement phase which inevitably precedes it. During this phase, congestion in the outer third of the vagina reaches a maximum. This produces a firm area of engorged tissue around the vaginal introitus, which Masters & Johnson described as the 'orgasmic platform'. Breast changes are also maximal at this time with an increase in breast size of 20–25% in many women who have not previously breastfed. As the plateau phase proceeds, congestion of the areolae gives the impression of loss of erection of the nipple and finally, just prior to orgasm, the clitoris is retracted firmly against the pubic bone, often seeming to disappear. Although this phase is described as a plateau, it none the less involves increments of sexual excitement which may then build up to the intensity required for orgasm.

Orgasm

Orgasm represents a peak of pleasurable sensation associated with the discharge of the sexual tension which is built up during the preceding phases. Physiological changes during orgasm are remarkably similar in both sexes, with the subjective feeling of pleasure being associated with involuntary rhythmic contraction of the genital muscles (at 0.8/s intervals). In women the pelvic floor muscles, including the orgasmic platform, are involved, while in the male the muscles at the base of the penis and in the penile urethra contract to produce ejaculation. In the male, this part of orgasm is preceded by emission in which the seminal fluid passes into the base of the urethra.

After ejaculation, the male experiences a refractory period. During this time, further stimulation will not produce further response and may even cause feelings of discomfort. The length of this refractory period increases with age (from a few minutes in the teenager to many hours in the elderly). Many women, and some men, do not have a refractory period, and further stimulation can cause further orgasms in this group. It is uncertain what proportion of the population have this ability.

Many of the more important myths of human sexuality surround the orgasm. One of the more damaging of these, from a clinical point of view, is the myth of the vaginal orgasm. Freud, in particular, promoted the idea that the psychologically more mature woman would be capable of achieving an orgasm in response to vaginal stimulation alone, and that this vaginal orgasm provided a higher level of experience than a climax produced by other forms of stimulation. It is now clear that the nature of an orgasm is not affected by the type of stimulation needed to produce it, although masturbatory orgasms may be somewhat more intense. Only a minority of women can achieve orgasm from coitus alone, and stimulation of the clitoris and other erogenous zones is a normal pathway to orgasm.

Resolution

Following orgasm, the body gradually returns to the non-aroused state, unless effective stimulation is continued. The speed of the resolution phase is related to age in men, and probably in women too. In some older women impairment of the resolution phase, especially if associated with orgasmic failure, may lead to pelvic congestion and non-specific symptoms of pelvic and low backache.

Masters & Johnson's original four-phase cycle of excitement, plateau, orgasm and resolution, however, ignores what is perhaps the least understood component of sexuality, namely desire or libido. Thus, Kaplan's (1979) triphasic model of desire, arousal and orgasm provides a better parallel between sexual dysfunction and the response cycle.

The more common categories of sexual dysfunction presenting among women are dyspareunia, vaginismus, orgasmic dysfunction and general sexual dysfunction, while the corresponding problems in the male are those of erectile difficulty, premature ejaculation, retarded ejaculation and dyspareunia. The relatively uncommon problem of retrograde ejaculation is also relevant to the gynaecologist because of its implications for fertility.

Female sexual dysfunction

Dyspareunia

Dyspareunia is defined as pain on intercourse and is perhaps one of the most common sexual difficulties presented to the gynaecologist, partly because of the assumption that there may be an underlying organic reason.

Dyspareunia is traditionally described as being superficial when the pain is solely at the vaginal introitus or deep when the pain is felt within the pelvis. As with all other sexual dysfunctions, dyspareunia may be primary (i.e. having been present since the first attempts at intercourse) or secondary (i.e. a problem which has arisen after previously painfree intercourse). Other features which are of importance in dyspareunia are whether the pain is sufficient to prevent intercourse, whether it is continuous or intermittent, and whether it continues after attempts at intercourse have ceased.

Vaginismus

Vaginismus is a condition characterized by the involuntary spasm of the pubococcygeus muscle, leading to an effective closure of the vaginal introitus. Attempts at penetration produce pain in the clenched muscle, thus aggravating the situation. Vaginismus may generalize to the point where any attempt at vaginal examination is impossible and the patient may take up the position of opisthotonos on the examination couch. Contrary to many people's belief, there is no association between vaginismus and an individual's ability to become aroused or to be orgasmic. Nor does vaginismus imply any particular personality or sexual attitudes on the part of the sufferer.

Orgasmic dysfunction

Orgasmic dysfunction is the inability to achieve an orgasm or climax. This may be associated with a general inability to become aroused. Alternatively, a woman may be able to achieve normal arousal and reach a plateau phase, but be unable to climax. Masters & Johnson (1970) divided the inability to achieve an orgasm according to whether this was only a problem during intercourse or whether the individual was also unable to achieve a climax by masturbation. Inability to reach orgasm by intercourse alone is a sufficiently common problem that most women would probably not regard it as a dysfunction.

General sexual dysfunction

General sexual dysfunction is the more common term used for an inability to become aroused and has a large overlap with hypoactive sexual desire. The most severe form of this is the woman who experiences no sexual interest, either spontaneously or in response to her partner, and gives a history of never having experienced sexual arousal or orgasm. It seems unusual for such women to report mere indifference to sexual activity and they are most likely to present with a degree of aversion to any sexual advance. Milder presentations overlap with the orgasmic dysfunctions described above.

Male sexual dysfunction

Erectile difficulty is a difficulty in achieving or inability to maintain an erection. It may be primary or secondary. It may also be situational, i.e. an individual who can achieve an erection with one partner may not be able to do so with another. It may or may not be associated with a low level of sexual interest. Paraphilias are those conditions where an individual responds to an unusual sexual object or an unusual form of stimulation. Most paraphilias hide an underlying low sexual drive and erectile difficulty.

Premature ejaculation

Premature ejaculation is a relative term and may be defined as the tendency for an individual to ejaculate appreciably more quickly than would be required for his own or his partner's satisfaction. This is clearly heavily influenced by expectations. Kinsey et al (1948), for instance, found that the average American male at that time would ejaculate within 2 min of penetration.

Extreme cases of premature ejaculation, where the man ejaculates before he can approach or penetrate his partner, can be more readily accepted as a problem.

Other ejaculatory dysfunctions

Retarded ejaculation involves normal arousal and plateau phases, but ejaculation either fails to occur or requires prolonged stimulation (more than is acceptable to the couple) to trigger it. Retrograde ejaculation also occurs where the man experiences normal feelings but the seminal fluid, instead of being passed forward through the penile urethra, is forced backwards into the bladder. Men are not always aware that this phenomenon is occurring, and in some individuals it may be situational. Conditions which alter the anatomy of the bladder neck (e.g. prostatectomy or spinal cord injury) will also produce retrograde ejaculation.

Dyspareunia

Dyspareunia in the male is less common than in the female and may be divided into pain on achieving an erection and pain on actual intercourse. These complaints are usually physical in origin.

Loss of sexual desire

Loss or lack of libido may be complained of in both men and women, though traditionally this is a problem which men find more difficult to present to the medical profession, perhaps partly because of society's myths about male sexual performance. The underlying basis for sexual desire in the human is poorly understood. Clearly the psychic and endocrine components are important but, particularly in the female, there is no clear consensus on the importance of hormonal changes.

AETIOLOGY

Like many problems in gynaecology, sexual difficulties were originally regarded as being almost exclusively psychological in origin. More recently, it has been suggested that up to 50% of erectile difficulties may have at least a partly organic cause. There are no obvious reasons why this should not also apply to arousal difficulties in women, though as yet there is little substantiating evidence for this. While recognizing that there is always some overlap between the two, it may be useful to look at organic and psychological factors in sexual dysfunction separately.

Organic factors

Although most sexual problems other than dyspareunia may have no organic basis, it is important to establish the organic elements, if any, of the problem. The distinction between organic and psychological will often be clear from the history. Otherwise physical examination of the relevant partner is mandatory. General physical examination should look for signs of genetic abnormality or systemic illness and where pain is part of the presenting complaint an attempt should be made to reproduce this on examination.

Normal sexual response assumes normal genitalia with an unimpaired blood supply and an intact innervation. Any changes in these obviously modify or prevent response.

Neurological

A variety of neurological conditions will have an impact on sexual functioning. Autonomic neuropathy in diabetes mellitus or demyelination in multiple sclerosis may impair one or other phase of the sexual response cycle. Spinal cord injuries will have a variable effect depending on the level at which the cord is damaged and whether the damage is full or partial. Relatively little is known about the effect of spinal cord injury in women. In men the vast majority with upper motor neuron lesions are able to achieve reflex erections in response to tactile stimulation. Orgasmic and ejaculatory capacity, however, are more variable.

Gynaecological cancer/surgery

Gynaecological or other cancers may cause sexual disability in a number of ways. Libido, particularly in women, is often closely linked to mood and can be suppressed by even mild levels of depression occurring either as part of the illness process or as a reaction to the diagnosis. Cancer surgery can often be mutilating and appreciably alter an individual's body image. Studies of women who have undergone radical surgery for gynaecological cancers have shown a significant deterioration both in body image and in sexual relationships. Radiotherapy, particularly for cervical cancer, may produce a degree of vaginal stenosis with reduced lubrication and soreness.

Post-hysterectomy

While a total hysterectomy normally leaves the length of the vagina unchanged, deep dyspareunia becomes relatively common when a vaginal cuff has been removed. This discomfort seems to be related to thrusting against a scarred vault in a vagina which no longer has the same capacity to balloon out on arousal.

The role of hysterectomy in the causation of psychosexual problems has long been controversial. However, it does seem that in the vast majority of women for whom hysterectomy is indicated, sexual relationships are likely to improve subsequently. Clearly there is no physical necessity for the presence of the uterus for sexual enjoyment, though there is anecdotal evidence that some women gain important erotic sensation from their uterus or cervix. Loss of libido following either hysterectomy or sterilization is unlikely to be organic.

Drugs

A wide variety of drugs have an impact on sexual function, either directly or indirectly. In general, the effects of drugs on male sexuality are far better documented than those effects on the female, partly because the male response is more easily studied. However, any drugs with a central stimulatory or sedative action may be expected to have an effect either on libido or arousal. Most hypotensive agents are associated with some sexual side-effects. Alcohol, often used to enhance sexual enjoyment, will produce a sexual dysfunction when abused. The aetiology of this is complex and is only partly organic.

EPIDEMIOLOGY

Because many people with sexual problems never present to any source of help, the main sources of information about the incidence of such problems come either from general population studies or from surveys carried out by women's magazines, etc. The latter source tends to be biased towards those experiencing difficulties. The issue is further complicated by our poor understanding of how sexual dysfunction, sexual difficulties and sexual dissatisfaction may be linked.

Population studies

Kinsey et al's (1953) study of sexual behaviour in the human female remains one of the most important in this area. They found that of the 5900 women interviewed, 50% had not experienced orgasm in their late teens. This figure decreased to 10% by the mid 30s. In their previous study (1948) on male sexual behaviour, the Kinsey team had found that male sexual function tended to deteriorate with age. In all, 1.6% of men had more or less permanent problems achieving an erection and this figure rose to 27% by the age of 70. A further 35% reported erectile difficulties on occasions, while 6% complained of premature ejaculation.

However, orgasmic dysfunction does not necessarily correlate with sexual dissatisfaction, while a normal physiological response does not necessarily rule out sexual problems. Dissatisfaction for men and women is more likely to be associated with sexual difficulties such as difficulty in relaxing or a general lack of interest. Social and cultural factors in sexual enjoyment have been poorly studied, but there is a general agreement in the literature that positive attitudes to sexual relationships and the ability to respond are positively associated in women with both social class and educational attainment.

Gynaecological clinic attendees

The incidence of sexual dysfunction in clinic populations has been the subject of only a limited number of studies. Clearly there will be a number of biasing factors in these, including the nature of the clinic and the attitude of the clinicians involved. Routine direct questioning about sexual problems will double the number presented to the clinician, yet in most clinics this approach is still not used. None the less, a Dutch study (Frenken & Van Tol 1987), interviewing a sample of Dutch gynaecologists, found that during the preceding week 1 patient in 14 presented with a sexual problem, most commonly dyspareunia or loss of sexual interest.

Clinics specifically for sexual difficulties clearly see a very selected population. However, overall, men presenting to such clinics tend to complain of problems with their genital responses while women are more likely to complain of a lack of interest or enjoyment, and there is some evidence that this trend is becoming more marked. It is important to note that in up to one-third of couples where one partner presents with a sexual dysfunction, a sexual problem will also be found in the other partner.

PRESENTATION

Patients' ability to share their sexual problems depend heavily on the attitude of the clinician. The majority of couples with sexual problems first present these to their general practitioner. In general, if these couples are referred on for specialist advice it is not usually to the gynaecologist. Other couples may find their general practitioner difficult to approach or may choose not to share such a highly personal matter in this setting, and for them marriage guidance clinics may be a more attractive alternative.

Bancroft (1989) has emphasized the value of having a co-ordinated range of services to meet the needs of couples with sexual problems, partly in order to offer an appropriate range of helping skills, and partly to allow for different patterns of presentation.

Sexual dysfunction frequently presents in the gynaecologist's clinic as a secondary rather than a main presenting problem. Despite the apparent increase in freedom in our society to talk about sex, particularly in the media, one should not underestimate the levels of naivety and ignorance which still exist. Couples who have never managed to achieve intravaginal intercourse, yet are unaware of this, may still be seen in infertility clinics.

Other problems may be more easily presented in certain contexts; for instance, a lack of sexual interest may be presented by the gynaecological patient who is asking whether it might be related to her hormones. This is particularly common in family planning clinics where the contraceptive pill may be blamed for reduced libido or in the woman presenting with the premenstrual syndrome or with menopausal problems. Over 40% of patients attending a London menopausal clinic acknowledged either loss of libido or dyspareunia when questioned directly (Studd et al 1977).

Sexual problems in some gynaecological patients will only be discovered at the time of physical examination. Here spasm of the pubococcygeus muscle may be apparent, leading to a possible diagnosis of vaginismus. Alternatively, deep pelvic pain may be elicited on bimanual examination and it is always appropriate to ask whether similar discomfort is experienced on intercourse.

INVESTIGATIONS

It has already been noted that the gynaecologist's ability to detect sexual problems will depend both on attitude and on a willingness to ask direct questions. Sexual dysfunction is frequently better dealt with within a context other than the gynaecology outpatient clinic. However, the clinician has three clear duties. First is the detection of the problem, and this has already been dealt with. The second is the taking of a careful sexual *problem* history and the third is the elucidation of underlying organic factors.

Taking a sexual problem history

The main barriers to taking a sexual problem history are usually embarrassment and discomfort, often both on the part of the patient and the clinician. In order to be able to carry out a sensitive interview in this area the clinician at least must be comfortable. Such comfort can be based on a combination of a good fundamental knowledge of human sexual functioning and experience in developing general interviewing and counselling skills. Specific information requires specific questioning and if the patient is indicating that she has a psychosexual dysfunction the questioning needs to be directed towards establishing the nature of the current problem. Focusing on the presenting complaint rather than proceeding directly to taking a more general sexual history has a number of advantages. Firstly, it reassures the patient that her complaint is being taken seriously. Secondly, it often provides the necessary information for distinguishing possible organic components.

When a clear picture of the problem as it exists has been obtained, a history of this problem should then be taken. This will include some information about the first time the problem occurred, whether it developed abruptly or has come on gradually, how long the patient has been aware of it, whether it is getting better or worse, whether it is situational (e.g. occurring with one partner and not another or in one sexual position and not another) and any obvious aggravating or ameliorating factors. In the case of deep dyspareunia, the standard eight questions which are asked about any complaint of pain should be included. Finally, it is worth trying to get some idea of the patient's own views of the cause of the problem and her partner's reaction to it. Attempts are often made to distinguish between sexual and 'marital' problems but unless the relationship is obviously grossly unsatisfactory there tends to be little advantage in this approach.

General physical examination

Careful inspection of the external and internal genitalia will exclude developmental abnormalities such as vaginal atresia or imperforate hymen in the female and hypospadias or undescended testes in the male. Normal secondary characteristics should also be present. A careful check of the vulva and vagina should be made, especially when there is a complaint of dyspareunia. It is important to rule out acute infections such as monilia, trichomonas or genital herpes. As well as chronic conditions such as cysts of Bartholin's gland, manual pelvic examination should look for evidence of pelvic inflammatory disease or endometriosis. A retroverted uterus can also be a source of deep dyspareunia, either because of the effect of thrusting the uterus against the base of the spine or because of direct thrusting against the ovaries which tend to prolapse into the pouch of Douglas. The important iatrogenic cause for superficial pain can be the presence of an episiotomy scar. Kolodny et al (1979) lists 37 possible causes of dyspareunia. Of these, 35 are organic and 2 are psychological, so the importance of careful examination cannot be overemphasized. Laparoscopy will also be appropriate in some cases of deep dyspareunia.

Hormones

Whilst testosterone is clearly the hormone responsible for both libido and sexual response in the male, the situation in the female is less clear. Testosterone does seem to play a role, but oestrogen also seems to be important.

TREATMENT

It is clear from what has been noted earlier in this chapter that there is no possibility of offering treatment for everyone experiencing sexual difficulties or dissatisfaction. Fortunately this is neither necessary nor is it the expectation of patients. Jack Annon (1976a,b) has devised a model by means of which the appropriate level of response can be selected for each problem presented to the clinician. This model, also known by the acronym PLISSIT, assumes that problems with an organic basis have already been filtered out. The term PLISSIT refers to the four levels of response: permission, limited information, specific suggestions and intensive therapy.

Permission

Patients often want to check with their doctor that certain aspects of their sexual life are acceptable. They may seek permission to be less sexually active, for example, in the puerperium or postmenopausally. They may have particular aspects of their behaviour or their partner's which concern them and about which they seek the approval of a professional. This brings us again to the clinician's comfort with his or her own sexuality. Clearly, it is very difficult to give permission to other people if you do not have that permission yourself.

Limited information

Limited information may need to be given to women about normal sexual response and about the times when it may change. Most women achieve orgasm more reliably by masturbation, partner manipulation, or oral sex than by intercourse, yet many are unaware of or feel uncomfortable with this. Since the work of Masters & Johnson, demonstrating the ability of some women to be multiply orgasmic, many women now feel that this is an expectation of them. They may need to know that this is an idiosyncratic response which only some women experience.

Women in their first pregnancy may need to know about the normal changes in libido and in the sensitivity of the erogenous zones during pregnancy and in the puerperium. Those women approaching the menopause may need to know about physiological changes in vaginal lubrication and how to prevent the development of vaginal atrophy.

Specific suggestions

Often the most useful specific suggestion, particularly for the gynaecologist whose time or experience is limited, is some appropriate reading for the patient. There are a variety of useful books varying from the general (Brown & Faulder 1979; Yaffé & Fenwick 1986a,b) to those designed for specific problems (e.g. Heiman et al 1986; Valins 1988).

Several specific suggestions are frequently offered in gynaecological clinics. If a couple are deriving less pleasure from intercourse following childbirth and there is evidence that this is related to looseness of the pubococcygeus muscle, then reteaching of Kegel's (pelvic floor) exercises may be helpful, as may the female superior position.

Suggestions about alternative positions or new stimulatory techniques may be helpful where there is an organic cause for dyspareunia which is untreatable.

Intensive therapy

Dyspareunia (without a discernible organic cause), the orgasmic dysfunctions and the male dysfunctions all need a structured form of therapy and unfortunately, because of the structure of provision of gynaecological services in the UK, this cannot normally be considered to be the province of the gynaecologist.

Modern intensive therapy usually involves some level of compromise between the psychoanalytic and the behavioural approach and most clinics now offer a form of treatment which is based loosely on the work of Masters & Johnson (1970), Annon (1976a,b) and Kaplan (1974, 1979). The features which these therapies, have in common are that they are client- and couple-centred. After varying levels of assessment of both the sexual problem and the couple's relationship, a behavioural framework is adopted. Any attempt at intercourse is usually 'banned' at this stage and sexual experiences are prescribed in very small steps. 'Progress', or lack of it, in taking these steps can then be examined in the context of the couple and their relationship, while trying to tackle those factors which are commonly involved in the maintenance of chronic sexual difficulties. These include a lack of information, a failure to communicate (especially on matters with a sexual or emotional content), goal orientation, sexual anxiety and spectatoring.

These factors have been well described by Masters & Johnson (1970) and Kaplan (1974, 1979) and are a common response to continuing sexual difficulties. Repeated sexual 'failure' leads to anxiety at every sexual encounter. This in turn leads to the individuals carefully watching their bodies' responses rather than allowing arousal to happen spontaneously. Couples who previously enjoyed a varied and imaginative sexual life often restrict the expressions of their sexuality further and further when a problem arises until their behaviour is highly stereotyped and geared only to achieving the 'goal' of sexual experience which by then has become the erection or the orgasm.

This type of sex therapy has been developed to try to produce a relatively brief but effective intervention for couples with sexual problems. Treatment sessions may typically be held at fortnightly intervals with a standard initial contract of up to 12 sessions.

Some forms of physical treatment have been developed which will to some degree over-ride those psychological elements responsible for the maintenance of problems. Thus intracavernosal injections of papaverine for erectile dysfunction or, more controversially, the use of testosterone supplementation in problems of female loss of libido may have a place.

RESULTS

Assessment of the outcome of treatment for sexual dysfunction is fraught with difficulties. Diagnostic classifications, based as they are on the physiological sexual response cycle, are problematic and often contain heterogeneous groups. Prognoses are also clearly likely to be affected by general health, age, and the state of the relationship when help is sought. Sexual difficulties may act as a guise for marital difficulties and these underlying relationship problems may have a major effect on the prognosis. If one individual in the couple is labelled as 'the patient' he or she may be under considerable pressure to seek help, yet there may be covert reasons for avoiding a successful resolution of the problem.

The second area of difficulty in assessing outcome is the uncertainty about what constitutes success. One couple may experience only slight alterations in coital or orgasmic frequency, yet may consider that therapy has produced a substantial improvement in their sexual health and the quality of their relationship. Others may have been assisted to achieve a 'Masters & Johnson-style' physiological sexual response but still find their partner unexciting and sex unrewarding.

These difficulties in measuring outcome are aggravated further by different ways of reporting results. Masters & Johnson (1970), for instance, report the proportion of failures on the grounds that failure is easier to measure than success.

If 'complete success' and 'much improvement' are taken together, then a number of studies, (e.g. Bancroft and Coles 1976; Hawton 1982; Heisler 1983; Warner & Bancroft 1986) all show 60–65% falling into one of these groups. However, drop-out rates vary and some results (e.g. Heisler 1983) account only for those who stayed in therapy.

Long-term follow-up is in more doubt. Masters & Johnson reported a 5% relapse rate among their 'non-failures' at 5 years but both recurrence of sexual difficulties and relationship breakdown are worryingly common in most other studies.

KEY POINTS

1. Although a psychosexual disorder may have an underlying organic basis, its presentation and prognosis are usually dependent on the expectations of both the individual and the society in which she lives.
2. Psychosexual disorders may be situational; that is to say, they may occur within the context of one relationship, but not another.
3. Dyspareunia is perhaps one of the most common sexual difficulties presented to the gynaecologist.
4. Inability to reach orgasm by intercourse alone is a sufficiently common problem that most women would probably not regard it as dysfunction.
5. Premature ejaculation is a relative term and may be defined as the tendency for an individual to ejaculate appreciably more quickly than would be required for his own or his partner's satisfaction.
6. Male dyspareunia is less common than in the female and may be divided into pain on achieving an erection and pain on actual intercourse.
7. A variety of neurological conditions will have an impact on sexual functioning.
8. Loss of libido following either a hysterectomy or sterilization is unlikely to be organic.
9. Patients' ability to share their sexual problems depend heavily on the attitude of the clinician.
10. Sexual dysfunction is frequently better dealt with within a context other than the gynaecology outpatient clinic.
11. Modern intensive therapy usually involves some level of compromise between the psychoanalytic and the behavioural approach.

REFERENCES

Annon J S 1976a The behavioural treatment of sexual problems. Volume 1: Brief therapy. Enabling Systems, Honolulu

Annon J S 1976b The behavioural treatment of sexual problems. Volume 2: Intensive therapy. Enabling Systems, Honolulu

Bancroft J 1989 Human sexuality and its problems. Churchill Livingstone, Edinburgh

Bancroft J, Coles L 1976 Three years' experience in a sexual problem clinic. British Medical Journal 1: 1575–1577

Brown P, Faulder C 1979 Treat yourself to sex: a guide for good loving. Penguin, Harmondsworth

Frenken J, Van Tol P 1987 Sexual problems in gynaecological practice. Journal of Psychosomatic Obstetrics and Gynaecology 6: 143–155

Hawton K 1982 The behavioural treatment of sexual dysfunction. British Journal of Psychiatry 140: 94–101

Heiman J, Lo Piccolo L, Lo Piccolo J 1986 Becoming orgasmic: a sexual growth program for women. Prentice-Hall International, London

Heisler J 1983 Sexual therapy in the National Marriage Guidance Council. NMGC, Rugby

Kaplan H S 1974 The new sex therapy. Bailliere Tindall, London

Kaplan H S 1979 Disorders of sexual desire and other new concepts and techniques in sex therapy. Brunner/Mazel, New York

Kinsey A C, Pomeroy W B, Martin C F 1948 Sexual behaviour in the human male. Saunders, Philadelphia

Kinsey A C, Pomeroy W B, Martin C F, Gebhard P H 1953 Sexual behaviour in the human female. Saunders, Philadelphia

Kolodny R C, Masters W H, Johnson V E 1979 Textbook of sexual medicine. Little, Brown, Boston

Masters W H, Johnson V E 1966 Human sexual response. Little, Brown, Boston

Masters W H, Johnson V E 1970 Human sexual inadequacy. Little, Brown, Boston

Studd J, Chakrovarti S, Oram D 1977 The climacteric. Clinics in Obstetrics and Gynaecology 4: 3–29

Valins L 1988 Vaginismus: understanding and overcoming the blocks to intercourse. Ashgrove Press, Bath

Warner P, Bancroft J 1986 Sex therapy outcome research: a reappraisal of methodology. 2. Methodological considerations — the importance of prognostic variability. Psychological Medicine 16: 855–863

Yaffé M, Fenwick E 1986a Sexual happiness for men. A practical approach. Dorling Kindersley, London

Yaffé M, Fenwick E 1986b Sexual happiness for women. A practical approach. Dorling Kindersley, London

FURTHER READING

Comfort A 1978 Sexual consequences of disability. George F. Stickley, Philadelphia

Gillan P 1987 Sex therapy manual. Blackwell, Oxford

Wagner G, Green R 1981 Impotence, physiological, psychological, surgical diagnosis and treatment. Plenum, New York

Index

Page numbers in *italics* indicate an illustration appearing on a different page from the text. **Abbreviations:** CIN: cervical intraepithelial neoplasia; GIFT: gamete intrafallopian transfer; GnRH: gonadotrophin releasing hormone; HRT: hormone replacement therapy; IUD: intrauterine device; IVF: in vitro fertilization; LH: luteinizing hormone; PMS: premenstrual syndrome; PID: pelvic inflammatory disease; UTI: urinary tract infection; VAIN: vaginal intraepithelial neoplasia; VIN: vulval intraepithelial neoplasia.